a LANGE medical book

CURRENT
Diagnosis & Treatment: Family Medicine

FIFTH EDITION

Jeannette E. South-Paul, MD, DHL (Hon), FAAFP

Andrew W. Mathieson UPMC Professor and Chair
Department of Family Medicine
University of Pittsburgh School of Medicine
Pittsburgh, Pennsylvania

Samuel C. Matheny, MD, MPH, FAAFP

Assistant Provost for Global Health Initiatives
Professor of Family and Community Medicine
University of Kentucky
Lexington, Kentucky

Evelyn L. Lewis, MD, MA, FAAFP, DABDA

Chief Medical Officer, Warrior Centric Health, LLC
Columbia, Maryland
Adjunct Associate Professor
Department of Family Medicine and Community Health
Rutgers, Robert Wood Johnson Medical School
Piscataway, New Jersey

Mc Graw Hill

New York   Chicago   San Francisco   Athens   London   Madrid
Milan   New Delhi   Singapore   Sydney   Toronto

CURRENT Diagnosis & Treatment: Family Medicine, Fifth Edition

1 2 3 4 5 6 7 8 9   LCR   25 24 23 22 21 20

ISBN 978-1-260-13489-6
MHID 1-260-13489-X
ISSN 1548-2189

Notice

Medicine is an ever-changing science. As new research and clinical experience broaden our knowledge, changes in treatment and drug therapy are required. The authors and the publisher of this work have checked with sources believed to be reliable in their efforts to provide information that is complete and generally in accord with the standards accepted at the time of publication. However, in view of the possibility of human error or changes in medical sciences, neither the authors nor the publisher nor any other party who has been involved in the preparation or publication of this work warrants that the information contained herein is in every respect accurate or complete, and they disclaim all responsibility for any errors or omissions or for the results obtained from use of the information contained in this work. Readers are encouraged to confirm the information contained herein with other sources. For example and in particular, readers are advised to check the product information sheet included in the package of each drug they plan to administer to be certain that the information contained in this work is accurate and that changes have not been made in the recommended dose or in the contraindications for administration. This recommendation is of particular importance in connection with new or infrequently used drugs.

This book was set in Minion Pro by Cenveo® Publisher Services.
The editors were Kay Conerly and Christie Naglieri.
The production supervisor was Catherine H. Saggese.
Project management was provided by Revathi Viswanathan, Cenveo Publisher Services.

This book is printed on acid-free paper.

We would like to dedicate this book to all family physicians and clinical partners, especially our colleagues in uniform, and the families who support them.

Jeannette E. South-Paul, MD, DHL (Hon), FAAFP
Samuel C. Matheny, MD, MPH, FAAFP
Evelyn L. Lewis, MD, MA, FAAFP, DABDA

Contents

Authors

Robert B. Allison, II, DO
Assistant Professor
Department of Family Medicine/WVU Medicine
Morgantown, West Virginia
Robert.Allison.m@wvumedicine.org
Common Geriatric Problems

Pamela Allweiss, MD, MSPH
Private practice
Lexington, Kentucky
pallweiss@gmail.com
Endocrine Disorders

Kelley Anderson, DO
Assistant Professor
Centre for Sports Medicine
University of Pittsburgh
Assistant Primary Care Sports Medicine Fellowship
    Director UPMC
Medical Advisor
UPMC Sports Concussion Program
Team Physician
Pittsburgh Ballet Theatre
Point Park University
Carnegie Mellon University
Pittsburgh, Pennsylvania
andersonka3@upmc.edu
Acute Musculoskeletal Complaints

Scott K. Andrews, MD, MBA
Assistant Professor
Department of Family Medicine
Pennsylvania State University College of Medicine
University Park, Pennsylvania
sandrews4@pennstatehealth.psu.edu
Physical Activity in Adolescents

Robert M. Arnold, MD
Distinguished Service Professor of Medicine
Chief, Section of Palliative Care and Medical Ethics
Director, Institute for Doctor-Patient Communication
University of Pittsburgh School of Medicine
Medical Director, UPMC Palliative and Supportive Institute
Pittsburgh, Pennsylvania
arnoldrm@upmc.edu
Hospice & Palliative Medicine

Cindy M. Barter, MD, MPH, IBCLC, CTTS, FAAFP
Residency Faculty
Hunterdon Family Medicine Residency Program
Flemington, New Jersey
cbarter@hhsnj.org
Abdominal Complaints

Layne D. Bennion, PhD
Assistant Professor of Psychology (Clinical Educator)/SOM
    Director of Academic Success
Uniformed Services University
Bethesda, Maryland
layne.bennion@usuhs.edu
*Combat-Related Posttraumatic Stress Disorder & Traumatic
    Brain Injury*

Natasha Robin Berman, MA, MS, MPH, LCGC
Licensed Certified Genetic Counselor
UPMC Children's Hospital of Pittsburgh
Pittsburgh, Pennsylvania
natasha.berman@chp.edu
Genetics for Family Physicians

Heather M. Bernard, MD
Clinical Fellow of Pediatrics
Harvard Medical School
General Academic Pediatric Fellow
Boston Children's Hospital
Boston, Massachusetts
heather.bernard@childrens.harvard.edu
Common Acute Infections in Children

Kevin Bernstein, MD, MMS, CAQSM, FAAFP
Family and Sports Medicine Physician
Naval Branch Health Clinic Mayport
Jacksonville, Florida
kevin.bernstein@gmail.com
Hypertension

John N. Boll, Jr., DO, FAAFP
Associate Director
UPMC Williamsport Family Medicine Residency
Williamsport, Pennsylvania
bolljn@upmc.edu
Chronic Pain Management

Scott R. Brown, DO
Faculty
UPMC Shadyside Family Medicine Residency
Fellow
UPMC Faculty Development Fellowship
Pittsburgh, Pennsylvania
brownsr4@upmc.edu
Skin Diseases in Infants & Children

Susan C. Brunsell, MD
Medstar Medical Group at The World Bank
Washington, DC
Susan.c.brunsell@medstar.net
Contraception

Kim A. Bullock, MD, FAAFP
Director
Community Health Division
Director
Community Health Leadership Development Fellowship
Associate Director
Service Learning
Associate Clinical Professor
Department of Family Medicine
Georgetown Medical School
Washington, DC
KAB75@georgetown.edu
Cultural & Linguistic Competence

Deepa Burman, MD, FAASM
Co-Director Pediatric Sleep Program UPMC Children's
    Hospital of Pittsburgh
Associate Professor of Pediatrics University of Pittsburgh
Pittsburgh, Pennsylvania
burmand@upmc.edu
Travel Medicine

Peter J. Carek, MD, MS
C. Sue and Louis C. Murray, M.D. Chair and Professor
Department of Community Health and Family Medicine
University of Florida College of Medicine
Gainesville, Florida
carek@ufl.edu
Endocrine Disorders

Robert J. Carr, MD
Vice President
Clinical Transformation
Western Connecticut Health Network
Danbury, Connecticut
Adjunct Associate Clinical Professor
University of Vermont School of Medicine
Burlington, Vermont
robert.carr@wchn.org
Urinary Incontinence

C. Randall Clinch, DO, MS
Professor
Department of Family & Community Medicine
Wake Forest University School of Medicine
Winston-Salem, North Carolina
crclinch@wakehealth.edu
Evaluation & Management of Headache

Tracey D. Conti, MD
Assistant Professor and Vice Chair
Department of Family Medicine
University of Pittsburgh School of Medicine
Pittsburgh, Pennsylvania
Program Director
UPMC McKeesport Family Medicine Residency
Vice Chair
UPMC McKeesport Department of Family Medicine
McKeesport, Pennsylvania
contitd@upmc.edu
Breastfeeding & Infant Nutrition

Barry Coutinho, MBBS
Clinical Assistant Professor
Department Family Medicine
University of Pittsburgh School of Medicine
Faculty
Family Medicine Residency,
UPMC Shadyside Hospital
Pittsburgh, Pennsylvania
coutinhobv@upmc.edu
Skin Diseases in Infants & Children

Lora Cox-Vance, MD, CMD
Chief, Geriatrics & Extended Care Services
Chillicothe VA Medical Center—VHA
Chillicothe, Ohio
coxla1999@gmail.com
Health Maintenance for Adults
Healthy Aging & Geriatric Assessment

Amy Crawford-Faucher, MD, FAAFP
Program Director
Forbes Family Medicine Residency Program
Vice Chair
Department of Family Medicine
Allegheny Health Network
Pittsburgh, Pennsylvania
Amy.CrawfordFaucher@ahn.org
Adolescent Sexuality
Interpersonal Violence

K. Michael Cummings, PhD, MPH
Professor
Department of Psychiatry & Behavioral Sciences
Co-lead Tobacco Research Hollings Cancer Center
Medical University of South Carolina
Charleston, South Carolina
cummingk@musc.edu
Tobacco Cessation

Anja Dabelić, MD, FAAFP
United States Navy Commander
Navy Medicine
Millington, Tennessee
Anja.dabelic@gmail.com
Respiratory Problems

Niladri Das, MD
Physician
Penn State Health Community Medical Group
Lancaster, Pennsylvania
ndas@pennstatehealth.psu.edu
Tickborne Disease

Alan K. David, MD
Professor of Family Medicine
Department of Family and Community Medicine
Medical College of Wisconsin
Milwaukee, Wisconsin
akdavid@mcw.edu
Anemia

Billy R. Davis, DO
Fellow of Addiction Medicine
Department of Medical Education
Baptist Memorial Hospital
Memphis, Tennessee
Bdavis@integratedaddictioncare.com
Heart Failure

James C. Dewar, MD
Family Physician
East Hills Primary Care
Conemaugh Health System
Johnstown, Pennsylvania
dewarjc2@gmail.com
Failure to Thrive

Stephanie B. Dewar, MD
Associate Professor of Pediatrics
University of Pittsburgh School of Medicine
Co-Director Pediatric Residency Program
UPMC Children's Hospital of Pittsburgh
Pittsburgh, Pennsylvania
dewar.stephanie@gmail.com
Common Acute Infections in Children
Failure to Thrive

Charles R. Doarn, MBA, FATA, FAsMA
Department of Environmental and Public Health
    Sciences, College of Medicine
University of Cincinnati
Cincinnati, Ohio
charles.doarn@uc.edu
Telemedicine

Jeanne Doperak, DO
Assistant Professor Sports Medicine University of Pittsburgh
Primary Care Sports Medicine Fellowship Director UPMC
Chief of Primary Care Sports Medicine Pittsburgh Children's
    Hospital
Team Physician University of Pittsburgh
Pittsburgh, Pennsylvania
doperakjm@upmc.edu
Acute Musculoskeletal Complaints

Tyler K. Drewry, MD, CAQSM
Sports Medicine Specialist and Associate Program Director
Beaumont Wayne Family Medicine Residency Program
Department of Family Medicine
Westland, Michigan
tyler.drewry@beaumont.org
Common Upper & Lower Extremity Fractures

Laura Dunne, MD, CAQSM, FAAFP
OAA Orthopedic Specialists
Sports Medicine Institute
Allentown, Pennsylvania
lauradunne@aol.com
Abdominal Complaints

William G. Elder, PhD
Clinical Professor and Chair
Department of Behavioral and Social Sciences
University of Houston College of Medicine
Houston, Texas
welder@Central.UH.EDU
Personality Disorders
Somatic Symptom Disorder (Previously Somatoform Disorder),
    Factitious Disorder, & Malingering

Patricia Evans, MD, MA
Assistant Professor
Department of Family Medicine
Georgetown University
Washington, DC
evansp@georgetown.edu
Abnormal Uterine Bleeding

Kelly Evans-Rankin, MD, CAQSM
Core Faculty
Family Medicine Residency Program
Bon Secour Mercy Health
Mercy Health-Anderson
Cincinnati, Ohio
kelly_lee_evans@yahoo.com
Common Upper & Lower Extremity Fractures

Michael A. Fitzgerald, DO
Department of Family & Community Medicine
University of Kentucky
Lexington, Kentucky
mafi243@uky.edu
Common Upper & Lower Extremity Fractures

Julie Gallo, DO
PGY-3
UPMC Horizon Family Medicine Residency
Farrell, Pennsylvania
gallojl@upmc.edu
Prenatal Care

Natalie E. Gentile, MD
Physician and Founder
Gentile Family Direct Primary Care
Pittsburgh, Pennsylvania
gentilefamilydpc@gmail.com
Nutrition and the Development of Healthy Eating Habits

Ronald M. Glick, MD
Associate Professor of Psychiatry
Physical Medicine and Rehabilitation and Family Medicine
Center for Integrative Medicine—UPMC Shadyside
Pittsburgh, Pennsylvania
glickrm@upmc.edu
Chronic Pain Management

Wanda C. Gonsalves, MD
Professor and Interim Dean of Natural, Applied and
    Health Sciences
Kentucky State University
Frankfort, Kentucky
wanda.gonsalves@uky.edu
Oral Health

Amanda C. Goodale, DO
Clinical Faculty
Bethesda Family Medicine Residency Program
TriHealth Primary Care Sports Medicine Fellowship Program
Cincinnati, Ohio
Amanda_Goodale@trihealth.com
Common Upper & Lower Extremity Fractures

Darci L. Graves, MPP, MA, MA
Former Instructor and Research Assistant
Office of Medical Education and Research
University of Missouri–Kansas City School of Medicine
Kansas City, Missouri
darci.graves@gmail.com
Cultural and Linguistic Competence

Mary P. Guerrera, MD, FAAFP, FAAMA, DABIHM
Professor Emeritus of Family Medicine and Director of
    Integrative Medicine
Department of Family Medicine
University of Connecticut School of Medicine
Farmington, Connecticut
guerrera@uchc.edu
Complementary & Integrative Health

Scott A. Harper, MD
Assistant Professor
Director of Medical Student Education
Department of Family & Community Medicine
Wake Forest School of Medicine
Winston-Salem, North Carolina
saharper@wakehealth.edu
Evaluation & Management of Headache

Garry W. K. Ho, MD, FACSM, FAMSSM, FAAFP, RMSK, CIC
Program Director
Virginia Commonwealth University (VCU)
Fairfax Family Practice Sports Medicine Fellowship Program
Associate Physician
Fairfax Family Practice Comprehensive Concussion Center,
    Fairfax, Virginia
Associate Professor
Department of Family Medicine
Virginia Commonwealth University School of Medicine
Richmond, Virginia
Associate Professor
Department of Family Medicine
Georgetown University School of Medicine
Washington, DC
gho@ffpcs.com
Neck Pain

Poh Choo How, MD, PhD
Assistant Clinical Professor
Department of Psychiatry and Behavioral Sciences
University of California Davis
Sacramento, California
phow@ucdavis.edu
Depression in Diverse Populations & Older Adults

Thomas M. Howard, MD, FACSM, RMSK
Flexogenix
Adjunct, Associate Professor
Department of Family Medicine
Campbell University
Jerry M Wallace School of Osteopathic Medicine
Cary, North Carolina
thmd2020@gmail.com
Neck Pain

Carla Jardim, MD, FAAP
Medical Director
Hunterdon Family Medicine
Delaware Valley
Faculty
Hunterdon Family Medicine Residency
Clinical Instructor in Family Medicine
UMDNJ Robert Wood Johnson
Flemington, New Jersey
cjardim@hhsnj.org
Abdominal Complaints

Jennie B. Jarrett, PharmD, BCPS, MMedEd, FCCP
Assistant Professor
College of Pharmacy
University of Illinois at Chicago
Chicago, Illinois
jarrett8@uic.edu
Pharmacotherapy Principles for the Family Physician

Martin Johns, MD
Program Director
UPMC Horizon Family Medicine Residency Family
    Medicine Residency
Farrell, Pennsylvania
johnsmg@upmc.edu
Prenatal Care

Bruce E. Johnson, MD
Professor of Medicine
Virginia Tech Carilion School of Medicine
Roanoke, Virginia
cotylurus@yahoo.com
Arthritis: Osteoarthritis, Gout, & Rheumatoid Arthritis

Wayne B. Jonas, MD
Executive Director
Samueli Integrative Health Programs
Alexandria, Virginia
wayne@hsventures.org
Complementary & Integrative Health

Katie B. Kaczmarski, PharmD, BCACP, AE-C
Clinical Assistant Professor
University of Illinois at Chicago
College of Pharmacy
Chicago, Illinois
kkaczm3@uic.edu
Pharmacotherapy Principles for the Family Physician

Peter J. Katsufrakis, MD, MBA
President and CEO
National Board of Medical Examiners
Philadelphia, Pennsylvania
pkatsufrakis@nbme.org
Sexually Transmitted Diseases

Michael King, MD, MPH, FAAFP
Program Director and Associate Professor
Family Medicine Residency Program
HCA Healthcare/USF Morsani College of Medicine GME
    Programs
Oak Hill Hospital
Brooksville, Florida
Michael.King@oakhillhospital.com
Heart Failure

Joe E. Kingery, DO, MBA, FACOFP
Associate Dean of Osteopathic Medical Education
Associate Professor and Chair of Family Medicine
University of Pikeville Kentucky College of
    Osteopathic Medicine
Pikeville, Kentucky
JoeKingery@Upike.edu
Urinary Tract Infections

N. Randall Kolb, MD
Associate Program Director, UPMC Shadyside Family
    Medicine Residency Program
Pittsburgh, Pennsylvania
kolbnr@upmc.edu
Tuberculosis

Mark A. Knox, MD
Associate Director
Hawaii Island Family Medicine Residency Program
Clinical Associate Professor
John A. Burns School of Medicine
Department of Family Medicine and Community Health
University of Hawaii
Hilo, Hawaii
mknox@hhsc.org
Skin Diseases in Infants & Children

Matthew Koperwas, MD
Teaching Physician
AHN Department of Geriatrics
Pittsburgh, Pennsylvania
mattkoperwas@gmail.com
Elder Abuse

Ronald J. Koshes, MD, DFAPA
Private Practice
Washington, DC
ronkoshes@aol.com
*Combat-Related Posttraumatic Stress Disorder &
    Traumatic Brain Injury*

Matthew D. Krasowski, MD, PhD
Clinical Professor
Department of Pathology
Vice Chair of Clinical Pathology and Laboratory Services
University of Iowa Hospitals and Clinics
Iowa City, Iowa
mkrasows@healthcare.uiowa.edu
Pharmacogenomics

COL Mary V. Krueger, DO, MPH
United States Army Medical Corps
Hospital Commander
Tripler Army Medical Center
Honolulu, Hawaii
Mary.Krueger@us.army.mil
Menstrual Disorders

Archana M. Kudrimoti, MD
Associate Professor and Director of Residency
Department of Family and Community Medicine
University of Kentucky
Lexington, Kentucky
archana.kudrimoti@uky.edu
Hearing & Vision Impairment in the Elderly

Paul R. Larson, MD, MS, MBA, CPE, FAAFP
Director
Global Health Education
UPMC St. Margaret Family Medicine Residency Program
Clinical Assistant Professor
Department of Family Medicine
University of Pittsburgh School of Medicine
Pittsburgh, Pennsylvania
larsonpr@upmc.edu
Health Maintenance for Adults

Evelyn L. Lewis, MD, MA, FAAFP, DABDA
Clinical Instructor
Rosalind Franklin University of Medicine and Science
North Chicago, Illinois
Chief Medical Officer, Warrior Centric Health
Ellicott City, Maryland
President and Chair
Warrior Centric Healthcare Foundation
Rockville, Maryland
Adjunct Associate Professor
Department of Family Medicine and Community Health
Rutgers, Robert Wood Johnson Medical School
Piscataway, New Jersey
elewismd2504@gmail.com
Combat-Related Posttraumatic Stress Disorder &
    Traumatic Brain Injury
Health & Healthcare Disparities
Nutrition and the Development of Healthy Eating Habits

Gordon Liu, MD, AAHIVS
HIV Primary Care Physician
Maple Leaf Medical Clinic
Toronto, Ontario, Canada
gliu@mlmedical.com
HIV Primary Care
Tuberculosis

Kristin L. Long, MD, MPH, FACS
Assistant Professor of Surgery
Department of Surgery, Section of Endocrine Surgery
University of Wisconsin School of Medicine and Public Health
Madison, Wisconsin
longk@surgery.wisc.edu
Hepatobiliary Disorders

Charles W. Mackett, III, MD, MMM
President
Indian River Medical Associates
Cleveland Clinic Indian River Hospital
Vero Beach, Florida
charles.mackett@irmc.cc
Adult Sexual Dysfunction

Martin C. Mahoney, MD, PhD, FAAFP
Professor
Department of Family Medicine
Jacobs School of Medicine and Biomedical Sciences
University at Buffalo
Professor of Oncology
Department of Internal Medicine and Department of
    Health Behavior
Roswell Park Cancer Institute
Buffalo, New York
martin.mahoney@roswellpark.org
Neonatal Hyperbilirubinemia
Tobacco Cessation

Robin Maier, MD, MA
Assistant Professor of Family Medicine
Department of Family Medicine
Director of Medical Student Education
Clerkship Director
University of Pittsburgh School of Medicine
Pittsburgh, Pennsylvania
maierrm@upmc.edu
Sexually Transmitted Diseases

Kimberly Mallin, MD
Associate Dean for Wellness and Inclusion
Professor and Director of AUA Health Clinic
American University of Antigua
Coolidge, Antigua
Kmallin@auamed.net
Substance Use Disorders

Robert Mallin, MD
University Provost
American University of Antigua
Coolidge, Antigua
rmallin@auamed.org
Substance Use Disorders

Mylynda B. Massart, MD, PhD
Assistant Professor
Department of Family Medicine
University of Pittsburgh School of Medicine
Pittsburgh, Pennsylvania
massartmb@upmc.edu
Genetics for Family Physicians

Samuel C. Matheny, MD, MPH, FAAFP
Assistant Provost for Global Health Initiatives
Professor of Family and Community Medicine
University of Kentucky
Lexington, Kentucky
matheny@uky.edu
Hepatobiliary Disorders

Victoria McCurry, MD
Clinical Assistant Professor
Department of Family Medicine
University of Pittsburgh
Pittsburgh, Pennsylvania
Mccurryvr@upmc.edu
Acute Coronary Syndrome

Philip J. Michels, PhD
Michels Psychological Services
LLC
Columbia, South Carolina
michelsfour@hotmail.com
Anxiety Disorders

Donald B. Middleton, MD
Professor
Department of Family Medicine
University of Pittsburgh School of Medicine
Vice President
Family Medicine Residency Education
UPMC St. Margaret
Pittsburgh, Pennsylvania
middletondb@upmc.edu
Routine Vaccines
Seizures
Well-Child Care

MAJ Patricia R. Millner, MD, FAAFP
United States Army Medical Corps
Family Medicine Residency Faculty
Tripler Army Medical Center
Honolulu, Hawaii
patricia.r.millner.mil@mail.mil
Menstrual Disorders

Karen Moyer, MD
Director of Family Medicine Obstetrics
UPMC St Margaret Family Medicine Residency Program
Pittsburgh, Pennsylvania
boylekm@upmc.edu
Preconception Care

Francis G. O'Connor, MD, MPH
Professor, Medical Director, Consortium for Health and
    Military Performance
Department of Military and Emergency Medicine
Uniformed Services University of the Health Sciences
Bethesda, Maryland
francis.oconnor@usuhs.edu
Low Back Pain in Primary Care: An Evidence-Based Approach

Richard A. Okragly, MD, FAMSSM
Program Director
Primary Care Sports Medicine Fellowship
TriHealth
Cincinnati, Ohio
Richard_Okragly@trihealth.com
Common Upper & Lower Extremity Fractures

Maureen O'Hara Padden, MD, MPH, FAAFP
Family Physician
Ascension Sacred Heart Medical Group
Pensacola, Florida
maureen.padden@ascension.org
Hypertension

Saranne E. Perman, MD
Assistant Professor of Family Medicine
Augusta University
Augusta, Georgia
spearman1@gmail.com
Hearing & Vision Impairment in the Elderly

Nicole Powell-Dunford, MD, MPH, FAAFP, FAsMA
Associate Professor
Department of Military and Emergency Medicine
Uniformed Services University of the Health Sciences
Bethesda, Maryland
School of Army Aviation Medicine
Ft Rucker, Alabama
Nicole.c.powell-dunford.mil@mail.mil
Cancer Screening in Women

Praneeth Pillala, MBBS
HIV Primary Care Physician
PCMH Restore Health
Bangalore, India
praneeth0353@gmail.com
HIV Primary Care

Ramakrishna Prasad, MD, MPH
Founder & Director
PCMH Restore Health
Chair
National Center for Primary Care Research and Policy
Academy of Family Physicians of India (AFPI)
Bangalore, India
dr.rk.prasad@gmail.com
Tuberculosis
HIV Primary Care

Annelle B. Primm, MD, MPH
Senior Medical Director
The Steve Fund
Baltimore, Maryland
annelleprimm@aol.com
Depression in Diverse Populations & Older Adults

Timothy Scott Prince, MD, MSPH, FACOEM, FACPM
Associate Professor
Department of Preventive Medicine and Environmental Health
University of Kentucky College of Public Health
Lexington, Kentucky
scott.prince@uky.edu
Travel Medicine

Wade M. Rankin, DO, CAQSM
Program Director
Family Medicine Residency Program
Bon Secour Mercy Health
Mercy Health-Anderson
Cincinnati, Ohio
wademrankin@hotmail.com
Common Upper & Lower Extremity Fractures

Brian V. Reamy, MD
Senior Associate Dean for Academic Affairs & Professor of
    Family Medicine
F. Edward Hébert School of Medicine
Uniformed Services University
Bethesda, Maryland
brian.reamy@usuhs.edu
Dyslipidemias

Eva B. Reitschuler-Cross, MD
Assistant Professor of Medicine
University of Pittsburgh School of Medicine
University of Pittsburgh Medical Center
Division of General Medicine
Section of Palliative Care and Medical Ethics
Pittsburgh, Pennsylvania
reitschulercrosseb@upmc.edu
Hospice & Palliative Medicine

Angelina Rodriguez, MD, FAAFP
Associate Program Director and Assistant Professor
Family Medicine Residency Program
HCA Healthcare/USF Morsani College of
    Medicine GME Programs
Oak Hill Hospital
Brooksville, Florida
Angelina.Rodriguez@hcahealthcare.com
Heart Failure

Jennifer E. Roper, MD
Assistant Professor
Department of Family and Community Medicine
Wake Forest University School of Medicine
Winston-Salem, North Carolina
jetovey@wakehealth.edu
Evaluation & Management of Headache

J. Scott Roth, MD, FACS
Professor of Surgery
Chief
Gastrointestinal Surgery
College of Medicine
University of Kentucky
Lexington, Kentucky
S.roth@uky.edu
Hepatobiliary Disorders

Kerry Sadler, MD
Family Physician
Naval Hospital Jacksonville
Jacksonville, Florida
kephilbin@gmail.com
Hypertension

Courtney M. Saint, DO
Family Medicine Attending
Branch Health Clinic Atsugi
Atsugi, Japan
Courtneysaint89@gmail.com
Hypertension

Steven Sanker, DO
Family Medicine/Sports Medicine Physician
TriHealth – Group Health Anderson
Cincinnati, Ohio
stephen_sanker@trihealth.com
Common Upper & Lower Extremity Fractures

Joseph Sapoval, DO
Family Physician
United States Naval Hospital Okinawa
Okinawa, Japan
joseph.sapoval@gmail.com
Hypertension

Ruth S. Shim, MD, MPH
Luke & Grace Kim Professor in Cultural Psychiatry
Department of Psychiatry and Behavioral Sciences
University of California, Davis
Sacramento, California
rshim@ucdavis.edu
Depression in Diverse Populations

Tiffany Simon, DO, MS
Chief Resident
Family Medicine Residency Program
HCA Healthcare/USF Morsani College of Medicine GME
    Programs
Oak Hill Hospital
Brooksville, Florida
tiffany.simon@hcahealthcare.com
Heart Failure

Stephanie Singh, DO
Sports Medicine/Primary Care Physician
VCU—Fairfax Family Practice and Sports Medicine
Fairfax, Virginia
scart019@gmail.com
Neck Pain

Suzan Skef, MD, MS
Assistant Professor
UPMC—St. Margaret Family Medicine Residency Program
Assistant Director of the Bloomfield-Garfield Family
    Health Center
Pittsburgh, Pennsylvania
skefs@upmc.edu
Acute Coronary Syndrome

Jeannette E. South-Paul, MD, DHL (Hon), FAAFP
Andrew W. Mathieson UPMC Professor and Chair
Department of Family Medicine
University of Pittsburgh School of Medicine
Pittsburgh, Pennsylvania
soutjx@upmc.edu or jes1239@pitt.edu
Osteoporosis
Health & Healthcare Disparities

Mark B. Stephens, MD, MS, FAAFP
Professor of Family and Community Medicine
Professor of Humanities
Penn State College of Medicine
University Park, Pennsylvania
mstephens3@pennstatehealth.psu.edu
Physical Activity in Adolescents

Nathaniel D. Stewart, MD
Family and Community Medicine
University of Kentucky
Lexington, Kentucky
Nat.Stewart@uky.edu
Hearing & Vision Impairment in the Elderly

Paul Stranges, PharmD, BCACP
University of Illinois at Chicago
Chicago, Illinois
pmstrang@UIC.EDU
Pharmacotherapy Principles for the Family Physician

Marian Swope, MD
Professor of Psychiatry
Program Director
Child and Adolescent Psychiatry
University of Kentucky College of Medicine
Lexington, Kentucky
maswop1@uky.edu
Behavioral Disorders in Children

Andrew B. Symons, MD, MS
Clinical Associate Professor and Vice Chair for Medical
    Student Education
Department of Family Medicine
Jacobs School of Medicine and Biomedical Sciences
University at Buffalo
Buffalo, New York
symons@buffalo.edu
Neonatal Hyperbilirubinemia

Teiichi Takedai, MD, FAAFP
Clinical Assistant Professor of Family Medicine
University of Pittsburgh School of Medicine
Faculty
UPMC Shadyside Family Medicine Residency
Pittsburgh, Pennsylvania
takedait@upmc.edu
Skin Diseases in Infants & Children

Mehret Birru Talabi, MD, PhD
Assistant Professor of Medicine
Associate Program Director
UPMC Rheumatology Fellowship
Division of Rheumatology and Clinical Immunology
University of Pittsburgh Department of Medicine
Pittsburgh, Pennsylvania
birrums@upmc.edu
Osteoporosis

Yelena Tarasenko, DO
Core Faculty
Family Medicine Residency Program
HCA Healthcare/USF Morsani College of Medicine
    GME Programs
Oak Hill Hospital
Brooksville, Florida
Yelena.Tarasenko@med.lecom.edu
Heart Failure

Belinda Vail, MD, MS, FAAFP
David M. Huben Professor and Chair
Department of Family Medicine and Community Health
University of Kansas School of Medicine
Kansas City, Kansas
bvail@kumc.edu
Diabetes Mellitus

Abigail K. Vargo, MD, MPH
Aerospace and Occupational Medicine Resident
School of Army Aviation Medicine
Fort Rucker, Alabama
abigail.k.vargo.mil@mail.mil
Cancer Screening in Women

Shannon Voogt, MD
Assistant Professor of Family Medicine
Department of Family & Community Medicine
University of Kentucky
Lexington, Kentucky
shannon.voogt@uky.edu
Abnormal Uterine Bleeding

David Yuan, MD, MS
Program Director, Geriatrics Fellowship
UPMC St. Margaret's
Pittsburgh, Pennsylvania
yuand@upmc.edu
Health Maintenance for Adults
Elder Abuse

Jacqueline S. Weaver-Agostoni, DO, MPH
Program Director, Family Medicine Residency
Co-Chair, UPMC Med Ed ARQC Committee
University of Pittsburgh Department of Family Medicine
UPMC Shadyside
Pittsburgh, Pennsylvania
agostonijs@upmc.edu
Acute Coronary Syndrome

**Charles W. Webb, DO, FAAFP, FAMSSM,
CAQ Sports Medicine**
Sports Medicine Physician
Department of Orthopedic Surgery & Sports Medicine
Legacy Medical Group
Portland, Oregon
thesportsdo@gmail.com
Low Back Pain in Primary Care: An Evidence-Based Approach

Richard Welsh, LCSW, MSW
Professor
Department of Psychiatry
University of Kentucky College of Medicine
Professor
College of Social Work
University of Kentucky
Lexington, Kentucky
rjwels0@email.uky.edu
Behavioral Disorders in Children

Katie L. Westerfield, DO, IBCLC, FAAFP
Assistant Professor of Family Medicine
Uniformed Services University of the Health Sciences
Bethesda, Maryland
1st Security Force Assistance Brigade
Fort Benning, Georgia
katie.l.westerfield.mil@mail.mil
Cancer Screening in Women

Katherine Wilhelmy, MD
Family Medicine Physician
Renaissance Family Practice
Pittsburgh, Pennsylvania
wilhelmykh2@upmc.edu
Elder Abuse

Stephen A. Wilson, MD, MPH, FAAFP
Chair
Department of Family Medicine
Boston University School of Medicine
Chief of Family Medicine
Boston Medical Center
Boston, Massachusetts
stephen.wilson@bmc.org
Health Maintenance for Adults
Acute Coronary Syndrome

Jeanette M. Witter, PhD
Assistant Professor
Department of Medical and Clinical Psychology
Uniformed Services University
Bethesda, Maryland
jeanette.witter@usuhs.edu
*Combat-Related Posttraumatic Stress Disorder &
    Traumatic Brain Injury*

Steven R. Wolfe, DO, MPH, FAAFP, AAHIVS
Dean
AHN/LECOM Clinical Campus
Clinical Professor
LECOM Department of Family Medicine
Associate Clinical Professor
Temple Department of Family Medicine
Osteopathic Program Director
Forbes Family Medicine Residency Program
Forbes Hospital, AHN
Monroeville, Pennsylvania
Swolfe1@wpahs.org
Caring for LGBTQIA Patients

Rachel K.F. Woodruff, MD, MPH
Assistant Professor
Wake Forest Department of Family and Community Medicine
Wake Forest University School of Medicine
    Winston-Salem, North Carolina
rkwoodru@wakehealth.edu
Evaluation & Management of Headache

Yaqin Xia, MD, MHPE
Assistant Professor
Department of Family Medicine
University of Pittsburgh School of Medicine
Pittsburgh, Pennsylvania
xiay@upmc.edu
Movement Disorders

Preface

The Fifth Edition of *Current Diagnosis & Treatment: Family Medicine* is a comprehensive, single source reference for practicing family physicians and trainees delivering primary care in a continuity environment for all patients across the lifespan. The text is organized according to the developmental lifespan beginning with infancy, childhood, and adolescence, including a focus on the reproductive years, and progressing through adulthood and the mature, senior years.

The text has been adapted from one edition to another to incorporate emerging areas that impact individual patients and/or populations and are likely to present in a primary care setting. Areas such as immunization updates, genetics in primary care, pharmacogenomics, and telemedicine are presented, as well as current approaches and treatments for the usual chronic diseases such as hypertension and diabetes mellitus.

OUTSTANDING FEATURES

- Evidence-based recommendation
- Culturally related aspects of each condition and alternative
- Conservative and pharmacologic therapies
- Complementary and alternative therapies when relevant
- Suggestions for collaborations with other healthcare providers
- Attention to the mental and behavioral health of patients as solitary as well as comorbid conditions
- Recognition of the impact of illness on the family
- Patient education information
- End-of-life issues

INTENDED AUDIENCE

Primary care trainees and practicing physicians will find this text a useful resource for common conditions seen in ambulatory practice. Detailed information in tabular and text format provides a ready reference for selecting diagnostic procedures and recommending treatments. Advanced practice nurses and physician's assistants will also find the approach provided here a practical and complete first resource for both diagnosed and undifferentiated conditions and an aid in continuing management.

Unlike smaller medical manuals that focus on urgent, one-time approaches to a particular presenting complaint or condition, this text was envisioned as a resource for clinicians who practice continuity of care and have established a longitudinal, therapeutic relationship with their patients. Therefore, each chapter includes recommendations for immediate as well as subsequent clinical encounters.

ACKNOWLEDGMENTS

We thank our many contributing authors for their diligence in creating complete, practical, and readable discussions of the many conditions seen on a daily basis in the average family medicine and primary care practice. Furthermore, the vision and support of our editors at McGraw-Hill for creating this resource for primary care have been outstanding and critical to its completion.

Jeannette E. South-Paul, MD, DHL (Hon), FAAFP
Samuel C. Matheny, MD, MPH, FAAFP
Evelyn L. Lewis, MD, MA, FAAFP, DABDA

Well-Child Care

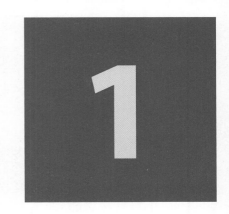

Donald B. Middleton, MD

ESSENTIALS OF WELL-CHILD CARE

Providing a comprehensive patient-centered medical home for children and assisting in the progressive transition to adulthood are integral components of family medicine. The provision of well-child care through a series of periodic examinations forms the foundation for the family physician to build lasting relationships with the entire family, a critical distinction between the family physician and other medical specialists.

Health care for infants and children has changed markedly over the past half century. Prior focus on infectious disease and illness prevention has shifted to largely behavioral and environmental concerns. Paramount among behaviors is the issue of screen time, including television, iPads, computers, and cell phones. Environmental concerns such as water purity continue to be problematic. Of course, safety should always be emphasized. However, family physicians should remember that the goal of child care is to allow the child and family to experience joyous childrearing. Too often a well-child visit focuses on difficulties and not on pleasantries. Part of making certain that the child has a happy childhood is to limit toxic experiences such as corporal punishment that have been linked to later adult difficulties such as early myocardial infarction. Limiting negative experiences necessitates investigation into whether the parents and other family members are doing well, part of every family physician's goals.

Enhanced nutrition, mandated safety standards, and expanded schedules for immunizations have significantly improved the health of US children, but serious childhood health problems persist. Inadequate prenatal care leading to poor birth outcomes, poor management of developmental delay, childhood obesity, lack of proper oral health, learning disabilities, and substance abuse are examples of ongoing dilemmas.

A key reference guide for childhood health promotion is the fourth edition of *Bright Futures: Guidelines for Health Supervision of Infants, Children, and Adolescents* (https://brightfutures.aap.org/clinical-practice/Pages/default.aspx), funded by the US Department of Health and Human Services. The guidelines give providers a comprehensive system of care that addresses basic concerns of childrearing such as nutrition, parenting, safety, dental care, and infectious disease prevention with focused attention on evidence-based health components and interventions. *Bright Futures* materials include interim history forms for parents, well-child chart notes for each recommended visit, and anticipatory guidance sheets to be given to parents at the visit's conclusion. It also lists and describes numerous community resources, some of which are designed to address medical or behavioral issues and some of which are designed to enhance childrearing.

One widely utilized, online schedule for routine well-child visits (Table 1–1) is the *Bright Futures/AAP* Periodicity Schedule (https://www.aap.org/en-us/Documents/periodicity_schedule.pdf). Following a prenatal visit, seven visits are suggested during the first year, five visits age 12 to 30 months, and then yearly visits until adulthood at age 21 years. Table 1–1 provides a structured framework for anticipatory guidance, examinations, and growth and developmental screening at appropriate intervals.

The most important components of a preventive well-child visit include: (1) developmental/behavioral assessment; (2) physical examination, including measurement of growth; (3) screening tests and procedures; and (4) anticipatory guidance. One specific goal of each visit is to identify concerns about a child's development and then intervene with early treatment and monitor closely for changes. An essential component is adherence to the most recent schedule of recommended immunizations from the Advisory Committee

Table 1–1. Schedule of routine well-care visits.

Recommendations for Preventive Pediatric Health Care

Bright Futures/American Academy of Pediatrics

American Academy of Pediatrics
DEDICATED TO THE HEALTH OF ALL CHILDREN®

Bright Futures.

Each child and family is unique; therefore, these Recommendations for Preventive Pediatric Health Care are designed for the care of children who are receiving competent parenting, have no manifestations of any important health problems, and are growing and developing in a satisfactory fashion. Developmental, psychosocial, and chronic disease issues for children and adolescents may require frequent counseling and treatment visits separate from preventive care visits. Additional visits also may become necessary if circumstances suggest variations from normal.

These recommendations represent a consensus by the American Academy of Pediatrics (AAP) and Bright Futures. The AAP continues to emphasize the great importance of continuity of care in comprehensive health supervision and the need to avoid fragmentation of care.

Refer to the specific guidance by age as listed in the *Bright Futures Guidelines* (Hagan JF, Shaw JS, Duncan PM, eds. *Bright Futures: Guidelines for Health Supervision of Infants, Children, and Adolescents*. 4th ed. Elk Grove Village, IL: American Academy of Pediatrics; 2017).

The recommendations in this statement do not indicate an exclusive course of treatment or serve as a standard of medical care. Variations, taking into account individual circumstances, may be appropriate.

The Bright Futures/American Academy of Pediatrics Recommendations for Preventive Pediatric Health Care are updated annually.

Copyright © 2020 by the American Academy of Pediatrics, updated March 2020.

No part of this statement may be reproduced in any form or by any means without prior written permission from the American Academy of Pediatrics except for one copy for personal use.

AGE	Prenatal	Newborn	3-5 d	By 1 mo	1 mo	2 mo	4 mo	6 mo	9 mo	12 mo	15 mo	18 mo	24 mo	30 mo	3 y	4 y	5 y	6 y	7 y	8 y	9 y	10 y	11 y	12 y	13 y	14 y	15 y	16 y	17 y	18 y	19 y	20 y	21 y
HISTORY Initial/Interval	●	●	●	●	●	●	●	●	●	●	●	●	●	●	●	●	●	●	●	●	●	●	●	●	●	●	●	●	●	●	●	●	●
MEASUREMENTS																																	
Length/Height and Weight		●	●	●	●	●	●	●	●	●	●	●	●	●	●	●	●	●	●	●	●	●	●	●	●	●	●	●	●	●	●	●	●
Head Circumference		●	●	●	●	●	●	●	●	●	●	●	●																				
Weight for Length		●	●	●	●	●	●	●	●	●	●	●																					
Body Mass Index													●	●	●	●	●	●	●	●	●	●	●	●	●	●	●	●	●	●	●	●	●
Blood Pressure		★	★	★	★	★	★	★	★	★	★	★	★	★	●	●	●	●	●	●	●	●	●	●	●	●	●	●	●	●	●	●	●
SENSORY SCREENING																																	
Vision		★	★	★	★	★	★	★	★	★	★	★	★	★	●	●	●	●	★	●	★	●	★	●	★	●	★	●	★	●	★	●	★
Hearing		●	←	→	★	★	★	★	★	★	★	★	★	★	★	●	●	●	★	●	★	●	←	●	→	●	←	●	→	★	★	★	★
DEVELOPMENTAL/BEHAVIORAL HEALTH																																	
Developmental Screening									●			●		●																			
Autism Spectrum Disorder Screening												●	●																				
Developmental Surveillance		●	●	●	●	●	●	●	●	●	●	●	●	●	●	●	●	●	●	●	●	●	●	●	●	●	●	●	●	●	●	●	●
Psychosocial/Behavioral Assessment		●	●	●	●	●	●	●	●	●	●	●	●	●	●	●	●	●	●	●	●	●	●	●	●	●	●	●	●	●	●	●	●
Tobacco, Alcohol, or Drug Use Assessment																							★	★	★	★	★	★	★	★	★	★	★
Depression Screening																								●	●	●	●	●	●	●	●	●	●
Maternal Depression Screening			●	●	●	●																											
PHYSICAL EXAMINATION		●	●	●	●	●	●	●	●	●	●	●	●	●	●	●	●	●	●	●	●	●	●	●	●	●	●	●	●	●	●	●	●
PROCEDURES																																	
Newborn Blood		●	●	★																													
Newborn Bilirubin		●																															
Critical Congenital Heart Defect		●																															
Immunization		●	●	●	●	●	●	●	●	●	●	●	●	●	●	●	●	●	●	●	●	●	●	●	●	●	●	●	●	●	●	●	●
Anemia							★		★	★	★	★	★	★	★	★	★	★	★	★	★	★	★	★	★	★	★	★	★	★	★	★	★
Lead								★	★	★ or ★		★	★ or ★		★	★	★	★															
Tuberculosis								★			★		★		★	★	★	★	★	★	★	★	★	★	★	★	★	★	★	★	★	★	★
Dyslipidemia													★			★			★		★	●	★	★	★	★	★	★	★	★	●	★	★
Sexually Transmitted Infections																							★	★	★	★	★	★	★	★	★	★	★
HIV																							←	★	→	★	★	★	★	★	★	★	★
Cervical Dysplasia																																	●
ORAL HEALTH								★	★	★		★	★	★	★	★	★	★															
Fluoride Varnish								←						→																			
Fluoride Supplementation								★	★	★	★	★	★	★	★	★	★	★	★	★	★	★	★	★									
ANTICIPATORY GUIDANCE	●	●	●	●	●	●	●	●	●	●	●	●	●	●	●	●	●	●	●	●	●	●	●	●	●	●	●	●	●	●	●	●	●

1. If a child comes under care for the first time at any point on the schedule, or if any items are not accomplished at the suggested age, the schedule should be brought up-to-date at the earliest possible time.

2. A prenatal visit is recommended for parents who are at high risk, for first-time parents, and those who request a conference. The prenatal visit should include anticipatory guidance, pertinent medical history, and a discussion of benefits of breastfeeding and planned method of feeding, per "The Prenatal Visit" (http://pediatrics.aappublications.org/content/124/4/1227.full).

3. Newborns should have an evaluation after birth, and breastfeeding should be encouraged (and instruction and support should be offered).

4. Newborns should have an evaluation within 3 to 5 days of birth and within 48 to 72 hours after discharge from the hospital to include evaluation for feeding and jaundice. Breastfeeding newborns should receive formal breastfeeding evaluation, and their mothers should receive encouragement and instruction, as recommended in "Breastfeeding and the Use of Human Milk" (http://pediatrics.aappublications.org/content/129/3/e827.full). Newborns discharged less than 48 hours after delivery must be examined within 48 hours of discharge, per "Hospital Stay for Healthy Term Newborns" (http://pediatrics.aappublications.org/content/125/2/405.full).

5. Screen, per "Expert Committee Recommendations Regarding the Prevention, Assessment, and Treatment of Child and Adolescent Overweight and Obesity: Summary Report" (http://pediatrics.aappublications.org/content/120/Supplement_4/S164.full).

6. Screening should occur per "Clinical Practice Guideline for Screening and Management of High Blood Pressure in Children and Adolescents" (http://pediatrics.aappublications.org/content/140/3/e20171904). Blood pressure measurement in infants and children with specific risk conditions should be performed at visits before age 3 years.

7. A visual acuity screen is recommended at ages 4 and 5 years, as well as in cooperative 3-year-olds. Instrument-based screening may be used to assess risk at ages 12 and 24 months, in addition to the well visits at 3 through 5 years of age. See "Visual System Assessment in Infants, Children, and Young Adults by Pediatricians" (http://pediatrics.aappublications.org/content/137/1/e20153596) and "Procedures for the Evaluation of the Visual System by Pediatricians" (http://pediatrics.aappublications.org/content/137/1/e20153597).

8. Confirm initial screen was accomplished, verify results, and follow up, as appropriate. Newborns should be screened, per "Year 2007 Position Statement: Principles and Guidelines for Early Hearing Detection and Intervention Programs" (http://pediatrics.aappublications.org/content/120/4/898.full).

9. Verify results as soon as possible, and follow up, as appropriate.

10. Screen with audiometry including 6,000 and 8,000 Hz high frequencies once between 11 and 14 years, once between 15 and 17 years, and once between 18 and 21 years. See "The Sensitivity of Adolescent Hearing Screens Significantly Improves by Adding High Frequencies" (https://www.sciencedirect.com/science/article/abs/pii/S1054139X16000483).

11. See "Identifying Infants and Young Children With Developmental Disorders in the Medical Home: An Algorithm for Developmental Surveillance and Screening" (http://pediatrics.aappublications.org/content/118/1/405.full).

12. Screening should occur per "Identification and Evaluation of Children With Autism Spectrum Disorders" (http://pediatrics.aappublications.org/content/120/5/1183.full).

13. This assessment should be family centered and may include an assessment of child social-emotional health, caregiver depression, and social determinants of health. See "Promoting Optimal Development: Screening for Behavioral and Emotional Problems" (http://pediatrics.aappublications.org/content/135/2/384) and "Poverty and Child Health in the United States" (http://pediatrics.aappublications.org/content/137/4/e20160339).

14. A recommended assessment tool is available at http://crafft.org.

15. Recommended screening using the Patient Health Questionnaire (PHQ)-2 or other tools available in the GLAD-PC toolkit and at (https://downloads.aap.org/AAP/PDF/Mental_Health_Tools_for_Pediatrics.pdf).

16. Screening should occur per "Incorporating Recognition and Management of Perinatal Depression Into Pediatric Practice" (https://pediatrics.aappublications.org/content/143/1/e20183259).

17. At each visit, age-appropriate physical examination is essential, with infant totally unclothed and older children undressed and suitably draped. See "Use of Chaperones During the Physical Examination of the Pediatric Patient" (http://pediatrics.aappublications.org/content/127/5/991.full).

18. These may be modified, depending on entry point into schedule and individual need.

KEY: ● = to be performed   ★ = risk assessment to be performed with appropriate action to follow, if positive   ←→ = range during which a service may be provided

BFNC-2020-PFEB
3-305/0220

(continued)

(continued)

19. Confirm initial screen was accomplished, verify results, and follow up, as appropriate. The Recommended Uniform Screening Panel (https://www.hrsa.gov/advisorycommittees/heritable-disorders/rusp/index.html), as determined by The Secretary's Advisory Committee on Heritable Disorders in Newborns and Children, and state newborn screening laws/regulations (https://www.babysfirsttest.org/newbornscreening/states) establish the criteria for and coverage of newborn screening procedures and programs.

20. Verify results as soon as possible, and follow up, as appropriate.

21. Confirm initial screening was accomplished, verify results, and follow up, as appropriate. See "Hyperbilirubinemia in the Newborn Infant ≥35 Weeks' Gestation: An Update With Clarifications" (http://pediatrics.aappublications.org/content/124/4/1193).

22. Screening for critical congenital heart disease using pulse oximetry should be performed in newborns, after 24 hours of age, before discharge from the hospital, per "Endorsement of Health and Human Services Recommendation for Pulse Oximetry Screening for Critical Congenital Heart Disease" (http://pediatrics.aappublications.org/content/129/1/190.full).

23. Schedules, per the AAP Committee on Infectious Diseases, are available at https://redbook.solutions.aap.org/SS/Immunization_Schedules.aspx. Every visit should be an opportunity to update and complete a child's immunizations.

24. Perform risk assessment or screening, as appropriate, per recommendations in the current edition of the AAP *Pediatric Nutrition: Policy of the American Academy of Pediatrics* (Iron chapter).

25. For children at risk of lead exposure, see "Prevention of Childhood Lead Toxicity" (http://pediatrics.aappublications.org/content/138/1/e20161493) and "Low Level Lead Exposure Harms Children: A Renewed Call for Primary Prevention" (http://www.cdc.gov/nceh/lead/ACCLPP/Final_Document_030712.pdf).

26. Perform risk assessments or screenings as appropriate, based on universal screening requirements for patients with Medicaid or in high prevalence areas.

27. Tuberculosis testing per recommendations of the AAP Committee on Infectious Diseases, published in the current edition of the AAP *Red Book: Report of the Committee on Infectious Diseases*. Testing should be performed on recognition of high-risk factors.

28. See "Integrated Guidelines for Cardiovascular Health and Risk Reduction in Children and Adolescents" (http://www.nhlbi.nih.gov/guidelines/cvd_ped/index.htm).

29. Adolescents should be screened for sexually transmitted infections (STIs) per recommendations in the current edition of the AAP *Red Book: Report of the Committee on Infectious Diseases*.

30. Adolescents should be screened for HIV according to the USPSTF recommendations (https://www.uspreventiveservicestaskforce.org/Page/Document/UpdateSummaryFinal/human-immunodeficiency-virus-hiv-infection-screening1) once between the ages of 15 and 18, making every effort to preserve confidentiality of the adolescent. Those at increased risk of HIV infection, including those who are sexually active, participate in injection drug use, or are being tested for other STIs, should be tested for HIV and reassessed annually.

31. See USPSTF recommendations (https://www.uspreventiveservicestaskforce.org/Page/Document/UpdateSummaryFinal/cervical-cancer-screening2). Indications for pelvic examinations prior to age 21 are noted in "Gynecologic Examination for Adolescents in the Pediatric Office Setting" (http://pediatrics.aappublications.org/content/126/3/583.full).

32. Assess whether the child has a dental home. If no dental home is identified, perform a risk assessment (https://www.aap.org/en-us/advocacy-and-policy/aap-health/initiatives/Oral-Health/Pages/Oral-Health-Practice-Tools.aspx) and refer to a dental home. Recommend brushing with fluoride toothpaste in the proper dosage for age. See "Maintaining and Improving the Oral Health of Young Children" (http://pediatrics.aappublications.org/content/134/6/1224).

33. Perform a risk assessment (https://www.aap.org/en-us/advocacy-and-policy/aap-health-initiatives/Oral-Health/Pages/Oral-Health-Practice-Tools.aspx). See "Maintaining and Improving the Oral Health of Young Children" (http://pediatrics.aappublications.org/content/134/6/1224).

34. See USPSTF recommendations (https://www.uspreventiveservicestaskforce.org/Page/Document/UpdateSummaryFinal/dental-caries-in-children-from-birthrough-age-5-years-screening). Once teeth are present, fluoride varnish may be applied to all children every 3–6 months in the primary care or dental office. Indications for fluoride use are noted in "Fluoride Use in Caries Prevention in the Primary Care Setting" (http://pediatrics.aappublications.org/content/134/3/626).

35. If primary water source is deficient in fluoride, consider oral fluoride supplementation. See "Fluoride Use in Caries Prevention in the Primary Care Setting" (http://pediatrics.aappublications.org/content/134/3/626).

Summary of Changes Made to the
Bright Futures/AAP Recommendations for Preventive Pediatric Health Care
(Periodicity Schedule)

This schedule reflects changes approved in October 2019 and published in March 2020.
For updates and a list of previous changes made, visit www.aap.org/periodicityschedule.

CHANGES MADE IN OCTOBER 2019

MATERNAL DEPRESSION

- Footnote 16 has been updated to read as follows: "Screening should occur per 'Incorporating Recognition and Management of Perinatal Depression Into Pediatric Practice' (https://pediatrics.aappublications.org/content/143/1/e20183259)."

CHANGES MADE IN DECEMBER 2018

BLOOD PRESSURE

- Footnote 6 has been updated to read as follows: "Screening should occur per 'Clinical Practice Guideline for Screening and Management of High Blood Pressure in Children and Adolescents' (http://pediatrics.aappublications.org/content/140/3/e20171904). Blood pressure measurement in infants and children with specific risk conditions should be performed at visits before age 3 years."

ANEMIA

- Footnote 24 has been updated to read as follows: "Perform risk assessment or screening, as appropriate, per recommendations in the current edition of the AAP *Pediatric Nutrition: Policy of the American Academy of Pediatrics* (Iron chapter)."

LEAD

- Footnote 25 has been updated to read as follows: "For children at risk of lead exposure, see 'Prevention of Childhood Lead Toxicity' (http://pediatrics.aappublications.org/content/138/1/e20161493) and 'Low Level Lead Exposure Harms Children: A Renewed Call for Primary Prevention' (https://www.cdc.gov/nceh/lead/ACCLPP/Final_Document_030712.pdf)."

HRSA
Health Resources & Services Administration

This program is supported by the Health Resources and Services Administration (HRSA) of the U.S. Department of Health and Human Services (HHS) as part of an award totaling $5,000,000 with 10 percent financed with non-governmental sources. The contents are those of the author(s) and do not necessarily represent the official views of, nor an endorsement, by HRSA, HHS, or the U.S. Government. For more information, please visit HRSA.gov.

AAP updates annually.
Copyright © 2020 by the American Academy of Pediatrics, updated March 2020.

on Immunization Practices and the Centers for Disease Control and Prevention (CDC) (see Chapter 7), available at https://www.cdc.gov/vaccines/schedules/index.html. The number one risk to children is accidental death. Each well-child visit should focus some attention on safety.

The purpose of well visits is to engage the caregivers to partner with the physician to optimize the physical, emotional, and developmental health of the child and family. Family physicians need to identify common normal variants as well as abnormal findings that may require referral. Parents should be encouraged to use these dedicated well visits to raise questions, share observations, and advocate for their child, as they know their child best. Parents should be advised to bring in a list of questions and maintain their own records, especially for immunizations and growth, for each child.

Supplemental visits may be required if the child is adopted or living with surrogate parents; is at high risk for medical disorders as suggested by conditions observed during pregnancy, delivery, neonatal history, growth pattern, or physical examination; or exhibits psychological disorders. Supplemental visits may also be required if the family is socially or economically disadvantaged or if the parents request or require additional education or guidance.

▶ General Considerations

Well-child care ideally begins in the preconception period. Family physicians have the opportunity to provide preconception counseling, especially to a woman who presents for gynecologic examination before pregnancy. Prospective parents should be counseled about appropriate nutrition, including 0.4 mg of folic acid supplementation daily for all women of childbearing age. Prior to conception, referral for genetic screening and counseling should be offered based on age, ethnic background, or family history. Prescription drug and supplement use should be reviewed. Exposure to cigarette smoke, alcohol, illicit drugs, or chemicals such as pesticides should be strongly discouraged. Clinicians should verify or complete immunization against hepatitis B, pertussis, tetanus, rubella, and varicella prior to pregnancy. A tetanus toxoid, reduced diphtheria toxoid, and reduced acellular pertussis vaccine (Tdap) should be given during each pregnancy, preferentially between age 27 and 36 weeks of gestation, regardless of prior Tdap vaccination, to optimize maternal transfer of antibodies to the fetus prior to delivery. These antibodies have proven to be effective in protecting the infant against pertussis during the first 2 months of life. During flu season, every pregnant woman should be given an influenza vaccination regardless of the trimester of pregnancy. Other necessary vaccinations should be given immediately postpartum. Clinicians should discuss prevention of infection from toxoplasmosis (often

transmitted by contact with kittens), cytomegalovirus, and parvovirus B19.

Medical problems such as diabetes, epilepsy, depression, or hypertension warrant special management prior to conception, especially because medications may need to be changed before pregnancy. The "prenatal" visit provides an opportunity to discuss cultural, occupational, and financial issues related to pregnancy; to gather information about preparations for the child's arrival; to discuss plans for feeding and child care; and to screen for domestic violence. The prenatal visit is a good opportunity to promote breastfeeding. A social history should include the family structure (eg, caregivers, siblings) and socioeconomic status, which serve to guide specific suggestions about child care.

Once the child is born, the prenatal and neonatal records should be reviewed for gestational age at birth; any abnormal maternal obstetric laboratory tests; maternal illnesses such as diabetes, preeclampsia, depression, or infections during pregnancy; maternal use of drugs or exposure to teratogens; date of birth; mode of delivery; Apgar scores at 1 and 5 minutes; and birth weight, length, and head circumference. All newborn infants should be given vitamin K intramuscularly and the first hepatitis B vaccine. Plans for emergencies such as fire should be in place. Repeated screening of parents during well-child visits for depression and tobacco use with an offer of counseling and treatment can have profound benefits for the child.

COMPONENTS OF PREVENTIVE WELL-CHILD CARE

▶ Developmental/Behavioral Assessment

A 2016 CDC report states that 16.7% of children and adolescents have a developmental delay or disorder. Young children who experience toxic stress such as maltreatment, neglect, poverty, or a depressed parent are at increased risk for later life health problems such as asthma, heart disease, cancer, and depression. During the prenatal and early childhood years, the neuroendocrine-immune network creates end-organ setpoints that lead to these disorders. Because well-timed adjustments to the child's environment can reduce the risk for later disease, the clinician should attempt to uncover toxic stressors at each preventive health visit. Whether happy times can reverse this process is unclear. Nonetheless, the physician should stress the wonderful parts of having a child as part of the family and give multiple compliments to the parents on how well they are doing raising the child.

Watching a newborn develop from a dependent being into a communicative child with a unique personality is an amazing process. Early identification of developmental disorders is critical for the well-being of children and their families. CDC advice on developmental screening is available at their website (https://www.cdc.gov/ncbddd/childdevelopment/ screening.html). A report from the United States during 2006–2008 found that about one in six children had a developmental disability. Unfortunately, primary care physicians fail to identify and appropriately refer many developmental problems, even though screening tools are available. The period of most easily identified development occurs during the first 3 years when formal developmental screens are recommended. However, clinicians must assess and document developmental surveillance for every preventive care visit and preferably at every other office visit regardless of purpose. Table 1–2 lists some developmental "red flags."

Surveillance includes asking parents if they have any concerns about their child's development, taking a developmental history, observing the child, identifying any risk factors for developmental delay, and accurately tracking the findings and progress. If the family shows concerns, reassurance and reexamination are appropriate if the child is at low risk.

As a result of concerns identified during surveillance and specifically at the 9-, 18-, and 24- or 30-month visits, a formal developmental screening tool should be administered to uncover problems such as those listed in Table 1–3. These visits occur when parents and clinicians can readily observe strides in the different developmental domains: fine and gross motor skills, language and communication, problem solving/adaptive behavior, and personal-social skills. Developmental tests screen children who are apparently normal, confirm or refute any concerns, and serve to

Table 1–3. Prevalence of developmental disorders.

Disorder	Cases per 1000
Attention deficit/hyperactivity disorder	75–150
Learning disabilities	75
Behavioral disorders	60–130
Mental retardation	25
Autism spectrum disorders	2–11
Cerebral palsy	2–3
Hearing impairment	0.8–2
Visual impairment	0.3–0.6

Data from Levy SE, Hyman SL. Pediatric assessment of the child with developmental delay. *Pediatr Clin North Am.* 1993;40:465; and Centers for Disease Control and Prevention. Prevalence of autism spectrum disorders—autism and developmental disabilities monitoring network, 14 sites, United States, 2002. *MMWR (Morbidity and Mortality Weekly Report).* 2007;6:1–40.

monitor children at high risk for developmental delay. Each test approaches the task of identifying children in a different way; no screening tool is universally deemed appropriate for all populations and all ages.

Table 1–4 lists several useful developmental screening tests. The historical gold standard, the Denver Developmental Screening Test–Revised, requires about 20–30 minutes of office time to administer by trained personnel. Proper use is not widespread in practice. The Parents' Evaluation of Developmental Status, the Ages and Stages Questionnaire, and the Child Development Review-Parent Questionnaire are all parent-completed tools that take <15 minutes to complete and are easily used in a busy clinical practice but are unfortunately proprietary. Shortened, customized lists of developmental milestones should not replace the use of validated developmental assessment tools, a list of which is available from the Early Childhood Technical Assistance Center (http://ectacenter.org/topics/earlyid/screeneval.asp).

If the screening tool results are concerning, the physician should inform the parents and schedule the child for further developmental or medical evaluation or referral to subspecialists such as neurodevelopmental pediatricians, pediatric psychiatrists, speech-language pathologists, or physical or occupational therapists. In approximately one-fourth of all cases, an etiology is identified through medical testing, such as genetic evaluation, serum metabolite studies, and brain imaging.

If screening results are within normal limits, the physician has an opportunity to focus on optimizing the child's

Table 1–2. Developmental "red flags."[a]

Age (months)	Clinical Observation
2	Not turning toward sights or sounds
4–5	No social smiling or cooing
6–7	Not reaching for objects
8–9	No reciprocating emotions or expressions
9–12	No imitative sound exchange with caregivers
18	No signs of complex problem-solving interactions (following 2-step directions)
18–24	Not using words to get needs met
36–48	No signs of using logic with caregivers No pretend play with toys

[a]Serious emotional difficulties in parents or family members at any time warrant full evaluation.
Data from Brazelton TB, Sparrow J. *Touchpoints: Birth to Three,* 2nd ed. Boston, MA: Da Capo Press; 2006.

Table 1–4. Developmental screening tools.

Test	Age	Time (minutes)	Source
Office Administered			
Denver II	0–6 years	30	www.denverii.com
Battelle Developmental Inventory Screening Tool (BDI-ST)	0–8 years	15	www.riverpub.com
Brigance Screens–II	0–90 months	15	www.curriculumassociates.com
Bayley Infant Neuro-developmental Screen (BINS)	3–24 months	10	www.pearsonassessments.com
Parent Administered			
Ages and Stages Questionnaires (ASQ)	4–60 months (every 4 months)	15	www.brookespublishing.com
Parents' Evaluation of Development Status (PEDS)	0–8 years	<5	www.pedstest.com
Child Development Inventory (CDI)	1.5–6 years	45	www.childdevrev.com
Language and Cognitive Screening			
Early Language Milestone (ELM)	0–3 years	5–10	www.proedinc.com
Capute Scales (Cognitive Adaptive Test/Clinical Linguistic Auditory Milestone Scale [CAT/CLAMS])	3–36 months	15–20	www.brookespublishing.com
Modified Checklist for Autism in Toddlers	16–48 months	5–10	www.firstsigns.com

Data from Mackrides PS, Ryherd SJ: Screening for developmental delay. *Am Fam Physician*. 2011 Sep 1;84(5):544–549.

potential. Parents can be encouraged to read to their children on a regular basis, sing and play music, limit television and other media device use altogether in toddlers and to no more than 2 hours daily for older children, and directly engage in age-appropriate stimulating activities such as exercise or game playing. The revised American Academy of Pediatrics (AAP) statement on media use is available on their website (https://www.aap.org/en-us/about-the-aap/aap-press-room/Pages/American-Academy-of-Pediatrics-Announces-New-Recommendations-for-Childrens-Media-Use.aspx). These standards do allow for some media time to communicate with other family members even at a young age. Clinicians should encourage the parents and patients to report on positive behaviors and activities at every visit.

At both the 18- and 24-month visits, clinicians should formally screen for autism spectrum disorders (ASDs). Increasing public awareness and concern about ASD has made this recommendation key. The Modified Checklist for Autism in Toddlers (M-CHAT) is a widely used, validated, autism-specific screening tool. Autistic disorder is a pervasive developmental disorder resulting in various social, language, and/or sensorimotor deficits with an incidence as high as 1 in 88 children. Early diagnosis and intervention may help many autistic persons achieve some degree of independent living. The differential diagnosis includes other psychiatric and developmental disorders; profound hearing loss; metabolic disorders, such as lead poisoning; and genetic disorders, such as fragile X syndrome and tuberous sclerosis. The measles-mumps-rubella (MMR) vaccine does not cause autism, but failure to take folic acid during pregnancy is linked to an increased risk.

The school years offer an excellent opportunity to evaluate the child's development through grades, standardized test results, and athletic or extracurricular activities. Participation in activities outside the home and school also helps gauge the child's development. For example, a critical event during adolescence is learning to drive a motor vehicle.

▶ **Physical Examination**

A general principle for well-child examinations (newborn to 4 years old) is to perform maneuvers from least to most invasive. Clinicians should first make observations about the child–parent(s) interaction, obtain an interval history, and then perform a direct examination of the child. Some parts of the examination are best accomplished when the infant is quiet, so they may be performed "out of order." Although most communication about the child's health is between the physician and the parent(s), clinicians should attempt to communicate directly with the patient to gauge whether he or she is developmentally appropriate and to develop familiarity directly with that patient.

A physical examination of the newborn should include the following:

- **General observation:** evidence of birth trauma, dysmorphic features, respiratory rate, skin discolorations, or rashes
- **Head, ears, eyes, nose, and throat (HEENT) examination:** mobile sutures, open fontanelles, head shape, ears, bilateral retinal red reflexes, clarity of lens, nasal patency, absence of cleft palate or lip, and palpation of clavicles to rule out fracture
- **Cardiovascular examination:** cardiac murmurs, peripheral pulses, capillary refill, and cyanosis
- **Pulmonary examination:** use of accessory muscles and auscultation of breath sounds
- **Abdominal examination:** masses, distention, and the presence of bowel sounds
- **Extremity examination:** number and abnormalities of digits, and screening for congenital dislocation of the hips using Ortolani and Barlow maneuvers
- **Genitourinary examination:** genitalia including testicle position or vaginal patency and anus
- **Neurologic examination:** presence of newborn reflexes (eg, rooting, grasping, sucking, stepping, and Moro reflex), resting muscle tone

To track the child's physical and developmental progress, a comprehensive interval history and physical examination are important at each encounter, even if the parents do not report concerns. The child's weight (without clothes or shoes), height, and head circumference (until 3 years of age) are measured and plotted on standard CDC growth charts at each visit. A child's rate of growth will usually follow one percentile (eg, 25th, 50th) from birth through school age. A child can appropriately cross percentiles upward (eg, a premature infant who then "catches up") or inappropriately (eg, a child who becomes obese). Any child who drops more than two percentiles over any period of time should be evaluated for failure to thrive (see Chapter 2).

By 15 months of age, children experience stranger anxiety and are much less likely to be cooperative. Clinicians can minimize the child's adverse reactions by approaching the child slowly and performing the examination while the child is in the parent's arms, progressing from least to most invasive tasks. Touching the child's shoe or accompanying stuffed animal first and then gradually moving up to the chest while distracting the child with a toy or otoscope light is often helpful. After the first year of life, the pace of the infant's growth begins to plateau. At the 15- to 18-month visit, the infant

most likely will be mobile and may want to stand during the examination. To engage the child, the clinician can ask where to do the examination or which body part to examine first. Teeth and oral evaluation should be accompanied by advice to seek a dental home.

Beginning at 2 years of age, the body mass index is plotted; at age 3 years, the child's blood pressure is measured. Eye examination for strabismus (also known as "cross-eye"; measured by the cover/uncover test) allows early treatment to prevent amblyopia. By age 3 or 4 years, documentation of visual acuity should be attempted. Hearing, now tested at birth, is informally evaluated until the age of 4 years, when audiometry can be attempted. At least 75% of speech in 3-year-olds should be intelligible. Speech delay should trigger referral. Physicians need to assess gait, spinal alignment, and injuries, looking particularly for signs of child abuse or neglect. Problems such as knock knees or bowlegs generally resolve over time on their own. Table 1–5 highlights the

Table 1–5. Highlights of physical examination by age.

Age of Child	Essential Components of Examination
2 weeks	Presence of bilateral red reflex Auscultation of heart for murmurs Palpation of abdomen for masses Ortolani/Barlow maneuvers for hip dislocation Assessment of overall muscle tone Reattainment of birth weight
2 months	Observation of anatomic abnormalities or congenital malformations (effects of birth trauma resolved by this point) Auscultation of heart for murmurs
4–6 months	Complete musculoskeletal examination (neck control, evidence of torticollis) Extremity evaluation (eg, metatarsus adductus) Vision assessment (conjugate gaze, symmetric light reflex, visual tracking of an object to 180°) Bilateral descent of testes Assessment for labial adhesions
9 months	Pattern and degree of tooth eruption Assessment of muscle tone Presence of bilateral pincer grasp Observation of crawling behavior
12 months	Range of motion of the hips, rotation, and leg alignment Bilateral descent of testes
15–18 months	Cover test for strabismus Signs of dental caries Gait assessment Any evidence of injuries

important components of the physical examination at each age. The examiner should comment on the child's psychological and intellectual development, particularly during adolescence, when mood and affect evaluations should be recorded.

► Screening Laboratory Tests

Every state requires newborns to undergo serologic screening for inborn errors of metabolism (Table 1–6), preferably at age 2–3 days. Funded by the Department of Health and Human Services, Baby's First Test (www.babysfirsttest.org) is an unbiased website that provides information for providers about the mandated screening requirements in each state. Examples of commonly screened conditions are hypothyroidism, phenylketonuria, maple syrup urine disease, congenital adrenal hyperplasia, and cystic fibrosis. Most institutions routinely screen newborns for hearing loss (US Preventive Services Task Force [USPSTF] recommendation for universal screening level B). The USPSTF assigned a level I (insufficient evidence) to universal screening of newborns for risk of chronic bilirubin encephalopathy with a transcutaneous bilirubin.

The AAP recommends screening for anemia with fingerstick hemoglobin or hematocrit at age 12 months. Although the USPSTF assigned a level I to screening for iron deficiency, it did recommend iron dietary supplementation for children age 6–12 months. Because of the high prevalence of iron deficiency anemia in toddlers (about 9%), repeat screenings may be necessary in high-risk situations. Measurement of hemoglobin or hematocrit alone detects only those patients with iron levels low enough to become anemic, so dietary intake of iron should be assessed. Pregnant adolescents should be screened for anemia. A positive screening test at any age is an indication for a therapeutic trial of iron. Thalassemia minor is the major differential consideration. A sickle cell screen is indicated in all African American children.

The AAP recommends universal lead screening at ages 12 and 24 months. Recently high levels of lead in the water supply have supported this recommendation. If the child is considered to be at high risk, annual lead screening begins at age 6 months. Risk factors include exposure to chipping or peeling paint in buildings built before 1950, frequent contact with an adult with significant lead exposure, having a sibling under treatment for a high lead level, and location of the home near an industrial setting likely to release lead fumes or in a city with lead pipes as part of the water supply system. Although many agencies require a one-time universal lead screening at 1 year of age because high-risk factors are often absent in children with lead poisoning, the USPSTF recommends against screening children at average risk and assigns a level I to screening for high-risk children, but these recommendations are under review in 2018.

Tuberculosis (TB) screening using a purified protein derivative (PPD) is offered on recognition of high-risk factors at any age. Routine testing of children without risk factors is not indicated. Children require testing if they have had contact with persons with confirmed or suspected infectious TB, have emigrated from endemic countries (Asia or the Middle East), or have any clinical or radiographic findings suggestive of TB. Human immunodeficiency virus (HIV)-infected children require annual PPD tests. Children at risk for HIV due to exposure to high-risk adults (eg, HIV positive, homeless, institutionalized) are retested every 2–3 years. Children without specific risk factors for TB but who live in high-prevalence communities may be tested at ages 6 months, 1 year, 4–6 years, and 11–12 years.

The AAP recommends universal dyslipidemia screening at ages 10 and 20 years. A cholesterol level may be obtained after age 2 years if the child has a notable family history. The National Cholesterol Education Program recommends screening in a child with a parent who has a total cholesterol of ≥240 mg/dL or a parent or grandparent with the onset of cardiovascular disease before age 55 years. Clinical evaluation and management of the child are to be initiated if the low-density lipoprotein cholesterol level is ≥130 mg/dL. The USPSTF assigns a level I to cholesterol screening during childhood.

The AAP recommends an HIV test for all 20-year-olds.

Table 1–6. Commonly screened components of newborn screening panels.[a]

Diseases Screened	Incidence of Disease in Live Births
Congenital hypothyroidism	1:4000
Duchenne muscular dystrophy	1:4500
Congenital adrenal hyperplasia	1:10,000–1:18,000
Phenylketonuria	1:14,000
Galactosemia	1:30,000
Cystic fibrosis	1:44,000–1:80,000 (depending on population)
Biotinidase deficiency	1:60,000

[a]Screening panel requirements vary in each state.
Data from Kaye CI and Committee on Genetics. *Newborn Screening Fact Sheets*. Technical report. Available at www.pediatrics.org/cgi/content/full/118/3/1304. See also *Baby's First Test* (http://babysfirsttest.org/) for complete listing of disease tests by state.

▶ Anticipatory Guidance

A. Nutrition

All mothers should be strongly encouraged to breastfeed their infants. A widely accepted goal is exclusive breastfeeding for at least the first 6 months of life. Vitamin D supplement (400 U/d) is indicated for breastfed children. Parents who choose to bottle-feed their newborn have several choices in formulas but should avoid cow's milk because of risks such as anemia. Commercial formulas are typically fortified with iron and vitamin D, and some contain fatty acids such as docosahexaenoic acid and arachidonic acid, which are not as yet proven to promote nervous system development. Soy-based or lactose-free formulas can be used for infants intolerant of cow's milk formulas.

An appropriate weight gain is 1 oz/d during the first 6 months of life and 0.5 oz/d during the next 6 months. This weight gain requires a daily caloric intake of ~120 kcal/kg during the first 6 months and 100 kcal/kg thereafter. Breast milk and most formulas contain 20 cal/oz. Initially, newborns should be fed on demand or, in some cases as for twins, on a partial schedule. Caregivers need to be questioned about the amount and duration of the child's feedings and vitamin D and fluoride intake at every visit.

Healthy snacks and regular family mealtimes may help reduce the risk of obesity. Fruit juice is best avoided altogether; water is preferred for hydration. Ideal calorie intake is somewhat independent of weight but does change according to activity level. Children age 1 year should take in about 900 kcal/d; age 2–3 years, 1000 kcal/d; age 4–8 years, 1200 kcal/d for girls and 1400 kcal/d for boys; age 9–13 years, 1600 kcal/d for girls and 1800 kcal/d for boys; and age 14–18, 1800 kcal/d for girls and 2200 kcal/d for boys.

Solid foods such as cereals or pureed baby foods are introduced at 4–6 months of age when the infant can support her or his head and the tongue extrusion reflex has extinguished. Delaying introduction of solid foods until this time appears to limit the incidence of food sensitivities. The child can also continue breast- or bottle-feeding, limited to 30 oz/d, because the solids now provide additional calories. Around 1 year of age, when the infant can drink from a cup, bottle-feeding should be discontinued to protect teeth from caries. No specified optimum age exists for weaning a child from breastfeeding. After weaning, ingestion of whole or 2% cow's milk may promote nervous system development.

Estimated to affect 1–2% of children, peanut allergy often is severe and lifelong. Infants with eczema should be started on pureed peanuts as early as 4–6 months. For full guidance, see the AAP statement on peanut supplements (http://www.aappublications.org/news/2017/05/09/Peanut050917).

Older infants can tolerate soft adult foods such as yogurt and mashed potatoes. A well-developed pincer grasp allows children to self-feed finger foods. With the eruption of primary teeth at 8–12 months of age, children may try foods such as soft rice or pastas.

With toddlers, mealtimes can be a source of both pleasure and anxiety as children become "finicky." The normal child may exhibit specific food preferences or be disinterested in eating. An appropriate growth rate and normal developmental milestones should reassure frustrated parents. Coping strategies include offering small portions of preferred items first and offering limited food choices. Eating as a family gives toddlers a role model for healthy eating and appropriate social behaviors during mealtimes.

B. Elimination

Regular patterns for voiding and defecation provide reassurance that the child is developing normally. Newborn infants should void within 24 hours of birth. An infant urinates approximately 6–8 times a day. Parents may count diapers in the first few weeks to confirm adequate feeding. The older child usually voids 4–6 times daily. Changes in voiding frequency reflect the child's hydration status, especially when the child is ill.

Routine circumcision of male infants is not currently recommended, so parents who are considering circumcision require additional guidance. Although a circumcised boy has a decreased incidence of urinary tract infections (odds ratio 3–5) and a decreased risk of phimosis and squamous cell carcinoma of the penis, some clinicians raise concerns about bleeding, infection, pain of the procedure, or damage to the genitalia (incidence of 0.2–0.6%). The decision about circumcision is based on the parents' personal preferences and cultural influences. When done, the procedure is usually performed after the second day of life, on a physiologically stable infant. Contraindications include ambiguous genitalia, hypospadias, HIV, and any overriding medical conditions. The denuded mucosa of the phallus appears raw for the first week after the procedure, exuding a small amount of serosanguineous drainage on the diaper. Infection occurs in <1% of cases. Mild soap and water washes are the best method of cleansing the area. By the 2-week checkup, the phallus should be completely healed with a scar below the corona radiata. The parents should note whether the infant's urinary stream is straight and forceful.

Newborns are expected to pass black, tarry meconium stools within the first 24 hours of life. Failure to pass stool in that period necessitates a workup for Hirschsprung disease (aganglionic colon) or imperforate anus. Later, the consistency of the stool is usually semisolid and soft, with a yellow-green seedy appearance. Breastfed infants typically defecate after each feeding or at least 2 times a day. Bottle-fed infants generally have a lower frequency of stooling. Occasionally, some infants may have only one stool every 2 or 3 days without discomfort. If the child seems to be grunting forcefully with defecation or is passing extremely hard stools, treatment with lubricants such as glycerin is recommended. Any appearance of blood in the stools is abnormal and warrants investigation. Anal fissure is a common cause and can be treated with lubricants.

With the introduction of solid foods and maturation of intestinal function, stool becomes more solid and malodorous. Treatment of mild to moderate constipation may include the use of Karo syrup mixed in with feedings (1–2 tsp in 2 oz of milk) or psyllium seed or mineral oil (15–30 mL) for older children. Older children and adolescents should ingest high-fiber foods such as fruits and vegetables and drink water to reduce the risk of constipation. Children who are severely constipated may require referral. Despite attention to these approaches, encopresis (stool retention with loose stool leaking) and enuresis (night or day time) remain significant issues in otherwise normal children.

C. Sleep Patterns

An important issue for parents is the development of proper sleeping habits for their child. Newborns and children experience different stages of sleep/wakefulness cycles, including deep, light, or rapid eye movement (REM) sleep; indeterminate state; wide-awake, alert state; fussiness; and crying. On average, a baby experiences a cycle every 3–4 hours, and the new parents' first job is to learn their baby's unique style. Newborns sleep an average of 18–20 hours in each 24-hour period.

At first, feeding the baby whenever he or she wakes up is the most appropriate response. Because of frequent feedings and because babies often have their days and nights "reversed," tiring nighttime awakenings are commonplace. When the baby is 3 or 4 weeks old, feedings can be delayed for a bit of play and interaction. The goals are to space out the baby's awake time to 3 or more hours between feedings and to induce a long sleep at night.

By 2–3 months, the baby's pattern of sleeping and feeding should be more predictable. Parents can institute some routines that allow the child to self-comfort. After feeding, rocking, and soothing, parents should be encouraged to lay the baby down in the crib when she or he is quiet but not asleep. A soothing, consistent bedtime ritual allows babies to learn to settle down by themselves and lays the foundation for other independent behaviors in the future. White noise may enhance sleep in some infants.

To reduce the risk of sudden infant death syndrome (SIDS), all newborn infants should be placed on their backs to sleep. Risk factors include prone and side positions for infant sleep, smoke exposure, soft bedding and sleep surfaces, and overheating. Cosleeping (bed sharing) slightly increases the overall risk of SIDS, especially for infants <11 weeks old. The issue of cosleeping is often difficult to address because it is viewed as a common and necessary practice in some cultures. Evidence also suggests that pacifier use and room sharing (without bed sharing) are associated with decreased risk of SIDS. Although the cause of SIDS is unknown, immature cardiorespiratory autonomic control and failure of arousal responsiveness from sleep are important factors. With the "Back to Sleep" campaign, prone sleeping among all US infants has decreased to <20%, and the incidence of SIDS has decreased to 40%.

An unintended consequence of the supine sleep position has been increased incidence of positional head deformity or plagiocephaly. Providers need to recognize physical examination distinctions between this cosmetic deformity and the more significant concern of craniosynostosis. Parents should be counseled early about strategies to minimize plagiocephaly, including use of supervised prone positioning ("tummy time") and avoidance of prolonged car seat or rocker use. Early referral and treatment (often the use of hockey-style helmets) in severe cases typically result in satisfactory outcomes.

Sleep disorders are extremely common in young children and adolescents. Good sleep hygiene offers the best solution to these difficulties. Advice should include a standard bedtime regimen including a mandated time to go to sleep and using the bed only for sleep or relaxing activities such as reading. Unfortunately, screen time often occurs in the bedroom, a habit that may interfere with good sleep hygiene.

D. Oral Health

The poor state of oral health in many children is a continued major concern. Tooth decay remains one of the most common chronic diseases of childhood, even more common than asthma (which can exacerbate decay through mouth breathing and drying of protective oral secretions). Medically and developmentally compromised children and children from low-income families are at highest risk. Affected children remain at higher risk for cavities throughout their childhood and adulthood. To minimize early-childhood caries, children should not be put to sleep with a bottle or by breastfeeding. Parents should also be discouraged from inappropriately using the bottle or "sippy cup" as a pacifier. Dietary sugars along with cariogenic bacteria, most often acquired from the mother, who should never clean off a pacifier by inserting it into her own mouth, lead to accelerated decay in the toddler's primary teeth. Ingestion of water after feeding may help reduce cavities.

Current recommendations encourage establishing regular dental care around 6–9 months of age in high-risk children and at 1 year of age for all others, but the number of infants with a dental visit by that age is low. Most children have been seen by age 3 years. Children should have regular biannual dental appointments. Primary prevention includes provision of a diet high in calcium and fluoride supplementation for those with an unfluoridated water supply (<0.6 ppm) from age 6 months through age 16 years. Once primary teeth erupt, parents should use a soft-bristled brush or washcloth with water to clean the teeth twice daily. A pea-sized amount of fluoride-containing toothpaste is adequate. Infants should drink from a cup and be weaned from the bottle at around 12–14 months of age. Pacifiers and thumb sucking are best limited after teeth have erupted. All children need limits on the intake of high-sugar drinks and juices, especially between meals. Fluoride applications at least 2 times per year on erupted teeth markedly reduce the incidence of caries (http://www.ada.org/goto/fluoride). Primary care physicians can offer this service especially when other dental care is limited.

E. Safety

Accidental injury and death are the major risks to a healthy child. Safety should be stressed at every well-child visit. Poison avoidance; choking hazard risks; fall risks; and water, pet, gun, and automobile safety are critical areas to review. The Injury Prevention Program (TIPP; available at https://patiented.solutions.aap.org/handout-collection.aspx?categoryid=32033) from the AAP provides an excellent framework for accident prevention.

▶ Issues in Normal Development

Anticipatory guidance can be helpful to caregivers in preparation for normal growth and development and when their child exhibits variations from ideal behavior. *Bright Futures* provides extensive information about anticipatory guidance throughout childhood and adolescence. Important anticipatory guidance topics include safety, school readiness, school refusal, bullying, physical activity, media (eg, TV, smartphones) use, drug addiction, sexuality, and intellectual pursuits. Selected behavioral issues that are commonly encountered in young children include infantile colic, temper tantrums, and reluctant toilet training.

A. Infantile Colic

Colic is a term often used to describe an infant who is difficult to manage or fussy despite being otherwise healthy. Colic may be defined as 3 or more hours of uncontrollable crying or fussing at least 3 times a week for at least 3 weeks. Many parents complain of incessant crying well before 3 weeks have passed. Other symptoms include facial expressions of pain or discomfort, pulling up of the legs, passing flatus, fussiness with eating, and difficulty falling or staying asleep. Symptoms classically worsen during the evening hours. Because the diagnosis depends on parental report, the incidence of colic varies from 5% to 20%. It occurs equally in both sexes and peaks around 3–4 weeks of age.

The cause of colic is unknown, but organic pathology is present in <5% of cases. Possible etiologies include an immature digestive system sensitive to certain food proteins, an immature nervous system sensitive to external stimuli, or a mismatch of the infant's temperament with those of caregivers. Feeding method is probably unrelated. Clinicians can provide reassurance to caregivers by informing them that colicky children continue to eat and gain weight appropriately, despite the prolonged periods of crying, and that the syndrome is self-limited and usually dissipates by 3–4 months of age. Colic has no definite long-term consequences; therefore, the main problem for caregivers is to cope with anxiety over the crying child. A stressed caregiver who is unable to handle the situation is at risk for abusing a child or becoming depressed.

No definitive treatment can be offered for colic. Little evidence supports the use of simethicone or acetaminophen drops. Switching to a hypoallergenic (soy) formula is effective when the child has other symptoms suggestive of cow's milk protein allergy. Breastfeeding mothers can attempt to make changes in their diets (eg, avoidance of cruciferous vegetables such as broccoli and cabbage) to see if the infant improves. Both clinicians and caregivers have proposed many "home remedies." Both reducing stimulation and movement such as a car ride or walk outdoors are recommended. Frequent burping, swaddling, massage, a crib vibrator, and background noise from household appliances or a white-noise generator are moderately effective. Rigorous study of these techniques is difficult, but clinicians can suggest any or all because the potential harm is minimal.

B. Temper Tantrums

A normal part of child development, temper tantrums encompass excessive crying, screaming, kicking, thrashing, head banging, breath holding, breaking or throwing objects, and aggression. Between the ages of 1 and 3 years, a child's growing sense of independence is in conflict with physical limitations and parental controls and hampered because of limited vocabulary and inability to express feelings or experiences. This power struggle sets the stage for the expression of anger and frustration through a temper tantrum. Tantrums can follow minor frustrations or occur for no obvious reason but are mostly self-limited. A child's tendency toward impulsivity or impatience or a delay in the development of motor skills or cognitive deficits and parental inconsistency—excessive restrictiveness, overindulgence, or overreaction—may increase the incidence of tantrums. Tantrums that produce a desired effect have an increased likelihood of positive reinforcement and recurrence.

As much as possible, parents should provide a predictable home environment. Consistency in routines and rules will help the child know what to expect. Parents should prepare the child for transitions from one activity to another, offer some simple choices to satisfy the child's growing need for control, acknowledge the child's wants during a tantrum, and act calmly when handling negative behaviors to avoid reinforcement. Physical (corporeal) punishment is not advised.

Most importantly, ignoring attention-seeking tantrums and not giving in to the demands of the tantrum will, in time, decrease recurrence. Children who are disruptive enough to hurt themselves or others must be removed to a safe place and given time to calm down in a nonpunitive manner. Most children learn to work out their frustrations with their own set of problem-solving and coping skills, thus terminating tantrums. Persistence of tantrums beyond age 4 or 5 years requires further investigation and usually includes referral or group education and counseling. On occasion, a temper tantrum can turn into a breath-holding spell. Although breath-holding spells are frightening, they rarely result in any consequence for the child. The best response to a breath-holding spell is to simply wait for the spell to subside.

C. Toilet Training

Some indicators of readiness for toilet use include an awareness of impending urination or defecation, prolonged dryness, and the ability to walk easily, to pull clothes on and off easily, to follow instructions, to identify body parts, and to initiate simple tasks. These indicators are not likely to be present until 18–30 months of age. Once the child becomes interested in bathroom activities or watching his or her parents use the toilet, parents should provide a potty chair. Parents can then initiate toilet training by taking the diaper off and seating the child on the potty at a time when she or he is likely to urinate or defecate. Routine sittings on the potty at specified times, such as after meals when the gastrocolic reflex is functional, may be helpful. The child who is straining or bending at the waist may be escorted to the bathroom for a toileting trial. If the child eliminates in the potty or toilet, praise or a small reward may reinforce that behavior. Stickers, storybooks, or added time with the parents can be used for motivation.

With repeated successes, transitional diapers or training pants may be used until full continence is achieved. The training process may take days to months, and caregivers can expect accidents. Accidents need to be dealt with plainly; the child should not be punished or made to feel guilty or forced to sit on the toilet for prolonged periods. Significant constipation can be treated medically, because it may present a barrier to training. About 80% of children achieve success at daytime continence by age 30 months.

As with many childrearing issues, consistency and a nurturing environment give the child a sense of security. Training should not start too early or during times of family stress. Parents can be asked to describe specific scenarios, so concrete anticipatory guidance may be given to deal with any barriers. Toilet training, as with most behavior modification, has a higher chance of success if positive achievements are rewarded and failures are not emphasized.

D. Media Use

Although increasingly difficult to accomplish, children should limit TV and computer use to no more than 2 hours per day. Excessive media use has worsened the obesity crisis and may delay normal developmental milestones. A family media use plan that prohibits such activities as using cell phones during family mealtimes and allows contact with distant relatives such as grandparents is paramount. Parents must be aware of the content of viewed programs, videogames, and websites to reduce childhood exposure to violence and socially inappropriate content such as drug use or electronic bullying. Safe use of handheld phones and computer devices should be routinely discussed with all parents and older children and adolescents.

E. Adolescent Concerns

Besides navigating their ways through identity development, school, sports, sexuality, and personal relationships, between 20% and 25% of adolescents will suffer from a mental disorder. Anxiety, mood disorders, particularly depression, and substance use disorders are most common. Behavioral concerns include ASD, attention deficit/hyperactivity disorder, oppositional defiant disorder, and conduct disorder. These problems tend to surface in early adolescence when the physical development of the child makes control of behavior more difficult. Management frequently requires consultation and a modicum of experience with appropriate medications.

▶ Medical Concerns Outside Normal Development

Beyond the normal variations in child development, the family physician may need to identify and treat significant medical problems. Early diagnosis and referral lead to prevention of potentially serious sequelae and improved quality of life. Some of the major abnormalities detected in the young child (Table 1–7) underscore the importance of regular and thorough well-child care visits with the family physician.

Table 1–7. Medical problems commonly diagnosed in childhood.

Problem	Definition	Prevalence	Risk Factors	Assessment	Treatment
Developmental dysplasia of hips	Spectrum of abnormalities that cause hip instability, ranging from dislocation to inadequate development of acetabulum	8–25 cases per 1000 births	Female gender; Breech delivery; Family history; Possibly birth weight >4 kg	Screening clinical examination at birth and well-child visits of marginal use. Diagnosis: ultrasound in infants <6 months; radiographs >6 months	Abduction splints in infants <6 months; open or closed reduction more effective in those >6 months; optimal treatment remains controversial; consider orthopedic referral
Congenital heart disease	Major—large VSDs, severe valvular stenosis, cyanotic disease, large ASDs; Minor—small VSDs, mild valvular stenosis, small ASDs	5–8 cases per 1000 newborns, 50% with major disease and 50% with minor disease	Maternal diabetes or connective tissue disease; congenital infections (eg, CMV, HSV, rubella); drugs taken during pregnancy; family history; Down syndrome	Major disease presents shortly after birth. Minor disease can present with murmur, tachycardia, tachypnea, pallor, peripheral pulses; ECG, CXR, echocardiogram	Cardiology evaluation; medication; surgical treatment options
Cryptorchidism	Testicles are absent (agenesis), vascular compromise) or undescended	2–5% of full-term and 30% of premature male infants; prevalence varies geographically	Disorders of testosterone secretion; abdominal wall defects; trisomies	Increased risk of inguinal hernia, testicular torsion, infertility, and testicular cancer	Hormonal or surgical treatment, or both; can start at age 6 months; complete before age 2 years
Pyloric stenosis	Hypertrophic (elongated, thickened) pylorus, progresses to obstruction of gastric outlet	3 cases per 1000 live births	Male infants; first-born infants; unconjugated hyperbilirubinemia	Diagnosis by clinical examination, ultrasound, or upper GI series; electrolyte abnormalities (metabolic alkalosis)	Surgical repair; fluid, electrolyte resuscitation
Hypospadias	Ventral location of urethral meatus (anywhere from proximal glans to perineum)	~1 case per 250 male births	Advanced maternal age; maternal diabetes mellitus; Caucasian ethnicity; delivery before 37 weeks' gestation	Check for other abnormalities (cryptorchidism) and intersex conditions (congenital adrenal hyperplasia)	Circumcision contraindicated; urology referral, usually within 3–6 months
Strabismus	Anomaly of ocular alignment (one or both eyes, any direction)	~2–4% of population	Family history; low birth weight; retinopathy of prematurity; cataract	Clinical tests: corneal light reflex, red reflex, cover test, and cover/uncover test	Child should be referred to pediatric ophthalmologist for early treatment to reduce visual loss (amblyopia)

ASD, atrial septal defect; CMV, cytomegalovirus; CXR, chest x-ray; ECG, electrocardiogram; GI, gastrointestinal; HSV, herpes simplex virus; VSD, ventricular septal defect.

Centers for Disease Control and Prevention. Developmental disabilities. Accessed at https://www.cdc.gov/ncbddd/developmentaldisabilities/index.html. Accessed November 12, 2019.

Chaudhary SS, Pomerantz W, Miller B, Agarwal M. Pediatric injury prevention programs: identify markers for success and sustainability. *J Trauma Acute Care Surg.* 2017;83:S184–S189. [PMID: 28557845]

Hagan JF, Shaw JS, Duncan PM, eds. *Bright Futures: Guidelines for Health Supervision of Infants, Children, and Adolescents.* 4th ed. Elk Grove Village, IL: American Academy of Pediatrics; 2017. Accessed at https://brightfutures.aap.org/materials-and-tools/Pages/default.aspx. Accessed November 12, 2019.

Johnson SB, Riley AW, Granger DA, Riis J. The science of early toxic stress for pediatric practice and advocacy. *Pediatrics.* 2013;131:319–327. [PMID: 23339224]

Kavan MG, Saxena SK, Rafiq N. General parenting strategies: practical suggestions for common child behavior issues. *Am Fam Physician.* 2018;97:642–648. [PMID: 29763275]

Patterson BL, Gregg WM, Biggers C, Barkin S. Improving delivery of EPSDT well-child care at acute visits in an academic pediatric practice. *Pediatrics.* 2012;130(4):e988–e995. [PMID: 22987871]

Silk H, McCollum W. Fluoride: the family physician's role. *Am Fam Physician.* 2015;92:174–176. [PMID: 26280136]

Turner K. Well-child visits for infants and young children. *Am Fam Physician.* 2018;98:347–353. [PMID: 30215922]

Failure to Thrive

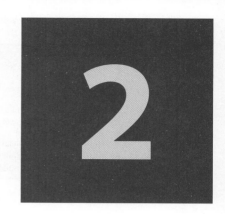

James C. Dewar, MD
Stephanie B. Dewar, MD

ESSENTIALS OF DIAGNOSIS

▶ Persistent weight loss over time.

▶ Growth failure associated with disordered behavior and development.

▶ Weight less than third percentile for age.

▶ Weight crosses two major percentiles downward over any period of time and continues to fall.

▶ Median weight for age of 76–90% (mild undernutrition), 61–75% (moderate undernutrition), or <61% (severe undernutrition).

General Considerations

Failure to thrive (FTT) is an old problem that continues to be an important entity for all practitioners who provide care to children. Growth is one of the essential tasks of childhood and is an indication of the child's general health. Growth failure may be the first symptom of serious organ dysfunction. Most frequently, however, growth failure represents inadequate caloric intake. Malnutrition during the critical period of brain growth in early childhood has been linked to delayed motor, cognitive, and social development. Developmental deficits may persist even after nutritional therapy has been instituted.

There is no unanimously established definition of FTT. Practitioners must also recognize the limitations of the different definitions of FTT. In a European study, 27% of well children met one criterion for FTT in the first year of life. This illustrates the poor predictive value of using a single measurement in diagnosis. Competing definitions of FTT include the following:

- **Persistent weight loss over time.** Children should steadily gain weight. Weight loss beyond the setting of an acute illness is pathological. However, the assessment and treatment for FTT need to be addressed *before* the child has had persistent weight loss.

- **Growth failure associated with disordered behavior and development.** This old definition is useful because it reminds the practitioner of the serious sequelae and important alarm features in children with undernutrition. Currently, FTT is more commonly defined by anthropometric guidelines alone.

- **Weight less than the third to fifth percentile for age.** This is a classic definition. However, this definition includes children with genetic short stature and whose weight transiently dips beneath the third percentile with an intercurrent illness.

- **Weight crosses two major percentiles downward over any period of time.** Thirty percent of normal children will drop two major percentiles within the first 2 years of life as their growth curve shifts to their genetic potential. These healthy children will continue to grow on the adjusted growth curve. Children with FTT do not attain a new curve, but continue to fall. The most accurate assessment for FTT is a calculation of the child's median weight for age. This quick calculation enables the clinician to assess the degree of undernutrition and plan an appropriate course of evaluation and intervention. The median weight for age should be determined using the most accurate growth chart for the area in which the child lives. The median should not be adjusted for race, ethnicity, or country of origin. Differences in growth are more likely due to inadequate nutrition in specific geographic or economically deprived populations. Determinations of nutritional status are as follows:

- **Mild undernutrition:** 76–90% median weight for age. These children are in no immediate danger and may be safely observed over time (Table 2–1).

Table 2–1. Degree of undernutrition.

Percentage of Median Weight for Age (%)	Degree of Undernutrition	Recommendation
76–90	Mild	Observe as outpatient
61–75	Moderate	Urgent outpatient evaluation Close weight follow-up
>61	Severe	Hospitalization Nutrition support In-hospital evaluation

- **Moderate undernutrition:** 75% median weight for age. These children warrant immediate evaluation and intervention with close follow-up in an outpatient setting.
- **Severe malnutrition:** <61% median weight for age. These children may require hospitalization for evaluation and nutritional support.

FTT is one of the most common diagnoses of early childhood in the United States. It affects all socioeconomic groups, but children in poverty are more likely to be affected and more likely to suffer long-term sequelae. Ten percent of children in poverty meet criteria for FTT. As many as 30% of children presenting to emergency departments for unrelated complaints can be diagnosed with FTT. This group of children is of most concern. They are least likely to have good continuity of care and most likely to suffer additional developmental insults such as social isolation, tenuous housing situations, and neglect. Because FTT is most prevalent in at-risk populations that are least likely to have good continuity of care, it is crucial to address growth parameters at every visit, both sick and well. Many children with FTT may not present for well-child visits. If that is the only visit at which the clinician considers growth, then many opportunities for meaningful intervention may be lost.

▶ **Pathogenesis**

All FTT is caused by undernutrition. The mechanism varies. The child may have increased caloric requirements because of organic disease. The child may have inadequate intake because not enough food is made available, or there may be mechanical difficulty in eating. Also, adequate calories may be provided, but the child may be unable to utilize them either because the nutrients cannot be absorbed across the bowel wall or because of inborn errors of metabolism.

When diagnosing FTT, it is essential to consider the etiology. Over the past few decades, FTT has been better understood as a mixed entity in which both organic disease and psychosocial factors influence each other. With this understanding, the old belief that a child who gains weight in the hospital has nonorganic FTT has been debunked.

A. Organic FTT

Organic causes are identified in 10% of children with FTT. In-hospital evaluations reveal an underlying organic etiology in about 30% of children. The data are misleading. More than two-thirds of these children are diagnosed with gastroesophageal reflux disease (GERD). The practitioner risks one of two errors in diagnosing GERD as the source of FTT. Physiologic reflux is found in at least 70% of infants. It may be a normal finding in an infant who is failing to thrive for other reasons. Further, undernutrition causes decreased lower esophageal segment (LES) tone, which may lead to reflux as an effect rather than a cause of FTT.

B. Nonorganic FTT

Nonorganic FTT, inadequate growth in which no physiologic disease is identified, constitutes 80% of cases. Historically, the responsibility for this diagnosis fell on the caregiver. The caregiver was either unable to provide enough nutrition or emotionally unavailable to the infant. In either circumstances, the result was inadequate feeding. Psychosocial stressors were thought to create a nonnurturing environment, preventing growth even when calories were available. Increased cortisol and decreased insulin levels in undernourished children inhibit weight gain.

C. Mixed FTT

Most FTT is *mixed*. There is a transaction between both physiologic and psychosocial factors that creates a cycle of undernutrition. For example, a child with organic disease may initially have difficulty eating for physiologic reasons. However, over time, the feedings become more challenging for both parents and child and are even less successful. The child senses the parents' anxiety and eats less and more fretfully than before. The parents, afraid to overtax the "fragile" child, may not give the child the time needed to eat. They may become frustrated that they are not easily able to accomplish this most basic and essential care for the child. Parents of an ill child may perceive that other aspects of care are more important than feeding, such as strict adherence to a medication or therapy regimen.

Children with organic disease underlying FTT often gain weight in the hospital when fed by emotionally uninvolved parties such as nurses, volunteers, or physicians. *Weight gain in the hospital should not be mistaken for parental neglect in the home.* The primary care provider should pay close attention to the psychosocial stressors on the feeding dyad.

Conversely, the child who seems to be failing to thrive for purely psychosocial reasons often has complicating organic issues. The undernourished child is lethargic and irritable, especially at feeding times. Undernutrition decreases LES tone and may worsen reflux. The undernourished child is more difficult to feed and retains fewer calories. Poor nutrition adversely affects immunity. Children with FTT often have recurrent infections that increase their caloric requirements and decrease their ability to meet them.

The mixed model reminds the clinician that FTT is an interactive process involving physiologic and psychosocial elements and, more importantly, both caregiver and child. A fussy child may be more difficult for a particular parent to feed. A "good" or passive baby may not elicit enough feeding. Physical characteristics also affect parent–child relationships; organic disease may not only make feeding difficult but may also engender a sense of failure or disappointment in the parent. It is crucial to remember that caregivers have unique relationships with each of their children. Therefore, a parent whose first child is diagnosed with FTT is not doomed to repeat the cycle with the second child. Conversely, an experienced caregiver who has fed previous children successfully may care for a child with FTT.

▶ Prevention

FTT may be prevented by good communication between the primary care provider and the family. The practitioner should regularly assess feeding practices and growth and educate parents about appropriate age-specific diets. As a general rule, infants who are feeding successfully gain about:

- 30 g/d at 0–3 months
- 20 g/d at 3–6 months
- 15 g/d at 6–9 months
- 12 g/d at 9–12 months
- 8 g/d at 1–3 years

In addition, growth parameters need to be recorded at every visit, sick or well. Weight should be documented for all children. Recumbent length is measured for children younger than 2 years old. Height is measured for children older than 3 years old. Between the ages of 2 and 3 years, either height or length may be recorded. Length measurements exceed heights by an average of 1 cm. With a good growth chart in hand, the primary care provider can monitor growth and intervene early if problems arise.

Clinicians should investigate the economic stresses on families to ensure adequate access to nutrition for the family.

▶ Clinical Findings

A. Symptoms and Signs

The importance of a complete, long-term growth curve in making the diagnosis of FTT cannot be overemphasized. In acute undernutrition, the velocity of weight gain decreases while height velocity continues to be preserved. The result is a thin child of normal height. Chronic undernutrition manifests as "stunting"; both height and weight are affected. The child may appear proportionately small. Review of a growth curve may reveal that weight was initially affected and increase the suspicion for FTT. In interpreting growth charts, it is important to remember that healthy children may cross up to two major percentile lines up to 39% of the time between birth and 6 months of age and up to 15% of the time between 6 and 24 months of age. Children with length above the 50th percentile seldom have endocrine disease.

Children should be plotted on an appropriate growth curve. Growth curves are gender specific and are available at the Centers for Disease Control and Prevention (CDC) website. Growth curves should not be used for specific countries of origin. Specific growth curves are available for children with genetic disorders such as trisomy 21 (Down syndrome) or Turner syndrome. However, these curves are not well validated. These curves draw from a small group of children, and the nutritional status of the participants was not assessed. These curves may be useful for the clinician in discussing an affected child's growth potential with the child's family.

B. History

1. General history—The clinician's most valuable tool in the diagnosis of FTT is the history. While taking the history, healthcare providers have the opportunity to establish themselves as the child's advocate and the parents' support. Care must be exercised to avoid establishing an adversarial relationship with the parents. It is useful to begin by asking the parents their perception of their child's health. Many parents do not recognize FTT until the clinician brings it to their attention.

The history and physical examination can uncover significant organ dysfunction contributing to growth failure. For example, the child who feeds poorly may have a physical impediment to caloric intake such as cleft palate or painful dental caries. Poor suck (ie, inadequate ability to suck) may also raise concerns for neurologic disease. Recurrent upper or lower respiratory tract infections may suggest cystic fibrosis, human immunodeficiency virus (HIV), or immunodeficiency. Sweating during feeding should prompt consideration of an underlying cardiac problem even in the absence of cyanosis. Chronic diarrhea can indicate malabsorption. Symptoms of chronic infection, eosinophilic disease, celiac disease, and pancreatic insufficiency should be elicited.

The healthcare provider must elicit more subtle aspects of past medical history as well, focusing particularly on developmental history and intercurrent illnesses. Delay in achievement of milestones should prompt a close neurologic examination. Inborn errors of metabolism and cerebral palsy can present with growth failure. A history of recurrent serious illness and FTT may be the only indicators of inborn errors of metabolism. Recurrent febrile illness without a clear source may also indicate occult urinary tract infection.

A history of snoring or sleep disturbances should prompt an evaluation for tonsillar and adenoidal hypertrophy, which has been identified as a cause of FTT.

Past medical history must include a complete perinatal history (Table 2–2). Children with lower birth weights and those with specific prenatal exposures are at higher risk for growth problems. Of all children with diagnosed FTT, 40% have birth weights below 2500 g; only 7% of all births are below 2500 g.

Low birth weight may be caused by infection, drug exposure, or other maternal and placental factors. The child with symmetric growth retardation is of particular concern. Infants exposed in utero to rubella, cytomegalovirus, syphilis, toxoplasmosis, or malaria are at high risk for low birth weight, length, and head circumference. These measurements portend poor catch-up growth potential. Short stature is often accompanied by developmental delay and mental retardation in these children.

Children with asymmetric intrauterine growth retardation (preserved head circumference) have better potential for catch-up growth and appropriate development. Fetal growth is affected by both maternal factors and exposure to toxins. Drugs of abuse such as tobacco, cocaine, and heroin have been correlated with low birth weight. Placental insufficiency caused by hypertension, preeclampsia, collagen vascular disease, or diabetes may result in an undernourished baby with decreased birth weight. Finally, intrauterine physical factors may reduce fetal growth; uterine malformation, multiple gestation, and fibroids may all contribute to smaller babies.

Maternal HIV infection is also a significant risk factor for FTT. Most children born to HIV-positive mothers have normal birth weights and lengths. However, children who are infected frequently develop FTT within the first year of life.

Family history is essential. A family history of atopy, eczema, or asthma raises the suspicion of eosinophilic enteritides. A family history of autoimmune disease should heighten the concern for celiac disease. Metabolic diseases are generally recessive, and an absence of family history should not be regarded as reassuring.

An examination of the family's relationships with the child and one another can uncover valuable information. Children described as "difficult" or "unpredictable" by their mothers have been noted to be slow or poor feeders by independent observers. Maternal depression and history of abuse are strong risk factors for FTT; addressing these issues is integral to establishing a functional feeding relationship between parent and child. Finally, a thorough assessment of economic supports may reveal that nutritious foods are unobtainable or difficult to access. Social financial supports are often inadequate to meet children's needs. Tenuous housing or homelessness may make it impossible to keep appropriate foods readily available.

2. Feeding history—A careful feeding history is part of the history of present illness. It often sheds more light on the problem than a battery of laboratory tests. When assessing an infant, it is essential to know what formula the infant is taking, in what volume, and how frequently. Caregivers should describe the preparation of formula. Caregivers may be inadvertently mixing dilute formula. In calculating caloric intake, the practitioner should remember that breast milk and formula have 20 cal/oz. Baby foods range from 40 to 120 calories per jar. An 80-cal/4-oz jar is a good average to use when making calculations.

The examiner should ask how long it takes the baby to eat; slow eating may be associated with poor suck or decreased stamina secondary to organic dysfunction. Parental estimation of the infant's suck may also be helpful. Parents should

Table 2–2. History taking.

Questions	Differential

Perinatal
  Infection
  Movement
	Congenital infection
	Genetic disorders

Feeding behavior
  Diaphoresis
  Poor suck, swallow
  Length of feedings
	Cardiac problem
	Neurologic, mechanical
	  (submucosal cleft)

Diet history
  Infant
    Breastfeeding: time of
      nursing, sensation of
      letdown, fullness of breasts
    Formula fed: assess how
      parents are mixing
      formula, feeding
      techniques
  Older children
    24-hour diet history
    Prospective 72-hour diet diary
    Dysphagia
	Inadequate milk production
	Inappropriate diet
	Inappropriate interaction to
	  stimulate feeding
	Inappropriate caloric intake
	Eosinophilic or allergic disorder
	  reflux

Growth history
  Onset in infancy
  Onset of FTT after addition
    of solids
  Onset after infancy, recent drop
	Genetic disorder: cystic fibrosis,
	  syndromic, metabolic, urinary
	  tract anomalies
	Celiac, eosinophilic
	Inflammatory bowel disease, celiac

Stooling history
  Diarrhea
  Constipation
	Malabsorption: celiac, inflammatory
	  bowel disease, eosinophilic
	  enteritis
	Maldigestion: pancreatic
	  insufficiency
	Cystic fibrosis, undernutrition, celiac

Voiding history	Poor stream in boys: posterior urethral valves

be asked about regurgitation after eating. The clinician should also inquire about feeding techniques. Bottle propping may indicate a poor parent–child relationship or an overtaxed parent.

The breastfed baby merits special mention. The sequelae of unsuccessful breastfeeding are profound. Infants may present with severe dehydration. Parents rarely recognize that the infant is failing to thrive. Mothers are often discharged from the hospital before milk is in and may be unsure about what to expect when initially learning how to breastfeed. The neonatal period is the most critical period in the establishment of breastfeeding. The primary care provider should educate the breastfeeding mother prior to hospital discharge. Milk should be in by day 3 or 4. The neonate should feed at least 8 times in a 24-hour period and should not be sleeping through the night. A "good" baby (an infant who sleeps through the night) should raise concerns of possible dehydration. Breastfed babies should have at least six wet diapers a day. Whereas formula-fed infants may have many stool patterns, the successful breastfed neonate should have at least four yellow seedy stools a day. After 4 weeks of life, the stool pattern may change to once a day or less.

Breastfed babies should be seen within the first week of life to evaluate infant weight and feeding success. Weight loss is expected until day 5 of life. Infants should regain their birth weight by the end of the second week of life. Any weight loss greater than 8% should elicit close follow-up. Weight loss greater than 10–12% should prompt an evaluation for dehydration. Primary care providers should ask about the infant's suck and whether the mother feels that her breasts are emptied at the feeding. The successful infant should empty the mother's breast and be content at the end of the nursing session. When breastfed infants are not gaining weight, it may be useful to observe the breastfeeding or obtain consultation with a lactation specialist.

The evaluation of older children also requires a thorough diet history. An accurate diet history begins with a 24-hour diet recall. Parents should be asked to quantify the amount of each food that their child has eaten. The 24-hour recall acts as a template for a 72-hour diet diary, the most accurate assessment of intake; the first 48 hours of a diet diary are the most reliable. All intakes must be recorded, including juices, water, and snacks. The child who consumes an excessive amount of milk or juice may not have the appetite to eat more nutrient-rich foods. A child needs no more than 16–24 oz of milk and should be limited to <12 oz of juice per day.

It is as important to assess mealtime habits as the meals themselves. Activity in the household during mealtime may be distracting to young children. Television viewing may preempt eating. Excessive attention to how much the child eats can increase the tension and ultimately decrease the child's intake. Most toddlers cannot sit for longer than 15 minutes; prolonging the table time in the hopes of increasing the amount eaten may only exacerbate the already fragile parent-child relationship. Many toddlers snack throughout the day, but some are unable to take in appropriate calories with this strategy.

The primary care provider should also discuss the family's beliefs about a healthy diet. Some families have dietary restrictions, either by choice or culturally, that affect growth. Many have read the dietary recommendations for a healthy adult diet, but a low-fat, low-cholesterol diet is not an appropriate diet for a toddler. Until the age of 2 years, children should drink whole milk, and their fat intake should not be limited.

C. Physical Examination

In addition to reviewing the growth curve, the clinician must complete a physical examination. A weight, length, or height, as appropriate for the child's age, and head circumference are indicated for all children. Growth parameters may be roughly interpreted using the following guidelines:

- **Acute undernutrition:** low weight, normal height, normal head circumference
- **Chronic undernutrition:** short height, normal weight for height, normal head circumference
- **Acute or chronic undernutrition:** short height, proportionately low weight for height, normal head circumference
- **Congenital infection or genetic disorder impairing growth:** short height, normal to low weight for height, small head circumference

The general examination provides a wealth of information. Vital signs should be documented. Bradycardia and hypotension are worrisome findings in the malnourished child and should prompt consideration of immediate hospitalization. It is important to document observations of the parent-child interaction. It is also useful to note both the caregiver's and the child's affects. Parental depression has been associated with higher risk of FTT. Occasionally the examiner may find subtle indications of neglect, such as a flat occiput, indicating that the child is left alone for long periods. However, a flat occiput may be a normal finding when caregivers follow current infant sleeping recommendations.

Children with undernutrition often have objective findings of their nutritional state. Unlike the genetically small child, children with FTT have decreased subcutaneous fat. If undernutrition has been prolonged, they will also have muscle wasting; in infants, it is easier to assess muscle wasting in the calves and thighs rather than in the interosseous muscles. It is also important to remember that infants suck rather than chew; therefore, they will not have the characteristic facies of temporal wasting. Nailbeds and hair should be carefully noted because nutritional deficiencies may cause pitting or lines in the nails. Hair may be thin or brittle. Skin should be examined for scaling and cracking, which may be seen with both zinc and fatty acid deficiencies. Presence of eczema may indicate allergic diathesis and eosinophilic enteritis.

The physical examination should be completed with special attention directed to the organ systems of concern uncovered in the history. However, examination of some organ systems may reveal abnormalities not elicited through history. A thorough abdominal examination is of particular importance. Organomegaly in the child with FTT suggests possible inborn errors of metabolism and requires laboratory evaluation. The examiner should note the genitourinary examination. Undescended testicles may indicate panhypopituitarism, and ambiguous genitalia may indicate congenital adrenogenital hyperplasia. A careful neurologic examination may reveal subtly increased or decreased muscle tone consistent with cerebral palsy and, therefore, increased caloric requirements or inability to coordinate suck and swallow, respectively.

Children with undernutrition have been repeatedly shown to have behavioral and cognitive delays. Unfortunately, the Denver Development Screen II is an inadequate tool to assess the subtle but real delays in these children. It has been suggested that the Bayley test may be a more sensitive tool when assessing these children. Even with nutritional and social support, behavioral and cognitive lags may not resolve. Children who have suffered FTT remain sensitive to undernutrition throughout childhood; one study found a significant decrease in fluency in children with a remote history of undernutrition when they did not eat breakfast. Children with a normal nutritional history were not found to be similarly affected.

The immune system is affected by nutritional status. Children with FTT may present with recurrent mucosal infections: otitis media, sinusitis, pneumonia, and gastroenteritis. Immunoglobulin A (IgA) production is extremely sensitive to undernutrition.

Undernourished children are frequently iron deficient, even in the absence of anemia. Iron and calcium deficiencies enhance the absorption of lead. In areas in which there is any concern for lead exposure, lead levels should be assessed as part of the workup for FTT.

D. Laboratory Findings

No single battery of laboratory tests or imaging studies can be advocated in the workup of FTT. Testing should be guided by the history and physical examination. Fewer than 1% of "routine laboratory tests" ordered in the evaluation of FTT provide useful information for treatment or diagnosis.

Tests that had been advocated as markers of nutritional status have limitations. Albumin has an extremely long half-life (21 days) and is a poor indicator of recent undernutrition. Prealbumin, which has been touted as a marker for recent protein nutrition, is decreased in both acute inflammation and undernutrition.

Children with more severe malnutrition may be lymphopenic (lymphocyte count <1500) or anergic.

Undernourished children are frequently iron deficient, even in the absence of anemia. Iron and calcium deficiencies enhance the absorption of lead. In areas in which there is any concern for lead exposure, lead levels should be assessed as part of the workup for FTT.

Laboratory evaluation is indicated when the history and physical examination suggest underlying organic disease. Children with developmental delay and organomegaly or severe episodic illness should have a metabolic workup, including urine organic and serum amino acids; there is a 5% yield in this subset of patients. Children with a history of recurrent respiratory tract infections or diarrhea should have a sweat chloride testing. A history of poorly defined febrile illnesses or recurrent "viral illness" may be followed up with a urinalysis, culture, and renal function to evaluate for occult urinary tract disease. In children with diarrhea, it may be useful to send stool for *Giardia* antigen, qualitative fat, white blood cell count, occult blood, ova and parasites, rotavirus, and α_1-antitrypsin. Rotavirus has been associated with a prolonged gastroenteritis and FTT. Elevated α_1-antitrypsin in the stool is a marker for protein enteropathy.

For children who develop FTT after the addition of solid foods, an evaluation for celiac disease is warranted regardless of whether diarrhea is present. Fifteen percent of celiac patients present with constipation. Tissue transglutaminase along with a total IgA level may be useful for diagnosis (Table 2–3).

Infectious diseases need to be specifically addressed. Worldwide, tuberculosis (TB) is one of the most common causes of FTT. A Mantoux test and anergy panel must be placed on any child with risk factors for TB exposure. The possibility of HIV must also be entertained. FTT is frequently a presenting symptom of HIV in the infant.

Table 2–3. Laboratory evaluation.

Complete blood count with differential	Anemia: possible inflammatory bowel disease or celiac Eosinophilia: possible eosinophilic enteritis
Complete metabolic panel	Low albumin: chronic inflammation Elevated transaminases: chronic undernutrition, metabolic disorder Bicarbonate: renal disease
Antigliadin antibody	Children <3 years to evaluate for celiac
Tissue transglutaminase with total immunoglobulin A	Older children to evaluate for celiac
Urinalysis	Chronic urinary tract infection
Sweat chloride	Cystic fibrosis

Differential Diagnosis

It is essential to differentiate a small child from the child with FTT. No criterion is specific enough to exclude those who are small for other reasons. Included in the differential diagnosis of FTT are familial short stature, Turner syndrome, normal growth variant, prematurity, endocrine dysfunction, and genetic syndromes limiting growth.

The child with FTT has a deceleration in weight first. Height velocity continues unaffected for a time. Children with familial short stature manifest a simultaneous change in their height and weight curves. Height velocity slows first (it can even plateau) in endocrine disorders such as hypothyroidism. The preterm infant's growth parameters need to be adjusted for gestational age; head circumference is adjusted until 18 months, weight until 24 months, and height through 40 months.

The family history is helpful in differentiating the child with FTT from the child with constitutional growth delay or familial short stature. Midparental height, which can be calculated from the family history, is a useful calculation of probable genetic potential:

- **For girls**: (father's height in inches − 5 + mother's height)/2 ± 2 inches
- **For boys**: (mother's height in inches + 5 + father's height)/2 ± 2 inches

If the child's current growth curve translates into an adult height that falls within the range of midparental height, reassurance may be offered.

It is most difficult to differentiate the older child with constitutional growth delay from the child with FTT. These children typically have reduced weight for height, as do children with FTT. However, unlike children with FTT, they ultimately gain both weight and height on a steady curve. Family history is often revealing in constitutional growth delay. Querying parents about the onset of their own pubertal signs may seem intrusive, but often gives the clinician the information needed to reassure parents about their child's growth.

Breastfeeding infants may be growing normally and not follow the CDC growth curves. After 4–6 months, their weight may decrease relative to their peers. After 12 months, their weight may catch up to that of age-matched formula-fed infants. However, a decrease in weight in early infancy is a symptom of unsuccessful breastfeeding, and FTT should be considered.

Complications

Developmental delay may persist in children with FTT well past the period of undernutrition. Studies have repeatedly shown that these children, as a group, have more behavioral and cognitive problems in school than their peers, even into adolescence. One caveat about these studies is that many investigators defined FTT by that classic definition: growth failure associated with disordered behavior and development. These studies do not doom every child with FTT to scholastic and social failure, but the clinician must be vigilant and act as the child's advocate. Formal developmental screening is especially important in the child with a history of FTT. Intervention should be offered early rather than waiting to see if the child catches up. Children with FTT are generally successful but may need specific supports on the road to achieving that success.

Treatment

A. Nutrition

The cornerstone of therapy is nutrition. The goal of treatment is catch-up growth. Children with FTT may need 1.5–2 times the usual daily calories to achieve catch-up growth. For an infant, this is roughly 150–200 cal/kg per day. There are many formulas for calculating caloric requirements. One simple estimate is:

$$\text{kcal/kg} = 120 \text{ kcal/kg} \times \text{median weight for current height/current weight (kg)}$$

It is important that this nutrition include adequate protein calories. Children with undernutrition require 3 g of protein per kilogram of body weight per day to initiate catch-up growth and may need as much as 5 g/kg. In severe malnutrition, the protein needs can double this amount. High-calorie diets should continue until the child achieves an age-appropriate weight for height. Infant formula can often be mixed in a more concentrated way to facilitate caloric intake at a lower volume.

It is almost impossible for any child to take in twice the usual volume of food. Some solutions are to offer higher-calorie formulas (24–30 cal/oz) to infants. For older children, it is possible to replace or add higher-calorie foods. Heavy cream may be substituted for milk on cereal or in cooking. Cheese may be added to vegetables. Instant breakfast drinks may be offered as snacks. It is advisable to enlist a dietician in designing a high-calorie diet for the child with FTT. Achieving an effective nutritional plan may require structured trials of meal timing and rewards, as well food types, colors, temperatures, and textures.

Tube feedings are sometimes indicated in the child with FTT. Some children may benefit from nighttime feedings through a nasogastric or a percutaneous endoscopic gastrostomy tube. This solution is particularly useful in children with underlying increased caloric requirements, for example, children with cystic fibrosis and cerebral palsy. Children with mechanical feeding difficulties may also require tube feeding for some period of time. Early intervention with an occupational or speech therapist is recommended for a child who is primarily tube fed. Without therapy, the child may develop oral aversions or fail to develop appropriate oral-motor coordination. Parents need to be educated at the onset of nutritional therapy. Catch-up growth is expected within the first month. However, some children may not show accelerated weight gain until after the first 2 weeks of increased nutrition. Children usually gain 1.5 times their daily expected weight gains during the catch-up phase. Children's weight improves well before their height increases. This change in body habitus does not indicate overfeeding; rather, it indicates successful therapy. It does not matter how quickly the child gains; the composition of weight gain will be 45–65% lean body mass.

B. Medications

Few medications are indicated in the treatment of FTT. Those few are nutritional supports. Children with FTT should be supplemented with iron. Zinc has also been shown to improve linear growth. It is sufficient to supplement children with a multivitamin containing zinc and iron. Vitamin D supplementation should also be considered. Vitamin D replacement is especially important in dark-skinned children and in children who are not regularly exposed to sunlight.

C. Social Support

Social support is essential. The services offered must be tailored to the family and the child. Certainly, frequent visits with the primary care provider are useful; weight gain can be measured and concerns addressed. Home visits by social services have been shown to decrease hospitalizations and improve weight gain. Children with developmental delay need early assessment and intervention by the appropriate therapists.

These interventions, if performed early in childhood, have long-lasting ramifications throughout the lifespan.

D. Indications for Referral or Hospital Admission

Most cases of FTT can and should be managed by the primary care provider. A trusting relationship between the clinician and the family is an invaluable asset in the treatment of FTT. Parents struggling with the diagnosis often believe that the healthcare system views them as neglectful. This anxiety creates barriers to open and honest communication about the child's feeding and developmental status. However, suspicions may be allayed when primary care providers enlist themselves as allies in the treatment.

The primary indication for referral is the treatment of an underlying organ dysfunction that requires specialized care. Referral is also warranted when the primary care provider feels that specialized testing is needed (eg, endoscopic biopsies for the further evaluation of celiac disease or eosinophilic enteritis). The clinician may also wish to reevaluate the child who fails to begin catch-up growth after 1–2 months of nutritional intervention.

Most children with FTT can be managed in the outpatient setting. A few may need hospitalization at some point during their evaluation. Indications for admission at initial evaluation are bradycardia or hypotension, which often indicate severe malnutrition. Children who are <61% of the median weight for their age should be admitted for nutritional support. Children with FTT who are admitted electively during the usual workweek have a shorter length of stay and less unhelpful lab and imaging studies. Children with hypoglycemia should be admitted. A low serum glucose is worrisome for severe malnutrition and metabolic disease.

If the clinician suspects abuse or neglect, the child should be admitted. About 10% of children with FTT are abused. These children ultimately experience poorer developmental outcomes than other children with FTT if unrecognized. When abuse is documented, social services must be involved.

Another group of children who may be considered for hospital admission are those who have failed to initiate catch-up growth with outpatient management. A hospital stay of several days will allow the clinician to observe feeding practices and enable the family to internalize the plan of care. Further testing for organ dysfunction may be indicated during this hospitalization. It can also be a time to enlist other health professionals in the treatment plan; occupational therapists and social workers are often helpful allies in the treatment of FTT.

Bonuck K, Parikh S, Bassila M. Growth failure and sleep disordered breathing: a review of the literature. *Int J Pediatr Otorhinolaryngol.* 2006;70:769–778. [PMID: 16460816]

Cole SZ, Lanham JS. Failure to thrive: an update. *Am Fam Physician.* 2011;83(7):829–834. [PMID: 21524049]

Ficicioglu C, Haack K. Failure to thrive: when to suspect inborn errors of metabolism. *Pediatrics.* 2009;124:972–979. [PMID: 19706585]

Frank DA. Failure to thrive. *Pediatr Clin North Am.* 1988;35(6): 1187–1206. [PMID: 3059294]

Jaffee AC. Failure to thrive: current clinical concepts. *Pediatr Rev.* 2011;32(3):100–107. [PMID: 21364013]

Maggioni A. Nutritional management of failure to thrive. *Pediatr Clin North Am.* 1995;42(4):791–810. [PMID: 7610013]

Olsen EM, Petersen J, Skovgaard AM, et al. Failure to thrive: the prevalence and concurrence of anthropometric criteria in a general infant population. *Arch Dis Child.* 2007;92(2):109–114. [PMID: 16531456]

Prasse K, Kikano G. An overview of pediatric dysphagia. *Clin Pediatr.* 2009;48(3):247–251. [PMID: 19023104]

Rudolph MC. What is the long term outcome for children who fail to thrive? A systematic review. *Arch Dis Child.* 2005;90(9): 925–931. [PMID: 15890695]

Thompson RT. Increased length of stay and costs associated with weekend admissions for failure to thrive. *Pediatrics.* 2013;131:e805. [PMID: 23439903]

Neonatal Hyperbilirubinemia

Andrew B. Symons, MD, MS
Martin C. Mahoney, MD, PhD, FAAFP

ESSENTIALS OF DIAGNOSIS

▶ Visible yellowing of the skin, ocular sclera, or both are present in neonatal jaundice; however, because visual estimates of total bilirubin are prone to error, quantitative testing (serum or transcutaneous) should be completed in infants noted to be jaundiced within the first 24 hours of life.

▶ Risk of subsequent hyperbilirubinemia can be assessed by plotting serum bilirubin levels onto a nomogram; all bilirubin levels should be interpreted according to the infant's age (in hours).

▶ General Considerations

Nearly every infant is born with a serum bilirubin level higher than that of the normal adult. Approximately 60% of newborns are visibly jaundiced during the first week of life. The diagnostic and therapeutic challenge for the physician is to differentiate normal physiologic jaundice from pathologic jaundice and to institute appropriate evaluation and therapy when necessary.

Several factors are considered as major predictors for the development of severe hyperbilirubinemia among infants of ≥35 weeks' gestation. Among the most significant clinical characteristics associated with severe hyperbilirubinemia are predischarge levels in the high-risk zone on the serum bilirubin nomogram (Figure 3–1) and jaundice noted within 24 hours of birth. Other risk factors include various forms of hemolytic disease (eg, ABO incompatibility, glucose-6-phosphate dehydrogenase [G6PD] deficiency), elevated end-tidal carbon monoxide, gestation age of 35–36 weeks, a sibling who required phototherapy, cephalohematoma or significant bruising, exclusive breastfeeding, East Asian race, maternal age ≥25 years, and male gender.

The American Academy of Pediatrics currently recommends universal predischarge bilirubin screening using total serum bilirubin (TSB) or total cutaneous bilirubin (TcB) measurements. Although the US Preventive Services Task Force (USPSTF, 2004) previously determined that the evidence is insufficient to recommend screening infants for hyperbilirubinemia to prevent chronic bilirubin encephalopathy, this policy was retired in 2009 because there was no new evidence available for review. The American Academy of Family Physicians continues to concur with the USPSTF 2004 statement. In clinical practice, however, testing is completed for the vast majority of infants.

American Academy of Pediatrics Subcommittee on Hyperbilirubinemia. Management of hyperbilirubinemia in the newborn infant 35 or more weeks of gestation. *Pediatrics*. 2004;114:297. [PMID: 15231951]

Muchowski KE. Evaluation and treatment of neonatal hyperbilirubinemia. *Am Fam Physician*. 2014;89(11):873–878. [PMID: 25077393]

US Preventive Services Task Force. Screening of infants for hyperbilirubinemia to prevent chronic bilirubin encephalopathy: US preventive services task force recommendation statement. *Pediatrics*. 2009;124(4):1172–1177. [PMID: 19786451]

▶ Pathogenesis

A. Physiologic Jaundice

The three classifications of neonatal hyperbilirubinemia are based on the following mechanisms of accumulation: increased bilirubin load, decreased bilirubin conjugation, and impaired bilirubin excretion. In the newborn, unconjugated bilirubin is produced faster and removed more slowly than in the normal adult because of the immaturity of the glucuronyl transferase enzyme system. The main source of unconjugated bilirubin is the breakdown of hemoglobin in senescent red blood cells. Newborns have an increased erythrocyte mass at birth (average hematocrit of 50% vs 33% in

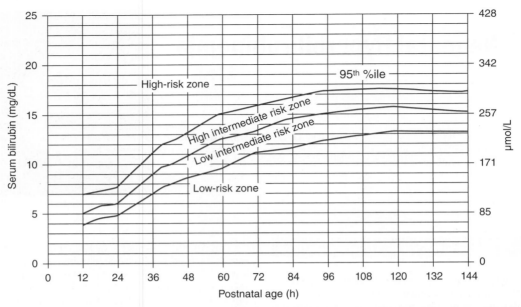

▲ **Figure 3–1.** Nomogram for designation of risk in 2840 well newborns of ≥36 weeks' gestational age with birth weight of ≥2000 g or ≥35 weeks' gestational age and birth weight of ≥2500 g based on the hour-specific serum bilirubin value. (Reproduced with permission from American Academy of Pediatrics Subcommittee on Hyperbilirubinemia: Management of hyperbilirubinemia in the newborn infant 35 or more weeks of gestation. *Pediatrics.* 2004 Jul;114(1):297–316.)

the adult) and a shorter lifespan for erythrocytes (90 days vs 120 days in the adult). The newborn cannot readily excrete unconjugated bilirubin, and much of it is reabsorbed by the intestine and returned to the enterohepatic circulation.

Increased production and decreased elimination of bilirubin lead to a *physiologic jaundice* in most normal newborns. Bilirubin is a very effective and potent antioxidant, and physiologic jaundice may provide a mechanism for protecting the newborn from oxygen free radical injury. The average full-term white newborn experiences a peak serum bilirubin concentration of 5–6 mg/dL (86–103 μmol/L), which begins to rise after the first day of life, peaks on the third day of life, and falls to normal adult levels by days 10–12. African American infants tend to have slightly lower peaks in serum bilirubin. In Asian infants, serum bilirubin levels rise more quickly than in white infants and tend to reach higher peaks on average (8–12 mg/dL; 135–205 μmol/L). This leads to a longer period of physiologic jaundice among Asian and Native American newborns. Preterm infants (<37 weeks' gestation) of all races may take 4–5 days to reach peak serum bilirubin levels, and these peaks may be twice those observed among full-term infants.

B. Breastfeeding and Breast Milk Jaundice

Infants who are breastfed may experience exaggerated bilirubin levels as a result of two separate phenomena associated with breastfeeding and breast milk.

Breastfed infants may experience relative starvation in the first few days of life, due to delayed release of milk by the mother and/or difficulties with breastfeeding. This nutritional inadequacy can result in increased enterohepatic circulation of bilirubin, leading to elevated serum bilirubin levels in the first few days of life. Termed *breastfeeding jaundice,* this finding is considered abnormal and can be overcome by offering frequent feedings (10–12 times per day) and by avoiding water supplementation in breastfed infants.

Breast milk is believed to increase the enterohepatic circulation of bilirubin; however, the specific factor(s) in breast milk that is (are) responsible for this action is (are) unknown. For the first 5 days of life, the serum bilirubin level in breastfed infants parallels that in nonbreastfed infants. Beginning at approximately day 6, *breast milk jaundice* occurs in breastfed infants as serum bilirubin either rises a little for a few days or declines more slowly. Approximately two-thirds of breastfed infants may be expected to have hyperbilirubinemia from 3 weeks to 3 months of age, with as many as one-third exhibiting clinical jaundice. Breast milk jaundice (unlike breastfeeding jaundice) is considered a form of normal physiologic jaundice in healthy, thriving breastfed infants.

C. Pathologic Jaundice

Exaggerated physiologic jaundice occurs at serum bilirubin levels between 7 and 17 mg/dL (between 104 and 291 μmol/L).

Bilirubin levels above 17 mg/dL in full-term infants are no longer considered physiologic, and further investigation is warranted.

The onset of jaundice within the first 24 hours of life or a rate of increase in serum bilirubin exceeding 0.5 mg/dL (8 μmol/L) per hour is potentially pathologic and suggestive of hemolytic disease. Conjugated serum bilirubin concentrations exceeding 10% of total bilirubin or 2 mg/dL (35 μmol/L) are also not physiologic and suggest hepatobiliary disease or a general metabolic disorder.

Differentiating between pathologic and physiologic jaundice requires consideration of historical as well as clinical factors. Important historical features increasing the likelihood that jaundice is pathologic include family history of hemolytic disease, ethnicity suggestive of inherited disease (eg, G6PD deficiency), onset of jaundice in the first 24 hours of life, and jaundice lasting >3 weeks. Clinical assessment requires careful attention to general appearance, vital signs, weight loss, feeding patterns, stool and urine appearance, activity levels, and hepatosplenomegaly, which may be indicative of inborn errors in metabolism, sepsis, or other conditions. A rapid rise in serum bilirubin levels and lack of response to phototherapy are also indicative of pathologic jaundice. Cholestatic jaundice, manifesting as pale-colored stool and dark urine, indicates the need to explore for the presence of biliary atresia or other pathology.

The primary concern with severe hyperbilirubinemia is the potential for neurotoxic effects as well as general cellular injury, which can occur at TSB levels exceeding 20–25 mg/dL. The term *kernicterus* refers to the yellow staining of the basal ganglia observed postmortem among infants who died with severe jaundice. (Bilirubin deposition in the basal ganglia can also be imaged using magnetic resonance techniques.) The American Academy of Pediatrics (AAP) has recommended that the term *acute bilirubin encephalopathy* be used to describe the acute manifestations of bilirubin toxicity seen in the first weeks after birth and that the term *kernicterus* be reserved for the chronic and permanent clinical sequelae of bilirubin toxicity.

Although kernicterus was a common complication of hyperbilirubinemia in the 1940s and 1950s due to Rh erythroblastosis fetalis and ABO hemolytic disease, it is rare today, with the use of Rh immunoglobulin and with the intervention of phototherapy and exchange transfusion. With early discharge to home, however, a small resurgence of kernicterus has been observed in countries in which this complication had essentially disappeared. The reported incidence of chronic kernicterus in the United States is ~1 case/27,000 live births and 1 case/44,000 live births in Canada.

Bilirubin can interfere with various metabolic pathways and may also impair cerebral glucose metabolism. The concentration of bilirubin in the brain and the duration of exposure are important determinants of the neurotoxic effects of bilirubin. Bilirubin can enter the brain when not bound to albumin, so infants with low albumin are at increased risk of developing kernicterus. Conditions that alter the blood-brain barrier such as infection, acidosis, hypoxia, sepsis, prematurity, and hyperosmolarity may affect the entry of bilirubin into the brain.

In infants without hemolysis, serum bilirubin levels and encephalopathy do not correlate well. In infants with hemolysis, TSB levels of >20 mg/dL are associated with worse neurologic outcomes, although some infants with concentrations of 25 mg/dL are normal. Kernicterus has been detected in 8% of infants with associated hemolysis who had TSB levels of 19–25 mg/dL, 33% of infants with levels of 25–29 mg/dL, and 73% of infants with levels of 30–40 mg/dL. It should be noted that the majority of cases of kernicterus described in recent years have been among neonates who had TSB levels of >30 mg/dL at the time of diagnosis, which is well above the recommended treatment thresholds of 15 or 20 mg/dL.

In its acute form, kernicterus (eg, acute bilirubin encephalopathy) may present in the first 1–2 days with poor sucking, stupor, hypotonia, and seizures, although 15% of affected infants may be asymptomatic. During the middle of the first week, hypertonia of extensor muscles, opisthotonus (backward arching of the trunk), retrocollis (backward arching of the neck), and fever may be observed. After the first week, the infant may exhibit generalized hypertonia. Some of these changes disappear spontaneously or can be reversed with exchange transfusion. In most infants with moderate (10–20 mg/dL) to severe (>20 mg/dL) hyperbilirubinemia, evoked neurologic responses return to normal within 6 months. A minority of infants (ranging between 6% and 23%) exhibit persistent neurologic deficits.

In its chronic form, kernicterus may present in the first year with hypotonia, active deep tendon reflexes, obligatory tonic neck reflexes, dental dysplasia, and delayed motor skills. After the first year, movement disorders, upward gaze, and sensorineural hearing loss may develop. It has been suggested that long-term effects of severe hyperbilirubinemia on intelligence quotient (IQ) are more likely in boys than in girls. In 1991, Seidman and colleagues studied 1948 subjects from Hadassah Hebrew University Medical Center in Jerusalem born in 1970–1971 and drafted into the Israeli army 17 years later and found a higher risk of lowered IQ (<85) among males with a history of TSB exceeding 20 mg/dL (odds ratio 2.96; 95% confidence interval 1.29–6.79).

Kuzniewicz M, Newman TB. Interaction of hemolysis and hyperbilirubinemia on neurodevelopmental outcomes in the collaborative perinatal project. *Pediatrics*. 2009;123:3. [PMID: 19255038]

Seidman DS, Paz I, Stevenson DK, et al. Neonatal hyperbilirubinemia and physical and cognitive performance at 17 years of age. *Pediatrics*. 1991;88:828. [PMID: 1896294]

Sgro M, Campbell DM, Kandasamy S, Shah V. Incidence of chronic bilirubin encephalopathy in Canada, 2007–2008. *Pediatrics*. 2012;130:4. [PMID: 22966025] van den Esker-Jonker B, den Boer L, Pepping RM, et al. Transcutaneous bilirubinometry in jaundiced neonates: a randomized controlled trial. *Pediatrics*. 2016;138(6):e20162414. [PMID: 27940715]

Weiss AK, Vora PV. Conjugated hyperbilirubinemia in the neonate and young infant. *Pediatr Emerg Care*. 2018;34:280–285. [PMID: 29601463]

▶ Clinical Findings

In 2004, the AAP issued an updated practice parameter for the management of hyperbilirubinemia among newborns of ≥35 weeks' gestation. Elements of these recommendations are summarized in the following sections and can be accessed in full at http://www.aap.org.

A. Symptoms and Signs

Clinically, jaundice usually progresses from head to toe. Visual estimates of total bilirubin are prone to error, especially in infants with pigmented skin. TSB or TcB levels should be measured in infants who develop jaundice within the first 24 hours, and all bilirubin levels should be interpreted according to the infant's age (in hours). TcB measurement devices may provide an alternative to frequent blood draws for the accurate assessment of serum bilirubin, although current guidelines indicate variability in the accuracy of TcB instruments from different manufacturers.

Evaluation of infants who develop abnormal signs such as feeding difficulty, behavior changes, apnea, and temperature changes is recommended regardless of whether jaundice has been detected in order to rule out underlying disease. Clinical protocols for evaluating jaundice, with assessments to be performed no less than every 8–12 hours in the newborn nursery, should be in place.

B. Laboratory Findings

When a pathologic cause for jaundice is suspected, laboratory studies should be promptly completed:

- When jaundice is noticed within the first 24 hours, clinicians should consider a sepsis workup, evaluation for rubella and toxoplasmosis infection, assessment of fractionated serum bilirubin levels, and blood typing to rule out erythroblastosis fetalis. Results of thyroid and galactosemia testing, obtained during the newborn metabolic screening, also should be reviewed.

- If the level of conjugated bilirubin is >2 mg/dL, a reason for impaired bilirubin excretion should be sought. If conjugated bilirubin is <2 mg/dL, hemoglobin levels and reticulocyte counts should be evaluated. A high hemoglobin concentration indicates polycythemia, whereas a low hemoglobin concentration with an abnormal reticulocyte count suggests hemolysis. If the reticulocyte count is normal, the infant must be evaluated for a nonhemolytic cause of jaundice.

- Infants with a poor response to phototherapy and those whose family history is consistent with the possibility of G6PD deficiency require further testing.

- Maternal prenatal testing should include ABO and Rh(D) typing and a serum screen for unusual isoimmune antibodies. If the mother has not had prenatal blood grouping or is Rh negative, a direct Coombs test, blood type, and Rh(D) typing of the infant's cord blood should be performed. Institutions are encouraged to save cord blood for future testing, particularly when the mother's blood type is group O.

C. Neonatal Jaundice after Hospital Discharge

Follow-up should be provided to all neonates discharged <48 hours after birth. This evaluation by a healthcare professional should occur within 2–3 days of discharge.

Approximately one-third of healthy breastfed infants have persistent jaundice beyond 2 weeks of age. A report of dark urine or light-colored stools should prompt a measurement of direct serum bilirubin. If the history and physical examination are normal, continued observation is appropriate. If jaundice persists beyond 3 weeks, a urine sample should be tested for bilirubin, and a measurement of total and direct serum bilirubin should be obtained.

American Academy of Pediatrics Subcommittee on Hyperbilirubinemia. Management of hyperbilirubinemia in the newborn infant 35 or more weeks of gestation. *Pediatrics*. 2004;114:297. [PMID: 15231951]

Maisels MJ, Bhutani VK, Bogen D, et al. Hyperbilirubinemia in the newborn infant ≥35 weeks' gestation: an update with clarification. *Pediatrics*. 2009;124:1193–1198. [PMID: 19786452]

▶ Prediction & Prevention

Shorter hospital stays after delivery limit the time for hospital-based assessment of infant feeding, instruction about breastfeeding, and the detection of jaundice. Hyperbilirubinemia and problems related to feeding are the main reasons for hospital readmission during the first week of life. Among 25,439 infants discharged between 2008 and 2009 from a large medical center in Israel, 143 (0.56%) were readmitted for phototherapy.

Because bilirubin levels usually peak on day 3 or 4 of life and because most newborns are discharged within 48 hours, most cases of jaundice occur at home. It is therefore important that infants be seen by a healthcare professional within a few days of discharge to assess for jaundice and overall well-being. This is important in near-term infants (35–36 weeks' gestation) who are at particular risk for hyperbilirubinemia because of both relative hepatic immaturity and inadequate nutritional intake.

Measuring TSB before discharge and then plotting this value on a nomogram (see Figure 3–1) can be useful for predicting the risk of subsequent moderately severe hyperbilirubinemia (>17 mg/dL) and identify neonates for whom close follow-up is warranted. A study of 17,854 live births reported that neonates in the high-risk group (95th percentile for TSB) at 18–72 hours of life had a 40% chance of developing moderately severe hyperbilirubinemia on discharge, whereas for those in the low-risk group (40th percentile for TSB), the probability for subsequently developing moderately severe hyperbilirubinemia was zero. Clinicians may consider use of one of several smart phone and web-based applications for determining an infant's risk of developing hyperbilirubinemia and thresholds for therapy.

Bromiker R, Bin-Nun A, Schimmel MS, Hammerman C, Kaplan M. Neonatal hyperbilirubinemia in the low-intermediate-risk category on the bilirubin nomogram. *Pediatrics.* 2012;130(3): e470–e475. [PMID: 22926183]
Kuzniewicz MW, Escobar GJ, Wi S, et al. Risk factors for severe hyperbilirubinemia among infants with borderline bilirubin levels: a nested case-control study. *J Pediatr.* 2008;153:2. [PMID: 18534217]

▶ **Treatment**

A. Suspected Pathologic Jaundice

Treatment decisions for both phototherapy (Figure 3–2) and exchange transfusion (Figure 3–3) are based on TSB levels; management options should be discussed with the parents or guardians of the infant. Intensive phototherapy should produce a decline in TSB of 1–2 mg/dL within 4–6 hours, and the decline should continue thereafter. If the TSB does not respond appropriately to intensive phototherapy, exchange transfusion is recommended. If levels are in a range that suggests the need for exchange transfusion (see Figure 3–3), intensive phototherapy should be attempted while preparations for exchange transfusion are made. Exchange transfusion is also recommended in infants whose TSB levels rise to exchange transfusion levels despite intensive phototherapy. In any of the preceding situations, failure of intensive phototherapy to lower the TSB level strongly suggests the presence of hemolytic disease or other pathologic processes and strongly warrants further investigation or consultation.

In infants with isoimmune hemolytic disease, administration of intravenous gamma globulin (0.5–1 g/kg over 2 hours) is recommended if the TSB is rising despite intensive phototherapy or the TSB is within 2–3 mg/dL of the exchange level. If necessary, this dose can be repeated in 12 hours.

Figure 3–2 summarizes the management strategy for hyperbilirubinemia in infants of ≥35 weeks' gestation. Management decisions regarding phototherapy and exchange transfusion (see Figure 3–3) are based on the infant's age, risk factors, and TSB levels.

B. Phototherapy and Exchange Transfusion

1. Phototherapy—This procedure involves exposing the infant to high-intensity light in the blue-green wavelengths.

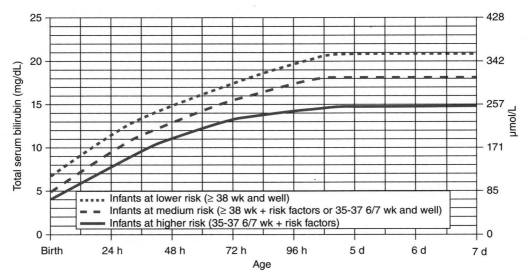

▲ **Figure 3–2.** Guidelines for phototherapy in hospitalized infants of ≥35 weeks' gestation. (Reproduced with permission from American Academy of Pediatrics Subcommittee on Hyperbilirubinemia: Management of hyperbilirubinemia in the newborn infant 35 or more weeks of gestation. *Pediatrics.* 2004 Jul;114(1):297–316.)

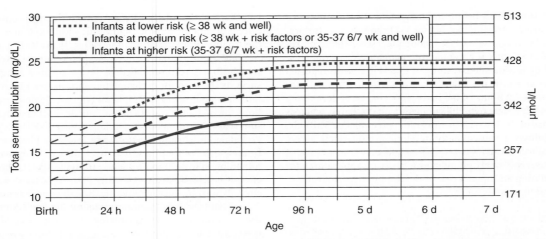

▲ **Figure 3–3.** Guidelines for exchange transfusion in infants of ≥35 weeks' gestation. (Reproduced with permission from American Academy of Pediatrics Subcommittee on Hyperbilirubinemia: Management of hyperbilirubinemia in the newborn infant 35 or more weeks of gestation. *Pediatrics.* 2004 Jul;114(1):297–316.)

Light interacts with unconjugated bilirubin in the skin, converting it to less toxic photoisomers that are excreted in the bile and urine without conjugation. The efficacy of phototherapy is strongly influenced by the energy output in the blue spectrum, the spectrum of the light, and the surface area of the infant exposed to phototherapy. Commonly used light sources for providing phototherapy are special blue fluorescent tubes, compact fluorescent tubes, and halogen spotlights; however, light-emitting diodes (LEDs) have been shown to be as efficacious as conventional sources, with less heat emission.

Eye protection is placed on the infant, and the bank of lights is placed 15–20 cm from the naked infant. Exposure is increased by placing a fiberoptic blanket under the infant, lightening units all around the infant, or a white sheet around the bassinet to serve as a reflecting surface. If slight warming of the infant is noted, the tubes can be moved away a bit. Phototherapy may be interrupted briefly for parental visits or breastfeeding.

In infants with TSB levels of >25 mg/dL, phototherapy should be administered continuously until a response is documented or until exchange therapy is initiated. If the TSB is not responding to conventional phototherapy (a *response* is defined as a sustained reduction in TSB of 1–2 mg/dL in 4–6 hours), the intensity should be increased by adding more lights; the intensity of the lights should also be increased while exchange transfusion is prepared. With commonly used light sources, overdose is impossible, although the infant may experience loose stools. Phototherapy is continued until the TSB level is lower than 14–15 mg/dL. The infant may be discharged after the completion of phototherapy. Rebound of TSB following cessation of phototherapy is usually <1 mg/dL.

2. Exchange transfusion—This procedure rapidly removes bilirubin from the circulation. Circulating antibodies against erythrocytes are also removed. Exchange transfusion is particularly beneficial in neonates with hemolysis. One or two central catheters are placed. Small aliquots of blood (8–10 mL per pass) are removed from the infant's circulation and replaced with equal amounts of donor red cells mixed with plasma. The procedure is repeated until twice the infant's blood volume is replaced (~160–200 mL/kg). Serum electrolytes and bilirubin are measured periodically during the procedure. In some cases, the procedure must be repeated to lower serum bilirubin levels sufficiently. Infusing salt-poor albumin at a dose of 1 g/kg 1–4 hours before exchange transfusion has been shown to increase the amount of bilirubin removed during the procedure.

Complications of exchange transfusion include thrombocytopenia, portal vein thrombosis, necrotizing enterocolitis, electrolyte imbalance, graft-versus-host disease, and infection. Mortality from exchange transfusion approaches 2%, and an additional 12% of infants may suffer serious complications. Therefore, exchange transfusion should be reserved for neonates who have failed intensive phototherapy and should be performed by clinicians and facilities with proper experience.

If exchange transfusion is being considered, the bilirubin/albumin ratio is used in conjunction with the TSB level and other factors in determining the need for exchange transfusion (see Figure 3–3).

C. Suspected Nonpathologic Jaundice

For the management of breastfeeding jaundice, interruption of breastfeeding in healthy full-term newborns is generally discouraged. Frequent breastfeeding sessions (at least 8–10 times in 24 hours) are advised. However, if the mother and physician wish, they may consider using supplemental formula feedings or temporarily interrupting breastfeeding and replacing it with formula feedings. Phototherapy may be initiated, depending on TSB levels.

As discussed previously, breast milk jaundice is seen initially after day 6 of life in the majority of healthy breastfed infants between 3 weeks and 3 months of age. This is a form of normal physiologic jaundice.

Bhutani VK, Johns L. Kernicterus in the 21st century: frequently asked questions. *J Perinatol.* 2009;29:S1. [PMID: 19177056]

Dijk PH, Hulzebos CV. An evidence-based view on hyperbilirubinaemia. *Acta Paediatrica.* 2012;101:s464 [PMID: 22404885]

Maisels MJ, McDonagh AF. Phototherapy for neonatal jaundice. *N Engl J Med.* 2008;358:920–928. [PMID: 18305267]

Murki S, Murki S, Malik GK, et al. Light emitting diodes versus compact fluorescent tubes for phototherapy in neonatal jaundice: a multi-center randomized controlled trial. *Indian Pediatr.* 2010;47:2. [PMID: 19578227]

▷ Conclusions

Because up to 60% of all newborns are noted to be clinically jaundiced, all family physicians who care for neonates will encounter this common clinical entity. In the overwhelming majority of cases, this jaundice is entirely benign. However, it is important that the family physician recognize cases in which jaundice could represent a pathologic process or the risk for development of severe hyperbilirubinemia.

Infants who are discharged prior to 48 hours of age, particularly those who are born at <35 weeks' gestation, should be seen in the office within 2 days of discharge to evaluate jaundice and overall clinical status.

Parental education should emphasize the need to monitor the infant for jaundice, the generally benign course of most cases of jaundice, and associated symptoms such as poor feeding, lethargy, dark urine, and light-colored stools. Family physicians should encourage parents to contact the office with specific questions and concerns. An example of a parent information sheet, available in English and Spanish, can be found at https://www.healthychildren.org/English/tips-tools/symptom-checker/Pages/symptomviewer.aspx?symptom=Jaundiced%20Newborn.

Maisels MJ, Bhutani VK, Bogen D, et al. Hyperbilirubinemia in the newborn infant ≥35 weeks' gestation: an update with clarification. *Pediatrics.* 2009;124(4):1193–1198. [PMID: 19786452]

Moyer VA, Ahn C, Sneed S. Accuracy of clinical judgment in neonatal jaundice. *Arch Pediatric Adolesc Med.* 2000;154:391–394. [PMID: 1076879]

Muchowski, KE. Evaluation and treatment of neonatal hyperbilirubinemia. *Am Fam Physician.* 2014;89(11):873–878. [PMID: 25077393]

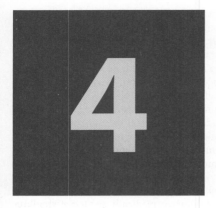

Breastfeeding & Infant Nutrition

Tracey D. Conti, MD

General Considerations

Nutrition is a critical capstone for the proper growth and development of infants. Breastfeeding of term infants by healthy mothers is the optimal mechanism for providing the caloric and nutrient needs of infants. Preterm infants can also benefit from breast milk and breastfeeding, although supplementation and fortification of preterm breast milk may be required. Barring some unique circumstances, human breast milk can provide nutritional, social, and motor developmental benefits for most infants. The American Academy of Pediatrics (AAP) recommends that infants be exclusively breastfed for about the first 6 months with continued breastfeeding alongside introduction of appropriate complementary foods for 1 year or longer. The World Health Organization also recommends exclusively breastfeeding up to 6 months of age with continued breastfeeding along with appropriate complementary foods up to 2 years of age or beyond.

According to the 2018 Breastfeeding Report Card published by the Centers for Disease Control and Prevention, among infants born in 2015 in the United States, four (83.2%) of five started to breastfeed, over half (57.6%) were breastfeeding at 6 months, and over one-third (35.9%) were breastfeeding at 12 months. Compared to rates for infants born in 2014, rates for infants born in 2015 increased for breastfeeding at 6 and 12 months. Efforts to alter knowledge, attitudes, and behaviors regarding breastfeeding must effectively address the numerous psychosocial barriers to breastfeeding and continuance. Healthcare providers are critical conduits for maternal and familial education. All members of the healthcare team, including physicians, midwives, and nurses, are valuable sources of important evidence-based information as well as psychological support for mothers in search of guidance regarding infant feeding practices. A 2015 systematic review and meta-analysis of 17 studies found that breastfed infants performed better on intelligence tests later in life than those who were not breastfed, even after controlling for maternal IQ. The literature has shown that infants who are breastfed have fewer episodes of diarrheal illness, ear infections, and allergies. Exclusive breastfeeding for at least 4 months in infants at risk for developing atopic disease decreases the cumulative incidence of atopic dermatitis. Lower rates of childhood obesity, type 2 diabetes, sudden infant death syndrome, and leukemia have also been associated with breastfeeding. There are likewise financial advantages to breastfeeding. Other somewhat controversial investigations suggest higher intelligence among breastfed infants.

There are also maternal benefits to breastfeeding. Mothers who breastfeed are less likely to develop premenopausal breast cancer. An association with decreased rates of type 2 diabetes and ovarian cancer also exists. Studies are also looking at the relationship between breastfeeding and rates of postpartum depression and cardiovascular disease. Most importantly, however, is the bonding relationship breastfeeding promotes between mother and infant.

The AAP Committee on Nutrition recommends breastfeeding for the first year of life with supplemental vitamin D at birth and the addition of supplemental iron at age 4 months and possible addition of fluoride at age 6 months for infants living in regions in which water is low in fluoride. Vitamin D supplementation is particularly applicable in regions with limited sunlight and for infants of mothers with decreased daily intake of cow's milk. Further recommendations include delaying introduction of cow's milk until after 1 year and delaying addition of reduced-fat milk until 2 years of age. To this end, new mothers should be encouraged to continue prenatal vitamins containing supplemental iron, calcium, and vitamin D. Supplemental solid foods should be considered at or around 6 months of age once the infant demonstrates appropriate readiness. Key practice recommendations are listed in Table 4–1.

Table 4–1. Key recommendations for practice.

Clinical Recommendation	Evidence Rating
Exclusive breastfeeding is recommended to reduce the risk of infant gastrointestinal infection and atopic dermatitis.	B
Primary care interventions to support breastfeeding are recommended.	B
Adequate milk supply during breastfeeding should be monitored through test weighing (the clothed infant is weighed under identical conditions before and after a feeding, and the two measurements are subtracted; 1 g of weight gain = 1 mL of milk intake).	C
Frenotomy to treat ankyloglossia in infants reduces breastfeeding-related nipple pain in the short term	C

American Academy of Pediatrics Section on Breastfeeding. Breastfeeding and the use of human milk. *Pediatrics*. 2012;129(3): e827–e841. [PMID: 22371471]

Centers for Disease Control and Prevention. Breastfeeding report card–United States, 2018. https://www.cdc.gov/breastfeeding/data/reportcard.htm. Accessed November 12, 2019.

Cramton R, Zain-Ul-Abideen M, Whalen B. Optimizing successful breastfeeding in the newborn. *Curr Opin Pediatr.* 2009;21: 386–396. [PMID: 19421060]

US Department of Health and Human Services. *Healthy People 2010 Objectives for Breastfeeding: Healthy People 2010 Midcourse Review.* Washington, DC: US Department of Health and Human Services.

Westerfield KL, Koenig K, Oh R. Breastfeeding: common questions and answers. *Am Fam Physician.* 2018;98(6):368–373. [PMID: 30215910]

World Health Organization. Breastfeeding. https://www.who.int/topics/breastfeeding/en/. Accessed November 12, 2019.

▶ **Breastfeeding Technique**

Preparation for breastfeeding should begin in the preconception period or at the first contact with the patient. Most women choose their method of feeding prior to conception. Psychosocial support and education may encourage breastfeeding among women who might not otherwise have considered it. Evidence for this strategy, however, is anecdotal and requires further investigation.

There are numerous potential supports available to women who are considering feeding behaviors. Practitioners are encouraged to identify members of the patient's support network and provide similar education to minimize the potential barriers posed by uninformed support individuals.

One commonly perceived physical barrier is nipple inversion. Women who have inverted nipples will have difficulty with the latch-on process (discussed later). Nipple shields are relatively inexpensive devices that can draw the nipple out. Manual or electric breast pumps may also be used to draw out inverted nipples, typically beginning after delivery.

Breastfeeding should begin immediately in the postpartum period, ideally in the first 30–40 minutes after delivery. This is easier to accomplish if the infant is left in the room with the mother before being bathed and before the newborn examination is performed. It is also safe to allow breastfeeding before administration of vitamin K and erythromycin ophthalmic ointment.

Clinical situations arise that preclude initiation of breastfeeding in the immediate postpartum period (eg, cesarean delivery, maternal perineal repair, maternal or fetal distress). In such cases, breastfeeding should be initiated at the earliest time possible. Only when medically necessary should a supplemental feeding be initiated. If mothers have expressed a desire to breastfeed, the practitioner should coordinate an interim feeding plan, emphasizing that bottle feeding not be started. Acceptable alternatives include spoon, cup, or syringe feeding.

Breastfed children commonly feed at least every 2–3 hours during the first several weeks postpartum. Infants should not be allowed to sleep through feedings; however, if necessary, feeding intervals may be increased to every 3–4 hours overnight. The production of breast milk is on a supply-demand cycle. Breast stimulation through suckling and the mechanism of breastfeeding signals the body to make more milk. When feedings are missed or breasts are not emptied effectively, the feedback loop decreases the milk supply. As the infant grows, feedings every 3–4 hours are acceptable. During growth spurts, the amount of milk needed for the rate of growth often exceeds milk production. Feeding intervals often must be adjusted to growth periods until the milk supply catches up.

Although feeding intervals may be increased during nighttime periods, a common question becomes when to stop waking the infant for night feedings. Anecdotal evidence suggests that after the first 2 weeks postpartum, in the absence of specific nutritional concerns, the infant can determine its own overnight feeding schedule. Typically, most infants will begin to sleep through the night once they have reached approximately 10 lb.

Positioning of the infant is critical for effective feeding in the neonatal period, allowing for optimal latch-on. In general, infant and mother should face each other in one of the following three positions: the cradle, the most common; the football; or the lay/side. The cradle hold allows the mother to hold the infant horizontally across the front of the chest. The infant's head can be on the left or right side of the mother depending on which side he or she is feeding. The infant's head should be supported with the crook of the mother's arm. The football hold is performed with the mother sitting on a bed or chair, the infant's bottom against the bed or chair and the infant's body lying next to the mother's side, and the infant's head cradled in her hand. The side position allows the mother to lay on her left or right side with the infant lying parallel to her. Again, the infant's head is cradled in the crook of the mother's elbow. This position is ideally suited for women after cesarean delivery because it reduces the pain associated with pressure from the infant on their incisions. It must be stressed that choice of position is based on mother and infant comfort. It is not unusual to experiment with any or all positions prior to determining the most desirable. It is likewise not uncommon to find previously undesirable positions more effective and comfortable as the infant grows and the breast-feeding experience progresses. All breastfeeding positions should allow for cradling of the infant's head with the mother's hand or elbow, allowing for better head control in the latch-on stage. The infant should be placed at a height (often achieved with a pillow) appropriate for preventing awkward positioning, maximizing comfort, and encouraging latch-on.

Many of the difficulties with breastfeeding result from improper latch-on. Latch-on problems are often the source of multiple breastfeeding complaints among mothers, ranging from engorgement to sore cracked nipples. Many women discontinue breastfeeding secondary to these issues. The latch-on process is governed by primitive reflexes. Stroking the infant's cheek will cause the infant to turn toward the side on which the cheek was stroked. This reflex is useful if the infant is not looking toward the breast. Tickling the infant's bottom lip will cause his or her mouth to open wide in order to latch on to the breast. The mother should hold her breast to help position the areola to ease latch-on. It is important that the mother's fingers be behind the areola so as not to provide a physical barrier to latch-on. Once the infant's mouth is opened wide, the head should be pulled quickly to the breast. The infant's mouth should encompass the entire areola to compress the milk ducts. If this is done improperly, the infant will compress the nipple, leading to pain and eventually cracking, with minimal or no milk expression. The mother should not experience pain with breastfeeding. If this occurs, the mother should break the suction by inserting a finger into the side of the infant's mouth and then latch the infant on again. This process should be repeated as many times as necessary until proper latch-on is achieved.

One issue that continually concerns parents is whether the infant is receiving adequate amounts of breast milk. Several clinical measures can be used to determine if infants are receiving enough milk. Weight is an excellent method of assessment. Pre- and postfeed measurement of an infant with a scale that is of high quality and measures to the ounce is a very accurate means of determining weight. The problem is that this type of scale is not available to most families. Weight can also be evaluated on a longer-term basis. Infants should not lose more than about 8% of their birth weight after delivery and should gain this weight back in 2 weeks. Most infants with difficulties, however, will decompensate before this 2-week period. Breastfed infants should

be evaluated 2–3 days after discharge, especially if discharged prior to 48 hours after delivery. A more convenient way to determine the adequacy of the infant's intake of milk is through clinical signs such as infant satisfaction after feeding and bowel and bladder amounts. In most cases, infants who are satisfied after feeding will fall asleep. Infants who do not receive enough milk will usually be fussy or irritable or continuously want to suck at the breast, their finger, and so on. Breastfed infants usually will stool after most feeds but at a minimum 5–6 times a day. After the first couple of days, the stool should turn from meconium-like to a mustard-colored seedy type. If breastfed infants are still passing meconium or do not have an adequate amount of stool, parents and the healthcare team should evaluate whether they are taking in enough milk. Infants should also urinate approximately 3 or 4 times a day. This may be hard to assess with the current era's superabsorbent diapers; therefore, careful examination of the diaper should be made.

▶ Problems Associated with Breastfeeding

An inadequate milk supply can lead to disastrous outcomes if not identified and treated. There are two types of milk inadequacies: the inability to make milk and the inability to keep the supply adequate. The first type of milk inadequacy is quite rare, but examples include surgeries in which the milk ducts are severed or Sheehan syndrome. There is no specific treatment to initiate milk production in affected women. The inability to maintain an adequate milk supply has numerous etiologies, ranging from dietary deficiencies to engorgement. The key in preventing adverse events is early recognition and effective treatment. One of the mainstays of treatment is working with the body's own feedback loop of supply and demand to increase the supply. As more milk is needed, more milk will be produced. This is effectively done by using a breast pump. Pumping should be performed after the infant has fed.

Engorgement is caused by inadequate or ineffective emptying of the breasts. As milk builds up in the breasts, they become swollen. If the condition is not relieved, the breasts can become tender and warm. Mastitis can also develop. The mainstay of treatment is emptying the breasts of milk, either by the infant or, if that is not possible, by mechanical means. Usually when the breast is engorged, the areola and nipple are affected, and proper latch-on becomes difficult if not impossible. A warm compress may be used to help with letdown, and the breast can be manually expressed enough to allow the infant to latch on. If this is not possible or is too painful, the milk can be removed with an electrical breast pump. Between feedings, a cold pack can be used to decrease the amount of swelling. There have been reports that chilled cabbage leaves used to line the bra can act as a cold pack that conforms to the shape of the breast and can reduce the pain and swelling. However, there is no evidence of any medicinal properties in the cabbage that affect engorgement. Mastitis, if occurring, is treated with antibiotics. Mothers can continue to breastfeed with the affected breast, so care should be taken to choose an antibiotic that is safe for the infant.

Sore nipples are a common problem for breastfeeding mothers. In the first few weeks, there may be some soreness associated with breastfeeding as the skin gets used to the constant moisture. There should not be pain with breastfeeding; if there is pain, it is usually secondary to improper latch-on, which resolves with correction. With severe cracking, there will occasionally be bleeding. Breastfeeding can be continued with mild bleeding, but if severe bleeding occurs, the breast should be pumped and the milk discarded to prevent gastrointestinal upset in the infant. There are some remedies that can be used in the event of cracking. Keeping the nipples clean and dry between feedings can help prevent and heal cracking. The mother's own milk or a pure lanolin ointment can also be used as a salve. Mothers should be warned not to use herbal rubs or vitamin E because of the risk of absorption by the infant. Another cause of sore nipples is candidal infection. This usually occurs when an infant has thrush. Sometimes treating the infant will resolve the problem, but occasionally, the mother will need to be treated as well. Taking the same nystatin liquid dose that the infant is using twice a day will resolve the infection. Again, keeping the nipples clean and dry can help.

Blebs, a small pimple or blister-like lesion on the nipple, can also be a cause of sore nipples. This occurs secondary to the opening of the milk duct being covered by new epithelial cells. Treatment includes moisturizing the nipples with lanolin and gentle exfoliation. This can be exacerbated by a candidal infection as well and would require the same treatment stated previously. If these lesions do not heal, they may require surgical debridement.

Another controversial issue in breastfeeding is silicone implants. Although only little research has been done on effects of silicone implants on lactation, there are a few areas of concern, including implants leaking material in breast milk, baby absorbing the silicone from the milk if it is spilled, and additional risks of infant exposure to the silicone. Due to its presence in the environment, it is difficult to distinguish between normal and abnormal maternal levels. It has been found that silicon is present in higher concentrations in cow's milk and formula than in milk of humans with implants. An additional study directly assayed the silicone polymer and found that levels in the milk of women with implants were not significantly different from those in other human milk samples. The AAP, in its policy statement on silicone breast implants and breastfeeding, concluded the following: "The Committee on Drugs does not feel that the evidence currently justifies classifying silicone implants as a contraindication to breastfeeding." Safety of breastfeeding by women with silicone breast implants has not been adequately studied, a fact these women should be told. The potential health risks of artificial feeding have been shown, and until there is better evidence, women with implants should be encouraged to breastfeed.

Other issues with breastfeeding include medications, nutrient supplementation, and mothers returning to work. These issues are broad in scope; in fact, whole books have been dedicated to these subjects. The most important issue to understand when considering medication use during pregnancy is that limited research has been done in this area and that there is insufficient information on most medicines to advocate their use. Healthcare providers should try to use the safest medications possible that will allow mothers to continue breastfeeding. If this is not possible, mothers should be encouraged to pump the milk and discard it to maintain the milk supply.

Nutrient supplementation is another controversial issue. Vitamin D is recommended for supplementation in either dark-skinned women or women who do not receive much sunlight. The iron found in breast milk, although in low concentrations, is highly absorbable. Infants who are breastfed do not need additional sources of iron until they are 4–6 months old. This is the time when most children are started on cereal. Choosing an iron-fortified cereal will satisfy the additional iron requirement.

Return to work is the major reason why women discontinue breastfeeding. Planning this return from birth and pumping milk for storage help women to continue breastfeeding. Employers who provide time and a comfortable place to pump milk at work will also improve breastfeeding rates. Although the goal is to increase the number of women who begin breastfeeding and continue it throughout the first year of the infant's life, many women cannot or do not choose to breastfeed. Their decision must be supported, and they must be educated on alternative methods of providing nutrition for their infant.

Johnston ML, Esposito N. Barriers and facilitators for breastfeeding among working women in the United States. *J Obstet Gynecol Neonatal Nurs.* 2007;36:9–20. [PMID: 17238942]

▶ Maternal Nutrition & Breastfeeding

There are many studies that look at maternal nutrition and breastfeeding. It is well known that adequate fluid intake is necessary for milk production. Studies seem to suggest that the benefits of infant nutrition outweigh the risk of any maternal effects of breastfeeding.

Often some maternal foods that are strong in flavor, such as garlic, broccoli, and onions, can provide a flavor to breast milk that is displeasing to the infant or can create increased flatulence. These food types should be avoided if they interfere with feeding. There are also women who are concerned about creating allergies based on food that is consumed while breastfeeding. Currently, there is lack of evidence that maternal dietary restrictions (eg, avoiding peanuts) during pregnancy or lactation play a significant role in prevention of atopic disease in infants. Antigen avoidance during lactation does not prevent atopic disease, with the possible exception of eczema, although more data are needed to substantiate conclusions.

Vegetarian Diet & Breastfeeding

The number of Americans choosing a vegetarian diet has increased dramatically over the past decade. With these increasing numbers, more research has been done in an effort to evaluate the feasibility of a vegetarian diet in infancy. A vegetarian diet is defined as a diet consisting of no meat. This definition does not encompass the variety of vegetarian diets that are consumed. A pure vegetarian or vegan consumes only plant food. In general, most pure vegetarians also do not use products that result from animal cruelty such as wool, silk, and leather. Lacto-ovo vegetarians consume dairy products and eggs in addition to plants, and lacto vegetarians consume only dairy products with their plant diet.

There is great variety in each of these diets and, therefore, great variety in the type and amount of food necessary for adequate nutrition. Milk from breastfeeding mothers who are vegetarians is adequate in all nutrients necessary for proper growth and development. Although all required nutrients can be found in any vegetarian diet, in infancy, the amount necessary may be difficult to provide without supplementation. The American Dietetic Association stated that a lacto-ovo vegetarian diet is recommended in infancy. If this diet is not desired by parents or is not tolerated by children, then supplementation may be necessary. Vitamin B_{12}, iron, and vitamin D are nutrients that may need to be supplemented, depending on environmental factors.

Contraindications to Breastfeeding

Although considered the optimal method of providing infant nutrition during the first year of life, breastfeeding may be contraindicated in some mothers. Scenarios that may preclude breastfeeding include mothers who actively use illicit drugs such as heroin, cocaine, alcohol, and phencyclidine (PCP); mothers with human immunodeficiency virus (HIV) infection or acquired immunodeficiency syndrome (AIDS); and mothers receiving pharmacotherapy with agents transmitted in breast milk and contraindicated in children, particularly potent cancer agents. Some immunizations for foreign travelers and military personnel may also be contraindicated in breastfeeding mothers. Infants with galactosemia should also not breastfeed.

Infant Formulas

The historical record reveals that methods of replacing, fortifying, and delivering milk and milk substitutes date back to the Stone Age. Evidence suggests that the original infant "formulas" of the early and mid-20th century consisted of 1:1 concentrations of evaporated milk and water with supplemental cod liver oil, orange juice, and honey. As the number of working mothers steadily increased during this time, the use of infant formulas became more popular.

In the past three decades, more sophisticated neonatal medical practices have led to the development of countless infant formula preparations to meet a wide variety of clinical situations. Formulas exist as concentrates and powders that require dilution with water and as ready-to-feed preparations. Commonly, formula preparations provide 20 cal/oz with standard dilutions of 1 oz concentrate to 1 oz water and 1 scoop powder formula to 2 oz water for liquid concentrates and powders, respectively. Formulas exist as cow's milk–based, soy-based, and casein-based preparations.

A. Cow's Milk–Based Formula Preparations

This is the preferred, standard non–breast milk preparation for otherwise healthy term infants who do not breastfeed or for whom breastfeeding has been terminated prior to 1 year of age. Cow's milk–based formula closely resembles human breast milk and is composed of 20% whey and 80% casein, with 50% more protein/dL than breast milk as well as iron, linoleic acid, carnitine, taurine, and nucleotides. Formulas containing docosahexaenoic acid and arachidonic acid have been recently marketed to promote eye and brain development. So far, no randomized trials have shown any benefit, although no harm has been established.

Approximately 32 oz will meet 100% of the recommended daily allowance (RDA) for calories, vitamins, and minerals. These formula preparations are diluted to a standard 20 cal/oz and are typically whey-dominant protein preparations with vegetable oils and lactose. There are also multiple lactose-free preparations. Most standard formula preparations do not meet the RDA for fluoride, and exclusively formula-fed infants may require 0.25 mg/d of supplemental fluoride.

B. Soy-Based Formula Preparations

Indicated primarily for vegetarian mothers and lactose-intolerant, galactosemic, and cow's milk–allergic infants, soy-based formulas provide a protein-rich formula that contains more protein per deciliter than both breast milk and cow's milk formula preparations. Because the proteins are plant based, vitamin and mineral composition is increased to compensate for plant-based mineral antagonists while supplementing protein composition with the addition of methionine. Soy-based formulas tend to have a sweeter taste owing to a carbohydrate composition that includes sucrose and corn syrup. There is no proven benefit of soy-based formulas for milk protein allergy. Soy-based formulas should not be used for preterm infants because they cause less weight gain and increase the risk of osteopenia of prematurity. ProSobee, Isomil, and I-Soyalac are common soy-based preparations.

C. Casein Hydrolysate–Based Formula Preparations

This poor-tasting, expensive formula preparation is indicated principally for infants with either milk and soy protein allergies or intolerance. Other indications include complex gastrointestinal pathologies. This formula, which contains casein-based protein and glucose, is not recommended for prolonged use in preterm infants owing to inadequate vitamin and mineral composition and proteins that may be difficult to metabolize. Standard preparations provide 20–24 cal/oz.

D. Premature Infant Formula Preparations

Indicated for use in preterm infants of <1800 g birth weight and with 3 times the vitamin and mineral content of standard formula preparations, these formulations provide 20–24 cal/oz. Premature infant preparations are approximately 60% casein and 40% whey, with 1:1 concentrations of lactose and glucose as well as 1:1 concentrations of long- and medium-chain fatty acids. Commercially available preparations include Enfamil Premature with Iron, Similac Natural Care Breast Milk Fortifier, and Similac Special Care with Iron. Similac Neo-Care, designed for preterm infants weighing >1800 g at birth, provides 22 cal/oz in standard dilution.

▶ Human Milk Fortifiers for Preterm Infants

Human milk fortifiers (HMFs) are indicated for preterm infants <34 weeks' gestation or <1500 g birth weight once feeding has reached 75% full volume. HMFs are designed to supplement calories, protein, phosphorus, calcium, and other vitamins and minerals.

Enfamil-HMF is mixed to 24 cal/oz by adding one 3.8-g packet to 25 mL of breast milk, increasing the osmolality to >350 mOsm/L. Increased osmolality may enhance gastrointestinal irritability and affect tolerance. Practitioners may recommend a lower osmolality for the first 48 hours, beginning with one packet of Enfamil-HMF in 50 mL of breast milk, producing 22 cal/oz. The maximum caloric density from this HMF is 24 cal/oz. Practitioners may add emulsified fat blends to increase caloric needs.

Similac Natural Care is a liquid milk fortifier that is typically mixed in a 1:1 ratio with breast milk. Other alternatives may include feedings with breast milk and fortifier. The osmolality of Similac Natural Care is lower than that of Enfamil—280 mOsm/L. This liquid fortifier may be preferable, particularly for infants whose mothers have low milk production.

Other specially formulated formulas are available including antireflux and hypoallergenic formulas. Reflux usually does not require treatment unless there is poor weight gain. Antireflux formulas decrease emesis and regurgitation, but long-term benefit in terms of growth and development has not been established. Hypoallergenic formulas have shown to promote slightly greater weight gain in the first year of life. They have also shown improvement in atopic symptoms.

Websites

American Academy of Pediatrics: Policy on Breastfeeding. https://www.aap.org/en-us/advocacy-and-policy/aap-health-initiatives/Breastfeeding/Pages/default.aspx

Breastfeeding Basics: Resources for breastfeeding products and information. https://www.breastfeedingbasics.com/

La Leche League International. https://www.llli.org/

Medela: Breastfeeding resources. http://www.medela.us/

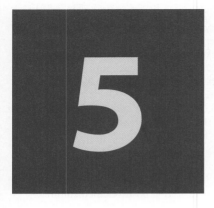

Common Acute Infections in Children

Stephanie B. Dewar, MD

Heather M. Bernard, MD

Infections are a major cause of illness in children. The widespread use of antibiotics and immunizations has greatly reduced morbidity and mortality from serious bacterial infections, but infections remain one of the most common types of problems encountered by physicians who care for children.

▼ GENERAL

FEVER WITHOUT A SOURCE

▶ General Considerations

Fever can be an indication of an infectious process in children of all ages. Other than fever, however, few young children display signs or symptoms indicative of an underlying disease. Even after a careful history and a complete physical examination, a portion of children will have no clear source of infection. Most of these children will have a viral infection; however, the physician must identify those children at risk for serious bacterial infection while minimizing the risks of laboratory evaluation, treatment with antibiotics, and hospitalization. A *serious bacterial infection* is defined as bacteremia, meningitis, urinary tract infection (UTI), pneumonia, bacterial enterocolitis, abscess, or cellulitis.

Children are generally divided into three groups for evaluation purposes: neonates (age ≤1 month), young infants (age <2–3 months), and young children (age 3 months to 3 years). There is no consensus statement or guideline available for physicians in the workup and management of febrile illnesses in children. Hamilton (2013) published a useful set of guidelines that are summarized in Table 5–1.

Neonates younger than 1 month of age can be the most challenging to diagnose because they are unable to localize infections. The rate of serious bacterial infection in nontoxic febrile neonates is between 11% and 25%. However, existing screening protocols lack the sensitivity and negative predictive value to identify infants at low risk for these infections. For this reason, it is generally accepted that all febrile infants younger than 1 month of age be admitted to the hospital, undergo a complete sepsis workup, and be treated with parenteral antibiotics pending the results of the workup. Most of these infants will be found to have a viral infection; however, some will have a serious bacterial infection such as UTI, in which *Escherichia coli* is the most common pathogen; bacteremia, with group B *Streptococcus, Enterobacter, Listeria, Streptococcus pneumoniae, E coli, Enterococcus,* or *Klebsiella* pathogens; or meningitis. The remainder may have nonbacterial gastroenteritis, aseptic meningitis, or bronchiolitis.

In evaluating infants age >1 month, those who are at low risk for a serious bacterial infection should be identified first. The criteria for low risk are being previously healthy, having no focal source of infection found on physical examination, and having a negative laboratory evaluation, defined as a white blood cell (WBC) count of 5000–15,000/mm^3, <1500 bands/mm^3, normal urinalysis, and, if diarrhea is present, <5 WBCs per high-power field in the stool. Chest radiography is included in some sets of criteria. Lumbar puncture should be performed if the patient is ill appearing, if neurologic signs are present, or if empiric antibiotics are to be used. Additional low-risk criteria are the appearance of being nontoxic and the likelihood of reliable follow-up (see Table 5–1). Low-risk, non–toxic-appearing infants may be treated as outpatients, with close follow-up. Empiric antibiotics are generally recommended but may be withheld if the infant can be followed closely. All toxic-appearing or non–low-risk infants should be hospitalized and treated with parenteral antibiotics.

Similar criteria may be used to evaluate children age 3 months to 3 years. The most common serious bacterial infections in this group are bacteremia and UTIs. UTIs are present in nearly 5% of febrile infants younger than 12 months of age, with an incidence slightly higher in girls and uncircumcised

Table 5–1. Evaluation and treatment of febrile children.

Infant age ≤1 month
Admit for evaluation (blood, urine, CSF, ± stool, ± CXR and treatment with empiric antibiotics (ampicillin and gentamicin or ampicillin and cefotaxime)

Infant age 2–3 months
Consider rapid influenza testing in flu season
Toxic or non–low risk: admit and evaluate as above and treat with ceftriaxone
Nontoxic, low risk:
  CBC and blood culture
  Urinalysis and urine culture
  Lumbar puncture if WBC >15,000/mm³ or <5000/mm³
  Consider empiric antibiotics
  Return for reevaluation within 24 hours
Low-risk criteria:
  Clinical
    Previously healthy, term infant with uncomplicated nursery stay
    Nontoxic appearance
    No focal bacterial infection on examination (except otitis media)
  Laboratory
    WBC count 5000–15,000/mm³, ≤1500 bands/mm³
    Negative Gram stain of unspun urine (preferred), or negative urine leukocyte esterase and nitrite, or ≤5 WBCs/HPF
    CSF ≤8 WBCs/mm³ and negative Gram stain

Child age 3 months to 3 years
Consider rapid influenza testing in flu season
Toxic: admit and evaluate as above and treat with ceftriaxone
Nontoxic:
  CBC and blood culture rarely recommended
  Urinalysis and urine culture obtained via catheterization or clean catch
  Lumbar puncture rarely recommended
  CXR if temperature >39°C, respiratory distress, tachypnea, rales, WBC count >20,000/mm³
Symptomatic treatment for fever
Consider empiric antibiotics
Return if fever persists for ≥48 hours or if condition deteriorates
Admit for inpatient monitoring if good outpatient follow-up not available

CBC, complete blood count; CSF, cerebrospinal fluid; CXR, chest x-ray; HPF, high-power field; IM, intramuscular; SaO₂, oxygen saturation; WBC, white blood cell.
Data from Hamilton JL, John SP: Evaluation of fever in infants and young children. *Am Fam Physician.* 2013 Feb 15;87(4):254–260.

boys and in those with higher temperatures. After 12 months of age, the prevalence of UTI is lower but should continue to be tested for in girls age ≤24 months. The rate of bacteremia is still significant and more likely if the temperature is ≥39°C (≥102.2°F). The most common organisms isolated are *S pneumoniae*, *Haemophilus influenzae* type b (Hib), and *Neisseria meningitidis*. The rate of infection with *H influenzae* and *S pneumoniae* has fallen since the introduction of the Hib and Prevnar vaccines. Occult pneumonia is rare in febrile children who have a normal WBC count and no signs

of lower respiratory infection, such as cough, tachypnea, rales, or rhonchi. As in younger infants, toxic-appearing or non–low-risk infants should be hospitalized and treated with parenteral antibiotics as the rate of serious bacterial infections in toxic-appearing children in this age group has been reported to be anywhere between 10% and 90% Low-risk, non–toxic-appearing children in this age group may be treated as outpatients. The use of empiric antibiotics pending culture results is left to the physician's discretion depending on the appearance of the child and availability for follow-up visit. There is general consensus that bacteremia is a risk factor for development of infectious complications, such as meningitis. However, pneumococcal bacteremia responds well to oral antibiotics, so these drugs can be used in children who appear well despite having positive blood cultures.

▶ **Clinical Findings**

A. Symptoms and Signs

Fever is defined as temperature of ≥38°C (≥100.4°F). Rectal measurement is the most accurate way to measure temperature. Teething is not a cause for elevated temperature. A history of any recent immunizations should be obtained in order to understand another possible cause for temperature elevation. A careful, complete physical examination is necessary to exclude focal signs of infection. The skin should be examined for exanthem, cellulitis, abscess, or petechiae. A petechial rash may herald a serious bacterial infection, most often caused by *N meningitidis*. Common childhood infections such as pharyngitis and otitis media should be sought, and a careful lung examination should be done to rule out pneumonia. The abdomen should be examined for signs of peritonitis or tenderness. A musculoskeletal examination should be done to rule out osteomyelitis or septic arthritis. The neurologic examination should be directed toward the level of consciousness and should search for focal neurologic deficits. Nuchal rigidity may be absent even in the presence of meningitis, especially in young infants. However, infants may demonstrate "paradoxical irritability," where they prefer to be left alone rather than held, as a subtle sign of meningeal irritation.

The most important clinical decision is which infants appear toxic and therefore need more aggressive evaluation and treatment. *Toxic* in the present context is defined as a picture consistent with the sepsis syndrome—lethargy, signs of poor perfusion, marked hypoventilation or hyperventilation, or cyanosis. *Lethargy* is defined as an impaired level of consciousness as manifested by poor or absent eye contact or by failure of the child to recognize parents or to interact with people or objects in the environment.

B. Laboratory Findings

The laboratory investigation includes WBC count and differential, urinalysis and urine culture, blood culture, lumbar puncture with routine analysis and culture, and chest x-ray if there are respiratory symptoms or an elevation of the WBC. If the child has diarrhea, stool cultures should be obtained.

▶ Treatment

All infants younger than 1 month of age should undergo complete sepsis evaluation and be treated in the hospital with intravenous (IV) antibiotics, either (1) ampicillin plus gentamicin or (2) ampicillin plus cefotaxime.

Ceftriaxone is an appropriate antibiotic for hospitalized older infants and children and for infants and children treated as outpatients as long as there is no evidence or concern for meningitis. In that case, the child should be admitted and vancomycin added to the therapy. In infants 2–3 months of age, a single intramuscular (IM) dose of ceftriaxone may be given. The child should be reevaluated in 24 hours and a second dose of ceftriaxone given. If blood cultures are found to be positive, the child should be admitted for further treatment. If the urine culture is positive and there is a persistent fever, the child should be admitted for treatment. If the child is afebrile and well, outpatient antibiotics may be used.

Table 5–1 presents guidelines that may be useful for investigating and treating febrile children.

Biondi E. Evaluation and management of febrile, well-appearing young infants. *Infect Dis Clin North Am.* 2015;29(3):575–585. [PMID: 26188607]

Hamilton J. Evaluation of fever in infants and young children. *Am Fam Physician.* 2013;87:254–260. [PMID: 23418797]

Huppler A. Performance of low-risk criteria in the evaluation of young infants with fever: review of the literature. *Pediatrics.* 2010;125(2):228–233. [PMID: 20083517]

INFLUENZA

ESSENTIALS OF DIAGNOSIS

▶ Nonspecific respiratory infection in infants and young children.

▶ In older children, respiratory symptoms: coryza, conjunctivitis, pharyngitis, dry cough.

▶ In older children, pronounced high fever, myalgia, headache, malaise.

▶ General Considerations

Influenza virus causes a respiratory infection of variable severity in children. Although influenza itself is a benign, self-limited disease, its sequelae, primarily pneumonia, can cause serious illness and occasionally death, especially in children age <2 years and with other medical conditions, including asthma.

▶ Pathogenesis

Influenza is caused by various influenza viruses. Types A and B cause epidemic illness, whereas type C produces sporadic cases of respiratory infections. Infection with influenza virus confers limited immunity that lasts several years, until the natural antigenic drift of the virus produces a pathogen that is genetically distinct enough to escape this protection. Because every virus is new for infants, the attack rate is highest in infants and young children, with 30–50% showing serologic evidence of infection in a normal year.

▶ Prevention

Annual influenza vaccination is the most effective way to prevent influenza and its complications. All people age >6 months should receive annual influenza vaccination. Children age 6 months to 8 years require two doses of flu vaccine the first season of vaccination, 1 month apart. Children age ≥9 years and those previously immunized need only receive one dose each year. The unit dose for children age 6–35 months is 0.25 mL. The unit dose for children age ≥36 months is 0.5 mL. The vaccine must be repeated annually. The vaccine should be given prior to the onset of influenza activity in the community and throughout the season. Physicians should begin offering the vaccine as soon as it is available. Parents of infants <6 months of age should be encouraged to have all members of the household vaccinated.

Chemoprophylaxis with an antiviral medication can reduce the risk of complications from influenza and should be initiated as early as possible for any patient with confirmed or suspected influenza who is hospitalized; has severe, complicated, or progressive illness; or is at high risk for complications, such as children age <2 years or those with chronic conditions, including asthma.

▶ Clinical Findings

A. Symptoms and Signs

Influenza in infants and young children causes a nonspecific respiratory infection often characterized by fever and cough. Occasionally the fever is high enough and the child toxic enough in appearance to prompt hospitalization and workup for sepsis. In older children and adolescents, the disease presents with the abrupt onset of respiratory symptoms, such as upper respiratory infection (URI) symptoms, conjunctivitis, pharyngitis, and dry cough. The features that distinguish influenza from the usual URI are high fever and pronounced myalgia, headache, and malaise. The acute symptoms typically last for 2–4 days, but the cough and malaise may persist for several days longer. Physical findings are nonspecific and include pharyngitis, conjunctivitis, cervical lymphadenopathy, and occasionally rales, wheezes, or rhonchi in the lungs.

B. Special Tests

Diagnosis of influenza is generally based on clinical criteria. The virus can be identified by nasopharyngeal swabs sent for rapid influenza diagnostic tests. These tests have high specificity (>90%) but low sensitivity (20–70%). Therefore, positive tests are generally reliable in a community when influenza activity is high and might be useful in deciding whether to institute antiviral therapy. Reverse transcription–polymerase chain reaction is the most accurate and sensitive test for detecting influenza viruses, but the time required for testing and the limited availability may limit its usefulness for medical management of individual patients.

▶ Complications

Otitis media and pneumonia are the most common complications from influenza in children. Up to 25% of children develop otitis media after a documented influenza infection. Influenza may cause a primary viral pneumonia, but the more serious pneumonic complications are caused by bacterial superinfection. Encephalopathy, transverse myelitis, myositis, myocarditis, pericarditis, and Reye syndrome, while rare, may also occur.

▶ Treatment

Antiviral treatment with a neuraminidase inhibitor (zanamivir or oseltamivir) is recommended for all persons with suspected or confirmed influenza who are at higher risk for complications because of age or underlying medical conditions. This would include children age <5 years, especially those <2 years old and those with underlying medical conditions, such as asthma, sickle cell disease, diabetes mellitus, cerebral palsy, epilepsy, or intellectual disability. The benefits of treatment are greater if initiated within 2 days of the onset of symptoms; however, anyone requiring hospitalization should be treated regardless of the length of symptoms. Oseltamivir can be used in children beginning at age 2 weeks at a dose of 3 mg/kg given twice daily up to age 1 year when dosing is based on age. Zanamivir can be used for children age ≥7 years. Zanamivir is administered via an inhaler device twice daily. Both are given as a 5-day course. Because of resistance in recent viral strains, amantadine and rimantadine are no longer recommended.

▶ Prognosis

Influenza is ordinarily a benign self-limited disease. Morbidity and mortality are related either to postinfluenza pneumonia or to exacerbation of underlying chronic illness caused by the virus.

Fiore AE, Fry A, Shay D, et al. Antiviral agents for the treatment and chemoprophylaxis of influenza: recommendations of the Advisory Committee on Immunization Practices (ACIP), 2011. *MMWR Morbid Mortal Wkly Rep.* 2011;60:1–25. [PMID: 21248682]

▼ EAR, NOSE, & THROAT INFECTIONS

OTITIS MEDIA

ESSENTIALS OF DIAGNOSIS

▶ Preexisting URI (93%).

▶ Fever (25%).

▶ Ear pain (depending on age).

▶ Bulging, immobile tympanic membrane that is dull gray, yellow, or red in color.

▶ Perforated tympanic membrane with purulent drainage (most diagnostic).

▶ General Considerations

Acute otitis media (AOM) is a common reason why children are prescribed antibiotics. Almost all children have had at least one episode of AOM by age 3 years. Although common, the number of visits for AOM has been decreasing in the United States. Much of this decrease is attributed to improved clinician understanding of AOM and the routine vaccination of children. Most of the advice on managing AOM presented here is applicable to children age >6 months who are otherwise healthy. Children with immune deficiencies, anatomic abnormalities, and ear-nose-throat surgeries may require more aggressive treatment.

▶ Pathogenesis

The middle ear is more prone to bacterial infection in children mainly because of the position and length of the eustachian tube. *S pneumoniae*, nontypeable *H influenzae*, and *Moraxella catarrhalis* are the most frequent bacterial pathogens, along with respiratory viruses. *S pneumoniae* is a frequent cause of recurrent or persistent otitis media.

▶ Prevention

Routine use of pneumococcal conjugate and influenza vaccines has decreased the incidence of AOM and the need for surgical treatment of AOM. Breastfeeding for at least 6 months also decreases the incidence of AOM in infants. Other modifiable risk factors include daycare attendance, tobacco exposure, air pollution exposure, pacifier use, and challenging living conditions.

Clinical Findings

A. Symptoms and Signs

Signs and symptoms must be used together to make an accurate diagnosis of AOM. Most patients have nonspecific antecedent upper respiratory symptoms. Onset of ear pain for <2 days is the most frequent specific symptom. Nonverbal children may hold, tug, or rub their affected ears. Caregivers may also note a purulent discharge from the ear. Frequent but less specific symptoms include fever, crying, and changes in behavior or sleep. When symptoms are present, mild bulging of the tympanic membrane (TM) or intense erythema of the TM confirms the diagnosis of AOM. Children with severe TM bulging or new otorrhea without otitis externa can be diagnosed with AOM on the basis of examination alone. Other signs that can indicate abnormal mobility or position of the TM include opacity, nonvisualization of the bony landmarks, and air/fluid levels. Clinicians should confirm the presence of a middle ear effusion through pneumatic otoscopy or tympanometry to finalize the diagnosis of AOM whenever possible.

Differential Diagnosis

The primary illness that may be confused with AOM is acute URI. Otitis externa can be distinguished from AOM by tenderness, redness, swelling, and exudates in the external auditory canal. More benign middle ear effusions that can occur after a previous AOM or from eustachian tube dysfunction from a URI or allergies should be distinguished from an episode of AOM by the lack of acute symptoms. These patients do not benefit from treatment with antibiotics.

Complications

Complications of otitis media fall into two main categories: suppurative and nonsuppurative. *Suppurative* complications may arise from direct extension of the infection into the surrounding bones or into the adjacent brain, such as mastoiditis, venous sinus thrombosis, and brain abscess. They may also arise from hematogenous spread of the bacteria from the middle ear, resulting in sepsis and meningitis. The most frequent suppurative complications are TM perforation or chronic suppurative AOM. In most children, TM perforation will resolve spontaneously in 3 months. *Nonsuppurative* complications are primarily those that arise from middle ear effusion and inflammation and scarring of the structures of the middle ear. This includes hearing loss, balance problems, and cholesteatoma formation.

Treatment

All children with AOM should be assessed for pain. The most frequently used medications are oral acetaminophen and ibuprofen. They have the advantage of being readily available, effective, and easy to administer. Topical anesthetics can work as well in children age >5 years. Caregivers should be instructed on the appropriate dosing of analgesics to maximize effectiveness and minimize side effects.

Antibiotic treatment for AOM is effective for reducing pain and hastening recovery. Overprescription of antibiotic therapy can have negative consequences for the patient and the population. It is important that antibiotic treatment be targeted for those patients who will benefit the most. Children age >6 months with severe signs of AOM or severe symptoms for at least 48 hours or temperature >39°C (102°F) should be prescribed antibiotics. Children younger than 24 months with bilateral AOM and less severe signs and symptoms should receive antibiotics. Unilateral AOM in children age 6–24 months without severe signs and symptoms can initially be treated with antibiotics or be observed. When children are older than 24 months and have nonsevere AOM, they also can be prescribed antibiotics or be observed. Children who are observed should have timely follow-up and administration of antibiotics if they do not improve or worsen in 48–72 hours. The decision surrounding AOM treatment should be made with the child's caregiver.

The choice of initial antibiotic therapy for most patients is amoxicillin dosed at 80–90 mg/kg daily. For penicillin-allergic children, most second- and third-generation cephalosporins have little cross-reactivity. Cefdinir, cefuroxime, and cefpodoxime are preferred unless there is a documented severe reaction. Macrolides or clindamycin can be used when amoxicillin and cephalosporins are not preferred, but they provide inferior antimicrobial coverage. The duration of therapy should be 10 days for children age <2 years or those with severe AOM. A 7-day course is sufficient for other patients.

Topical antibiotic treatment can be used in AOM with perforation. Quinolones have been shown to be effective. IM or IV ceftriaxone once daily can be used, but the optimal dosing is not known. One to three doses are likely to be effective. Children who have AOM and purulent conjunctivitis, have previously received amoxicillin in the past 30 days, or have failed treatment with amoxicillin before have a greater chance of failure with amoxicillin. They should be treated with amoxicillin-clavulanate. Caregivers of children with AOM who receive antibiotics should be instructed to report if the patient fails to improve in 48–72 hours. These children should be reassessed and considered for a change in therapy.

Prophylactic antibiotics are no longer recommended for reducing recurrent episodes of AOM. Tympanostomy can be useful for children with recurrent AOM. *Recurrent* AOM is defined as three episodes in 3 months or four episodes in 6 months with the most recent episode in the latest 6 months. Surgery has been shown to be effective in reducing episodes of AOM and improving quality of life.

Prognosis

In general, children with otitis media recover uneventfully. Middle ear effusions may persist for ≤3 months.

Granath A. Recurrent acute otitis media: what are the options for treatment and prevention? *Curr Otorhinolaryngol Rep.* 2017;5(2):93–100. [PMID: 28616364]

Lieberthal A, Carroll AE, Chonmaitree T, et al. The diagnosis and management of acute otitis media. *Pediatrics.* 2013;131(3): 2012–3488. [PMID: 23439909]

Pettinger TK, Force RW. Tubes for otitis media do not improve developmental outcomes. *J Fam Pract.* 2003;52:939–940. [PMID: 14653978]

BACTERIAL PHARYNGITIS

Sore throat is a common problem in pediatrics, leading to millions of physician office visits each year. The most important diagnosis to make is infection with group A β-hemolytic streptococci (GABHS; or group A *Streptococcus* [GAS]), which is responsible for approximately 25% of cases of pharyngitis. Antibiotic treatment has only a modest effect on the course of the disease, but treatment with antibiotics reduces the risk of rheumatic fever.

Many viruses cause the majority of cases of pharyngitis, including some cases of exudative pharyngitis. Adenoviruses can cause pharyngoconjunctival fever, with exudative pharyngitis and conjunctivitis. Herpesviruses and coxsackie viruses can cause ulcerative stomatitis and pharyngitis. Most viruses, however, cause signs and symptoms that overlap with those of GAS.

Infectious mononucleosis can cause pharyngitis and is described in detail later. Rarely, *Neisseria gonorrhoeae* can cause acute pharyngitis in children and should be considered in sexually active teenagers and abused children. Group C and G *Streptococcus* can also cause pharyngitis. This can often be epidemic and foodborne.

Group A Streptococcal Infection

ESSENTIALS OF DIAGNOSIS

▶ Moderate to severe tonsillar swelling often with exudates.

▶ Moderate to severe tender anterior cervical lymphadenopathy.

▶ Scarlatiniform rash (depending on the strain of bacteria).

▶ Absence of moderate to severe viral symptoms (cough, nasal congestion).

General Considerations

Approximately 20–30% of all cases of sore throat in children are due to GAS infection. The infection is uncommon in children age <3 years unless there is close contact with a contagious person. It occurs most often from November to May in temperate climates.

Clinical Findings

A. Symptoms and Signs

Clinical symptoms and signs overlap those of viral pharyngitides and URIs. The Centor criteria (C – cough absent, E – exudate, N – nodes, T – temperature (fever), OR – young OR old modifier) have been validated for adults but not for children. Attia and colleagues (1999) proposed a predictive model for GAS after examining a large number of signs and symptoms. The findings most highly correlated with GABHS are (1) moderate to severe tonsillar swelling, (2) moderate to severe tender anterior cervical lymphadenopathy, (3) scarlatiniform rash, and (4) the absence of moderate to severe coryza. If conditions 1 through 4 are present, the likelihood of GAS is 95%. In the absence of conditions 1 through 3 but in the presence of moderate to severe coryza, the likelihood of GABHS is <15%. When conditions 1 through 3 are present, the probability of GAS is ~65%

B. Laboratory Findings

A positive throat culture is the standard test to confirm GAS pharyngitis but may take 24–48 hours for a positive test. Rapid antigen detection tests (RADTs) and throat culture should be used in the ambulatory setting to complement clinical evaluation. Positive RADTs confirm the presence of GAS. Negative RADTs should be confirmed by throat culture because of the higher false-negative rates with this test. Another complicating factor is the inability of either rapid antigen testing or culture to distinguish between a true streptococcal infection and a viral infection in a child who is an otherwise asymptomatic GAS carrier. Carrier rates among asymptomatic children may be as high as 20%, depending on the age of the child and the season of the year.

Complications

Complications of GAS fall into two main categories: nonsuppurative and suppurative. The nonsuppurative complications are rheumatic fever and poststreptococcal glomerulonephritis.

Acute rheumatic fever follows about 3% of cases of untreated GABHS. The cause is immunologic and still not fully understood. There is great geographic variability in the incidence of this disease. The risk of rheumatic fever can be reduced by treatment of GAS, even if treatment is delayed for ≤9 days, but a full 10 days of treatment are required.

Poststreptococcal glomerulonephritis is caused by a poorly understood antigen-antibody reaction. Unlike rheumatic fever, the risk of glomerulonephritis is not reduced by treatment of GAS. Hematuria following URIs should prompt further investigation.

The major suppurative complications are peritonsillar abscess (see later), cervical lymphadenitis, and mastoiditis.

Treatment

Treatment of acute GAS pharyngitis with antibiotics may expedite resolution of symptoms and prevent complications as well as prevent transmission. Only confirmed cases of GAS pharyngitis should be treated with antibiotics to avoid drug side effects and prevent the development of antibiotic-resistant strains of bacteria. Penicillin and amoxicillin are the strongly preferred treatments. Narrow-spectrum cephalosporins, clindamycin, and macrolides can be used as alternative medications when indicated by drug intolerance or allergy. All antibiotics should be dosed for 10 days, except azithromycin, which has a 5-day course of treatment.

The painful throat symptoms of pharyngitis can be lessened by local treatment with topical anesthetics or warm saline rinses in older children. Treatment with acetaminophen or ibuprofen may reduce systemic symptoms such as fever and may be used for symptoms in younger children.

A test for cure is not recommended for patients who respond to treatment. Some studies show lower than expected rates of GAS eradication even after clinical response and high asymptomatic carrier rates. At present, these conditions are not considered to present enough risk to warrant the expense and risk of GAS eradication except in rare epidemic outbreaks of nonsuppurative complications. Asymptomatic household or school contacts of infected children should not be tested or empirically treated. Children should not return to school or daycare until they have been treated with antibiotics for at least 24 hours and their symptoms are controlled.

Prognosis

Streptococcal pharyngitis is ordinarily a benign, self-limited disease. Morbidity and mortality are related primarily to the previously mentioned complications. Antibiotic treatment can minimize many but not all of these.

Attia M, Zaoutis T, Eppes S, et al. Multivariate predictive models for group A beta-hemolytic streptococcal pharyngitis in children. *Acad Emerg Med.* 1999;6:8–13. [PMID: 9928970]

Centers for Disease Control and Prevention. *CDC Academic Detailing Sheet.* Bethesda, MD: Centers for Disease Control and Prevention; 2006.

Pichichero ME. Pathogen shifts and changing cure rates for otitis media and tonsillopharyngitis. *Clin Pediatr.* 2006;45:493–502. [PMID: 16893853]

Shulman S, Bisno AL, Clegg HW, et al. Clinical practice guideline for the diagnosis and management of group A streptococcal pharyngitis: 2012 update. Infectious Disease Society of America. *Clin Infect Dis.* 2012;55(10):1279–1282. [PMID: 23091044]

INFECTIOUS MONONUCLEOSIS

ESSENTIALS OF DIAGNOSIS

▶ Fever.
▶ Pharyngitis.
▶ Generalized lymphadenopathy.

General Considerations

Infectious mononucleosis is a clinical syndrome often caused by Epstein-Barr virus (EBV). Although ordinarily a benign illness, it has several important, if unusual, complications.

Pathogenesis

Although EBV is by far the most common cause of mononucleosis, 5–10% of mononucleosis-like illnesses are caused by cytomegalovirus (CMV), *Toxoplasma gondii,* or other viruses, including human immunodeficiency virus (HIV). EBV infects 95% of the world's population. It is transmitted in oral secretions. The incubation period is 30–50 days. Viral shedding is highest for 1 year after the acute infection, but infection is lifelong. Most infants and young children have unapparent infections, or infections that are indistinguishable from other childhood respiratory infections. In developed countries, about one-third of infections occur in adolescence or early adulthood, and of those infected, about one-half develop clinically apparent disease. Infection occurs earlier in other countries but is rare before the age of 1 year.

The infection begins in the cells of the oral cavity and then spreads to adjacent salivary glands and lymphoid tissue. Eventually the virus infects the entire reticuloendothelial system, including the liver and spleen.

Prevention

Because the virus is ubiquitous and is shed intermittently by many adults, there is no effective prevention for this illness. No vaccine is presently available.

Clinical Findings

A. Symptoms and Signs

After the incubation period, there is a 1- to 2-week prodromal period of nonspecific respiratory symptoms, including fever and sore throat. Typical symptoms include fever, sore throat, myalgia, headache, nausea, and abdominal pain.

Physical findings include pharyngitis, often with exudative tonsillitis and palatal petechiae similar to those of streptococcal pharyngitis. Lymphadenopathy is seen in 90% of cases, most often in the anterior and posterior cervical chains and less often in the axillary and inguinal chains. Epitrochlear adenopathy may also be present. Splenomegaly is found in ~50% of cases and hepatomegaly in 10–25%. Symptomatic hepatitis, with or without jaundice, may occur but is unusual. Various rashes, most often maculopapular, are seen in less than half of patients, but nearly all patients develop a rash if they are given ampicillin or amoxicillin.

B. Laboratory Findings

At the onset of the illness, the WBC count is usually elevated to 12,000–25,000/mm³; 50–70% of these cells are lymphocytes, and 20–40% are atypical lymphocytes. Although 50–80% of patients have elevated hepatic transaminases, jaundice occurs in only ~5%.

The most commonly performed diagnostic test is a rapid heterophile antibody test. The diagnosis may be ambiguous because this test is 25% negative during the first week of symptoms and ≤10% negative in the second week of symptoms. In children age <12 years, heterophile antibody testing is positive in only 25–50% of infected patients. The test may remain positive for 1 year or more after acute infection. A positive test in the presence of typical clinical symptoms is highly sensitive and specific. Heterophile tests are usually negative when viruses other than EBV are causing symptoms. In the early days of the infection, looking for atypical lymphocytes in a complete blood count may be a reasonable approach. Definitive diagnosis of EBV infection may require testing for IgM and IgG levels. These levels change over time as evidenced in Figure 5–1. Testing for other causes of infectious mononucleosis is usually performed only when there is identified specific risk of exposure or transmission to vulnerable populations such as pregnant women.

C. Imaging Studies

No imaging studies are routinely useful in this illness. Ultrasound shows splenomegaly more accurately than physical examination but is usually performed only to assess the risk of splenic rupture in patients who are active in sports.

▶ Differential Diagnosis

Streptococcal pharyngitis is the chief illness in the differential diagnosis. Strep testing can identify asymptomatic carriers that complicate the diagnosis. Children with mononucleosis generally have more widespread lymphadenopathy than those with GAS pharyngitis. Symptoms consistent with infectious mononucleosis can also occur with HIV, CMV, human herpesvirus 6, and toxoplasmosis.

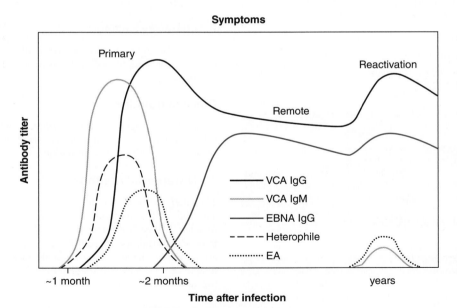

▲ **Figure 5–1.** Levels of antibodies specific to Epstein-Barr virus (EBV) during infectious mononucleosis and convalescence. EBNA, EBV nuclear antigen; IgG, immunoglobulin G; IgM, immunoglobulin M; VCA, viral capsid antigens. (Reproduced with permission from Gulley ML, Tang W: Laboratory assays for Epstein-Barr virus-related disease. *J Mol Diagn.* 2008 Jul;10(4):279–292.)

Complications

Mononucleosis is normally a benign illness. The most serious complication is spontaneous splenic rupture. This occurs in 0.5–1% of patients, almost always during the first 3 weeks of the illness. The risk of splenic rupture is elevated with trauma, and all patients with this illness should avoid contact sports for at least 3 weeks. Clinical symptoms should be resolved, and the athlete should feel well enough to participate before returning to play. Those with documented splenomegaly should not resume athletic activity until resolution has been confirmed by ultrasound.

Other complications are unusual and include rare cases of airway obstruction (1%), hepatitis (rare), and a variety of neurologic complications (1–5%), including meningitis, encephalitis, and cranial, autonomic, or peripheral neuritis. Hemolytic anemia may occur in ~3% of cases. Aplastic anemia is rare. Mild neutropenia and thrombocytopenia are common early in the disease, but severe cytopenias are rare.

Treatment

Treatment is symptomatic and supportive with fluids and analgesics. Systemic corticosteroids can be used to lessen symptom severity and hasten recovery in more serious cases. Upper airway obstruction and severe hematologic complications generally warrant the use of steroids. A commonly recommended regimen is a daily dose of prednisone 1–2 mg/kg (≤60 mg) for 1 week. Antiviral medications have not shown a consistent benefit.

Prognosis

Symptoms typically last 2–4 weeks. Fatigue may be the last symptom to resolve. Most patients resume normal activities within 2 months.

Bell AT, Fortune B. What test is the best for diagnosing infectious mononucleosis? *J Fam Pract.* 2006;55:799–800. [PMID: 16948964]

Luzuriaga K, Sullivan JL. Infectious mononucleosis. *N Engl J Med.* 2010;362:1993–2000. [PMID: 20505178]

Putakian M, O'Connor FG, Stricker P, et al. Mononucleosis and athletic participation: an evidence-based review. *Clin J Sports Med.* 2008;18:309–315. [PMID: 18614881]

PERITONSILLAR ABSCESS

 ESSENTIALS OF DIAGNOSIS

► Severe sore throat.

► Odynophagia.

► High fever.

► Unilateral pharyngeal swelling with deviation of the uvula.

General Considerations

Peritonsillar abscess is the most common deep-space head and neck infection in children, accounting for almost half of these infections. It is most commonly caused by infection with GAS. The exact cause is unknown, but it is assumed that the infection usually spreads from the tonsil itself into the deep spaces behind the tonsil, where it produces a collection of pus. It can occur in children of all ages, as well as in adults, but it affects older children and adolescents more than younger children. It is usually unilateral.

Clinical Findings

A. Symptoms and Signs

Most children with peritonsillar abscess have had symptoms of pharyngitis for 1–7 days before presenting with symptoms related to the abscess. Many of these children have been treated with antibiotics for pharyngitis before developing the abscess. The most common symptoms are severe throat or neck pain, painful swallowing, high fever, and poor oral intake. The most common physical signs are cervical adenopathy, uvular deviation, and muffled voice with trismus. There is usually unilateral tense swelling of the anterior tonsillar pillar on the affected side. Symptoms are less clear and the examination more difficult in younger children, and young children who cannot cooperate may have to be examined under sedation.

B. Laboratory Findings

The WBC count is usually elevated, with a left shift. Throat cultures for streptococci are positive in only ~16% of specimens.

C. Imaging Studies

Computed tomography and ultrasound studies of the neck often show the abscess, but the diagnosis is generally made by history and physical examination.

Differential Diagnosis

The chief disease in the differential diagnosis is epiglottitis. This infection is uncommon in an era of widespread immunization against *H influenzae* type b, but the clinical picture may be identical in young children. Examination in the operating room under sedation may be necessary to establish the diagnosis, especially if the patient manifests tripoding, drooling, and stridor.

Complications

Prompt treatment is necessary, because untreated abscesses may spread into other deep spaces in the head and neck. The airway may be compromised by swelling, especially in younger children. If the abscess ruptures into the throat, aspiration of pus may cause pneumonia.

Treatment

The initial treatment consists of IV antibiotics effective against streptococci and staphylococci, such as ampicillin/sulbactam or clindamycin. The abscess may subsequently require drainage, either by incision or by needle aspiration. This is generally done by an otolaryngologist or a surgeon familiar with the anatomy of the neck. Tonsillectomy may subsequently be necessary. Once cultures of the pus indicate the causative organism, treatment may be focused according to its antibiotic sensitivities. Systemic corticosteroids may speed recovery, but the evidence is limited to children age >12 years.

Prognosis

Children generally recover uneventfully once appropriate treatment has begun, but they may be at increased risk for a second infection.

Galioto N. Peritonsillar abscess. *Am Fam Physician*. 2008;77(2): 199–202. [PMID: 18246890]

Ozbek C, Aygenc E, Tuna EU, et al. Use of steroids in the treatment of peritonsillar abscess. *J Laryngol Otol*. 2004;118:439. [PMID: 15285862]

Schraff S, McGinn JD, Derkay CS. Peritonsillar abscess in children: a 10-year review of diagnosis and management. *Int J Pediatr Otorhinolaryngol*. 2001;57:213–218. [PMID: 11223453]

▼ INFECTIONS OF THE LOWER RESPIRATORY TRACT

CROUP (ACUTE LARYNGOTRACHEITIS)

ESSENTIALS OF DIAGNOSIS

- ▶ URI prodrome.
- ▶ Barking cough.
- ▶ Symptoms worst on the first or second day, with gradual resolution.
- ▶ Lungs clear.
- ▶ Inspiratory stridor, respiratory distress, cyanosis in severe cases.

General Considerations

Croup (laryngotracheitis and spasmodic croup) is an illness of infants and children age <6 years. It is most common between 7 and 36 months of age, and slightly more common in boys than in girls. About 5% of children will have croup during their second year of life.

Pathogenesis

Croup is caused by an infection of the upper airways—the larynx, trachea, and the upper levels of the bronchial tree. Obstruction of these airways caused by edema produces most of the classic symptoms of the disease. Nearly all cases of croup are caused by viruses; parainfluenza viruses are the most common agents, along with adenovirus, respiratory syncytial virus (RSV), and (rarely) *Mycoplasma pneumoniae*.

Clinical Findings

A. Symptoms and Signs

Most children with croup present after several days of prodromal URI symptoms, which are followed by the rapid onset of a barking, "seal-like" cough, and inspiratory stridor. This is somewhat frightening to both patients and parents; however, respiratory distress is generally only mild to moderate. The symptoms are generally worst on the first or second day, peak at night, and gradually resolve over the next several days. If the symptoms progress beyond this point, the child may develop worsening respiratory distress, more pronounced and more constant stridor, and cyanosis.

The lungs are usually clear. The degree of subcostal and intercostal retractions, the degree of stridor, and the presence of cyanosis are important clues to the severity of the illness. If the child is cyanotic and in respiratory distress, manipulation of the pharynx (eg, attempts to examine the pharynx using a tongue depressor) may trigger respiratory arrest. This maneuver should therefore be avoided unless the clinician is in a position to manage the child's airway by endotracheal intubation only with an experienced team.

B. Laboratory Findings

Laboratory studies are rarely useful in the evaluation of routine croup. The WBC count is usually normal or slightly elevated; however, counts of >15,000/mm^3 may be seen. The blood oxygen saturation may be normal or decreased, depending on the severity of the disease.

C. Imaging Studies

The chest x-ray is usually normal, but anteroposterior soft tissue x-rays of the neck may show subglottic narrowing, creating the classic "steeple" sign.

Differential Diagnosis

Croup must be differentiated from other respiratory illnesses that cause obstruction in the region of the larynx. Epiglottitis generally lacks the URI prodrome and the croupy cough. The child prefers to sit forward, may be drooling and reluctant to lie down, and may have a high fever. Lateral neck film will demonstrate a swollen epiglottis. Children who have both foreign body and angioneurotic edema have onset of symptoms suddenly and lack fever or other signs of infection. Children with bacterial tracheitis have persistent worsening of symptoms and signs of upper airway obstruction despite treatment. There may be evidence of soft densities on lateral neck radiograph consistent with purulent exudate within the trachea.

Complications

Approximately 15% of children with croup experience complications. These are usually related to extension of the infection to other parts of the respiratory tract, such as otitis media or viral pneumonia. Bacterial pneumonia is unusual, but bacterial tracheitis may occur. Children with severe croup may develop complications of hypoxemia, if this is not adequately treated. Death is unusual and is generally due to laryngeal obstruction.

Treatment

Croup scoring systems may be useful for research purposes, but they do not present validated criteria for determining the best course of treatment for an individual child. High fever, toxic appearance, worsening stridor, respiratory distress, cyanosis or pallor, hypoxia, and restlessness or lethargy are all symptoms of more severe disease and should prompt the physician to admit the child for inpatient treatment.

Many children with croup may be treated at home. The mainstay of treatment has long been held to be cool, moist air, although research has not confirmed the effectiveness of this treatment. Corticosteroids have been shown to decrease the croup score and the time spent in emergency departments and hospitals. A single IM dose of dexamethasone, at 0.6 mg/kg, may be effective in reducing the severity of moderate to severe croup in patients treated at home. Because the onset of action for dexamethasone is ~6 hours, a single dose of racemic epinephrine may be given before the child is sent home. The physician might also consider an oral course of steroids for home treatment, but this has not been shown to be as effective as the IM route.

Patients who require hospitalization often receive supplemental oxygen in order to correct hypoxemia. Racemic epinephrine is the mainstay of treatment for patients with significant respiratory distress. Numerous studies have confirmed its effectiveness. The drug is administered via nebulizer and face mask. Its duration of action is 1–2 hours. Although racemic epinephrine is the drug most commonly used, L-epinephrine is equally effective, less expensive, and more widely available. Numerous studies have shown systemic dexamethasone to be effective in reducing both the severity and duration of the disease and the need for intubation. Because of its long action, the drug can be given as a single dose, which remains effective for the remainder of the course of the disease. The dose is 0.6 mg/kg IM, and it should be given as early as possible in the course of hospitalization. Nebulized steroids and oral dexamethasone are more effective than placebo but less effective than IM dexamethasone. Children hospitalized for treatment of croup should be observed carefully for any signs of respiratory distress. Intubation and mechanical ventilation are necessary in a small percentage of children with this disease.

Prognosis

The natural history of croup is that recurrences are common. However, as children grow, the airways grow larger and are less affected by edema, and symptoms tend to become less severe over time.

Cherry J. Croup. *N Engl J Med.* 2008;358:384–391. [PMID: 18216359]

BRONCHIOLITIS

 ESSENTIALS OF DIAGNOSIS

▶ URI symptoms.

▶ Wheezing.

▶ Cough.

▶ Dyspnea.

▶ Tachypnea.

General Considerations

Bronchiolitis is a disorder of the lower respiratory tract that occurs most often in infants and young children. It is seen most commonly in the first 2 years of life, with more than one-third of children affected. The peak age is ~6 months. It is the leading cause of infant hospitalization and is most commonly caused by RSV. Older children and adults may contract the same infection, but because they have larger airways, they do not experience the same degree of airway obstruction. An older sibling or a parent is often the source of the infant's infection.

Pathogenesis

Bronchiolitis is generally the result of a viral etiology. RSV causes more than half of cases; others are caused by parainfluenza virus, influenza, and human metapneumovirus. Pathologically, edema and accumulated cellular debris cause obstruction of small airways. This obstruction causes a ventilation-perfusion mismatch with wasted perfusion, a right-to-left shunt, and hypoxemia early in the course of the disease.

Prevention

Palivizumab is available in the United States for prevention of RSV disease in high-risk infants. The drug has been shown to decrease hospitalization rates among high-risk infants with and without chronic lung disease. The decision to use this drug is based on the age of the child at the onset of RSV season and the child's medical history. The American Academy of Pediatrics (AAP) recommends prophylaxis with palivizumab for the following groups:

- Children age <2 years with chronic lung disease who have required medical treatment in the preceding 6 months
- Infants with cyanotic or complicated congenital heart disease who are receiving medication to control congestive heart failure and will require surgery and those with moderate to severe pulmonary hypertension
- Infants who were born before 29 weeks' gestation who are younger than 12 months of age

Palivizumab is given at a dose of 15 mg/kg IM once every 30 days during the local RSV season, in five doses or less.

Clinical Findings

A. Symptoms and Signs

Bronchiolitis is an acute infectious illness that begins with URI symptoms. It may progress to respiratory distress, wheezing, cough, and dyspnea. The infant may be irritable and feed poorly, but there are rarely any other systemic symptoms. The temperature may be elevated or below normal.

Physical examination shows the child to be tachypneic, with a respiratory rate as high as 60–80 breaths per minute, and often in severe respiratory distress. Nasal flaring, retractions, and the use of accessory muscles of respiration may be evident. Examination of the lungs often shows a prolonged expiratory phase with diffuse wheezes. Diffuse fine inspiratory crackles may be present. The lungs are often hyperinflated with shallow respirations, and breath sounds may be nearly inaudible if the obstruction is severe.

B. Laboratory Findings

Pulse oximetry may reveal hypoxemia and aid in the decision concerning need for hospitalization. A nasopharyngeal swab may be done for RSV rapid viral antigen testing; however, results may have little impact on management.

C. Imaging Studies

The use of chest radiography is not routinely recommended but may show signs of hyperinflation with scattered areas of consolidation. These may represent postobstructive atelectasis or inflammation of alveoli. It may not be possible to exclude early bacterial pneumonia solely on the basis of radiographic findings.

Differential Diagnosis

The differential diagnosis for the wheezing infant includes viral bronchiolitis along with other pulmonary infections (eg, pneumonia, chlamydia, tuberculosis), laryngotracheomalacia, foreign body, gastroesophageal reflux, congestive heart failure, vascular ring, allergic reaction, cystic fibrosis, mediastinal mass, bronchogenic cyst, and tracheoesophageal fistula.

Complications

Complications such as bacterial pneumonia and respiratory failure are more common and more severe in children with underlying cardiac or pulmonary disease. Fewer than 400 deaths occur annually, but deaths are highest in infants age <6 months and in those who are premature or have underlying cardiopulmonary disease or immunodeficiency.

Treatment

The treatment of bronchiolitis is primarily supportive, with the focus on providing adequate hydration and oxygenation while the patient recovers from the illness. This may require hospitalization. Some patients may benefit from routine suctioning of the nasopharynx, especially prior to attempting to take oral feeds. Bronchodilators such as albuterol or racemic epinephrine may transiently improve the clinical status of patients with bronchiolitis but have not been shown to decrease the need for hospitalization, shorten the length of hospitalization, or decrease the time to illness resolution. Their use is not routinely recommended, but they may be used only after proven benefit in a trial of therapy in each patient. Corticosteroids and leukotriene receptor antagonists have not been shown to decrease the length of illness or need for hospitalization and thus are not routinely recommended. Nebulized hypertonic saline may reduce the length of hospitalization but is not currently routinely recommended. Patients with evidence of lobar pneumonia on chest radiograph may benefit from a course of antibiotics. Ribavirin is no longer recommended for children with bronchiolitis.

Prognosis

There appears to be a relationship between bronchiolitis and reactive airway disease, although the exact connection is unclear. Some studies have shown an increased incidence of airway hyperreactivity that may persist for years in children who have had bronchiolitis.

Kimberlin DW, ed. *Red Book: 2018-2021 Report of the Committee on the Infectious Diseases*, 31st ed. Elk Grove Village, IL: American Academy of Pediatrics; 2018:688–691.

Seehusen DA. Effectiveness of bronchodilators for bronchiolitis treatment. *Am Fam Physician*. 2011;83(9):1045–1047. [PMID: 21534515]

Zorc JJ, Hall CB. Bronchiolitis: recent evidence on diagnosis and management. *Pediatrics.* 2010;125(2):342–349. [PMID: 20100768]

PERTUSSIS

ESSENTIALS OF DIAGNOSIS

▶ URI symptoms.

▶ Paroxysms of coughing, often with "whoops" on inspiration.

▶ Posttussive emesis

▶ Dyspnea.

▶ Seizures.

▶ General Considerations

Pertussis is a bacterial infection that affects airways lined with ciliated epithelium. The disease is most common in unimmunized infants and in adults, because immunity wanes 5–10 years after the last immunization. Pertussis causes serious disease in children and mild or asymptomatic disease in adults. Infants age <6 months have greater morbidity than older children, and those age <2 months have the highest rates of pertussis-related hospitalization, pneumonia, seizures, encephalopathy, and death. Pertussis is highly contagious, with attack rates as high as 100% in susceptible individuals exposed at close range.

▶ Pathogenesis

The most common cause of pertussis is *Bordetella pertussis,* but adenoviruses, *Bordetella parapertussis, Mycoplasma pneumoniae, Chlamydia trachomatis,* and RSV can cause a similar disease. The organisms attack ciliated epithelium, producing toxins and resulting in inflammation and necrosis of the walls of small airways. This leads to plugging of airways, bronchopneumonia, and hypoxemia.

▶ Prevention

The key to prevention of pertussis is immunization. Unfortunately, immunization does not confer complete protection. A total of 17,972 cases of pertussis were still reported in 2016. Up to 80% of immunized household contacts of symptomatic cases acquire infection as a result of waning immunity. All infants and toddlers should be routinely immunized as previously recommended by the Centers for Disease Control and Prevention. In addition, since 2006, a vaccine combining acellular pertussis vaccine with tetanus and diphtheria toxoids (Tdap) has been available for use in children age >7 years for all subsequent doses of vaccine, including the recommended adolescent booster dose given at age ≥11 years. Tdap is also recommended for all adults to replace the next booster dose of tetanus and diphtheria vaccine and for adults (including those who are age 65 years or older) who have close contact with infants <12 months of age.

▶ Clinical Findings

A. Symptoms and Signs

Children age <2 years show the most typical symptoms of the disease, paroxysms of coughing, inspiratory "whoops" (which give the disease its more common name of whooping cough), vomiting induced by coughing, and dyspnea lasting <1 month. Some will have seizures. Children age >2 years have lower incidences of all these symptoms and a shorter duration of disease, whereas adults often have atypical symptoms. High fever is unusual in all ages.

Pertussis has an incubation period lasting 7–10 days with a range of 5–21 days. The disease progresses through the following three stages:

1. The *catarrhal stage,* which is characterized by symptoms typical of a common cold.

2. The *paroxysmal stage,* which lasts 2–4 weeks, occasionally longer. During this stage, episodes of coughing increase in severity and number. The typical paroxysm is 5–10 hard coughs in a single expiration, followed by the classic whoop as the patient inspires. Young infants seldom manifest the whoop. Coughing to the point of vomiting is common. Fever is absent or minimal.

3. During the *convalescent stage,* the paroxysms gradually decrease in frequency and number. The patient may experience a cough for several months after the disease has otherwise resolved.

Pertussis can usually be diagnosed in the paroxysmal stage, but it requires a certain level of suspicion. A cough lasting >2 weeks and associated with posttussive vomiting should prompt the physician to consider the diagnosis.

B. Laboratory Findings

A high WBC count (20,000–50,000/mm³) with an absolute lymphocytosis is suggestive of pertussis in infants and young children but is often absent in adolescents and adults.

Culture is considered the gold standard for diagnosis of pertussis. The organism can be obtained for culture by a nasopharyngeal swab but may be difficult to grow secondary to its fastidious nature. False negatives may occur in a previously immunized person, if antimicrobial therapy has been started, if >3 weeks has elapsed since the onset of the cough, or if the specimen is not handled appropriately.

Polymerase chain reaction assays on nasopharyngeal samples are increasingly available for detection of pertussis.

These have improved sensitivity and quicker turnaround time than cultures.

Convalescent serology may be helpful to confirm the diagnosis, especially later in the illness. An elevated IgG antibody to pertussis toxin after 2 weeks of the onset of cough is suggestive of recent B pertussis infection.

Direct fluorescent antibody staining is no longer recommended.

Differential Diagnosis

Any illness that causes cough should be considered in the differential diagnosis. Older children and children who have been immunized against the disease may have milder, atypical symptoms, and the only clue to the disease may be the long duration of symptoms.

Complications

Complications of pertussis among infants include pneumonia, seizures, encephalopathy, hernia, subdural bleeding, conjunctival bleeding, and death. A mortality rate of approximately 1% is seen in infants age <2 months, and a rate of 0.5% is seen in those age 2–11 months. Complications among adolescents and adults include syncope, sleep disturbances, incontinence, rib fractures, and pneumonia. Adults have increased complications with increasing age.

Treatment

Treatment is primarily supportive, involving hydration, pulmonary toilet, and oxygen. Young infants and children may require hospitalization, especially those age <6 months. Hospitalized patients should be placed in droplet isolation until antibiotics have been given for at least 5 days or until 3 weeks after the onset of the cough if antibiotics are not administered.

Antibiotics given during the catarrhal phase may shorten the course of the illness. Once the cough is established, antibiotics are recommended to limit the spread of the organism to others but will not shorten the course of illness. Azithromycin or erythromycin is recommended for treatment and can be used to eliminate the bacteria from the respiratory tract. Clarithromycin may also be used in patients age >1 month, and trimethoprim-sulfamethoxazole may be used in infants age >2 months as alternatives. Any infant age <1 month who is treated with a macrolide should be monitored for development of infantile hypertrophic pyloric stenosis. All household contacts of patients with pertussis should receive chemoprophylaxis and be monitored for development of the illness.

During a pertussis outbreak, public health authorities may recommend starting the series at 6 weeks of age with doses 2 and 3 in the primary series administered at intervals as short as 4 weeks. Partially immunized children age <7 years should complete the immunization series at the minimum intervals, and completely immunized children age <7 years should receive one booster dose, unless they have received one in the preceding 3 years. Unimmunized or boosted older children and adults should receive Tdap.

Prognosis

The prognosis of pertussis depends primarily on the age of the patient. Mortality is rare in adults and children. The mortality rate for children age <6 months is highest, but with proper care, it may be minimized. Most mortality is due to pneumonia and cerebral anoxia.

Kimberlin DW, ed. *Red Book: 2018-2021 Report of the Committee on the Infectious Diseases*, 31st ed. Elk Grove Village, IL: American Academy of Pediatrics; 2018:620–634.

PNEUMONIA

ESSENTIALS OF DIAGNOSIS

► Fever.
► Acute respiratory symptoms.
► Tachypnea.

General Considerations

Pneumonia, infection of the lung parenchyma, occurs more often in young children than in any other age group. Although rates are decreasing worldwide, pneumonia remains the leading cause of morbidity and mortality in children beyond the neonatal period. The diagnosis can generally be made clinically, and the majority of patients can be treated successfully with oral antibiotics and recover at home. Occasionally, the child may require hospitalization. Although it is the leading cause of hospitalization among children in the United States, only a small percentage will experience a complicated course.

Pathogenesis

Viruses are a leading cause of pneumonia in children of all ages. Bacterial infections are more common in developing countries and in children with complicated infections.

Age is an important consideration in determining the potential etiology of pneumonia. Neonates age <20 days are most likely to have infections with pathogens that cause other neonatal infection syndromes, including group B streptococci, gram-negative enteric bacteria, CMV, and *Listeria monocytogenes.*

Children between the ages of 3 weeks and 3 months may have infections caused by *C trachomatis,* normally acquired from exposure at the time of birth to infection in the mother's genital tract. In addition, RSV, parainfluenza, and B pertussis and S pneumoniae also cause pneumonia at this age.

Respiratory viruses such as RSV, adenovirus, parainfluenza, human metapneumovirus, influenza, and rhinovirus are the most common causes of pneumonia in children between the ages of 4 months and 4 years. S pneumoniae and nontypeable H influenzae are common bacterial causes. M pneumoniae mainly affects older children in this age group. Tuberculosis should be considered in children who live in areas of high tuberculosis prevalence.

M pneumoniae is the most common cause of pneumonia in children age 5–15 years. Chlamydia pneumoniae is also an important cause in this age group. Pneumococcus is the most likely cause of lobar pneumonia. As in younger children, Mycobacterium tuberculosis should be considered in areas of high prevalence.

▶ Prevention

The only significantly effective form of prevention is immunization. Children should be immunized with vaccines for H influenzae type b, S pneumoniae, and pertussis. Children age >6 months should be immunized against influenza annually. Parents and caretakers of infants age <6 months should be immunized against influenza and pertussis. High-risk infants should receive immune prophylaxis against RSV.

▶ Clinical Findings

A. Symptoms and Signs

The hallmark symptoms of pneumonia are fever and cough; however, although these symptoms can be nonspecific. Young infants are particularly likely to have nonspecific signs and symptoms. Tachypnea and hypoxia are important findings. Hypoxia is defined by an oxygen saturation <90%. Tachypnea is defined by a respiratory rate of >60 breaths per minute in infants age <2 months, >50 in infants age 2–12 months, and >40 in children age >12 months. The absence of tachypnea is associated with a lower likelihood of pneumonia. Additionally, increased work of breathing, such as subcostal or intercostal retractions, nasal flaring, and grunting, is strongly associated with a diagnosis of pneumonia and may indicate more severe disease. Auscultatory findings are variable and include decreased breath sounds, wheezes, rhonchi, and crackles. Moreover, auscultatory findings can be difficult to assess and can subjective. The absence of these various pulmonary findings is helpful in predicting that a child will not have pneumonia, but their presence is only moderately predictive of the presence of pneumonia.

B. Laboratory Findings

Laboratory findings are seldom helpful in the diagnosis of pneumonia. A WBC count of >17,000/mm^3 indicates a higher likelihood of bacteremia, although blood cultures are rarely positive except in complicated infections, and oxygen desaturation indicates more severe disease. Sputum culture is the most accurate way to ascertain the cause of the infection, although obtaining a sputum sample from a child is not always possible.

C. Imaging Studies

Although a chest radiograph is not necessary for the pediatric patient who is well enough to be treated in the outpatient setting, it is generally recommended for children with hypoxia or significant respiratory distress or who have failed initial antibiotic therapy. These patients are at increased risk of complications of pneumonia, including parapneumonic effusions, necrotizing pneumonia, and pneumothorax. Of note, radiography findings may lag behind the clinical findings associated with pneumonia. Routine follow-up chest radiographs are not necessary for children who recover uneventfully.

▶ Differential Diagnosis

The differential diagnosis of pneumonia includes asthma, foreign body aspiration, bronchiolitis, cystic fibrosis, viral myocarditis, and congenital heart disease.

▶ Treatment

The appropriate treatment of childhood pneumonia depends on the age of the child and severity of the illness. Neonates should all be treated as inpatients. Infants age 3 weeks to 3 months may be treated as outpatients if they are not febrile or hypoxemic, do not appear toxic, or have an alveolar infiltrate or a large pleural effusion. Older infants and children may be treated as outpatients if they do not appear seriously ill.

The choice of antibiotics depends on the age of the child and the most likely cause of infection. Neonates should be treated with ampicillin and gentamicin, with or without cefotaxime, as appropriate for a neonatal sepsis syndrome. High-dose amoxicillin should be used in children between 2 months and 5 years of age if a bacterial etiology is suspected. Otherwise, treatment may be withheld if a viral infection is considered to be the most likely cause. For children sick enough to require hospitalization, IV ampicillin is appropriate. For children who appear septic or who manifest alveolar infiltrates or large pleural effusions, cefotaxime or ceftriaxone should be used. If Staphylococcus aureus is suspected, either vancomycin or clindamycin should also be provided.

Macrolides are also appropriate first-line choices for school-aged children and adolescents who are evaluated and treated as outpatients and with findings compatible with atypical pathogens. Doxycycline may be used in children age >8 years. Children who are ill enough to require inpatient treatment should be treated with a macrolide, plus either cefotaxime or ceftriaxone. The recommended duration of treatment is 10 days, depending on the clinical response.

Influenza antiviral therapy should be given to children who have moderate to severe pneumonia consistent with influenza, particularly during community outbreaks.

Prognosis

Worldwide, pneumonia is an important cause of death in children. In developed countries, however, the death rate for childhood pneumonia has dropped dramatically with the development of antibiotics.

Bradley J, Byington CL, Shah SS, et al. Executive summary: the management of community-acquired pneumonia in infants and children older than 3 months of age: clinical practice guidelines by the Pediatric Infectious Disease Society and the Infectious Disease Society of America. *Clin Infect Dis.* 2011;53(7):617–630. [PMID: 21890766]

Jain S, Williams DJ, Arnold SR, et al. Community-acquired pneumonia requiring hospitalization among U.S. children. *N Engl J Med.* 2015;372(9):835–845. [PMID: 25714161]

Shah SN, Bachur RG, Simel DL, Neuman MI. Does this child have pneumonia? The rational clinical examination systematic review. *JAMA.* 2017;318(5):462–471. [PMID: 28763554]

Walker CLF, Rudan I, Liu L, et al. Global burden of childhood pneumonia and diarrhea. *Lancet.* 2013;381(9875):1405–1416. [PMID: 23582727]

▼ GASTROINTESTINAL & GENITOURINARY INFECTIONS

GASTROENTERITIS

ESSENTIALS OF DIAGNOSIS

► Diarrhea.

► Vomiting may be present or absent.

General Considerations

Diarrheal diseases are among the most common illnesses and perhaps the leading cause of death among children worldwide. It is estimated that there are 1 billion illnesses and 3–5 million deaths from these illnesses each year. In the United States, there are an estimated 20–35 million cases of diarrhea annually, with 1.5 million outpatient visits to physicians and >200,000 hospitalizations but only 300 deaths per year. Gastroenteritis may be caused by any of a large number of viruses, bacteria, or parasites. Most infections are caused by ingestion of contaminated food or water.

Pathogenesis

Four families of viruses can cause gastroenteritis. All are spread easily through fecal-oral contact, and many are associated with localized outbreaks in hospitals, daycare centers, and schools. Rotavirus is a common cause of gastroenteritis during winter months. It primarily affects children between 3 months and 2 years of age, and by age 4 or 5 years, nearly all children have serologic evidence of infection. Norwalk virus is the most common cause of gastroenteritis among older children and, along with astroviruses and enteric adenoviruses, causes year-round, often localized outbreaks of disease.

Bacteria may cause either inflammatory or noninflammatory diarrhea. Common causes of inflammatory diarrhea are *Campylobacter jejuni,* enteroinvasive or enterohemorrhagic *E coli, Salmonella* species, *Shigella* species, and *Yersinia enterocolitica.* Noninflammatory diarrhea may be caused by enteropathogenic or enterotoxigenic *E coli* or by *Vibrio cholerae.*

The most common parasitic cause of diarrhea in the United States is *Giardia lamblia.* Numerous other parasites, including *Cryptosporidium* and *Entamoeba histolytica,* along with helminthes such as *Strongyloides stercoralis,* may cause diarrhea. Most parasitic infections cause chronic diarrhea and are beyond the scope of this chapter.

Prevention

The most effective prevention measure is for children to have access to uncontaminated food and water. Careful hand washing and good sanitation practices also help prevent the spread of infection among children. An increased rate of breastfeeding has been shown to decrease the incidence of gastroenteritis among all children in small communities.

In 2006, the Advisory Committee on Immunization Practices (ACIP) recommended that the new oral rotavirus vaccine (RotaTeq) be given to all children at 2, 4, and 6 months of age. This immunization schedule has been shown to be effective for two seasons after administration, but no studies have been done to establish whether it is effective for longer. It should be noted that, unlike the initial rotavirus vaccine, which was withdrawn from the market, the new vaccine has not been shown to be associated with an increased rate of intussusception. In 2008, a second oral vaccine (Rotarix) was licensed as a two-dose series, given at 2 and 4 months of age. The ACIP does not express a preference for one vaccine over the other.

Clinical Findings

A. Symptoms and Signs

The cardinal sign of gastroenteritis is diarrhea, with or without vomiting. Systemic symptoms and signs may include fever and malaise. Fever and severe abdominal pain are more common with inflammatory diarrhea. The estimated degree of dehydration should be established before beginning treatment.

In most children with viral gastroenteritis, fever and vomiting last <2–3 days, although diarrhea may persist for ≤5–7 days. Most cases of diarrhea caused by foodborne toxins last 1–2 days. Many, but not all, bacterial infections persist for longer periods of time.

B. Laboratory Findings

Stool cultures for bacteria and examination for parasites should be analyzed if the stool is positive for blood or leukocytes, if diarrhea persists for >1 week, or if the patient is immunocompromised. The presence of fecal leukocytes indicates an inflammatory infection, although not all such infections produce a positive test. Blood indicates a hemorrhagic or inflammatory infection. In a child who appears significantly dehydrated, serum electrolytes should be tested, especially if the child is hospitalized for fluid therapy.

▶ Complications

Diarrheal diseases are for the most part benign, self-limited infections. Mortality is caused primarily by dehydration, shock, and circulatory collapse. Bacterial pathogens may spread to remote sites and cause meningitis, pneumonia, and other infections. *E coli* O157:H7 may cause hemolytic-uremic syndrome.

▶ Treatment

The keys to treatment of gastroenteritis are rehydration, or avoidance of dehydration, and early refeeding. Children who are severely (>9%) dehydrated or who appear toxic or seriously ill should be hospitalized for rehydration and treatment. Otherwise, children may be managed at home. Vomiting is the chief obstacle to rehydration or maintenance of hydration. Children who are vomiting should be given frequent (every 1–2 minutes) very small amounts (≤5 mL) of rehydration solution to avoid provoking further attacks of emesis (Table 5–2).

Children who have diarrhea but are not dehydrated should continue on whatever age-appropriate foods they were taking before the illness. In those who are dehydrated but not severely so, oral rehydration has been shown to be the preferred method of rehydration. Juices, water flavored with drink mix, and sports drinks do not have the recommended concentrations of carbohydrates and electrolytes and should be avoided. The World Health Organization's or UNICEF's reduced-osmolarity rehydration solution is the preferred therapy. Children who are mildly (<3%) dehydrated should be given 50 mL/kg of solution, plus replacement of ongoing losses from stool or emesis, over each 4-hour period. Children who are moderately (3–9%) dehydrated should be given

Table 5–2. Evaluation of dehydration in children.

Although the degree of dehydration is often misjudged by clinicians, the following scale is one of several that can be helpful in estimating the severity in infants and young children:
<3%—usually subclinical
Mild to moderate dehydration (3–9%):
Thirsty, eager to drink
Decreased tears
Slightly dry mucous membranes
Sunken eyes
Cool extremities
Decreased urine output
Severe dehydration (>9%):
Thready/absent pulses
Prolonged capillary refill
Prolonged or absent capillary refill
Cold extremities
Apathetic, lethargic, unconscious
Minimal urine output

Data from Granado-Villar D, Cunill-De Sautu B, Granados A: Acute gastroenteritis. *Pediatr Rev.* 2012 Nov;33(11):487–494.

100 mL/kg, plus losses, over each 4-hour period. Refeeding with age-appropriate foods should begin as soon as the child is interested in eating. Therapy with antidiarrheal and antiemetic medications has been shown to have minimal effect on the volume of diarrhea. Additionally, these drugs have an unacceptably high rate of side effects, and their use is not recommended.

Even when diagnosed, many bacterial infections do not require treatment. *Campylobacter* (erythromycin) and *Shigella* (trimethoprim-sulfamethoxazole or cephalosporin) infections may require treatment. Infections with *Salmonella* should not be treated with antibiotics unless the child is age <3 months or manifests bacteremia or disseminated infection. Treatment of *E coli* O157:H7 infection does not reduce the severity of the illness and may increase the likelihood of hemolytic-uremic syndrome. Other *E coli* infections should be treated only if they are severe or prolonged. *Giardia* infections should be treated.

Probiotics such as *Lactobacillus* may reduce the duration of the diarrhea, especially if caused by rotavirus, and are most effective when started early in the illness.

▶ Prognosis

With proper rehydration and refeeding, morbidity and mortality from viral gastroenteritis are minimal. Morbidity and mortality from bacterial infections are dependent on the virulence of the organism and complications from distant spread or remote effects, such as hemolytic-uremic syndrome.

Committee on Infectious Diseases American Academy of Pediatrics. Prevention of rotavirus diseases: updated guidelines for use of rotavirus vaccine. *Pediatrics*. 2009;123(5):1412–1420. [PMID: 19332437]

URINARY TRACT INFECTIONS

ESSENTIALS OF DIAGNOSIS

▶ Common bacterial cause of febrile illness in young children.

▶ Symptoms are often nonspecific in young children.

▶ Urinalysis is not always reliable; appropriate culture is needed for final diagnosis

General Considerations

Urinary tract infections (UTIs) are the most common serious bacterial infection in children age <2 years. Among febrile young children, between 3% and 5% have a UTI, and among infants, UTIs account for approximately 5% of unfocused febrile illnesses. UTI is the most frequent site of serious bacterial infections in young children. UTI may also be a marker for urinary tract anomalies in young children. UTIs may lead to renal scarring, which may cause hypertension and renal insufficiency later in life.

Pathogenesis

In the first 8–12 weeks of life, some UTIs may be caused by hematogenous spread of bacteria from a remote source. Otherwise, the infections are caused by bacteria ascending the urethra into the bladder. From the bladder, bacteria may ascend the ureters to cause pyelonephritis.

The most common pathogens responsible for UTIs are enteric bacteria. *E coli* is found in 70–90% of infections. *Pseudomonas aeruginosa* is the most common nonenteric gram-negative pathogen, and *Enterococcus* species are the most common gram-positive organisms seen. Group B *Streptococcus* is occasionally found in neonates. *S aureus* is rarely seen in children who do not have indwelling catheters and suggests seeding from a distant focus, such as renal abscess, osteomyelitis, or endocarditis.

Clinical Findings

A. Symptoms and Signs

The most important factors in prevalence of UTI are the patient's age and gender. In newborns, preterm infants are several times more likely to have a UTI than full-term infants. In febrile infant girls, the most important factors are nonblack race, age <12 months, fever ≥39°C, fever for ≥2 days, and no other source of infection. More than two of these risk factors should prompt serious consideration of UTI. In infant boys, circumcision is the most important risk factor. Nonblack race, fever ≥39°C, fever for ≥2 days, and no other source of infection are other important risk factors. Circumcised febrile infant boys have a significant risk of UTI with more than two of the other risk factors. Comparatively, uncircumcised febrile infant boys with more than one of the other risk factors are at significant risk of UTI. Uncircumcised febrile infant boys have a >1% risk of UTI. The usual age at which children experience a first symptomatic infection is 1–5 years. In this age group, girls are 10–20 times more likely to have a UTI than boys. Two-thirds of young children with a febrile UTI have acute pyelonephritis.

Among children age <2 years, symptoms are often lacking or nonspecific. Parents may become suspicious if the child appears to be in pain while urinating, but otherwise, fever may be the only presenting complaint. Among children who have developed language skills, typical UTI symptoms, such as dysuria, urgency, and urinary frequency, may be seen.

B. Laboratory Findings

To be most reliable, urine must be collected by a clean catch, catheterization, or suprapubic aspiration. Urine collected in an adhesive collection bag is often contaminated. Bag urinalysis is mostly helpful when negative. Bag urine culture is helpful retrospectively only if negative. The final diagnosis of UTI depends on an appropriately collected culture result of ≥50,000 colony-forming units (CFUs) per milliliter of a uropathogen combined with a urinalysis suggestive of pyuria.

Urine should be analyzed for pyuria and bacteriuria. Dipstick urinalysis is a component of urine evaluation. A positive urine nitrite test is very specific, but a negative test is not helpful for bacteriuria. Leukocyte esterase testing is very sensitive but not as specific for UTI. Fever from other conditions, vigorous activity, or contamination can produce a positive leukocyte esterase test. Both pyuria and bacteriuria signal the presence of a UTI. Pyuria in the absence of bacteriuria is nonspecific and can occur in various noninfectious, inflammatory conditions. Bacteriuria without pyuria could be secondary to external contamination or asymptomatic bacteriuria. Microscopic urinalysis for pyuria is positive if there are ≥5 WBCs per high-powered field in a spun urine sample. An "enhanced" or unspun urinalysis using a counting chamber is positive if there are ≥10 WBCs/mm³. Significant bacteriuria correlating to a UTI is confirmed by the presence of bacteria on examination of least 10 oil immersion fields of gram-stained unspun fresh urine.

Urine collected for analysis should be sent for culture. A culture is considered positive if there is growth of a single uropathogen of at least 50,000 CFUs/mL. *Lactobacillus*, coagulase-negative *Staphylococcus*, and *Corynebacterium* are seldom considered pathogens. The diagnosis of asymptomatic bacteriuria should be considered for positive cultures without evidence of pyuria. The sensitivity and specificity of laboratory urine testing for UTI increase significantly as more components of the evaluation are concordant. Relying on a single test to diagnose UTI is not preferred. In febrile infants determined not to be low risk, the AAP recommends obtaining a urine specimen through catheterization or suprapubic aspiration for urinalysis and culture. In acute care settings, recent studies suggest that a two-step diagnostic method can be used for children age 6–24 months. As a second option, the AAP guidelines support obtaining a urine sample via the most accessible methods to send for urinalysis. Samples suggestive of a UTI (positive leukocyte esterase, nitrites, pyuria, or bacteriuria) should prompt the clinician to obtain a sterile sample via catherization or suprapubic aspiration for confirmatory urinalysis and urine culture testing.

C. Imaging Studies

The goal of imaging is to diagnose the presence of urinary tract anomalies that require further evaluation.

Children of any age with a UTI who have a family history of renal or urologic disease, poor growth, or hypertension should undergo a renal and bladder ultrasound. Renal and bladder ultrasound should be performed on febrile infants age ≤24 months with their first UTI. Older children with recurrent febrile UTIs should also be studied. This evaluation should include assessment of the renal parenchyma and renal size. If a child is not seriously ill or responds quickly to treatment, it may be preferable to delay the ultrasound until UTI treatment is completed to ensure the most accurate assessment of ureter and kidney size. More seriously ill children should be imaged in the first 2 days of treatment to assess for serious complications such as abscess formation.

The optimal treatment of vesicoureteral reflux (VUR) is not presently known. Recent evidence contraindicates a voiding cystourethrogram (VCUG) on all children with a first febrile UTI. VCUG should be performed on children with recurrent febrile UTIs or if ultrasound findings are suggestive of ongoing VUR (renal scarring or poor renal growth or hydronephrosis) or obstructive uropathy. VCUG should be performed after the patient's symptoms have resolved.

▶ Differential Diagnosis

UTI should be considered in any child who presents with a febrile illness in whom the cause of the fever cannot be readily ascertained by physical examination. In premenarcheal girls, chemical urethritis may cause dysuria. Prolonged exposure to bubble baths is a frequent source. Trauma can also cause dysuria, including sexual abuse. Systemic symptoms of infection are absent in these children. In older children, sexually transmitted diseases (STDs) can cause acute urinary symptoms.

▶ Complications

Acute complications of UTI include sepsis, renal abscess, and disseminated infection, including meningitis. Recurrent pyelonephritis can cause renal scarring, which can lead to hypertension or renal insufficiency later in life.

▶ Treatment

A. Acute Infection

Infants age <2 months with UTI should be hospitalized and treated with IV antibiotics as indicated for sepsis until cultures identify the causative organism and the best antibiotic for treatment. Infants age 2 months to 2 years may be treated as outpatients with oral antibiotics unless they appear toxic, are dehydrated, or are unable to retain oral intake. Older children can usually be treated as outpatients unless they appear seriously ill. The initial choice of antibiotic may be a sulfonamide, trimethoprim-sulfamethoxazole, a cephalosporin, or amoxicillin-clavulanate. Nitrofurantoin, which is excreted in the urine but does not reach therapeutic blood levels, should not be used to treat febrile children with a UTI. Ideally, the choice of antimicrobial agent should be driven by local patterns of infection and susceptibility. The duration of treatment should be 7–14 days. Treatment courses of ≤3 days have been shown to be inferior in children.

If the child responds clinically to treatment within 2 days, no further immediate follow-up is needed. A child who is not improving after 2 days of treatment should be reevaluated. Retesting and hospital treatment should be considered. Antibiotic treatment should be guided by the patient's urine culture results as they become available.

B. Prevention of Recurrent Infection

Prevention of long-term sequelae focuses on prevention of recurrent infection. Caregivers should be made aware to have patients promptly evaluated for future unexplained febrile illnesses. Delays in treatment of febrile UTIs are associated with increased risk of renal scarring. Infants and children with abnormal ultrasounds or grade III–V VUR should be considered for consultation with a pediatric urologist. In children with structurally normal urinary tracts, treatment of chronic constipation has been shown to decrease the recurrence of UTI, as has behavioral correction of voiding dysfunction associated with incomplete emptying of the bladder. Improving hygiene, especially in girls, has not been shown to decrease UTI rates. Based on retrospective studies, circumcision of boys has been claimed to be associated with decreased UTI rates.

For some children with recurrent UTIs, long-term prophylactic antibiotic treatment may be effective in reducing the frequency of infections. However, there are no clear guidelines as to when this treatment should be considered.

DeMuri GP, Wald ER. Imaging and antimicrobial prophylaxis following the diagnosis of urinary tract infection in children. *Pediatr Infect Dis J*. 2008;27:553–554. [PMID: 18520594]

Farhat W, McLorie G. Urethral syndromes in children. *Pediatr Rev*. 2001;22:17. [PMID: 11139643]

Hoberman A, Charron M, Hickey RW, et al. Imaging studies after a first febrile urinary tract infection in young children. *N Engl J Med*. 2003;348:195. [PMID: 12529459]

Keren R. Imaging and treatment strategies for children after first urinary tract infection. *Curr Opin Pediatr*. 2007;19:705–710. [PMID: 18025941]

La Scola C, De Mutiis C, Hewitt IK, et al. Different guidelines for imaging after first UTI in febrile infants: yield, cost, and radiation. *Pediatrics*. 2013;131:e665. [PMID: 23439905]

Lavelle JM, Blackstone MM, Funari MK, et al. Two-step process for ED UTI screening in febrile young children: reducing catheterization rates. *Pediatrics*. 2016;138(1):pii:e20153023. [PMID: 27255151]

Roberts KB, Wald ER. The diagnosis of UTI: colony count criteria revisited. *Pediatrics*. 2018;141(2):e20173239. [PMID: 29339563]

Shah G, Upadhyay J. Controversies in the diagnosis and management of urinary tract infections in children. *Pediatr Drugs*. 2005;7:339–346. [PMID: 16356021]

Shaikh N, Hoberman A, Keren R, et al. Recurrent urinary tract infections in children with bladder and bowel dysfunction. *Pediatrics*. 2016;137(1):e20152982. [PMID: 26647376]

Shaikh N, Mattoo TK, Keren R, et al. Early antibiotic treatment for pediatric febrile urinary tract infection and renal scarring *JAMA Pediatr*. 2016;170(9):848–854. [PMID: 27455161]

Shaikh N, Morone NE, Bost JE, et al. Prevalence of urinary tract infection in childhood: a meta-analysis. *Pediatr Infect Dis J*. 2008;27:302–308. [PMID: 18316994]

Subcommittee on Urinary Tract Infection. Reaffirmation of AAP clinical practice guideline: the diagnosis and management of the initial urinary tract infection in febrile infants and young children 2-24 months of age: *Pediatrics*. 2016;138(6):e20163026. [PMID: 27940735]

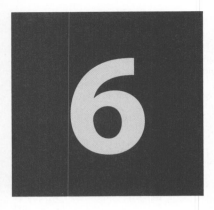

Skin Diseases in Infants & Children

Mark A. Knox, MD

Barry Coutinho, MBBS

Teiichi Takedai, MD, FAAFP

Scott R. Brown, DO

▼ INFECTIONS OF THE SKIN

IMPETIGO

ESSENTIALS OF DIAGNOSIS

▶ Nonbullous: yellowish crusted plaques.

▶ Bullous: bullae, with minimal surrounding erythema, rupture to leave a shallow ulcer.

▶ General Considerations

Impetigo is a bacterial infection of the skin. More than 70% of cases are of the nonbullous variety.

▶ Pathogenesis

Most cases of nonbullous impetigo are caused by *Staphylococcus aureus*, although group A β-hemolytic streptococci are found in some cases. *S aureus* that produces exfoliative toxin is the cause of bullous impetigo; methicillin-resistant *S aureus* (MRSA) has been isolated from patients. Impetigo can develop in traumatized skin, or the bacteria can spread to intact skin from its reservoir in the nose.

▶ Clinical Findings

Nonbullous impetigo usually starts as a small pustule or vesicle that ruptures easily, followed by the classic small (<2-cm), honey-colored, crusted plaque. The infection may be spread to other parts of the body by fingers or clothing. There is usually little surrounding erythema, itching occurs occasionally, and pain is usually absent. Without treatment, the lesions resolve without scarring in 2 weeks.

Bullous impetigo is usually seen in infants and young children. Lesions begin on intact skin on almost any part of the body; common locations include the diaper area, axillae, and skin folds. Flaccid, thin-roofed vesicles develop, which rupture to form shallow ulcers with surrounding "collarette" of scale.

▶ Differential Diagnosis

Nonbullous impetigo is unique in appearance. Bullous impetigo is similar in appearance to pemphigus and bullous pemphigoid. Growth of staphylococci from fluid in a bulla confirms the diagnosis.

▶ Complications

Cellulitis follows ~10% of cases of nonbullous impetigo but rarely follows bullous impetigo. Either type may rarely lead to septicemia, septic arthritis, or osteomyelitis. Scarlet fever and poststreptococcal glomerulonephritis, but not rheumatic fever, may follow streptococcal impetigo. Treating impetigo has not been shown to prevent poststreptococcal glomerulonephritis.

▶ Treatment

Localized disease is effectively treated with topical 2% mupirocin or 1% retapamulin ointment for 5 days. Ozenoxacin 1% cream is a newer, second-line option. Patients with widespread lesions or evidence of cellulitis should be treated with systemic antibiotics effective against staphylococci and streptococci. If infection with MRSA is a possibility, trimethoprim-sulfamethoxazole or clindamycin should be considered; fluoroquinolones must not be used due to risks of widespread MRSA resistance and musculoskeletal adverse effects.

▶ Patient Education

Further information is available at the following link:
https://kidshealth.org/en/parents/impetigo.html.

FUNGAL INFECTIONS

▶ General Considerations

Fungal infections of the skin and skin structures may be generally grouped into three categories: dermatophyte infections, other tinea infections, and candidal infections.

▶ Pathogenesis

Dermatophytoses are caused by a group of related fungal species—primarily *Microsporum*, *Trichophyton*, and *Epidermophyton*—that require keratin for growth and can invade hair, nails, and the stratum corneum of the skin. Some of these organisms are spread from person to person; some are zoonotic, spreading from animals to people; and some infect people from the soil. Other fungi can also cause skin disease, such as *Malassezia furfur* in tinea versicolor. Finally, *Candida albicans*, a common resident of the gastrointestinal tract, can cause diaper dermatitis and thrush.

▶ Clinical Findings

A. Symptoms and Signs

1. Dermatophytoses

A. TINEA CORPORIS—Infection of the skin produces one or more characteristic gradually spreading lesions with an erythematous raised border and central areas that are generally scaly but relatively clearer and less indurated than the margins of the lesions. The central clearing helps differentiate these lesions from those of psoriasis. Small lesions may resemble those of nummular eczema. The lesions may have a somewhat serpiginous border, but they are usually more or less round in shape, hence the common name of "ringworm." They can range in size from one to several centimeters.

B. TINEA CAPITIS—Fungal infection of the scalp and hair is the most common dermatophytosis in children. This presents as areas of alopecia with generally regular borders. Typically, the hair shafts break off a few millimeters from the skin surface, distinguishing this from alopecia areata. The infection may also produce a sterile inflammatory mass in the scalp, called a *kerion*, which may be confused with a bacterial infection.

2. Nondermatophyte infections

A. TINEA VERSICOLOR—Tinea versicolor is normally seen in adolescents and adults. The causative organism, *M furfur*, is part of the normal skin flora. The infection most often becomes evident during warm weather, when new lesions develop. A warm, humid environment, excessive sweating, and genetic susceptibility are important factors for developing this infection. Because treatment does not eradicate the fungus from the skin, it often recurs annually, during the summer months, in susceptible individuals. In chronically warm climates, it is a perennial problem, with new crops of lesions developing unpredictably throughout the year. The lesions are characteristically scaly macules, usually reddish brown in light-colored skin but often hyper- or hypopigmented in people with more pigmented skins. They can be found almost anywhere on the body but are seen most commonly on the torso. The lesions are rarely pruritic. The individual lesions may enlarge and coalesce to form larger lesions with irregular borders.

3. Candidal infections

A. THRUSH—Thrush is a common oral infection in infants. Isolated incidents of this disease are common in immunocompetent infants, but recurrent infections in infants or infections in children and adolescents may indicate an underlying immune deficiency. The infection presents as thick white plaques on the tongue and buccal mucosa. These can be scraped off only with difficulty, revealing an erythematous base.

A. CANDIDAL DIAPER DERMATITIS—This infection is most common in infants age 2–4 months. *Candida* is a common colonist of the gastrointestinal tract, and infants with diaper dermatitis should be examined for signs of thrush. The fungus does not ordinarily invade the skin, but the warm, humid environment of the diaper area provides an ideal medium for growth. The infection is characterized by an intensely erythematous plaque with a sharply demarcated border. Advancing from the border are numerous satellite papules, which enlarge and coalesce to enlarge the affected area.

B. Special Tests

Dermatophyte and other tinea infections are usually diagnosed clinically. Examination of potassium hydroxide (KOH) preparations of scrapings from the affected area, which show hyphae, confirms the diagnosis. KOH preparation of tinea versicolor reveals the classic "spaghetti and meatballs" pattern with hyphae and spores. Fungal cultures may be helpful when the diagnosis is suspected but cannot otherwise be confirmed. Diagnosis of candidal infections is generally made by clinical findings.

▶ Treatment

Tinea corporis is treated with topical antifungal medications. The azoles, including miconazole, clotrimazole, and ketoconazole, and the allylamines such as terbinafine and butenafine creams are all effective. Nystatin treats candida infections only. Rarely, widespread infection requires systemic therapy.

Topical therapy is ineffective in tinea capitis, although applications of shampoo containing 2% ketoconazole or 1%

or 2.5% selenium sulfide 2–3 times a week for 10 minutes have been shown to reduce fungal spore shedding and may reduce transmission. Oral griseofulvin and terbinafine are both accepted first-line therapies. Terbinafine has the advantage of a shorter course, typically 4–6 weeks, but is not approved for use in children under 4 years old. Although not approved by the US Food and Drug Administration (FDA) for this use, fluconazole and itraconazole are also effective. Oral ketoconazole must not be used because of risks of serious hepatotoxicity.

Ely JW, Rosenfeld S, Seabury Stone M. Diagnosis and management of tinea infections. *Am Fam Physician*. 2014;90:702–710. [PMID: 25403034]

Tinea versicolor can be treated with topical selenium sulfide lotion or any of the previously listed topical creams. These are preferred over oral medications in children due to the risk of hepatotoxicity and other adverse effects.

Candidal infections are most often treated with nystatin. Diaper dermatitis responds well to topical nystatin cream. If intense inflammation is present, topical steroids for a few days may be helpful. Thrush is usually treated with nystatin suspension. Up to 2 weeks may be needed for complete resolution of the infection.

Prognosis

All of these infections in immunocompetent children respond well to treatment. However, left untreated, they can cause widespread and significant skin disease.

Patient Education

Further information is available at the following links:
https://familydoctor.org/condition/ringworm/
https://www.mayoclinic.org/diseases-conditions/tinea-versicolor/symptoms-causes/syc-20378385
https://familydoctor.org/condition/diaper-rash/

▼ PARASITIC INFESTATIONS

SCABIES

ESSENTIALS OF DIAGNOSIS

► Intense generalized pruritus.
► Small erythematous papules.
► Burrows are pathognomonic but may not be seen.

Pathogenesis

Scabies is a common infestation caused by the mite *Sarcoptes scabiei*. The disease is acquired by physical contact with an infected person. Transmission of the disease by contact with infested linens or clothing is less common, because the mites can live off the body for only 2–3 days. The female mite burrows between the superficial and deeper layers of the epidermis, laying eggs and depositing feces as she goes along. After 4–5 weeks, her egg laying is complete, and she dies in the burrow. The eggs hatch, releasing larvae that move to the skin surface, molt into nymphs, mature to adults, mate, and begin the cycle again. Pruritus is caused by an allergic reaction to mite antigens.

Clinical Findings

A. Symptoms and Signs

Diagnosis is based primarily on clinical suspicion, as physical findings are highly variable and the disease can mimic a wide variety of skin conditions. The classic early symptom is intense generalized pruritus, especially at night. The usual finding is 1- to 2-mm erythematous papules, often in a linear pattern. The finding of burrows connecting the papules is diagnostic but is not always seen. Consider scabies in patients with diffuse itching with visible lesions in typical predilection sites and pruritus in close contacts. In infants, the disease may involve the entire body—including the face, scalp, palms, and soles—and pustules and vesicles are common. In older children and adolescents, the lesions are most often seen in the interdigital spaces, wrist flexors, umbilicus, groin, and genitalia. Severe infestation may produce widespread crusted lesions.

B. Special Tests

Superficial scrapings under mineral oil may show entire mites, eggs, or fecal pellets. However, success in finding these is limited, and a negative examination does not rule out the disease. Dermoscopy to look for the "arrowhead sign," which represents the mite at the end of a burrow, can be helpful as a noninvasive test, with fewer false negatives.

Treatment

Permethrin 5% cream, applied to the entire body (excluding the face in older children), is the preferred treatment in subjects age ≥2 months. It is applied for 8–14 hours and then washed off and repeated in 1 week. Treatment will kill mites and eliminate the risk of contagion within 24 hours. However, pruritus may continue for several days to 2 weeks after treatment. The entire family should be treated at the same time, and all clothing and bedding should ideally be machine washed in hot water (>60°C) and dried in a hot dryer. A single 200-μg/kg oral dose of ivermectin, repeated in 2 weeks, is an effective treatment option in patients who weigh >15 kg, with no serious adverse reactions.

Rosumeck S, Nast A, Dressler C. Ivermectin and permethrin for treating scabies. *Cochrane Database Syst Rev.* 2018;4:CD012994. [PMID: 29608022]

 Patient Education

Further information is available at the following link:
https://kidshealth.org/en/parents/scabies.html.

LICE (PEDICULOSIS)

ESSENTIALS OF DIAGNOSIS

▶ Pruritus.

▶ Visualization of lice on the body or nits in hair.

Pathogenesis

Three varieties of lice cause human disease. *Pediculus humanus corporis* causes infestations on the body, and *Pediculus humanus capitis* causes infestation on the head. *Pthirus pubis*, or crab lice, infest the pubic area. All are spread by physical contact with an infested person; fomite transmission is rare. Body lice can be a vector for other disease, such as typhus, trench fever, and relapsing fever. Infestation with pubic lice is highly correlated with infection by other sexually transmitted diseases. Nits are the eggs of the louse. They are cemented to hairs, are usually <1 mm in length, and are translucent. Body lice lay their nits in the seams of clothing. The nits can remain viable for ≤1 month and will hatch when exposed to body heat when the clothing is worn again.

Prevention

Body lice are associated primarily with poor hygiene and can be prevented by regular bathing and washing of clothing and bedding. Patients with hair lice must not share clothing, hair accessories, combs, brushes, or towels.

Clinical Findings

The cardinal symptom of louse infestation is pruritus, which develops as a delayed hypersensitivity reaction. Excoriations in the infested area are common. The lice themselves can usually be seen easily. Head and pubic lice are easily seen, but body lice are present on the body only when feeding.

Treatment

A. Head Lice

The first-line treatment is permethrin 1% cream rinse or lotion, applied for 10 minutes, then rinsed off with warm water. It may be repeated after 7 days. Alternative treatments can be used if permethrin fails after two treatments. These include other insecticidal agents such as a single application of spinosad 0.9% topical suspension in children age ≥4 years, topical ivermectin 0.5% lotion in patients age ≥6 months, malathion 0.5% lotion, or pyrethrins 0.3%/piperonyl butoxide 4% shampoo. Noninsecticidal agents include benzyl alcohol 5% lotion and dimethicone solution. Another agent, isopropyl myristate solution, is not yet available in the United States.

Nit removal combs can be used as alternatives or adjuncts to topical pediculicides but have variable cure rates, and studies have not been of high quality. "No-nit" policies are not recommended at schools and daycares because their presence does not indicate an active infestation. Children should not be kept out of school during treatment because the likelihood of transmission is low.

B. Body and Pubic Lice

Permethrin 1% lotion and pyrethrins 0.3%/piperonyl butoxide 4% shampoo are first-line agents, with malathion 0.5% lotion or oral ivermectin as alternatives. Pediculosis pubis is usually sexually transmitted, so the possibility of sexual abuse must always be considered in children.

In all cases of lice, clothing and bedding should be heat-washed to at least 54°C to prevent recurrence.

Gunning K, Kiraly B, Pippitt K. Lice and scabies: treatment update. *Am Fam Physician.* 2019;99(10):635–642. [PMID: 31083883]

 Patient Education

Further information is available at the following link:
https://familydoctor.org/condition/head-lice/.

INFECTIOUS DISEASES WITH SKIN MANIFESTATIONS

BACTERIAL INFECTIONS

Scarlet Fever (Scarlatina)

ESSENTIALS OF DIAGNOSIS

▶ Symptoms of streptococcal pharyngitis.

▶ "Sandpaper" rash.

▶ Circumoral pallor.

▶ "Strawberry" tongue (red or white).

General Considerations

Scarlet fever is a rash representing a hypersensitivity reaction of the skin against an infection caused by certain strains of group A streptococci. The infection most commonly begins as a typical streptococcal pharyngitis, but it can also follow streptococcal cellulitis.

Clinical Findings

A. Signs and Symptoms

The classic feature of scarlet fever is the rash. It develops 12–48 hours after the onset of pharyngitis symptoms, usually beginning in the neck, axillae, or groin, which becomes generalized within 24 hours. The rash is a fine, faintly erythematous exanthem that is often more easily felt than seen, giving it the name of "sandpaper" rash. The rash itself is seldom present on the face, but there is often flushing of the face except for the area around the mouth (circumoral pallor). The tongue is often erythematous and swollen. In the early stages of the disease, the tongue may have swollen papillae protruding through a white coating (white "strawberry" tongue). Later in the illness, the coating desquamates, leaving the tongue red and the papillae swollen, red "strawberry" tongue. Confluent petechiae may develop in antecubital fossae (Pastia lines). After about 1 week, desquamation begins on the face and progresses downward over the body, involving the hands and feet, and may last 4–6 weeks.

B. Laboratory Findings

Rapid antigen test has a sensitivity of 86% for diagnosing group A β-hemolytic streptococcal pharyngitis.

Differential Diagnosis

Kawasaki disease and any of the viral exanthems may be confused with scarlet fever.

Complications

Scarlet fever is generally a benign disease. In severe cases, bacteremia and sepsis may occur, and rheumatic fever may follow an untreated infection. Glomerulonephritis may also be a sequela.

Treatment

Treatment for scarlet fever is the same as the treatment for primary streptococcal infection.

Patient Education

Further information is available at the following link:
https://www.mayoclinic.org/diseases-conditions/scarlet-fever/symptoms-causes/syc-20377406.

VIRAL INFECTIONS

Roseola (Exanthem Subitum)

 ESSENTIALS OF DIAGNOSIS

► Sudden onset of high fever.
► Most cases between the ages of 7 and 13 months. (Rare at age <3 months or >2 years.)
► Development of rash as fever breaks after 3–4 days.

Pathogenesis

Human herpesvirus 6 (HHV6) causes the clear majority of cases of clinical roseola, although other viruses cause some cases as well. Infections occur year-round.

Clinical Findings

A. Signs and Symptoms

The hallmark of roseola is the abrupt onset of high fever, often between 39.4°C and 41.1°C (103°F and 106°F). Febrile seizures can occur in 6–25% of patients. Despite the high fever, children are usually alert and nontoxic. Other symptoms include mild diarrhea, mild signs of the upper respiratory infection, mild cervical lymph node swelling, and eyelid swelling. The fever breaks suddenly after 3–4 days, which is followed by the appearance of a rash. This is usually a blanching macular or maculopapular rash that starts on the neck and trunk and spreads to the face, scalp, and extremities. The rash resolves within 3 days, but it may be more transient.

B. Laboratory Findings

Laboratory tests are usually unnecessary, although relative neutropenia and mild atypical lymphocytosis may be seen.

Differential Diagnosis

Differential diagnoses include rubella, rubeola (measles), enteroviral infection (hand-foot-mouth syndrome), or erythema infectiosum. In the early stages of the disease, many children with high fever and seizures are admitted to the hospital for workup of suspected meningitis or sepsis. After the rash appears, the diagnosis is obvious in retrospect. Later onset of the rash is often misinterpreted as a drug allergy.

Complications

Febrile seizures can occur in 6–15% of patients. It is unknown whether it is due to the direct effect of the virus or the result of the indirect effect of elevated temperature. Rare cases of encephalitis (<1%) have been reported.

Treatment & Prognosis

Treatment is entirely symptomatic. Unless the patient develops one of the rare complications listed earlier, roseola is a benign, self-limited infection. Antipyretics (acetaminophen) may be used for fever during the initial febrile phase of the illness.

Patient Education

Further information is available at the following link:
https://www.mayoclinic.org/diseases-conditions/roseola/symptoms-causes/syc-20377283.

Varicella (Chickenpox)

ESSENTIALS OF DIAGNOSIS

▶ Prodrome of upper respiratory–like symptoms.

▶ Rash consists of small vesicles on an erythematous base.

▶ Vesicles rupture with crusting.

General Considerations

Prior to widespread immunization of children, approximately 90% of adults in the United States manifested with serologic evidence of varicella infection, regardless of whether they had clinically apparent disease.

Pathogenesis

Varicella-zoster virus is a herpesvirus. After resolution of the initial infection, the virus produces a latent infection in the dorsal root ganglia. Reactivation produces herpes zoster or "shingles."

Prevention

Childhood immunization should prevent most from developing the disease. The vaccine is given in two doses—the first between 12 and 15 months of age, and the second between 4 and 6 years of age. Varicella-zoster immune globulin can help prevent infection in immunocompromised children, nonimmune pregnant women who are exposed to the virus, and newborns exposed to maternal varicella.

Centers for Disease Control and Prevention. Updated recommendations for use of VariZIG–United States, 2013. *MMWR Morb Mortal Wkly Rep.* 2013;62(28):574–576. [PMID: 23863705]

Clinical Findings

The usual incubation period of varicella is about 14–16 days. Most children experience a prodromal phase of upper respiratory–like symptoms for 1–2 days before the onset of the rash. Fever is usually moderate. Almost all infected children will develop a rash. The extent of the rash is highly variable. Lesions usually begin on the trunk or the head but can eventually involve the entire body. The classic lesion is a pruritic erythematous macule that develops a clear central vesicle. After 1–2 days, the vesicle ruptures, forming a crust. New lesions develop daily for 3–7 days, and typically lesions are scattered over the body in various states of evolution at the same time. Ulcerative lesions on the buccal mucosa are common. The infection is contagious from the onset of the prodrome until the last lesions have crusted over.

Differential Diagnosis

Varicella usually presents as an unmistakable clinical picture, but the rash may be missed in children with mild disease.

Complications

In immunocompetent children, the most common complication is bacterial superinfection of the lesions, causing cellulitis or impetigo. Other, more serious complications are most common in children age <5 years or adults age >20 years. Meningoencephalitis and cerebellar ataxia can occur. These normally resolve within 1–3 days without sequelae. Viral hepatitis is common but normally subclinical. Varicella pneumonia is uncommon in healthy children, and it usually resolves after 1–3 days but may progress to respiratory failure in rare cases.

Treatment

Treatment is ordinarily symptomatic, including antipruritic medications if needed. Aspirin should be avoided to prevent development of Reye syndrome. Oral acyclovir should be considered for healthy persons at increased risk for moderate to severe varicella (>12 years of age, chronic cutaneous or pulmonary disease, chronic salicylate user). Patients with signs of disseminated varicella, such as encephalitis and pneumonia, should be treated with intravenous acyclovir.

Prognosis

Varicella is normally a benign, self-limited disease. Complications in immunocompetent children are rare.

Patient Education

Further information is available at the following link:
https://familydoctor.org/condition/chickenpox/.

Measles

ESSENTIALS OF DIAGNOSIS

▶ Cough, runny nose, and conjunctivitis.

▶ Koplik spots.

▶ Onset of rash associated with high fever up to 103–105°F.

▶ Maculopapular rash starting on the face at the hairline and spreading downward.

General Considerations

Measles was declared eliminated from the United States in 2000 but has had a resurgence in 2019, mostly due to unvaccinated individuals. It also occurred from people infected in other countries who arrived in the United States. It tends to spread and cause outbreaks in communities where groups of people are unvaccinated. Evidence shows that there is no association of the measles-mumps-rubella (MMR) vaccine with autism spectrum disorder (ASD), nor is there increased risk in children who have an older sibling with ASD.

Pathogenesis

Measles is a highly contagious single-stranded RNA virus of the Paramyxoviridae family. It is transmitted by airborne droplets and can live for up to 2 hours in the airspace of the cough or sneeze from the infected person. Humans are the only host. It is contagious from 5 days before the appearance of the rash to 4 days after.

Prevention

Immunity is achieved by administration of the combination MMR vaccine usually given at 12–15 months of age, with a second dose given at 4–6 years of age or at least 28 days following the first dose. It may be administered to children as young as 6 months of age as an outbreak control measure, but these patients should then receive revaccination at 12–15 months and 4–6 years of age. For postexposure prophylaxis, intramuscular immunoglobulin should be given to all infants younger than 12 months of age; MMR vaccine can be given in place of immunoglobulin for infants age 6–11 months.

American Academy of Pediatrics. Section 3: summaries of infectious diseases, in *AAP Redbook*. Itasca, IL: American Academy of Pediatrics; 2018.

Clinical Findings

Measles is an acute viral disease characterized by fever, cough, coryza, and conjunctivitis, followed by a red maculopapular rash beginning on the face and spreading cephalocaudally and centrifugally. The rash blanches with pressure for the first 3–4 days and resolves in 3–6 days, fading in the order it appears. The pathognomonic enanthems of clustered white lesions usually appear opposite the lower first and seconds molars and are known as Koplik spots. They may present during the prodromal phase 2–3 days before the rash. They have been described as "grains of salt on a reddish background" and often fade as the rash develops.

Differential Diagnosis

The differential includes rubella, atypical measles, roseola infantum, erythema infectiosum (fifth disease), infectious mononucleosis, acute human immunodeficiency virus (HIV), and enteroviral infections.

Complications

Common complications include otitis media, bronchopneumonia, laryngotracheobronchitis, and diarrhea. One out of 1000 cases will develop acute encephalitis, which often results in permanent brain damage. One to three out of 1000 cases will die from respiratory and neurologic complications. This includes patients at higher risk such as infants and children <5 years old and patients with immune compromise such as from leukemia or HIV infection. A rare, fatal, and late complication occurring 7–10 years after infection is subacute sclerosing panencephalitis, which is a degenerative disease of the central nervous system.

Treatment

Medical care is supportive to relieve symptoms; there is no specific antiviral therapy. Complications such as secondary bacterial infections should be appropriately treated. Vitamin A administered once daily for 2 days is recommended by the World Health Organization for treatment of severe cases in hospitalized children.

Prognosis

The disease is self-limiting, and improvement usually occurs 3–4 days after the rash appears, although cough can last up to 2 weeks.

Patient Education

Further information is available at the following link:
https://www.cdc.gov/measles/about/parents-top4.html.

Erythema Infectiosum (Fifth Disease)

 ESSENTIALS OF DIAGNOSIS

▶ Prodrome of mild upper respiratory–like symptoms.
▶ Rash begins as erythema of cheeks ("slapped cheek appearance") and then becomes more generalized—macular at first, then reticular.
▶ Rash lasts 1–3 weeks.

General Considerations

Erythema infectiosum (fifth disease) is a common childhood infection that rarely causes clinically significant disease.

Pathogenesis

The disease is caused by parvovirus B19. It appears sporadically but often in epidemics in communities. Children are infectious during the prodromal stage, which is inapparent or mild and usually indistinguishable from an upper respiratory infection. The rash is an immune-mediated phenomenon that occurs after the infection; therefore, children with the rash are not infectious and should not be restricted from school or other activities.

Clinical Findings

Erythema infectiosum begins with a prodromal stage of upper respiratory symptoms, headache, and low-grade fever. This stage may be clinically inapparent.

The rash occurs in three phases, often transient enough to go unnoticed. The first stage is facial flushing, described as a "slapped cheek" appearance. Shortly afterward, the rash becomes generalized over the body, initially as a faint erythematous, often confluent, macular rash. In the third stage, central regions of the macules clear, leaving a distinctive faint reticular rash. After 1–6 weeks, the rash resolves but may reappear with sun exposure, heat, or stress.

Differential Diagnosis

Erythema infectiosum is usually clinically recognizable, but it may be confused with other viral exanthems.

Complications

Arthritis occurs in approximately 8% of cases, more commonly in teens and young adults. Thrombocytopenic purpura and aseptic meningitis are rare complications.

Fetal hydrops and fetal demise may be seen in fetuses whose mothers contracted the infection. It is estimated that ≤5% of infected fetuses will be affected by the virus.

Treatment & Prognosis

Treatment is symptomatic and includes nonsteroidal anti-inflammatory drugs for arthralgia and antihistamines for pruritus. Except for rare complications in children, this is a benign infection. Fetal complications are unusual.

Patient Education

Further information is available at the following link:
https://familydoctor.org/condition/fifth-disease/.

ATOPIC DERMATITIS

 ESSENTIALS OF DIAGNOSIS

▶ Pruritus is the cardinal symptom.
▶ Lesions are excoriated, scaly, and may become lichenified.

General Considerations

Atopic dermatitis is a common skin disorder in children, affecting 25% of children and 2–3% of adults. It appears during the first year of life in 60% of cases and during the first 5 years in 85%.

Pathogenesis

The cause of atopic dermatitis is unclear. It has a strong association, both in the individual and in families, with allergic rhinitis and asthma, as well as elevated IgE levels, and is classified as an atopic disorder. Food allergies, primarily to cow's milk, wheat, eggs, soy, fish, and peanuts, have been implicated in 20–30% of cases. In recent years, however, there has been a shift in thinking about cause and effect. Rather than being a primary allergic disorder that leads to changes in skin architecture, many authorities now consider atopic dermatitis to be primarily an epidermal barrier defect, which allows allergens, including food allergens, to penetrate the skin and stimulate an immune response. Risk factors include a family history of atopic dermatitis, numerous genetic mutations, and multiple environmental factors including living in an urban environment or regions with low exposure to ultraviolet radiation, small family size, and a "Western diet," among others.

Bieber T. Atopic dermatitis. *N Engl J Med.* 2008;358:1483–1494. [PMID: 18385500]

Clinical Findings

Pruritus is the hallmark of the disease, usually preceding the skin lesions, which generally develop as a reaction to scratching. The skin becomes excoriated, develops weeping and crusting, and later may become scaly or lichenified. Secondary bacterial infection is common. In infants, the lesions usually involve the face but may appear in a generalized pattern over much of the body. In young children, the extensor surfaces of the extremities are often involved. In older children and adults, the disease often moves to involve the flexion areas of the extremities instead. The disease typically is chronic, although remissions and relapses are common.

The United Kingdom Working Party's diagnostic criteria are the most studied criteria for the diagnosis of atopic dermatitis. The criteria require pruritic skin plus at least three of the following criteria: (1) visible dermatitis on flexural areas; (2) history of skin crease involvement such as the elbows, knees, ankles, or neck; (3) history of dry skin within the past 12 months; (4) history of asthma or allergic rhinitis; and (5) onset before age 2 years.

Differential Diagnosis

Atopic dermatitis may be confused with seborrheic dermatitis, especially in infants, in whom facial lesions are common.

Atopic dermatitis seldom follows the distribution of oil glands, as is typical with seborrheic dermatitis. It may also be confused with impetigo, psoriasis, contact dermatitis, scabies, and cutaneous fungal infections.

Complications

The most common complication is secondary bacterial infection. Low-grade bacterial infection should be considered as a factor in lesions that do not respond well to usual therapies. Additionally, persistent pruritus and resultant excoriation can lead to scarring and sleep disturbances.

Treatment

The management of atopic dermatitis is focused on relieving flares and preventing relapses. Patients should be advised to use topical steroids to resolve flares and emollients to preserve the epidermal skin barrier. Moisturizers should be applied regularly and soon after bathing to improve skin hydration. The lowest potency preparation and shortest duration of steroid therapy that are effective should be used, especially on the face and the diaper area, which are more sensitive to the skin atrophy associated with the prolonged use of higher-potency steroids. Intermittent use (1–2 times/week) of topical steroids as maintenance therapy on areas that commonly flare is a useful proactive way to prevent relapses. The use of high-potency steroids over large areas of the body has the potential for significant systemic absorption and suppression of the hypothalamic-pituitary-adrenal axis. Systemic steroids are useful for severe acute flares. Antipruritic medications, including first-generation H_1 antihistamines, may be useful, but these all have significant sedative side effects.

Tacrolimus and pimecrolimus, topical immune modulators, are less effective than high-potency topical steroids but appear to have the same efficacy as moderate-potency corticosteroids. They play a role in moderate to severe atopic dermatitis and in patients who are at risk for atrophy from topical steroids. Approved by the FDA in 2016, topical crisaborole (Eucrisa) is another nonsteroid medication indicated for mild to moderate atopic dermatitis. The American Academy of Dermatology recommends cyclosporine, azathioprine, and dupilumab for the most refractory cases.

Therapies with insufficient evidence to warrant routine use include second-generation H_1 antihistamines, homeopathy, Chinese herbal preparations, and probiotics.

Eichenfield LF, Tom WL, Berger TG, et al. Guidelines of care for the management of atopic dermatitis. *J Am Acad Dermatol.* 2014;71(1):116–132. [PMID: 24813302]

Williams HC, Burney PG, Pembroke AC, Hay RJ. The U.K. Working Party's Diagnostic Criteria for Atopic Dermatitis. III. Independent hospital validation. *Br J Dermatol.* 1994;131(3): 406–416. [PMID: 7918017]

Prognosis

Although it is fairly easy to control, atopic dermatitis is a chronic skin disorder. It becomes less severe in 70% of children as they grow into school age, but often relapses, and persistence of some disease into adulthood is common.

Patient Education

Further information is available at the following link:

https://www.aad.org/diseases/eczema/atopic-dermatitis-coping#overview.

▼ INFLAMMATORY DISORDERS OF THE SKIN

SEBORRHEIC DERMATITIS

 ESSENTIALS OF DIAGNOSIS

- ► Inflamed lesions with yellowish or brownish crusting.
- ► Lesions may be localized or generalized.

General Considerations

Seborrheic dermatitis is a common inflammatory disorder of the skin. It is most common in infancy and adolescence, when the sebaceous glands are more active. It generally resolves or becomes less severe after infancy, but localized lesions or mild, generalized scalp disease may be seen throughout adulthood.

Pathogenesis

The exact cause of seborrheic dermatitis is unknown. Infection with *Malassezia* yeasts has been implicated, and the disease may be caused by an abnormal inflammatory or immune response to the fungus.

Clinical Findings

The typical lesions of seborrheic dermatitis are inflammatory macular lesions, usually with brownish or yellowish scaling. Inflammation may begin during the first month of life, and it usually becomes evident within the first year. In infants, the lesions may be generalized, but in older children, lesions are most common in areas where sebaceous glands are concentrated, such as the scalp, face, thorax, and axillae. Marginal blepharitis may be seen. Cradle cap is a common variant seen in infants, either by itself or in association with other lesions. This is seen as scaling and crusting of the scalp, often with extremely heavy buildup of scale in untreated infants.

Differential Diagnosis

Atopic dermatitis is the main element in the differential diagnosis. The disease may also be confused with psoriasis and other cutaneous fungal infections.

Complications

Secondary infection, either bacterial or fungal, is a common complication.

Treatment

Topical treatment with antifungal creams or shampoo such as 2% ketoconazole is the mainstay of treatment. Low-potency topical steroids may be used for intense inflammation. Scalp lesions usually respond to antiseborrheic shampoos, such as selenium sulfide. Cradle cap is treated by soaking the scales with mineral oil and then gently débriding them with a toothbrush or washcloth. Following débridment, cleansing with baby shampoo is normally adequate for control; antiseborrheic or antifungal shampoos can be used in more extensive cases but are rarely necessary.

Clark GW, Pope SM, Jaboori KA. Diagnosis and treatment of seborrheic dermatitis. *Am Fam Physician*. 2015;91(3):185–190. [PMID: 25822272]

Prognosis

Seborrheic dermatitis generally resolves or lessens in severity after infancy, but localized lesions or mild, generalized scalp disease may be seen throughout adulthood.

Patient Education

Further information is available at the following link:
https://familydoctor.org/condition/seborrheic-dermatitis/.

ACNE VULGARIS

ESSENTIALS OF DIAGNOSIS

► Comedones, open or closed.
► Papules, pustules, or nodules.

General Considerations

Acne vulgaris is an extremely common skin disease in older children and adolescents. The prevalence of this disorder increases with age: 30–60% of 10–12-year-olds and 80–95% of 16- to 18-year-olds are affected.

Pathogenesis

Acne is caused by the interaction of several factors in the pilosebaceous unit of the skin. The basic abnormality is excessive sebum production caused by sebaceous gland hyperplasia and generally related to androgenic influences. Hyperkeratinization of the hair follicle results in obstruction of the follicle and the formation of a microcomedone. Sebum and cellular debris accumulate, forming an environment that can become colonized by *Propionibacterium acnes*. The presence of the bacteria provokes an immune response that includes the production of inflammatory mediators. Lesions are most commonly seen in areas of the body that have the highest concentration of sebaceous glands. The face is the most common site for lesions to develop, but the chest, back, neck, and upper arms may be affected as well. Comparatively, similar inflammatory lesions about the axilla and groin suggest hidradenitis suppurativa.

Although the androgenic influences that cause the increase in sebum production are generally related to puberty, numerous factors can cause or aggravate acne. Mechanical obstruction or irritation (eg, by shirt collars) can be a factor. Cosmetics can occlude follicles and trigger eruptions. Medications, most commonly anabolic steroids, corticosteroids, lithium, and phenytoin, can cause or aggravate acne. Hyperandrogenic states, such as polycystic ovarian syndrome, are often associated with acne. Emotional stress has been shown to exacerbate the problem as well. Finally, the role of diet has long been controversial. No specific foods have been found to aggravate acne, despite common assumptions. However, acne is almost uniformly a disease of Western cultures, and some authorities are studying the role of the high-glycemic-index Western diet in its development. This diet leads to higher levels of insulin-like growth factor, which has androgenic effects.

Clinical Findings

Several types of lesions characterize this disease, and they can occur in varying combinations and degrees of severity. Microcomedones can evolve into visible comedones, either open ("blackheads") or closed ("whiteheads"). Inflammatory papules and pustules may develop. Nodules are pustules with diameters of >5 mm. Hyperpigmentation and scarring may develop at the sites of more severe lesions.

Multiple classification systems have been devised to characterize this disorder. The disease may be classed as comedonal, papulopustular (inflammatory), and nodulocystic (also inflammatory, but more severe). The American Academy of Dermatology defines three levels of severity. In mild acne, there are a few to several papules and pustules, but no nodules. In moderate acne, there are several to many papules and pustules and a few to several nodules. In severe disease, there are extensive papules and pustules, along with many nodules.

Differential Diagnosis

The diagnosis is usually straightforward. The physician should consider drug-induced acne if the patient is taking any medications. Severe acne in athletes raises the possibility of anabolic steroid use. In women, severe acne, hirsutism, and other signs of virilization suggest an underlying hyperandrogenic condition, such as polycystic ovarian syndrome. Other conditions to be considered in the differential include rosacea, periorificial dermatitis, folliculitis, adenoma sebaceum of tuberous sclerosis, and keratosis pilaris.

Complications

The primary morbidity of acne is psychosocial. This can be a serious problem for the adolescent patient. Hyperpigmentation and scarring may result from more severe disease, especially from nodulocystic acne.

Treatment

The various treatments for acne are aimed at reducing infection and inflammation, normalizing the rate of desquamation of follicular epithelium, or correcting hormone excesses or other systemic factors. Treatments work better in combination than singly. Treatment choice is generally based on acne severity, location, and confounding factors.

A. Topical Antibiotics

Antibiotics are directed at the infectious component of acne. By reducing infection, they also have a beneficial effect on the inflammatory component of the disease. *P acnes* has been developing antibiotic resistance worldwide, and this may be responsible for some treatment failures.

Available topical antibiotic preparations include erythromycin, clindamycin, benzoyl peroxide, topical dapsone, and azelaic acid. Available evidence shows that erythromycin and clindamycin work better in combination with benzoyl peroxide than either agent alone, and this also limits the development of resistance. However, topical erythromycin has less efficacy than clindamycin due to bacterial resistance. The different strengths of benzoyl peroxide appear to be about equally effective.

B. Topical Retinoids

Retinoids are derivatives of vitamin A. They prevent the formation of comedones by normalizing the desquamation of the follicular epithelium. Tretinoin has been in use much longer than the other agents, adapalene and tazarotene. All agents have the main adverse effect of excessive drying, burning, and inflammation of the skin. This can be ameliorated by changing to a lower concentration of the agent or by periodically skipping a day of application. Topical adapalene, tretinoin, and benzoyl peroxide can be safely used in the management of preadolescent acne in children. Although tretinoin has been rated pregnancy category C, and there are no clear indications of teratogenicity, the role of topical retinoids in pregnancy is a matter of debate. Tazarotene has been designated pregnancy category X.

All agents are available in various strengths and vehicles. The choice of vehicle is determined by the patient's skin type.

C. Oral Antibiotics

It is generally believed that oral antibiotics are more effective than topical agents and therefore more useful in severe disease. However, because few, if any, good-quality comparisons of the two modalities exist, it is impossible to be certain of this. Tetracycline is the mainstay of oral antibiotic treatment. Side effects are minimal—primarily gastrointestinal upset. Doxycycline may be taken with food to minimize gastric upset, but this agent is more photosensitizing than tetracycline. Minocycline is a more effective agent against *P acnes* than the other tetracyclines, but it is more expensive and has a higher incidence of serious side effects, such as vertigo and lupus-like syndrome. It is generally best reserved for disease that does not respond to first-line agents. All tetracyclines bond to calcium in bone and teeth and can cause staining of dental enamel. They should not be given to children younger than 10 years of age. Azithromycin is not FDA approved for acne but can be considered as an alternative when tetracyclines cannot be used. The use of oral erythromycin should be restricted due to its increased risk of resistance. Systemic antibiotic use should be limited to the shortest possible duration and reevaluated at 3–4 months to minimize the development of bacterial resistance. Monotherapy with systemic antibiotics is not recommended.

D. Isotretinoin

Isotretinoin is a metabolite of vitamin A that reduces sebaceous gland size, decreases sebum production, and normalizes desquamation of follicular epithelium. It is effective for severe nodular acne and for acne unresponsive to other treatments. Adverse effects are common, including dry eyes, dry skin, headache, and mild elevation in liver enzymes and serum lipids. Benign intracranial hypertension is less common but must be considered if the patient develops headaches. Despite commonly held beliefs, evidence does not support the idea that depression is a side effect of this drug. Isotretinoin is extremely teratogenic, with major malformations occurring in 40% of infants exposed during the first trimester, so it must be used only after a negative pregnancy test—preferably after two negative tests—and with strict attention to contraception. Enrollment in the iPLEDGE program is a prerequisite to prescription of isotretinoin in the United States. This agent may also require close monitoring of liver function tests, as well as cholesterol and triglyceride levels, in certain patient populations.

E. Hormonal Therapy

Because of their net antiandrogenic effect, combined oral contraceptives are effective in reducing the severity of acne in women. Although some newer brands have been explicitly marketed for this indication, they have not been proved superior to older, less expensive brands. Spironolactone, an aldosterone antagonist, is not FDA approved for use in acne, but is often used for its antiandrogenic effects as well.

F. Combination Therapy

Agents for the treatment of acne work best in combination. The choice of agents can be tailored to the severity of the disease. Because of the time required for complete turnover of the epithelium, at least 6–8 weeks of treatment should be given before assessing the effectiveness of the regimen. If the disease is not adequately controlled, the regimen may be intensified (eg, by increasing the concentration of a retinoid, changing from a topical to an oral antibiotic, or adding another agent). Patients should be advised that total suppression of lesions may not be possible; otherwise, the patient's assessment can be used as a guide to decide whether more intensive treatment is necessary.

There are several guidelines for combination therapy:

- For patients with comedones only, retinoids are the first line of therapy. These are applied once a day to the entire area involved.

- For most patients with mild to moderate acne, combination treatment with topical antibiotics plus topical retinoids is the first-line treatment.

- For moderate to severe inflammatory acne, oral antibiotics can be added to, or substituted for, topical agents.

- For severe nodulocystic acne or for disease unresponsive to other regimens, isotretinoin is the treatment of choice.

G. Other Treatments

Intralesional steroids may be used as an adjunct for treating acne nodules. Laser and photodynamic therapy are newer options for acne treatment, with initial studies showing that they may be effective.

▶ Prognosis

Although in general, acne diminishes at the end of adolescence, it may persist into adult life.

▶ Patient Education

Further information is available at the following link: https://www.aad.org/self-care.

Zaenglein AL, Pathy AL, Schlosser BJ, et al. Guidelines of care for the management of acne vulgaris. *J Am Acad Dermatol.* 2016;74(5):945–973. [PMID: 26897386]

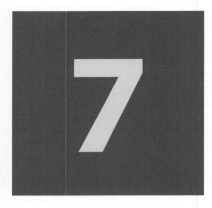

Routine Vaccines

Donald B. Middleton, MD

Routine vaccination is among the most significant of all medical advances and is a cornerstone for all preventive medical goals. Although many vaccine-preventable diseases (VPD) such as *Haemophilus influenzae* type b (Hib) infection are now rarely encountered, others such as pertussis persist despite widespread vaccination. Despite demonstrated vaccine effectiveness, concerns about vaccine efficacy, safety, and duration of protection continue to interfere with universal acceptance of some vaccines, and misinformation abounds. Important facets of vaccination include the patient's age and underlying medical conditions, disease burden, vaccine efficacy and adverse reactions, and official recommendations.

▶ General Rules for Vaccination

To achieve optimal protection, every clinician should vaccinate all patients in accordance with the timeline of the Centers for Disease Control and Prevention (CDC) universal vaccine schedules, found at https://www.cdc.gov/vaccines/schedules/index.html. The schedules are updated annually, so rather than printing any here, the reader is referred to CDC's website. Full compliance with CDC schedules now protects individuals against 16 VPDs, many of which have multiple types such as the 3 types of polio, 4 types of influenza, or 5 types of meningococcus. With few exceptions, notably rabies vaccine, all vaccine doses count for all time, even if separated by years, as long as minimal intervals are met. Prolonged delay between vaccine doses does not necessitate restarting a vaccine series, but a dose should not be given ≥4 days before the recommended age. A handy information source is the *Shots Immunizations App by AAFP and STFM* at https://www.aafp.org/patient-care/public-health/immunizations/shots-app.html, which is also downloadable to any iPhone/Android device. A useful childhood CDC Catch-Up Vaccine Scheduler is available at https://www.vacscheduler.org/index.html. Correct storage and management of vaccines are critical to effectiveness. These issues are covered in CDC publications and online at https://www.cdc.gov/vaccines/hcp/admin/storage/index.html. A discussion of specific vaccine products can be found on the Immunization Action Coalition website, which offers an exceptionally broad range of information in an easy-to-use format at http://www.immunize.org/.

HEPATITIS B VACCINE

Five hepatitis B vaccines (HepB) are available in the United States: Engerix-B or Recombivax HB, both monovalent vaccines given at birth and in a three-dose series at times 0, 1–2, and 6 months; Pediarix, a pentavalent vaccine given at age 2, 4, and 6 months (maximum age 6 years); Heplisav-B, given at time 0 and 1 month and at a minimum age of 18 years; and Twinrix, a bivalent vaccine given at time 0, 1, and 6 months and at a minimum age of 18 years. All children should be immunized against HBV. Adults with diabetes mellitus or other specific conditions like hepatitis C or travel or workplace risk (healthcare workers) should also be vaccinated (see https://www.cdc.gov/vaccines/hcp/vis/vis-statements/hep-b.html).

▶ Rationale for Routine Hepatitis B Vaccination

The estimated number of persons in the United States chronically infected with hepatitis B virus (HBV) is 1.25 million, 36% of whom acquired HBV during childhood. HBV infection becomes chronic in 90% of infected infants, 30–60% of those infected before the age of 4 years, and 5–10% of those infected as adults. Each year in the United States, HBV kills ≥2000 people. Up to 25% of infants infected with HBV will eventually die of HBV-related cirrhosis or liver cancer. Under universal hepatitis B vaccination, reported new cases of HBV fell to 3218 in 2016 (estimated real burden, 20,900). The source of HBV infection (usually blood or sexual contact) is not identified in 30–40% of cases. Hepatitis B surface antigen (HBsAg) has been found in impetigo, in saliva, on toothbrush holders of persons chronically infected with HBV, and on used blood sugar testing stylets. Infants and children can transmit HBV.

Efficacy for HepB is high. After the third dose of HepB, >95% of children seroconvert. Immunosuppression and prematurity with low birth weight are associated with lower rates of seroconversion, so HepB vaccination should be delayed in preterm infants weighing <2 kg until 1 month of age or hospital discharge, whichever is first, unless the mother is HBsAg-positive or has unknown HBsAg status, in which case HepB should be given within 12 hours of birth.

Adverse Reactions

Of all children given HepB, 3–9% have pain at the injection site; 8–18% have mild, transient systemic adverse events such as fatigue and headache; and 1–6% have temperature higher than 37.7°C (99.8°F). HepB does *not* cause immunologic dysfunction or diabetes mellitus.

Recommendations

The comprehensive US HBV vaccination policy includes the following: (1) routine vaccination of infants starting with monovalent HepB within 24 hours of birth, with dose 2 given at age 1–2 months and dose 3 at age 6–12 months; (2) catch-up immunization of adolescents not previously or fully vaccinated; and (3) immunization of unvaccinated adults age 19–59 years with diabetes mellitus (type 1 and type 2) as soon as possible after a diagnosis of diabetes is confirmed. Routine postvaccination testing is not indicated except for hepatitis B surface antibody (anti-HBs) and HBsAg testing at age 9–18 months for infants born to HBsAg-positive mothers and anti-HBs for healthcare workers. An adequate anti-HBs response is a titer of ≥10 mIU/mL. Postvaccination anti-HBs levels diminish over time, so low or absent serum antibody levels do not accurately predict susceptibility to HBV. Immunologic memory and the long incubation period of HBV infection enable most immunized persons to mount a protective anamnestic immune response. However, renal failure on dialysis necessitates higher antigen-content vaccines to maintain antibody level of ≥10 mIU/mL, measured annually.

HEPATITIS A VACCINE

All infants should receive two doses of hepatitis A vaccine (HepA), given at ages 12–15 and 18–21 months. Side effects include localized swelling and redness. Anyone wanting to be protected from hepatitis A virus should be given HepA at time 0 and 6 months. Hepatitis A is not a benign disease. Reported cases from 2016 to February 7, 2020, totaled 31,093, with 18,989 hospitalizations (61%) and 314 deaths (see https://www.cdc.gov/hepatitis/outbreaks/2017March-HepatitisA.htm). Homelessness and drug abuse are major causes of this increase.

PERTUSSIS VACCINE

A total of 15,609 cases of pertussis and 5 deaths were reported in the United States in 2018, representing hundreds of thousands of unreported infections (https://www.cdc.gov/pertussis/surv-reporting.html). Waning immunity after childhood pertussis vaccination, partial vaccine-induced protection, and alterations in pertussis surface proteins are apparent reasons for disease perpetuation. Most pertussis-related hospitalizations and deaths occur in infants too young to be fully vaccinated (see Pregnancy). Infants age <12 months suffer a case fatality rate of 0.6% but often have prolonged illness or hospital stays. Adults can suffer school or job loss, fractured ribs, or even strokes from chronic prolonged, powerful coughing.

Transmission is by respiratory droplets or by contact with freshly contaminated objects; 70–100% of susceptible household contacts and 50–80% of susceptible school contacts become infected following pertussis exposure. Contagion lasts from 1 week after exposure to 3 weeks after the onset of symptoms. Adults including healthcare workers and adolescents are the primary sources of pertussis infection for young infants. Intense, paroxysmal cough and malaise can last for months, with significant disruption of daily activities. Complications of pertussis include pneumonia, the leading cause of death, and seizures. Encephalopathy, due to hypoxia or minute cerebral hemorrhages, occurs in approximately 1% of cases, is fatal in about one-third of these, and causes permanent brain damage in another one-third.

Rationale for Vaccination

Before routine pertussis vaccination, peaks in whooping cough incidence occurred approximately every 3–4 years, infecting virtually all children. In the United States between 1925 and 1930, 36,013 persons died from pertussis-related complications. With widespread pertussis vaccination, the incidence of pertussis dropped by >95%, although it has been increasing in recent years, partly as a result of improved diagnostic techniques and a higher index of suspicion.

Adverse Reactions

Minor adverse reactions associated with diphtheria, tetanus, and acellular pertussis (DTaP) or tetanus toxoid, reduced diphtheria toxoid, and reduced acellular pertussis (Tdap) vaccination include injection site edema, fever, and fussiness. Previously reported uncommon adverse reactions with DTaP are no longer considered to be connected to the vaccine. Anaphylactic reaction to DTaP is a contraindication to further doses of DTaP/Tdap. Rarely, temporary swelling of the entire limb or a sterile abscess has occurred after DTaP vaccination.

Recommendations

All children should be vaccinated against pertussis at 2, 4, and 6 months of age with boosters at 15–18 months and 4–6 years (five total doses; maximum age, 6 years). Only four doses are needed if the fourth dose is given after the child's fourth birthday. All available pertussis-containing vaccines also vaccinate against tetanus and diphtheria. DTaP vaccines have efficacy rates ranging from 80 to 89%, but effectiveness wanes over time. Every adolescent and adult should receive one lifetime dose of Tdap. The Advisory Committee on Immunization Practices (ACIP) recommends a Tdap dose during each pregnancy, preferably at week 27–36 of gestation, regardless of prior Tdap administration (see Pregnancy). As of 2019, the CDC permits Tdap vaccine in place of tetanus and diphtheria (Td) to be used as the 10-year booster for tetanus protection.

DIPHTHERIA AND TETANUS

All persons need to be vaccinated against these two rare but dangerous diseases. Routine vaccination includes five DTaP vaccines doses during childhood, one Tdap in adolescence, and a Td or Tdap booster dose every 10 years thereafter for life. Guidelines for diphtheria and tetanus including wound control can be found at https://www.cdc.gov/mmwr/volumes/67/rr/pdfs/rr6702a1-H.pdf. As of 2019, Tdap may be used for all doses in tetanus prophylaxis for wounds and all doses of the catch-up immunization schedule for patients age ≥7 years (https://www.aafp.org/news/health-of-the-public/20191030acip.html).

PNEUMOCOCCAL CONJUGATE VACCINE

Prior to the introduction of pneumococcal conjugate vaccine, *Streptococcus pneumoniae,* a gram-positive diplococcus with >90 different polysaccharide capsules, caused ~17,000 cases of invasive disease (bacteremia, meningitis, or infection in a normally sterile site) each year in the United States, including 200 deaths annually among children age <5 years. Respiratory tract droplets spread infection. *S pneumoniae* remains a common cause of community-acquired pneumonia, sinusitis, otitis media, and bacterial meningitis.

▶ Rationale for Vaccination

Two vaccines protect against pneumococcus: the 23-valent polysaccharide vaccine (PPSV23) and the 13-valent conjugate vaccine (PCV13). PPSV23 does not produce an anamnestic response and thus may not induce long-lasting immunity and is not effective in children age <2 years. PCV13 elicits a T-cell reaction, leading to an anamnestic response, and thus it is effective in infants and induces long-lasting immunity. This vaccine reduces nasopharyngeal carriage rates and transmission of *S pneumoniae,* leading to herd immunity, including in older unvaccinated adults. PCV13's efficacy against invasive pneumococcal disease (IPD) is estimated at 94% for vaccine serotypes. Efficacy against clinical pneumonia is 11%; against clinical pneumonia with radiographic infiltrate, 33%;

and against pneumonia with radiographic consolidation of ≥2.5 cm (most typical of *S pneumoniae*), 73%. PPSV23 covers 11 different disease-causing pneumococcal types not in PCV13 and also reduces IPD.

▶ Adverse Reactions

No serious adverse reactions are associated with PCV13: 10–14% of vaccinees develop redness and 15–23% develop tenderness at the injection site. Fever of ≤38°C (≤100.4°F) occurs in 15–24% of vaccinees. PPSV23 causes injection site redness, pain, and swelling in ≤60%, but if given in too short a dose-spacing sequence (<5 years), it may induce serious skin reactions.

▶ Recommendations

The ACIP recommends four doses of PCV13 (age 2, 4, 6, and 12–15 months) for routine infant immunization. All children age 2–5 years who have not received PCV13 and all children age 6–17 years with chronic renal failure or nephrotic syndrome, functional or anatomic asplenia (eg, sickle cell disease or splenectomy), or immunosuppressive conditions (eg, congenital immunodeficiency or human immunodeficiency virus [HIV]), or who are receiving chemotherapy with alkylating agents, antimetabolites, or long-term systemic corticosteroids should receive one dose of PCV13. Children age ≥2 years with the conditions listed previously should receive a dose of PPSV23 in addition to PCV13 (see ACIP recommendations at https://www.cdc.gov/pneumococcal/vaccination.html). One-time PPSV23 revaccination after 5 years is recommended for immunocompromised or asplenic persons. The ACIP recommends that adults age ≥19 years with immunocompromising conditions including cancer, functional or anatomic asplenia, cerebrospinal fluid leaks, or cochlear implants receive a dose of PCV13 followed in 8 weeks by PPSV23. At least two higher valence conjugated pneumococcal vaccines are in development. See Adult Vaccines section for other age- and risk-based recommendations.

HAEMOPHILUS INFLUENZAE TYPE B VACCINE

All infants should receive either three doses of PRP-OMP (PedvaxHIB) at age 2, 4, and 12–15 months or four doses of other types of Hib vaccine at age 2, 4, 6, and 12–15 months. Combination vaccines that contain Hib serve to reduce the overall number of injections. Hib vaccine is not necessary above age 5 years except for splenic dysfunction or bone marrow transplant. Side effects are generally mild, including localized redness, pain, and swelling and low-grade fever.

POLIOVIRUS VACCINE

Poliovirus spreads to 73–96% of susceptible household contacts, primarily via the fecal-oral route (oral-oral possible). The incubation period ranges from 3 to 35 days. Up to 90%

Mumps produces excruciating, bilateral parotitis and sometimes pancreatitis, orchitis, cerebellar ataxia, or death. From January 1 to July 14, 2018, officials from 47 states reported 1,559 mumps cases to the CDC. Mumps outbreaks are common in camps, schools, and colleges and on teams. In 2018 officials from Alaska reported an as yet unabated mumps outbreak of 391 cases. Rubella causes posterior cervical adenopathy, arthralgia, and minimal rash, but it can also result in devastating congenital rubella syndrome. Clearly, continued emphasis on measles, mumps, and rubella (MMR) vaccine is warranted.

Rationale for Vaccination

The first dose of MMR protects 70–95% of children, necessitating a second vaccine dose to immunize 95–99% of vaccinees. To avoid interference from transplacentally conferred maternal antibodies, MMR vaccine is ideally given at age 12 months. Herd immunity with vaccination rates >95% is necessary to protect infants too young to be immunized. Measles immunity is probably lifelong in almost all persons who initially seroconvert; the rate of waning immunity is <0.2% per year.

Adverse Reactions

Pain, irritation, and redness at the injection site are common but mild. Reactions to MMR vaccine include fever (usually <38.8°C [102°F]) between days 7 and 12. The measles component can cause transient rash between days 5 and 20 or transient thrombocytopenia (1 in 25,000 to 2 million doses). Adverse reactions to rubella vaccine include generalized lymphadenopathy in children and transient arthralgia in young women, and adverse reactions to mumps vaccine include transient orchitis in young men. MMR does *not* cause autism.

Recommendations

The MMR vaccine is given routinely subcutaneously to all healthy children at age 12–15 months with a second dose at age 4–6 years. A second dose separated from the first by ≥3 months satisfies the requirements for the two-dose series. MMR is especially important for students planning to attend college. Combination MMR-V vaccine is approved for both the 1-year and 4- to 6-year doses, but because of a miniscule increase in febrile reactions in 1-year-olds, it is preferred only for the 4- to 6-year dose.

VARICELLA VACCINE

Varicella-zoster virus (VZV) causes chickenpox. The hospitalization rate was 5 cases per 1000 population. Because transmission rates are as high as 90% and communicability via aerosol droplets begins 1–2 days prior to rash onset, prevention of spread requires universal vaccination. Complications include secondary skin infection (impetigo and invasive group A streptococcal disease), pneumonia, and other severe disorders. VZV persists in the dorsal root ganglia and can reawaken to cause shingles later in life. The lifetime risk for herpes zoster (shingles) is 10–50%.

Rationale for Vaccination

Because VZV vaccination reduces hospitalization, routine vaccination is cost effective; each $1 spent on universal immunization avoids approximately $5 in costs. Varicella vaccine contains live attenuated virus and is 97% effective against moderate to severe disease. Postvaccination breakthrough disease is usually mild, producing fewer than 30 pox lesions. A two-dose vaccination strategy was adopted to reduce breakthrough cases.

Adverse Reactions

Following subcutaneous injection, local pain and erythema occur in 2–20% of vaccinees after the first dose and ≤47% after the second dose. Later, 5–40 days after administration, 4–10% of vaccinees develop a median of five varicella-like, short-lived (2–8 days) lesions. A brief, low-grade fever develops in 12–30% of vaccinees. Vaccine virus can rarely be transmitted to healthy immunocompetent persons. Persons with previously unrecognized prior immunization or VZV infection are not at increased risk from a dose of vaccine. Shingles is extraordinarily uncommon among vaccinees.

Recommendations

The ACIP recommends the first dose for age 12–15 months and the second dose for age 4–6 years with catch-up vaccination through 18 years of age for previously uninfected or unvaccinated children. Serologic tests are not required. Immunocompromised persons require no special precautions to avoid vaccinees except avoidance of direct contact with a vaccine-induced rash. (See Adults Vaccines section for shingles protection.)

Postexposure Prophylaxis

VZV vaccine is effective in modifying varicella if given within 3–5 days of exposure to wild varicella. Artificial varicella-zoster immune globulin (VariZIG) is recommended for exposed immunosuppressed patients, for pregnant women, and for infants of mothers who develop varicella 5 days before to 2 days after delivery (the period of in utero infection risk) and may be effective if given within 10 days of exposure.

MENINGOCOCCAL CONJUGATE VACCINE (MENACYW AND MENB)

In the pre–conjugate vaccine era, *Neisseria meningitidis,* the most common cause of bacterial meningitis in children and young adults in the United States, caused approximately

2200–3000 cases of invasive disease annually. Death occurs in ~10% of cases, and sequelae such as limb loss, neurologic disabilities, and hearing loss occur in 11–19%.

Many types, pathologic and benign, of *N meningitidis* commonly colonize the throat. It is transmitted via respiratory tract droplets and occurs sporadically most often in children age <5 years with a second bump in incidence in older teenagers and young adults. Serogroup B accounts for >30% of meningococcal disease, mostly in children age <2 years. Serogroup Y accounts for approximately 30% of sporadic cases, whereas serogroups A and C cause most outbreaks. A 2018 outbreak was serogroup W. In the prevaccine era, the incidence of meningococcal disease for college freshmen living in dormitories was 5.1 per 100,000, compared with 0.7 per 100,000 for other undergraduates and 1.4 per 100,000 in 18- to 23-year-olds in the general population. Quadrivalent meningococcal serogroups A, C, Y, and W (MenACWY) and monovalent MenB vaccines are probably both effective to stem meningococcal outbreaks.

▶ Vaccine Types

MenACWY is recommended for all adolescents at age 11–12 years, with a booster dose at age 16 years and catch-up vaccination for ages 13–18 years; for all persons age 2–55 years with high-risk medical indications, including asplenia or terminal complement deficiencies; and for travelers to hyperendemic areas such as sub-Saharan Africa. It provides long-term immunity and should replace polysaccharide vaccine. Two MenACWY brands exist for somewhat different age ranges: see the package inserts; the phone application *Shots Immunizations App by AAFP and STFM at* https://www.aafp.org/patient-care/public-health/immunizations/shots-app.html, which is embedded in the American Academy of Family Medicine phone app; or CDC information for details. MenACWY is available for infants at high risk; see CDC or *Shots* for details. Consideration should be given to vaccination against meningococcus group B with MenB at age 16 years. Two distinct, noninterchangeable MenB vaccines are available.

Following intramuscular injection, the most common adverse events are mild local pain, headache, and fatigue. Mild to moderate systemic reactions such as fever, fussiness, and drowsiness are infrequent.

ROTAVIRUS VACCINE

Prior to the introduction of rotavirus vaccine, rotavirus caused 2–3 million cases of gastroenteritis, 60,000 hospitalizations, and a reported 20–60 deaths annually in the United States. Two live oral rotavirus vaccines are licensed in the United States: pentavalent (RV5) and monovalent (RV1). The vaccines reduce hospitalization for rotavirus gastroenteritis by 85–100% and reduce rotavirus of any severity by 74–87%. The duration of immunity is not clear

but appears to wane in the second season after administration, at which point children are better able to tolerate infection if it occurs.

Beginning at age 6 weeks, all infants should receive either three doses of RV5 or two doses of RV1 by age 32 weeks. Doses are given 2 months apart. Side effects include vomiting, diarrhea, irritability, and fever. Intussusception after either RV1 or RV5 is rare.

HUMAN PAPILLOMA VIRUS VACCINE

To prevent anogenital cancers and genital warts, all children and adolescents age ≥9 years and adult women and men age ≤26 years should receive nine-valent human papillomavirus (HPV) vaccine. CDC recommends two doses 6 months apart at age 11–12 years (maximum age for first dose, ≤14 years) and three doses at time 0, 1–2, and 6 months for initial dose at age ≥15 years. Immunocompromised persons need three doses regardless of age at first dose. Using shared clinical decision making, HPV vaccine is now approved for men and women up to age 45 years (see https://www.cdc.gov/mmwr/volumes/68/wr/pdfs/mm6832a3-H.pdf). Side effects include local pain and swelling and syncope, necessitating 15–20 minutes of postvaccination observation in children and adolescents. The HPV vaccine's effectiveness is reflected in the 29% decrease in cervical cancer incidence rates for females age 25–34 years during the post-HPV vaccine availability period in 2011–2014 compared to the pre-HPV vaccine availability period of 2003–2006 and in the markedly reduced oral vaccine-type HPV carriage in vaccinated men.

ADULT VACCINES

All adults need annual influenza vaccine, at least one lifetime Tdap vaccine unless pregnant (see Pregnancy) followed by Td or Tdap vaccine every 10 years, three doses of HPV vaccine for unvaccinated persons age 21–26 years, two doses of shingles (recombinant) vaccine at age ≥50 years, and one PPSV23 at age ≥65 years. Using shared clinical decision making, PCV13 may be used in certain individuals age ≥65 years but is no longer routinely indicated at this age (https://www.cdc.gov/mmwr/volumes/68/wr/mm6846a5.htm). Younger immunocompromised adults such as those with cancer or HIV need PCV13, followed 8 weeks later by PPSV23. Individuals age 19–64 years who smoke or who have significant underlying medical disorders such as diabetes mellitus, asthma, chronic obstructive pulmonary disease, liver failure, or heart failure need PPSV23. The maximum number of adult lifetime doses is one PCV13 dose and three PPSV23 doses, spaced ≥5 years apart. Adults age ≥50 years, who almost universally have had chickenpox regardless of history, should be vaccinated with recombinant zoster vaccine, with two doses given at time 0 and 2–6 months. This vaccine is ~95% effective in preventing shingles and therefore postherpetic neuralgia. Live zoster vaccine is still approved for those age ≥60 years. Nonimmune individuals should also receive chickenpox, measles, mumps, and rubella vaccines. Some travel or underlying medical conditions are indications for hepatitis B, hepatitis A, Hib, or meningococcal vaccine. CDC updates schedules for adults annually. Schedules for adults, age-based indications, and medical or behavioral indications can be found at https://www.cdc.gov/vaccines/schedules/hcp/imz/adult.html. See Chapter 15 for more information on adult vaccines and schedules.

Shared Clinical Decision Making

CDC currently recommends that three vaccines be discussed using shared clinical decision making: MenB for adolescents, HPV for persons age 27–45 years, and PCV13 for persons age ≥65 years. Information about the advisability of using these vaccines is available in the *Morbidity and Mortality Weekly Report* and at the Immunization Action Coalition website.

Pregnancy

All women, pregnant or not, should receive annual flu vaccine. It can be given in any trimester. ACIP recommends a Tdap dose during each pregnancy, preferably at week 27–36 of gestation, regardless of prior Tdap administration to optimize transplacental antipertussis antibody to protect newborns through the first 2 months of life until they can be vaccinated. In a 2018 report among 675,167 mother-infant pairs, infants whose mothers received prenatal Tdap had a rate of pertussis 43% lower than infants whose mothers did not receive prenatal Tdap.

American Academy of Family Physicians. Shots Immunization App by AAFP and STFM. https://www.aafp.org/patient-care/public-health/immunizations/shots-app.html. Accessed February 17, 2020.

Centers for Disease Control and Prevention. Chapter 11: human papillomavirus. Hamborsky J, Kroger A, Wolfe S, eds. *Epidemiology and Prevention of Vaccine-Preventable Diseases*. 13th ed. Washington, DC: Public Health Foundation; 2015. https://www.cdc.gov/vaccines/pubs/pinkbook/supplement.html. Accessed February 17, 2020.

Centers for Disease Control and Prevention. Vaccines and Immunizations. www.cdc.gov/vaccines. Accessed February 17, 2020. Provides profuse information.

Immunization Action Coalition. Homepage. www.immunize.org. Accessed February 17, 2020. Provides profuse information.

Kimberlin DW, ed. *Red Book: 2018-2021 Report of the Committee on Infectious Diseases*. 31st ed. Itasca, IL: American Academy of Pediatrics, 2018.

Kroger AT, Duchin J, Vázquez M. General best practice guidelines for immunization. Best Practices Guidance of the Advisory Committee on Immunization Practices (ACIP). https://www.cdc.gov/vaccines/hcp/acip-recs/general-recs/index.html. Published 2017. Accessed August 23, 2018.

Behavioral Disorders in Children

Richard Welsh, LCSW, MSW
Marian Swope, MD

ATTENTION DEFICIT/HYPERACTIVITY DISORDER

 ESSENTIALS OF DIAGNOSIS

► Neurodevelopmental abnormalities with an early age of onset.
► Deficits on measures of attention and cognitive function.
► Hyperactivity.
► Impulsivity.

General Considerations

Up to 20% of school-aged children in the United States have behavioral problems, at least half of which involve attention and/or hyperactivity difficulties. Attention deficit/hyperactivity disorder (ADHD) is the most common and well-studied of the childhood behavioral disorders.

Clinical Findings

Individuals diagnosed with ADHD are likely to experience significant difficulties with executive functioning, which impairs academic performance, social relationships, self-control, and memory. Brown (2005) outlines six executive function deficits that are observed in individuals diagnosed with ADHD: (1) organizing and prioritizing (difficulty getting started on tasks); (2) focusing and sustaining attention (easily distracted); (3) regulating alertness, sustaining effort (drowsiness); (4) managing frustration (low frustration tolerance or disproportionate emotional reactions); (5) working memory (difficulty retrieving information); and (6) self-regulation (difficulty inhibiting verbal and behavior responses).

Brown TE. *Attention Deficit Disorder: The Unfocused Mind in Children and Adults.* New Haven, CT: Yale University Press; 2005.

There is no single diagnostic test or tool for ADHD. The diagnostic criteria included in the *Diagnostic and Statistical Manual of Mental Disorders,* fifth edition (DSM-5) are the current basis for the identification of individuals with ADHD. There is rarely a need for extensive laboratory analysis, but screening for iron deficiency and thyroid dysfunction is reasonable.

The American Academy of Child and Adolescent Psychiatry and the American Academy of Pediatrics (AAP), with input from members of the American Academy of Family Physicians, have formulated evidence-based practice guidelines to aid in the improvement of current diagnostic and treatment practices.

American Academy of Child and Adolescent Psychiatry. https://www.aacap.org. Accessed November 12, 2019.
American Academy of Pediatrics. https://www.aap.org/. Accessed November 12, 2019.

Differential Diagnosis

The diagnosis is made by parent interview, direct observation, and the use of standardized and scored behavioral checklists such as the Connors Parent and Teacher Rating Scales, Child Behavior Checklist, Vanderbilt ADHD Diagnostic Parent and Teacher Scales, and Achenbach Child Behavior Checklist, along with computerized tests (Gordon Diagnostic Testing, Connors Continuous Performance Task, and Test of Variables of Attention) measuring impulsivity and inattention that are specific for ADHD and should include input from both parents and teachers.

Complications

ADHD is often associated with other Axis I diagnoses. From 35% to 60% of referred ADHD children have oppositional defiant disorder (ODD), and 25–50% will develop conduct disorder (CD). Of these, 15–25% progress to antisocial personality disorder in adulthood. Of all referred ADHD children, 25–40% have a concurrent anxiety disorder. As many as 50% of referred children with ADHD eventually develop a mood disorder, most commonly depression, diagnosed in adolescence. The diagnosis of bipolar disease in childhood increases the risk of a concurrent label of ADHD because of the overlap of behaviors. About half the children with Tourette syndrome have ADHD.

There is a definite association among ADHD, academic problems, and learning disabilities. Between 20% and 50% of children with ADHD have at least one type of learning disorder.

► Treatment

A. Pharmacotherapy

1. Stimulants—Stimulant medications are the most frequently researched and the safest and most effective treatments for the symptoms of ADHD, but they are not a "cure." The fact that stimulants are controlled substances (schedule II) with an abuse potential justifies the close scrutiny of their use. About 65% of children with ADHD show improvement in the core symptoms of hyperactivity, inattention, and impulsivity with their first trial of a stimulant, and ≤95% will respond when given appropriate trials of various stimulants. The management of these medications can be complex, and treatment failures may more often be the result of improper treatment strategies than effective medication.

Perhaps the most important step is the choice of medications. Stimulants most commonly used include methylphenidate (Ritalin, Concerta, Metadate CD, Ritalin LA, Methylphenidate ER, Daytrana), dexmethylphenidate (Focalin), dextroamphetamine (Dexedrine, Vyvanse), and mixed amphetamine salts (Adderall). Novel drug delivery systems have been developed for stimulants, and these formulations have become routine in clinical practice.

Recently developed methylphenidate and amphetamine products include liquid, chewable, and orally disintegrating versions of each. Newer methylphenidate formulations include Quillivant, Quillichew, Cotempla XR ODT, Aptensio XR, and Jornay PM. Recent dextroamphetamine formulations include ProCentra and Zenzedi; recent amphetamine formulations include Adzenys ER and XR ODT, Evekeo, Dynavel XR, and Mydayis.

Absolute contraindications to the use of stimulants include concomitant use of monoamine oxidase (MAO) inhibitors, psychosis, glaucoma, underlying cardiac conditions, existing liver disorders, and a history of stimulant drug dependence. Adverse cardiovascular effects of stimulants have consistently documented mild increases in pulse and blood pressure of unclear clinical significance. Caution should be used in treating patients who have a family history of early cardiac death of arrhythmias or a personal history of structural abnormalities, palpitations, chest pain, and shortness of breath or syncope of unclear origin either before or during treatment with stimulants.

Because stimulants are Schedule II controlled substances, prescriptions with no refills are usually written monthly; however, several states allow 3-month prescriptions. Growth and vital signs should be checked and documented, and it is vital to monitor the medication effects and the child's progress. Issues to address include (1) adequacy and timing of the dosage, (2) compliance with the regimen, (3) changes in school or non–school-related activities that may affect medical therapy, and (4) maintenance of appropriate growth. An initial drop-off in weight gain may occur during titration phase, but over 2 years, this reverses, resulting in no long-term sustained growth suppression from stimulant use. Drug holidays are no longer standard procedure, but parents may opt for their children to have periods off the medications to minimize potential unknown drug effects or to assess the continuing need for the medication.

2. Nonstimulants—Many nonstimulant medications are being used for ADHD, alone and in combination with neurostimulants. Nonstimulant agents are less widely studied and are summarized here to inform the physician about their use. They vary from the tricyclic antidepressants to α-agonists (Tenex, Intuniv and Clonidine, Kapvay) to the highly selective catecholamine reuptake inhibitor atomoxetine (Strattera). Nonstimulants are often used to treat both ADHD and comorbid states, and their effectiveness alone is generally less than that of the neurostimulants. Fear and misunderstanding about the effects of neurostimulants make these nonstimulant agents attractive to parents.

B. Psychotherapeutic Interventions

1. Behavioral modification—Behavioral modifications are designed to improve specific behaviors, social skills, and performance in specific settings. Behavioral approaches require detailed assessment of the child's responses and the conditions that elicited them. Strategies are then developed to change the environment and the behaviors while maintaining and generalizing the behavioral changes. The most prudent approach to the treatment of ADHD is multimodal. The combination of psychosocial interventions and medications produces the best results.

2. Educational interventions—The education of children with ADHD is covered by three federal statutes: the Individuals with Disabilities Education Act (IDEA), Section 504 of the Rehabilitation Act of 1973, and the Americans with Disabilities Act (ADA) of 1990. The diagnosis of ADHD alone does not suffice to qualify for special education services. The ADHD must impair the child's ability to learn. A 1991 Department of Education Policy Clarification

Memorandum specifies three categories by which ADHD children may be eligible for special education: (1) health impaired (other documented condition such as Tourette syndrome), (2) specific learning disability (could be ADHD alone if there is a significant discrepancy between a child's cognitive ability or intelligence and his or her academic performance), and (3) seriously emotionally disturbed. It is therefore vital to document all comorbid conditions in these children.

3. Parent education and training—Parental understanding of ADHD is vital to successful treatment. Parents must know the difference between nonadherence and inability to perform. They need to understand that ADHD is not a choice but a result of nature. Many parents respond well to referral to local and national support groups such as Children and Adults with Attention Deficit/Hyperactivity Disorder (CHADD) or the Attention Deficit Disorder Association (ADDA).

Parent training programs such as developed by Russell Barkley and others provide confused and overwhelmed parents with specific management strategies shown to be effective in reducing noncompliance. In these group training sessions, parents are taught skills in how to more effectively communicate with their children, learn how to consequate noncompliance, and learn how to enhance school performance.

Treatment is less effective when both the parent and the child have ADHD. Since ADHD is inherited, treatment must address both the parent's and the child's ADHD. If parental ADHD is suspected, but not addressed, consistent management of the child cannot be achieved.

Additionally, marital dysfunction and divorce are not uncommon with couples who have children with ADHD or when one of the parents has ADHD.

4. Coaching—Coaching is a relatively new field that offers an adjunct to medical interventions.

Coaching differs from traditional counseling or psychotherapy. Instead, it focuses on teaching practical daily life skills such as time management and organization.

Unfortunately, coaches do not have to be licensed. However, many licensed mental health practitioners offer coaching services. The International Coach Federation does provide approved specialized training and ADHD certification. Other resources include the Institute for the Advancement of ADHD Coaching and the Professional Association of ADHD Coaches.

▶ Prognosis

Follow-up studies of children with ADHD show that adult outcomes vary greatly. There are three general outcome groups. The largest group is the 50–60% of affected children who continue to have concentration, impulsivity, and social problems in adulthood. About 30% of affected children function well in adulthood and have no more difficulty than controlled normal children. The final group represents about 10–15%, who, in adulthood, have significant psychiatric or antisocial problems. Predictors for bad outcomes include comorbid CD, low IQ, and concurrent parental pathology.

OPPOSITIONAL DEFIANT DISORDER

ESSENTIALS OF DIAGNOSIS

▶ Age-inappropriate display of angry, irritable, and oppositional behaviors that has occurred for at least 6 months.

▶ Behaviors are *not* part of a psychotic or mood disorder, nor is the diagnosis made if the criteria for CD are met.

▶ Physical aggression is *not* typical, nor are significant problems with the law.

▶ Progression to CD is rare.

▶ Not associated with any known physical or biochemical abnormality.

▶ General Considerations

The cause is generally related to social, parental, and child factors. A correlation exists between ODD and living in crowded conditions such as high-rise buildings with inadequate play space. There are strong correlations between the way parents act and oppositional behavior. Mothers, especially, demonstrate high levels of anxiety and depression. Family relationships, especially the marital relationship, tend to be strained. This sets up a vicious cycle as the child becomes increasingly insecure and more difficult to handle, conditions that prompt the parents to react with more rejection and anger.

▶ Prevalence

The reported prevalence of ODD varies from 2% to 16% of children and adolescents. Studies show an increasing rate of diagnosis from late preschool or early school-aged children to grade school to middle school to high school and then a decrease in college-aged individuals. Unlike gender differences in CD and ADHD, gender differences are minimal in ODD, and boys are only slightly more likely to receive a diagnosis of ODD than girls. Conclusive data on racial or cultural differences do not exist, but worldwide, ODD and CD are more prevalent among families of low socioeconomic status who tend to live in close quarters.

▶ Clinical Findings

Common manifestations of ODD include persistent stubbornness, résistance to directions, and unwillingness to negotiate and compromise with others. Defiant behaviors include persistent testing of limits, arguing, ignoring orders, and denying blame for most misdeeds. Hostility usually takes the form of verbal abuse and aggression. The most common setting is the home, and behavioral problems may not be evident to teachers or others in the community. Because the symptoms of the disorder are most likely to be manifested toward individuals that the patient knows well, they are rarely apparent during clinical examination. Children and adolescents with ODD do not see themselves as the problem, but instead view their behavior as a reasonable response to unreasonable demands.

Differential Diagnosis

Diagnosis is made by parent, patient, or teacher history and direct observation.

Behavioral checklists are available that can identify the pattern of ODD. They include the Child Behavioral Checklist. It is rare that any medical testing or neuropsychiatric testing is necessary, unless comorbid states are present. The DSM-5 presents specific diagnostic criteria for ODD.

Complications

ODD is common among children and adolescents with ADHD. The combination of ADHD, ODD, family adversity, and low verbal IQ are predictors of progression to more serious CD and antisocial behaviors as adults. However, although ≤50% of ADHD children have ODD behaviors, only ~15% of those diagnosed with ODD have ADHD.

Approximately 15% of ODD children have anxiety disorders, and approximately 10% have depression or mood disorders. Addressing these problems can often help with the oppositional behaviors.

Treatment

A. Behavioral Therapy

The vast majority of patients with ODD and their families can be managed with behavioral therapies, especially parental training and family therapy.

B. Medications for Oppositional Defiant Disorder

Medication for youth with ODD should not be the sole intervention and are primarily adjunctive, palliative, and noncurative. Medications may be beneficial in the context of other diagnoses and, as such, may be helpful adjuncts to a treatment package for symptomatic treatment and to treat comorbid conditions. For example, stimulants and atomoxetine may be useful in treating ODD in the context of another principal diagnosis such as ADHD. ODD behaviors in the context of an anxiety disorder or a depressive disorder may be successfully treated with a selective serotonin reuptake inhibitor. Aggressive and oppositional behaviors complicate a wide range of other diagnoses in this age range.

Therefore, medications should target specific syndromes as much as possible.

Loeber R, Burke JD, Lahey BB, et al. Oppositional defiant and conduct disorder: a review of the past 10 years, part 1. *J Am Acad Child Adolesc Psychiatry*. 2000;39:1468–1484. [PMID: 11128323]

Steiner H, Remsing L, Work Group on Quality Issues. Practice parameter for the assessment and treatment of children and adolescents with oppositional defiant disorder. *J Am Acad Child Adolesc Psychiatr*. 2007;46(1):126–141. [PMID: 17195736]

C. Pharmacotherapy for Comorbid Conditions

There is no accepted pharmacologic treatment for oppositional behaviors, but comorbid conditions such as ADHD or depression must be properly addressed and appropriately treated. For children who do not respond to nonmedical interventions or are extremely impaired, it is best to consult a pediatric psychiatrist. Medications used for ODD, comorbid with other conditions, include clonidine, lithium, carbamazepine, valproic acid, and risperidone; all have significant risks, and their use should be monitored carefully.

Prognosis

The most serious consequence of ODD is the development of more dangerous conduct problems. Although the majority of children with ODD will not develop CD, in some cases, ODD appears to represent a developmental precursor of CD. This seems to hold true for boys more than for girls. For children in whom such symptoms subsequently decrease with maturity, the prognosis is good. If oppositional behaviors progress and begin to involve the violation of others' rights, then the child will probably progress to CD.

American Academy of Child and Adolescent Psychiatry. *ODD: A Guide for Families*. https://www.aacap.org/App_Themes/AACAP/docs/resource_centers/odd/odd_resource_center_odd_guide.pdf. Accessed November 12, 2019.

Lavigne JV, Cicchetti C, Gibbons RD, et al. Oppositional defiant disorder with onset in pre-school years: longitudinal stability and pathways to other disorders. *J Am Acad Child Adolesc Psychiatry*. 2001;40:1393–1400. [PMID: 11765284]

CONDUCT DISORDER

ESSENTIALS OF DIAGNOSIS

► A repetitive and persistent pattern of behavior in which the basic rights of others and major age-appropriate societal norms are violated.

► Behaviors may be characterized by aggression toward people and animals, destruction of property, deceitfulness or theft, and serious violation of rules.

General Considerations

Conduct disorder (CD) constitutes a public health concern by contributing to school and gang violence, weapon use, substance abuse, and high dropout rates. It is therefore important to identify these behaviors and intervene as early as possible.

The risk of CD is higher in children whose biological or adoptive parents have antisocial personality disorder, and siblings of children with CD have a higher risk for developing the condition as well. CD is also more common in children whose biological parents have ADHD, CD, alcohol dependence, mood disorders, and schizophrenia.

There is no doubt that the caregiver–child interaction contributes to disruptive behavior. Factors in these relationships include (1) low levels of parental involvement in the child's activities, (2) poor supervisions, and (3) harsh and inconsistent disciplinary practices. The child views behavioral problems as strategies to secure attention and become closer to the caregiver or parent. Neighborhood and peer factors also contribute to the incidence of CD. Poverty, living in crowded conditions in a high-crime neighborhood, and having a "deviant" peer group all increase the risk of CD.

Prevalence

The prevalence of CD varies from 1% to 10% overall, depending on the studied population, with ranges of 6–16% in boys and 2–9% in girls younger than 18 years. CD tends to increase from middle childhood to adolescence. Although certain behaviors (eg, physical fighting) decrease with age, the most serious aggressive behaviors (eg, robbery, rape, and murder) increase during adolescence. The differing incidence of CD in boys and girls does not occur until after age 6 years, and boys and girls with CD manifest different behaviors. Boys exhibit more fighting, stealing, vandalism, and school discipline problems, whereas girls are more likely to lie, be truant, run away, and abuse substances.

Clinical Findings

There are four main groupings of behaviors in CD: (1) aggression toward people or animals, (2) destruction of property, (3) deceitfulness or theft, and (4) serious violation of rules. Behavioral disorders must be differentiated from normal reactions to abnormal circumstances. The DSM-5 states that the diagnosis of CD should not be made when behaviors are in response to the social context. Screening questions might include asking about troubles with police, involvement in physical fights, suspensions from school, running away from home, sexual activity, and the use of tobacco, alcohol, and drugs.

Differential Diagnosis

A clear majority (75%) of children with CD have at least one other psychiatric diagnosis. Of all children with CD, 30–50% also have ADHD. A significant proportion of children present with symptoms of both ADHD and CD, and both conditions should be diagnosed when this occurs. Comorbid ADHD and CD are consistently reported to be more disabling than either disorder alone. Finally, children with comorbid ADHD and CD appear to have a much worse long-term outcome than those with either disorder alone.

Other psychiatric diagnoses commonly seen in association with CD include anxiety disorders, mood disorders, substance abuse, schizophrenia, somatoform disorder, and obsessive-compulsive disorder. This is not surprising, considering that these diagnoses are more common in the parents of children with CD.

Intermittent explosive disorder features sudden aggressive outbursts that are usually unprovoked. These individuals do not intend to hurt anyone but say that they "snapped" and, without realizing it, attacked another person. Intermittent explosive disorder is distinguished from CD in that these episodes are the only signs of behavioral problems and these individuals do not engage in other rule violations. The treatise by Green (2010) is an excellent reference for diagnosis and treatment recommendations.

Green R. *The Explosive Child*. New York, NY: Harper Collins; 2010.

Treatment

A key element in the initial treatment of these children is to obtain parental involvement. Although many parents of children with CD have problems themselves, they do not want their children to follow their path. All parties need to be aware of the possibility of a poor prognosis without the interventions of the caregiver.

A. Behavioral Interventions

Behavioral interventions are similar to those for ODD. Collaborative resources such as school counselors, residential care, juvenile court designated workers, and the Department of Social Services can provide wraparound services for children and adolescents who are generally unmotivated and resistive to any type of intervention that may be necessary.

B. Psychopharmacology

Psychopharmacologic interventions alone are insufficient to treat youth with CD. Medications are best seen as adjunctive treatments. Very often, youths with CD have other diagnoses. Because aggression, mood lability, and impulsivity may be seen in a wide range of comorbid diagnoses, these symptoms may be targets for pharmacologic interventions. Antidepressants, anticonvulsants, lithium carbonate, α-agonists, and antipsychotics have been used clinically. The potential side effects of various classes of medications may potentially outweigh their benefits.

Steiner H. Practice parameters for the assessment and treatment of children and adolescents with conduct disorder. *J Am Acad Child Adolesc Psychiatry*. 1997;36(10):122S–139S. [PMID: 9334568]

▶ **Prognosis**

The social burden and public health concerns associated with CD make diagnosis and treatment of this condition very important. About 40% of children with early-onset CD are diagnosed in adulthood with antisocial personality disorder or psychopathology. Overall, approximately 30% of children with CD continue to demonstrate a repetitive display of illegal behaviors. Antisocial behavior rarely begins in adulthood, and the family cycle of such behaviors is difficult to break.

American Academy of Child and Adolescent Psychiatry. Conduct disorder. https://www.aacap.org/AACAP/Families_and_Youth/Facts_for_Families/FFF-Guide/Conduct-Disorder-033.aspx. Accessed November 12, 2019.

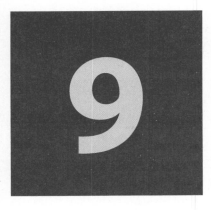

Seizures

Donald B. Middleton, MD

ESSENTIALS OF DIAGNOSIS

- ▶ Occurrence of an aura.
- ▶ Alteration in or impaired consciousness or behavior.
- ▶ Abnormal movement.
- ▶ Interictal trauma or incontinence.
- ▶ Eyewitness account.
- ▶ Presence of fever.
- ▶ Postictal confusion, lethargy, sleepiness, or paralysis.
- ▶ Diagnostic electroencephalogram.
- ▶ Abnormality on neuroimaging.

▶ General Considerations

Despite an alarming appearance, a single seizure rarely causes injury or permanent sequelae or signals the onset of epilepsy. The lifetime risk for seizure is about 10%, but only 2% of the population develops unprovoked, recurrent seizures (epilepsy). *Epilepsy* is usually defined as repetitive, often stereotypic seizures, but even a single seizure coupled with a significant abnormality on neuroimaging or a diagnostic electroencephalogram (EEG) can signify epilepsy. Seizure incidence is high in childhood, decreases in midlife, and then peaks in the elderly. The annual number of new seizures during childhood is 50,000–150,000, only 10,000–30,000 of which constitute epileptic seizures. In 2010, active epilepsy afflicted 1% of all adults in the United States and 1.9% of those with family incomes below $35,000. During childhood, the incidence of partial seizures is 20 per 100,000; generalized tonic-clonic seizures, 15 per 100,000; and absence seizures, 11 per 100,000. About 25% of new-onset seizures occur in adults age ≥65 years.

After a single seizure, about 30% of children get a medical evaluation, but >80% of children with a second seizure obtain medical assistance. Approximately 50% of adults with epilepsy have seen a neurologist. A recognizable, treatable seizure etiology; a negative family history; a normal physical examination; a lack of head trauma; a normal EEG; and normal neuroimaging indicate a low risk for seizure recurrence. Each year, approximately 3% of 6-month-old to 6-year-old children have a febrile seizure, the most common childhood seizure entity. The likelihood of these children developing epilepsy is extremely low even if the febrile seizure recurs.

▶ Pathogenesis

A seizure results from an abnormal, transient outburst of involuntary neuronal activity. Common etiologies are structural, genetic, infectious, metabolic, immune, or unknown defects. Anoxic degeneration, focal neuron loss, hippocampal sclerosis (common in temporal lobe epilepsy), and neoplasia are examples of pathologic central nervous system (CNS) changes that can produce seizures. Why a seizure spontaneously erupts is unclear.

Seizures are either generalized (a simultaneous discharge from the entire cortex) or focal (partial, a discharge from a focal point within the brain) or both. Generalized seizures impair consciousness and, except for some petite mal (absence) spells, cause visible abnormal movement, usually intense muscle contractions termed *convulsions*. Because generalized convulsions occur most commonly in the absence of a focal defect, the initiating mechanism of a generalized seizure is less well understood than that of a focal seizure, which often initiates from a CNS lesion. Focal seizures may either impair consciousness (complex) or not (simple) and can start with almost any neurologic complaint, termed the *aura*, including abnormal smells, visions, movements, feelings, or behaviors such as nonresponsiveness. Focal seizures can progress to and thus mimic generalized seizures, a fact that sometimes obscures the true nature of the problem because the commotion of the convulsion dominates recall of events.

The etiology of epilepsy in childhood is 68% idiopathic, 20% congenital, 5% traumatic, and 4% postinfectious, but only 1% each vascular, neoplastic, and degenerative. The latter three are much more common in adulthood: 16% vascular, 11% neoplastic, and 3% degenerative. Complex partial seizures, the most difficult type to control, afflict 21% of children; generalized tonic-clonic seizures, the easiest to control, 19%; myoclonic seizures, often difficult to recognize because of limited motor activity, 14%; absence seizures, rare in adults, 12%; simple partial seizures, 11%; other generalized seizures, 11%; simultaneous multiple types, often syndrome associated, 7%; and other types, 5%. In adults, 39% of epilepsy cases are complex partial seizures, 25% generalized, 21% simple partial, and 15% other types.

The majority of convulsions are due to an inciting event such as head trauma; CNS infection; drug ingestion including some common over-the-counter drugs such as antihistamines; or metabolic abnormalities such as hypoglycemia, hyponatremia, or alcohol withdrawal. The cause of many reactive seizures remains unknown. Nonspecific etiologies such as stress or sleep deprivation are often assumed to lower the seizure threshold. Impact seizures are common after head trauma, but the 5-year risk for epilepsy is only 2%. On the other hand, 15–30% of children with depressed skull fractures develop epilepsy. Syncopal episodes from any cause with diminished CNS perfusion can result in minor twitching or even major tonic-clonic seizures that do not portend epilepsy.

Unprovoked seizures are more likely to be epilepsy. The majority of epileptic seizures have no known cause and thus are termed *cryptogenic*. Those with identifiable causes such as prior head trauma are called *symptomatic*. If genetic inheritance is at fault, the epilepsy is *idiopathic*. Genetic predisposition to epilepsy has been determined for many entities, including tuberous sclerosis and juvenile myoclonic epilepsy, which affects 1–3 per 1000 persons and is linked to 15 different chromosomal loci. A genetic predisposition to seize given the proper stimulus is probably distributed throughout the population.

Table 9–1 presents a scheme of seizure description to guide treatment and predict outcome. Some forms of epilepsy are specially categorized as epilepsy syndromes (eg, infantile spasms [West syndrome] or benign childhood epilepsy with centrotemporal spikes [rolandic epilepsy]). Table 9–2 lists a general classification of epilepsy syndromes.

▶ Prevention

Primary prevention begins in pregnancy. Pregnant women must avoid addictive drug use (alcohol, cocaine, benzodiazepines), trauma (automobile safety), and infection (young kittens with toxoplasmosis). Birth trauma and cerebral

Table 9–1. Classification of seizures.

I. Generalized
  A. Convulsive: tonic, clonic, tonic-clonic
  B. Nonconvulsive: absence (petit mal), atypical absence, myoclonic, atonic
II. Partial (focal or localization related)
  A. Simple (consciousness preserved): motor, somatosensory, special sensory, autonomic, psychic
  B. Complex (consciousness impaired): at onset, progressing to loss of consciousness
  C. Evolving to secondary generalized
III. Unclassified
  A. Syndrome-related: West syndrome (infantile spasms), Lennox-Gastaut syndrome, neonatal seizures, others
  B. Other etiology

anoxia, the leading causes of cerebral palsy, are unfortunately persistent difficulties despite efforts to reduce incidence. Family history may reveal significant errors of metabolism (Gaucher disease) or genetic disorders, some of which are amenable to treatment. Strict compliance with childhood immunizations to prevent CNS infection, especially pertussis, pneumococcal, or *Haemophilus influenzae* type b infection; attention to safety throughout life beginning in infancy (using car seats, wearing bicycle helmets, supervision when swimming or in the bathtub, wearing seatbelts); and avoidance of addictive drugs (alcohol, cocaine, phencyclidine) are examples of appropriate primary seizure prevention strategies. Annual influenza vaccination decreases the potential for febrile illness and secondary seizures, especially in persons with epilepsy. A full night's sleep, regular exercise, and a well-rounded diet are important in the primary prevention of seizures.

Secondary prevention requires attention to the triggers, such as drugs that lower seizure threshold or cause seizures de novo (Table 9–3). Some children seize after prolonged fasting, possibly from hypoglycemia (eg, the unfed infant who seizes on Sunday morning when the parents oversleep, known as the "Saturday night seizure"). Stimulation from light or noise, startle responses, faints, metabolic derangements, and certain videogames, television shows, or computer programs can cause seizures. Avoidance of any known precipitant reduces the future likelihood of another event. Although a convulsion can cause significant injury on its own, accident prevention is paramount. Individuals with newly diagnosed epilepsy should not drive until seizure-free for 6 months, swim or take baths alone, or engage in potentially dangerous activities such as climbing on a roof. Patient education and referral to sources such as the Epilepsy Foundation (http://www.epilepsyfoundation .org/) play important roles in keeping patients and families healthy and active.

Table 9–2. Abbreviated classification of epilepsies and epileptic syndromes.

I. Localization-related (focal, local, partial) epilepsies and syndromes
   A. Idiopathic (genetic) with age-related onset
      1. Benign childhood epilepsy with centrotemporal spikes (rolandic or BECTS)
      2. Childhood epilepsy with occipital paroxysms
      3. Primary reading epilepsy
   B. Symptomatic (remote or preexisting cause)
   C. Cryptogenic (unknown etiology)
II. Generalized epilepsies and syndromes
   A. Idiopathic with age-related onset, in order of age at onset
      1. Benign neonatal familial convulsions
      2. Benign neonatal convulsions
      3. Benign myoclonic epilepsy in infancy
      4. Childhood absence epilepsy (pyknolepsy)
      5. Epilepsy with grand mal seizures on awakening
      6. Other
   B. Cryptogenic and/or symptomatic epilepsies in order of age at onset
      1. Infantile spasms (West syndrome)
      2. Lennox-Gastaut syndrome
      3. Other
   C. Symptomatic
      1. Nonspecific etiology
      2. Specific syndromes
         a. Diseases presenting with or predominantly evidenced by seizures
III. Epilepsies and syndromes undetermined as to whether they are focal or generalized
   A. With both types
      1. Neonatal seizures
      2. Severe myoclonic epilepsy in infancy
      3. Acquired epileptic aphasia (Landau-Kleffner syndrome)
   B. Without unequivocal generalized or focal features
      1. Sleep-induced grand mal
IV. Special syndromes
   A. Situation-related seizures
      1. Febrile convulsions
      2. Related to other identifiable situations: stress, hormonal changes, drugs, alcohol, sleep deprivation
   B. Isolated, apparently unprovoked epileptic events
   C. Epilepsies characterized by specific modes of seizure precipitation
   D. Chronic progressive epilepsia partialis continua of childhood

Data from Berg AT, Berkovic SF, Brodie MJ, et al: Revised terminology and concepts for organization of seizures and epilepsies: report of the ILAE Commission on Classification and Terminology, 2005–2009. *Epilepsia.* 2010 Apr;51(4):676–685.

▶ Clinical Findings

A. Symptoms and Signs

The clinician must decide whether a neurologic event could be a seizure and, if so, what evaluations are necessary (Table 9–4) and whether treatment is required to prevent

Table 9–3. Drugs linked to seizures.

A. Over-the-counter drugs
   1. Antihistamines: cold remedies
   2. Ephedra: common in diet supplements
   3. Insect repellents and insecticides: benzene hexachloride
   4. "Health" and "diet" drugs: ginkgo
B. Prescription drugs
   1. Antibiotics: penicillins, imipenem, fluoroquinolones; acyclovir; ganciclovir; metronidazole; mefloquine; isoniazid
   2. Asthma treatments: aminophylline, theophylline, high-dose steroids
   3. Chemotherapeutic agents: methotrexate, tacrolimus, cyclosporine
   4. Mental illness agents: tricyclics, selective serotonin reuptake inhibitors, methylphenidate, lithium, antipsychotics, bupropion
   5. Anesthetics and pain relievers: meperidine, propoxyphene, tramadol; local (lidocaine) or general anesthesia
   6. Antidiabetic medications: insulin and oral agents
   7. Antiepilepsy drugs: carbamazepine
   8. Miscellaneous: some β-blockers, immunizations, radiocontrast
C. Drugs of abuse
   1. Alcohol
   2. Cocaine
   3. Phencyclidine
   4. Amphetamine
   5. LSD (lysergic acid diethylamide)
   6. Marijuana overdose
D. Drug withdrawal
   1. Benzodiazepines: diazepam, alprazolam, chlordiazepoxide; flumazenil in benzodiazepine-dependent patients
   2. Barbiturates
   3. Meprobamate
   4. Pentazocine may precipitate withdrawal from other agents
   5. Alcohol
   6. Narcotics
   7. Antiepileptic drugs: rapid drop in levels

Data from Koppel BS. Toxins and drugs reported to induce seizures. https://www.epilepsy.com/learn/professionals/resource-library/tables/toxins-and-drugs-reported-induce-seizures. Accessed February 7, 2020.

recurrence. The consequences of diagnosing a seizure include consideration of the effects on the family, school, driving, activities, work, and plans such as pregnancy. The primary tool for seizure assessment is the history, including (1) age at onset; (2) family history; (3) developmental status; (4) behavior profile; (5) intercurrent distress, including fever, vomiting, diarrhea, headache, or other illness; (6) precipitating events, including exposure to flashing lights, toxins, or trauma; (7) sleep pattern; (8) diet; and (9) licit (smoking, alcohol) and illicit drug use. A critical feature pointing to a partial seizure is the occurrence of an aura, although a brief aura can also accompany a generalized seizure. Any symptom can constitute an aura, which usually requires more extensive evaluation for a focal CNS lesion. Because 20% of childhood seizures occur only at night, a description of early-morning

Table 9–4. Historical evaluation of possible seizure.

I. Behavior: mood or behavior changes before and after the seizure
II. Preictal symptoms or aura
   A. Vocal: cry or gasp, slurred or garbled speech
   B. Motor: head or eye turning, chewing, posturing, jerking, stiffening, automatisms (eg, purposeless picking at clothes or lip smacking), jacksonian march, hemiballism
   C. Respiration: change in or cessation of breathing, cyanosis
   D. Autonomic: drooling, dilated pupils, pallor, nausea, vomiting, urinary or fecal incontinence, laughter, sweating, swallowing, apnea, piloerection
   E. Sensory changes
   F. Consciousness alteration: stare, unresponsiveness, dystonic positioning
   G. Psychic phenomena: delusion, déjà vu, daydreams, fear, anger
III. Postictal symptoms
   A. Amnesia
   B. Paralysis: ≤24 hours, may be focal without focal CNS lesion
   C. Confusion, lethargy, or sleepiness
   D. Nausea or vomiting
   E. Headache
   F. Muscle ache
   G. Trauma: tongue, broken tooth, head, bruising, fracture, laceration
   H. Transient aphasia

Data from the National Institute for Health and Clinical Excellence (NICE). *The Epilepsies: The Diagnosis and Management of the Epilepsies in Adults and Children in Primary and Secondary Care.* London, United Kingdom: National Institute for Health and Clinical Excellence (NICE); 2012 (Clinical Guideline 137).

Table 9–5. Some causes of seizures.

Cause	Examples
Reflex	
Visual	Photic stimulation, colors, television, videogames
Auditory	Music, loud noise, specific voice or sound
Olfactory	Smells
Somatosensory	Tap, touch, immersion in water, tooth brushing
Cognitive	Math, card games, drawing, reading
Motor	Movement, swallowing, exercise, eye convergence, eyelid fluttering
Other	Startle, eating, sudden position change, sleep deprivation
Genetic	Neurofibromatosis, Klinefelter syndrome, Sturge-Weber syndrome, tuberous sclerosis
Structural	Hippocampal sclerosis, neoplasia, cerebral atrophy (dementia)
Congenital	Hamartoma, porencephalic cyst
Cerebrovascular	Arteriovenous malformation, stroke
Infectious	Syphilis, tuberculosis, toxoplasmosis, HIV infection, meningitis, encephalitis
Metabolic	Porphyria, phenylketonuria, electrolyte disorder (eg, hypoglycemia, hypocalcemia, hypomagnesemia), hyperosmolality, hyperventilation, drugs
Trauma	Depressed skull fracture, concussion
Other	Collagen vascular disease (systemic lupus erythematosus), eclampsia, demyelinating disease (multiple sclerosis), blood dyscrasias (sickle cell disease, idiopathic thrombocytopenia), mental disease (autism)

behavior, including transient neurologic dysfunction or disorientation, is important. Reports of preictal, ictal, and postictal events from both the patient and witnesses help clarify the seizure type and therapy.

Mental retardation and cerebral palsy are among the most common conditions associated with epilepsy. Other cognitive disorders linked to epilepsy include attention deficit/hyperactivity disorder, learning disorders, and dementia. Associated psychological difficulties such as depression; psychoses; anxiety disorders, including panic attacks; eating disorders, such as anorexia nervosa; or personality disorders are common in epilepsy and often make recognition or control of seizures difficult. In adults, sleep apnea can cause recurrent seizures. The myriad causes of seizures (Table 9–5) require diligence to elucidate.

1. Generalized seizures—Tonic-clonic (grand mal) seizures are both the most common and the most readily recognized. A short cry just before the seizure, apnea, and cyanosis are usual. The majority of these seizures are reactive, do not recur, last <3 minutes (usual maximum 15 minutes), and have no major sequelae. Following a convulsion, Todd postictal paralysis can persist for ≤24 hours even without an underlying structural lesion. When myoclonic or tonic-clonic

epilepsy begins between ages 8 and 18 years, prospects for permanent remission are poor: about 90% relapse when antiepileptic drug (AED) treatment is stopped. About 3% of children have febrile seizures, which are most often tonic-clonic.

Typical absence spells (petit mal) are brief (10- to 30-second) losses of consciousness and unresponsive stare with occasional blinking, chewing, or lip smacking without collapse. Common between ages 3 and 20 years, these spells often can be precipitated by photic stimulation or hyperventilation and interrupt normal activity only briefly. Up to 50% of petit mal seizures evolve into tonic-clonic seizures, especially if the onset is during adolescence. Approximately 10% of epileptic children have atypical absence spells with some motor activity of the extremities, duration >30 seconds, and postictal confusion. Many of these children are mentally handicapped. Both types of absence spells can occur up to hundreds of times per day, creating havoc with school performance and recreational activities.

2. Focal (partial) seizures—Benign epilepsy with centrotemporal spikes (BECTS) accounts for 15% of all epilepsy, has an onset between ages 2 and 14 years, and often presents in the early morning with guttural noises and tonic or clonic face or arm contractions. An aura of numbness or tingling in the mouth can precede arrest of speech and excessive salivation in a conscious child. Although not dangerous, nocturnal BECTS may generalize into grand mal convulsions. Approximately 20% of these children have only one episode; 25% develop repetitive seizures unless treated. By age 16 years, almost all are seizure free.

The classic, albeit rare, simple partial seizure is the jacksonian march, an orderly progression of clonic motor activity, distal to proximal, indicating a focal motor cortex defect. The arm on the side to which the head turns may be extended while the opposite arm flexes, creating the classic fencer's posture. Many of these seizures generalize into clonic-tonic convulsions.

Myoclonic jerks consist of single or repetitive contractions of a muscle or muscle group and account for 7% of seizures in the first 3 years of life. Benign occipital epilepsy has an onset between ages 1 and 14 years, with a peak incidence between ages 4 and 8 years, and consists of migraine-like headaches with vomiting, loss of vision, visual hallucinations, or illusions. Episodes usually stop during adolescence.

Complex partial seizures usually begin after age 10 years and last 1–2 minutes each. Consciousness may be lost at onset or gradually; postictal confusion occurs in 50–75%. Behavior alteration, including hissing, random wandering, sleepwalking, and irrelevant speech; affective changes such as fearfulness or anger; and autonomic dysfunction such as vomiting, pallor, flushing, enuresis, falling, and drooling demonstrate the variety of manifestations. Especially common are changes in body or limb position, ictal confusion, and a dazed expression. The child always exhibits amnesia for these events.

Syndromes usually present with several different types of seizures closely linked in time. Myoclonic jerks, grand mal seizures, and absence spells in a mentally deficient individual suggest Lennox-Gastaut syndrome.

Videos of seizures are on many websites including https://epilepsyontario.org/research-and-resources/seizure-videos/ and https://www.clinicalneurologyvideos.com/classification-of-seizures-videos.

B. Physical Findings

Fever is the most important physical finding. A stiff neck coupled with a fever mandates a lumbar puncture. Focal infection such as pneumonia or otitis media can cause febrile seizures. Keeping current with immunizations is the best preventive measure. The presence of a rash may guide the differential. Many febrile seizures are linked to viral infections like herpesvirus 6, the cause of roseola with its typical rash.

Abnormal neurologic findings such as focal paralysis or facial asymmetry point to the need for imaging studies. Seizures often complicate cerebral palsy or stroke. Failure to return to baseline alertness in short order should trigger more intensive evaluation. Café-au-lait spots (neurofibromatosis), adenoma sebaceum and hypopigmented spots (tuberous sclerosis), port-wine stain (Sturge-Weber), or cutaneous telangiectasia (Louis-Bar) on the skin or cherry red spots in the eyes (Tay-Sachs) clue the diagnosis. Primary or metastatic cancer is a particularly important consideration in smokers or those with unexplained weight loss, human immunodeficiency virus (HIV) infection, or lymphadenopathy.

Trauma such as a fractured tooth or broken bone provides definitive evidence of seizure activity. Trauma is generally absent if syncope is at fault. Other significant complications of seizures include lacerations, dislocations, concussion, aspiration pneumonia, arrhythmias, pulmonary edema, myocardial infarction, drowning, and death. Well-intentioned but misdirected bystanders who attempt to stop the seizure or stop the tongue from "being swallowed" can lead to trauma. Lacerations or fractures can suggest child abuse; shaken baby syndrome with CNS hemorrhage can present with a seizure.

C. Laboratory Findings

The decision to perform tests is based on (1) the patient's age (patients <6 months require action); (2) history of preceding illness, especially diabetes mellitus, gastroenteritis, and dehydration; (3) history of substance abuse or drug exposure; (4) type of seizure (eg, complex partial seizures); (5) failure to return to normality following a seizure; and (6) interictal abnormal neurologic examination. Table 9–6 lists the usual evaluations. The majority of evidence fails to support routine testing, especially for first-time, tonic-clonic seizures.

Routine blood tests are more often abnormal in patients with isolated seizures than in those with epilepsy, but electrolytes are universally normal in a normal-appearing child with a new-onset nonfebrile seizure. Glucose, magnesium, and calcium levels and complete blood counts (CBCs) usually are normal, but persons taking carbamazepine, diuretics, or other medications can develop hyponatremia. A high creatine phosphokinase or prolactin level (performed within 10–30 minutes of the seizure) may indicate prior generalized seizure activity with the exception of absence and myoclonic types. Other helpful evaluations include toxicology screens, pregnancy tests, and psychometric studies. Lumbar puncture is required for suspected meningitis, which is unusual in a fully immunized person. Meningococcal meningitis is most likely to affect young infants, first-year college students

Table 9–6. Recommendations for evaluation of a first seizure.

Study	Recommendation	Strength of Recommendation[a]
Electroencephalogram	All patients (somewhat in debate)	A
Blood tests (electrolytes, glucose, blood urea nitrogen, creatinine, calcium, magnesium)	Individual basis: especially indicated for age ≤6 months; continued illness; history of vomiting, diarrhea, dehydration, or diuretic use	A
Toxicology screening	Possible drug or substance of abuse exposure	C
Lumbar puncture	Possible meningitis or central nervous system (CNS) infection; continued CNS dysfunction	B
CNS imaging Computed tomography (CT) Magnetic resonance imaging (MRI)	Value limited largely to head trauma Best performed for: Prolonged postictal paralysis or failure to return to baseline Persistent significant cognitive, motor, or other unexplained neurologic abnormality Age <12 months Perhaps with partial seizures An EEG indicative of nonbenign seizure disorder	A A
Prolactin level	Variable benefit; 10–30 minutes after a seizure	B
Creatine kinase level	Variable benefit	C

[a]A, supported by clinical studies and expert opinion; B, expert opinion; limited evidence for support; C, limited to specific situations; insufficient evidence for or against this evaluation.

residing in a dormitory room, or travelers returning from the Middle East.

An EEG is diagnostic in 30–50% of first-time seizures; accuracy improves to 90% with repetitive testing. A focally abnormal EEG suggests the need for neuroimaging. An EEG is not necessary for a single febrile seizure. Up to a one-third of seizure victims with normal EEGs eventually are proven to have epilepsy. Awake, asleep, sleep-deprived, hyperventilation, and light-stimulated EEG tracings are best at uncovering an abnormality. Because tracings within 48 hours of a seizure may be falsely abnormal (generalized slowing is common), the optimal timing for an EEG is in debate. EEG patterns are particularly diagnostic in absence spells, BECTS, and juvenile myoclonic epilepsy. Video EEG recording can verify a seizure diagnosis or detect psychogenic seizures, and 24-hour EEG monitoring often reveals an unexpectedly high seizure frequency.

Many experts advise that an EEG is indicated for all patients with first nonfebrile seizures or repetitive febrile seizures, ~5% of whom develop epilepsy. However, obtaining an EEG after the first seizure may not be worthwhile because obtaining an EEG in some children is difficult and ~2% of normal children have abnormal EEGs. If the EEG is abnormal, treatment with an AED often causes new dilemmas. Seizure reoccurrence is ~50% with an abnormal EEG and <25% with a normal EEG. Neuroimaging deserves similar consideration,

but in the absence of other abnormalities, an underlying brain tumor in children and adolescents is rare while seizures are not. In an international review of 3291 children with brain tumors, only 35 otherwise normal children (1%) had a seizure as the initial difficulty. However, neuroimaging for the onset of epilepsy before age 3 years reveals etiologic relevant abnormalities in 40% of infants. The key is to perform a complete physical examination and provide follow-up. In older children and adolescents with normal exams, parental or patient acquiescence with a decision to delay evaluation until a second seizure occurs is generally advisable. Routine neuroimaging in adults is advisable but is complicated by the finding of incidental, nonpathologic lesions.

If neuroimaging is done, magnetic resonance imaging (MRI) is preferred over computed tomography (CT) scanning. Although abnormalities are detected in up to one-third of MRIs, only 1–2% of these findings influence either treatment or prognosis, especially in otherwise normal children. Table 9–7 lists recommended evaluations for neuroimaging for each seizure type. Conversely, some studies have found that ~25% of adults with new-onset seizures have epileptogenic lesions on MRI. With focal seizures, ~50% have a focal lesion, including ~15% with tumors.

In sum, neuroimaging is most useful for focal neurologic abnormalities; those with a history of infection, deteriorating behavior or school function, or trauma; the young infant;

Table 9–7. Imaging recommendations for childhood seizures.

Seizure Type	Imaging Study
Neonatal	Cranial ultrasound preferred CT acceptable
Partial	MRI preferred CT acceptable

Generalized
  Neurologically normal
  Neurologically abnormal
	MRI or CT but low yield
	MRI preferred
	CT acceptable

Intractable or refractory	MRI preferred SPECT acceptable PET acceptable
Febrile	No study
Posttraumatic (seizures within 1 week of trauma)	CT preferred MRI acceptable

CT, computed tomography; MRI, magnetic resonance imaging; PET, positron emission tomography; SPECT, single-photon emission computed tomography.

those with persistent focal seizures (except BECTS); focal EEG abnormalities; persons age >18 years; or those with status epilepticus (27% have abnormal MRI findings). Prior to CNS surgery to treat epilepsy, MRI or cerebral angiography and positron emission tomography (PET) scans are needed to assess the feasibility and extent of the procedure.

Differential Diagnosis

Seizure mimics in infants include gastroesophageal reflux, brief shuddering, benign nonepileptic myoclonus like the Moro reflex; in toddlers, breath-holding spells, night terrors, and benign paroxysmal vertigo; and in older persons, tics, behavior problems, hysteria, panic attacks, transient global amnesia, and hyperventilation. Persons with psychogenic seizures (pseudoseizures) must be evaluated for psychiatric disturbances, especially depression or suicidal ideation. Psychogenic seizures account for 20% of referrals to epilepsy centers and often coexist with true seizures. Malingering to avoid stressful situations such as school (bullying is a risk factor) and true conversion reactions are in the differential. Malingering patients may use soap to simulate frothing at the mouth, bite their tongues, or urinate or defecate voluntarily to simulate seizures. The differential diagnosis includes drugs of abuse, narcolepsy, migraine, Tourette syndrome, shuddering attacks, hereditary tremors, and cough-induced or vasovagal syncopal convulsions. Syncopal seizures, uncovered through tilt-table testing, are best treated with control of syncope, not as seizures. Cardiac entities such as prolonged QT interval (electrocardiogram) or aortic stenosis or hypertrophic cardiomyopathy (echocardiogram) should be considered in those with a family history of fainting or suggestive physical findings. Specialist consultation, video EEG recording, 24-hour EEG recording, and watchful waiting almost always provide the correct diagnosis eventually.

Treatment

Four components constitute the cornerstones of epilepsy treatment: (1) avoidance of participating factors; (2) lifestyle modifications, including daily sleep regimens and exercise; (3) AEDs; and (4) surgery for localized seizure foci.

A. First Aid and Initial Care

Acute assistance for a seizure requires placing the patient prone, removing eyeglasses, loosening clothing and jewelry, and clearing the area of harmful objects, but *not* putting any object into the patient's mouth or attempting to apply any restraint. If a patient is diabetic, sublingual glucose (tablets or solution) or sucrose may help. After the seizure, the patient should be placed on one side and observed until awake. Families should call for medical assistance if a seizure lasts longer than 3 minutes, the patient requests assistance or is injured, or a second seizure occurs. After a tonic-clonic seizure, vigorous stimulation may reduce postictal apnea and perhaps sudden death. To reduce the risk of sudden death, patients with epilepsy should be encouraged to sleep in the *supine* position. Hospitalization is necessary only if the patient is at high risk, lives alone without appropriate supervision, or remains ill. Postictal confusion, sleepiness, headache, muscle soreness, and lethargy are common. Patients and families appreciate an explanation of what transpired, information as to how to avoid further difficulties, and definite follow-up arrangements. Avoidance of seizure-provoking activities and provocative drugs or behaviors is appropriate treatment for reactive seizures.

B. Pharmacotherapy

Reactive seizures with correctable causes or unprovoked seizures that are benign or infrequent do not require AEDs. Many experts do not use AEDs for a single seizure; medication side effects include worsening seizure severity or frequency, organ damage, and even death. AEDs do not positively affect long-term prognosis or always provide complete seizure control; 20–30% of those on AEDs still have significant seizure activity.

All primary care physicians should have a command of basic AED use and side effect profiles. In addition to carbamazepine, phenytoin, and valproic acid, three other AEDs approved for generalized tonic-clonic and partial epilepsy are worth attention: (1) lamotrigine approved for those age >2 years, (2) levetiracetam for those age >1 month and for myoclonic epilepsy in those age >12 years, and (3) topiramate for persons age >2 years. Table 9–8 provides information on

Table 9–8. Drugs for the treatment of seizures.

Drug	Seizure Type	Pediatric Dosage (mg/kg)		Adult Starting Daily Dose (Maximal Dose [mg])	Number of Daily Doses	Therapeutic Level (µg/mL)	Dosage Forms			Notes
		Starting Dose	Usual Daily Dose				Pill (mg)	Liquid		
Lamotrigine	GM, CPS, SPS	0.15–0.6	1–15	100 (700)	2	Variable	CT: 2, 5, 25; T: 25, 100, 150, 200	—		Gen/Tr (some forms)
Topiramate	GM, CPS, SPS	1–3	5–9	25 (400)	2	Variable	C: 15, 25; T: 25, 50, 100, 200	—		Tr only
Phenytoin	GM, CPS, SPS	5 orally, 10–20 intravenously	5–15	100 TID (700) (1500 loading dose)	1–3	10–20	C:100; EC: 30, 100; CT: 50	S:125 mg/5 mL (use not recommended)		Gen/Tr (some forms)
Carbamazepine	GM, CPS, SPS	5–10	15–30	200 TID (2000)	2–4	4–12	T: 200; CT:100; ET: 100, 200, 300, 400	S:100 mg/5 mL		Gen/Tr (some forms)
Valproic acid	GM, PM, CPS, SPS, M	10–15	15–60	250 BID (3000)	2–4	50–120	C: 250; CS: 125; ET: 500; DT: 125, 250, 500	SY: 250 mg/5 mL		Gen/Tr (some forms)
Ethosuximide	PM	10–20	10–40	250 BID (2000)	1–2	40–100	C: 250	SY: 250 mg/5 mL		Gen/Tr (some forms)
Clonazepam	M	0.01–0.03	0.025–0.2	0.5 TID (20)	2–3	18–80	T: 0.5, 1, 2	—		Gen/Tr
Gabapentin	Additive only; GM, CPS, SPS	10–15	25–50	100 TID (4800)	3	>2	C: 100, 300, 400, 800; T: 100, 300, 400, 600, 800	Sol: 250 mg/5 mL		Tr
Primidone	GM, CPS, SPS	10	10–30	100 QHS (1500)	2–4	5–15	T: 50, 250	—		Gen/Tr (some forms)
Levetiracetam	GM, CPS, SPS, M	10	20–60	500 BID (3000)	1–2	Not established	T: 250, 500, 750, 1000; ET: 500, 750	Sol: 300 mg/5 mL		Gen/Tr

BID, twice a day; C, capsule; CPS, complex partial seizure; CS, capsule sprinkles; CT, chewable tablet; DT, delayed-release tablet; EC, extended-release capsule; ET, extended-release tablet; Gen, generic; GM, grand mal; M, myoclonic; PM, petit mal; QHS, every night at bedtime; S, suspension; Sol, solution; SPS, simple partial seizure; SY, syrup; T, tablet; TID, three times a day; Tr, trade.

selected AEDs. Some drugs (acetazolamide, adrenocortico-tropic hormone, brivaracetam, clobazam, eslicarbazepine, ezogabine, felbamate, lacosamide, nitrazepam, oxcarbaze-pine, perampanel, pyridoxine [vitamin B_6], rufinamide, tiagabine, vigabatrin, and zonisamide) usually require spe-cialist guidance, whereas others, including gabapentin, pregabalin, clonazepam, ethosuximide, and primidone, are often well known to primary care physicians.

The selection of AED is based on the seizure type, which is unfortunately inaccurately identified ~25% of the time. The least toxic AED, usually carbamazepine, lamotrigine, valproate, or levetiracetam, is initiated. Primary general-ized seizures respond best to monotherapy with levetirace-tam or valproate, which control seizures in 80% of cases. Lamotrigine and carbamazepine are also good choices to control tonic-clonic or partial convulsions. Ethosuximide is ideal for absence spells, with lamotrigine and valproate as alternatives. Sometimes difficult to control, juvenile myo-clonic epilepsy responds best to valproate or levetiracetam. Gabapentin or pregabalin can be added when control of sei-zures is inadequate. Any new symptom or sign in a patient on an AED must trigger a search in a standard reference for AED side effects (Table 9–9). These are sometimes serious and often unfamiliar to primary care physicians. Many of the newer agents are also expensive. Generic lamotrigine, topira-mate, levetiracetam, and valproate are inexpensive. Because of its side effects, phenytoin has fallen from favor but is still frequently prescribed because it is among the cheaper

effective AEDs. For a patient on phenytoin, whenever any drug is added to or withdrawn from the medical regimen, a serum phenytoin level should be obtained, usually 5–7 days later. Phenobarbital should not be used. For home treatment of acute repetitive seizures, rectal diazepam gel (0.2–0.5 mg/kg) and buccal or intranasal midazolam liquid (0.25–1 mg/kg) are safe and effective.

Use of one drug to control seizures—increased to its maximum dose or to just below toxicity—is best. If one drug proves to be ineffective, another AED is started while the current AED is withdrawn slowly over ≥1 week. Polyther-apy is fraught with drug side effects and often loss of seizure control, but to achieve satisfactory control, it is necessary to administer two drugs in 25% of patients. Complex focal seizures are difficult to control, hence the large numbers of agents available to treat this condition. Neurologic consulta-tion is often a superior choice to random new drug use.

Serum AED levels to guide dosage should be obtained: (1) as a check on compliance; (2) to detect toxicity, especially with multiagent regimens or in the young or mentally handi-capped; (3) when the drug regimen is changed; (4) for poor seizure control; and (5) when a problem develops that can affect drug levels. Table 9–10 provides a scheme for monitor-ing the effects of three common AEDs: valproate, phenytoin, and carbamazepine. Valproate levels often fail to predict either toxicity or seizure control. The recommended time for measurement is just before the next dose is taken (trough level) or during an acute event to check compliance. Leveti-racetam has become a favored AED because it has no known drug interactions. The therapeutic range for levetiracetam is 12–46 µg/mL, with >46 µg/mL considered potentially toxic.

Whether seizure-free patients require periodic drug level monitoring is unclear. Growing children may need levels more often, but after informing patients and parents about the plan, allowing a seizure-free child to "grow out" of the AED like a slow taper of medication seems reasonable. In some circumstances such as pregnancy or salicylate use, free AED (non–protein bound) serum levels may be a better guide to dosing, especially for phenytoin and valproate.

Whether routine checks of hematologic or liver functions can prevent organ damage is also unclear. All patients and parents should be warned to be alert for fever, jaundice, itch-ing, bruising, and bleeding as signs of toxicity. Many phy-sicians follow CBCs, liver and renal tests, and serum AED levels periodically, once or twice a year.

Some AEDs, especially carbamazepine, phenytoin, prim-idone, and topiramate, may interfere with oral contracep-tives. Midcycle bleeding indicates possible oral contraceptive failure. Management includes alternative contraceptive methods, a higher estrogen content product, or a noninter-acting AED such as gabapentin, levetiracetam, or valproate. Some AEDs may increase the risk of suicide, but the overall risk is low. In one large study, suicidal ideation was found in 0.43% of patients on AEDs compared to 0.22% on placebo,

Table 9–9. Side effects of selected antiepileptic drugs.

Drug	Common Side Effects
Phenytoin	Hirsutism, coarse facial appearance, gum hyperplasia, nystagmus
Carbamazepine	Hyponatremia (in ≤10% of patients)
Valproic acid	Hair loss, weight gain, edema, pancreatitis, thrombocytopenia
Lamotrigine	Life-threatening rash (as high as ~1 out of 50 children; first 2 months of treatment)
Phenobarbital	Personality change
Topiramate	Renal stones, weight loss
Zonisamide	Renal stones
Ethosuximide	Abdominal pain, abnormal behavior
Levetiracetam	Dizziness, behavioral changes, severe rash
Gabapentin	Nausea, lethargy, behavioral changes

Reproduced with permission from Treatment Guidelines from The Medical Letter, June 2013; vol. 11 (126):9–18. www.medicalletter.org.

Table 9–10. Recommended monitoring parameters for antiepileptic drugs.

Drug	Monitoring
Carbamazepine	Complete blood count (CBC) with platelets at baseline, then twice monthly for first 2 months, and annually or as clinically indicated Blood chemistries with emphasis on hepatic and renal function and electrolytes at baseline, then at 1 months, and annually or as clinically indicated Electrocardiogram (ECG) at baseline for patients >40 years and as clinically indicated
Phenytoin	CBC at baseline and as clinically indicated Blood chemistries with emphasis on hepatic and renal functions at baseline, annually, and as clinically indicated ECG at baseline for patients >40 years and as clinically indicated Phenytoin level in 1 weeks, then in 1 month, and annually or as clinically indicated in older patients
Valproic acid	CBC with platelets at baseline, then twice monthly for first 2 months, and annually or as clinically indicated Blood chemistries with emphasis on hepatic function at baseline, then at 1 month, and annually or as clinically indicated Prothrombin time, international normalized ratio, and partial prothrombin time at baseline and annually Valproic acid level weekly for 2 weeks, then annually or as clinically indicated in older patients

Data from the National Institute for Health and Clinical Excellence (NICE). *The Epilepsies: The Diagnosis and Management of the Epilepsies in Adults and Children in Primary and Secondary Care.* London, United Kingdom: National Institute for Health and Clinical Excellence (NICE); 2012 (Clinical Guideline 137).

but another study found no direct link. Some AEDs (phenobarbital, carbamazepine, phenytoin) may adversely affect bone density, necessitating preventive vitamin D and calcium supplements.

No specific seizure-free time interval predicts resolution of epilepsy. A single seizure type, normal neurologic examination, normal intelligence quotient (IQ), and normal EEG all predict good outcomes if the AED is stopped. In one study of 1013 patients free of seizures for 2 years, 40% had a recurrence following drug withdrawal, compared with 12% of those who maintained AED treatments. Freedom from drug side effects and daily medication must be weighed against this 28% difference with potential loss of job or driving ability or possible injury. A recent abnormal EEG makes the decision to stop therapy more difficult. Most AEDs should be slowly withdrawn over at least 6–12 weeks. During withdrawal, recurrence of the aura signals that the risk of seizure recurrence is high. Once children grow into young adulthood, assuming a 2- to 5-year period without seizures, attempts to stop AED treatment ought to be strongly considered.

During pregnancy, since many AEDs can cause fetal malformations, the AED that controls seizures the best, except possibly valproate, should be continued. Lamotrigine and levetiracetam are the safest, with rates of malformation similar to placebo. A fetal sonogram can identify malformations. Folic acid, 4 mg daily, and vitamins D and K during the last 4 weeks of pregnancy minimize fetal problems. Serum AED levels during pregnancy are helpful. Women who take AEDs can safely breastfeed.

C. Referral or Hospitalization

Poorly controlled or complicated seizures or progressive developmental delay should prompt neurologic consultation. Hospitalization is necessary for prolonged or complicated seizures, status epilepticus, inadequate family resources, or parental or physician concern. In general, seizures are not dangerous and do not cause CNS damage, but persons with repetitive seizures must be guarded from injury (eg, helmets) and other complications.

D. Surgery and Other Treatments

Treatments that require referral and extensive evaluation prior to institution include vagal nerve stimulation, ketogenic diet, and surgery. Vagal nerve stimulation is less invasive than surgery and controls or reduces seizures in ~40% of patients with previously refractory epilepsy. The ketogenic diet reduces episodes by ~50%, but compliance is difficult.

Many experts believe that surgical correction for epilepsy is underutilized. At least 20% of patients with epilepsy are inadequately controlled with AEDs alone, and some, even if controlled, may benefit from surgery because of reduced seizure frequency or AED side effects. Surgery for specific epilepsy types, including temporal lobe lesion resection, results in 80% seizure-free outcomes. Indications for surgery include recurrent uncontrolled seizures, focal EEGs, consistent focal abnormalities on neuroimaging, or major AED side effects. Unfortunately, PET or single-photon emission CT (SPECT) imaging often reveals unsuspected abnormalities that may preclude surgical correction.

E. Family Counseling

Family members, caregivers, teachers, and coworkers need instruction in proper seizure first aid. Helpful information and group support are available from the American Epilepsy Society (http://www.aesnet.org), the Epilepsy Foundation of America (http://www.epilepsyfoundation.org/), or local epilepsy foundations. Vocational help and assistance to defray medical costs, such as drug manufacturer patient assistance programs, are often needed. A close physician-patient relationship, adequate sleep and exercise, stress reduction, and avoidance of alcohol or sedative drugs serve the interests of patients and their families.

A seizure per se does not lower IQ or cause brain damage. Although the negative consequences of epilepsy to daily life should not be underestimated, most otherwise normal patients lead full, productive lives. Scheduling activities for each day may help. Some children respond better to home schooling until seizures are controlled. Untreated epilepsy is often but not always debilitating. Children with epilepsy are significantly more likely to suffer from depression, attention deficit/hyperactivity disorder, developmental delay, autism, and headaches. For those who develop psychological dysfunction, especially depression, psychiatric consultation or medication is usually helpful.

F. Alternative Therapies

Few alternative therapies have evidence-based support. Pyridoxine (vitamin B_6) and magnesium have scientific grounding for specific seizure disorders. Beneficial claims for acupuncture, chiropractic, or naturopathic manipulation are unfounded. Food allergies do not cause convulsions unless they cause anaphylaxis. Most alternative therapy sources advise avoidance of alcohol, caffeine, and aspartame, the first two of which are logical. Proof that taurine, folic acid, vitamin B_{12}, manganese, zinc, dimethylglycine, megavitamins, or various nonketogenic diets reduce seizure frequency or medication requirements is absent or marginal. Herbal remedies such as passionflower, skullcap, valerian, belladonna, causticum, cicuta, or cuprum metallicum have not been adequately studied. However, any nontoxic technique to reduce stress and bring order to a patient's life may help. Some patients have learned to control seizures with self-relaxation or special techniques such as looking at a particular piece of jewelry as an aura comes on. Those who wish to augment medical treatment with noninvasive treatments may be permitted to do so after physician review for safety and follow-up to see if the treatments appear to help over time.

▶ Febrile Convulsions

The most common childhood seizure disorder, febrile convulsions, affects 3% of children between ages 6 months and 6 years. After age 14 years, febrile seizures are rare. Despite a recurrence rate of 30%, only 3% of these individuals develop epilepsy. Those with a family history of epilepsy, abnormal neurologic or developmental status, or a prolonged (>15 minute) focal seizure have at least a 15% incidence of epilepsy. Commonly, a toddler with an upper respiratory infection, enterovirus, or roseola suddenly seizes during an afternoon nap. Usually short tonic-clonic convulsions, such seizures are multiple in one-third of cases. Postictal sleepiness can last several hours. Laboratory tests are unnecessary

unless the child is age <6 months or meningitis is suggested by failure to arouse, continued focal seizures, or physical findings (stiff neck, bulging fontanel, rash). Seizures that occur in the office or emergency department are suggestive of more serious infection.

Treatment consists of reassurance to worried parents that the worst has passed and that these seizures leave no permanent brain damage. Controlling fever with warm baths to reduce shivering, acetaminophen (10–15 mg/kg every 4 hours), or ibuprofen (5–10 mg/kg every 6 hours) may reduce immediate risk of recurrence. If begun at the onset of fever, buccal or intranasal midazolam, 0.25–1 mg/kg; oral or rectal valproic acid, 20 mg/kg every 8 hours for 1–3 days; or diazepam, 0.5 mg/kg every 8 hours for 1–3 days can reduce recurrence. Intravenous (IV) lorazepam is the drug of choice for prolonged febrile seizures. Hospitalization is best if seizures are prolonged beyond 30 minutes or are recurrent or complicated, if follow-up is inadequate, or if parents or the physician want observation. Chronic treatment is advised only for the child with multiple recurrences, persistent neurologic abnormality, or worrisome EEG findings.

▶ Status Epilepticus

Any recurrent or prolonged seizure uninterrupted by consciousness for >5 minutes is termed *status epilepticus* (SE), classified as either convulsive or nonconvulsive. SE carries a low risk of permanent residual brain damage that can be minimized through rapid treatment. Approximately 5% of children with febrile convulsions and 20% of all persons with epilepsy have SE at least once. Newly diagnosed epileptic patients often develop SE. Although any seizure type, including myoclonic or simple partial seizures, can cause SE, most commonly consciousness is severely impaired. A persistent grand mal seizure is readily identified as SE, but diagnosing SE in a comatose patient with no abnormal motor movement can be difficult without an EEG. Confused but ambulating persons may be in a state of absence or complex partial SE. Diagnosis is based on EEG findings. Death is usually related to a serious underlying etiology rather than SE itself.

Management requires stabilization of vital signs. Adolescents and adults should be given 100 mg of thiamine IV, 50 mL of 50% glucose (children: 2–4 mL/kg of 25% glucose), and naloxone, 0.4–2 mg (children: 0.01 mg/kg) every 2–3 minutes as needed. Lorazepam, 0.1 mg/kg (maximum of 4 mg) IV push at 2 mg/min, is successful in stopping 80% of SE episodes in 2–3 minutes. A second dose in 10 minutes is frequently successful in the remaining 20%. For prehospital treatment or lack of IV access, intramuscular (IM) midazolam, 5–10 mg (children: 0. 2mg/kg), is effective for cessation of seizures, prevention of hospitalization, and prevention of intensive care unit admissions (strength of recommendation: B; one large randomized controlled trial). If neither the IV nor IM route is feasible, rectal diazepam or intranasal or buccal midazolam are drugs of choice. Poorly controlled SE responds to phenytoin, 20 mg/kg IV push at 50 mg/min, while monitoring the electrocardiogram and blood pressure, or its safer prodrug, fosphenytoin, given at 30 mg/kg IV push at 150 mg/min. Other alternatives are phenobarbital, levetiracetam, and propofol. Some SE in children younger than 18 months of age responds to pyridoxine, 50 mg IV. For other information, see the flowchart from the American Epilepsy Society in the references. Once the SE is controlled, a search for the underlying cause should be conducted.

Neonatal Seizures

Neonatal seizures are difficult to recognize. In the first month of life, clonic-tonic seizure activity is uncommon. Focal rhythmic twitches, recurrent vomiting, poor feeding and responsiveness, high-pitched crying, posturing, chewing, apnea, cyanosis, and excessive salivation should raise alarm. Diligent inquiry into family history, prenatal history, and maternal habits is warranted. Neurologic consultation is advisable. Often difficult to control, these seizures may have a dismal outcome. Treatment for maternal drug addiction with resultant neonatal drug withdrawal seizures, which usually leave no residual defects, includes paregoric, methadone, phenytoin, phenobarbital, and various benzodiazepines. Table 9–11 lists suggested evaluations.

Eclampsia

The AED of choice is magnesium sulfate, 4–6 g IV, given over 15 minutes, followed by 2 g/h as a continuous IV infusion. Calcium gluconate (1 g IV) may be administered to counteract magnesium toxicity.

Prognosis

Clinical practice guidelines for management of patients with seizure disorders are presented in Table 9–12. Overall,

Table 9–11. Evaluation of neonatal seizures.

I. History
  A. Pregnancy related
    1. Infection: toxoplasmosis, rubella, cytomegalovirus, herpes, syphilis (TORCHS) titers; IgM level
    2. Maternal addiction: smoking, alcohol, cocaine, heroin, barbiturates
    3. Maternal behavior: inadequate prenatal care, lack of folic acid
  B. Delivery related
    1. Anoxia
    2. Trauma
  C. Family history: chromosomal disorders, errors of metabolism

II. Physical findings
  A. Recognizable patterns of malformation: eyes, ears, hands, facies, head shape
  B. Neurologic evaluation: motor, sensory, cranial nerves
  C. Odor: phenylketonuria
  D. Dermatologic signs: crusted vesicles, abnormal creases, hypopigmentation, nevi
  E. Ocular: chorioretinitis, cataracts, coloboma, cherry red spot

III. Laboratory evaluation
  A. Neuroimaging: cranial ultrasound, magnetic resonance imaging (MRI), computed tomography (CT) scan
  B. Chest radiograph
  C. Cerebral spinal fluid: culture, cell count, Gram stain, India ink, VDRL, glycine, glucose, protein, xanthochromia
  D. Blood test: cultures, complete blood count, electrolytes, renal function, glucose, magnesium, calcium, karyotype, glycine, lactate, ammonia, long-chain fatty acid levels
  E. Urine: culture, glucose, protein, cells

VDRL, Venereal Disease Research Laboratory.
Data from the National Institute for Health and Clinical Excellence (NICE). *The Epilepsies: The Diagnosis and Management of the Epilepsies in Adults and Children in Primary and Secondary Care.* London, United Kingdom: National Institute for Health and Clinical Excellence (NICE); 2012 (Clinical Guideline 137).

Table 9–12. Clinical practice guidelines for management of patients with seizure disorders.

Clinical Scenario	Guideline
Febrile seizure	Children with febrile seizures, even if recurrent, should rarely be treated with antiepileptic drugs (AEDs)
Provoked seizure	Long-term prophylactic AED treatment for children with head injuries or correctable causes of seizure is not indicated
Unprovoked, tonic-clonic epileptic seizure	AED treatment should generally not be commenced routinely after a first unprovoked tonic-clonic seizure if the history and physical examination are otherwise normal
Generalized epilepsy	The choice of first AED should be determined, where possible, by the seizure type and potential adverse effects
Focal seizure	When appropriate monotherapy fails to reduce seizure frequency, combination therapy should be considered; use of >2 drugs usually requires consultation
Monitoring for adverse effects of AEDs	Routine AED level monitoring is generally not required
Withdrawal of AEDs	Withdrawal of AED treatment should be considered for individuals who have been seizure free for ≥2 years, especially if a recent EEG is normal
Prolonged or serial seizure	Prolonged or serial seizures can be treated with intravenous lorazepam or intranasal or buccal midazolam or rectal diazepam

roughly one-third of patients have a second seizure, and about 75% of these patients experience a third seizure. No adverse outcomes are likely even with ≤10 untreated seizures. A study of 220 children indicated that 92% of those treated for idiopathic seizures remained seizure free for as long as 5 years. Eventually, about 70% of epileptic children and 60% of adults become seizure free after treatment.

Sudden unexpected death in epilepsy occurs in 1–2 persons per 1000 per year, peaking at age 50–59 years. Tonic-clonic seizures, treatment with three or more AEDs, and an IQ of <70 are risk factors for sudden death; choice of AED and AED serum levels are not.

American Epilepsy Society. New guideline for treatment of prolonged seizures in children and adults. https://www.aesnet.org/about_aes/press_releases/guidelines2016. Accessed August 20, 2018.

Brophy GM, Bell R, Claassen J, et al; Neurocritical Care Society Status Epilepticus Guideline Writing Committee. Guidelines for the evaluation and management of status epilepticus. *Neurocrit Care.* 2012;17(1):3–23. [PMID: 22528274]

Centers for Disease Control and Prevention. Epilepsy in adults and access to care–United States, 2010. *MMWR.* 2012;61:909–913. [PMID: 23151949]

Dang LT, Silverstein FS. Drug treatment of seizures and epilepsy in newborns and children. *Pediatr Clin North Am.* 2017;64:1291–1308. [PMID: 29173786]

Devinsky O. Sudden, unexpected death in epilepsy. *N Engl J Med.* 2011;365:1801–1811. [PMID: 22070477]

National Institute for Health and Clinical Excellence. *The Epilepsies: The Diagnosis and Management of the Epilepsies in Adults and Children in Primary and Secondary Care.* London, United Kingdom: National Institute for Health and Clinical Excellence; 2012 (Clinical Guideline 137).

Patel H, Dunn DW, Austin JK, et al. Psychogenic nonepileptic seizures (pseudoseizures). *Pediatr Rev.* 2011;32:e66–e72. [PMID: 21632872]

Patel N, Ram D, Swiderska N, et al. Febrile seizures. *BMJ.* 2015;18:h4240:1–7. [PMID: 26286537]

Russ SA, Larson K, Halfon N. A national profile of childhood epilepsy and seizure disorder. *Pediatrics.* 2012;129:256–264. [PMID: 22271699]

Scheffer IE, Berkovic S, Capovilla G, et al. ILAE classification of the epilepsies: position paper of the ILAE Commission for Classification and Terminology. *Epilepsia.* 2017;58:512–521. [PMID: 28276062]

The Medical Letter. Drugs for epilepsy. *Med Lett Drugs Ther.* 2017;59(1526):121–130. [PMID: 28746301]

Wilden JA, Cohen-Gadol AA. Evaluation of first nonfebrile seizures. *Am Fam Physician.* 2012;86:334–340. [PMID: 22963022]

Physical Activity in Adolescents

Mark B. Stephens, MD, MS, FAAFP
Scott K. Andrews, MD, MBA

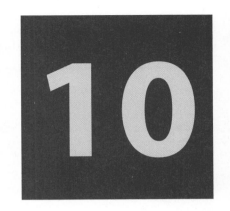

"Do it, move it, make it happen. No one ever sat their way to success."

—Unknown

The United States continues to struggle with the medical and economic consequences of physical inactivity and obesity. Declines in physical activity over the past several decades have mirrored a rise in rates of obesity among children and adolescents. Longitudinal data from the National Health and Nutrition Examination Surveys (NHANES) show that the percentage of overweight and obese adolescents in the United States has increased from 5% to 21% since the mid-1980s. Overweight and obese youth are less likely to engage in physical activity and are more likely to report chronic health problems compared with peers of normal weight. Overweight and obese adolescents are more likely to struggle with orthopedic problems and behavioral health issues. They are also more likely to be obese as adults.

During adolescence, levels of spontaneous physical activity drop significantly from high points in childhood. This likely correlates with increased rates of obesity among adolescents (21%), compared with children ages 6–11 (18%) and ages 2–5 (14%). The number of US adolescents meeting recommended activity levels also remains low and has not changed significantly over the past decade (Table 10–1). Adolescents spend much of their time engaged in sedentary activities. In 2010, children and adolescents (ages 8–18 years) were reported to spend an average of >4 hours watching television, >2 hours listening to music, and >2 hour using computers or playing video games each day. With the recent proliferation of smartphone technology, most teens now have access to a smartphone. In this context, 95% of teens report daily internet use, and 45% of teens report that they are online "almost constantly." In contrast, adolescents currently average a mere 12 minutes per day of vigorous physical activity. Data continue to suggest that one-third of US high school students are not regularly active and one-half of high school seniors are not enrolled in physical education classes. Interestingly, teens active in school sporting activities are also more likely to be active as adults. Health-related behaviors, such as dietary habits and physical activity patterns, solidify during adolescence and persist into adulthood. Recognizing adolescents who are insufficiently active, overweight, or obese can help to promote a lifetime of healthy habits.

Hales CM, Carroll MD, Fryar CD, et al. Prevalence of obesity among adults and youth: United States 2015-2016. *NCHS Data Brief.* 2017;288:1–8. [PMID: 29155689]

HealthPeople.gov. Nutrition, physical activity, and obesity. https://www.healthypeople.gov/2020/leading-health-indicators/2020-lhi-topics/Nutrition-Physical-Activity-and-Obesity/data. Accessed August 23, 2018.

Herman KM, Craig CL, Gauvin L, et al. Tracking of obesity and physical activity from childhood to adulthood: the Physical Activity Longitudinal Study. *Int J Pediatr Obes.* 2009;4(4):281–288. [PMID: 19922043]

Kaiser Family Foundation Study. Generation M2: Media in the lives of 8- to 18-year-olds. http://kaiserfamilyfoundation.files.wordpress.com/2013/01/8010.pdf. Accessed August 23, 2018.

Pew Research Center. Teens, social media and technology 2018. http://www.pewinternet.org/2018/05/31/teens-social-media-technology-2018/. Accessed August 23, 2018.

Singh A, Mulder C, Twisk JW, et al. Tracking of childhood overweight into adulthood: a systematic review of the literature. *Obes Rev.* 2008;9(5):474–488. [PMID: 18331423]

DEFINITIONS

The following definitions apply to the discussion of physical activity and obesity (Table 10–2). *Physical fitness* refers to a general state of well-being that allows an individual to perform activities of daily living in a vigorous manner. Physical fitness includes health-related characteristics and skill-related characteristics. Health-related components of physical fitness include cardiorespiratory endurance, muscular strength, muscular endurance, flexibility, and body

Table 10–1. Trends in moderate to vigorous physical activity and sedentary behavior among US high school students, 2011 national overview.

General Behaviors

13.8% of students had not participated in ≥60 minutes of any kind of physical activity that increased their heart rate and made them breathe hard some of the time on at least 1 day during the 7 days before the survey (ie, did not participate in ≥60 minutes of physical activity on any given day)

28.7% of students had been physically active doing any kind of physical activity that increased their heart rate and made them breathe hard some of the time for a total of ≥60 minutes per day on each of the 7 days before the survey (ie, were physically active for ≥60 minutes on all 7 days)

51.8% of students went to physical education (PE) classes on ≥1 day in an average week when they were in school (ie, attended PE classes)

31.5% of students attended PE classes 5 days in an average week when they were in school (ie, attended PE classes daily)

Sedentary Behaviors

31.1% of students played videogames or computer games or used a computer for nonschool work activity for ≥3 days on an average school day (ie, used computers ≥3 hours per day)

32.4% of students watched television ≥3 hours per day on an average school day

Data from the National Youth Risk Behavior Surveys, Centers for Disease Control and Prevention.

Table 10–2. Definitions of physical activity, physical fitness, and exercise.

Physical activity	Any body movement that results in the expenditure of energy
Physical fitness	A general state of overall well-being that allows individuals to conduct the majority of their activities of daily living in a vigorous manner
Health-related physical fitness	Aerobic capacity (cardiorespiratory endurance) Body composition Muscular strength Muscular endurance Flexibility
Skill-related physical fitness	Power Agility Speed Balance Coordination Reaction time
Exercise	A structured routine of physical activity specifically designed to improve or maintain one of the components of health-related physical fitness

composition. Skill-related components of physical fitness include power, speed, agility, and balance. Historically, physical education programs have emphasized skill-related activities and athletic ability. From a public health perspective, however, the health-related components of physical fitness are more important in terms of overall morbidity and mortality from chronic diseases related to physical inactivity.

Physical activity refers to any body movement resulting in the expenditure of energy. Physical activity occurs in a broad range of settings. Leisure-time activities, occupational activities, routine activities of daily living, and dedicated exercise programs all represent valid forms of physical activity. Physical activity varies along a continuum of intensity from light (eg, housework) to moderate (eg, jogging) to more vigorous (eg, strenuous bicycling). *Exercise* refers to a structured routine of physical activity that is specifically designed to improve or maintain one of the components of health-related physical fitness. Historically, society has placed more emphasis on formal exercise programs as the primary means of achieving physical fitness rather than promoting physical activity in a more general sense.

Body mass index (BMI) is the anthropometric measurement of choice for assessing body composition in children, adolescents, and adults. BMI is calculated by dividing an individual's weight (in kilograms) by the square of the individual's height (in meters). BMI correlates with other measures of body fat including skinfold measurements, densitometry, and bioelectrical impedance. Charts and digital tools for the office (http://www.nhlbi.nih.gov/guidelines/obesity/BMI/bmicalc.htm) and for mobile devices are available for rapid calculation of BMI. Normative values for underweight, normal weight, overweight, and obesity for adolescents have been established and are presented in Table 10–3. BMI-for-age charts have replaced standard weight-for-height charts as the preferred mechanism for tracking weight in children and adolescents (Figures 10–1 and 10–2). *Overweight* adolescents

Table 10–3. Definitions of overweight and obesity for adolescents and adults.

Definition	Clinical Parameter
Obesity (adults)	BMI >30
Overweight (adults)	BMI 25.1–29.9
Obesity (adolescents)	BMI >95th percentile for age
Overweight (adolescents)	95th < BMI > 85th percentile for age
Underweight (adolescents)	BMI <5th percentile for age

BMI, body mass index.
Data from Centers for Disease Control and Prevention. Body mass index. http://www.cdc.gov/nccdphp/dnpa/bmi/bmi-for-age.htm. Accessed November 11, 2019.

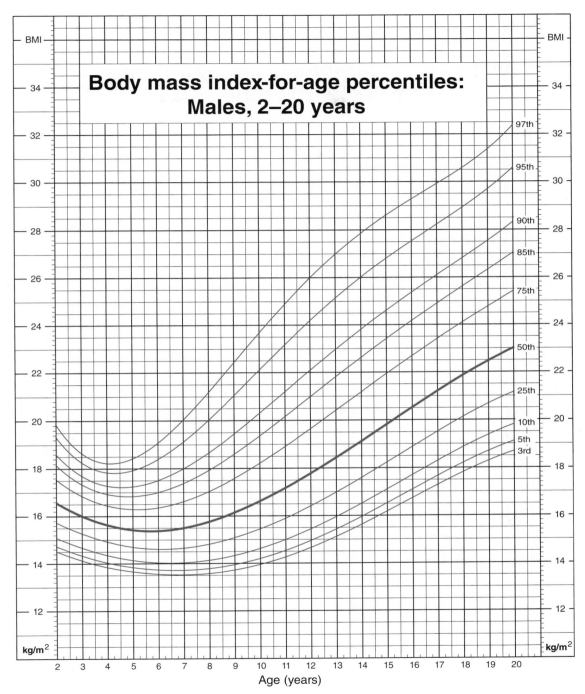

▲ **Figure 10–1.** Body mass index for age: males. (Reproduced with permission from Centers for Disease Control and Prevention, Atlanta, GA. http://www.cdc.gov/growthcharts/data/set1clinical/cj41l023.pdf. Accessed November 11, 2019.)

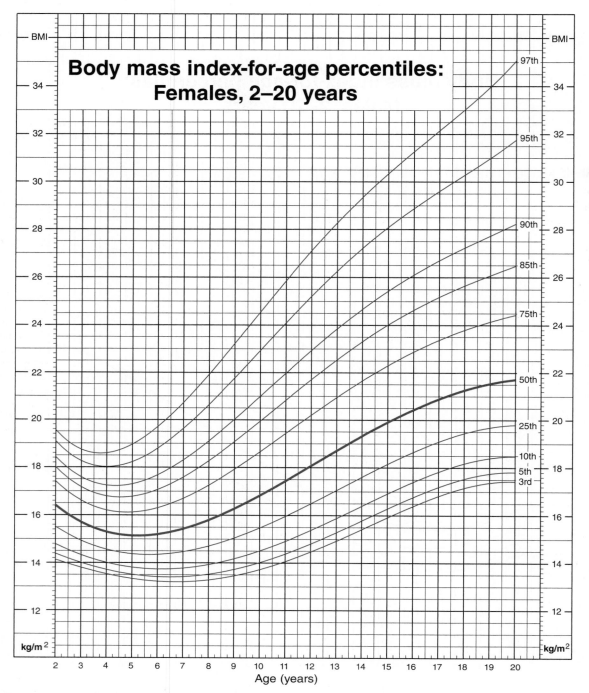

▲ **Figure 10–2.** Body mass index for age: females. (Reproduced with permission from Centers for Disease Control and Prevention, Atlanta, GA. http://www.cdc.gov/growthcharts/data/set1clinical/cj41l024.pdf. Accessed November 11, 2019.)

are those who fall between the 85th and 95th percentiles of BMI for age. *Obese* adolescents are above the 95th percentile of BMI for age.

Centers for Disease Control and Prevention. Defining childhood obesity. https://www.cdc.gov/obesity/childhood/defining.html. Accessed August 23, 2018.

Whitlock EP, Williams SB, Gold R, et al. Screening and interventions for childhood overweight: a summary of evidence for the US Preventive Services Task Force. *Pediatrics*. 2010;116(1):125–144. [PMID: 15995013]

RISKS ASSOCIATED WITH PHYSICAL INACTIVITY

Physical inactivity is a primary risk factor for cardiovascular disease and all-cause mortality. A sedentary lifestyle also contributes to increased rates of diabetes, hypertension, hyperlipidemia, osteoporosis, cerebrovascular disease, and colon cancer. Adolescents who are less physically active are more likely to smoke cigarettes, less likely to consume appropriate amounts of fruits and vegetables, and less likely to routinely wear a seatbelt. They are also more likely to spend increased time engaged in sedentary technology-related behaviors.

Physical activity also serves numerous preventive functions. In addition to preventing chronic diseases such as hypertension, diabetes, and cardiovascular disease, sufficient levels of physical activity on a regular basis are associated with lower rates of mental illness. Teens that spend more time engaged in sedentary technology-related behaviors have higher rates of depression. High use of digital media has also been linked with attention deficit/hyperactivity disorder. Physically active adolescents have lower levels of stress and anxiety and have higher self-esteem than sedentary peers. Active adolescents also have fewer somatic complaints and are more confident about their own future health. They also have improved relationships with parents and authority figures and a better body image. Physical activity has also been associated with improved cognitive function and academic achievement in youth.

Donnelly JE, Hillman CH, Castelli D, et al. Physical activity, fitness, cognitive performance and academic achievement in children: a systematic review. *Med Sci Sports Exerc*. 2016;48(6):1197–1222. [PMID: 27182986]

Gopinath B, Hardy LL, Baur LA, et al. Physical activity and sedentary behaviors and health-related quality of life in adolescents. *Pediatrics*. 2012;130(1):e167–e174. [PMID: 22689863]

Ra CK, Cho J, Stone MD, et al. Association of digital media use with subsequent symptoms of attention-deficit/hyperactivity among adolescents. *JAMA*. 2018;320(3):255–263. [PMID: 30027248]

FACTORS INFLUENCING PHYSICAL ACTIVITY

Despite overwhelming evidence supporting the health-related benefits of physical activity, young Americans are persistently sedentary. A complex interaction of social, cultural, environmental, and familial factors associated with "modern living" contribute to low rates of physical activity.

▶ Social Factors

Socioeconomic status is one of the strongest predictors of physical activity in both adolescents and adults. Lower socioeconomic status is associated with lower levels of spontaneous physical activity. Youth of higher socioeconomic status engage in more spontaneous physical activity, are more frequently enrolled in physical education classes, and are more likely to be active during physical education classes when compared with peers of lower socioeconomic status. This relationship persists when controlling for age, gender, and ethnicity. While school-based programs help to increase the number of children engaged in moderate to vigorous physical activity and increase the duration of participation in physical activity, a similar effect has not been noted in school-based programs for adolescents.

Social mobility also plays an important role in shaping levels of physical activity. Specifically, achieved levels of social positioning are more strongly associated with positive health behaviors and increased levels of physical activity than the social class of origin. Youth with active friends are more likely to be active. Youth with sedentary friends are more likely to be sedentary. There are also significant differences in patterns of spontaneous physical activity when youth attending public schools are compared with youth attending private secondary schools. Adolescents are more likely to enroll in physical education classes in public schools. In private schools, adolescents are more likely to participate in organized team sports. Participation in organized sports in adolescence is associated with higher levels of physical activity in adulthood.

As a consequence of modern life, most Americans have become increasingly reliant on automated transportation. This has had a negative impact on the simplest form of physical activity: walking. Historically, most children and adolescents walked to school. This is no longer the case. Despite the fact that one-third of American schoolchildren live <1 mile from their school, fewer than 25% of these children walk or bike to school. The number of children walking to school in the United States has decreased by 66% since 1977.

▶ Cultural & Ethnic Factors

Cohort studies consistently suggest that there are inherent cultural differences in levels of spontaneous physical activity. Data from the Youth Risk Behavior Surveillance System (http://www.cdc.gov/HealthyYouth/yrbs/index.htm) and the National Longitudinal Study of Adolescent to Adult Health (http://www.cpc.unc.edu/projects/addhealth) show that minority adolescents engage in the lowest levels of both leisure time and structured (physical education class) activity.

Hispanic youth are more likely to view themselves as overweight when compared with African Americans and non-Hispanic whites. Adolescents who view themselves as overweight are significantly less likely to be physically active than normal-weight peers. They are also less likely to engage in other healthy behaviors. Compared with non-Hispanic whites, African American and Hispanic youth are at significantly higher risk for being overweight and obese. NHANES suggests the prevalence of obesity is 14% for non-Hispanic whites and 11% for non-Hispanic Asians, compared to 22% for non-Hispanic blacks and 26% for Hispanic youth.

There are also important cultural differences in perceptions about the inherent value of exercise. Not all cultures promote leisure time as a good opportunity for fitness activities. Exercise as an isolated activity can be viewed as either selfish or as a poor use of time. Cultural and ethnic differences also exist in television viewing and use of screen time. Hispanic and African American adolescents spend significantly more time watching television or on mobile digital media than do non-Hispanic whites.

▶ Gender-Related Factors

There are significant differences in levels of spontaneous physical activity between male and female adolescents. Boys are generally more active than girls from childhood through adolescence. Levels of physical activity decline for both boys and girls during adolescence, but there is a disproportionate decline for girls. The reasons for this are unclear. Factors that are positively associated with an increased likelihood of physical activity among female adolescents include perceived competence at a particular activity, perceived value of the activity, favorable physical appearance during and after the activity, and positive social support for the activity.

▶ Environmental Factors

Many of the barriers to physical activity are environmental. Of these, mobile digital technology (primarily smartphones), television, and videogaming (collectively referred to as "screen-time" activities) are important for adolescents. It is estimated that between the ages of 8 and 18, youth spend up to 8 hours a day engaged in sedentary technology-related behaviors. This translates to nearly half of waking hours spent in front of a video device. By contrast, adolescents spend <1% of their time (an estimated 12–14 minutes per day) engaged in vigorous physical activity. The impact of smartphones, videogaming, social media, and other personal computing devices and handheld gaming devices on the activity levels of youth has been extraordinary. To address this, the American Academy of Pediatrics (AAP) has released a position statement recommending that youth age 2–5 years engage in no more than 1 hour per day of screen time and that children age 6 and older have consistent limits on screen time and the types of media used. The AAP recommends a family media plan to curb inappropriate and excessive use of smartphones and other electronic devices (https://www.healthychildren.org/English/media/Pages/default.aspx#wizard).

Mobile technology and television are not the only environmental issue contributing to adolescent inactivity and obesity. Poor community planning has resulted in a paucity of safe gymnasiums or playing fields for adolescents to access and use during their leisure time. Erosions in public infrastructure such as poorly maintained sidewalks and poorly controlled crossings (eg, lack of traffic lights and/or crossing guards) also contribute to decreased physical activity in children and adolescents. Thoughtful community planning and healthy urban design are meaningful ways to embed physical activity into the fabric of community life. An additional factor contributing to increased obesity is a lack of access to healthy foods. Within the urban environment, in particular, there is an abundance of readily available, inexpensive, and calorically dense foods. These so-called food swamps and food deserts are directly associated with poor dietary habits in adolescents.

▶ Familial Factors

Finally, there are factors inherent within individual families that shape how active young individuals will be. Children and adolescents with overweight parents are more likely to be overweight. Paradoxically, parental levels of physical activity do not accurately predict their children's levels of physical activity. Children and youth from larger families are more active than children from small families. Children whose parents watch a great deal of television are more likely to spend time watching television themselves. Children whose parents are available to provide transportation to organized sporting activities are more likely to be physically active. Interestingly, individuals *forced* to exercise as children are less likely to be physically active as adults.

American Academy of Pediatrics Council on Communications and Media. Media use in school-aged children and adolescents. *Pediatrics*. 2016;138(5):e2016592. [PMID: 27940794]

Booth VM, Rowlands AV, Dollman J. Physical activity temporal trends among children and adolescents. *J Sci Med Sport*. 2015;18:418–425. [PMID: 25041963]

Dobbins M, Husson H, DeCorby K, et al. School-based physical activity programs for promoting physical activity and fitness in children and adolescents aged 6 to 18. *Cochrane Database Syst Rev*. 2013;2:CD007651. [PMID: 23450577]

Forshee RA, Anderson PA, Storey ML. The role of beverage consumption, physical activity, sedentary behavior and demographics on body mass index of adolescents. *Int J Food Sci Nutr*. 2004;55:463–478. [PMID: 15762311]

Gordon-Larsen P, McMurray RG, Popkin BM. Determinants of adolescent physical activity and inactivity patterns. *Pediatrics*. 2000;105(6):E83. [PMID: 10835096]

Hager ER, Cockerham A, O'Reilly N, et al. Food swamps and food deserts in Baltimore City, MD: associations with dietary behaviours among urban adolescent girls. *Public Health Nutr.* 2017;20(14):2598–2607. [PMID: 27652511]

Hales CM, Carroll MD, Fryar CD, et al. Prevalence of obesity among adults and youth: United States 2015-2016. *NCHS Data Brief.* 2017;288:1–8. [PMID: 29155689]

Mantjes JA, Jones AP, Corder K, et al. School related factors and 1 yr change in physical activity amongst 9–11 year old English school children. *Int J Behav Nutr Phys Act.* 2012;9:153. [PMID: 23276280]

Pew Research Center. Teens, social media and technology 2018. http://www.pewinternet.org/2018/05/31/teens-social-media-technology-2018/. Accessed August 23, 2018.

Pinto Pereira SM, Li L, Power C. Early life factors and adult leisure time physical inactivity-stability and change. *Med Sci Sports Exerc.* 2015;47(9):1841–1848. [PMID: 25563907]

Singh GK, Kogan MD, Siahpush M, van Dyck PC. Independent and joint effects of socioeconomic, behavioral, and neighborhood characteristics on physical inactivity and activity levels among US children and adolescents. *J Commun Health.* 2008; 33(4):206–216. [PMID: 18373183]

Tammelin T, Näyhä S, Laitinen J, et al. Physical activity and social status in adolescence as predictors of physical inactivity in adulthood. *Prevent Med.* 2003;37:375. [PMID: 14507496]

Whitt-Glover MC, Taylor WC, Floyd MF, et al. Disparities in physical activity and sedentary behaviors among US children and adolescents: prevalence, correlates, and intervention implications. *J Public Health Policy.* 2009;30(suppl 1):S309–S334. [PMID: 19190581]

Yang X, Telama R, Viikari J, et al. Risk of obesity in relation to physical activity tracking from youth to adulthood. *Med Sci Sports Exercise.* 2006;38:919–925. [PMID: 16672846]

ASSESSMENT

There are several ways to assess physical activity levels in adolescents: (1) direct observation, (2) activity or heart rate monitors, and (3) self-report questionnaires. Of these methods, direct observation and electronic assessment (accelerometry, actigraphy) provide the most accurate and objective measurements. However, direct observation is labor intensive, and higher technology solutions are often prohibitively expensive. Several cost-effective alternatives are available.

The Patient-Centered Assessment and Counseling for Exercise Plus (PACE+) Nutrition program has been developed to help clinicians assess physical activity levels as well as to provide patients with proper advice regarding physical activity and proper nutrition. As part of this program, a two-question self-report screening tool has been developed as a self-assessment tool for estimating adolescent physical activity. The combination of BMI and the PACE+ activity measure provides a rapid clinical assessment of physical activity status, weight status, and health risks. Two other simple screening tools, the World Health Organization Health Behavior in School-Aged Children (WHO HBSC; http://www.hbsc.org/methods/index.html) and International Physical Activity Questionnaire (IPAQ short version; https://sites.google.com/site/theipaq/questionnaire_links) are also available tools for assessing adolescent physical activity levels. Additional electronic monitoring devices, including heart rate monitors, accelerometers, and pedometers, can provide objective assessments of physical activity levels in adolescents. Fitness bands and smartphone applications are also increasingly available tools that can help to assess physical activity levels.

Case MA, Burwick HA, Volpp, KG, et al. Accuracy of smartphone applications and wearable devices for tracking physical activity data. *JAMA.* 2015;313(6):625–626. [PMID: 25668268]

Prochaska JJ, Sallis JF, Long B. A physical activity screening measure for use with adolescents in primary care. *Arch Pediatr Adolesc Med.* 2001;155:554. [PMID: 11343497]

Sirard JR, Pate RR. Physical activity assessment in children and adolescents. *Sports Med.* 2001;31:439. [PMID: 11394563]

GUIDELINES & CLINICAL INTERVENTIONS

It is known that risk factors for chronic disease track from childhood through adolescence into adulthood. Overweight adolescents are more likely to become overweight adults. Multiple guidelines are available to help clinicians promote appropriate levels of physical activity for their adolescent patients (Table 10–4).

▶ American College of Sports Medicine/American Heart Association Guidelines

The most recent American College of Sports Medicine (ACSM)/American Heart Association (AHA) guidelines for physical activity in individuals age >18 years recommend a minimum of 30 minutes of moderate-intensity activity 5 days a week or 20 minutes of vigorous activity 3 days a week. Moderate-intensity aerobic activity is equivalent to a brisk walk, while vigorous-intensity activity is exemplified by jogging. Individuals can further improve their health in a dose-response relationship by exceeding these minimum recommendations for physical activity.

Garber, CE, Blissmer B, Deschenes MR, et al. Quantity and quality of exercise for developing and maintaining cardiorespiratory, musculoskeletal, and neuromotor fitness in apparently healthy adults: guidance for prescribing exercise. *Med Sci Sports Exerc.* 2011;43(7):1334–1359. [PMID: 21694556]

▶ International Consensus Conference on Physical Activity Guidelines for Adolescents; American Academy of Pediatrics

Convened in 1993, this expert panel recommends that adolescents be physically active on most, if not all, days of the week. Adolescents should strive for activity 3–5 days per week for ≥20 minutes at levels requiring moderate to

Table 10–4. Guidelines for physical activity in adolescence.

Guideline Source	Recommendation
International Consensus Conference on Physical Activity Guidelines for Adolescents/American Academy of Pediatrics Statement (2012)	1. Physical activity 3–5 days/week 2. Activity sessions of ≥20 minutes requiring moderate to vigorous physical exertion 3. Emphasis on consideration of familial, social, and community factors when promoting activity
ACSM/AHA consensus statement	1. All Americans should strive to be physically active on most, preferably all, days of the week according to individual abilities 2. Goal of accumulating 30 minutes of moderate to vigorous physical activity each day 3. Sedentary individuals benefit from even modest levels of physical activity 4. Sufficient levels of activity can be accumulated through independent bouts of activity throughout the day
National Strength and Conditioning Association (2009)	1. A properly designed and supervised resistance training program is relatively safe for youth 2. A properly designed and supervised resistance training program can enhance the muscular strength and power of youth 3. A properly designed and supervised resistance training program can improve the cardiovascular risk profile of youth 4. A properly designed and supervised resistance training program can improve motor skill performance and may contribute to enhanced sports performance of youth 5. A properly designed and supervised resistance training program can increase a young athlete's resistance to sports related injuries 6. A properly designed and supervised resistance training program can help improve the psychosocial well-being of youth 7. A properly designed and supervised resistance training program can help promote and develop exercise habits during childhood and adolescence
Healthy People 2020 (2012)	1. Increase the proportion of adolescents who meet current federal physical activity guidelines for aerobic physical activity and for muscle-strengthening activity 2. Increase the proportion of the nation's public and private schools that require daily physical education for all students 3. Increase the proportion of adolescents who participate in daily school physical education 4. Increase the proportion of children and adolescents who do not exceed recommended limits for screen time 5. Increase the proportion of the nation's public and private schools that provide access to their physical activity spaces and facilities for all persons outside of normal school hours (ie, before and after the school day, on weekends, and during summer and other vacations) 6. Increase the proportion of physician office visits that include counseling or education related to physical activity 7. Increase the proportion of trips made by walking 8. Increase the proportion of trips made by bicycling
Physical Activity Guidelines for Americans (2008)	1. Accumulate 60 minutes of moderate to vigorous activity every day 2. Children and adolescents should perform cardiovascular activities on 3 days of the week and muscle-strengthening or bone-strengthening activities on 3 days of the week 3. All activities should be age- and developmentally appropriate to avoid the risk for overtraining

ACSM, American College of Sports Medicine; AHA, American Heart Association.

vigorous exertion. Activity should routinely occur as part of play, games, sporting activities, work, recreation, physical education, or planned exercise sessions. These guidelines also emphasize the importance of considering family, school, and community factors when counseling adolescents about physical activity. The AAP further recommends that adolescents accumulate 60 minutes of moderate to vigorous physical activity every day for children over 6 years of age. Activity should be moderate in intensity and should be varied in type to include recreation, sports, or home-based, community-based, and school-based activities. Activities that are unstructured and enjoyable have the best rates of compliance.

American Academy of Pediatrics. Energy out: daily physical activity recommendations. https://www.healthychildren.org/English/healthy-living/fitness/Pages/Energy-Out-Daily-Physical-Activity-Recommendations.aspx. Accessed August 23, 2018.

Twisk JW. Physical activity guidelines for children and adolescents: a critical review. *Sports Med.* 2001;31:617. [PMID: 1147523]

Healthy People 2020

Healthy People 2020 contains national health objectives for promotion of adolescent general health as well as adolescent physical activity. Of the 15 objectives outlined in *Healthy People 2020*, 8 are specifically targeted to promote physical activity in adolescents (see Table 10–4).

US Department of Health and Human Services. *Healthy People 2020*. https://www.healthypeople.gov/2020/topics-objectives/topic/physical-activity. Accessed August 23, 2018.

Dietary Guidelines for Americans

The 2015–2020 dietary guidelines emphasize sound clinical nutritional advice as part of a holistic approach to health and wellness. This approach emphasizes the inherent relationship between physical activity, dietary choices, and resultant weight issues. The current guidelines specifically recommend physical activity as a routine complement to sound dietary practice. The guidelines also emphasize the avoidance of sugar-sweetened beverages, particularly for adolescents. As part of a healthy lifestyle, adolescents should aim to accumulate at least 60 minutes of moderate physical activity every day.

US Department of Health and Human Services, US Department of Agriculture. *2015-2020 Dietary Guidelines for Americans*. 8th ed. December 2015. https://health.gov/dietaryguidelines/2015/guidelines/. Accessed August 23, 2018.

Physical Activity Guidelines for Americans Midcourse Report

Updating the 2008 activity guidelines, a subsequent report provides several key recommendations: (1) all adolescents should perform ≥60 minutes of moderate to vigorous physical activity every day and participate in vigorous physical activity at least 3 days a week; (2) as part of the daily physical activity, children and adolescents should engage in muscle-strengthening or bone-strengthening activities on 3 days of the week; and (3) all activities should be age- and developmentally appropriate to avoid overuse injury.

2018 Physical Activity Guidelines Advisory Committee. *2018 Physical Activity Guidelines Advisory Committee Scientific Report*. Washington, DC: US Department of Health and Human Services; 2018.

US Department of Health and Human Services. *2008 Physical Activity Guidelines for Americans*. https://health.gov/paguidelines/. Accessed August 23, 2018.

US Department of Health and Human Services. *Physical Activity Guidelines for Americans Midcourse Report. Strategies to Increase Physical Activity among Youth*. http://www.health.gov/paguidelines/midcourse/pag-mid-course-report-final.pdf. August 23, 2018.

National Strength & Conditioning Association

The National Strength and Conditioning Association (NSCA) guidelines offer 10 recommendations for long-term development of athletic development in children and adolescents. These recommendations highlight the importance of tailoring training programs based on individual growth and development, injury prevention, and the promotion of overall physical and psychosocial well-being.

Lloyd RS, Cronin JB, Faigenbaum AD, et al. National Strength and Conditioning Association position statement on long-term athletic development. *J Strength Cond Res*. 2016;30(6):1491–1509. [PMID: 26933920]

PROMOTING PHYSICAL ACTIVITY: THE KEY ROLE OF FAMILY PHYSICIANS

Healthcare professionals play a central role in promoting physical activity among adolescents. Adolescents have the lowest utilization of healthcare services of any segment of the population. They do, however, trust their physician as a reliable source of healthcare information. Clinicians should use this opportunity to provide sound preventive advice during each adolescent visit. Based on current guidelines, physicians should *ask* adolescents about their current levels of physical activity and *advise* adolescents about appropriate levels of physical activity at every visit. As a goal, adolescents should strive for 60 minutes of moderate to vigorous physical activity while incorporating activities to improve muscle and bone health.

When reviewing guidelines or recommending lifestyle changes with adolescent patients, it is important to promote the concept of physical activity rather than physical fitness. Adolescents should be aware that cumulative bouts of physical activity are just as effective as sustained periods of exercise for attaining health-related benefits. To promote a lifetime of healthy behaviors, physical activity should be enjoyable and sustainable. Social support from family, peers, and/or the local community is also extremely helpful.

Dobbins M, Husson H, DeCorby K, et al. School-based physical activity programs for promoting physical activity and fitness in children and adolescents aged 6 to 18. *Cochrane Database Syst Rev*. 2013;2:CD007651. [PMID: 23450577]

Huang J, Sallis J, Patrick K. The role of primary care in promoting children's physical activity. *Br J Sports Med*. 2009;43:19–21. [PMID: 19001016]

Joy EA. Practical approaches to office-based physical activity promotion for children and adolescents. *Curr Sports Med Rep*. 2008;7(6):367–372. [PMID: 19005361]

Ma J, Wang Y, Stafford RS. U.S. adolescents receive suboptimal preventive counseling during ambulatory care. *J Adolesc Health*. 2005;36:441e1. [PMID: 15841517]

Smith BJ, van der Ploeg HP, Buffart LM, et al. Encouraging physical activity—five steps for GP's. *Aust Fam Physician*. 2008; 37(1–2):24–28. [PMID: 18239748]

Van Sluijs E, McMinn AM, Griffin SJ. Effectiveness of interventions to promote physical activity in children and adolescents: systematic review of controlled trials. *Br Med J*. 2007;335(7622): 703–712. [PMID: 17884863]

SPECIAL CONSIDERATIONS

▶ Performance-Enhancing Supplements

The use of performance-enhancing supplements is common among adolescents. One-half of the US population consumes some form of nutritional supplement on a regular basis, resulting in over $36 billion in annual sales. The most common reasons for using dietary nutritional supplements include preventing illness, improving performance, warding off fatigue, and enhancing personal appearance.

Estimates suggest that roughly 5% of all adolescents have used some form of performance-enhancing nutritional supplements. Adolescents, in particular, are vulnerable to the allure of performance-enhancing products to promote gains in strength and/or muscle mass, improve athletic performance, enhance their appearance, and improve self-esteem.

Creatine is a popular performance-enhancing supplement among adolescents. It has been reported to increase energy during short-term intense exercise; increase muscle mass, strength, and lean body mass; and decrease lactate accumulation during intense exercise. While supplementation with exogenous creatine can raise intramuscular creatine stores, it is not clear how effective creatine is as a performance aid. In general, creatine supplementation may be useful for activities requiring short, repetitive bouts of high-intensity exercise. There is conflicting evidence, however, as to whether it is effective in increasing muscle strength or muscle mass. There are no scientific data regarding the safety or effectiveness of long-term use of creatine in adolescents.

Anabolic-androgenic steroids (AASs) are another category of performance-enhancing substances used by adolescents. Testosterone is the prototypical androgenic steroid hormone. Many synthetic modifications have been made to the basic molecular structure of testosterone in an attempt to promote the anabolic, muscle-building effects of testosterone while minimizing androgenic side effects. Androstenedione is one of several oral performance-enhancing supplements that are precursors to testosterone. The effectiveness of androstenedione as a performance-enhancing supplement is debatable. To date, the largest controlled trial examining its effectiveness showed no significant gains in muscular strength compared with a standard program of resistance training. The Anabolic Steroid Control Act of 2004 expanded the definition of anabolic steroids to include androstenedione and tetrahydrogestrinone (THG) as controlled substances, making their use as performance-enhancing drugs illegal.

Despite this ban, it is estimated that 3–10% of adolescents have used anabolic steroids. Importantly, adolescents who use anabolic steroids are more likely to engage in high-risk personal health behaviors such as tobacco use and excessive alcohol consumption. Users of other nutritional performance-enhancing supplements have also been shown to engage in similarly predictable high-risk behaviors. The American Academy of Family Physicians and the AAP discourage the use of anabolic steroids for anything other than medical indications.

Given the prevalence of performance-enhancing supplement use among adolescents and the health-risk behaviors that often accompany the use of these products, family physicians should be prepared to provide appropriate preventive counseling whenever possible. The preparticipation physical examination represents an excellent opportunity for clinicians to provide information about performance-enhancing products to young athletes. When counseling adolescents about the use of performance-enhancing products, it is helpful to ask the following questions:

1. Is the product *safe* to use?
2. *Why* does the adolescent want to use a particular product?
3. Is the product *effective* in helping to meet the desired goal?
4. Is the product *legal*?

Many adolescents will either experiment with or regularly use performance-enhancing products. Adolescents often trust peers, coaches, mainstream media sources, and family regarding the safety and effectiveness of supplements. Family physicians have the responsibility to ensure that adolescents are aware of potential health risks and bans from competition that can accompany use of performance-enhancing products. As such, the use of performance-enhancing supplements in adolescents should be discouraged.

Evans MW, Ndetan H, Perko M, et al. Dietary supplement use by children and adolescents in the United States to enhance sport performance: results of the National Health Interview Survey. *J Prim Prevent*. 2012;33(1):3–12. [PMID: 22297456]

LaBotz M, Griesemer BA, Council on Sports Medicine and Fitness. Use of performance-enhancing substances. *Pediatrics*. 2016;138(1):e1–e12. [PMID: 27354458]

Stephens MB, Olsen C. Ergogenic supplements and health-risk behaviors. *J Fam Pract*. 2001;50:696. [PMID: 11509164]

▶ Female Athlete Triad

Although many adolescents engage in insufficient physical activity, there is a segment of the population for whom too much exercise leads to specific physiologic side effects. The term *female athlete triad* refers to the combination of disordered eating, amenorrhea, and osteoporosis that can accompany excessive physical training in young female athletes. Athletes particularly at risk include those who participate in gymnastics, ballet, figure skating, distance running, or any other sport that emphasizes a particularly lean physique.

The preparticipation physical examination is an excellent opportunity for clinicians to also screen for and prevent the female athlete triad. Screening questions for female athletes should include careful menstrual, dietary (including a history of disordered eating practices), and exercise histories. When elicited, a history of amenorrhea (particularly in a previously menstruating woman) should be taken seriously. The ACSM recommends that these women be considered at risk for the athlete triad and that a formal medical evaluation be undertaken within 3 months.

DeSouza MJ, Nattiv A, Joy E, et al. 2014 Female Athlete Triad Coalition Consensus Statement on the treatment and return to play of the female athlete triad. *Br J Sports Med.* 2014;48(4):289. [PMID: 24463911]

▶ Exercise & Sudden Death

Exercise is a high-risk activity for selected adolescents who are at risk for sudden cardiac death during physical activity. Highly publicized events among well-known athletes have focused significant media attention on this issue. Although the incidence of sudden cardiac death in young athletes is low, proper screening is essential. Here, again, the preparticipation physical examination is an excellent clinical opportunity to identify adolescents at risk for sudden cardiac death during physical activity.

When screening for sudden death in young athletes, the medical history should include questions about exercise-related syncope or near-syncope, shortness of breath, chest pain, and palpitations. A family history of premature death or premature cardiovascular disease is important to elicit. It is also important to ascertain a prior history of a cardiac murmur or specific knowledge of an underlying cardiac abnormality (either structural, valvular, or arrhythmic). On physical examination, blood pressure should be recorded. The precordial fields should be auscultated in the supine, squatting, and standing positions. Murmurs that increase from squatting to standing or that increase with the Valsalva maneuver are of potential concern and merit further evaluation. The equality of the femoral pulses should be noted. Although routine use of modalities such as electrocardiograms, stress testing, and/or echocardiograms as screening efforts are not routinely recommended, if there is any suspicion that the athlete might have a symptomatic arrhythmia or be at risk for sudden cardiac death, that individual should be withheld from physical activity pending formal cardiology consultation and evaluation.

Dave S, Feinstein R. Cardiovascular clearance for sports participation. *Curr Probl Pediatr Adolesc Health Care.* 2018;18:30051–30058. [PMID: 20049477]

Mirabelli MH, Singh J, Mendoza M. The preparticipation sports evaluation. *Am Fam Physician.* 2015;92(5):371–376. [PMID: 26371570]

Nutrition and the Development of Healthy Eating Habits

Natalie E. Gentile, MD

Evelyn L. Lewis, MD, MA, FAAFP, DABDA

A major topic pertinent to the health and wellness of children and adolescents is the development of healthy lifestyle habits beginning at an early age. In this chapter, we explore the factors that influence these habits, the consequences of poor dietary patterns, and how the provider can educate the child or adolescent and family to successfully adopt healthy eating.

A great deal of dieting occurs in Western culture as part of normal eating. In fact, estimates suggest that anywhere from 15% to 80% of the population may be dieting at a given time. The term *dieting* in lay culture has been used to describe a wide variety of behaviors ranging from healthful (eg, eating more vegetables, cutting out processed foods) to extreme (eg, self-induced vomiting, laxative misuse). Further, consideration of dieting in the context of an individual's weight status is an important factor in evaluating whether dieting is pathologic (in underweight or nonoverweight individuals) versus appropriate (in overweight individuals). Dieting can also be related to eating disorders (EDs). For example, it has been suggested that dieting typically precedes ED onset in cases of bulimia nervosa (BN), whereas for binge eating disorder (BED), binge eating has been reported as preceding the onset of dieting in approximately half of cases.

The provider needs to be aware of the risk factors for EDs, including eating behaviors that lead to development of obesity, and how to recognize these in patients. More than 8 million Americans suffer from EDs. Approximately 90% of them are young women; however, middle-aged women, children, and men are also affected. The prevalence of EDs appears to vary by the population being studied.

BED appears to afflict adults of all socioeconomic strata and education level equally. Furthermore, BED is often diagnosed in middle-aged adults. Finally, it should be noted that BED is the most prevalent ED in the United States, affecting 6–10% of young women. Recent research suggests that individuals diagnosed with an ED not otherwise specified (EDNOS) did not differ significantly from those with anorexia nervosa (AN) and BED in terms of eating or general pathology. However, individuals with BN exhibited greater eating and general psychopathology compared to EDNOS. Clinicians should monitor possible progression of EDNOS to full-syndrome AN, BN, or BED, especially given the paucity of treatment recommendations for EDNOS.

Obesity may be the sequela of disordered eating behaviors or may be the impetus for their development. One issue that is now at the forefront of the family medicine community is the epidemic of childhood obesity. Among children age 2–19 years, obesity is defined as a body mass index (BMI) at or above the 95th percentile of sex-specific BMI for age, and severe obesity is defined as a BMI at or above 120% of the 95th percentile. Nearly one in five children in the United States are now considered obese. Childhood obesity increases the risk of obesity in adulthood and subsequent development of chronic illness, including but not limited to a wide range of renal and cardiovascular disease.

Broaching the topic of weight with children and adolescents is further complicated by the psychological effects of obesity. Irrespective of gender, obese children have lower quality of life scores and higher risk of poor body image and depression. During the office visit, the provider runs the risk of weight stigmatization, a significant nonintended consequence. Similar to the effects of being obese, experiencing weight stigmatization is linked to increased prevalence of disordered eating behavior, depression, and low self-esteem in children. It goes without saying then that decreasing weight stigmatization can improve mental health in these patients.

INFLUENCES ON DIETARY HABITS

There are several factors, including gender, societal pressures, familial habits, ethnicity, and socioeconomic status, that influence the complex decision that children and adolescents make every time they are presented with the opportunity to eat.

Females are most likely to restrict their food intake to control their weight or lose weight, but increasingly males are also engaging in dieting behavior. Perhaps most worrisome is the prevalence of dieting among adolescents and even children. Data suggest that 40% of 9-year-old girls have dieted, and even 5-year-olds voice concern about their diet that appear to be linked to cultural standards for body image.

African American women are also more likely to develop BN or BED than AN, and a recent study by Marques and colleagues found a strong association between BED and obesity in this population. Age- and sex-specific estimates suggest that about 0.5–1% of adolescent girls develop AN, whereas 5% of older adolescent and young adult women develop BN. This population also exhibits a high frequency of coexistence between AN and BN. It has been reported that as many as 50% of AN patients may exhibit bulimic behaviors, whereas 30–80% of patients with BN have a history of AN.

Familial eating patterns are often passed down through generations. These eating habits are often formed in early childhood and influence food choices for the rest of the child's life. In addition, what a child or adolescent perceives as a "normal" weight or body size may be tied to what his or her family members look like.

Adolescents and children currently are under more pressure than ever from the influence of social media. Body image has taken on a whole new meaning as this population has constant access to photographs of people from all over the world. With the advent of social media platforms such as Instagram, Facebook, and Snapchat, children and adolescents can now post and view actual photos of themselves; in addition, many of these photos are doctored with filters that enhance the images. This falsification and idealization of body image leads to unrealistic expectations for the viewer of what they should or could look like. This has led to an unprecedented environment of appearance norms that are often not achievable for the average child or adolescent, leading to lower self-esteem and self-worth. This has been shown in young women in particular, who associate negative body image with viewing of other young women who are more attractive through social media. The populations at highest risk for AN and BN are female adolescents and young adults, and screening should occur throughout adolescence, especially at ages 14 and 18 years. This correlates with the transition to high school and college and the associated stressors.

With regard to ethnicity, data suggest that BN is more prevalent among Hispanics and African Americans than among non-Hispanic whites. Hispanics are more likely to develop binge eating and BED than AN and BN. Several studies have shown that other abnormal eating behaviors may be as common or even more common among African Americans (eg, purging by laxatives vs vomiting, binge eating). The predominance of non-Hispanic whites among cases of AN may contribute to cultural bias in diagnosis, with less recognition of EDs among ethnic minorities. Compared to adults, the prevalence of EDs among adolescents is characterized by a different racial and ethnic pattern. Among adolescents, a recent study by Swanson and colleagues of racial and ethnic differences in ED prevalence within a nationally representative sample suggest that non-Hispanic white adolescents report a greater prevalence of AN compared to other racial and ethnic groups. However, Hispanic adolescents report the highest prevalence of BN in comparison to non-Hispanic white and black adolescents. Further, there is a trend for greater prevalence of BED among ethnic minorities, relative to AN and BN. Among high school students, Hispanic and non-Hispanic white girls tend to report similar levels of eating disordered attitudes and cognitions, such as excessive shape and weight concern and extreme dieting, which may be risk factors for full-syndrome disorders. African American girls, however, report lower body weight concerns and behaviors than girls of other ethnicities. Among adolescent boys, nearly all ethnic minorities report more ED symptoms and weight concerns compared to white boys. How subthreshold disturbances and risk factors manifest into differential prevalence of full-syndrome disorders across cultures is not well understood.

High prevalence of obesity appears to disproportionately affect those of racial and ethnic minorities. Approximately 75% of African American and Mexican American adults, compared to approximately 68% of non-Hispanic white adults, are considered overweight or obese. Similarly, approximately 22% of African American and Hispanic children, compared with 14% of non-Hispanic white children, are overweight. Given the high rates of obesity in ethnic minority populations, experts have postulated that BED is a significant problem among these groups.

It is traditionally believed that AN and BN tend to affect adolescent girls of middle to upper socioeconomic status. However, some recent data suggest a lack of association between socioeconomic status and the presentation of any ED.

POPULAR DIETARY PATTERNS

Given the vast number of dietary patterns popularized in the media, the provider can expect that children and adolescents will have questions about certain types of diets. The mainstream patterns of eating that will likely be addressed include vegetarian/vegan, ketogenic, paleo, intermittent fasting, Mediterranean, and gluten-free. A broad overview of these diets will be reviewed here.

Vegetarians restrict or avoid meat intake, whereas vegans restrict or avoid intake of any animal products including eggs, dairy, poultry, meat, and sometimes honey. This eating pattern may or may not be associated with religious beliefs (eg, Seventh-Day Adventists) and/or environmental concerns.

The ketogenic diet refers to a focus on high-fat and low-carbohydrate intake. It differs from the Paleo diet in that it does not emphasize high-protein intake. The Paleo diet also emphasizes restriction of high glycemic index carbohydrates and incorporation of high-protein and high-fiber foods.

Intermittent fasting refers to cycling between periods of eating and periods of little to no caloric intake.

The Mediterranean diet is similar in many ways to the vegan diet with promotion of plant-based foods. There is some incorporation of small amounts of animal protein like fish or seafood.

Historically associated with those who have celiac disease, the gluten-free diet has now been popularized as a weight loss diet for the general population. This diet avoids all food containing gluten. In addition to being found in wheat, barley, some oats, and rye, gluten is also used in many processed foods, pastas, cereals, and breads. In general, this is the diet of choice for patients with celiac disease or gluten sensitivity. In the general population though, one should be aware that just because a product is labeled as "gluten-free," this does not equate with "healthy." There are many processed products on the market that are gluten-free but lack essential nutrients such as fiber, B vitamins, and iron. Those who avoid gluten do not necessarily take in few calories or make healthier food choices, and some studies show that the lack of whole grains in this type of diet is associated with an increased risk of heart disease.

DIETARY RECOMMENDATIONS

Dietary recommendations should focus heavily on incorporating as many whole, plant foods as possible. Generally, this includes whole grains, fruits, vegetables, and legumes. Water should be the primary source of hydration with minimal to no intake of dairy or juice products. The provider can encourage families to "crowd out" less healthful foods by incorporating those that are more healthful. A general guideline for children and adolescents is teaching them how to fill their plate at each meal. Equally as important is discussing the quality and source of each food group being eaten. For example, whole grains, vegetables, and fruits are excellent and healthful sources of carbohydrates, whereas one may consume a "lower-carb" processed food with less health benefits. Similarly, studies have shown that diets low in carbohydrates, when coupled with plant-based fat and protein sources, are associated with lower heart disease incidence, but the same does not hold true for those coupled with animal-based sources of fat and protein.

▶ Protein

Dietary protein, once digested into amino acids, plays a major role throughout the entire body, with amino acids found in enzymes, hormones, and cellular function components. The body can make several amino acids endogenously, but nine of the amino acids must be obtained through the diet. These nine amino acids are histidine, isoleucine, leucine, lysine, methionine/cysteine, phenylalanine/tyrosine,

threonine, tryptophan, and valine. Protein is found in both plant and animal sources, including meat, fish, eggs, dairy, poultry, legumes, grains, nuts, seeds, and vegetables (http://www.nationalacademies.org/hmd/Activities/Nutrition/ObesitySolutions/2019-APR-1.aspx). Recommended daily intake is higher in pregnancy and lactation, approximately 70 g/d. In general, it is recommended that males have a slightly higher intake of protein (~50 g/d) than females (40 g/d). With regard to protein, Americans get about twice as much as they actually need. The type of protein chosen is important to discuss with families. A protein source should take up no more than one-quarter of the plate and ideally be from a plant-based source, such as beans, nuts, or legumes. Other sources include fish and lean meats. Red and processed meats (eg, bacon or deli meat) should be minimized, if not avoided. In 2015, the World Health Organization (WHO) made a statement that red meats and processed meats are known carcinogens. Type of protein (animal vs plant) is associated with BMI, even from the prenatal stages. Some studies suggest that intake of animal protein during pregnancy is associated with an increased risk of obesity in subsequent offspring.

▶ Fat

Dietary fat is an energy source that aids in absorption of fat-soluble vitamins. Omega-6 fatty acids in particular are structural components of lipid membranes and assist in skin function. Omega-3 fatty acids play a critical role in nerve function. Saturated fat, *trans* fat, and dietary cholesterol have no essential function in the body other than an additional energy source. The body is able to synthesize cholesterol and saturated fatty acids to meet its functional needs. Fat is readily available in many foods including oils, meat, butter, some fish, nuts, seeds, and baked goods. Saturated fat is found in animal products such as meat and butter, as well as some oils. Cholesterol is only found in animal fats. Intake of saturated fat, *trans* fat, or cholesterol is associated with an increase in low-density lipoprotein concentrations. A moderate amount of plant oils can be used sparingly, including olive oil or canola oil. Oils high in *trans* fats, such as partially hydrogenated oils (eg, shortening, oils used in frying foods), should be minimized or avoided.

▶ Carbohydrates

Carbohydrates are a major dietary nutrient that provides energy for bodily functions, and the category includes sugars, fiber, and starches. Pregnant and lactating women need a higher intake of carbohydrates, approximately 200 g/d. Men, women, and children should get approximately 130 g/d. Sugars and starches provide energy via their breakdown into glucose. These are typically considered sources of simple carbohydrates. Naturally occurring sugars, found primarily in fruit, should be the primary source of sugar in the diet. Added sugars, found in packaged and refined foods such as pastries, candy, soda, and syrups, should be minimized in the diet. The primary sources of starch that should be included in the diet are beans, vegetables, and whole grains. Fiber, divided into soluble and insoluble types, is not broken down. Fiber helps with proper bowel function and is associated with blood glucose regulation. Given that foods containing fiber tend to be filling, it is likely that overall food consumption is lowered due to satiety when foods high in fiber are consumed. Soluble fiber plays a role in blood glucose regulation. Insoluble fiber helps with bulking of the stools. Fiber intake is associated with a risk reduction in coronary artery disease. Fiber is found in sufficient amounts in whole grains, beans, legumes, most vegetables, fruits, nuts, and seeds. The majority of Americans only get 15 g of daily fiber, but the recommendation is around 30–40 g. The primary sources of carbohydrate in the diet should be from whole fruits, whole vegetables, and whole grains. One-quarter of the plate should be whole, unrefined grains, such as brown rice, whole-wheat pasta, and quinoa. These grains help with blood sugar control and, depending on the type of grain chosen, also can provide protein. The refining process, which removes the bran and germ components from the whole grain, results in a longer shelf life for food products but at the cost of the B vitamins, fiber, and iron in these products. Therefore, refined grains tend to be enriched with iron and B vitamins, but not fiber. Half of the plate should be a colorful variety of fruits and vegetables. This provides fiber, essential vitamins, and minerals including calcium.

▶ Sodium

A small amount of sodium is required in the diet for nerve and muscle function as well as electrolyte balance. Excess sodium intake is associated with heart disease, stroke, and hypertension. Sodium in the standard American diet is found in processed foods and foods made in restaurants. Food made in the home or added salt accounts for a very small proportion of the typical intake. The recommended daily amount of sodium intake is <2300 mg. The average American consumes excess sodium, at least 3400 mg/d.

▶ Resources for Promoting Dietary Recommendations

One example of a simple method for families to remember healthy lifestyle methods is the Let's Go! 5-2-1-0 Program (5-2-1-0), which has been effective in preventing and treating obesity in many community settings across the country. These guidelines encourage incorporating the daily habits of 5 fruits and vegetables, 2 hours or less of screen time, 1 hour of physical activity, and 0 sugary beverages. The MaineHealth website for 5-2-1-0 (https://mainehealth.org/lets-go) is an excellent resource for families to learn about more detailed ways to incorporate these guidelines into their children's lives.

Another excellent guide for families is the Harvard Healthy Eating Plate through the Nutrition Source with Harvard School of Public Health (Figure 11–1). This site provides guidelines and examples of the different food groups to include in the daily diet and helps families make healthier choices (https://www.hsph.harvard.edu/nutritionsource/healthy-eating-plate/).

Although the focus in counseling should primarily be on what foods to incorporate more, as discussed earlier, it can be mentioned that patients would be best served by minimizing intake of refined, processed foods and foods containing refined sugars. The concept of energy density can be discussed with families. This is defined as the number of calories per unit of weight in food and drink. For example, fiber and water are high in weight with a low number of calories, making them low in energy density. On the contrary, fatty foods are higher in energy density. A general rule to guide food choices would be to minimize high energy density foods in the diet and maximize those low in energy density, or higher in water and fiber.

Engaging children and teens in the process of selecting and preparing the foods they consume facilitates their ability to develop and maintain a healthy relationship with food. In addition, it is imperative that parents be encouraged to lead by example with regard to healthy eating habits.

Given the association between lifestyle habits, nutrition, and lifestyle-related disease development later in life, the family physician is in an ideal position to counsel children, teens, and their families about nutrition recommendations. This is particularly important when considering lifestyle-related diseases. This includes chronic conditions such as diabetes, heart disease, and hypertension. Equally important as the physical diseases are the mental, behavioral, and psychosocial consequences.

Ideally, the primary care provider will be aware of community resources for children, teens, and families that offer healthy living education or activities, such as those offered at local facilities like the YMCA or community education centers. In addition to physical activity, sleep, and emotional support, proper nutrition is an integral contributor to the overall physical and emotional well-being of children and adolescents.

The family medicine provider needs to have the tools at hand to counsel patients and families about nutrition, including knowing the appropriate guidelines and community resources. Ideally, family medicine visits will focus on prevention in addition to treatment of weight issues in children and adolescents, but this requires that the provider have an understanding of the factors that influence eating patterns in these patients.

Leading this discussion in the family medicine office visit can at times be a delicate subject and lead to emotional responses from parents and/or patient embarrassment. It is important to emphasize that healthy eating habits and weight

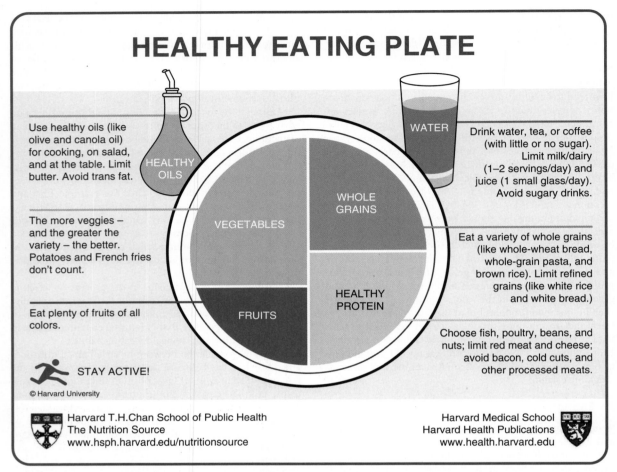

▲ **Figure 11–1. Healthy Eating Plate.** (Copyright © 2011 Harvard University. For more information about The Healthy Eating Plate, please see The Nutrition Source, Department of Nutrition, Harvard T.H. Chan School of Public Health, http://www.thenutritionsource.org and Harvard Health Publications, health.harvard.edu.)

management lead to longevity and healthy bodily processes, with minimal emphasis on physical appearance or meeting social standards.

Ashmore JA, Friedman KE, Reichmann SK, Musante GJ. Weight-based stigmatization, psychological distress, & binge eating behavior among obese treatment-seeking adults. *Eat Behav.* 2008;9(2):203–209. [PMID: 18329599]

Bouvard V, Loomis D, Guyton KZ, et al. Carcinogenicity of consumption of red and processed meat. *Lancet Oncol.* 2015;16(16):1599–1600. [PMID: 26514947]

Cohen R, Newton-John T, Slater A. The relationship between Facebook and Instagram appearance-focused activities and body image concerns in young women. *Body Image.* 2017;23: 183–187. [PMID: 29055773]

Eisenberg ME, Neumark-Sztainer D, Story M. Associations of weight-based teasing and emotional well-being among adolescents. *Arch Pediatr Adolesc Med.* 2003;157(8):733–738. [PMID: 12912777]

Flegal KM, Carroll MD, Kit BK, Ogden CL. Prevalence of obesity and trends in the distribution of body mass index among US adults, 1999-2010. *JAMA.* 2012;307(5):491–497. [PMID: 22253363]

Flegal KM, Carroll MD, Ogden CL, Curtin LR. Prevalence and trends in obesity among US adults, 1999-2008. *JAMA.* 2010;303(3):235–241. [PMID: 20071471]

Friedman KE, Ashmore JA, Applegate KL. Recent experiences of weight-based stigmatization in a weight loss surgery population: psychological and behavioral correlates. *Obesity (Silver Spring).* 2008;16(Suppl 2):S69–S74. [PMID: 18978766]

Friedman KE, Reichmann SK, Costanzo PR, Musante GJ. Body image partially mediates the relationship between obesity and psychological distress. *Obes Res.* 2002;10(1):33–41. [PMID: 11786599]

Gouveia MJ, Frontini R, Canavarro MC, Moreira H. Quality of life and psychological functioning in pediatric obesity: the role of body image dissatisfaction between girls and boys of different ages. *Qual Life Res.* 2014;23(9):2629–2638. [PMID: 24817248]

Hales CM, Fryar CD, Carroll MD, Freedman DS, Ogden CL. Trends in obesity and severe obesity prevalence in US youth and adults by sex and age, 2007-2008 to 2015-2016. *JAMA.* 2018;319(16):1723–1725. [PMID: 29570750]

Halton TL, Willett WC, Liu S, et al. Low-carbohydrate-diet score and the risk of coronary heart disease in women. *N Engl J Med.* 2006;355(19):1991–2002. [PMID: 17093250]

Harvard T.H. Chan School of Public Health. The Nutrition Source. Diet Reviews. https://www.hsph.harvard.edu/nutritionsource/healthy-weight/diet-reviews/. Accessed November 11, 2019.

Hogue JV, Mills JS. The effects of active social media engagement with peers on body image in young women. *Body Image.* 2019;28:1–5. [PMID: 30439560]

Holland G, Tiggemann M. A systematic review of the impact of the use of social networking sites on body image and disordered eating outcomes. *Body Image.* 2016;17:100–110. [PMID: 26995158]

Janesick AS, Shioda T, Blumberg B. Transgenerational inheritance of prenatal obesogen exposure. *Mol Cell Endocrinol.* 2014;398(1-2):31–35. [PMID: 25218215]

Kim JW, Chock TM. Body image 2.0: associations between social grooming on Facebook and body image concerns. *Comput Human Behav.* 2015;48:331–339. [No PMID]

MaineHealth. Let's Go! 5-2-1-0. https://mainehealth.org/lets-go. Accessed November 11, 2019.

Marques L, Alegria M, Becker AE, et al. Comparative prevalence, correlates of impairment, and service utilization for eating disorders across US ethnic groups: implications for reducing ethnic disparities in health care access for eating disorders. *Int J Eat Disord.* 2011;44:412–420. [PMID: 20665700]

Maslova E, Hansen S, Grunnet LG, et al. Maternal protein intake in pregnancy and offspring metabolic health at age 9-16 y: results from a Danish cohort of gestational diabetes mellitus pregnancies and controls. *Am J Clin Nutr.* 2017;106(2):623–636. [PMID: 28679553]

Maslova E, Rytter D, Bech BH, et al. Maternal protein intake during pregnancy and offspring overweight 20 y later. *Am J Clin Nutr.* 2014;100(4):1139–1148. [PMID: 25099541]

Mustillo S, Worthman C, Erkanli A, et al. Obesity and psychiatric disorder: developmental trajectories. *Pediatrics.* 2003;111(4 Pt 1): 851–859. [PMID: 12671123]

Myers TA, Crowther JH. Social comparison as a predictor of body dissatisfaction: A meta-analytic review. *J Abnorm Psychol.* 2009;118(4):683–698. [PMID: 19899839]

Nehus E, Mitsnefes M. Childhood obesity and the metabolic syndrome. *Pediatr Clin North Am.* 2019;66(1):31–43. [PMID: 30454749]

Ogden CL, Carroll MD, Kit BK, Flegal KM. Prevalence of obesity and trends in body mass index among US children and adolescents, 1999-2010. *JAMA.* 2012;307(5):483–490. [PMID: 22253364]

Puhl RM, Moss-Racusin CA, Schwartz MB. Internalization of weight bias: Implications for binge eating and emotional well-being. *Obesity (Silver Spring).* 2007;15(1):19–23. [PMID: 17228027]

Sanderson K, Patton GC, McKercher C, Dwyer T, Venn AJ. Overweight and obesity in childhood and risk of mental disorder: a 20-year cohort study. *Aust N Z J Psychiatry.* 2011;45(5): 384–392. [PMID: 21500955]

Swanson SA, Crow SJ, Le Grange D, et al. Prevalence and correlates of eating disorders in adolescents: results from the National Comorbidity Survey Replication Adolescent Supplement. *Arch Gen Psychiatry.* 2011;68:714–723. [PMID: 21383252]

US Department of Health and Human Services and US Department of Agriculture. *2015–2020 Dietary Guidelines for Americans.* 8th ed. December 2015. https://health.gov/dietaryguidelines/2015/guidelines/. Accessed November 11, 2019.

US National Library of Medicine. Medical Encyclopedia. Medline Plus. https://medlineplus.gov/encyclopedia.html. Accessed November 11, 2019.

Van Horn L. Achieving nutrient density: a vegetarian approach. *J Am Diet Assoc.* 2011;111(6):799. [PMID: 21616188]

Yin J, Quinn S, Dwyer T, Ponsonby AL, Jones G. Maternal diet, breastfeeding and adolescent body composition: a 16-year prospective study. *Eur J Clin Nutr.* 2012;66(12):1329–1334. [PMID: 23047715]

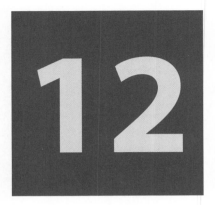

Adolescent Sexuality

Amy Crawford-Faucher, MD, FAAFP

Adolescence, generally between 12 and 19 years, is a time of complex physical, cognitive, psychosocial, and sexual changes, and physical development occurs in advance of cognitive maturity. Not until maturity is reached in all of these realms does the adolescent acquire mature decision-making skills and the ability to make healthy decisions regarding sexual activity. Sexuality involves more than just anatomic gender or physical sexual behavior, but incorporates how individuals view themselves as male, female, or other; how they relate to others; and the ability to enter into and maintain an intimate relationship on a giving and trusting basis. Adolescent sexual development forms the basis for further adult sexuality and future intimate relationships. Adolescents who are sexually active before having achieved the capacity for intimacy are at risk for unwanted or unhealthy consequences of sexual activity.

DEVELOPMENT

▶ Physical Changes

Rapid changes in their bodies often make adolescents feel uncomfortable and self-conscious. Puberty usually starts between 9 and 12 years for girls and between 11 and 14 years for boys. In girls, these hormonal changes result in the development of breasts, growth of pubic and axillary hair, body odor, and menstruation (often irregular or unpredictable for the first 18–24 months). Boys develop increased penis and testicular size; facial, pubic, and axillary hair; body odor; and a deepened voice, and experience nocturnal ejaculations ("wet dreams"). As adolescents are learning to adjust and grow comfortable with their changing bodies, questions concerning body image are common (eg, penis size, breast size and development, distribution of pubic hair, and changing physique in general).

▶ Cognitive Changes

The shift from concrete thinking to abstract thinking (the cognitive development of formal operations) begins in early adolescence (11–12 years) and usually reaches full development by 15–16 years, so 10- to 14-year-olds should not be expected to function with full capacity for abstract thinking. In contrast to younger children, adolescents:

- Show an increased ability to generate and hold in mind more than one complex mental representation.
- Show an appreciation of the relativity and uncertainty of knowledge.
- Tend to think in terms of abstract rather than only concrete representations; they think of consequences and the future (abstract) versus a sense of being omnipotent, invincible, infallible, and immune to mishaps (concrete).
- Show a far greater use of strategies for obtaining knowledge, such as active planning and evaluation of alternatives.
- Are self-aware in their thinking and able to reflect on their own thought processes and evaluate the credibility of the knowledge source.
- Understand that fantasies are not acted out.
- Have the capacity to develop intimate, meaningful relationships.

▶ Psychosocial Changes

Core psychosocial developmental tasks of adolescence include the following:

- Becoming emotionally and behaviorally independent rather than dependent, especially in developing independence from the family.
- Acquiring educational and other experiences needed for adult work roles and developing a realistic vocational goal.
- Learning to deal with emerging sexuality and to achieve a mature level of sexuality.

- Resolving issues of identity and achieving a realistic and positive self-image.
- Developing interpersonal skills, including the capacity for intimacy, and preparing for intimate partnerships with others.

Psychosocial development includes both internal (introspective) and external forces. Peers, parents or guardians, teachers, and coaches all influence adolescent expectations, evaluations, values, feedback, and social comparison. Failure to accomplish the developmental tasks necessary for adulthood results in identity or role diffusion: an uncertain self-concept, indecisiveness, and clinging to the more secure dependencies of childhood.

As part of this maturation process, it is natural for adolescents to explore sexual relationships and sexual roles in their social interactions. The adolescent's task is to successfully manage the conflict between sexual drives and the recognition of the emotional, interpersonal, and biological results of sexual behavior.

Sexual Changes

Gender, sexual identity, and sexual orientation are distinct concepts and can be complex. Gender identity, the sense of maleness, femaleness, a combination of the two, or neither male nor female, is established by around age 2 years and solidifies as adolescents experience and integrate sexuality into their identity. Sexual identity is the awareness of self as a sexual being who can be involved in a sexual relationship with others. Sexual orientation is who an individual is sexually and romantically attracted to. Sexual orientation emerges during adolescence and includes behavior, sexual attraction, erotic fantasy, emotional preference, social preference, and self-identification. The task of adolescence is to integrate sexual orientation into sexual identity. Although society assumes heterosexual orientation, it is more realistically a continuum from completely heterosexual to completely homosexual (see Chapter 62).

Societal attitudes against nonheterosexual individuals are associated with significant psychological distress for gay, lesbian, bisexual, and transgendered (GLBT) persons and have a negative impact on mental health, including a greater incidence of depression and suicide (as many as one-third have attempted suicide at least once), lower self-acceptance, and a greater likelihood of hiding sexual orientation. When GLBT adolescents disclose their orientation to their families, they may experience overt rejection at home as well as social isolation among their peers. GLBT adolescents may lack role models and access to support systems. They are more likely to run away and become homeless, which puts them at higher risk for unsafe sex, drug and alcohol use, and exchanging sex for money or drugs. Negative attitudes within society toward GLBT individuals lead to antigay violence (see Chapter 58).

Adolescents with questions or concerns about sexual orientation need the opportunity to discuss their feelings, their experiences, and their fears of exposure to family and friends. GLBT adolescents need reassurance about their value as a person, support regarding parental and societal reactions, and access to role models. Parents, Families, and Friends of Lesbians and Gays (PFLAG) is a nationwide organization whose purpose is to assist parents with information and support (see Chapter 62).

Problems with sexual identity may manifest in extremes—sexually acting out or repression of sexuality. Frequent sexual activity and various sexual partners are negative risk factors for physical or psychological health and can suggest poor integration of sexual identity in adolescents.

American Academy of Child and Adolescent Psychiatry. *Normal Adolescent Development, Part I. Facts for Families*, no. 57. https://www.aacap.org/AACAP/Families_and_Youth/Facts_for_Families/FFF-Guide/Normal-Adolescent-Development-Part-I-057.aspx. Accessed April 19, 2013.
Christie D, Viner R. Adolescent development. *Br Med J.* 2005; 330(7486):301–304. [PMID: 15695279]
Leibowitz SF, Tellingator C. Assessing gender identity concerns in children and adolescents: evaluation, treatments and outcomes. *Curr Psychiatry Rep.* 2012;14(2):111–120. [PMID: 22367419]

SEXUAL BEHAVIOR & INITIATION OF SEXUAL ACTIVITY

Early- to middle-stage adolescents begin to experience sexual urges that may be satisfied by masturbation. Masturbation is the exploration of the sexual self and provides a sense of control over one's body and sexual needs. Masturbation starts in infancy, providing children with enjoyment of their bodies. Parents are typically uncomfortable observing this behavior. In early adolescence, masturbation is an important developmental task, allowing the adolescent to learn what forms of self-stimulation are pleasurable and integrating this with fantasies of interacting with another. Sexual curiosity intensifies. With older adolescents, the autoeroticism of masturbation develops into experimentation with others, including intercourse.

Typical reasons for sexual activity in early to mid-adolescence are curiosity, peer pressure, seeking approval, physical urges, and rebellion. Sexual activity can be misinterpreted by the adolescent as evidence of independence from the family or individuation. Adolescent girls may misinterpret sexual activity as a measure of a meaningful relationship. When sexual activity is used to satisfy needs such as self-esteem, popularity, and dependence, it delays or prevents development of a capacity for intimacy and is associated with casual and less responsible sexual activity. Appropriate education, parental support, and a positive sexual self-concept are associated with a later age of first intercourse, a higher consistent use of contraceptives, and a lower pregnancy rate.

Parental supervision and establishing limits, living with both parents in a stable environment, high self-esteem, higher family income, and orientation toward achievement are associated with delayed initiation of sexual activity.

Commitment to a religion or affiliation with certain religious denominations appears to influence sexual behavior. For example, an adolescent's frequent attendance at religious services is associated with a greater likelihood of abstinence. On the other hand, for adolescents who are sexually active, frequency of attendance is associated with decreased contraceptive use by girls and increased use by boys.

Evidence suggests that school attendance reduces adolescent sexual risk-taking behavior. Worldwide, as the percentage of girls completing elementary school has increased, adolescent birth rates have decreased. In the United States, adolescents who have dropped out of school are more likely to initiate sexual activity earlier, fail to use contraception, become pregnant, and give birth. Among those who remain in school, greater involvement with school, including athletics for girls, is related to less sexual risk taking, including later age of initiation of sex and lower frequency of sex, pregnancy, and childbearing.

Schools structure students' time, creating an environment that discourages unhealthy risk taking, particularly by increasing interactions between children and adults. They also affect selection of friends and larger peer groups. Schools can increase belief in the future and help adolescents plan for higher education and careers, and they can increase students' sense of competence, as well as their communication and refusal skills. Evaluation of school-based sex education programs that typically emphasize abstinence, but also discuss condoms and other methods of contraception, indicates that the programs either have no effect on—or, in some cases, result in—a delay in the initiation of sexual activity. There is strong evidence that providing information about contraception does not increase adolescent sexual activity by hastening the onset of sexual intercourse, increasing the frequency of sexual intercourse, or increasing the number of sexual partners. More importantly, providing this information results in increased use of condoms or contraceptives among adolescents who were already sexually active.

Factors associated with early age of first intercourse and lack of contraceptive use are early pubertal development, a history of sexual abuse, lower socioeconomic status, poverty, lack of attentive and nurturing parents, single-parent homes, cultural and familial patterns of early sexual experience, lack of school or career goals, and dropping out of school. Additional factors include low self-esteem, concern for physical appearance, peer group pressure, and pressure to please partners.

Compared with those not sexually active, sexually active male adolescents used more alcohol, engaged in more fights, and were more likely to know about human immunodeficiency virus (HIV) and acquired immunodeficiency syndrome (AIDS). Similarly, sexually active female adolescents used more alcohol and cigarettes. Both sexually active male and female adolescents had higher levels of stress. Alcohol and drug use is associated with greater risk taking, including unprotected sexual activity.

Kirby DB, Baumler E, Coyle KK, et al. The "safer choices" intervention: its impact on the sexual behaviors of different subgroups of high school students. *J Adolesc Health.* 2004;35:442–452. [PMID: 15581523]

SCOPE OF THE PROBLEM

▶ Prevalence & Consequences of Sexual Activity

Approximately 47% of all US adolescents have ever had sex. Most teens become sexually active in their later teen years; 70% have had sexual intercourse by the time they turn 19. Approximately 33% of all 15- to 19-year-olds have had sexual intercourse in the past 3 months. For adolescents who want to have intercourse, the primary reasons given are sexual curiosity (50% of boys; 24% of girls) and affection for their partner (25% of boys; 48% of girls). For adolescents who agree to have intercourse but do not really want to, the primary reasons given are peer pressure (~30%), curiosity (50% of boys; 25% of girls), and affection for their partner (>33%). With little sex education, adolescents are poorly prepared to openly discuss their need for contraception, negotiate safe sex, and negotiate the types of behavior in which they are willing to participate. Sexual behavior that contradicts personal values is associated with emotional distress and lower self-esteem. As adolescents are learning to develop appropriate interpersonal skills, damage to self-esteem can be significant when sexual activity is exchanged for attention, affection, peer approval, or reassurance about their physical appearance. Furthermore, early unsatisfactory sexual experiences can set up patterns for repeated unsatisfactory sexual experiences into adulthood.

▶ Unintended Pregnancy

The rates of teen pregnancy, birth, and abortion have all decreased in the past 25 years, likely due to a combination of delayed initiation of sexual activity and increased use of contraception. Despite these advances, however, at least 70% of teen pregnancies in the United States are not planned. With similar rates of adolescent sexual activity between the United States and Europe, American teens have the highest rate of adolescent pregnancy among developed nations, at 18.8 per thousand. Compared to American teens, European teens are more likely to use contraception and to use the most reliable contraception.

Unintended pregnancy is socially and economically costly. Medical costs include lost opportunity for preconception care and counseling, increased likelihood of late or no pre-natal care, increased risk for a low-birth-weight infant, and increased risk for infant mortality. The social costs include reduced educational attainment and employment oppor-tunity, increased welfare dependence, and increased risk of child abuse and neglect. In addition to the adolescent being confronted with adult problems prematurely, the parents' ability to lead productive and healthy lives and to achieve academic and economic success is compromised.

In 2013, 25% of adolescent pregnancies ended in abor-tion. Adolescents who terminate pregnancies are less likely to become pregnant over the next 2 years; more likely to graduate from high school; and more likely to show lower anxiety, higher self-esteem, and more internal control than adolescents who do not terminate pregnancies. For an ado-lescent, postponement of childbearing improves social, psy-chological, academic, and economic outcomes of life (see Chapter 16).

▶ Sexually Transmitted Infections

Adolescents and young adults (15–24 years old) have the highest rates of sexually transmitted diseases and account for 50% of new sexually transmitted disease diagnoses each year. Additionally, 21% of new HIV cases are diagnosed in young people age 13–24 years; four of five of these cases are in young males. Education about transmission and increased access and use of condoms can help prevent sexually trans-mitted diseases.

▶ Sexual Abuse

About 68,000 children are victims of sexual abuse each year. Sexual abuse contributes to sexual and mental health dys-function as well as public health problems such as substance abuse. Victims of sexual abuse may have difficulty estab-lishing and maintaining healthy relationships with others. Additionally, they may engage in premature sexual behavior, frequently seeking immediate release of sexual tension, and have poor sexual decision-making skills.

Delinquency and homelessness are associated with a history of physical, emotional, and sexual abuse, as well as negative parental reactions to sexual orientation. Homeless-ness is associated with exchanging sex for money, food, or drugs. Additionally, homeless adolescents are at high risk for repeated episodes of sexual assault.

Centers for Disease Control and Prevention. *Sexually Transmitted Diseases Surveillance. STDs in Adolescents and Young Adults.* Atlanta, GA: Centers for Disease Control and Prevention; 2017.
Guttmacher Institute. Facts on American teens' sexual and repro-ductive health. http://www.schoolhealthcenters.org/wp-content/uploads/2011/07/Reproductive-health.pdf.Accessed May 6, 2019.
Marin JA, Hamilton BE, Oserman MJK, et al. Births: Final data for 2017. *National Vital Statistics Reports*; vol 67 no. 8. Hyattsville, MD: NCHS; 2018.

US Department of Health and Human Services, Administration for Children and Families, Administration on Children, Youth and Families, Children's Bureau. Child maltreatment 2017. https://www.acf.hhs.gov/sites/default/files/cb/cm2017.pdf. Accessed November 11, 2019.
US Department of Health and Human Services, Office of Ado-lescent Health. Trends in teen pregnancy and childbearing. 2018. https://www.hhs.gov/ash/oah/adolescent-development/reproductive-health-and-teen-pregnancy/teen-pregnancy-and-childbearing/trends/index.html. Accessed May 6, 2019.

SOURCES OF INFORMATION

▶ The Family

While parents are not the primary source of information about sexuality, they do influence their adolescent's sexual attitudes; parent-adolescent communication can mitigate the strength of peer influence on sexual activity. Warm parent-child relationships with parental supervision and monitor-ing can lead to decreased sexual activity. However, parental control can be associated with negative effects if it is exces-sive or coercive. Adolescent sexuality can be very threatening to adults, who may not have resolved their own issues con-cerning sexuality. With escalating stresses, the self-esteem of parents may decline, making them either highly impulsive or overly controlling or rigid. Heightened levels of anxiety contribute to blocked communication.

▶ The Family Physician

Because many parents are uncomfortable discussing sexual-ity with their children, family physicians must be proactive in initiating and facilitating conversations about the topic.

Providing a handout (Table 12–1) for parents might help facilitate home discussions about sexuality. If information is not available at home, the family physician is uniquely posi-tioned to serve as a resource and should take a proactive approach by creating the proper environment for discussion, initiating the topic of sexuality, and providing anticipatory guidance for both adolescents and their families (Table 12–2).

A. Creating the Environment

- Ensure confidentiality for the preadolescent or adolescent for discussions about sexuality.

- Interview adolescents without the parent or guardian in the room to help create a trusting environment.

- Provide an office letter to the parent to outline policies regarding confidentiality and accessibility for adolescents.

Many states have laws regarding the ability of adolescents to seek health care for specific issues—such as contraception, mental health, substance abuse, and pregnancy—without parental presence or approval. Family physicians need to be familiar with the nuances of these laws in their practicing state.

Table 12–1. How to talk to your child about sex.

1. **Be available.** Watch for clues that show they want to talk. If your child doesn't ask, look for ways to bring up the subject. For example, you may know a pregnant woman, watch the birth of a pet, or see a baby getting a bath. Use a TV program or film to start a discussion. Libraries and schools have good books on sex that are geared to different ages.
2. **Answer their questions.** Answer honestly and without showing embarrassment, even if the time and place do not seem appropriate. A short answer may be best for the moment. Then return to the subject later. Not knowing enough about the subject to answer a question can be an opportunity to learn with your child. Tell your child that you'll get the information and continue the discussion later, or do the research together. Answer the question that is asked, but don't overload the child with too much information at once.
3. **Identify components accurately.** Use correct names for body parts and their functions to show that they are normal and okay to talk about.
4. **Practice talking about sex.** Discuss sex with your partner, another family member, or a friend. This will help you feel more comfortable when you do talk with your child.
5. **Talk about sex more than once.** Children need to hear things repeatedly over the years, because their level of understanding changes as they grow older. Make certain that you talk about feelings and not just actions. It is important not to think of sex only in terms of intercourse, pregnancy, and birth. Talk about feeling oneself as man or woman; relating to others' feelings, thoughts, and attitudes; and feelings of self-esteem.
6. **Respect their privacy.** Privacy is important, for both you and your child. If your child doesn't want to talk, say, "OK, let's talk about it later," and do. Don't forget about it. Avoid searching a child's room, drawers, or purse for "evidence," or listening in on a telephone or other private conversation.
7. **Listen to your children.** They want to know that their questions and concerns are important. Laughing at or ignoring children's questions may stop them from asking again. They will get information, accurate or inaccurate, from other sources. Listen, watch their body language to know when they are ready for you to talk, and repeat back to them what you think you heard.
8. **Share your values.** If your jokes, behaviors, or attitudes don't show respect for sexuality, then you cannot expect your child to be sexually healthy. Children learn attitudes about love, caring, and responsibility from you, whether you talk about it or not. Tell your child what your values are about sex and about life. Parents need to know what their children value in their lives, and children need to know that their parents are concerned about their health and future well-being.
9. **Help teach your child how to make decisions.** It is important for you to: (a) have your child identify the problem, (b) analyze the situation, (c) search for options or solutions, (d) think about possible consequences to these options, (e) choose the best option, (f) take action, and then (g) watch for the results.

Data from http://www.plannedparenthood.org/parents/ and http://www.familydoctor.org/familydoctor/en/teens/puberty-sexuality/questions-and-answers-about-sex.html. Accessed November 11, 2019.

Table 12–2. Office approach to adolescent health care.

1. Establish comfortable, friendly relationships that permit discussion in an atmosphere of mutual trust well before sensitive issues arise. Ensure confidentiality before the need arises. Establish separate discussions with parents and adolescents as a matter of routine.
2. Take a firm, proactive role to initiate developmentally appropriate discussions of sexuality. Recognize and use teachable moments regarding sexuality.
3. Provide anticipatory guidance and resources to facilitate family discussions about sexuality and cue families and preteens about upcoming physical and psychosocial developmental changes.
4. Enhance communication skills. Use reflective listening. With a nonjudgmental manner, accept what adolescents have to say without agreeing or disagreeing.
5. Use a positive approach when discussing developmental changes and needed interventions, complimenting pubertal changes.
6. Increase knowledge of family systems and the potential impact of physicians on the family.
7. Discuss topics about sexuality incrementally over time to improve assimilation and decrease embarrassment. Avoid scientific terms. Keep answers to questions thorough yet simple. Be cautious about questions that might erode trust.
8. Know your limitations. Use other professional staff and referrals when necessary.

Data from Croft CA, Asmussen L. A developmental approach to sexuality education: implications for medical practice. *J Adolesc Health.* 1993 Mar;14(2):109–114.

B. Proactive Approach

- Provide anticipatory guidance to parents of adolescents when they present for their own health needs.
- Cue preteens about the upcoming physical changes of puberty.
- Discuss sexuality topics incrementally, in developmentally appropriate forms (Table 12–3).

C. Asking the Question

Family physicians can initiate the topic of sexuality with adolescents during health maintenance or perhaps even acute care visits. For instance, physicians might ask their adolescent patients whom they are dating and to whom they are attracted. Because abstract thinking is still undergoing development, adolescents need explicit examples to understand ideas. History taking must be specific and directive. Instructions should be concrete. Answers to questions should be simple and thorough.

Concerns in early adolescence typically relate to body image and what is "normal," both physically and socially. Information and reassurance about pubertal changes are critical parts of physical examinations. Conversations may include addressing concerns about obesity, acne, and body image that affect self-perception of acceptability and attractiveness. Discussions about how to handle peer pressure are always helpful. The adolescent's understanding of safer sexual practices as well as the ability to negotiate the behavior in which they are willing or unwilling to participate should be explored.

Although it is important to avoid making assumptions about sexual orientation, an adolescent who presents with depression and suicidal ideation should be questioned about this. Hiding one's orientation increases stress. It is important to be aware of community resources for GLBT adolescents such as psychologists and counselors, GLBT community support groups, and organizations such as PFLAG.

Table 12–3. Adolescent sexual development.

	8–12 Years	≥13 Years
Sexual knowledge	Knows correct terms for sexual parts, commonly uses slang; understands sexual aspects of pregnancy; increasing knowledge of sexual behavior (eg, masturbation, intercourse); knowledge of physical aspects of puberty by age 10	Understands sexual intercourse, contraception, and sexually transmitted diseases (STDs)
Body parts and function	Should have complete understanding of sexual, reproductive, and elimination functions of body parts; all need anticipatory guidance on upcoming pubertal changes for both sexes, including menstruation and nocturnal emissions	Important to discuss health and hygiene, as well as provide more information about contraceptives, STDs/HIV, and responsible sexual behaviors; access to health care is important
Gender identity	Gender identity is fixed; encouragement to pursue individual interests and talents regardless of gender stereotypes is important	Discuss men and women's social perception; males tend to perceive social situations more sexually than females and may interpret neutral cues (eg, clothing, friendliness) as sexual invitations
Sexual abuse prevention	Assess their understanding of an abuser and correct misconceptions; explain how abusers, including friends, relatives, and strangers, may manipulate children; help them identify abusive situations, including sexual harassment; practice assertiveness and problem-solving skills; teach them to trust their body's internal cues and to act assertively in problematic situations	Teach them to avoid risky situations (eg, walking alone at night, unsafe parts of town); discuss dating relationships, particularly date/acquaintance rape and its association with alcohol and drug use, including date rape drugs; encourage parents to provide transportation home immediately if their teenagers are ever in difficult or potentially dangerous situations and also to consider enrolling their children in a self-defense class (eg, karate)
Sexual behavior	Sex games with peers and siblings: role play and sex fantasy, kissing, mutual masturbation, and simulated intercourse; masturbation in private; shows modesty, embarrassment;hides sex games and masturbation from adults; may fantasize or dream about sex; interested in media sex; uses sexual language with peers; considers making decisions in the context of relationships; should be provided with information about contraceptives, STDs/HIV, and responsible sexual behaviors	Pubertal changes continue;most girls menstruate by 16, boys are capable of ejaculation by 15; dating begins; sexual contacts are common—mutual masturbation, kissing, petting; sexual fantasy and dreams; sexual intercourse may occur in ≤70% by age 19; encourage parents to share attitudes and values; provide access to contraceptives; respect need and desire for privacy; set clear rules about dating and curfews
Developmental issues;[a] most sexual concerns are related to the developmental tasks	Early adolescence (Tanner I, II): physical changes, including menstruation and nocturnal emissions; often ambivalent over issues of independence and protection and family relationships; egocentric; beginning struggles of separation and emerging individual identity; seemingly trivial concerns to adults can reach crisis proportions in young adolescents; common concerns include fears of too slow or too rapid physical development, especially breasts and genitalia; concern and curiosity about their bodies; sexual feelings and sexual behavior of their peer group as well as adults around them; although masturbation is very healthy and normal, reassurance may be needed given persistence of myths and mixed messages	Middle adolescence (Tanner III, IV): peer approval; experimentation and risk-taking behavior arise from developmental task of defining oneself socially; sexual intercourse may be viewed as requisite for peer acceptance; curiosity, need for peer approval, self-esteem, and struggle for independence from parents can lead to intercourse at this stage; feelings of invincibility lead to sexual activity that is impulsive and lacking discussion about sexual decision making, such as contraception, preferences for behavior, relationship commitment, or safe sex; increasing insistence on control over decisions; increasing conflict with parents

(Continued)

Table 12–3. Adolescent sexual development. (*Continued*)

8–12 Years	≥13 Years
Developmental tasks: 1. Independence and separation from the family 2. Development of individual identity 3. Beginning to shift from concrete to abstract thinking	Developmental tasks: 1. Development of adult social relationships with both sexes 2. Continued struggle for independence 3. Continued development of individual identity 4. Continued shifting from cognitive to abstract thinking Late adolescence (Tanner V): With cognitive maturation, issues regarding peer acceptance and conflicts with parents regarding independence lessen; intimacy, commitment, and life planning, including thoughts of future parenthood; self-identity continues to solidify, moral and ethical values, exploration of sexual identity; crises over sexual orientation may surface at this stage; increasing ability to recognize consequences of own behavior Developmental tasks: 1. Abstract (futuristic) thinking 2. Vocational plans 3. Development of moral and ethical values 4. Maturation toward autonomous decision making

^aThese are general categories; adolescents vary in their physical, psychosocial, and cognitive development.
Data from Gordon BN, Schroeder CS. *Sexuality: A Developmental Approach to Problems.* New York, NY: Plenum Press; 1995; and Alexander B, McGrew MC, Shore W. Adolescent sexuality issues in office practice. *Am Fam Physician.* 1991;Oct;44(4):1273–1281.

Caring for adolescents can be exciting and challenging. Physicians should recognize that their own projections of unfinished sexual issues from their adolescence may surface in caring for adolescent patients. This can make discussions, particularly about sensitive subjects such as drugs, alcohol, nicotine, and sex, difficult. Recognizing and addressing these issues or referring adolescents to colleagues with greater experience and comfort with these matters would be appropriate.

The role of family physicians is to provide a supportive, sensitive, and instructive environment in which they neither ignore nor judge adolescent sexual activity but reassure, listen to, clarify, and provide correct information about this important aspect of adolescent development. Ideally the goal should be to delay sexual activity until adolescents have the knowledge and tools needed to make healthy decisions about sex. However, identifying adolescents at risk, educating them about safer sex, establishing sexual limits, and providing information about support and educational resources for adolescents who are currently sexually active are critical activities for the family physician.

Martino SC, Elliott MN, Corona R, et al. Beyond the big talk: the roles and breadth and repetition in parent-adolescent communication about sexual topics. *Pediatrics.* 2008;121; e612–e618. [PMID: 18310180]

Websites

For Patient Information

American Academy of Family Physicians. Information from your family doctor: Sex: Making the right decision. https://familydoctor.org/sex-making-the-right-decision

American Academy of Family Physicians. Adolescent health care, sexuality and contraception. https://www.aafp.org/about/policies/all/adolescent-sexuality.html

Parents, Families, and Friends of Lesbians and Gays (PFLAG). http://www.pflag.org

For Provider Information

Gay and Lesbian Medical Association (GLMA). http://www.glma.org

Menstrual Disorders

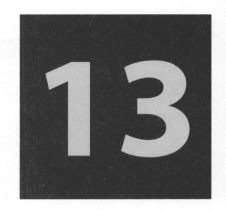

Mary V. Krueger, DO, MPH

Patricia R. Millner, MD, FAAFP

Menstrual disorders are a heterogeneous group of conditions that are both physically and psychologically debilitating. Although they were once considered nuisance problems, it is now recognized that menstrual disorders take a significant toll on society, in days lost from work, as well as the pain and suffering experienced by individual women. These disorders may arise from physiologic (eg, pregnancy), pathologic (eg, stress, excessive exercise, weight loss, endocrine or structural abnormalities), or iatrogenic (eg, secondary to contraceptive use) conditions.

Irregularities in menstruation may manifest as complete absence of menses, abnormal uterine bleeding, dysmenorrhea, or premenstrual syndrome. Vaginal bleeding is addressed in Chapter 34. Since it is essential to know what is normal in order to define that which is abnormal, normal menstrual parameters are listed in Table 13–1.

AMENORRHEA

ESSENTIALS OF DIAGNOSIS

▶ Primary amenorrhea: the absence of menses by 16 years of age in a patient with or without secondary sex characteristics, or absence of menses by 14 years of age in a patient without secondary sex characteristics, or girls without onset of period after 2 years of onset of secondary sexual characteristics.

▶ Secondary amenorrhea: absence of menses for at least 3 months in a woman with previously normal menses, or fewer than nine cycles in a year in a woman with previously irregular menses.

▶ General Considerations

Amenorrhea is a symptom, not a diagnosis, and may occur secondary to a number of endocrine, physiologic, and anatomic abnormalities. Classifying amenorrhea into primary and secondary amenorrhea can aid in evaluation and simplify diagnosis.

▶ Primary Amenorrhea

The clinician must be sensitive to the fact that the adolescent patient may be uncomfortable discussing her sexuality, especially in the presence of a parent. The most common causes of primary amenorrhea are gonadal dysgenesis, hypothalamic hypogonadism, pituitary disease, and anatomic abnormality.

▶ Clinical Findings

A. Signs and Symptoms

The history and physical exam are the most important steps in diagnosing primary amenorrhea. Key elements of the history are listed in Table 13–2. This targeted history will help narrow the differential and eliminate unnecessary testing. Physical examination should focus on appearance of secondary sexual characteristics and pelvic examination findings—specifically the presence or absence of a uterus. Body mass index should also be calculated and compared with prior visits to assess both for rapid weight loss or weight gain. Presence or absence of breast development and presence or absence of the uterus and cervix are decision points for further testing and diagnostic categories.

B. Laboratory Findings

Choice of laboratory examination should be guided by history and physical findings, and examinations are listed here based on etiology. A pregnancy test should be performed on all individuals presenting for primary amenorrhea that have secondary sexual characteristics and functional anatomy. Although the initial cycles after menarche are often anovulatory, pregnancy can occur before the first

Table 13–1. Normal menstrual parameters.

Age of menarche	<16 years old
Age of menopause	>40 years old; mean age 52
Length of menstrual cycle	22–45 days
Length of menstrual flow	3–7 days
Amount of menstrual flow	<80 mL

recognized menstrual cycle. Patients with a normal pelvic examination but absent breast development should have serum follicle-stimulating hormone (FSH) measured to distinguish peripheral (hypergonadotropic hypogonadism) from central (hypogonadotropic hypogonadism) causes of amenorrhea. A high FSH suggests gonadal dysgenesis. A karyotype should be performed to differentiate patients with Turner syndrome (45,X), which is most common, from other variations. It is important to identify patients with a 46,XY karyotype, since these individuals have a high peripubertal risk for gonadoblastoma and dysgerminoma. If the uterus is absent, serum testosterone and karyotype should be performed. Elevated testosterone in the presence of a Y chromosome indicates androgen insensitivity and the presence of functional testicular tissue that should be excised to prevent later neoplastic transformation. If uterus is present, consider outflow obstruction versus workup for secondary amenorrhea. In patients with both normal breast development and a

Table 13–2. Key historical elements in the evaluation of primary amenorrhea.

• Recent medical history
• History of head trauma (damage to the hypothalamic-pituitary axis)
• History of weight loss and amount of regular physical activity (female athlete triad)
• Timeline of development of secondary sexual characteristics (if present)
• Past medical history
  • Diabetes
  • Juvenile rheumatoid arthritis
  • Inflammatory bowel disease
  • Malignancy
  • Chronic infection
	• Family history
	  • Time of menarche in the patient's mother and sister(s)
	  • Family history of gonadal dysgenesis
	• Medications
	  • Medication or supplement use (particularly hormonal)
	  • Social history
	  • Sexual activity
	  • History of psychosocial deprivation/abuse
	• Symptoms
	  • Anosmia (Kallmann syndrome)
	  • Monthly abdominal pain (imperforate hymen, transverse vaginal septum)
	  Headache
	  Visual changes
	  Lactation (in the absence of pregnancy)

Table 13–3. Etiologies of primary amenorrhea.

Physiologic Constitutional delay Pregnancy
Pathologic **Absent breast development, normal pelvic examination findings** Hypothalamic failure Anorexia nervosa, excessive weight loss, excessive exercise, stress Chronic illness (juvenile rheumatoid arthritis, diabetes, irritable bowel syndrome)
Gonadotropin deficiency Kallmann syndrome (associated with anosmia) Pituitary dysfunction after head trauma or shock Infiltrative or inflammatory processes Pituitary adenoma Craniopharyngioma
Gonadal failure Gonadal dysgenesis (ie, Turner syndrome)
Normal breast development, normal pelvic examination findings Hypothyroidism Hyperprolactinemia
Normal breast development, abnormal pelvic examination findings Testicular feminization Anatomic abnormalities (uterovaginal septum, imperforate hymen)

pelvic examination, serum prolactin and thyroid-stimulating hormone (TSH) should be measured to rule out hyperprolactinemia and hypothyroidism. If these values are in the normal range, investigation should proceed according to the secondary amenorrhea algorithm. The etiologies for primary amenorrhea are listed in Table 13–3, and the workup for patients with primary amenorrhea is listed in the algorithm in Figure 13–1.

C. Imaging Studies

Radiographic studies are targeted toward the diagnosis suggested by history, physical, and laboratory studies. Magnetic resonance imaging (MRI) is indicated in patients with suspected pituitary pathology. Computerized visual field testing may be added if examination or MRI indicates optic chiasm compression. Pelvic imaging should be performed in patients with suspected pelvic anomalies or outflow obstructions and when it is difficult to establish if a uterus is present on physical exam. Transverse vaginal septum, imperforate hymen, or vaginal agenesis can be detected or confirmed through imaging.

▶ Treatment

A. Medical Therapy

Successful treatment of primary amenorrhea is based on correct diagnosis of the underlying etiology. The patient should

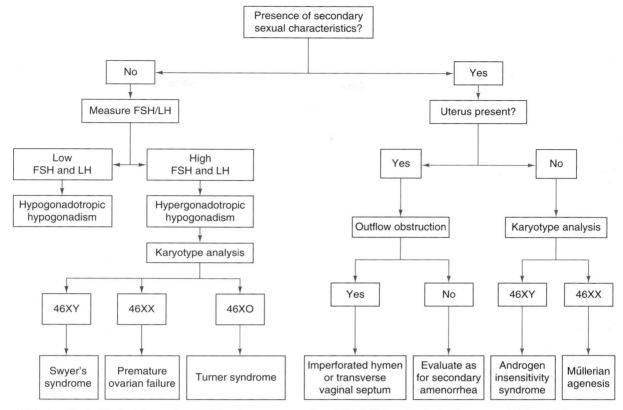

▲ **Figure 13–1.** Workup for patients with primary amenorrhea. FSH, follicle-stimulating hormone; LH, luteinizing hormone. (Reproduced with permission from DeCherney AH, Nathan L, Laufer N, et al: *Current Diagnosis & Treatment: Obstetrics & Gynecology*, 12th ed. McGraw Hill LLC; 2019.)

be counseled as to the cause of her amenorrhea, implications for future fertility, risks of malignancy (if applicable), and treatment options. Patients with functional hypothalamic amenorrhea due to physical or psychological stress can reverse this by weight gain, resolution of emotional issues, or decrease in intensity of exercise. For patients with hypothyroidism, thyroid replacement should be started at a low dose and titrated up, with caution to avoid overreplacement. Patients with pituitary adenomas should be treated with the dopamine agonists bromocriptine or cabergoline, with the former having the best established safety record and being approved for use in pregnancy. Cyclical estrogen-progesterone and combined estrogen-progesterone oral contraceptive pills, patches, or vaginal ring can be used in patients with gonadal dysgenesis or hypoestrogenic state. Only providers experienced in this field should perform induction of puberty in patients with constitutional delay. Estrogen is responsible for epiphyseal closure as well as the adolescent growth spurt; mistimed administration could have significant effects on

the final achieved height in these patients. For patients who desire fertility, ovulation induction with clomiphene citrate, exogenous gonadotropins, or pulsatile gonadotropin-releasing hormone (GnRH) may be required.

B. Surgical Intervention

Structural anomalies should be addressed surgically. In patients with congenital absence of a uterus, investigation should be undertaken for associated renal anomalies. Gonadectomy should be performed after puberty in patients with Y chromosome material to prevent the development of subsequent gonadal neoplasia.

C. Behavioral Modification

Patients with hypothalamic failure due to rapid weight loss, excessive exercise, or stress should receive counseling to address the underlying cause of these problems.

▶ Secondary Amenorrhea

The most common type of amenorrhea, secondary amenorrhea, is diagnosed when a woman with previously normal menses goes at least 3 months without a period or when a woman with previously irregular menses has less than nine cycles in a year.

▶ Clinical Findings

A. Signs and Symptoms

Pertinent history in the evaluation of secondary amenorrhea includes the following: (1) previous menstrual history (timing and quality of menses); (2) pregnancies (including terminations and complicated deliveries); (3) symptoms of endocrine disease; (4) medication history; (5) weight loss or gain; (6) exercise level; (7) history of instrumentation or surgery to genital tract; and (8) masculinizing characteristics noticed by patient or family. Physical examination should assess pubertal development and secondary sexual characteristics while looking for evidence of hyperandrogenism. These latter findings may include oily skin, acne, striae, clitoromegaly, and hirsutism.

B. Laboratory Findings

After the exclusion of pregnancy, initial labs should include fasting glucose, TSH, and prolactin levels. In the absence of significant abnormalities in these values, a progestin challenge test should be performed to assess the patient's estrogen status. In a progestin challenge test, the patient is given 10 mg of oral medroxyprogesterone daily for 10 days. If there is withdrawal bleeding after completing this 10-day course, endogenous estrogen is present. If no bleeding occurs after 10 days of oral medroxyprogesterone, there is either a hypoestrogenic state or possibly outflow obstruction occurring. FSH should be measured on women who do not experience withdrawal bleeding within 2 weeks. A high FSH value (>30 IU/L) is indicative of ovarian failure, whereas normal or low values indicate either an acquired uterine anomaly (Asherman syndrome) or hypothalamic-pituitary failure. Ovarian failure is confirmed with a low serum estradiol level (<30 pg/mL). A serum luteinizing hormone (LH) and FSH should be drawn on women who do not experience withdrawal bleeding after the progesterone challenge and have a normal estrogen level. An elevated LH value is highly suggestive of polycystic ovarian syndrome (PCOS), especially in a woman with clinical features of virilization. If the LH level is normal, an LH/FSH ratio should be determined. This ratio is elevated (>2.5) in women with PCOS even when FSH and LH values are within normal limits. This diagnosis can be confirmed by measurement of serum testosterone and dehydroepiandrosterone sulfate (DHEA-S), which should be normal or just mildly elevated in PCOS. An increased testosterone/DHEA-S ratio is suggestive of an adrenal source.

This finding warrants further study with determination of 17-hydroxyprogesterone. This level is elevated in late-onset congenital adrenal hyperplasia and Cushing syndrome. Cushing syndrome may be excluded with a 24-hour urinary free cortisol and dexamethasone suppression testing. The workup for patients with secondary amenorrhea can be seen in the algorithm in Figure 13–2.

C. Imaging Studies

Hysterosalpingogram is indicated with history of uterine instrumentation and/or suggestion of anatomic anomaly as source of amenorrhea. Computed tomography (CT) scanning of the adrenal glands and ultrasound of the ovaries should be performed in women with clinical features of virilization and increased testosterone (>200 ng/dL) or DHEAS-S (>7 μg/mL). A CT or MRI of the pituitary should be performed if pituitary pathology is suspected.

▶ Differential Diagnosis

The differential diagnosis of secondary amenorrhea can be broken down into those etiologies with and those without evidence of hyperandrogenism.

A. With Evidence of Hyperandrogenism

1. Polycystic ovary syndrome—PCOS is the most common reproductive female endocrine disorder, occurring in 5–15% of women, and is characterized by heterogeneous signs and symptoms of ovarian dysfunction with possible associated virilization. PCOS is associated with an increased risk of type 2 diabetes, abdominal obesity, hypertension, hypertriglyceridemia, and cardiovascular events.

2. Autonomous hyperandrogenism—Tumors of adrenal or ovarian origin may secrete androgens. Virilization is more pronounced than in PCOS and may manifest as frontal balding, increased muscle bulk, deep voice, clitoromegaly, and severe hirsutism.

3. Late-onset or mild congenital adrenal hyperplasia—This rare condition may be diagnosed with the finding of an increased 17-hydroxyprogesterone level in the setting of secondary amenorrhea and hyperandrogenism.

B. Without Evidence of Hyperandrogenism on Examination

1. Medication use—History should be reviewed for use of contraceptives, particularly progesterone-only preparations. These may take the form of oral contraceptives, implants, injectables, or intrauterine devices. It is important to inform women on progestin-only pills that 20% of patients will become amenorrheic within the first year of use. Rates are even higher for those using injectable progesterone, with 55% of women at 1 year and 68% of women at 2 years reporting amenorrhea.

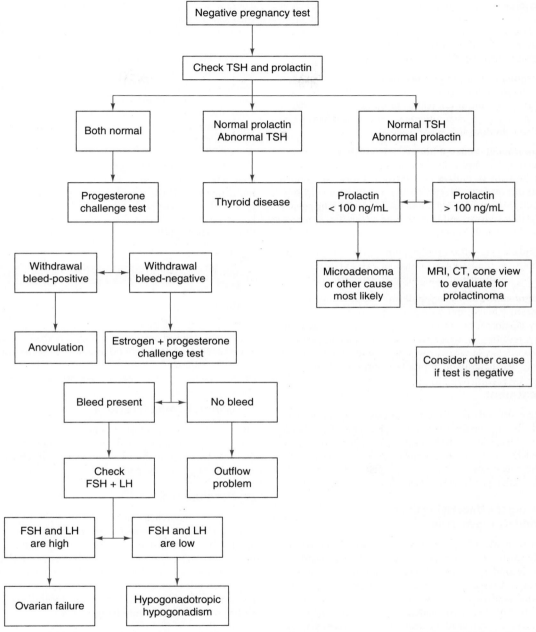

▲ **Figure 13–2.** Workup for patients with secondary amenorrhea. CT, computed tomography; FSH, follicle-stimulating hormone; LH, luteinizing hormone; MRI, magnetic resonance imaging; TSH, thyroid-stimulating hormone. (Reproduced with permission from DeCherney AH, Nathan L, Laufer N, et al: *Current Diagnosis & Treatment: Obstetrics & Gynecology*, 12th ed. McGraw Hill LLC; 2019.)

2. Functional hypothalamic amenorrhea—Amenorrhea in this setting, seen in patients who have experienced rapid weight loss, severely restricted calorie intake, stress or rigorous exercise, may be part of the female athlete triad of amenorrhea, disordered eating, and osteoporosis.

3. Hypergonadotropic hypogonadism—Premature ovarian failure (cessation of ovarian function before 40 years of age) may be autoimmune or idiopathic, or may occur secondarily to radiotherapy or chemotherapy (cyclophosphamide is associated with destruction of oocytes).

4. Hyperprolactinemia—Pituitary adenomas may present with amenorrhea and galactorrhea and are responsible for 20% of cases of secondary amenorrhea. Prolactin secreted by these tumors acts directly on the hypothalamus to suppress GnRH secretion. Dopamine receptor–blocking agents, hypothalamic masses, and hypothyroidism are less common causes of hyperprolactinemia.

5. Thyroid disease—Profound hypothyroidism or hyperthyroidism affects the feedback control of LH, FSH, and estradiol on the hypothalamus, causing menstrual irregularities.

6. Hypogonadotropic hypogonadism—Head trauma, severe hypotension (shock), infiltrative or inflammatory processes, pituitary adenoma, or craniopharyngioma may damage the pituitary, resulting in decreased or absent gonadotropin (LH and FSH) release. These patients will often display symptoms relating to deficiency of other pituitary hormones as well.

▶ Treatment

Treatment depends on correct diagnosis of the underlying etiology. As in primary amenorrhea, the goals of treatment are to establish a firm diagnosis, to restore ovulatory cycles and treat infertility (when possible), to treat hypoestrogenemia and hyperandrogensim, and to assess and address risks associate with a persistent hypoestrogenemic state.

A. Treating the Underlying Causes of Secondary Amenorrhea

Patients with identified hypothyroidism should be treated with thyroxine replacement. Patients with hyperprolactinemia secondary to prolactinoma may be treated with either surgical resection or dopamine agonist therapy. Bromocriptine is often used in women who desire to conceive, since there is no increased incidence of congenital malformations, and it has been used successfully for >20 years. Patients found to have empty sella or Sheehan syndrome should be treated with replacement of pituitary hormones.

Women whose amenorrhea is secondary to absent ovarian function before 40 years of age have premature ovarian failure. Those who experience ovarian failure before 30 years of age should undergo karyotype testing to screen for Y chromosome elements, which are associated with malignancies.

These patients are at a high risk of osteoporosis and cardiovascular disease because of their hypoestrogenemic state. Estrogen replacement should be considered, with progesterone for patients with an intact uterus, to prevent these sequelae.

Women with adrenal or ovarian androgen-secreting tumors should undergo appropriate surgical intervention. Likewise, women found to have Asherman syndrome as a cause for their amenorrhea should undergo lysis of adhesions followed by endometrial stimulation with estrogen. These patients are at increased risk of placenta accreta in subsequent pregnancies.

Patients with PCOS may achieve resumption of menses with weight loss. Metformin, a biguanide insulin sensitizer, has been used to treat PCOS, with reports of success in inducing both ovulation and fertility and improving laboratory markers for cardiovascular risk.

DYSMENORRHEA

ESSENTIALS OF DIAGNOSIS

▶ Affects 50% of all women, and between 20% and 90% of all adolescent women.

▶ Primary defined as painful menses in absence of pelvic disease; secondary defined as painful menses caused by pelvic disease.

▶ General Considerations

Dysmenorrhea is the most common gynecologic complaint and is a leading cause of morbidity in women of reproductive age, resulting in absence from work and school, as well as nonparticipation in sports.

▶ Pathogenesis

Primary dysmenorrhea is caused by the release of prostaglandin $F_2\alpha$ from the endometrium at the time of menstruation and rarely occurs until ovulatory menstrual cycles are established. Prostaglandins induce smooth muscle contraction in the uterus, causing pressure within the uterus to exceed that of the systemic circulation. Ischemia ensues, causing an anginal equivalent in the uterus. The cause of secondary dysmenorrhea varies with the underlying disease.

▶ Clinical Findings

A. Symptoms and Signs

Symptoms of primary dysmenorrhea include pain beginning with the onset of menstruation and lasting 12–72 hours, characterized as crampy and intermittent in nature, with radiation to the low back or upper thighs. Headache, nausea, vomiting, diarrhea, and fatigue may accompany the pain. Symptoms are usually worst on the first day of menses and then gradually resolve. The patient may report that her dysmenorrhea began gradually, with the first several years of menses, and then intensified as her periods became regular and consistently ovulatory. Conversely, patients with *secondary amenorrhea* report symptoms beginning after age 20 and lasting 5–7 days and progressive worsening of pain with time. These patients may also report pelvic pain that is not associated with menstruation.

B. Physical Findings

A pelvic examination with cervical smear and cultures should be performed in all patients presenting with a chief complaint of dysmenorrhea. Findings of cul-de-sac induration and uterosacral ligament nodularity on pelvic examination are indicative of endometriosis. Adnexal masses could indicate endometriosis, neoplasm, hydrosalpinx, or scarring from chronic pelvic inflammatory disease. Likewise, uterine abnormalities or tenderness should raise the examiner's index of suspicion for the underlying pathology as the cause for dysmenorrhea.

C. Laboratory Findings

Any woman with acute onset of pelvic pain should have a pregnancy test. Women with a history consistent with primary dysmenorrhea do not require additional initial labs. In those who fail to respond to therapy for primary dysmenorrhea or in those whom a diagnosis of secondary dysmenorrhea is suspected, a complete blood count and an erythrocyte sedimentation rate may help in detection of the underlying infection or inflammation.

D. Imaging Studies

Patients with abnormal findings on pelvic examination who do not respond to therapy for primary dysmenorrhea or who have a history suggestive of pelvic pathology should undergo pelvic ultrasound.

E. Special Examinations

For patients in whom endometriosis is suggested, diagnostic laparoscopy may be indicated. Because of the high rates of treatment and diagnostic failure with laparoscopy, some authors recommend empirically treating patients with a presumptive diagnosis of endometriosis with GnRH analogs for 3 months. Proponents argue that this provides both diagnostic and therapeutic functions, while forgoing surgical complications.

▶ Treatment

A. Medical Therapies

Treatment for primary dysmenorrhea focuses on reducing endometrial prostaglandin production. This can be accomplished with nonsteroidal anti-inflammatory drugs, which inhibit prostaglandin synthesis, or with contraceptives that suppress ovulation. It is recommended to allow at least three full cycles to assess efficacy of either of these approaches. In patients who do not experience success with these means, an alternate diagnosis, such as endometriosis, should be considered. Medical therapies are listed in Table 13–4 with respect to their degree of efficacy.

B. Physical Modalities

Physical modalities using heat, acupuncture/acupressure, and spinal manipulation have been proposed for inclusion in the treatment of dysmenorrhea. A heated abdominal patch was demonstrated to have efficacy similar to ibuprofen (400 mg) for the treatment of dysmenorrhea, with quicker, but not greater, relief observed with the combination of ibuprofen and heat. Acupuncture relieved pain in 91% of patients with dysmenorrhea, compared to 36% relief for control patients in a study with sham acupuncture. A systematic review of spinal manipulation in the treatment of dysmenorrhea failed to find evidence for the effectiveness of this approach.

C. Supplements and Herbals

A number of supplements and herbal formulations have been touted as relieving the symptoms of dysmenorrhea. While some small trials have showed promising results, the data are not strong enough at this time to recommend widespread use. A systematic review of Chinese herbal therapy for treatment of dysmenorrhea showed promising results with self-designed formulas in small studies, but not with commonly used herbal health products. Results were limited by poor methodologic quality and small sample size.

D. Behavior Modification

Strenuous exercise and caffeine intake are both lifestyle factors that can modulate prostaglandin-induced uterine contractions. Strenuous exercise can increase uterine tone, resulting in increased periods of uterine "angina" with accompanying increases in prostaglandins. Decreasing strenuous exercise in the first few days of a woman's menses may reduce her dysmenorrhea. Conversely, caffeine decreases uterine tone by increasing uterine cyclic adenosine monophosphate levels.

E. Surgical Therapy

If a patient continues to have significant dysmenorrhea with this treatment, further testing for causes of secondary dysmenorrhea should be considered, and surgical options, such as interruption of pelvic nerve pathways, should be explored when applicable.

Table 13–4. Medications for the treatment of primary dysmenorrhea.

	Medication	Mechanism of Action	Primary Side Effects/ Complications	Strength of Recommendation[a]	Comments
Effective	NSAIDs: diclofenac, ibuprofen, mefenamic acid, naproxen, ASA	Inhibits prostaglandin synthesis (fenamates also block prostaglandin action)	GI upset, GI bleed	A	Most effective when started before onset of pain; fenamates show enhanced action in some studies due to dual mechanism of action
	Danazol	Suppression of menses	Amenorrhea, vaginal dryness, jaundice, eosinophilia	B	Significant side effects; primarily for severe endometriosis
	Hormonal contraceptives: oral, injectable, implantable, intravaginal administration	Reduced prostaglandin release during menstruation	Irregular menses, mood swings, acne, DVT	B	Use with caution in patients >35 years old and smokers; not for patients desiring fertility
	COX-2 inhibitors	Inhibits prostaglandin synthesis	Cardiovascular risk, acute renal failure	B	Contains sulfa moiety; consider safer, less expensive NSAIDs first
	Levonorgestrel intrauterine device (Mirena)	Thins uterine lining through inhibition	Hypertension, acne, weight gain	B	Effective for 5 years
Probably effective	Leuprolide acetate (Lupron)	Suppression of menses	Weight gain, hirsutism, elevation of BP	B	Very expensive with significant side effects. Not first line.
	Depo-medroxyprogesterone acetate (Depo-Provera)	Suppression of menses	Amenorrhea, hypermenorrhea	B	Weight gain may be significant
	Glyceryl trinitrate patches	Tocolytic	Headache	B	Less effective than NSAIDs; more side effects, low tolerability
Uncertain efficacy	Nifedipine (Procardia)	Induction of uterine relaxation	Hypotension, peripheral edema	C	Moderate to good pain reduction but high rate side effects
	Transdermal contraceptive patch	Reduced prostaglandin release during menstruation	Local irritation, irregular menses	B	Less effective than OCPs, efficacy varies with patient weight

ASA, acetylsalicylic acid; BP, blood pressure; COX-2, cyclooxygenase-2; DVT, deep vein thrombosis; GI, gastrointestinal; NSAID, nonsteroidal anti-inflammatory drug; OCPs, oral contraceptive pills.
[a]A, consistent, good-quality, patient-oriented evidence; B, inconsistent or limited-quality patient-oriented evidence; C, consensus, disease-oriented evidence, usual practice, opinion, or case series.

PREMENSTRUAL SYNDROME

ESSENTIALS OF DIAGNOSIS

▶ A cluster of affective, cognitive, and physical symptoms that occur before the onset of menses, during the luteal phase of the menstrual cycle.

▶ Absence of a symptom-free week in the time period immediately following menses suggests that a chronic psychiatric disorder may be present.

▶ General Considerations

Although 40% of women experience premenstrual syndrome (PMS) symptoms significant enough to interfere with daily life, 5% of women experience severe impairment. Evaluation, diagnosis, and treatment of PMS should be undertaken prudently, as it is often mistaken for other disorders and sometimes treated with counterproductive and even harmful approaches. The clinician must be sensitive in addressing issues of reduced self-worth, frustration, and depression that may be present in women suffering from this condition.

Pathogenesis

PMS is assumed to be secondary to interactions between the ovarian hormones, estrogen and progesterone, and central neurotransmitters. Serotonin is the central neurotransmitter most often implicated in the manifestations of PMS. This would explain the cyclical mood changes that are synchronized with the changes in ovarian hormone levels. Systemic symptoms, such as bloating, may be produced through the peripheral effects of these hormones. Trace elements and nutrients are also speculated to have a role in the pathogenesis of PMS symptoms, but their role is less clear.

Clinical Findings

A. Symptoms and Signs

Symptoms may include irritability, bloating, depression, food cravings, aggressiveness, and mood swings. Abraham's classification of premenstrual syndrome (Table 13–5) helps the clinician to organize history taking for patients with PMS.

Factors associated with an increased risk of PMS include stress, alcohol use, exercise, smoking, and the use of certain medications. It is not clear whether some of these factors are causative or are forms of self-medication used by sufferers. A prospective symptom diary kept for at least 2 months is helpful in assessing the relation of symptoms to the luteal phase of menses. The absence of a symptom-free week early in the follicular phase, the time period just after menses, suggests that a chronic psychiatric disorder may be present. A record of symptoms that are temporally clustered before menses and that decline or diminish 2–3 days after the start of menses is highly suggestive of PMS. Patients with PMS experience fluid retention and fluctuating weight gain in relation to their menses. Mild edema may or may not be evident on physical examination.

B. Laboratory Findings

There are no laboratory evaluations recommended in the diagnosis of PMS. Nutrient deficiency tests are not recommended because they do not adequately assess the patient's physiologic state.

C. Radiologic Studies

There are no radiologic studies recommended in the assessment of PMS.

Treatment

The treatment goals for PMS are to minimize symptoms and functional impairment while optimizing the patient's overall health and sense of well-being. Therapy should take an integrative approach, including education, psychological support, exercise, diet, and pharmacologic intervention, if necessary. By providing education about the prevalence and treatability of PMS, the clinician can destigmatize the disease and encourage the patient to take ownership of the treatment plan.

Many first-line treatments for PMS, although not based on well-designed prospective trials, also have general health benefits, are inexpensive, and have few side effects. These include dietary modifications, as recommended by the American Heart Association, and moderate exercise at least 3 times a week. Patients should begin to see the results of these lifestyle changes 2–3 months after initiation. Patients should be counseled to expect improvement in their symptoms, rather than cure. Multiple approaches may be required before finding the optimal treatment.

For patients with continued symptoms, secondary treatment strategies may be employed. Dietary supplements, specifically vitamin B_6, calcium, and magnesium, have been suggested to correct possible deficiencies. Current therapies are listed in Table 13–6, with their levels of supporting evidence, primary benefits, and potential side effects.

Alternative therapies include herbal medicine, dietary supplements, relaxation, massage, reflexology, manipulative therapy, and biofeedback. Although some small trials have shown promising results, there is no compelling evidence from well-designed studies supporting the use of these therapies in the treatment of PMS. A systematic review in 2016 suggested that transcutaneous electrical nerve stimulation (TENS) and heat therapy interventions may be potentially effective in reducing and managing the pain in primary dysmenorrhea; however, high-quality research is too limited to

Table 13–5. Abraham's classification of symptoms of premenstrual syndrome.

A: Anxiety
  Nervous tension
  Mood swings
  Irritability
  Anxiety

C: Cravings
  Headache
  Craving for sweets
  Increased appetite
  Heart pounding
  Fatigue
  Dizziness or faintness

D: Depression
  Depression
  Forgetfulness
  Crying
  Confusion
  Insomnia

H: Water-related symptoms
  Weight gain
  Swelling of extremities
  Breast tenderness
  Abnormal bloating

Table 13–6. Selected pharmacologic and supplemental therapies for PMS.

Medication	Mechanism of Action	Indication(s) for Use in PMS	Dosing	Primary Side Effects/ Complications	Evidence Supporting Use
Mefenamic acid	Inhibits prostaglandin synthesis; competes for prostaglandin binding sites	Pain relief	500 mg loading dose, then 250 g PO QID for ≤7 days	Diarrhea, nausea, vomiting, drowsiness with prolonged use: decreased renal blood flow and renal papillary necrosis	RCCT
GnRH agonists (nafrelin, leuprolide)	LH and FSH transient stimulation then prolonged suppression	Severe PMS; relief of all symptoms in 50% of patients	Nafrelin: 200 mg intranasal BID; leuprolide: 3.75 mg depot IM every 4 weeks or 0.5 mg SQ daily	Vaginal dryness, accelerated bone loss (drugs can be given with additional back therapy to avoid these symptoms), hot flashes	Controlled clinical trial
Danazol	Suppresses LH and FSH	Severe PMS	200 mg PO daily in luteal phase	Acne, weight gain, hirsutism, virilization	RCCTs
Alprazolam (second-line since it appears to treat only depressive symptoms and has high addictive potential)	Depressant effect on central nervous system	Depression caused by PMS	0.25 mg PO TID during late luteal phase of cycle	Drowsiness, increased appetite, withdrawal (discontinue if patient exhibits withdrawal symptoms)	RCCT
Selective serotonin reuptake inhibitors: fluoxetine, sertraline, paroxetine, venlafaxine, citalopram	Serotonin reuptake inhibitor	Depression, anger, and anxiety caused by PMS	Varies with drug: all month or just during luteal phase (start day 14, end at start of menses)	Nervousness, insomnia, drowsiness, nausea, anorexia	EBM review
Diuretics (metolazone, spironolactone)	Reduction in retained fluid	Bloating, edema, breast tenderness (especially in women with >1.5 kg premenstrual weight gain)	Metolazone: 2.4 mg/d PO; spironolactone: 25 mg PO QID	Electrolyte imbalance	EBM review
Bromocriptine	Dopamine agonist	Breast tenderness and fullness	2.5 mg PO BID-TID	Postural hypotension, nausea	Use not supported by RCCTs
Hormonal contraceptives	Suppression of estrogen and progesterone	General symptoms	Varies by formulation	Varies by formulation	Use not supported by RCCTs for treatment of PMS
Vitamin B_6	Precursor in coenzyme for the biosynthesis of dopamine and serotonin	Depression and general symptoms	50 mg PO QD or BID	Ataxia, sensory neuropathy	EBM review
γ-Linoleic acid	Prostaglandin E1 precursor that inhibits prostaglandin production and metabolism	Breast tenderness, bloating, weight gain, edema	3 g/d in late luteal phase of menstrual cycle	Headache, nausea	Efficacy not supported
Calcium	Restoration of calcium homeostasis	Depression, anxiety, and dysphoric states	800–1600 mg QD in divided doses	Bloating, nausea	RCCT

BID, twice a day; EBM, evidence-based medicine; FSH, follicle-stimulating hormone; GnRH, gonadotropin-releasing hormone agonist; IM, intramuscular; LH, luteinizing hormone; PMS, premenstrual syndrome; PO, oral; QD, once a day; QID, four times a day; RCCT, randomized controlled clinical trials; SQ, subcutaneous; TID, three times a day.

make a more definitive statement; the risks of using TENS with heat therapy are low, and therefore, it can and should be considered in clinical practice.

Cho SH, Hwang EW. Acupuncture for primary dysmenorrhoea: a systematic review. *Br J Obstet Gynecol.* 2010;117:509–521. [PMID: 20184568]

Hall J. Menstrual disorders and pelvic pain. In Kasper D, Fauci A, Hauser S, et al (eds): *Harrison's Principles of Internal Medicine.* 19th ed. New York, NY: McGraw-Hill Education; 2015.

Hoffman B, Schorge J, Bradshaw KD, et al: *Williams Gynecology.* 3rd ed. New York, NY: McGraw-Hill Education; 2016:249–274, 369–387.

Igwea SE, Tabansi-Ochuogu CS, Abaraogu UO. TENS and heat therapy for pain relief and quality of life improvement in individuals with primary dysmenorrhea: a systematic review. *Complement Ther Clin Pract.* 2016;24:86–91. [PMID: 27502806]

Morley C, Tang T, Yasmin E, Norman R, Balen H. Insulin-sensitising drugs (metformin, rosiglitazone, pioglitazone, D-chiro-inositol) for women with polycystic ovary syndrome, oligo amenorrhea and subfertility. *Cochrane Database Syst Rev.* 2017;11:CD003053. [PMID: 29183107]

Simon A, Chong W, DeCherney A. *Current Diagnosis & Treatment Obstetrics and Gynecology.* 11th ed. New York, NY: McGraw-Hill Education; 2013:611–619, 889–899.

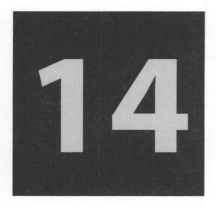

Sexually Transmitted Diseases

Robin Maier, MD, MA

Peter J. Katsufrakis, MD, MBA

ESSENTIALS OF DIAGNOSIS

▶ Privacy, confidentiality, and legal disease reporting concerns affect detection and treatment.

▶ Suspicion or diagnosis of one sexually transmitted disease (STD) should prompt screening tests for others.

▶ Diagnosis of an STD should always include identification and treatment of partners and education to reduce risk of future infection.

▶ General Considerations

Sexually transmitted diseases (STDs) include sexually transmitted infections and the clinical syndromes they cause. There are an estimated 20 million new STDs in the United States annually, and the three nationally reported STDs (chlamydia, gonorrhea, and syphilis) reached 2 million in 2016, the highest number ever.

Although all sexually active individuals are susceptible to infection, adolescents and young adults are most commonly affected. Reasons for this include (1) an attitude of invincibility, (2) lack of knowledge about the risks and consequences of STDs, and (3) barriers to healthcare access.

This chapter emphasizes the clinical presentation, diagnostic evaluation, and treatment of STDs commonly found in the United States. Readers of this chapter should be able to:

• Differentiate common STDs on the basis of clinical information and laboratory testing.

• Treat STDs according to current guidelines.

• Intervene in patients' lives to reduce risk of future STD acquisition.

The discussion draws greatly from the most recent Centers for Disease Control and Prevention (CDC) guidelines for treatment of STDs. The authors are indebted to the individuals who worked to develop these recommendations.

Federal and state laws create disease-reporting requirements for many diseases that can be spread sexually. Gonorrhea; chlamydia; chancroid; syphilis; hepatitis A, B, C; and human immunodeficiency virus (HIV; including acquired immunodeficiency syndrome [AIDS]) are all nationally notifiable. Clinicians should contact their local health department for pertinent reporting information.

Privacy and confidentiality concerns are different for STDs than for general medical information. Patients generally experience greater anxiety about information pertaining to a possible diagnosis of an STD, and this may limit their willingness to disclose clinically pertinent information. Conversely, legal requirements for disease reporting and health department partner notification programs can inadvertently compromise patient confidentiality if not handled with the utmost professionalism. Furthermore, although minors generally require parental consent for nonemergent medical care in all states, minors can be diagnosed and treated for STDs without parental consent. Additionally, many US states' legislations may permit physicians to prescribe treatment for the heterosexual partners of men or women with chlamydia or gonorrhea without examining the partner. Thus, laws in different jurisdictions create additional options and complexities in treating STDs. Practitioners need to be familiar with local requirements.

Centers for Disease Control and Prevention. CDC fact sheet: reported STDs in the United States, 2016. https://www.cdc.gov/nchhstp/newsroom/docs/factsheets/STD-Trends-508.pdf. Accessed November 11, 2019.

Centers for Disease Control and Prevention. *Sexually Transmitted Disease Surveillance 2016*. Atlanta, GA: US Department of Health and Human Services; 2017.

Centers for Disease Control and Prevention; Workowski KA, Bolan GA. Sexually transmitted disease treatment guidelines, 2015. *MMWR Recomm Rep.* 2015;64(RR-3):1–140. [PMID: 26042815]

Prevention

Intervening in patients' lives to reduce their risk of disease due to STDs is no less important than reducing risk due to smoking, inadequate exercise, poor nutrition, and other health risks. STD risk assessment should prompt providers to undertake discussion of risk reduction and thus disease prevention. Physicians' effectiveness depends on their ability to obtain an accurate sexual history employing effective counseling skills. Specific techniques include creating a trusting, confidential environment; obtaining permission to ask questions about STDs; demonstrating a nonjudgmental, optimistic attitude; and combining information collection with patient education, using clear, mutually understandable language (see Chapter 17). Prevention is facilitated by an environment of open, honest communication about sexuality.

A. Counseling

The US Preventive Services Task Force (USPSTF) recommends high-intensity behavioral counseling to prevent sexually transmitted infections (STIs) for all sexually active adolescents and for adults at increased risk for STIs, for example, adults with current STIs or infections within the past year who have multiple current sexual partners or who are members of a population with a high rate of STIs. Recommendations for changes in behavior should be tailored to the patient's specific risks and needs; simple suggestions such as keeping condoms available have been shown to be effective. Brief counseling using personalized risk reduction plans and culturally appropriate videos can significantly increase condom use and prevent new STDs and can be conducted even in busy public clinics with minimal disruption to clinic operations. Effective interventions to reduce STDs in adolescents can extend beyond the examination room and include school-based and community-based education programs. Characteristics of successful interventions include multiple sessions, most often in groups, with total duration from 3 to 9 hours, or two 20-minute counseling sessions before and after HIV testing. Individuals with chronic infections (eg, herpes simplex virus [HSV] and human papillomavirus [HPV]) will need counseling tailored to help them accurately understand their infection and effectively manage symptoms and transmission risk.

Lin JS, Whitlock E, O'Connor E, Bauer V. Behavioral counseling to prevent sexually transmitted infections: a systematic review for the U.S. Preventive Services Task Force. *Ann Intern Med.* 2008;149(7):497–508, W96–W99. [PMID: 18838730]

US Preventive Services Task Force. *Final Recommendation Statement: Sexually Transmitted Infections: Behavioral Counseling.* December 2016. https://www.uspreventiveservicestaskforce.org/Page/Document/RecommendationStatementFinal/sexually-transmitted-infections-behavioral-counseling1. Accessed November 11, 2019.

B. Condoms

For sexually active patients, male condoms are effective in reducing the sexual transmission of HIV infection. When used correctly and consistently, male latex condoms can reduce the risk of other STIs, including chlamydia, gonorrhea, and *Trichomonas*. Condoms may afford some protection against transmission of HSV and may mitigate some adverse consequences of infection with HPV, as their use has been associated with higher rates of regression of cervical intraepithelial neoplasia and clearance of HPV in women.

Effectiveness depends on correct, consistent use. Patients should be instructed to use only water-based lubricants. Providers may need to demonstrate how to place a condom on the penis via a suitable model, especially for persons who may be inexperienced with condom use.

Spermicide is not recommended for STI/HIV prevention. Some may confuse contraception with disease prevention; nonbarrier methods of contraception such as hormonal contraceptives or surgical sterilization do not protect against STDs. Women employing these methods should be counseled about the role of condoms in prevention of STDs.

Centers for Disease Control and Prevention. Condoms and STDs: fact sheet for public health personnel. https://www.cdc.gov/condomeffectiveness/latex.html. Accessed July 30, 2018.

C. Vaccination

Vaccination for hepatitis B virus (HBV) is indicated for all unvaccinated adolescents, all unvaccinated adults at risk for HBV infection, and all adults seeking protection from HBV infection. Other settings where all unvaccinated persons should receive vaccination include correctional facilities, drug abuse treatment and prevention services centers, healthcare settings serving men who have sex with men, and HIV testing and treatment facilities. Additionally, individuals with chronic liver disease (including chronic HBV or hepatitis C infection), end-stage renal disease, diabetes mellitus, and potential occupational or travel exposure should be vaccinated. The prevalence of past exposure to HBV in homosexual men and injection drug users may render prevaccination testing cost effective, although it may lower compliance. For this reason, if prevaccination testing is employed, patients should receive their first vaccination dose when tested. If employed, HBV core antibody testing is an effective screen for immunity.

Vaccination for hepatitis A virus (HAV) is indicated for homosexual or bisexual men, persons with chronic liver disease (including hepatitis B and C), and intravenous (IV) drug users; additionally, some individuals with occupational or travel exposure should be vaccinated. In cases of sexual or household contact with someone with HAV, hepatitis A vaccine or immune globulin should be administered as soon as possible after exposure. (For additional information on hepatitis A and B, see Chapter 31.)

Vaccination is a major defense against HPV, which causes cervical, vaginal, vulvar, and anal cancers and genital warts in women, and anal cancer and genital warts in men. Universal vaccination of females age 11–12 years against HPV is recommended with any of three vaccines (bivalent Cervarix, quadrivalent Gardasil, or nonavalent Gardasil-9), as is catch-up vaccination for females age 13–26 years. Universal vaccination of males age 11–12 years against HPV is recommended with either the quadrivalent or nonavalent vaccines, as is catch-up vaccination for all males age 13–21 years and for high-risk males up to age 26. It is permissible to vaccinate any male up to age 26.

Centers for Disease Control and Prevention. Advisory Committee on Immunization Practices (ACIP) recommended immunization schedules for persons aged 0 through 18 years and adults aged 19 years and older–United States, 2018. *MMWR Suppl.* 2013;62(1):1. [PMID: 23364301]

D. Partner Treatment

Following treatment of an individual patient, treatment of asymptomatic partners of a diagnosed patient is commonly employed in STD treatment. For patients with multiple partners, it may be difficult to identify the source of infection. Partner treatment should be recommended for sexual contacts occurring prior to diagnosis within the time intervals indicated for each disease:

- Chancroid, 10 days
- Granuloma inguinale, 60 days
- Lymphogranuloma venereum, 60 days
- Syphilis, 3 months plus the duration of symptoms for patients diagnosed with primary syphilis (even if the contact tests seronegative); 6 months plus the duration of symptoms for patients diagnosed with secondary syphilis, and 1 year for patients with early latent syphilis
- Chlamydial infection, 60 days
- Gonorrhea, 60 days
- Epididymitis, 60 days
- Pelvic inflammatory disease (PID), 60 days
- Pediculosis pubis, 30 days
- Scabies, 30 days

Although in general physicians must examine a patient directly before prescribing treatment, when prior medical evaluation and counseling are not feasible or resource limitations constrain evaluation and diagnosis, other partner management options may be considered. One of these is partner-delivered therapy, in which patients diagnosed with chlamydia or gonorrhea deliver the prescribed treatment to their partners; this option is affected by state laws and regulations.

Repeat testing at 3 months following treatment is indicated for persons with chlamydia or gonorrhea, due to the increased incidence of reinfection. Patients should also be instructed to avoid sexual contact for the duration of therapy to prevent further transmission. Patients taking single-dose azithromycin for chlamydia infection should be instructed to avoid sexual contact for 7 days. Patients must also be instructed to avoid contact with their previous partner(s) until both patient and partner complete treatment.

E. Screening

Some form of STD screening, such as questions asked during the history interview or included in routine history forms, should be a universal practice for *all* patients, with periodic and regular updating. Content, frequency, and additional screening should be determined by individual patient circumstances, local disease prevalence, and research documenting effectiveness and cost benefit. Table 14–1

Table 14–1. US Preventive Services Task Force (USPSTF) recommendations for sexually transmitted disease (STD) screening.[a]

Infection	Recommendation
Chlamydia	Screen *all* pregnant women and sexually active women aged ≤24 years; screen all sexually active or pregnant women aged ≥25 years who are at increased risk for sexually transmitted infection (eg, having a prior history of STD, having new or multiple sex partners, inconsistent condom use, or who exchange sex for money or drugs)
Gonorrhea	Screen all sexually active women, including those who are pregnant, for gonorrhea infection if they are at increased risk for infection (eg, aged <25 years), previous gonorrhea, or other STD, new or multiple sex partners, inconsistent condom use, sex work, and drug use
Hepatitis B	Screen all pregnant women at their first prenatal visit
HIV	Screen all pregnant women Screen all adolescents and adults age 15–65 years for HIV Screen younger adolescents and older adults believed to be at increased risk for HIV infection
Syphilis	Screen all pregnant women Screen persons at increased risk for syphilis infection (eg, men who have sex with men and engage in high-risk sexual behavior, commercial sex workers, persons who exchange sex for drugs, and those in adult correctional facilities)

[a]The USPSTF does not presently recommend routine screening for hepatitis C, human papillomavirus, or herpes simplex.
Data from US Preventive Services Task Force. Rockville, MD.

summarizes current recommendations for STD screening from the USPSTF.

F. Prophylactic Treatment

Preexposure prophylaxis is treatment of patients at high risk for contracting HIV with antiviral medication (tenofovir and emtricitabine) in order to reduce their chance of developing HIV, by more than 90% (for sexual exposures) or 70% (for IV drug exposures). Consistency in daily medication is very important for efficacy. Please see Chapter 55, on HIV, for more detail.

Centers for Disease Control and Prevention. CDC Vital Signs Fact Sheet: Daily pill can prevent HIV: reaching people who could benefit from PrEP. https://www.cdc.gov/vitalsigns/hivprep/index.html. Accessed August 1, 2018.

1. Chlamydia and gonorrhea—Annual screening of all sexually active women age <25 years is recommended, as is screening of older women with risk factors (eg, those who have a new sex partner or multiple sex partners).

The benefits of *Chlamydia trachomatis* screening in women have been demonstrated in areas where screening programs have reduced both the prevalence of infection and rates of PID. Evidence is insufficient to recommend routine screening for *C trachomatis* in sexually active young men, based on feasibility, efficacy, and cost-effectiveness. However, screening of sexually active young men should be considered in clinical settings with a high prevalence of chlamydia (eg, adolescent clinics, correctional facilities, and STD clinics).

2. Pregnancy—Recommendations for screening pregnant women vary somewhat depending on the source. According to the CDC, pregnant women should receive a serologic test for syphilis, hepatitis B surface antigen, and HIV at the onset of prenatal care. High-risk women should repeat HIV and syphilis testing early in the third trimester and should repeat hepatitis B surface antigen and syphilis testing again at delivery. Furthermore, pregnant women at risk for HBV infection should be vaccinated for hepatitis B.

Providers of obstetric care should test for *Neisseria gonorrhoeae* at the onset of care if local prevalence of gonorrhea is high or if the woman is at increased risk, and testing should be repeated in the third trimester if the woman is at continued risk. Providers should test for chlamydia at the first prenatal visit. Women age <25 years and those at increased risk for chlamydial infection (ie, those who have multiple partners or who have a partner with multiple partners) should also be tested again in the third trimester. Women at risk for hepatitis C infection should be screened at the initial visit. Evidence does not support routine testing for bacterial vaginosis. For asymptomatic pregnant women at high risk for preterm delivery, the current evidence is insufficient to assess the balance of benefits and harms of screening

for bacterial vaginosis. Symptomatic women should be evaluated and treated.

3. HIV—HIV screening is recommended for patients age 15–65 years in all healthcare settings after the patient is notified that testing will be performed unless the patient declines. CDC recommends that younger adolescents and older adults at increased risk also be screened. Repeat annual testing for HIV is indicated for any high-risk patient, including patients with a diagnosed STD or with a history of behaviors that could expose them to HIV. Testing is also indicated for patients who present with a history and findings consistent with the acute retroviral syndrome (ARS), the symptoms of which are listed in Table 14–2. The best choice for screening test is an HIV1/HIV2 antigen/antibody combined immunoassay, followed by an HIV1/HIV2 antibody differentiation assay. When the initial immunoassay is positive but the follow-up antibody differentiation assay is negative, RNA testing should be done to identify whether the patient may be in an acute infection stage.

Early diagnosis of ARS may present a very narrow window of opportunity to alter the course of HIV infection in the recently infected patient and to block the source of most presumed new HIV transmissions. Symptoms are common and nonspecific, rendering diagnosis difficult without a high index of suspicion; they include fever, malaise, lymphadenopathy, pharyngitis, and skin rash. Appropriate testing should include a combined antigen/antibody immunoassay or HIV RNA combined with an antibody test. If the

Table 14–2. Acute retroviral syndrome: associated signs and symptoms.

More common
Fever
Myalgia
Arthralgia
Headache
Photophobia
Diarrhea
Sore throat
Lymphadenopathy
Maculopapular rash
Less common
Acute meningoencephalitis
Peripheral neuropathy
Fatigue
Night sweats
Weight loss
Decreased libido
Muscle wasting

Data from Primary HIV Infection. In *DynaMed* [database online]. EBSCO Publishing (available at https://www.dynamed.com/condition/overview-of-hiv-infection; accessed October 27, 2019).

immunoassay is either indeterminant or negative, then RNA testing should be done. Home tests will not detect acute HIV infection. Individuals with positive HIV tests should be referred immediately to an expert in HIV care.

All HIV-infected individuals pose particular challenges for STD risk reduction. Reducing high-risk behaviors of known HIV-infected patients is a top priority, both to decrease the further spread of HIV and to limit the exposure of HIV patients to additional STDs. Persons with HIV also have substantial medical, psychological, and legal needs that are beyond the scope of this chapter.

4. Hepatitis C—Guidelines were published in 2013 that recommend offering hepatitis C screening to all persons regardless of risk born between 1945 and 1965, in addition to all patients at high risk for hepatitis C exposure.

5. Other STDs—Accepted national guidelines directing universal screening for other STDs do not exist. If undertaken, additional screening should be guided by local disease prevalence and an individual patient's risk behaviors.

Centers for Disease Control and Prevention; Workowski KA, Bolan, GA. Sexually transmitted disease treatment guidelines, 2015. *MMWR Recomm Rep.* 2015;64(RR-3):1–140. [PMID: 26042815]
US Preventive Services Task Force. USPSTF A and B Recommendations. July 2018. https://www.uspreventiveservicestaskforce.org/Page/Name/uspstf-a-and-b-recommendations/. Accessed November 11, 2019.

SEXUALLY TRANSMITTED INFECTIONS & SYNDROMES

ESSENTIALS OF DIAGNOSIS

▶ Presenting clinical syndromes often guide diagnosis and treatment.

▶ History and findings can justify presumptive treatment while awaiting laboratory confirmation of a diagnosis.

Patients who are infected with STDs rarely present with accurate knowledge of their microbiological diagnosis. More commonly, patients present with clinical syndromes consistent with one or more diagnoses, so that providers frequently employ syndromic evaluation and treatment. This approach is useful for several reasons, including the fact that more than one disease may be present, and has been employed commonly in resource-poor settings with limited access to advanced diagnostic technology. The following recommendations for testing strategies and use of empiric treatment pending laboratory results should be adapted to take into consideration local availability of specific tests, the probability of the diagnosis based on the history and examination,

disease-associated morbidity, the risk of further transmission while awaiting diagnosis, and the likelihood that an untreated patient will return for laboratory test results and treatment. Treatment information is summarized in Table 14–3, and additional treatment information appears within the text description of specific diseases where applicable.

GENITAL ULCER DISEASES

ESSENTIALS OF DIAGNOSIS

▶ Herpes is the most common cause of genital ulcers in the United States.

▶ Most persons infected with herpes simplex virus type 2 (HSV2) have *not* been diagnosed with genital herpes.

▶ All persons with genital ulcers need laboratory evaluation for syphilis and HSV (rapid plasma reagin [RPR] or Venereal Disease Research Laboratories [VDRL] darkfield microscopy, and culture or polymerase chain reaction [PCR] tests for HSV).

▶ General Considerations

In the United States, HSV is the most common cause of genital ulcer disease (GUD); syphilis is less common, and other causes such as chancroid, lymphogranuloma venereum, and granuloma inguinale are very uncommon. Because this is not true throughout the world, physicians treating international travelers or recent arrivals to the United States may need to consider a broad spectrum of potential etiologies. The approach to diagnosis needs to include consideration of the likelihood of the different etiologies based on the patient's history, physical examination, and local epidemiology. Furthermore, all types of GUD are associated with increased risk of HIV transmission, making HIV testing a necessary part of GUD evaluation.

Herpes Simplex

At least 50 million persons in the United States have genital HSV2 infection.

The majority of persons infected with HSV2 have not been diagnosed with genital herpes. Many such persons have mild or unrecognized infections but shed virus intermittently in the genital tract. The majority of genital herpes infections are transmitted by persons unaware that they have the infection or who are asymptomatic when transmission occurs. HSV1 is causing an increasing proportion of anogenital herpes, especially in some populations, such as young women and men who have sex with men (MSM).

Table 14–3. STD treatment guidelines for adults and adolescents.

Disease	Recommended Regimens	Dose, Route
Chlamydia (nonpregnant)	Azithromycin **or** doxycycline	1 g orally, single dose 100 mg PO BID × 7 days
Chlamydia (in pregnancy)	Azithromycin **or** amoxicillin	1 g orally, single dose 500 mg PO TID × 7 days
Gonorrhea	Ceftriaxone **plus** chlamydia treatment listed above, as appropriate for pregnancy status	250 mg IM, single dose
Pelvic inflammatory disease (nonpregnant, outpatient)	Ceftriaxone **plus** doxycycline ± metronidazole	250 mg IM, single dose 100 mg PO BID × 14 days 500 mg PO BID × 14 days
Pelvic inflammatory disease (nonpregnant, inpatient)	Doxycycline **plus** cefoxitin **or** cefotetan	100 mg PO every 12 hours 2 g IV every 6 hours 2 g IV every 12 hours
Pelvic inflammatory disease (in pregnancy)	Hospitalize and treat parenterally	
Cervicitis	Treat for chlamydia and consider concurrent gonorrhea treatment if prevalence is high	
Nongonococcal urethritis	Treat for chlamydia	
Epididymitis (initial therapy)	Ceftriaxone **plus** doxycycline	250 mg IM, single dose 100 mg PO BID × 10 days
Epididymitis (if gonorrhea negative, or likely caused by enteric organism)	Levofloxacin **or** ofloxacin	500 mg PO daily × 10 days 300 mg PO BID × 10 days
Trichomoniasis	Metronidazole **or** tinidazole (avoid during pregnancy)	2 g PO, single dose 2 g PO, single dose
Vulvovaginal candidiasis (choice between over-the-counter [OTC] intravaginal, prescription intravaginal, or oral treatment) (*Note:* During pregnancy, only 7-day topical azole treatments are recommended.)	**OTC intravaginal** butoconazole **or** clotrimazole **or** miconazole **or**	2% cream 5 g intravaginally × 3 days 1% cream 5 g intravaginally × 7–14 days **or** 2% cream 5 g intravaginally × 3 days 2% cream 5 g intravaginally × 7 days **or** 4% cream 5 g intravaginally × 3 days **or** 100 mg vaginal suppository, one daily × 7 days **or** 200 mg vaginal suppository, one daily × 3 days **or** 1200 mg vaginal suppository, once

(*Continued*)

Table 14–3. STD treatment guidelines for adults and adolescents. (*Continued*)

Disease	Recommended Regimens	Dose, Route
	tioconazole	6.5% ointment 5 g intravaginally, once
	Prescription intravaginal	
	butoconazole	2% cream (single-dose bioadhesive product), 5 g
	or	intravaginally, once
	nystatin	100,000-unit vaginal tablet, daily × 14 days (less effective)
	or	
	terconazole	0.4% cream 5 g intravaginally × 7 days
		or
		0.8% cream 5 g intravaginally × 3 days
		or
		80 mg vaginal suppository, daily × 3 days
	Oral treatment	
	fluconazole	150 mg oral tablet once
	(contraindicated in pregnancy)	
Bacterial vaginosis (nonpregnant)	Metronidazole	500 mg PO BID × 7 days
	or	(no alcohol for 9 days)
	metronidazole gel 0.75%	One applicator vaginally daily × 5 days
	or	
	clindamycin cream 2%	One applicator vaginally at bedtime × 7 days (oil-based, can weaken latex condoms)
Bacterial vaginosis (in pregnancy)	Metronidazole	500 mg PO BID × 7 days
	or	or
		250 mg PO 3× daily for 7 days
	clindamycin	300 mg PO BID × 7 days
Chancroid	Azithromycin	1 g PO single dose
	or	
	ceftriaxone	250 mg IM single dose
	or	
	ciprofloxacin	500 mg PO BID × 3 days
	(contraindicated in pregnancy)	
	or	
	erythromycin base	500 mg PO 3 × daily for 7 days
Lymphogranuloma venereum (nonpregnant)	Doxycycline	100 mg PO BID × 21 days
Lymphogranuloma venereum (in pregnancy)	Erythromycin base	500 mg PO 4 × daily for 21 days
Human papillomavirus (HPV) external genital/peri-anal warts (may choose either patient-applied or provider-administered treatments) (*Note:* Podofilox, imiquimod, sinecatechins, and podophyllin are all contraindicated in pregnancy.)	**Patient-applied** podofilox 0.5% soln or gel or imiquimod 5% cream or sinecatechins 15% ointment **Provider-administered** cryotherapy (liquid nitrogen or cryoprobe) or podophyllin resin 10–25% in a compound tincture of benzoin or TCA or BCA 80–90% or surgical removal	
HPV cervical warts	Biopsy and consultation	

(Continued)

Table 14–3. STD treatment guidelines for adults and adolescents. (*Continued*)

Disease	Recommended Regimens	Dose, Route
HPV vaginal warts	Cryotherapy with liquid nitrogen (not cryoprobe) **or** TCA or BCA 80–90%	
HPV urethral meatus warts (*Note:* Podophyllin is contraindicated in pregnancy.	Cryotherapy with liquid nitrogen **or** podophyllin 10–25% in compound tincture of benzoin	
HPV anal warts	Cryotherapy with liquid nitrogen **or** TCA or BCA 80–90% **or** surgical removal	
Herpes simplex virus (HSV) first episode (*Note:* Acyclovir is preferred in pregnancy.)	Acyclovir **or** famciclovir **or** valacyclovir	400 mg PO 3 × daily for 7–10 days **or** 200 mg PO 5 × daily for 7–10 days 250 mg PO 3 × daily for 7–10 days 1 g PO BID for 7–10 days
HSV episodic therapy for recurrent episodes (*Note:* Acyclovir is preferred in pregnancy.)	Acyclovir **or** famciclovir **or** valacyclovir	400 mg PO 3 × daily for 5 days **or** 800 mg PO BID × 5 days **or** 800 mg PO 3 × daily for 2 days 125 mg PO BID × 5 days **or** 1000 mg PO BID × 1 day **or** 500 mg PO once, followed by 250 mg PO BID for 2 days 500 mg PO BID × 3 days **or** 1 g PO daily × 5 days
HSV suppressive therapy (*Note:* Acyclovir is preferred in pregnancy.)	Acyclovir **or** famciclovir **or** valacyclovir	400 mg PO BID 250 mg PO BID 500 mg PO daily **or** 1 g PO daily
Syphilis: primary, secondary, and early latent	Benzathine penicillin G (*Note:* Nonpregnant patients without HIV coinfection can consider doxycycline or tetracycline as an alternative.)	2.4 million units IM
Syphilis: late latent and unknown duration	Benzathine penicillin G (*Note:* Nonpregnant patients without HIV coinfection can consider doxycycline or tetracycline as an alternative.)	7.2 million units, administered as 3 doses of 2.4 million units IM, at 1-week intervals

(*Continued*)

Table 14–3. STD treatment guidelines for adults and adolescents. (*Continued*)

Disease	Recommended Regimens	Dose, Route
Neurosyphilis	Aqueous crystalline penicillin G	18–24 million units daily, administered as 3–4 million units IV every 4 hours × 10–14 days (*Note:* Penicillin allergy requires desensitization.)
Pediculosis pubis: "crab lice" (*Note:* Wash clothes and bedding.)	Permethrin 1% cream rinse **or** Pyrethrins with piperonyl butoxide	Apply to affected areas and wash off after 10 minutes Apply to affected areas and wash off after 10 minutes
Scabies (*Note:* Wash clothes and bedding.)	Permethrin 5% cream **or** ivermectin (contraindicated in pregnancy)	Apply to entire body from neck down; wash off after 8–14 hours 0.2 mg/kg PO once and repeated after 2 weeks

BCA, bichloroacetic acid; BID, twice a day; IM, intramuscular; IV, intravenous; PO, oral; soln, solution; TCA, trichloroacetic acid; TID, three times a day. Data from Workowski KA1, Berman S; Centers for Disease Control and Prevention (CDC): Sexually transmitted diseases treatment guidelines, 2010. *MMWR Recomm Rep.* 2010 Dec 17;59(RR-12):1–110.

▶ Clinical Findings

A. Symptoms and Signs

A first episode of genital herpes classically presents with blisters and sores, with local tingling and discomfort. Visible lesions may be preceded by a prodrome of tingling or burning. Some patients also report dysesthesia or neuralgic pain in the buttocks or legs and malaise with fever. The clinical spectrum of disease can include atypical rashes, fissuring, excoriation, and discomfort of the anogenital area; cervical lesions; urinary symptoms; and extragenital lesions. Even patients who initially show mild symptoms can develop overt disease with significant symptoms. In immunocompromised persons, HSV can manifest as large, chronic, hyperkeratotic ulcers. If lesions persist despite antiviral therapy, acyclovir-resistant HSV should be suspected.

Both HSV1 and HSV2 cause genital disease, although HSV1 produces fewer clinical recurrences and may be less severe. Symptoms during recurrences are generally less intense and shorter in duration. Infectious virus is shed intermittently and unpredictably in some asymptomatic patients. Latex condoms, when used correctly and consistently, may reduce the risk of genital HSV transmission.

B. Laboratory Findings

Diagnosis of HSV is based on either culture of the vesicle base or ulcer or PCR test for HSV DNA. PCR assays for HSV DNA are more sensitive and have been increasingly used. Cytologic detection of cellular changes of HSV infection is insensitive and nonspecific, both in genital lesions (Tzanck smear) and cervical Papanicolaou (Pap) smears, and so should not be relied on. Type-specific serologic assays may be useful in patients with recurrent symptoms and negative HSV cultures, those with a clinical diagnosis of genital herpes without laboratory confirmation, or patients who have a partner with genital herpes. Serologic assays for HSV can be considered for patients at high risk for STDs, for patients with HIV, and for MSM patients, but it is important to note that these assays are very difficult to interpret, since they generally do not distinguish between oral HSV and genital HSV, and so patients should be counseled ahead of time regarding this complexity.

▶ Treatment

Treatment of HSV can be episodic (ie, in response to an episode of disease) or suppressive, with daily medication continuing for months or years. Treatment for an initial outbreak consists of 7–10 days of oral medication (see Table 14–3). Episodic treatment is effective when medication is started during the prodrome or on the first symptomatic day. No benefit will be seen if treatment of recurrences is delayed; thus, patients should be given a prescription to have available for use when needed.

Suppressive therapy is traditionally indicated for patients with frequent recurrences, although this may be individualized with respect to the stress and disability caused by recurrences. Available experience suggests that long-term suppression is safe and is not associated with development of antiviral resistance; data have shown safety with acyclovir up to 6 years and valacyclovir up to 1 year. Suppressive therapy seems to reduce but not eliminate asymptomatic shedding. Daily treatment with valacyclovir (500 mg) has been shown to decrease the rate of HSV2 transmission in discordant heterosexual couples in which the source partner has a history of genital HSV2 infection. Suppression does not change the natural history of a patient's infection; however, because the frequency of recurrences diminishes with time, suppression may be particularly useful during the time period immediately following initial infection. Available therapies appear to be safe in pregnant women, although data for valacyclovir and famciclovir are limited.

Syphilis

▶ General Considerations

Syphilis cases reported to the CDC had declined since the early 1950s until reaching a low of 2.1 cases per 100,000 population in 2000–2001. However, increases in syphilis rates have been noted nearly every year since then, and in 2016, the CDC received reports of 27,814 cases of primary and secondary syphilis, or 8.7 cases per 100,000 population. Men account for 90% of the reported cases, and of the cases in which sex of sex partner was known, more than 80% of the men with new-onset primary or secondary syphilis were MSM.

▶ Clinical Findings

A. Symptoms and Signs

Syphilis infection is characterized by stages, and accurate staging is vital to determine appropriate therapy. *Primary syphilis* is characterized by the appearance of a painless, indurated ulcer—the chancre—occurring 10 days to 3 months after infection with *Treponema pallidum*. The chancre usually heals by 4–6 weeks, although associated painless bilateral lymphadenopathy may persist for months.

Secondary syphilis has variable manifestations but usually includes symmetric mucocutaneous macular, papular, papulosquamous, or pustular lesions with generalized nontender lymphadenopathy. In moist skin areas such as the perianal or vulvar regions, papules may become superficially eroded to form pink or whitish condylomata lata. Constitutional symptoms such as fever, malaise, and weight loss occur commonly. Less common complications include meningitis, hepatitis, arthritis, nephropathy, and iridocyclitis.

Latent syphilis is diagnosed in persons with serologic evidence of syphilis infection *without* other current evidence of disease. "Early" latent syphilis is defined as infection for <1 year. A diagnosis of early latent syphilis is demonstrated by seroconversion, a definitive history of primary or secondary syphilis findings within the past year, or documented exposure to primary or secondary syphilis in the past year. Asymptomatic patients with known infection of >1 year or in whom infection of <1 year cannot be conclusively demonstrated are classified as having late latent syphilis or latent syphilis of unknown duration, respectively. These two categories of syphilis are treated equivalently. The magnitude of serologic test titers cannot reliably differentiate early from late latent syphilis.

Neurosyphilis can occur at any stage of infection and is difficult to diagnose, as no single test can be used in all instances. The cerebrospinal fluid (CSF) VDRL test is highly specific but insensitive. The diagnosis depends on a combination of serologic tests, elevated CSF cell count or protein, or a reactive VDRL. CSF fluorescent treponemal antibody absorption (FTA-abs) is less specific but highly sensitive. CSF pleocytosis (>5 white blood cells [WBCs]/mm^3) is usually evident, although HIV infection and other conditions may also cause increased WBCs in the CSF.

Tertiary syphilis is characterized by a self-destructive immune response to a persistent low level of pathogens. It can manifest as neurosyphilis, cardiovascular syphilis including aortitis, or in the form of gummas, granulomas, or psoriasiform plaques.

Patients are infectious during primary, secondary, and early latent stages of syphilis.

B. Laboratory Findings

Positive darkfield examination or direct fluorescent antibody tests of lesion exudates definitively diagnose primary syphilis. More typically, syphilis is diagnosed by positive serologic results of both a nontreponemal test (VDRL or RPR) and a treponemal test (*T pallidum* particle agglutination [TPPA] or FTA-abs).

Nontreponemal tests may be falsely positive because of other medical conditions (eg, some collagen vascular diseases). When positive because of syphilis, their titers generally rise and fall in response to *T pallidum* infection and treatment, respectively, and usually return to normal (negative) following treatment, although some individuals remain "serofast" and have persistent low positive titers. Treponemal tests usually yield persistent positive results throughout the patient's life following infection with *T pallidum*. Treponemal test titers do not correlate with disease activity or treatment.

Lumbar puncture is indicated for (1) neurologic or ophthalmologic signs or symptoms, (2) active aortitis or gumma, or (3) treatment failure (a fourfold increase in titer or a failure to decline fourfold or more within 12–24 months).

▶ Treatment

Treatment for syphilis as described in Table 14–3 is based on current CDC guidelines. Follow-up testing of patients diagnosed with syphilis is a vital part of care, as it determines the effectiveness of therapy and provides useful information to differentiate potential future serofast patients from those with recurrent infection.

The nontreponemal test titer should have fallen fourfold or more (eg, from 1:32 to ≤1:8) for persons with primary or secondary syphilis in 6–12 months after therapy. If it does not, consider this a possible treatment failure or an indication of reinfection (although current data suggest that

15–20% of patients who have received treatment will fail to fall fourfold or more within 12 months). In evaluating such a potential treatment failure, the patient should, at minimum, receive continued serologic follow-up and repeat HIV serology if previously negative. Lumbar puncture should also be considered, and if the results are normal, the patient can be treated with 2.4 million units of benzathine penicillin weekly for 3 weeks and followed as described previously.

Chancroid

Chancroid has declined in the United States and worldwide. In 2016, a total of seven cases of chancroid were reported in only six states in the United States. These data should be interpreted with caution, however, because *Haemophilus ducreyi* is difficult to culture, and thus, this condition may be substantially underdiagnosed.

Definitive diagnosis is difficult, requiring identification of *H ducreyi* on special culture medium that is seldom readily available. Presumptive diagnosis rests on the presence of painful genital ulcer(s) with a negative HSV test and negative syphilis serology, with or without regional lymphadenopathy.

Treatment consists of oral antibiotics, as listed in Table 14–3. Healing of large ulcers may require >2 weeks. If patients do not show clinical improvement after 7 days, consider the accuracy of the diagnosis, medication nonadherence, antibacterial resistance, or a combination of these. Fluctuant lymphadenopathy may require drainage via aspiration or incision.

Although definitive diagnosis generally rests on laboratory testing, history and examination often lead to a presumptive diagnosis. Table 14–4 summarizes findings for different causes of GUD.

Other Causes of GUD

Granuloma inguinale or donovanosis is caused by *Calymmatobacterium granulomatis*, which is endemic in some tropical nonindustrialized parts of the world and is rarely reported in the United States. The bacterium does not grow on standard culture media; diagnosis rests on demonstration of so-called Donovan bodies in a tissue specimen. Infection causes painless, progressive, beefy red, highly vascular lesions without lymphadenopathy. Treatment is often prolonged, and relapse can occur months after initial treatment and apparent cure.

Lymphogranuloma venereum is caused by serovars L1, L2, and L3 of *C trachomatis*. The small ulcer arising at the site of infection is often unnoticed or unreported. The most common clinical presentation is painful unilateral lymphadenopathy. Rectal exposure in women and in MSMs may result in proctocolitis (mucus or hemorrhagic rectal discharge, anal pain, constipation, fever, or tenesmus). Diagnosis rests on clinical suspicion, epidemiologic information, exclusion of other etiologies, and *C trachomatis* tests. In addition to antibiotics, treatment may require aspiration or incision and drainage of buboes; nevertheless, patients may still experience scarring.

Centers for Disease Control and Prevention. *Sexually Transmitted Disease Surveillance 2016*. Atlanta, GA: US Department of Health and Human Services; 2017.

Centers for Disease Control and Prevention; Workowski KA, Bolan GA. Sexually transmitted disease treatment guidelines, 2015. *MMWR Recomm Rep*. 2015;64(RR-3):1–140. [PMID: 21160459]

Domantay-Apostol GP, Handog EB, Gabriel MT. Syphilis: the international challenge of the great imitator. *Dermatol Clin*. 2008;26(2):191–202. [PMID: 18346551]

Table 14–4. Differentiation of common causes of genital ulcers.[a]

Parameter	Herpes	Syphilis	Chancroid	Lymphogranuloma Venereum	Granuloma Inguinale
Ulcer(s) appearance	Often purulent	"Clean"	Purulent	May be purulent	"Beefy," hemorrhagic
Number	Usually multiple	Single[b]	Often multiple	Single or multiple	Multiple
Pain	Yes	No	Yes	Ulcer: no Nodes: yes	No
Preceded by	Papule, then vesicle	Papule	Papule	Papule; ulcer often unnoticed	Nodule(s)
Adenopathy	Painful with primary outbreak	Painless	Painful; may suppurate	Painful; may suppurate	No, unless secondary bacterial infection
Systemic symptoms	Often with primary outbreak	Rarely	Occasionally	Usually not	No

[a]A diagnosis based solely on medical history and physical examination is often inaccurate.
[b]Up to 40% of patients with primary syphilis have more than one chancre.

Kapoor S. Re-emergence of lymphogranuloma venereum. *J Euro Acad Dermatol Venereol.* 2008;22(4):409–416. [PMID: 18363909]

Mattei P, Beachkofsky TM, Gilson RT, Wisco OJ. Syphilis: a reemerging infection. *Am Fam Physician.* 2012;86(5):433–440. [PMID: 22963062]

URETHRITIS

 ESSENTIALS OF DIAGNOSIS

▶ Coinfection with *C trachomatis* is common in those with *N gonorrhoeae*, justifying treatment for both.

▶ Nucleic acid amplification tests (NAATs) have largely supplanted cell culture tests for diagnosis.

In 2016, population studies showed a rate of *Chlamydia* infection of 497.3 cases per 100,000 and a rate of gonorrhea infection of 145.8 cases per 100,000 in the United States. Rates for chlamydia infection are higher in women, and gonorrhea infection rates are higher in men. Both of these pathogens are highest in the adolescent and young adult age groups.

STDs causing urethritis are typically diagnosed in men, although women may also experience urethritis as a consequence of an STD. For clinical management, urethritis can be divided into nongonococcal urethritis (NGU) and urethritis due to *N gonorrhoeae* infection.

Nongonococcal Urethritis

One frequent cause of NGU is *C trachomatis*. In 2016, 1,598,354 chlamydia cases were reported, and although significant, these numbers likely dramatically underestimate actual cases of *C trachomatis* infection. The spectrum of *C trachomatis*–caused disease includes extragenital manifestations, among them ophthalmic infection and a reactive arthritis.

Causes of nonchlamydial NGU may include *Mycoplasma genitalium, Ureaplasma urealyticum, Trichomonas vaginalis,* HSV, and adenovirus. Diagnosis of NGU can be based on (1) purulent urethral discharge; (2) Gram stain of urethral secretions with ≥2 WBCs per oil immersion field and no gram-negative intracellular diplococci (which, if present, would indicate gonorrhea); and (3) first-void urine with positive leukocyte esterase or ≥10 WBCs/high-power field (HPF). NAATs (chlamydia or gonorrhea) offer greater convenience and better sensitivity than culture and represent the best tests currently available.

In patients presenting with recurrent urethritis, clear diagnostic criteria as outlined earlier for NGU should be followed. In evaluating recurrent urethritis, the physician should assess medication compliance and potential reexposure and perform wet mount, culture, or ideally NAAT for *T vaginalis.* Studies have shown that the most common cause for recurrent urethritis in men (especially after treatment with doxycycline) is *M genitalium,* which can be treated empirically with azithromycin, or with moxifloxacin if the patient has already failed azithromycin treatment. Obviously a positive trichomonal test result would prompt appropriate trichomonal treatments for both patient and partner. See Table 14–3.

Treatment of NGU generally employs azithromycin or doxycycline, with alternatives as listed in Table 14–3. If findings of urethritis are present, treatment is generally indicated pending results of diagnostic tests. Because diagnostic testing typically does not look for all potential causes of urethritis, patients with negative tests for gonorrhea and *C trachomatis* may also benefit from treatment. Empiric treatment of symptoms without documentation of urethritis findings is recommended only for patients at high risk for infection who are unlikely to return for a follow-up evaluation. Such patients should be treated for gonorrhea and chlamydia. Partners of patients treated empirically should be evaluated and treated. If treatment is not offered at the initial visit, diagnostic testing should employ the most sensitive test available, with follow-up treatment as indicated by test results and symptom persistence.

Gonorrhea

▶ General Considerations

In 2016, 468,514 cases of gonorrhea were reported in the United States. Gonorrhea rates reached a historic low in 2009 at 98.1 cases per 100,000 population. Since then, rates have risen slowly nearly every year to reach a 2016 rate of 145.8 cases per 100,000 population. Reported cases are more common in the South (166.8 cases per 100,000 population vs 145.8 cases per 100,000 for the country) and more common in men than in women (170.7 vs 121.0 cases per 100,000, respectively). As recently as 2012, reported gonorrhea cases in women were more prevalent than in men, but recent rates of reported male gonorrheal infections have increased more rapidly than in women. It is unclear from the data whether this is related to increased testing or whether it might be related to sexual preference for partner, since those data are not collected.

▶ Clinical Findings

A. Symptoms and Signs

If symptomatic, gonorrhea typically causes dysuria and a purulent urethral discharge; however, it may also cause asymptomatic infection or disseminated systemic disease, including pharyngitis, skin lesions, septic arthritis, tenosynovitis, arthralgias, proctitis, perihepatitis, endocarditis, and meningitis. In these cases, there is usually minimal genital inflammation.

Clinical differentiation between gonorrhea and *Chlamydia* may be difficult. Characteristically, urethral exudate in gonorrhea is thicker, more profuse, and more purulent in appearance than the exudate caused by *C trachomatis*, which is often watery with mucus strands. However, differentiation of etiology based on clinical appearance is notoriously unreliable.

B. Laboratory Findings

NAAT (including PCR) has largely supplanted culture for diagnosis because of enhanced sensitivity and excellent specificity. NAAT tests can be performed on endocervical swabs, vaginal swabs, urethral swabs, and urine samples. In addition, some laboratories have established performance specifications for the use of NAAT testing for gonorrhea on rectal and pharyngeal swabs. However, the use of NAAT testing in nongenital sites is rendered more challenging by the potential for cross-reactivity with nongonorrheal *Neisseria* species.

Diagnostic evaluation identifies disease etiology and may facilitate the public health missions of contact tracing and disease eradication. For an individual patient, however, the physician may treat empirically if follow-up cannot be ensured and test methodology is insensitive. Decisions about diagnostic testing should consider both public health goals and how information obtained will influence patient (and partner) treatment.

▶ Treatment

When treating for gonorrhea, practitioners should treat also for *C trachomatis*, as coinfection is common. Quinolone-resistant *N gonorrhoeae* strains are now widely disseminated throughout United States and the world. Since April 2007, quinolones have no longer been recommended in the United States for treatment of gonorrhea and associated conditions such as PID. As of October 2012, oral cephalosporins are no longer a recommended treatment for gonorrheal infection. Decreased susceptibility of *N gonorrhoeae* to cephalosporins and other antimicrobials is expected to continue to spread; therefore, state and local surveillance for antimicrobial resistance is crucial for guiding local therapy recommendations. Ceftriaxone 250 mg intramuscularly with 1 g of oral azithromycin is currently effective for the treatment of uncomplicated gonorrhea at all anatomic sites.

Treatment failures should be followed by (repeat) culture and sensitivity testing, and any resistance should be reported to the public health department.

Centers for Disease Control and Prevention. *Sexually Transmitted Disease Surveillance 2016.* Atlanta, GA: US Department of Health and Human Services; 2017.
Centers for Disease Control and Prevention; Workowski KA, Bolan, GA. Sexually transmitted disease treatment guidelines, 2015. *MMWR Recomm Rep.* 2015;64(RR-3):1–140. [PMID: 21160459]

US Preventive Services Task Force. Evidence summary: chlamydia and gonorrhea: screening. September 2016. https://www.uspreventiveservicestaskforce.org/Page/SupportingDoc/chlamydia-and-gonorrhea-screening/evidence-summary3. Accessed November 11, 2019.

EPIDIDYMITIS

The cause of epididymitis varies with age. In men age ≤35 years, it is most commonly due to gonorrhea or *C trachomatis* or to gram-negative enteric organisms in men who engage in unprotected insertive anal intercourse. In men age >35 years who do not report insertive anal intercourse, epididymitis is seldom sexually transmitted and is more likely caused by gram-negative enteric organisms; increased risk in this case is found in patients who have undergone recent urologic surgery or who have anatomic abnormalities. Patients usually present with unilateral testicular pain and inflammation with onset over several days. The clinician must differentiate epididymitis from testicular torsion, since the latter is a surgical emergency requiring immediate correction. The laboratory evaluation of suspected epididymitis includes Gram stain, NAATs for gonorrhea and chlamydia, and first-void urinalysis with microscopy. In the case of chronic epididymitis (>6 weeks), tuberculosis should additionally be suspected, and urology consult is recommended in the absence of clear infectious cause.

PROCTITIS, PROCTOCOLITIS, & ENTERITIS

Proctitis, proctocolitis, and enteritis may arise from anal intercourse or oral-anal contact. Depending on organism and anatomic location of infection and inflammation, symptoms can include pain, tenesmus, rectal discharge, and diarrhea. Etiologic agents of proctitis include *C trachomatis* (lymphogranuloma venereum [LGV]), *N gonorrhoeae*, *T pallidum*, and HSV. Other agents may cause proctocolitis or enteritis, including *Giardia lamblia*, *Campylobacter*, *Shigella*, and *Entamoeba histolytica*. In HIV-infected patients, additional etiologic agents include cytomegalovirus, *Mycobacterium avium-intracellulare*, *Salmonella*, *Cryptosporidium*, *Microsporidium*, and *Isospora*. Symptoms may also arise as a primary effect of HIV infection.

Diagnosis involves examination of stool for ova, parasites, occult blood, and WBCs; stool culture and anoscopy or sigmoidoscopy; and testing for HSV (PCR or culture), gonorrhea (NAAT or culture), chlamydia (NAAT), syphilis (darkfield if available or blood testing), and HIV. If rectal swab is positive for *Chlamydia*, then PCR analysis for LGV should be completed.

Treatment should generally be based on results of diagnostic studies. However, if the onset of symptoms occurs within 1–2 weeks of receptive anal intercourse and there is evidence of purulent exudates or polymorphonuclear neutrophils on Gram stain of anorectal smear, the patient can be treated presumptively for gonorrhea and chlamydial infection. If painful perianal ulcers are present or mucosal ulcers are detected on anoscopy, presumptive therapy should include a regimen for genital herpes. If bloody discharge, perianal ulcers, or mucosal ulcers are present and if either HIV or chlamydia testing is positive, a regimen for LGV should be prescribed (waiting for LGV results should not postpone treatment in these cases).

VAGINITIS

ESSENTIALS OF DIAGNOSIS

▶ A careful history, examination, and laboratory testing should be performed to determine the etiology of vaginal complaints. Information on sexual behaviors and practices, gender of sex partners, menses, vaginal hygiene practices (eg, douching or use of douche products), and other medications should be elicited.

▶ Examination of vaginal discharge by wet mount, potassium hydroxide (KOH) preparation, pH, and odor.

▶ Disease-specific point-of-care test or vaginal fluid culture if indicated.

Patients with vaginitis may present with vaginal discharge, vulvar itching, irritation, or all of these, and sometimes with complaints of abnormal vaginal odor. Common etiologies include *Candida albicans*, *T vaginalis*, and bacterial vaginosis. Diagnostic evaluation typically includes physical examination and evaluation of a saline wet mount and KOH preparation. Differences between common causes of vaginitis are summarized in Table 14–5 and described next.

Vulvovaginal Candidiasis

Vulvovaginal candidiasis (VVC) is typically caused by *C albicans*, although occasionally other species are identified. More than 75% of all women will have at least one episode of VVC during their lifetime. The diagnosis is presumed if the patient has vulvovaginal pruritus and erythema with or without a white discharge and is confirmed by wet mount or KOH preparation showing yeast or pseudohyphae or culture showing a yeast species.

VVC can be classified as uncomplicated or complicated. Uncomplicated VVC encompasses sporadic, nonrecurrent, mild to moderate symptoms due to *C albicans* that, in an otherwise healthy patient, are responsive to routine therapy. Complicated VVC implies recurrent or severe local disease in a patient with impaired immune function (eg, diabetes or HIV) or infection with resistant yeast species. Recurrent VVC is defined as four or more symptomatic episodes annually.

Treatment is summarized in Table 14–3. Uncomplicated candidiasis should respond to short-term or single-dose therapies as listed. Complicated VVC may require prolonged treatment. Treatment of women with recurrent vulvovaginal candidiasis should begin with an intensive regimen (7–14 days of topical therapy or a multidose fluconazole regimen) followed by 6 months of maintenance therapy to reduce the likelihood of subsequent recurrence. Symptomatic candidal vaginitis is more frequent in HIV-infected women and correlates with severity of immunodeficiency.

Vulvovaginal candidiasis is seldom acquired through sexual intercourse. There are no data to support treatment of sex partners. Some male sex partners have balanitis and may benefit from topical antifungal agents.

Trichomoniasis

Vaginitis due to *T vaginalis* presents with a thin, yellow, or yellow-green frothy malodorous discharge and vulvar irritation that may worsen following menstruation. However, many women have minimal or no symptoms at all. It is recommended that highly sensitive and specific tests for *Trichomonas* be used, including approved NAAT testing methods, antigen detection methods, DNA hybridization probe tests, or culture. Diagnosis can sometimes be made via prompt examination of a freshly obtained wet mount, which reveals the motile trichomonads, although sensitivity

Table 14–5. Common causes of vaginitis.

Diagnostic Test	Findings Characteristics of		
	Candida albicans	*Trichomonas vaginalis*	Bacterial Vaginosis
pH	<4.5	>4.5	>4.5
KOH to slide	Yeast or pseudohyphae		Amine or "fishy" odor
Saline to slide	Yeast or pseudohyphae	Motile *T vaginalis* organisms	"Clue" cells
Culture	Yeast species	*T vaginalis*	Nonspecific (not recommended)

of this method is low (51–65%). Although culture and NAAT are more sensitive, they may not be as readily available, and results are delayed. Point-of-care tests (eg, Osom *Trichomonas* Rapid Test and Affirm VPIII) are also available and tend to be more sensitive than vaginal wet prep. Partners of women with *Trichomonas* infection require treatment.

Bacterial Vaginosis

Bacterial vaginosis arises when normal vaginal bacteria are replaced with an overgrowth of anaerobic bacteria. Although not thought to be an STD, it is associated with having multiple sex partners or a new sex partner.

Diagnosis can be based on the presence of three of four clinical criteria: (1) a thin, homogeneous vaginal discharge; (2) a vaginal pH value of >4.5; (3) a positive "whiff" test (fishy odor when KOH is added to vaginal discharge); and (4) the presence of clue cells in a wet mount preparation.

Treatment is recommended for women with symptoms. Potential benefits of therapy include reducing the risk for infectious complications associated with bacterial vaginosis during pregnancy and reducing the risk for other infections. Routine treatment of sex partners is not recommended.

Cervicitis

Cervicitis is characterized by purulent discharge from the endocervix, which may or may not be associated with vaginal discharge or cervical bleeding. The diagnostic evaluation should include testing for chlamydia, gonorrhea, bacterial vaginosis, and *Trichomonas*. Absence of symptoms should not preclude additional evaluation and treatment, as approximately 70% of chlamydial infections and 50% of gonococcal infections in women are asymptomatic.

Nucleic acid amplification tests are the preferred diagnostic test for gonorrhea and *Chlamydia* and can be performed on vaginal, cervical, or urine specimens. Empiric treatment should be considered in areas with high prevalence of *C trachomatis* or gonorrhea or if follow-up is unlikely.

Centers for Disease Control and Prevention; Workowski KA, Bolan GA. Sexually transmitted disease treatment guidelines, 2015. *MMWR Recomm Rep.* 2015;64(RR-3):1–140. [PMID: 21160459]

PELVIC INFLAMMATORY DISEASE

ESSENTIALS OF DIAGNOSIS

▶ Diagnosis is challenging, requiring the clinician to balance underdiagnosis with overtreatment.

▶ Consequences of untreated PID can include chronic pain, infertility, and death.

Pelvic inflammatory disease (PID) is defined as inflammation of the upper genital tract, including pelvic peritonitis, endometritis, salpingitis, and tubo-ovarian abscess due to infection with gonorrhea, *C trachomatis*, or vaginal or bowel flora; etiology is often polymicrobial. Diagnosis is challenging because of often vague symptoms, lack of a single diagnostic test, and the invasive nature of technologies needed to make a definitive diagnosis. Lower abdominal tenderness and uterine, adnexal, or cervical motion tenderness with signs of lower genital tract inflammation increase the specificity of a PID diagnosis. Other criteria enhance the specificity of the diagnosis (but reduce diagnostic sensitivity):

- Fever >38.3°C (>101°F)
- Abnormal cervical or vaginal discharge
- Abundant WBCs in saline microscopy of vaginal secretions
- Elevated sedimentation rate
- Elevated C-reactive protein
- Cervical infection with gonorrhea or *C trachomatis*

Definitive diagnosis rests on techniques that are not always readily available, some of which are rarely used to make the diagnosis. These include laparoscopic findings consistent with PID, evidence of endometritis on endometrial biopsy, and ultrasonographic findings showing thickened fluid-filled tubes with or without free pelvic fluid or tubo-ovarian complex, or pelvic infection suggested by Doppler studies.

Determination of appropriate therapy should consider pregnancy status, severity of illness, and patient compliance. Less severe disease can generally be treated with oral antibiotics in an ambulatory setting, whereas pregnant patients and those with severe disease may need hospitalization. Options are listed in Table 14–3.

Centers for Disease Control and Prevention; Workowski KA, Bolan GA. Sexually transmitted disease treatment guidelines, 2015. *MMWR Recomm Rep.* 2015;64(RR-3):1–140. [PMID: 21160459]

HPV INFECTION & EXTERNAL GENITAL WARTS

ESSENTIALS OF DIAGNOSIS

▶ Diagnosis of genital warts is usually made by visual inspection. Biopsy may be indicated if diagnosis is uncertain.

▶ Treatment is directed toward genital warts or to precancerous lesions caused by HPV. In the absence of lesions, treatment is not recommended for subclinical genital HPV infection, which often clears spontaneously.

General Considerations

It is estimated that >79 million Americans are infected with HPV, with 14 million new infections occurring annually. The vast majority of sexually active people who have not been vaccinated against HPV will get HPV sometime in their lives, although most never know it. Over 100 types of HPV have been identified, and >40 types cause genital lesions. Types 6, 11, and others typically produce benign exophytic warts, whereas types 16, 18, 31, 33, 35, and others are associated with dysplasia and neoplasia. Most precancers and cancers of the cervix, anus, vagina, vulva, penis, and oropharynx are caused by oncogenic strains of HPV; thus, cervical and anogenital squamous cancer can be considered STDs. In 2009, 34,788 new HPV-related cancers were reported in the United States.

Clinical Findings

Diagnosis of anogenital warts is almost always based on physical examination with bright light and magnification and rarely requires biopsy. Biopsy should be considered for warts that are >1 cm; indurated, ulcerated, or fixed to underlying structures; atypical in appearance; pigmented; or resistant to therapy. Application of 3–5% acetic acid as an aid to visualization is seldom useful, and the resulting nonspecific acetowhite reaction may lead to overdiagnosis of genital warts.

HPV is the primary cause of cervical cancer, and screening guidelines for cervical cancer screening, including the use of HPV testing, are reviewed in Chapter 26. Genital warts are not an indication for screening more frequently.

Because of the increased incidence of anal cancer in HIV-infected homosexual and bisexual men and high-risk women, screening for anal cytologic abnormalities may be considered. However, there are limited data on the natural history of anal intraepithelial neoplasias, the reliability of screening methods, the safety of and response to treatments, and the programmatic considerations that would support this screening approach.

Treatment

The therapeutic goal in treatment of external genital warts is elimination of warts. Treatment strives to eliminate symptoms, and a potential theoretical benefit is reduced likelihood of transmission. Clinicians should be certain of the diagnosis prior to instituting therapy and should not apply treatments to skin tags, pearly penile papules, sebaceous glands, or other benign findings that do not require (and will not respond to) genital wart treatment.

No evidence suggests any treatment is superior to others. The possibility of spontaneous resolution may justify no treatment, if that is the patient's wish.

Treatments can be categorized as provider-applied or patient-applied. Physicians should familiarize themselves with at least one or two treatments in each category, as described in Table 14–3. Most treatments work via tissue destruction. Imiquimod uses a different mechanism; by inducing production of interferon, it may be more effective than other therapies in treating some genital warts or other skin conditions, including molluscum contagiosum. Patients unresponsive to an initial course of treatment may require another round of treatment, more aggressive treatment, or referral to a specialist. Most anogenital warts will clear within 3 months of initiation of treatment.

Although most HPV infections will clear spontaneously within 2 years and cause no harm, patients with HPV need to understand the possibility of chronic infection, including its natural history and treatment options, and should receive adequate education and counseling to achieve optimal treatment outcomes. The chronic nature of HPV infection combined with the serious, albeit relatively infrequent, complication of cancer creates significant challenges to patient coping and provider counseling.

Centers for Disease Control and Prevention. Genital HPV infection–fact sheet. https://www.cdc.gov/std/hpv/stdfact-hpv.htm. Accessed August 15, 2018.
Centers for Disease Control and Prevention; Workowski KA, Bolan GA. Sexually transmitted disease treatment guidelines, 2015. *MMWR Recomm Rep.* 2015;64(RR-3):1–140. [PMID: 21160459]

MOLLUSCUM CONTAGIOSUM

Molluscum contagiosum appears in individuals of all ages and from all races but has been reported more commonly in the white population and in males. Lesions are due to infection with poxvirus, which is transmitted through direct skin contact, as occurs among children in a nursery school and among adults during sexual activity. Diagnosis is typically based on inspection, which reveals dimpled or umbilicated flesh-colored or pearly papules several millimeters in diameter; if needed, a smear of the core stained with Giemsa reveals cytoplasmic inclusion bodies. Lesions usually number fewer than 10–30, but may exceed 100, especially in HIV-infected patients who may have verrucous, warty papules, as well as mollusca of >1 cm diameter. Lesions usually resolve spontaneously within months of appearance but can be treated with cryotherapy, cautery, curettage, or removal of the lesion's core, with or without local anesthesia.

Villa L, Varela JA, Otero L, et al. Molluscum contagiosum: a 20-year study in a sexually transmitted infections unit. *Sex Transm Dis.* 2010;37(7):423–424. [PMID: 20414149]

HEPATITIS

Vaccines for prevention of viral hepatitis and indications were described previously. Diagnostic and treatment considerations of viral hepatitis are reviewed in Chapter 32.

ECTOPARASITES

Pediculosis pubis results from infestation with "crab lice" or *Pthirus pubis*. Affected patients usually present with pubic or anogenital pruritus and may have identified lice or nits. The physician should be able to identify lice or nits with careful examination, and their absence calls into question the diagnosis despite compatible history. In addition to antiparasitic treatments for the patient, bedding and clothing should be thoroughly decontaminated. Patients should be tested for other STDs and reexamined after 1 week.

Scabies, resulting from infestation with *Sarcoptes scabiei*, usually presents with pruritus not necessarily limited to the genital region. The intensity of pruritus may be increased at bedtime and may be out of proportion to modest physical findings of erythematous papules, burrows, or excoriation from scratching. A classic finding on physical examination is the serpiginous burrow present in the web space between fingers, although this finding is frequently absent in individuals with scabies.

Scabies can be sexually transmitted in adults; sexual contact is not the usual route of transmission in children. Pruritus may persist for weeks after treatment. Retreatment should be deferred if intensity of symptoms is diminishing and no new findings appear. Consider retreatment after 2 weeks in patients who continue to have symptoms or on whom live mites are observed. In HIV-infected patients with uncomplicated scabies, treatment is the same as for HIV-uninfected patients. However, HIV-infected patients are at risk for a more severe infestation with Norwegian scabies, which should be managed with expert consultation.

> Centers for Disease Control and Prevention; Workowski KA, Bolan GA. Sexually transmitted disease treatment guidelines, 2015. *MMWR Recomm Rep.* 2015;64(RR-3):1–140. [PMID: 21160459]

GENERAL PRINCIPLES OF THERAPY

ESSENTIAL FEATURES

▶ Presumptive treatment while awaiting laboratory test results is common practice.

▶ Coexisting HIV infection may modify STD treatment regimens.

▶ Patient education and partner treatment are essential to reduce disease spread.

Treatments may be empirically targeted to agents most likely causing the presenting clinical syndrome or targeted to a specific infection diagnosed definitively. Regardless, there are overarching concerns affecting STD treatment that pertain to adherence and treatment success, HIV status, partner treatment, test of cure, and pregnancy.

Adherence considerations favor shorter or single-dose regimens. Whenever possible, choose the shortest, simplest regimen to maximize the chance of compliance.

With HIV coinfection, treatments are generally the same as for uninfected patients unless stated otherwise. One potential difference is that HSV often causes more significant and prolonged symptoms in HIV-infected than in uninfected patients, so that HIV-infected patients may require longer treatment or higher medication dosages, or both. Syphilis treatment is the same as for HIV-uninfected patients regardless of stage. However, careful follow-up is important, as treatment failure or progression to neurosyphilis may be more common in the presence of HIV.

Ulcerative and nonulcerative STDs can increase the risk of HIV transmission.

Pregnancy imposes constraints and special considerations for therapy. Where applicable, these are noted in the treatment recommendations in Table 14–3.

As described previously, patients often present with a clinical syndrome potentially attributable to more than one infectious agent, and optimally focused therapy depends on microbiological identification. However, delaying therapy may allow symptoms to continue, resulting in untreated infection or continued spread (if the patient fails to return for follow-up or heed advice to avoid sexual contact until cured) and contribute to increased long-term morbidity. Consequently, it may be desirable to treat at the initial presentation for the infectious agents considered most likely.

> Centers for Disease Control and Prevention; Workowski KA, Bolan GA. Sexually transmitted disease treatment guidelines, 2015. *MMWR Recomm Rep.* 2015;64(RR-3):1–140. [PMID: 21160459]

SEXUAL ASSAULT

Management of victims of sexual assault encompasses much more than treatment or prevention of STDs. Providers must heed legal requirements and effectively manage the psychological trauma, while not compromising the best course of medical care.

Proper medical management of sexual assault victims includes collection of evidence, diagnostic evaluation, counseling, and medical therapies to treat infection and unintended pregnancy. The diagnostic evaluation should include the following:

• NAATs for *N gonorrhoeae* and *C trachomatis* from specimens collected from any sites of penetration or attempted penetration

• NAATs or sensitive point-of-care testing for *T vaginalis*; wet mount for detection of *Candida* or bacterial vaginosis, as well as sperm, which are motile for approximately 6 hours

- Serum tests for syphilis, hepatitis B, and HIV
- Pregnancy testing

Evaluation for STDs may be repeated in 1–2 weeks after the initial evaluation to detect organisms that may have been undetected, unless the patient was treated prophylactically. Follow-up exam can be scheduled in 1–2 months to examine patient for the development of anogenital warts, especially in the setting of other STDs. Repeat testing for syphilis and HIV should be performed at 6 weeks and 3 months, with repeat testing for HIV at 6 months (using test methods that detect acute HIV infection).

Prophylactic treatment for STDs may be offered or recommended because compliance with follow-up visits is poor. Hepatitis B vaccine should be administered according to the routine schedule; hepatitis B immune globulin is not necessary unless the perpetrator is known to be infected with HBV. Azithromycin 1 g orally, plus ceftriaxone 250 mg intramuscularly, plus metronidazole 2 g orally may be offered to treat *C trachomatis, N gonorrhoeae,* and *Trichomonas* (metronidazole can be deferred a few hours if the patient has had alcohol recently). Gastrointestinal side effects, especially when combined with postcoital oral contraceptive pills, may make this regimen intolerable, and alternative therapies or watchful waiting may be preferable.

HPV vaccination should be given to female survivors age 9–26 and males age 9–21 if they have not been vaccinated previously. HPV vaccine can be offered to MSM up to age 26. First dose is given at the time of the initial examination, and follow-up doses are scheduled as usual.

Need for and benefit from HIV postexposure prophylaxis is difficult to predict. If instituted, the greatest benefit results from initiation of therapy as soon after exposure as possible and certainly within 72 hours. For guidance in deciding whether to begin postexposure HIV prophylaxis and in selecting appropriate treatment and monitoring, providers may contact the National Clinician's Post-Exposure Prophylaxis Hotline (PEPline) at 888-HIV-4911 (888-448 4911).

After the neonatal period, STDs in children most commonly result from sexual abuse. In addition to vaginal gonococcal infection, pharyngeal and anorectal infection may occur. Specific diagnostic techniques should rely only on existing guidelines because data on NAATs for chlamydia and gonorrhea in this setting are limited and performance may be test dependent. Specimen preservation is essential for future testing when needed.

Centers for Disease Control and Prevention; Workowski KA, Bolan GA. Sexually transmitted disease treatment guidelines, 2015. *MMWR Recomm Rep.* 2015;64(RR-3):1–140. [PMID: 21160459]

Health Maintenance for Adults

Stephen A. Wilson, MD, MPH, FAAFP
Paul R. Larson, MD, MS, MBA, CPE, FAAFP
David Yuan, MD, MS
Lora Cox-Vance, MD, CMD

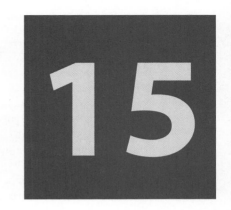

On average, each day longer you live, the longer you are likely to live, yet the closer to dying you become. The goal of health maintenance (HM) is to help people live as long and as healthy as possible.

General Considerations

In this chapter, the findings and positions of the US Preventative Services Task Force (USPSTF) are emphasized because it generates the most comprehensive and evidence-based recommendations of any organization. Hence, knowing the USPSTF grading system for its recommendations is important (Table 15–1). The USPSTF is sponsored by the Agency for Healthcare Research and Quality (AHRQ) and is the leading independent panel of private-sector experts in prevention and primary care.

This chapter describes prevention and then presents HM by the following age groups: 18–39, 40–49, 50–59, 60–74, and ≥75 years. USPSTF Grade A and B recommendations are emphasized. Due to multiple recent studies that call into question prior and current recommendations concerning the use of aspirin for prevention of heart disease, at the time of publication, we are unable to offer clear guidance and suggest accessing the USPSTF website for these evolving recommendations. HM involves three types of prevention: primary, secondary, and tertiary (Figure 15–1).

Prevention

A. Primary Prevention

Targets individuals who may be *at risk* to develop a medical condition and intervenes to prevent the onset of that condition (eg, childhood vaccination programs, water fluoridation, smoking prevention programs, clean water, and sanitation). The disease does *not* exist. The *goal is to prevent development* of disease.

B. Secondary Prevention

Targets individuals who have developed an *asymptomatic* disease and institutes treatment to prevent complications (eg, routine Papanicolaou [Pap] smears; screening for hypertension, diabetes, or hyperlipidemia). The disease does exist, but the person is unaware (*asymptomatic*). The *goal is to identify and treat* people with disease.

C. Tertiary Prevention

Treatment targets individuals with a *known* disease, with the goal of limiting or preventing future complications (eg, rigorous treatment of diabetes mellitus, post-myocardial infarction treatment with β-blockers and aspirin). The disease exists and there are symptoms. The *goal is to prevent complications.*

Secondary and tertiary prevention require some type of screening. This raises important issues: (1) who should be screened, (2) for which disease(s), and (3) with what test(s) (Table 15–2).

1. The disease—The disease must have a period of being detectable before the symptoms start so that it can be found and treated; for instance, colon cancer has no early symptoms but can be detected with screening. The disease cannot appear too quickly, such as a cold and certain lung cancers. The disease must be common in the target population; for instance, stomach cancer is not screened for in the United States (uncommon), but it is screened for in Japan, where is it is more common.

2. The test—*Ideally*, the screening test will identify all people with disease, and only people with disease will test positive. In *reality*, screening tests are acceptable if they do the job well enough (ie, are sensitive enough to have few false negatives and specific enough to have few false positives). Screening tests should also be cost efficient, easy, reliable, and as painless as possible.

Table 15–1. US Preventive Services Task Force (USPSTF) grade definitions.

Grade	Definition	Suggestions for Practice
A	USPSTF recommends the service. There is high certainty that the net benefit is substantial.	Offer or provide this service.
B	USPSTF recommends the service. There is high certainty that the net benefit is moderate or moderate certainty that the net benefit is moderate to substantial.	Offer or provide this service.
C	USPSTF recommends against routinely providing the service. There may be considerations that support providing the service in an individual patient. There is at least moderate certainty that the net benefit is small.	Offer or provide this service only if other considerations support the offering or providing the service in an individual patient.
D	USPSTF recommends against the service. There is moderate or high certainty that the service has no net benefit or that the harms outweigh the benefits.	Discourage the use of this service.
I statement	USPSTF concludes that the current evidence is insufficient to assess the balance of benefits and harms (risks) of the service. Evidence is lacking, of poor quality, or conflicting, and the balance of benefits and risks cannot be determined.	Read the clinical considerations section of USPSTF recommendation statement. If the service is offered, patients should understand the uncertainty about the balance of benefits and harms.

3. Treatment—When screening for disease, treatment must be available, be acceptable, and have benefits that outweigh the risk. Mortality is the most often used end point. If a group of people who are screened and then treated live longer or better than a group of people who are not screened, then the screening test may be good for that population. If the two groups of people die at the same rate, there is usually no point in screening for the disease.

SCREENING

A. Health Maintenance: Across the Ages— What *Not* to *Do*

Conditions for which the USPSTF recommends *against routine screening* in *asymptomatic* adults are as follows:

- Aspirin to prevent myocardial infarction in men age <45 years
- Asymptomatic bacteriuria in men and nonpregnant women

- Bacterial vaginosis in asymptomatic pregnant women at low risk for preterm delivery
- *BRCA*-related cancers in women not at increased risk
- Cancers: cervix (if hysterectomy), ovary, pancreas, prostate, testicular
- Carotid artery stenosis
- Chronic obstructive pulmonary disease
- Electrocardiography (ECG)
- Genital herpes
- Gonorrhea in low-risk men and women
- Heart disease in low-risk patients using ECG, electron-beam computed tomography
- Hemochromatosis
- Hepatitis B

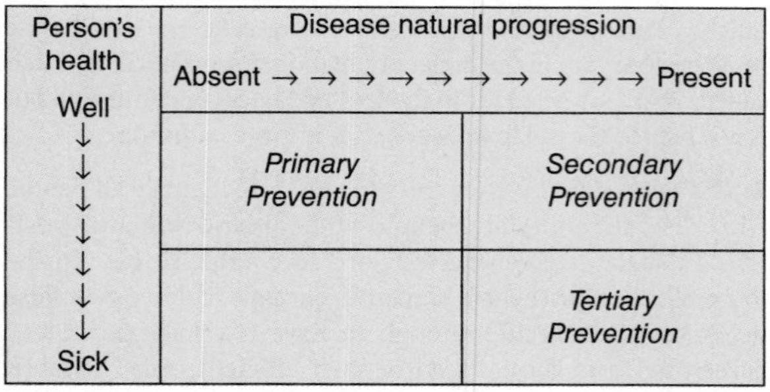

Person's health	Disease natural progression	
Well ↓ ↓ ↓ ↓ ↓ ↓ ↓ ↓ Sick	Absent → → → → → → → → → → Present	
	Primary Prevention	*Secondary Prevention*
		Tertiary Prevention

▲ **Figure 15–1.** The three types of disease prevention.

Table 15–2. Wilson-Jungner criteria for appraising the validity of a screening program.

1. The condition being screened for is an important health problem.
2. The natural history of the condition is well understood.
3. There is a detectable early stage.
4. The earlier the stage, the more beneficial is the treatment.
5. A suitable test is available for the early stage.
6. The test is acceptable.
7. Intervals for repeating the test are determined.
8. Adequate health service provision is made for the extra clinical workload resulting from screening.
9. The risks, both physical and psychological, are less than the benefits.
10. The costs are balanced against the benefits.

- Routine aspirin or nonsteroidal anti-inflammatory drugs for primary prevention of colorectal cancer for average risk
- Stress echocardiogram
- Syphilis
- Vitamin supplements with β-carotene to prevent cancer and cardiovascular disease (CVD)

B. Health Maintenance: Across the Ages— Insufficient Evidence

Conditions for which the USPSTF found *insufficient* evidence to promote routine screening in asymptomatic adults at low risk:

- Abuse of elderly and vulnerable adults
- Cancers: bladder, oral, skin
- *Chlamydia* in men
- Clinical breast examination beyond screening mammography in women age ≥40 years
- Dementia
- Diabetes mellitus if blood pressure <135/80 mmHg
- Drug abuse
- Family violence
- Gestational diabetes mellitus
- Glaucoma
- Peripheral artery disease with the ankle-brachial index
- Scoliosis
- Suicide risk
- Thyroid disease
- Vitamin supplementation with A, C, E, and multivitamins to prevent cancer and heart disease
- Vitamin D and calcium supplementation to prevent fractures: men, premenopausal women

C. Health Maintenance: Hypertension, Chlamydia, Lipid Disorders, Depression, and Tobacco

Table 15–3 summarizes USPSTF grade A and grade B screening and counseling recommendations for average-risk 18- to 39-year-olds. Addressing these areas of HM and prevention either continues into or starts with the onset of adulthood and continues on a disease-specific basis throughout adulthood. These issues are addressed across the continuum of life with further age-specific recommendations, which are discussed throughout this chapter.

1. Hypertension—Hypertension is the most common condition seen in family medicine. It contributes to many adverse health outcomes, including premature death, heart

attack, renal insufficiency, and stroke. Blood pressure measurement identifies individuals at increased risk and is considered elevated with a systolic blood pressure (SBP) >120 mmHg or a diastolic blood pressure (DBP) >80 mmHg on at least two occasions separated by at least 1 week. Treatment of hypertension decreases the incidence of CVD events. The Eighth Report of the Joint National Committee on Prevention, Detection, Evaluation, and Treatment of High Blood Pressure (JNC8) has established guidelines for the treatment of hypertension based on age and the presence of comorbid disease:

- 18–60 years of age: target SBP <140 mmHg and DBP <90 mmHg
- 60 years of age or older without heart disease: target SBP <150 mmHg and DBP <90 mmHg
- 18 years of age or older with diabetes mellitus or chronic kidney disease (defined as an estimated or measured glomerular filtration rate <60 mL/min/1.73 m² in individuals younger than 70 years): target SBP <140 mmHg and DBP <90 mmHg
- Of any age with albuminuria (>30 mg of albumin per gram of creatinine): target SBP <140 mmHg and DBP <90 mmHg

JNC8 also recommends screening every 2 years in persons with blood pressure <120/80 mmHg and every year in persons with SBP of 120–139 mmHg or DBP of 80–90 mm Hg. The USPSTF recommends confirming hypertension diagnosed in a clinical setting with measurements obtained elsewhere prior to initiating pharmacotherapy. Treatment is addressed in Chapter 35.

In 2017, the America College of Cardiology and American Heart Association offered new definitions for hypertension:

- Normal: <120/80 mmHg
- Elevated: SBP between 120 and 129 mmHg and DBP <80 mmHg
- Stage 1: SBP between 130 and 139 mmHg *or* DBP between 80 and 89 mmHg
- Stage 2: SBP at least 140 mmHg *or* DBP at least 90 mmHg
- Hypertensive crisis: SBP >180 mmHg and/or DBP >120 mmHg, with patients needing prompt changes in medication if there are no other indications of problems or immediate hospitalization if there are signs of organ damage

The American Academy of Family Physicians (AAFP) and the American College of Physicians have preferentially continued to endorse the JNC8 definitions.

2. Cervical cancer—Cervical cancer screening is discussed in detail in Chapter 27.

3. Chlamydia screening—The USPSTF recommends screening for *Chlamydia* infection in all sexually active

Table 15–3. Health promotion and preventive screening for adults age 18–39.

Grade	US Preventive Services Task Force Recommendations
A	Asymptomatic bacteriuria: screening—pregnant women
A	Cervical cancer: screening—women age 21–65 (Pap smear every 3 years) or 30–65 (in combination Pap smear cytology with human papillomavirus testing)
A	Folic acid: supplementation—women planning or capable of pregnancy
A	HIV: screening—adolescents and adults
A	HIV: screening—pregnant women
A	Hepatitis B virus: screening—pregnant women
A	High blood pressure: screening and home monitoring—adults
A	Rh(D) blood typing: screening—pregnant women, first pregnancy related visit
A	Syphilis: screening—pregnant women
A	Syphilis: screening—men and women at increased risk
A	Tobacco use: behavioral and pharmacotherapy interventions for adults who are not pregnant
A	Tobacco use: behavioral interventions for pregnant women
B	Alcohol misuse: screening and behavioral counseling interventions in primary care—adults, including pregnant women
B	Aspirin use for the prevention of morbidity and mortality from preeclampsia: preventive medication—pregnant women who are at high risk for preeclampsia
B	*BRCA*-related cancer: risk assessment, genetic counseling, and genetic testing—women at increased risk
B	Breastfeeding: primary care preventions—all pregnant women and new mothers
B	Chlamydia: screening—sexually active women
B	Depression: screening—adolescents age 12–18 years
B	Depression: screening—general adult population, including pregnant and postpartum women
B	Gestational diabetes mellitus: screening—pregnant women after 24 weeks of gestation
B	Gonorrhea: screening—sexually active women
B	Healthful diet and physical activity for cardiovascular disease (CVD) disease prevention: counseling—adults with CVD risk factors
B	Hepatitis B: screening—nonpregnant adolescents and adults at high risk
B	Hepatitis C virus infection: screening—adults age 18–79 years
B	Intimate partner violence: screening—women of childbearing age
B	Latent tuberculosis infection: screening—asymptomatic adults at increased risk for infection
B	Obesity: screening for and management of—all adults
B	Osteoporosis to prevent fractures: screening—postmenopausal women younger than 65 years at increased risk of osteoporosis
B	Perinatal depression: preventive interventions—pregnant and postpartum women
B	Preeclampsia: screening—pregnant women
B	Rh(D) blood typing: screening—antibody testing unsensitized Rh(D)-negative pregnant women
B	Sexually transmitted infections: behavioral counseling—sexually active adolescents and adults
B	Skin cancer prevention: behavioral counseling—young adults, adolescents, children, and parents of young children
B	Weight loss to prevent obesity-related morbidity and mortality: behavioral interventions—adults age 18 and older with a body mass index ≥ 30

women age 24 and younger, or women age 25 and older at increased risk. The optimal screening interval for nonpregnant women is unknown. The Centers for Disease Control and Prevention recommends at least annual screening for women at increased risk. *Chlamydia trachomatis* infection is the most common sexually transmitted bacterial infection in the United States. In women, genital infection may result in urethritis, cervicitis, pelvic inflammatory disease, infertility, ectopic pregnancy, and chronic pelvic pain. Infection during pregnancy is related to adverse pregnancy outcomes, including miscarriage, premature rupture of membranes, preterm labor, low birth weight, and infant mortality. The benefits of screening and subsequent treatment in high-risk pregnant and nonpregnant individuals are substantial.

The USPSTF concluded that the current evidence is insufficient to assess the benefits and harms of screening for chlamydia in men. The USPSTF also identified no evidence of the benefits of screening women age 25 or older who are *not* at increased risk for *Chlamydia* infection. In this low-risk population, the certainty is moderate that the benefits outweigh the harms of screening to only a small degree. Nucleic acid amplification tests for *Chlamydia* have high specificity and sensitivity as screening tests and may be used on specimens collected via urine or swabs (vaginal or cervical).

Screening of pregnant women for *Chlamydia* infection is recommended for all women at the first prenatal visit. For those who remain at increased risk or acquire a new risk factor (eg, a new sexual partner), screening should be repeated during the third trimester.

4. Lipid disorders—In 2016, the USPSTF concluded that current evidence is insufficient to assess the balance of benefits and harms of screening for lipid disorders in children and adolescents age 20 years old or younger. High levels of total cholesterol and low-density lipoprotein-cholesterol and low levels of high-density lipoprotein cholesterol are known independent risk factors for CVD. However, the risk is highest in those age 40–75 years with a combination of risk factors. Therefore, the use of statin pharmacotherapy for the primary prevention of CVD in adults must be based on a careful review of the complete risk factor profile. Dyslipidemia and the use of statin pharmacotherapy for CVD risk reduction are discussed in Chapter 22.

5. Depression screening—Depression is common and a leading cause of disability in both adolescents and adults. Screening for depression improves the accurate identification of depressed patients in primary care settings. The USPSTF recommends screening for depression in the general adult population, including pregnant and postpartum women. Screening should be implemented with adequate systems in place to ensure accurate diagnosis, effective treatment, and appropriate follow-up. There are several formal screening tools available but insufficient evidence to recommend one tool over another. All positive screens should trigger a full diagnostic interview. Depression screening is discussed in Chapter 56.

6. Tobacco use counseling—Cessation of tobacco use may be the single most important lifestyle intervention for the maintenance and improvement of health. All adults should be asked about tobacco use. Those who use tobacco products should be advised to stop and provided with US Food and Drug Administration (FDA)-approved tobacco cessation interventions. Tobacco use, including cigarette smoking, is the leading cause of preventable death in the United States, resulting in >400,000 deaths annually from CVD, respiratory disease, and cancer. Smoking during pregnancy results in the deaths of approximately 1000 infants annually and is associated with an increased risk for premature birth and intrauterine growth retardation. Environmental tobacco smoke may contribute to death in up to 38,000 people annually.

Electronic nicotine delivery systems (ENDS), also called electronic cigarettes, e-cigarettes, vaping devices, or vape pens, are battery-powered devices used to smoke or "vape" a flavored solution. The popularity of ENDS is rising rapidly, with the rate of adults trying an e-cigarette more than doubling between 2010 and 2013. More youth currently use e-cigarettes than combustible cigarettes. Most adult ENDS users also smoke conventional cigarettes. Following the 2016 "Deeming Rule," the FDA expanded regulatory authority to the ENDS industry.

Cessation of tobacco use is associated with a corresponding reduction in the risk of heart disease, stroke, and lung disease. Tobacco cessation at any point during pregnancy yields substantial health benefits for the expectant mother and baby.

Smoking cessation interventions, including brief (<10 minutes) behavioral counseling sessions and pharmacotherapy delivered in primary care settings, are effective in increasing the proportion of smokers who successfully quit and remain abstinent for 1 year. Even minimal counseling interventions (<3 minutes) are associated with improved quit rates. One of several screening strategies aimed at engaging patients in smoking cessation discussions is the "5A" behavioral counseling framework:

1. **A**sk about tobacco use.
2. **A**dvise to quit through clear personalized messages.
3. **A**ssess willingness to quit.
4. **A**ssist to quit.
5. **A**rrange follow-up and support.

The USPSTF concludes that the current evidence is insufficient to recommend ENDS for tobacco cessation in adults, including pregnant women. Behavioral therapy and pharmacotherapy interventions with established effectiveness and safety are provided in Chapter 61.

D. Health Maintenance: Age 18–39 Years

Table 15–3 summarizes USPSTF Grade A and Grade B screening and counseling recommendations for average-risk 18- to 39-year-olds. High-risk screenings are addressed below. Screening and counseling specifically for those age 18–39 years at *increased* risk are as follows (USPSTF grade in parentheses):

- Human immunodeficiency virus (HIV): Adolescents and adults age 15–65 years, younger adolescents, and older adults who are at increased risk should also be screened (A). Everyone in this age range should be screened once due to the prevalence of undiagnosed HIV in the population. Subsequent screening is based on high-risk behavior: men who have sex with men, intravenous drug users, those who have multiple sex partners without use of barrier protection, those diagnosed with sexually transmitted infections, and those who exchange sex for money or goods.
- Syphilis: Those who engage in high-risk sexual behaviors (A).
- *BRCA* mutation testing for breast and ovarian cancer should be offered to women with an increased risk of a harmful mutation in one of the genes (B). Risk factors include:
  - Breast cancer diagnosed before age 50 years
  - Cancer in both breasts
  - Both breast and ovarian cancers in either the woman or her family
  - Multiple breast cancers in the patient's family
  - Two or more primary types of *BRCA1-* or *BRCA2-* related cancers in any single family member
  - History of male breast cancer in the patient's family
  - Ashkenazi Jewish ethnicity
- Gonorrhea: Women who are pregnant or at increased risk (B).
- Healthy diet: Adults who are overweight or obese and have additional risk factors for CVD (B).
- Intimate partner violence: Women of childbearing age (B).
- Sexually transmitted infections: Behavioral counseling for sexually active adolescents and adults at increased risk (B).
- Skin cancer: Behavioral counseling for children, adolescents, and young adults regarding minimizing exposure to ultraviolet radiation from ages 6 months to 24 years (B).

E. Health Maintenance: Ages 40–49 with Emphasis on Breast Cancer and Lipid Screening

Tables 15–4, 15–5, and 15–6 summarize USPSTF recommendations for average-risk 40- to 49-year-olds.

1. Breast cancer—Please see Tables 15–5 and 15–6 and Chapter 27 for discussion of screening for breast cancer.

2. Lipid screening—All women age ≥45 years should be screened for lipid disorders. Women age 20–44 years should be screened if they are at increased risk for coronary heart disease (CHD). *Increased risk*, for this recommendation, is defined by the presence of any of the following risk factors: diabetes, previous personal history of CHD or noncoronary atherosclerosis (eg, abdominal aorta aneurysm, peripheral artery disease, carotid artery stenosis), a family history of CVD before age 50 years in male relatives or age 60 years in female relatives, tobacco use, hypertension, or obesity (body mass index >30). (Further discussion of dyslipidemia is found in the earlier section on HM for ages 18–39 years and in Chapter 22.)

3. Diabetes mellitus (type 2)—Patients between age 40 and 70 years who are overweight or obese should be screened.

F. Health Maintenance: Ages 50–59

Table 15–7 summarizes USPSTF recommendations for average-risk 50- to 59-year-olds, including changes in recommendations for prostate and diabetes screening and statin therapy.

1. Colorectal cancer screening—This should occur from age 50 to 75 years using a variety of tests, as follows:

> *Sensitivity*—Hemoccult II < fecal immunochemical tests < Hemoccult SENSA ≈ flexible sigmoidoscopy < colonoscopy

> *Specificity*—Hemoccult SENSA < fecal immunochemical tests ≈ Hemoccult II < flexible sigmoidoscopy = colonoscopy

Screening with fecal occult blood testing, sigmoidoscopy, or colonoscopy reduces mortality, assuming 100% adherence to any of the following regimens: (1) annual high-sensitivity fecal occult blood testing, (2) sigmoidoscopy every 5 years combined with high-sensitivity fecal occult blood testing every 3 years, or (3) screening colonoscopy at intervals of 10 years. Evidence is insufficient regarding screening with fecal DNA or computed tomography (CT) colonography.

2. Hypertension—Screen every 2 years if blood pressure is <120/80 mmHg and every year with SBP of 120–139 mmHg or DBP of 80–90 mmHg.

3. Prostate cancer screening in men age 55–69 years and age 70 years and older—As discussed earlier, an effective screening test should detect disease early, and early treatment should improve morbidity and mortality. There is inconclusive and varying evidence that treatment of prostate cancers detected by screening improves outcomes. Recognition that most men *with prostate cancer* do not die from it and of the limitations of currently available prostate

Table 15–4. Health promotion and preventive screening for adults age 40–49.

Intervention	Target Group[a] and Screening Interval[b]	Grade	Recommendation
Physical exam blood pressure (BP)	Every 1–2 years depending on BP	A	Screen every 2 years in persons with BP <120/80 mmHg and every year in persons with BP 120–130/80–90 mmHg
Testing Lipid disorders	Men >35, every 5 years Women >45 if risk for CHD, every 5 years	A	For women, the risk factors include diabetes, previous personal history of CHD or noncoronary atherosclerosis, a family history of cardiovascular disease before 50 in males and 60 in females, tobacco, hypertension, obesity (BMI >30)
Cervical cancer screening	Every 3–5 years	A	Screen for cervical cancer in women who have been sexually active and have a cervix. Pap smear every 3 years or Pap smear + HPV testing every 5 years
HIV	If high risk	A	Risks include men having sex with men; unprotected sex with multiple partners; injection drug use; sex worker; history of sex with partners who are HIV positive, bisexual, or injection drug users; history of STI; transfusion between 1978 and 1985
Syphilis	If high risk	A	Risks include men who have sex with men and engage in high-risk sexual behavior, commercial sex workers, persons who exchange sex for drugs, and those in adult correctional facilities
Chlamydia	If high risk	A	Risks factors include a history of *Chlamydia* or other STI, new or multiple sexual partners, inconsistent condom use, and exchanging sex for money or drugs
Counsel Tobacco use		A	Ask all adults about tobacco use and provide tobacco cessation interventions for those who use tobacco products
Testing Mammogram	Against routine screening in normal-risk women age 40–49 years	C	Offer mammography to an individual patient if she is at higher risk of breast cancer (http://www.cancer.gov/bcrisktool/), then screen biennially
Diabetes mellitus type 2	All with sustained BP >135/80 mmHg	B	Screen asymptomatic adults with sustained BP >135/80 mmHg
Counsel Obesity: BMI >30		B	Clinicians screen all adult patients for obesity and offer intensive counseling and behavioral interventions to promote sustained weight loss for obese adults
Alcohol misuse		B	Screen for risky or hazardous drinking and provide behavioral counseling interventions to reduce alcohol misuse by adults
Depression	If there are systems in place to ensure accurate diagnosis, effective treatment, and follow-up	B	Screening adults for depression in clinical practices that have systems in place to assure accurate diagnosis, effective treatment, and follow-up
Statin use for the primary prevention of CVD	Adults age 40–75 years	B	Prescribe if no history of CVD, one or more CVD risk factors, and a calculated 10-year CVD event risk of 10% or greater
STI	If high risk	B	Screen adults with STI in past year or multiple current sexual partners

[a]Target group: if none noted, includes men and women age 40–49 years.
[b]Screening interval: if none noted, unknown.
BMI, body mass index; CHD, coronary heart disease; CVD, cardiovascular disease; HIV, human immunodeficiency virus; HPV, human papillomavirus; STI, sexually transmitted infection.
Data from US Preventive Services Task Force. Rockville, MD. Recommendations for primary care practice.

Table 15–5. Insufficient evidence for clinical breast examinations (CBEs) and breast self-examinations.

Intervention	Target Group	Grade	Recommendation
Clinical breast exam	Women	I	Could not determine benefits of CBE alone or the incremental benefit of adding CBE to mammography
Breast self-exam	Women	D	Against teaching breast self-examination

Data from US Preventive Services Task Force. Rockville, MD. Breast cancer: screening.

screening tests has led to fluidity regarding the best prostate screening practices. As new data become available, the guidelines from major organizations become more similar with some nuances.

In May 2018, the USPSTF published final recommendations on prostate-specific antigen (PSA)-based screening for prostate cancer. For men age 55–69 years, the decision to undergo periodic PSA-based screening for prostate cancer should be an individual one. Before deciding whether to be screened, men should have an opportunity to discuss the potential benefits and harms of screening with their clinician and to incorporate their values and preferences in the decision (C recommendation). The USPSTF recommends against PSA-based screening for prostate cancer in men age 70 years and older (D recommendation).

The American Cancer Society (ACS) recommendations, published in 2010, recommend that asymptomatic men who have at least a 10-year life expectancy have an opportunity to make an informed decision with their healthcare provider about screening for prostate cancer after they receive information about the uncertainties, risks, and potential benefits associated with prostate cancer screening.

Table 15–6. US Preventive Services Task Force (2016) breast cancer screening recommendations in women using film mammography.

Population	Ages 40–49 Years	Ages 50–74 Years	Ages ≥75 Years
Recommendation	Do not screen routinely. Individualize decision to begin biennial screening according to the patient's context, risk, and values. (Grade: C)	Screen every 2 years (Grade: B)	No recommendation Grade: I (insufficient evidence)
Risk assessment	Recommendation applies to women age ≥40 years not at increased risk because of known preexisting breast cancer or a previously diagnosed high-risk breast lesion, genetic mutation (eg, *BRCA1*, *BRCA2*, other familial breast cancer syndrome), or history of chest radiation. Increasing age is the most important risk factor for most women.		
Screening tests	Standardization of film mammography has led to improved quality. Refer patients to facilities certified under the Mammography Quality Standards Act (MQSA). (Grade: B) Digital breast tomosynthesis (DBT) (Grade: I) Dense breasts: ultrasound, magnetic resonance imaging, DBT, or other methods instead of otherwise negative screening mammogram (Grade: I)		
Timing of screening	Evidence indicates that biennial screening is optimal. This preserves most of the benefit of annual screening and cuts the risk nearly in half. A longer interval may reduce the benefit.		
Benefit/risk balance	There is convincing evidence that screening with film mammography reduces breast cancer mortality, with a greater absolute reduction for women age 50–74 years than for younger women. Harms (risks) of screening include psychological risks, additional medical visits, imaging, and biopsies in women without cancer; inconvenience due to false-positive screening results; and risks of unnecessary treatment, and radiation exposure. Risks seem moderate for each age group. False-positive results are a greater concern for younger women; treatment of cancer that would not become clinically apparent during a woman's life (overdiagnosis) is an increasing problem as women age.		

Data from US Preventive Services Task Force. Rockville, MD. Breast cancer: screening.

Table 15–7. Health promotion and preventive screening for adults age 50–59.

USPSTF Grade	Recommended Health Promotion or Screening
A[a]	Cervical cancer: Screen sexually active women age ≥21 years until age 65 years
A	Colorectal cancer: Screen adults age 50–75 years
A	HIV: Screen adults and adolescents age 15-65 years once, more frequently for those with high-risk behaviors
A	High blood pressure: Screen and home monitor
A	Lipid disorders in adults: Screen men age ≥35 years
A	Lipid disorders in adults: Screen women ≥45 years, increased risk for CHD
A	Syphilis: Screen men and women at increased risk
A[a]	Tobacco smoking cessation: Behavioral and pharmacotherapy interventions—adults who are not pregnant
B	Aspirin use to prevent CVD and CRC: Preventive medication—adults age 50–59 years with a ≥10% 10-year CVD risk
B	Alcohol unhealthy use: Screen and behavioral counseling
B	*BRCA* mutation testing for breast and ovarian cancer: Women, increased risk
B	Breast cancer: Preventive medication discussion—women, increased risk
B[a]	Breast cancer: Screening with mammography for women age 50–74 years
B[a]	Chlamydia: Screening—sexually active women at increased risk
B[a]	Depression: Screen adults age ≥18 years, including pregnant and postpartum women, when staff-assisted depression care supports *are* in place
B	Diabetes mellitus (type 2) and abnormal blood glucose: Screening – Adults age 40–70 years who are overweight or obese – Adults with sustained blood pressure ≥135/80 mmHg
B	Gonorrhea: Sexually active women
B	Healthy diet and physical activity for CVD disease prevention: Counseling—adults with CVD risk factors (hypertension, dyslipidemia, impaired fasting glucose, or the metabolic syndrome.)
B	Hepatitis C virus infection: Screening—adults age 18–79 years
B	Latent tuberculosis infection: Screening—asymptomatic adults at increased risk for infection
B	Lung cancer: Annual screening for lung cancer with low-dose computed tomography in adults age 55–80 years who have a 30-pack-year smoking history and currently smoke or have quit within the past 15 years; screening should be discontinued once a person has not smoked for 15 years or develops a health problem that substantially limits life expectancy or the ability or willingness to undergo curative lung surgery
B	Obesity: Screening and intensive counseling for obese men and women
B	Osteoporosis to prevent fractures: Screening – Postmenopausal women younger than 65 years old at increased risk of osteoporosis – Women age 65 years and older
B	Sexually transmitted infections: Behavioral counseling—sexually active adults at increased risk
B	Statin use for the primary prevention of CVD: Preventive medicine—adults age 40–75 years with no history of CVD, one or more CVD risk factors, and a calculated 10-year CVD event risk of 10% or greater
B	Weight loss to prevent obesity-related morbidity and mortality: Behavioral interventions—if BMI ≥30
C[a]	Prostate cancer screening: Men age 55–69 years

BMI, body mass index; CHD, congestive heart disease; CRC, colorectal cancer; CVD, cardiovascular disease; USPSTF, US Preventive Services Task Force.
[a]See earlier discussions and tables.

The American Urological Association guidelines, published in 2013 and reviewed and confirmed in 2018, are as follows:

- The panel recommends against PSA screening in men under age 40 years (Evidence Strength Grade C).

- The panel does not recommend routine screening in men between age 40 and 54 years at average risk (Evidence Strength Grade C).

- For men age 55–69 years, the panel recognizes that the decision to undergo PSA screening involves weighing the benefits of reducing the rate of metastatic prostate cancer and prevention of prostate cancer death against the known potential harms associated with screening and treatment. The panel strongly recommends shared decision making for men age 55–69 years who are considering PSA screening and proceeding based on a man's values and preferences (Evidence Strength Grade B).

- The panel does not recommend routine PSA screening in men age 70+ years or any man with less than a 10- to 15-year life expectancy (Evidence Strength Grade C).

Prostate cancer is the most common nonskin cancer in US males. Of those who live to be 90 years old, one of six US males will be diagnosed with prostate cancer within their lifetime. Risk factors for development of prostate cancer include advanced age, family history, and race. Nearly 70% of prostate cancer diagnoses occur in men age 65 and older. The risk of developing prostate cancer is nearly 2.5 times greater in men with a family history of prostate cancer in a first-degree relative. Rates of prostate cancer occurrence are lower in Asian and Hispanic males than in white males. African American men are at twice the risk of white men. Although US men have an approximately 16% lifetime risk of being diagnosed with prostate cancer, they have only about a 3% risk of dying from it.

Digital rectal examination (DRE) and PSA testing are the most commonly used prostate cancer screening tools. DRE is limited in that it allows only a portion of the prostate gland to be palpated and has poor interrater reliability Sensitivity of DRE is low, estimated between 53% and 59%, and has a positive predictive value (PPV) of only 18–28%. The PPV of PSA for prostate cancer screening is also low, at about 30%. Other proposed prostate cancer screening methods include using a PSA cutoff of 4 ng/mL, measuring PSA velocity, and measuring percent free PSA. No currently available data demonstrate a mortality benefit with any of these methods.

Both DRE and PSA screening can lead to detection of clinically insignificant prostate cancers, exposing patients to undue psychological distress and potentially harmful procedures and treatments including biopsy and radical prostatectomy. DRE and PSA screening can also miss aggressive prostate cancers.

4. Lung cancer screening—The USPSTF assigns a B recommendation to annual screening for lung cancer with low-dose CT in adults age 55–80 years who have a 30-pack-year smoking history and currently smoke or have quit within the past 15 years. Screening should be discontinued once a person has not smoked for 15 years or develops a health problem that substantially limits life expectancy or the ability or willingness to undergo curative lung surgery. This has been a controversial recommendation because of concerns about radiation exposure (high false-positive findings on initial screen leading to more CT scanning; the 25-year recommendation is based on studies of 3 years of screening), cost-benefit concerns, and the unsure role of screening in people who continue to smoke (eg, whether a negative screen will impede the desire to quit, whether a false-positive screen will result in increased quit rates). The AAFP has not endorsed this recommendation. Like all USPSTF recommendations, it will be reevaluated as new data emerge.

G. Health Maintenance: Ages 60–74

Table 15–8 summarizes USPSTF recommendations for average-risk 60- to 74-year-olds by sex. (See earlier discussions in this chapter on prostate, breast, and lung cancers and lipids.)

Table 15–8. Health promotion and preventive screening USPSTF recommendations for adults age 60–74.

Blood pressure: Screen annually (A)
Colorectal cancer: Screening[a] (A)
Pap smear: Women every 3–5 years until age 65 (A); after age 65 (D)
Tobacco: Counsel about quitting (A)
Alcohol: Counsel to reduce alcohol misuse (B)
Abdominal aortic aneurysm: Ultrasound once in men age 65–75 who have ever smoked (B)
Aspirin use for prevention: See prior tables and discussion (B)
Cholesterol: Screen every 5 years until age 75 (B)
Depression: Screening—general adult population, including pregnant and postpartum women (B)
Diabetes mellitus (type 2) and abnormal blood glucose: Screening—adults age 40–70 years who are overweight or obese (B)
Falls prevention in community-dwelling older adults: Exercise—adults age 65 or older (B)
Hepatitis C virus infection: Screening—adults age 18–79 years (B)
Lung cancer: Screening—adults age 55–80 years with a 30-pack-year smoking history and who currently smoke or have quit within the past 15 years (B)
Mammogram: Women every 1–2 years (B)
Osteoporosis screening: All women age ≥65 years and high-risk women starting at age 60: screen using DEXA or bone densitometry testing (B)
Statin use for the primary prevention of CVD: Preventive medicine—adults age 40–75 years with no history of CVD, one or more CVD risk factors, and a calculated 10-year CVD event risk of 10% or greater (B)
Weight and BMI: Screen for obesity using BMI (B)

BMI, body mass index; CVD, cardiovascular disease; DEXA, dual-energy x-ray absorptiometry; USPSTF = United States Preventive Services Task Force.

1. Screening for abdominal aortic aneurysm (AAA), men only

- One-time screening for AAA by ultrasonography in men age 65–75 who have ever smoked (B).
- No recommendation for or against screening for AAA in men age 65–75 years who have never smoked (C).
- Against routine screening for AAA in women (D), due to false-positive rate and lower prevalence of AAA.

2. Screening for osteoporosis in postmenopausal women

- All women age ≥65 years should be screened routinely for osteoporosis (B).
- Women at increased risk[1] for osteoporotic fractures should begin screening at age 60 years (B).
- No recommendation for or against routine osteoporosis screening in postmenopausal women age <60 years or in women age 60–64 years who are not at increased risk for osteoporotic fractures (C).

Screening should occur every 3 years even if treatment is initiated.

3. Osteoporosis risk assessment tools

- Foundation on Osteoporosis Research and Education 10-year risk calculator at https://riskcalculator.fore.org/default.aspx
- FRAX World Health Organization Fracture Risk Assessment Tool at http://www.shef.ac.uk/FRAX/tool.jsp?country=9
- The Osteoporosis Risk Assessment Instrument uses age, weight, and the use of estrogen as an aid to selecting postmenopausal patients for bone density testing (Cadarette and colleagues, 2000).

Cadarette SM, Jaglal SB, Kreiger N, McIsaac WJ, Darlington GA, Tu JV. Development and validation of the Osteoporosis Risk Assessment Instrument to facilitate selection of women for bone densitometry. *Can Med Assoc J.* 2000;162(9):1289–1294. [PMID: 10813010]

H. Health Maintenance: Age ≥75

Perhaps the most important aspect of HM in people age ≥75 years is lifestyle. HM recommendations for this age group are summarized in Table 15–9 and discussed here.

In patients age ≥75 years, HM decisions become more complex. The focus remains both primary and secondary prevention; however, there are relatively few studies evaluating the utility and impact of HM interventions in this population. Therefore, it becomes increasingly important to work with geriatric patients to make informed, individualized HM decisions. Among patients age ≥75 years, there exist wide variations in the number and severity of comorbid conditions, functional status, life expectancy, and patients' overall goals of care and preferences. Each of these factors must be considered when discussing HM interventions in older patients. Consideration of both benefits and risks of any HM intervention is also essential.

Guidelines regarding cancer screening in patients age ≥75 years especially require individualized, patient-specific discussions and decisions. The USPSTF suggests that the benefits of colon cancer screening in adults age 75–85 years do not outweigh the risks and explicitly recommends against it in patients age >85 years. The American College for Gastroenterology recommends colon cancer screening beginning at age 50 and does not suggest when to discontinue screening.

For breast cancer screening, the USPSTF recommends neither for nor against mammography in women age ≥75 years. The American Geriatric Society recommends screening mammography every 3 years after age 75 with no upper age limit for women with an estimated life expectancy of ≥4 years. The ACS and USPSTF agree that older women with previously negative Pap results do not benefit from ongoing screening for cervical cancer after the age of 75.

Prostate cancer screening remains a controversial topic, with USPSTF advising against the use of PSA for prostate cancer. A detailed discussion of prostate cancer and prostate cancer screening is provided earlier in this chapter.

The American Geriatric Society recommends screening all older adults for a history of falls within the past year, and the USPSTF recommends the use of exercise, physical therapy, and vitamin D supplementation in community-dwelling older adults at increased risk for falls. The USPSTF recommends neither for nor against screening for vision impairment, hearing impairment, or dementia in asymptomatic patients age ≥75 years.

I. Health Maintenance: Adult Immunizations

Tables 15–10 and 15–11 summarize the vaccination recommendations for adults.

American Cancer Society. Cancer facts and figures 2014. http://www.cancer.org/research/cancerfactsstatistics/cancerfactsfigures2014/index. Accessed November 11, 2019.

American Cancer Society. Prostate cancer screening guidelines. https://www.cancer.org/health-care-professionals/american-cancer-society-prevention-early-detection-guidelines/prostate-cancer-screening-guidelines.html. Accessed November 11, 2019.

---

[1]Risk factors: Low body weight (<70 kg) is the single best predictor of low bone mineral density. The next best is no current use of estrogen therapy. Others supported by less evidence include smoking, weight loss, family history, decreased physical activity, alcohol or caffeine use, or low calcium and vitamin D intake.

Table 15–9. Health promotion and preventive screening for adults age ≥75 years.

Condition for Screening	USPSTF Recommendations (Grade)	Alternate Recommendations from Other Organizations
Tobacco abuse	Recommended (A)	
Alcohol unhealthy use	Recommended (A)	
Hypertension	Recommended (A)	
Hyperlipidemia	Recommended (A)	
Aspirin for prevention of cardiovascular disease[a]	Recommended (A), in men age ≤79 years	
Aspirin for prevention of ischemic stroke[a]	Recommended (A), in women age ≤79 years	
Depression	Recommended (B), if supportive care available	
Diabetes	Recommended (B), for blood pressure ≥135/80 mmHg	
Falls	Recommended (B); use of exercise, physical therapy, vitamin D supplementation if high risk, community-dwelling	AGS: All older adults should be screened for falls within the past year
Hepatitis C	Recommended (B); screen people age 18–79 years	
Nutrition screening and counseling	Recommended (B), for patients with risk factors for cardiovascular disease	
Obesity	Recommended (B)	
Colon cancer	Not recommended routinely (C); consider in select patients age 75–85 years; recommendation against (D) in patients age >85 years	ACG: Indefinite screening after age 50
Prostate cancer	Recommendation against (D); PSA	AUA[a], ACS: DRE and PSA annually for men aged ≥50 years with life expectancy ≥10 years
Breast cancer	Neither for nor against (I)	AGS: Mammogram every 3 years for adults age ≥75 years if life expectancy ≥4 years[a]
Cervical cancer	Recommendation against (I)	
Cognitive impairment	Neither for nor against (I)	
Vision impairment	Neither for nor against (I)	

ACG, American College for Gastroenterology; ACS, American Cancer Society; AGS, American Geriatrics Society; AUA, American Urologic Association; DRE, digital rectal examination; PSA, prostate-specific antigen; USPSTF, US Preventive Services Task Force.
[a]See earlier discussions and tables.

American College of Cardiology Foundation/American Heart Association Task Force on Practice Guidelines. 2009 focused update incorporated into the ACC/AHA 2005 Guidelines for the Diagnosis and Management of Heart Failure in Adults. *Circulation.* 2009;119:e391–e497. [PMID: 19324966]

American Urological Association. Early detection of prostate cancer. https://www.auanet.org/guidelines/prostate-cancer-early-detection-guideline. Accessed November 11, 2019.

Centre for Metabolic Bone Diseases, University of Sheffield. FRAX. Fracture Risk Assessment Tool. https://www.sheffield.ac.uk/FRAX/. Accessed November 11, 2019.

James PA, Oparil S, Carter BL, et al. 2014 evidence-based guideline for the management of high blood pressure in adults. Report from the panel members appointed to the eighth joint national committee (JNC 8). *JAMA.* 2014;311(5):507–520. [PMID: 24352797]

Table 15–10. Recommended adult immunization by age group, Centers for Disease Control and Prevention, United States, 2019.

Vaccine	19–21 years	22–26 years	27–49 years	50–64 years	≥65 years
Influenza inactivated (IIV) or Influenza recombinant (RIV) **or** Influenza live attenuated (LAIV)	1 dose annually				
	1 dose annually				
Tetanus, diphtheria, pertussis (Tdap or Td)	1 dose Tdap, then Td booster every 10 yrs				
Measles, mumps, rubella (MMR)	1 or 2 doses depending on indication (if born in 1957 or later)				
Varicella (VAR)	2 doses (if born in 1980 or later)				
Zoster recombinant (RZV) *preferred* **or**				2 doses	
Zoster live (ZVL)				1 dose	
Human papillomavirus (HPV) Female	2 or 3 doses depending on age at initial vaccination				
Human papillomavirus (HPV) Male	2 or 3 doses depending on age at initial vaccination				
Pneumococcal conjugate (PCV13)				1 dose	
Pneumococcal polysaccharide (PPSV23)			1 or 2 doses depending on indication		1 dose
Hepatitis A (HepA)	2 or 3 doses depending on vaccine				
Hepatitis B (HepB)	2 or 3 doses depending on vaccine				
Meningococcal A, C, W, Y (MenACWY)	1 or 2 doses depending on indication, then booster every 5 yrs if risk remains				
Meningococcal B (MenB)	2 or 3 doses depending on vaccine and indication				
Haemophilus influenzae type b (Hib)	1 or 3 doses depending on indication				

Recommended vaccination for adults who meet age requirement, lack documentation of vaccination, or lack evidence of past infection

Recommended vaccination for adults with an additional risk factor or another indication

No recommendation

Table 15–11. Recommended adult immunization by medical condition and other indications, Centers for Disease Control and Prevention, United States, 2019.

Vaccine	Pregnancy	Immuno-compromised (excluding HIV infection)	HIV infection CD4 count <200	HIV infection CD4 count ≥200	Asplenia, complement deficiencies	End-stage renal disease, on hemodialysis	Heart or lung disease, alcoholism[1]	Chronic liver disease	Diabetes	Health care personnel[2]	Men who have sex with men
IIV or RIV	1 dose annually → (all columns)										
LAIV	CONTRAINDICATED	CONTRAINDICATED	CONTRAINDICATED	CONTRAINDICATED	PRECAUTION →					1 dose annually	1 dose annually
Tdap or Td	1 dose Tdap each pregnancy	1 dose Tdap, then Td booster every 10 yrs → (remaining columns)									
MMR	CONTRAINDICATED	CONTRAINDICATED	CONTRAINDICATED	1 or 2 doses depending on indication → (remaining columns)							
VAR	CONTRAINDICATED	CONTRAINDICATED	CONTRAINDICATED	2 doses → (remaining columns)							
RZV (preferred)	DELAY	2 doses at age ≥50 yrs → (remaining columns)									
or ZVL	CONTRAINDICATED	CONTRAINDICATED	CONTRAINDICATED	CONTRAINDICATED	1 dose at age ≥60 yrs → (remaining columns)						
HPV Female	DELAY	3 doses through age 26 yrs →									2 or 3 doses through age 26 yrs
HPV Male		3 doses through age 26 yrs →			2 or 3 doses through age 21 yrs →						2 or 3 doses through age 26 yrs
PCV13	1 dose → (applicable columns)										
PPSV23	1, 2, or 3 doses depending on age and indication → (applicable columns)										
MenACWY	1 or 2 doses depending on indication, then booster every 5 yrs if risk remains → (applicable columns)										
MenB	PRECAUTION	2 or 3 doses depending on vaccine and indication → (applicable columns)									
Hib		3 doses HSCT[3] recipients only			1 dose						

Legend:
- Recommended vaccination for adults who meet age requirement, lack documentation of vaccination, or lack evidence of past infection
- Recommended vaccination for adults with an additional risk factor or another indication
- Precaution—vaccine might be indicated if benefit of protection outweighs risk of adverse reaction
- Delay vaccination until after pregnancy if vaccine is indicated
- Contraindicated—vaccine should not be administered because of risk for serious adverse reaction
- No recommendation

1. Precaution for LAIV does not apply to alcoholism. 2. See notes for influenza; hepatitis B; measles, mumps, and rubella; and varicella vaccinations. 3. Hematopoietic stem cell transplant.

Note: See Table 15–10 for abbreviations.

National Cancer Institute. Who should consider genetic testing for *BRCA1* and *BRCA2* mutations? https://www.cancer.gov/about-cancer/causes-prevention/genetics/brca-fact-sheet#who-should-consider-genetic-testing-for-brca1-and-brca2-mutations. Accessed November 11, 2019.

National Cancer Institute Surveillance, Epidemiology, and End Results Program. Cancer Stat Fact Sheets—Cancer of the Prostate, 2006. http://seer.cancer.gov/statfacts/html/prost.html. Accessed March 20, 2019.

US Preventive Services Task Force. Final recommendation statement: prostate cancer: screening. May 2018. https://www.uspreventiveservicestaskforce.org/Page/Document/RecommendationStatementFinal/prostate-cancer-screening1. Accessed November 11, 2019.

US Preventive Services Task Force. Guide to clinical preventive services, recommendations for adults. https://www.uspreventiveservicestaskforce.org/. Accessed March 20, 2019.

Walter L, Covinsky K. Cancer screening in elderly patients: a framework for individualized decision making. *JAMA*. 2001; 285(21):2750–2756. [PMID: 11386931]

Websites

Agency for Healthcare Research and Quality, Clinical Guidelines and Recommendations. http://www.ahrq.gov/CLINIC/uspstf/uspsprca.htm

American Cancer Society, American Cancer Society Guidelines for the Early Detection of Cancer. http://www.cancer.org/healthy/findcancerearly/cancerscreeningguidelines/american-cancer-society-guidelines-for-the-early-detection-of-cancer

American Society for Colposcopy and Cervical Pathology. http://www.asccp.org/default.aspx

Centers for Disease Control and Prevention, Recommended Adult Immunization Schedule by Medical Condition and Other Indications, United States, 2019. https://www.cdc.gov/vaccines/schedules/hcp/imz/adult-conditions.html

Electronic Nicotine Delivery Systems (ENDS). https://www.aafp.org/dam/AAFP/documents/patient_care/tobacco/ends-fact-sheet.pdf

Electronic Preventive Services Calculator. https://epss.ahrq.gov/PDA/index.jsp

FORE 10-Year Fracture Risk Calculator version 2.0. http://riskcalculator.fore.org/default.aspx

FRAX World Health Organization Fracture Risk Assessment Tool. https://www.sheffield.ac.uk/FRAX/

National Cancer Institute, Who should consider genetic testing for BRCA1 and BRCA2 mutations? https://www.cancer.gov/about-cancer/causes-prevention/genetics/brca-fact-sheet#who-should-consider-genetic-testing-for-brca1-and-brca2-mutations

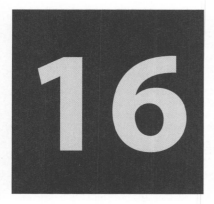

Preconception Care

Karen Moyer, MD

In 2017, the number of births in the United States was 3,853,472, 2% less than in 2016 and the lowest in 30 years. Although most infants are born healthy, it is of critical importance that the infant mortality rate in the United States ranks 26th among developed nations and is the only developed country where maternal morbidity and mortality are rising, despite advances in perinatal care.

Many factors contribute to the current maternal and infant morbidity and mortality rate in the United States. Birth rates are declining for women under 40, but rising for women over 40. Older age at conception brings with it a higher likelihood of other concomitant chronic medical conditions, pregnancy-related conditions like preeclampsia, increased risk for genetic disorders, and increased risk of preterm birth. Racial and socioeconomic disparities in access to care, rising rates of substance abuse and obesity, and increasing rates of mental health conditions have also been implicated.

In 2016, the Clinical Workgroup of the National Preconception Health and Health Care Initiative proposed nine core measures to be assessed at initiation of prenatal care that would serve as a measure of a woman's preconception wellness: (1) pregnancy intention, (2) access to care, (3) multivitamin with folic acid use, (4) tobacco avoidance, (5) absence of uncontrolled depression, (6) healthy weight, (7) absence of sexually transmitted infections, (8) optimal glycemic control, and (9) teratogen avoidance in chronic conditions. These recommendations are based on the idea that healthier women have healthier pregnancy outcomes.

Given that over 50% of pregnancies in the United States are unintended, to improve outcomes for women and infants, we must transform the way we provide preconception care. Instead of separating preconception care into its own silo and only addressing these issues at a preconception or first prenatal visit, we must challenge ourselves to provide preconception care at every visit for women of childbearing age. We must integrate assessment of folic acid intake, social

risk factors and mental health, review of medication lists, management of chronic medical conditions, and counseling on family planning routinely into ongoing primary care. This could be during a visit for routine health maintenance, an examination for school or work, at premarital or family planning visits, after a negative pregnancy test, or during well-child care for another family member. Maternal chronic health conditions and social behaviors ideally need to be addressed prior to pregnancy. Medications need to be prescribed thoughtfully to all women of childbearing age, and provision of comprehensive prenatal care and interconception care and access to reliable family planning methods are essential for all women throughout their reproductive lives.

Frayne D, Verbiest S, Chelmow D, et al. Health care system measures to advance preconception wellness: consensus recommendations of the clinical workgroup of the national preconception health and health care initiative. *Obstet Gynecol.* 2016;127(5):863–872. [PMID: 27054935]

Hamilton BE, Martin JA, Osterman MJK, et al. Births: preliminary data for 2017. *Vital Statistics Rapid Release; No 4.* Hyattsville, MD: National Center for Health Statistics; 2018. https://www.cdc.gov/nchs/data/vsrr/report004.pdf. Accessed November 11, 2019.

Robbins C, Boulet SL, Morgan I et al. Disparities in preconception health indicators: behavioral risk factor surveillance system, 2013-2015, and pregnancy risk assessment monitoring system, 2013-2014. *MMWR Surveill Summ.* 2018;67(1):1–16. [PMID: 29346340]

NUTRITION

A woman's nutritional status before pregnancy can also have a profound effect on reproductive outcomes. Obesity is the most common nutritional disorder in developed countries. Obese women are at increased risk for prenatal complications such as hypertensive disorders of pregnancy, gestational diabetes, blood clots, urinary tract infections, and stillbirth. They are more likely to deliver large-for-gestational-age infants and, as a result, have a higher incidence of intrapartum complications. Maternal obesity is also associated with a range of congenital malformations, including neural tube defects, cardiovascular anomalies, cleft palate, hydrocephalus, and limb reduction anomalies. Because dieting is not recommended during pregnancy, obese women should be encouraged to achieve a healthy weight prior to conception.

On the other hand, underweight women are more likely than women of normal weight to give birth to low-birth-weight infants. Low birth weight may be associated with an increased risk of developing cardiovascular disease and diabetes in adult life (the "fetal origin hypothesis"). Therefore, at each visit, the patient's weight and height should be assessed. A history should be documented in the medical record and include inquiries regarding anorexia, bulimia, pica, vegetarian eating habits, and use of megavitamin supplements.

Since the mid-1980s, multiple studies conducted in various countries have shown a reduced risk of neural tube defects (NTDs) in infants whose mothers used folic acid supplements. The strongest evidence was provided by the Medical Research Council Vitamin Study in the United Kingdom, which showed a 72% reduction of recurrence of NTDs with a daily dose of 4 mg of folic acid started 4 weeks prior to conception and continued through the first trimester of pregnancy.

Since 1992, the CDC has recommended that all women of childbearing age take at least 0.4 mg of folic acid daily starting 1–3 months prior to conception and continuing through the first trimester of pregnancy. However, only two in five women report actually taking folic acid prior to conception. Folic acid supplementation is recommended in order to avoid NTDs, including spina bifida, anencephaly, and encephalocele, which affect approximately 4000 pregnancies each year in the United States. Although anencephaly is almost always lethal, spina bifida is associated with serious disabilities including paraplegia, bowel and bladder incontinence, hydrocephalus, and intellectual impairment. Good or excellent sources of natural folate include broccoli, spinach, peas, Brussels sprouts, corn, lentils, and oranges.

Patients who have experienced a previous pregnancy affected by an NTD and those taking medications that decrease folate absorption (valproic acid, carbamazepine) should take 4 mg of folic acid 1–3 months prior to pregnancy and continuing through the first trimester. A vitamin with 0.4 mg of folic acid should be continued through the remainder of the pregnancy. Some studies suggest that women with a body mass index (BMI) >35 should also be offered high-dose folic acid continuing through the first trimester of pregnancy.

Women taking triamterene, trimethoprim, and sulfasalazine and patients with medical conditions that decrease folic acid absorption (pregestational diabetes, celiac disease, inflammatory bowel disease, or intestinal bypass surgery) should be advised to take 1 mg of folic acid daily starting 1–3 months prior to planned conception and continuing through the first trimester of pregnancy.

Prenatal folic acid may also have beneficial effects on child neurodevelopment. A study in 2013 revealed that maternal use of folic acid around the time of conception was associated with a lower risk of autistic disorder in children. However, some recent studies are looking at a possible association between continued folic acid supplementation past the first trimester and increased risks of childhood allergies and asthma.

Vitamin A is a known teratogen at high doses. Supplemental doses exceeding 5000 IU/d should be avoided by women who are, or may become, pregnant. The form of vitamin A that is teratogenic is retinol, not β-carotene, so large consumption of fruits and vegetables rich in β-carotene is not a concern.

Vitamin D deficiency is associated with preterm birth and preeclampsia. It is recommended that all women during pregnancy and lactation consume at least 600 IU/day of vitamin D. Current evidence is insufficient to recommend routine screening for vitamin D deficiency in all pregnant women, but for women at risk of deficiency, the serum 25-hydroxyvitamin D level can be used for assessment. An optimal serum level for pregnancy has not been determined, but most experts agree that a serum level of 20 ng/mL is needed to avoid bone problems. Doses of 1000–2000 IU/d of vitamin D have been deemed safe in pregnancy if needed for repletion.

Calcium deficiency has been linked to increased risk for hypertensive disorders of pregnancy. The recommended dose of calcium for women age 19–50 is 1000 mg daily, and this includes pregnancy. Dietary consumption, as opposed to supplementation, is preferred in order to reduce the risk of calcium-induced nephrolithiasis.

Iron-deficiency anemia in pregnancy is common given the increased need for serum iron for fetal red cell development. However, there is no known benefit to iron supplementation in pregnancy in the absence of anemia. Women can either be screened for anemia in pregnancy (as is common practice in the United States) or take 30 mg of supplemental iron daily.

American College of Obstetricians and Gynecologists. Vitamin D: Screening and supplementation during pregnancy. Committee Opinion No. 495. *Obstet Gynecol.* 2011;118:197–198. [PMID: 21691184]

Fox NS. Do's and don'ts in pregnancy: truths and myths. *Obstet Gynecol.* 2018;131:713–721. [PMID: 29528917]

McStay CL, Prescott SL, Bower C, et al: Maternal folic acid supplementation during pregnancy and childhood allergic disease outcomes: a question of timing. *Nutrients.* 2017;9:123. [PMID: 28208798]

MRC Vitamin Study Research Group. Prevention of neural tube defects: results of the Medical Research Council Vitamin Study. *Lancet* 1991;338:131. [PMID: 1677062]

Stothard KJ, Tennant PW, Bell R, et al. Maternal overweight and obesity and the risk of congenital anomalies: a systematic review and meta-analysis. *JAMA.* 2009;301(6):636–650. [PMID: 19211471]

Suren P, Roth C, Bresnahan M, et al. Association between maternal use of folic acid supplements and risk of autism spectrum disorders in children. *JAMA.* 2013;309(6):570–577. [PMID: 23403681]

Wilson RD, Genetics Committee, Audibert F, et al. Pre-conception folic acid and multivitamin supplementation for the primary and secondary prevention of neural tube defects and other folic acid-sensitive congenital anomalies. *J Obstet Gynaecol Can.* 2015;37(6):534–549. [PMID: 26334606]

EXERCISE

An increasing number of women opt to continue with their exercise programs during pregnancy. Among a representative sample of US women, 42% reported exercising during pregnancy. Walking was the leading activity (43% of all activities reported), followed by swimming and aerobics (12% each).

Moderate aerobic and strength-conditioning exercise is encouraged before, during, and after pregnancy for women who have no medical or obstetric complications. Exercise may actually reduce pregnancy-related discomforts, improve or maintain maternal cardiovascular fitness, help with weight management, reduce the risk of gestational diabetes in obese women, and improve mild to moderate depressive symptoms.

Women should try to achieve an average of 20–30 minutes of moderate intensity exercise 4–5 times a week. Women do not need to adhere to a specific target heart rate, but rather should gauge moderate-intensity exercise by the ability to still hold a conversation while exercising. Exercise in extremes of temperature should be avoided. Modifications in position (to avoid the supine position) and degree of impact (stepping rather than jumping for example) should be taken. In addition, any activity that increases the risk of falling or abdominal trauma should be avoided during pregnancy. Scuba diving is contraindicated during pregnancy because the fetus is at risk for decompression sickness. Absolute contraindications to exercise during pregnancy are significant heart or lung disease, incompetent cervix, premature labor or ruptured membranes, placenta previa, persistent second- or third-trimester bleeding, preeclampsia, or pregnancy-induced hypertension.

American College of Obstetricians and Gynecologists. Physical activity and exercise during pregnancy and the postpartum period. Committee Opinion No. 650. *Obstet Gynecol.* 2015; 126:e135–e142. [PMID: 26595585]

Fox NS. Do's and don'ts in pregnancy: truths and myths. *Obstet Gynecol.* 2018;131:713–721. [PMID: 29528917]

HOT TUBS

The rise in core body temperature that can be associated with hot tub use has been associated with a twofold increased risk for miscarriage prior to 20 weeks. There is also a linear relationship between frequency of hot tub use and risk of miscarriage (hazard ratios of 1.7 for less than once a week, 2.0 for once a week, and 2.7 for more than once a week).

Fox NS. Do's and don'ts in pregnancy: truths and myths. *Obstet Gynecol.* 2018;131:713–721. [PMID: 29528917]

ORAL HEALTH

Oral health care is an important part of a woman's general health across her life span. A joint report from the American College of Obstetricians and Gynecologists, the American Dental Association, and the National Maternal and Child Oral Health Resource Center recommends that routine dental care and procedures should continue during pregnancy. Cleanings, dental extractions, root canals, restorations and fillings, and even radiographs can be continued (assuming the abdomen and thyroid are shielded).

Fox NS. Do's and don'ts in pregnancy: truths and myths. *Obstet Gynecol.* 2018;131:713–721. [PMID: 29528917]

MEDICAL CONDITIONS

▶ Diabetes

Congenital anomalies occur 2–6 times more often in the offspring of women with diabetes mellitus and have been associated with poor glycemic control during early pregnancy. Preconception care with good diabetic control during early embryogenesis has been shown to reduce the rate of congenital anomalies to essentially that of a control population. To provide optimal maternal and fetal outcomes, women with risk factors for preexisting diabetes (BMI >25, family history of diabetes in a first-degree relative, hypertension, high-risk ethnicity, history of gestational diabetes) should be screened prior to conception or at the first prenatal visit. In a meta-analysis of 18 published studies, the rate of major anomalies was lower among preconception care recipients (2.1%) than nonrecipients (6.5%). Continued glucose control during pregnancy has been shown to reduce the frequency of hypertensive disorders of pregnancy, shoulder dystocia, large-for-gestational-age infants, and cesarean sections and decrease neonatal fat mass.

According to the American Diabetes Association recommendations, the goal for blood glucose management in the preconception period and in the first trimester is to reach the lowest hemoglobin A1c level possible without undue risk of hypoglycemia to the mother. Hemoglobin A1c levels that are <1% above the normal range are desirable. Suggested goals for glucose measurements are as follows: fasting capillary glucose <95 mg/dL; before meals 80–110 mg/dL; 1 hour after meals <140 mg/dL; and 2 hours after meals <120 mg/dL.

Lifestyle modification with a diet low in simple carbohydrates, nutritional counseling, and exercise are still first-line treatments for diabetic management, but when these measures do not provide adequate glucose control, the American Diabetes Association (ADA) and American College of Obstetrics and Gynecology (ACOG) recommend medical management with insulin. NPH insulin has been the mainstay for intermediate- to long-acting insulins (although insulin glargine and detemir have been described). Insulin lispro and aspart are typically used over regular insulin for short-acting coverage because the onset of action is more rapid, which allows for ease of timing with meals.

Insulin does not cross the placenta. The oral hypoglycemic agents glyburide and metformin do cross the placenta and are not currently recommended for treatment of diabetes in pregnancy due to inferior glucose control when compared to insulin, as well as concerns for neonatal exposure and lack of long-term safety data.

Although standard for use in nonpregnant diabetic patients, angiotensin-converting enzyme inhibitors and angiotensin receptor blockers should be avoided in pregnancy and preconception. These drugs can result in fetal renal impairment, anuria leading to oligohydramnios, intrauterine growth restriction, hypocalvaria, persistent patent ductus arteriosus, and stillbirth. Informed decision making with the patient should be used in terms of medication choice for any woman who is a diabetic and of childbearing age. If a woman and her doctor decide that she should use one of these mediations for renal protection or hypertension, she should have a plan to prevent pregnancy while on the medication, but also be advised to discontinue use and call her physician in the event of an unplanned pregnancy.

Prior to conception, a baseline dilated eye examination is recommended, because diabetic retinopathy can worsen during pregnancy. This is particularly important for those with type 1 diabetes.

After delivery, note should be made in the medical record of any woman who develops gestational diabetes in pregnancy regarding continued screening for type 2 diabetes. These women have a 15–70% risk of developing type 2 diabetes later in life and a sevenfold increased risk compared with women without a history of gestational diabetes. Screening for type 2 diabetes is recommended every 1–3 years in this population.

American College of Obstetricians and Gynecologists. Gestational diabetes mellitus. Practice Bulletin No. 180. *Obstet Gynecol.* 2017;130:e17–e31. [PMID: 28644329]

Garrison A. Screening, diagnosis, and management of gestational diabetes mellitus. *Am Fam Physician.* 2015;91(7):460–467. [PMID: 25884746]

▶ Thyroid Disorders

Following diabetes, thyroid disorders are the most common endocrine disorder in women of reproductive age. Approximately 2.5% of pregnant women in the United States have overt or subclinical hypothyroidism. Before 12 weeks' gestation, the fetal thyroid is unable to produce hormones and the fetus is dependent on maternal thyroxine that crosses the placenta. During pregnancy, maternal thyroid hormone requirements increase as early as the fifth week of gestation, typically before the first obstetrical visit. Inadequately treated maternal hypothyroidism is associated with decreased fertility and miscarriage, anemia, impaired cognitive function in the offspring, and pregnancy complications, including gestational hypertension, low birth weight, placental abruption, preeclampsia, and preterm birth.

Treatment of overt hypothyroidism with levothyroxine should be optimized before conception to achieve a thyroid-stimulating hormone (TSH) level of <2.5 mIU/L in order to reduce the incidence of infertility, miscarriage, and preterm birth and to improve fetal intellectual development. Patients should be advised of the need for increased dosage if they become pregnant (typically two extra doses of their medication per week). However, treatment seems to have little impact on the incidence of hypertensive disorders and placental abruption. Treatment of subclinical hypothyroidism in pregnancy and preconception is not recommended due to lack of evidence that medication treatment improves pregnancy outcomes or cognitive function in children up to 3 years old.

The Endocrine Society and ACOG also do not recommend universal screening of pregnant women for thyroid disease. A randomized trial of >4000 women did not show any difference in adverse outcomes with universal screening. The current recommendation is to screen only pregnant women with a personal history of thyroid disease or symptoms of thyroid dysfunction with a serum TSH level.

Only about 0.2% of pregnant women have hyperthyroidism. Overt hyperthyroidism that is inadequately treated is associated with maternal heart failure, placental abruption, preeclampsia, preterm delivery and fetal goiter, intrauterine growth restriction, small for gestational age, and stillbirth. Women with overt hyperthyroidism, should be counseled prior to pregnancy regarding treatment options (medications, radioactive iodine ablation, or subtotal thyroidectomy). Propylthiouracil (PTU) is the preferred medication antenatally and in the first trimester due to the risk of birth defects with methimazole. However, after the first trimester, a switch to methimazole should be considered due to the risk of liver failure with PTU. The goal of treatment is to maintain serum free thyroxine (T_4) levels in the high normal to slightly above normal range. Free T_4 levels should be measured every 2–4 weeks and doses adjusted accordingly.

Studies of women with subclinical hyperthyroidism have not shown the same adverse maternal and fetal outcomes. Therefore, treatment of subclinical hyperthyroidism in pregnancy is not currently recommended.

American College of Obstetricians and Gynecologists. Thyroid disease in pregnancy. Practice Bulletin No. 148. *Obstet Gynecol.* 2015;125:996–1005. [PMID: 25798985]
Carney LA, Quinlan JD, West JM. Thyroid disease in pregnancy. *Am Fam Physician.* 2014;89(4):273–278. [PMID: 24695447]

▶ Hypertension

Hypertensive disorders, which include chronic hypertension, gestational hypertension, and preeclampsia, affect 12–22% of pregnancies in the United States and are associated with increased risk of preterm birth, small-for-gestational-age and intrauterine growth-restricted infants, placental abruption, maternal cardiovascular disease, and stroke. Combined, these disorders are responsible for 18% of maternal deaths.

Ideally women with chronic hypertension should be evaluated and treated prior to conception for any secondary causes of hypertension including renal disease, endocrine disorders, sleep apnea, substance use, and coarctation of the aorta. Lifestyle modification should be undertaken for obesity. If no secondary causes of hypertension exist and lifestyle modifications are not effective, then management with antihypertensive medications is warranted for women with blood pressures consistently >150/100 mm Hg.

Blood pressure goals before pregnancy are the same as those for any other nonpregnant patient. However, in pregnancy, treating mild to moderately elevated blood pressure does not lead to any improvement in outcomes for mom or baby and, in fact, can cause placental hypoperfusion and growth restriction. So if a patient presents early in pregnancy and has stopped her blood pressure medication, it may be reasonable to prescribe a home blood pressure cuff and just monitor her blood pressures initially. Many women on low-dose antihypertensives are able to be maintained off all medication in the first and second trimesters (due to the physiologic drop in blood pressure that occurs in the second trimester). Often it is not until the third trimester that blood pressures start to rise again and medications may need to be restarted.

Angiotensin-converting enzyme inhibitors and angiotensin receptor blockers should be avoided in pregnant women and in the preconception period as they have been associated with neonatal renal failure, oligohydramnios, and death. For the same reasons, they should not be considered first-line treatment for hypertension in women of childbearing age in general. Short-acting β-blockers like labetalol, calcium channel blockers like nifedipine, and α-blockers like methyldopa all have good safety profiles and are effective for treatment. Diuretics do not have a teratogenic effect but are not first-line

treatment for hypertension and also exacerbate the intravascular volume depletion that accompanies preeclampsia.

American College of Obstetricians and Gynecologists. Executive summary: hypertension in pregnancy. *Obstet Gynecol.* 2013;122:1122–1131. [PMID: 24150027]
Leeman L, Dresang LT, Fontaine P. Hypertensive disorders of pregnancy. *Am Fam Physician.* 2016;93(2):121–129. [PMID: 26926408]

▶ Asthma

Asthma affects 4–8% of all pregnancies and, if left uncontrolled, can be associated with premature birth, preeclampsia, low birth weight, growth restriction, increased need for cesarean section, and increased maternal morbidity and mortality. Ideally, patients should strive to have good control of asthma symptoms prior to pregnancy and then monitor those symptoms over the course of the pregnancy. About one-third of women experience improvement in symptoms during pregnancy, one-third experience a worsening of symptoms, and one-third remain unchanged.

The goals for symptom control in pregnancy are the same as in the nonpregnant state: use of rescue inhalers less than twice a week, nighttime awakenings less than twice per month, and lack of activity impairment due to symptoms. A stepwise approach to treatment is recommended in order to use the lowest amount of drug necessary to control symptoms, but it is safer for pregnant women to be treated for asthma than to experience exacerbations and hypoxia.

Medications used prior to and during pregnancy are similar. Short- and long-acting β-agonists and inhaled and oral steroids should be used just as they are in the nonpregnant state for symptom control. Likewise, control of allergy symptoms with environmental modifications, antihistamines, leukotriene receptor antagonists, and allergy shots if needed is also appropriate. Caution is advised with the newer antimuscarinic agents in pregnancy because there are limited data regarding their use, although the available data do not suggest a teratogenic effect.

American College of Obstetricians and Gynecologists. Asthma in pregnancy. ACOG Practice Bulletin No. 90. *Obstet Gynecol.* 2008;111:457–464. [PMID: 18238988]

▶ Epilepsy

Epilepsy occurs in 1% of the population and is the most common serious neurologic problem seen in pregnancy. There are approximately 1 million women of childbearing age with epilepsy in the United States, approximately 20,000 of whom deliver infants every year. Much can be done to achieve a favorable outcome of pregnancy in women with epilepsy. Ideally, this should start before conception. Menstrual disorders, ovulatory dysfunction, and infertility are relatively common problems in women with epilepsy and should be addressed.

Women with epilepsy must make choices about contraceptive methods. Certain antiepileptic drugs (AEDs), such as phenytoin, carbamazepine, phenobarbital, primidone, and topiramate, induce hepatic cytochrome P450 enzymes, leading to an increase in the metabolism of the estrogen and progestin present in the oral contraceptive pills. This increases the risk of breakthrough pregnancy. The American Academy of Neurology recommends the use of oral contraceptive formulations with ≥50 μg of ethinyl estradiol or mestranol for women with epilepsy who take enzyme-inducing AEDs.

Both levonorgestrel implants (Norplant) and the progestin-only pill have reduced efficacy in women taking enzyme-inducing AEDs. Other AEDs that do not induce liver enzymes (eg, valproic acid, lamotrigine, vigabatrin, gabapentin, and felbamate) do not cause contraceptive failure.

Because many AEDs interfere with the metabolism of folic acid, all women with epilepsy who are planning a pregnancy should receive folic acid supplementation at a dose of 4–5 mg/d. Withdrawal of AEDs can be considered in any woman who has been seizure free for at least 2 years and has a single type of seizure, normal neurologic examination and intelligence quotient, and an electroencephalogram that has normalized with treatment. Because the risk of seizure relapse is greatest in the first 6 months after discontinuing AEDs, withdrawal should be accomplished before conception. If withdrawal is not possible, monotherapy should be attempted to reduce the risk of fetal malformations. Offspring of women with epilepsy are at increased risk for intrauterine growth restriction, congenital malformations that include craniofacial and digital anomalies, and cognitive dysfunction. The term *fetal anticonvulsant syndrome* encompasses various combinations of these findings and has been associated with use of virtually all AEDs. Some recent studies have indicated a higher risk for birth defects, as well as for language impairment in association with valproic acid compared with other AEDs, mainly carbamazepine and lamotrigine.

GENETIC CARRIER SCREENING

Carrier screening refers to genetic testing performed on an individual who does not have any phenotypic evidence of disease but who may carry a variant allele. If an individual is found to be a carrier for a specific condition, their partner should also be offered testing. If both partners are carriers, then genetic counseling should be offered. The ideal time for carrier screening and genetic counseling is before a couple attempts to conceive, especially if the history reveals advanced maternal age, previously affected pregnancy, consanguinity, or family history of genetic disease. This allows the couple to ascertain their reproductive risk and consider a full range of reproductive options.

ACOG considers it reasonable to offer cystic fibrosis and spinal muscular atrophy carrier screening to all couples regardless of race or ethnicity as both of these conditions have high carrier rates in the general population. In addition, it is also becoming increasingly difficult to assign a single ethnicity to individuals. Cystic fibrosis is the most common autosomal recessive genetic disorder in the non-Hispanic white population, with a carrier rate of 1:29. It is characterized by the production of thickened secretions throughout the body, but particularly in the lungs and the gastrointestinal tract. Spinal muscular atrophy has a carrier status of 1:54 and is characterized by degeneration of spinal cord motor neurons, which leads to atrophy of skeletal muscles and overall weakness.

Certain ethnic groups have a relatively high carrier incidence for other genetic disorders and should be offered screening for those particular disorders. For example, Ashkenazi Jews have a 1 in 30 chance of being a carrier for Tay-Sachs disease, a severe degenerative neurologic disease that leads to death in early childhood. Carrier status can easily be determined by a serum assay for the level of the enzyme hexosaminidase A. Screening for Tay-Sachs disease is recommended prior to conception, because testing on serum is not reliable in pregnancy and the enzyme assay on white blood cells that is used in pregnancy is more expensive and labor intensive. Couples of Ashkenazi Jewish ancestry should also be offered carrier screening for Canavan disease and familial dysautonomia before conception or during early pregnancy.

Other common genetic disorders for which there is reliable carrier screening are sickle cell disease in African Americans, β-thalassemia in individuals of Mediterranean descent, and α-thalassemia in Southeast Asians. Sickle cell carriers can be detected with solubility testing (Sickledex) for the presence of hemoglobin S. However, ACOG recommends hemoglobin electrophoresis screening in all patients considered at risk for having a child affected with a sickling disorder. Solubility testing is described as inadequate because it does not identify carriers of abnormal hemoglobins such as the β-thalassemia trait or the HbB, HbC, HbD, or HbE traits. A complete blood count with indices is a simple screening test for the thalassemias and will show a mild anemia with a low mean corpuscular volume.

Fragile X syndrome is the most common cause of mental retardation after Down syndrome and is the most common inherited cause of mental retardation. It affects approximately 1 in 3600 men and 1 in 4000–6000 women and results from a mutation in a gene on the long arm of the X chromosome. In addition to mental retardation, fragile X syndrome is characterized by physical features such as macro-orchidism, large ears, a prominent jaw, and autistic behaviors. Preconception screening should be offered to women with a known family history of fragile X syndrome or a family history of unexplained mental retardation, developmental delay, or autism.

Any patient who has a specific genetic disorder that runs in her family should be offered carrier screening for that particular disorder if it is available. Of note, carrier screening does not replace newborn screening, nor does newborn screening replace the value of carrier screening.

American College of Obstetricians and Gynecologists. Carrier screening for genetic conditions. Committee Opinion No. 691. *Obstet Gynecol* 2017;129:e41–55. [PMID: 28225426]

American College of Obstetrics and Gynecology, Committee on Genetics. ACOG Committee Opinion, no. 486, April 2011. Update on carrier screening for cystic fibrosis. *Obstet Gynecol.* 2011;117(4):1028. [PMID: 21422883]

IMMUNIZATIONS

All women of childbearing age should receive age- and risk-appropriate immunizations including influenza; pneumovax; tetanus, diphtheria, and pertussis; and hepatitis A and B. However, the live vaccines (rubella and varicella) are contraindicated in pregnancy. If a woman is receiving a live vaccine, her pregnancy plans should be assessed and a urine pregnancy test obtained.

Rubella vaccine should be offered to any woman with a negative rubella titer and advice given to avoid conception for 1 month due to the theoretical risk to the fetus. Rubella infection in pregnancy can result in miscarriage, stillbirth, or an infant with congenital rubella syndrome (CRS). The risk of developing CRS abnormalities (hearing impairment, eye defects, congenital heart defects, and developmental delay) is greatest if the mother is infected in the first trimester of pregnancy. However, inadvertent immunization of a pregnant woman with rubella vaccine should not suggest the need to terminate a pregnancy because there is no evidence that the vaccine alone causes any malformations or CRS.

If a woman does not have a clear history of varicella infection (chickenpox), it is reasonable to assess her varicella titer. Women who are seronegative should be offered vaccination. The recommended regimen for patients age >13 years is two doses at least 4 weeks apart. Patients should avoid becoming pregnant for at least 1 month after the second dose. If a pregnant woman acquires varicella before 20 weeks' gestation, the fetus has a 1–2% risk of developing fetal varicella syndrome, which is characterized by skin scarring, hypoplasia of the limbs, eye defects, and neurologic abnormalities. Infants born to mothers who manifest varicella 5 days before to 2 days after delivery may experience a severe infection and have a mortality rate as high as 30%.

LIFESTYLE CHANGES

▶ Caffeine

Caffeine is present in many beverages, in chocolate, and in over-the-counter medications such as cold and headache medicines. One cup of coffee contains approximately 120 mg of caffeine, a cup of tea has 40 mg of caffeine, and the average soft drink contains 45 mg of caffeine per 12-oz serving. Consumption of caffeine during pregnancy is quite common, but its metabolism is slowed. Cigarette smoking increases caffeine metabolism, leading to increased caffeine intake.

Several epidemiologic studies have suggested that high caffeine intake (the equivalent of 10 cups of coffee a day) may be associated with decreased fertility, increased spontaneous abortions, and decreased birth weight. As a result, in 1980, the US Food and Drug Administration (FDA) advised pregnant women to avoid caffeine during pregnancy. However, an extensive literature review of the effects of caffeine concluded that pregnant women who consume moderate amounts of caffeine (≤5–6 mg/kg daily) spread throughout the day and do not smoke or drink alcohol have no increase in reproductive risks.

▶ Substance Use

Substance use remains a major health problem in the United States. Among pregnant women age 15–44 years, 5.4% report using illicit drugs. Women of reproductive age are often not aware of the importance of pregnancy planning and reliable birth control in the setting of substance use. Pregnant women with substance use disorders face not only guilt and shame, but also potential legal issues and fear of losing custody of their child. Those feelings are amplified when met by judgmental or punitive actions by healthcare providers, and subsequently, women tend to avoid care at a time when medical care is most needed.

Many women will actually discontinue substance use on their own when they find out they are pregnant, but relapse rates postpartum are high. All patients should be questioned about substance use and encouraged to discontinue use. For women who are unable to discontinue use on their own, pregnancy should be looked at as an opportunity to do so and a discussion of maternal and child risk, counseling, referral, and access to recovery programs should be the goal of the discussion, rather than reprimand.

A. Tobacco

Based on 2016 CDC data, 7.2% of women smoked during pregnancy, subjecting themselves and their infants to numerous adverse health effects. Prevalence was highest for women age 20–24 years (10.7%), non-Hispanic American Indian or Alaska Native women (16.7%), and those with a high school degree (12.2%). Smoking also varied by state and was highest in West Virginia (25.1%), Kentucky (18.4%), Montana (16.5%), Vermont (15.5%), and Missouri (15.3%). Smoking during pregnancy has been associated with spontaneous abortion, prematurity, low birth weight, intrauterine growth restriction, placental abruption, and placenta previa, as well as an increased risk for sudden infant death syndrome, developmental delay, asthma, behavioral problems, and childhood obesity. Accumulating evidence also indicates that maternal tobacco use is associated with birth defects such as oral clefts and foot deformities. Paradoxically, smoking during pregnancy has reportedly been associated with a reduced risk of preeclampsia. However, the smoking-related adverse outcomes of pregnancy outweigh this benefit.

Cessation of smoking either before pregnancy or in early pregnancy is associated with improved maternal and child health and should be the recommended goal for all pregnant women. The use of nicotine replacement products (nicotine patch, lozenge, or gum) to facilitate smoking cessation is considered acceptable in pregnancy because it reduces exposure to other toxins contained in cigarettes, such as tar, lead, carbon monoxide, and arsenic, and has been shown to increase rates of smoking cessation compared with no pharmacotherapy. Nicotine gum is rated category C during pregnancy, whereas nicotine patches, inhaler, and nasal spray are category D. If the nicotine patch is used, it can be removed at night to limit fetal nicotine exposure. Bupropion showed a positive effect on quit rates as well and has a low risk of teratogenicity but should be reserved for heavy smokers who are unable to quit with counseling and therapy alone. Varenicline has not been studied in pregnancy and should not be used for prenatal smoking cessation.

Electronic nicotine delivery systems (ENDS), including electronic cigarettes, vaporizers, vape pens, and hookah pens, were introduced in 2007 and have been marketed as a safer alternative to smoking. This has led to an increased use in the general population as well as in pregnancy. ENDS are not currently approved by the FDA for smoking cessation, and in fact, the nicotine consumed by electronic cigarette users has been shown to be comparable to, or higher than, that consumed by traditional smokers. Given that nicotine readily crosses the placenta and that nicotine exposure alone has been linked with adverse outcomes, one would presume that the known detrimental effects of nicotine on mothers and infants would to apply to this population of users as well. However, there are limited data on the health consequences of ENDS for even the average adult, let alone pregnant women and their unborn children. ENDS do limit the exposure to other toxins contained in traditional cigarettes such as tar, arsenic, and carbon monoxide, but none are approved by the FDA for smoking cessation, and they expose users to propylene glycol, glycerin, and flavoring that are not contained in traditional cigarettes. The effects of inhaling these substances are unknown. The ideal situation is that women quit all forms of nicotine in pregnancy.

B. Alcohol

In 1981, the surgeon general of the United States recommended that women abstain from drinking alcohol during pregnancy and when planning a pregnancy, because such drinking may harm the fetus. Alcohol is rapidly absorbed, and so infants are exposed to the same alcohol levels as the mother. Nevertheless, approximately 1 in 13 pregnant women will drink alcohol during pregnancy and 1 in 71 will binge drink.

Heavy alcohol use (more than one drink per day or more than four drinks at any one time) has been associated with increased rates of infertility, spontaneous abortion, menstrual symptoms, hypertension, stroke, breast cancer, and overall mortality. In pregnancy, heavy alcohol use has been associated with miscarriage, stillbirth, low birth weight, preterm delivery, and infant morbidity and mortality. Evidence for low to moderate alcohol use in pregnancy and lactation has been inconclusive or shown no increased risk.

The most severe consequence of exposure to alcohol during pregnancy is fetal alcohol syndrome (FAS), characterized by a triad of prenatal or postnatal growth retardation, central nervous system (CNS) neurodevelopmental abnormalities, and facial anomalies (short palpebral fissures, smooth philtrum, thin upper lip, and midfacial hypoplasia). FAS is the major preventable cause of birth defects and intellectual disability in the Western world. In the United States, the prevalence of FAS is estimated to be between 0.5 and 2 cases per 1000 births.

Some ethnic groups are disproportionately affected by FAS. American Indians and Alaska Native populations have a prevalence of FAS 30 times higher than white populations. It also appears that binge drinking produces more severe outcomes in offspring than more chronic exposure, possibly because of in utero withdrawal and its concomitant effects.

Physicians should counsel their patients that they cannot predict a safe level of alcohol consumption during pregnancy for a particular woman and that the harmful effects on the developing fetal brain can occur at any time during pregnancy.

C. Marijuana

Marijuana is the most frequently used illicit drug in pregnancy (best estimates are 7.1% of women) and is also perceived by 65% of pregnant women to have "no risk" in pregnancy. Although marijuana does not appear to be teratogenic in humans or have a significant association with congenital malformations, data are mixed in terms of risk for low birth weight, stillbirth, preterm birth, and neonatal intensive care unit admissions. Some studies also suggest an association with increased hyperactivity, impulsivity, and inattention symptoms in children up to age 10, as well as possible lasting effects on long-term memory, short-term olfactory memory, social interaction, and aggression in adolescence. Providers should be aware of limitations of the existing literature though, including lack of quantification of marijuana exposure, ascertainment of exposure through self-report (which tends to underestimate exposure), and confounding factors such as education level and concurrent tobacco use.

Most women report using marijuana to treat other medical conditions such as depression, anxiety, nausea, vomiting, sleep disorders, and chronic pain. Cannabinoids have been shown to have efficacy for many of these symptoms in nonpregnant or cancer patients, but there are no current data to support its use in pregnant women. Furthermore, as mentioned earlier, the risks to the fetus have not been reliably established.

There is also a lack of data on marijuana use and breastfeeding. Tetrahydrocannabinol (THC) has been detected in breast milk at an average of 2.5% of the maternal dose and peaks an hour after use, but has been documented in concentrations up to 8 times that of maternal serum levels. The bioavailability of marijuana in the breast milk is unknown.

Current ACOG recommendations are for women to cease marijuana use during pregnancy and breastfeeding. The American Academy of Pediatrics recommends against breastfeeding in women using marijuana regularly, but suggests it should be considered on a case-by-case basis for women using marijuana only occasionally. The authors of the most recent article published in *Obstetrics and Gynecology* add the opinion that if women continue to use marijuana despite counseling on cessation, then it is reasonable to provide lactation support given the other known benefits of breastfeeding.

D. Cocaine and Methamphetamines

Stimulant drug use during pregnancy has been associated with spontaneous abortion, premature labor, intrauterine growth restriction, placental abruption, microcephaly, limb reduction defects, and urogenital malformations. Infants exposed to stimulant drugs may have trouble feeding and sleeping and experience increased muscle tone. These symptoms typically resolve spontaneously within a few weeks of birth. A meta-analysis of 36 studies concluded that cocaine exposure in utero has not been demonstrated to affect physical growth and that it does not appear to independently affect developmental scores from infancy to age 6 years, but can be associated with childhood behavioral abnormalities. Women using stimulant drugs should be advised not to breastfeed.

E. Benzodiazepines

Research on the effects of benzodiazepines in pregnancy and lactation is limited to prescribed benzodiazepine use. However, because benzodiazepines require albumin for serum transport and fetal albumin levels are low until the third trimester, it is thought that adverse outcomes of benzodiazepines would be caused mainly by exposure in the third trimester. Current research does not show an increased risk for malformations (odds ratio, 1.06). Some studies have shown associations with oral clefts, anal atresia, and cardiovascular malformations, but they did not account for concurrent use of other psychotropic drugs and illegal substance use.

Benzodiazepines do transfer into the breast milk, and some studies indicate the potential for increased irritability and sedation of the infant with breastfeeding, but again, the data are limited.

F. Opioids

In a recent sample of commercially insured women, 14.4% reported filling a prescription for an opioid at some point in their lives. Those who were prescribed chronic opioids tended to continue that use into pregnancy. Although opioids are not teratogenic, they are associated with growth restriction, placental insufficiency, oligohydramnios, premature rupture of membranes, preterm labor, preeclampsia, postpartum hemorrhage, cesarean delivery, low APGAR scores, and fetal demise. Maternal risks include increased risks of infection, overdose, poor nutrition and self-care, and increased length of hospital stay.

Infants born to opioid-dependent mothers are at risk for a syndrome of withdrawal known as neonatal abstinence syndrome (NAS) within 2–7 days of delivery. Neonatal withdrawal is characterized by CNS hyperirritability, respiratory distress, gastrointestinal dysfunction, poor feeding, high-pitched cry, yawning, and sneezing. Neonatal risks also include microcephaly, poor infant growth, neurobehavioral problems, and sudden infant death syndrome.

Methadone has long been used to treat opioid dependence in pregnancy because of its long half-life, but buprenorphine is a reasonable treatment option as well. Both have been shown to be clinically safe and effective and to improve relapse rates and maternal and infant outcomes. Rates of NAS are similar for infants exposed to both drugs, but infants exposed to methadone seem to have more severe withdrawal symptoms for a longer period of time. Maternal rates of attrition are higher with buprenorphine, but there are fewer maternal withdrawal symptoms and a lower risk of overdose. The American Society of Addiction Medicine recommends breastfeeding for mothers on both drugs because relatively low amounts of the drug are present in breast milk. The known benefits of breastfeeding outweigh the risk of exposure, and there are additional soothing effects of breastfeeding on NAS.

Benowitz N, Dempsey D. Pharmacotherapy for smoking cessation during pregnancy. *Nicotine Tobac Res.* 2004;6(suppl 2):S189. [PMID: 15203821]

Christian MS, Brent RL. Teratogen update: evaluation of the reproductive and developmental risks of caffeine. *Teratology.* 2001;64:51. [PMID: 11410911]

Drake P, Driscoll AK, Mathews TJ. Cigarette smoking during pregnancy: United States, 2016. *NCHS Data Brief, No. 305.* Hyattsville, MD: National Center for Health Statistics; 2018.

McLafferty LP, Becker M, Dresner N, et al. Guidelines for the management of pregnant women with substance use disorders. *Psychosomatics.* 2016;57:115–130. [PMID: 26880374]

Metz D, Borgelt LM. Marijuana use in pregnancy and while breastfeeding. *Obstet Gynecol.* 2018;132(5):1198–1210. [PMID: 30234728]

Substance Abuse and Mental Health Services Administration. *Results from the 2013 National Survey on Drug Use and Health: Summary of National Findings.* NSDUH Series H-48, HHS Publication No. (SMA) 11-4863. Rockville, MD: Substance Abuse and Mental Health Services Administration; 2014.

Whittington JR, Simmons PM, Phillips AM, et al. The use of electronic cigarettes in pregnancy: a review of the literature. *Obstet Gynecol Surv.* 2018;73(9):544–549. [PMID: 30265741]

SEXUALLY TRANSMITTED DISEASES

Since 2013, the United States has experienced a 22% increase in cases of chlamydia, a 67% increase in cases of gonorrhea, and a 76% increase in cases of syphilis. Screening for these and other sexually transmitted infections such as HIV, hepatitis C, and Zika virus is important in the context of possible pregnancy.

Chlamydia and gonorrhea are two of the most prevalent sexually transmitted diseases (STDs), and both are often asymptomatic in women. Untreated, they can lead to pelvic inflammatory disease (PID) 10% of the time. PID can lead to chronic inflammation and injury to the fallopian tubes, causing infertility and risk for tubal pregnancy.

In pregnancy, both chlamydia and gonorrhea have been associated with premature rupture of membranes, preterm labor, postpartum endometritis, and congenital infection. Infants whose mothers have untreated chlamydia infection have a 30–50% chance of developing inclusion conjunctivitis and a 10–20% chance of developing pneumonia. Inclusion conjunctivitis typically develops 5–14 days after delivery and is usually mild and self-limiting. Pneumonia due to chlamydia usually has a slow onset without fever and can have a protracted course if untreated. Long-term complications may be significant. Ophthalmia neonatorum is the most common manifestation of neonatal gonococcal infection. It occurs 2–5 days after birth in ≤50% of exposed infants who did not receive ocular prophylaxis. Corneal ulceration may occur, and unless treatment is initiated promptly, the cornea may perforate, leading to blindness.

Congenital syphilis occurs when the spirochete *Treponema pallidum* is transmitted from a pregnant woman with syphilis to her fetus. Untreated syphilis during pregnancy may lead to spontaneous abortion, nonimmune hydrops (edema), stillbirth, neonatal death, and serious sequelae in liveborn infected children. In 2017, a total of 918 cases of congenital syphilis were reported in the United States. This represents a 153% increase from 2013 and a 44% increase from 2016.

All women at high risk for HIV should be screened prior to pregnancy. In untreated HIV-infected pregnant women, the risk of mother-to-child transmission varies from 16% to 40%. It is possible to dramatically reduce the transmission rates by using highly active antiretroviral therapy during pregnancy, by offering elective cesarean delivery at 38 weeks if the viral load at term is higher than 1000 copies/mL, and by discouraging breastfeeding. Therefore, universal HIV screening in pregnancy is recommended. With the above measures, in developed countries, transmission rates as low as 1–2% have been achieved.

Any woman with prior or ongoing risk factors for hepatitis C should be screened prior to pregnancy. There is debate among expert clinical panels as to whether universal screening in pregnancy is warranted. Although the vertical transmission of hepatitis C in pregnancy is only about 5%, knowing a patient's hepatitis C status in labor can help to guide care for the mother and her infant. Trials on the safety and efficacy of treatment of hepatitis C in pregnancy are ongoing.

Zika virus is a mosquito-borne infection that can also be transmitted sexually and can lead to microcephaly and other neurologic complications in the fetus, including issues with motor development, vision, and hearing. All women should be asked about possible Zika virus exposure for themselves and their partner before and during a pregnancy. The CDC recommends that if a woman travels to an area with risk for Zika that the couple should use condoms or abstain from intercourse for at least 2 months after her last exposure or symptom, if she is symptomatic. Men who have been exposed to Zika virus should use condoms or abstain from intercourse for 3 months from the last exposure or symptom to avoid sexual transmission through the semen. Pregnant women should be advised against traveling to areas at risk for Zika virus.

Centers for Disease Control and Prevention. 2017 sexually transmitted diseases surveillance. https://www.cdc.gov/std/stats17/2017-STD-Surveillance-Report_CDC-clearance-9.10.18.pdf. Accessed November 11, 2019.

Oduyebo T, Polen KD, Walke HT, et al. Update: interim guidance for health care providers caring for pregnant women with possible Zika virus exposure—United States (including U.S. territories), July 2017. *MMWR Morb Mortal Wkly Rep.* 2017;66:781–793. [PMID: 28749921]

Polen KD, Gilboa SM, Hills S, et al. Update: interim guidance for preconception counseling and prevention of sexual transmission of Zika virus for men with possible zika virus exposure—United States, August 2018. *MMWR Morb Mortal Wkly Rep.* 2018;67:868–871. [PMID: 30091965]

MEDICATIONS

Medication use in pregnancy is almost ubiquitous. Therefore, it is important that physicians are able to discuss the risks and benefits of both over-the-counter and prescription medications during pregnancy. Of 9546 geographically and ethnically diverse nulliparous women in the 2015 nuMom2b study by Hess and colleagues, 97% reported taking at least one medication in pregnancy, 96% reported taking a medication in the first trimester, and 30% reported taking five or more medications during pregnancy. The most commonly prescribed medications were for nausea, vomiting, and gastrointestinal distress, followed by antibiotics.

Since 1979, the FDA has defined five risk categories (A, B, C, D, and X) that have been used by manufacturers to rate their products for use during pregnancy and lactation. Those ratings were used for many years but were thought to be oversimplified and misleading for providers in many ways. As of June 30, 2015, all new medications approved by the FDA are being labeled under a new Pregnancy and Lactation Labeling Rule. This new labeling consists of sections 8.1 (Pregnancy, Labor, and Delivery), 8.2 (Lactation Including Nursing Mothers), and 8.3 (Females and Males of Reproductive Potential). The new labeling includes more narrative, but also a more complete, statements of the known risks based on available animal and human data. For example, section 8.1 includes a pregnancy exposure registry, a risk summary, clinical considerations, and data. Section 8.2 provides information about the amount of drug in breast milk and potential effects on the infant. Section 8.3 addresses medication use for men and women in the preconception period, the need for pregnancy testing, contraception recommendations, and risk of infertility related to that drug. By June of 2020, all existing drug labeling will gradually be converted to the new rule as well. Labeling for over-the-counter drugs will remain unchanged. Online resources such as http://www.sickkids.ca/motherisk/index.html, www.reprotox.org, http://dailymed.nlm.nih.gov, and http://ww5.lactmed.com are also available to help physicians with up-to-date information on drugs in pregnancy and lactation.

In addition to prescription and over-the-counter medications, about 11% of women report using dietary and herbal supplements during pregnancy. Unfortunately, there are limited human data on the safety of these products in pregnancy. The Natural Medicines Comprehensive Database (http://naturaldatabase.therapeuticresearch.com) reviews the available evidence, but these products are not required to be registered by the FDA, and therefore, no action is required if a product is found to be unsafe after marketing.

► Anticoagulants

Warfarin (Coumadin) readily crosses the placenta and is a known human teratogen. The critical period for fetal warfarin syndrome is exposure during weeks 6–9 of gestation. This syndrome primarily involves nasal hypoplasia and stippling of the epiphyses. Later drug exposure may also be associated with intracerebral hemorrhage, microcephaly, and intellectual disability. In patients who require prolonged anticoagulation therapy, discontinuing warfarin in early pregnancy and substituting heparin or low-molecular-weight heparin will reduce the incidence of congenital anomalies because these drugs do not cross the placenta.

► Isotretinoin

Isotretinoin is indicated for severe recalcitrant nodular acne unresponsive to conventional therapy. As many as 50% of fetuses exposed to the drug develop severe congenital anomalies of the ears, CNS, heart, and thymus. In 2005, the FDA approved a computer-based risk management program called iPledge to prevent fetal exposure to isotretinoin (report available at http://www.ipledgeprogram.com). Female patients of childbearing age must have two negative pregnancy tests and use two appropriate forms of contraception before starting therapy. They also have to wait at least a month before considering pregnancy after completing a course of isotretinoin.

Haas DM, Marsh DJ, Dang DT, et al. Prescription and other medication use in pregnancy. *Obstet Gynecol.* 2018;131(5):789–798. [PMID: 29630018]
Pernia S, DeMaagd G. The new pregnancy and lactation labeling rule. *Pharmacy Ther.* 2016;41(11):713–715. [PMID: 27904304]
Servey J, Chang J. Over-the-counter medications in pregnancy. *Am Fam Physician.* 2014;90(8):548–555. [PMID: 25369643]

OCCUPATIONAL EXPOSURES

Occupational exposures should be assessed for all women of childbearing age. The three most common occupational exposures reported to affect pregnancy are video display terminals, organic solvents, and lead. However, physicians should assess the risk for infectious or traumatic exposures in the workplace as well.

► Video Display Terminals

In 1980, a cluster of four infants with severe congenital malformations was reported in Canada. The cluster was linked to exposure to video display terminals (VDTs) during their pregnancy at a newspaper department in Toronto. Many epidemiologic studies have since investigated the effects of electromagnetic fields emitted from VDTs on pregnancy outcome. Most studies found only equivocal or no associations of VDTs with birth defects, preterm labor, and low birth weight. Thus, it is reasonable to advise women that there is no evidence that using VDTs will jeopardize pregnancy.

► Organic Solvents

Organic solvents constitute a large group of chemically heterogeneous compounds that are widely used in industry and common household products. Occupational exposure to organic solvents can result from many industrial applications, including dry cleaning, painting, varnishing, degreasing, printing, and production of plastics and pharmaceuticals. Smelling the odor of organic solvents is not indicative of a significant exposure, because the olfactory nerve can detect levels as low as several parts per million, which are not necessarily associated with toxicity. A recent meta-analysis of epidemiologic studies demonstrated a statistically significant relationship between exposure to organic solvents in the first trimester of pregnancy and fetal malformations. There was also a tendency toward an increased risk for spontaneous abortion. Women who plan to become pregnant should minimize their exposure to organic solvents by routinely using ventilation systems and protective equipment.

▶ Lead

Despite a steady decline in average blood levels of lead in the US population in recent years, approximately 0.5% of women of childbearing age may have blood levels of lead of >10 μg/dL. The vast majority of exposures to lead occur in artists using glass staining and in workers involved in paint manufacturing for the automotive and aircraft industries. Other occupational sources of exposure to lead include smeltering, printing, and battery manufacturing. The most worrisome consequence of low to moderate lead toxicity is neurotoxicity. A review of the literature suggested that low-dose exposure to lead in utero may cause developmental deficits in the infant. However, these effects seem to be reversible if further exposure to lead is avoided. It is crucial to detect and treat lead toxicity prior to conception because the chelating agents used (dimercaprol, ethylenediaminetetraacetate, and penicillamine) can adversely affect the fetus if used during pregnancy.

DOMESTIC VIOLENCE

Domestic violence is increasingly recognized as a major public health issue. In the United States, 1.5 million women are raped or physically assaulted by an intimate partner every year. Domestic violence crosses all socioeconomic, racial, religious, and educational boundaries. Even physicians are not immune; in a survey, 17% of female medical students and faculty had experienced abuse by a partner in their adult life, an estimate comparable to that of the general population. Victims of domestic violence should be identified preconceptionally, because the pattern of violence often escalates during pregnancy. The prevalence of domestic violence during pregnancy ranges from 0.9% to 20.1%, with most studies identifying rates between 3.9% and 8.3%. Whereas violence in nonpregnant women is directed at the head, neck, and chest, the breasts and the abdomen are frequent targets during pregnancy. Physical abuse during pregnancy is a significant risk factor for low birth weight and maternal complications of low weight gain, infections, anemia, smoking, and alcohol or drug use. If it is identified that a patient is the victim of domestic violence, the physician should assess her immediate safety and make timely referrals to local community resources and shelters.

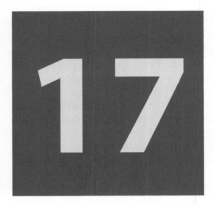

Prenatal Care

Martin Johns, MD
Julie Gallo, DO

Many family physicians assist pregnant women and deliver their infants as a routine part of their practice. According to a 2017 study by the Robert Graham Center, there has been a steady decline in the number of family medicine physicians practicing obstetrics. About 8% of family physicians are practicing obstetrics, and an even smaller number are practicing high-volume obstetrics. The shortage of obstetricians and family medicine physicians delivering babies has put a strain on the access to maternal and fetal care, particularly in rural areas. Practicing maternity care provides an opportunity to establish relationships with an entire family, developing lifelong continuity of care. During pregnancy, women have incentive to initiate preventive care, adopt a healthier lifestyle, quit smoking, and abstain from alcohol consumption. The goal of prenatal care is to promote a healthy pregnancy while minimizing risk to both mother and baby.

▶ General Considerations

Pregnant women receive 13–15 office visits for a typical low-risk pregnancy when care begins in the first trimester. After her initial visit, a woman will see her provider every 4 weeks until 28 weeks' gestation, every 2–3 weeks between 28 and 36 weeks' gestation, and weekly visits from 36 weeks' gestation until delivery. Women at higher risk for complications, or those who develop complications in pregnancy, may be seen more frequently. The World Health Organization (WHO) guidelines from November 2016 for antenatal care recommend a minimum of eight visits: one visit in the first trimester, two visits in the second trimester, and five visits in the third trimester. Eight or more visits for antenatal care can reduce perinatal deaths by up to 8 per 1000 births when compared to four visits.

A 2015 Cochrane review comparing fewer prenatal visits with the standard schedule demonstrated that in high-income countries there was no difference in perinatal mortality in the reduced visit group; this confirmed similar findings to the WHO that there was increased perinatal mortality in the reduced visit group in low- and middle-income countries. Women in all countries were less satisfied with the reduced-visit schedule.

Barreto T, Peterson L, Petterson S, Bazemore A. Family physicians practicing high-volume obstetric care have recently dropped by one-half. *Am Fam Physician.* 2017;95(12):762. [PMID: 28671420]

Carroli G, Dowswell T, Duley L, et al. Alternative versus standard packages of antenatal care for low-risk pregnancy. *Cochrane Database Syst Rev.* 2015;7:CD000934. [PMID: 26184394]

World Health Organization. WHO recommendations on antenatal care for a positive pregnancy experience. http://www.who.int/reproductivehealth/publications/maternal_perinatal_health/anc-positive-pregnancy-experience/en/. Accessed November 11, 2019.

PRENATAL VISITS

▶ Initial Visit

The initial visit should include a detailed history and physical exam, establish an accurate estimated date of confinement/estimated due date/expected date of delivery, and identify risk factors that will require additional testing and monitoring (Table 17–1).

Patient history obtained at this visit includes past medical history, past surgical history, family medical history, and social history. Mothers should also be asked to provide details about previous pregnancies including dates of prior pregnancies; lengths of gestation; methods of delivery; complications during pregnancy; labor courses; events in the postpartum period; and sex, size, and viability of infants. Additional gynecologic history including age of menarche, menstrual history, prior sexually transmitted diseases, gynecologic surgeries, and treatments for infertility should be discussed. Any travel history, specifically to areas endemic with malaria, tuberculosis, and/or Zika virus, is to be noted.

Table 17–1. Initial prenatal visit: basic components.

1. History of current pregnancy: assessment of gestational age and symptoms
2. Prior obstetrical history
3. Gynecologic history
4. Past medical history; chronic illnesses, surgeries, medications, allergies, immunizations
5. Social history: alcohol, drugs, tobacco, occupation, home situation
6. Screen for depression and intimate partner violence
7. Family/genetic history: ethnic background, genetic and congenital defects (include the father's children with other mothers)
8. Physical exam: general and pelvic with attention to uterine size
9. Testing: routine and other tests if indicated by history or exam (see Table 17–5)
10. Risk assessment
11. Patient education and anticipatory guidance

History of the current pregnancy begins by establishing the first day of the last menstrual period (FDLMP). According to Naegele's rule, the average pregnancy is 280 ± 14 days from a reliable last menstrual period (LMP). Using Naegele's rule, estimated due date can be calculated with the following formula: FDLMP + 1 year − 3 months + 7 days. Criteria for a reliable LMP include previous regular menstrual cycles of 28–35 days in length, an LMP that is normal in length, and a normal amount of menstrual flow when off hormonal contraception for 3 months.

If dates are uncertain, you may consider early ultrasound (US). A US-determined crown-rump length in the first trimester (up to and including 13 6/7 weeks' gestation) is accurate ±5–7 days and helps establish the estimated gestational age (EGA). Accuracy improves when the US is performed earlier in the first trimester. Dating based on an US beginning in the second trimester should be considered suboptimally dated.

Exploring the patient's medical history for any chronic problems is important. Preexisting medical conditions such as hypertension, thyroid disease, diabetes, asthma, and depression can impact the outcome of the pregnancy. Reviewing medications taken prior to the onset of pregnancy and any ongoing medication usage requires timely risk assessment. Patients must be converted from medications that are contraindicated in pregnancy to medications that are recognized as safe. These medication adjustments should occur during the initial visit, if not before. Allergies to medications should be reviewed and updated to limit exposure to the mother.

Family history should be reviewed with the patient, including a history of genetic or familial congenital abnormalities. It is particularly important to determine the ethnic background of the patient and the father of the baby because certain ethnicities have a greater likelihood of congenital diseases. Patients from at-risk groups such as Ashkenazi Jews,

Cajuns, and Amish should be offered screening if not done as part of preconception counseling. While gathering family history, it is important to ascertain whether the father has previously sired other children with any genetic or congenital defects.

Asking the patient about tobacco, alcohol, and drug use should always be addressed during the initial visit. Cessation of these substances should be encouraged and patients referred to support sources in the community to help with efforts to quit. Patients with active use of opioids should be referred for conversion to methadone or buprenorphine (Subutex) and outpatient maintenance programs. The practitioner should confirm current job status to determine whether any adaptations will be needed as the pregnancy progresses. Screening for depression with a standard "two-question screen" or the Patient Health Questionnaire (PHQ)-2 should be done at the initial visit and at least once each trimester to reduce the risk of postpartum depression. Patients who answer at least one question positive will then be administered the PHQ-9 (the standardized nine-item PHQ) to determine the presence or absence of depression. Patients who meet criteria for depression should be offered counseling and pregnancy-safe medication if needed. Pregnant women are at increased risk of intimate partner violence. Mothers should be screened for domestic/intimate partner violence using the HITS (Hurt, Insult, Threaten and Scream) screening tool or other validated screening methods.

A thorough physical examination should be performed to document blood pressure, weight, and height. A baseline body mass index (BMI) allows the clinician to counsel on the recommended weight gain during this pregnancy. A pelvic exam is performed to rule out any abnormalities that would preclude vaginal delivery. Bimanual exam facilitates comparison of uterine size with EGA as well as determination of the presence of other anatomic abnormalities like fibroids or malpositioning. First-trimester uterine size should be consistent with EGA on the basis of LMP or other dating parameters. If uterine size is significantly inconsistent with the historically determined EGA, the practitioner should perform an US to determine the discrepancy. Clinical pelvimetry is unreliable in determining the likelihood of vaginal delivery and is not recommended in the United States. Exam with a speculum should be done to identify cervical infection and to complete Papanicolaou (Pap) test screening if not up to date.

After the initial history and physical examination, the practitioner provides trimester-appropriate patient education, including physiologic changes during pregnancy and expectations of the birthing process, and determines patients' risk for less-than-optimal outcomes. The healthy patient with minimal risk can receive usual counseling, routine laboratory testing, and routine follow-up. Patients with an increased risk for genetic diseases or congenital abnormalities can be referred to genetics consultants for further evaluation. Patients with obstetrical or chronic medical problems should be referred to maternal-fetal medicine specialists to help with management or transfer of care.

▶ Subsequent Visits

Follow-up visits allow the maternity practitioner to determine the presence of any problems that would increase risk, address patient concerns, and cultivate the relationship with the patient (Table 17–2). In addition to eliciting patient questions or concerns, the practitioner should evaluate for the following symptoms (possible causes in parentheses):

1. Vaginal bleeding (spontaneous abortion, threatened abortion, placenta previa, placental abruption, ectopic pregnancy)
2. Dysuria (urinary tract infection)
3. Cramping (threatened abortion, preterm labor)
4. Headache or visual changes (preeclampsia, migraine)
5. Nausea and vomiting (multiple gestation, preeclampsia after first trimester, molar pregnancy)
6. Vaginal discharge (sexually transmitted infections, rupture of membranes)
7. Abdominal pain (ectopic pregnancy, threatened abortion, biliary colic, preeclampsia)

The presence of any of these symptoms should prompt further investigation to determine the cause and appropriate intervention. Additionally, the practitioner should ask about fetal movement, which is normally noted between 18 and 20 weeks. Once present, any decrease in frequency should prompt further investigation immediately.

Social issues identified in the initial visit should be reevaluated at subsequent visits. Patients with ongoing tobacco, alcohol, or drug use should be queried at each visit and counseled to quit. Screening for depression should be done each trimester. Patients with a history of intimate partner violence should be assessed frequently because the risk increases as pregnancy progresses.

At each visit, blood pressure and weight are documented. Practitioner-based intervention or referral to a nutritionist

is indicated for patients with excessive weight gain. Blood pressures of ≥140/90 mmHg after 20 weeks of pregnancy documented on two occasions at least 4 hours apart suggest preeclampsia and necessitate further workup including urine testing. Physical exam should include measurement of fundal height, fetal heart tones, and presentation and size of fetus by Leopold's maneuvers. Fundal height is a reliable predictor of gestational age and is measured from the pubic symphysis to the top of the fundus. The fundus can be palpated at the umbilicus at 20 weeks. With growth and progression of pregnancy, the fundus will be 1 cm above the umbilicus for each week of pregnancy correlating to week 20 to 36. For a uterus that is rotated, one should measure in the midline directly across from the uterine fundus. If uterine size varies by >3 cm above or below the EGA, one should look for a cause. Consider polyhydramnios and macrosomia if above the expected fundal height, or oligohydramnios and intrauterine growth restriction if below the expected fundal height. By 34–36 weeks, fetal presentation can be determined. If breech is suspected or presentation is uncertain, an abdominal US should be performed to clarify presentation. For persistent breech presentation, referral for external version should be considered at 37–38 weeks to reduce risk of a cesarean section. Additional examination of other body systems should be guided by patient complaints elicited during the interview.

American College of Obstetricians and Gynecologists. ACOG Committee Opinion No. 524: opioid abuse, dependence, and addiction in pregnancy. *Obstet Gynecol.* 2012;119(5):1070–1076. [PMID: 22525931]

American College of Obstetricians and Gynecologists. ACOG statement on opioid use during pregnancy. https://www.acog.org/About-ACOG/News-Room/Statements/2016/ACOG-Statement-on-Opioid-Use-During-Pregnancy. Accessed November 11, 2019.

American College of Obstetricians and Gynecologists, Task Force on Hypertension in Pregnancy Hypertension in Pregnancy. Report of the American College of Obstetricians and Gynecologists' Task Force on Hypertension in Pregnancy. *Obstet Gynecol.* 2013;122(5):1122–1131. [PMID: 24150027]

Kirkham C, Harris S, Grzybowski S. Evidence-based prenatal care: part I. General prenatal care and counseling issues. *Am Fam Physician.* 2005;71(7):1307–1316. [PMID: 15832534]

Kirkham C, Harris S, Grzybowski S. Evidence-based prenatal care: part II. Third-trimester care and prevention of infectious disease. *Am Fam Physician.* 2005;71(8):1555–1560. [PMID: 15864896]

Table 17–2. Subsequent visits.

1. Patient concerns
2. Focused symptoms review
3. Ongoing alcohol, tobacco, or drug use identified at first visit
4. Depression and intimate partner violence screens each trimester
5. Vitals: blood pressure, weight
6. Exam: fundal height, fetal heart tones, estimated fetal weight, and presentation
7. Testing (see Table 17–5)
8. Risk assessment
9. Patient education and anticipatory guidance

VACCINATIONS

Vaccinations are reviewed at the first prenatal visit. Ideally, a patient will be up to date on expected vaccines prior to the initiation of pregnancy. At least 1 month prior to pregnancy, the measles, mumps, rubella (MMR) vaccine should be completed. Initial blood work will include rubella titers to confirm

Table 17–3. Vaccinations in pregnancy.

1. Indicated: Influenza (inactivated), Tdap
2. Contraindicated: Influenza (live attenuated influenza vaccine), MMR, varicella-zoster, BCG
3. Decision determined with risk versus benefit: Hepatitis A, hepatitis B, meningococcal B, yellow fever
4. No recommendation/inadequate data: PCV13, PPSV23

BCG, Bacillus Calmette-Guérin; MMR, measles, mumps, rubella; PCV, pneumococcal conjugate vaccine; PPSV, pneumococcal polysaccharide vaccine.
Reproduced with permission from Centers for Disease Control and Prevention.

immune status. Between 27 and 36 weeks' gestation, women should be offered vaccination with the tetanus, diphtheria, and pertussis (Tdap) vaccine to provide short-term protection against pertussis (whooping cough) in the infant and reduce risk of maternal pertussis in the postpartum period. Tdap should be administered in each pregnancy. Patients not immune to rubella will need to be identified to ensure that they receive this attenuated live virus vaccine postpartum, as this vaccine is contraindicated in pregnancy. Fathers-to-be and others who will have close contact with the infant after delivery should be encouraged to be immunized with Tdap as well. During the flu season, all pregnant patients without a contraindication to the flu vaccine should be immunized with the current influenza vaccine strain regardless of trimester. Pregnant women are at increased risk for severe complications of influenza. It is important to understand the vaccines that are indicated and contraindicated during pregnancy for the safety of mother and baby (Table 17–3).

Centers for Disease Control and Prevention. Maternal vaccines: part of a healthy pregnancy. August 5, 2016. https://www.cdc.gov/vaccines/pregnancy/pregnant-women/index.html. Accessed May 31, 2018.
Centers for Disease Control and Prevention. Pregnancy and whooping cough. https://www.cdc.gov/pertussis/pregnant/mom/get-vaccinated.html. Accessed May 31, 2018.

ULTRASOUND

The use of US in prenatal care has revolutionized the diagnosis and treatment of fetal conditions during gestation. Additionally, most mothers-to-be expect to have a US at 18–20 weeks' EGA to determine the gender of the fetus while completing the anatomic screen (covered by most insurers regardless of clinical indication). Studies have shown that routinely performed US does not improve outcome versus clinically indicated US for suspected abnormalities in the mother or fetus (Table 17–4). Abnormalities identified on US will require follow-up or referral to obstetrical and/or

Table 17–4. Common maternal and fetal indications for ultrasound studies.

Maternal Indications	Fetal Indications
Uncertain last menstrual period	Fetal number
Uncertain dating	Fetal presentation
Vaginal bleeding	Decreased fetal movement
Pelvic pain	Fetal viability
Threatened abortion	Aneuploidy
Ectopic pregnancy	Abnormal α-fetoprotein
Uterine abnormalities	Polyhydramnios/oligohydramnios
Diabetes	Intrauterine growth restriction
Hypertensive disorders	Macrosomia
Placenta previa	Biophysical profile
Placental abruption	Postdates (missed due dates)
Size not equal to estimated gestational age	Follow-up abnormalities on routine anatomic scan

Data from Ewigman BG, Crane JP, Frigoletto FD, et al: Effect of prenatal ultrasound screening on perinatal outcome. RADIUS Study Group. *N Engl J Med.* 1993 Sep 16;329(12):821–827.

maternal-fetal medicine consultants for management as clinically indicated.

Preboth M. ACOG guidelines on antepartum fetal surveillance. *Am Fam Physician.* 2000;62(5):1184–1188. [PMID: 10997537]

PRENATAL TESTING

▶ Routine Tests in Prenatal Care

Women undergo a standard battery of diagnostic tests as part of routine prenatal care. Routine prenatal testing and the gestational ages at testing are listed in Table 17–5.

▶ Screening for Gestational Diabetes

Gestational diabetes mellitus (GDM) affects approximately 6% of pregnancies in the United States and causes significant maternal and fetal morbidity. The prevalence of GDM varies in direct proportion to the prevalence of type 2 diabetes in a given population or racial or ethnic group and increases with the same risk factors seen for type 2 diabetes such as obesity and increased age. Women with GDM have higher rates of preeclampsia, operative deliveries, shoulder dystocia, and subsequent development of type 2 diabetes. These outcomes may be improved with appropriate diagnosis and treatment of diabetes during pregnancy. The US Preventive Services Task Force recommends that all women should be screened for GDM between 24 and 28 weeks' gestation. The most common approach in the United States is a 1-hour glucose challenge test followed by diagnostic testing for women

Table 17–5. Routine prenatal tests.

Test	Indication	When Obtained	Additional Notes
Blood type and Rh status	Prevention of alloimmunization	Initial visit	
Antibody screen	Prevention of fetal hydrops	Initial visit	RhD-negative women with a negative antibody screen should receive RhoGam at 28 weeks' gestation
Hemoglobin	Anemia	Initial visit	Women with anemia should receive iron supplementation and repeat testing after 6 weeks; consider repeat testing at 28 weeks universally
Hemoglobin electrophoresis	Hemoglobinopathy screening	Initial visit	Testing based on race alone is not reliable in areas of ethnic diversity
Cystic fibrosis screening	Testing for heterozygous carriers of common cystic fibrosis genes	Initial visit	Although not necessary to test universally, information on testing should be made available to all patients
Human immunodeficiency virus	Prevention of neonatal transmission	Initial visit	Repeat at 36 weeks for women at highest risk for infection (commercial sex workers) or in areas of high prevalence
Rapid plasma reagin	Prevention of congenital syphilis	Initial visit	Repeated at 26–28 weeks
Rubella antibody titer	Prevention of congenital rubella syndrome in future pregnancies	Initial visit	Best obtained prior to pregnancy when vaccination is safe; vaccination should occur postpartum if patient is not immune
Hepatitis B	Prevention of neonatal hepatitis B	Initial visit	Infants born to chronic carriers of hepatitis B should receive hepatitis B immune globulin (HBIg) and vaccination against hepatitis B within 12 hours of life
Gonorrhea	Prevent neonatal transmission	Initial visit	Repeat at 36 weeks for women at high risk for reinfection or in areas of high prevalence
Chlamydia	Decrease preterm labor, prevent neonatal transmission	Initial visit	Repeat at 36 weeks for women at high risk for reinfection or in areas of high prevalence
Urine culture	Detect asymptomatic bacteriuria	11–16 weeks	Treatment of positive cultures with antibiotics should be followed by repeat testing to demonstrate eradication
1-Hour glucose (50 g)	Screening for gestational diabetes	24–28 weeks	Women at increased risk for diabetes due to obesity, prior history of gestational diabetes, or strong family history of diabetes should be tested early and then retested at 28 weeks
Group B β-*Streptococcus* culture	Screening for the presence of group B β-*Streptococcus*	35–36 weeks	Bacteria antibiotic sensitivities should be obtained for women allergic to penicillin to guide intrapartum antibiotic therapy; clindamycin is preferred if bacteria are sensitive

with abnormal test results. The glucose challenge test measures plasma glucose 1 hour after a 50-g oral glucose load. Women with abnormal 1-hour testing then require a diagnostic 3-hour oral glucose tolerance test (OGTT). This test uses a 100-g oral glucose load after an overnight fast, with fasting, 1-, 2-, and 3-hour measurements. Two or more abnormal values on OGTT are diagnostic of GDM.

Women at high risk for GDM due to obesity, a prior history of GDM, or a strong family history of diabetes should be screened for diabetes as early in pregnancy as possible with a 1-hour 50-g oral glucose test and a hemoglobin A1c. Abnormal 1-hour testing should be followed by a 3-hour OGTT. High-risk women whose test results are negative before 24 weeks'

gestation should be rescreened at 24–28 weeks' gestation with a 1-hour 50-g glucose test.

Women diagnosed with GDM should monitor their blood sugars four times a day with fasting and postprandial checks. They should receive nutrition and exercise counseling. If this fails to control blood sugars, medications should be initiated for maternal and fetal benefits. Additional fetal monitoring is recommended for women requiring medication to control GDM, usually beginning at 32 weeks.

Women diagnosed with GDM are at a high risk for the development of type 2 diabetes over the next several years after their pregnancy. They should receive counseling on lifestyle measures to reduce the risk of type 2 diabetes.

Follow-up screening for type 2 diabetes begins at the 6-week postpartum visit with a 2-hour 75-g oral glucose test. If negative, the American Diabetes Association recommends that women continue to be screened for diabetes every 3 years.

Committee on Practice Bulletins—Obstetrics. Practice Bulletin no. 190: Gestational diabetes mellitus. *Obstet Gynecol.* 2018; 131(2):e49–e64. [PMID: 29370047]

Correa A, Bardenheier B, Elixhauser A, et al. Trends in prevalence of diabetes among delivery hospitalizations, United States, 1993-2009. *Matern Child Health J.* 2015;19:635–642. [PMID: 24996952]

Garrison A. Screening, diagnosis, and management of gestational diabetes mellitus. *Am Fam Physician.* 2015;91(7):460–467. [PMID: 25884746]

Moyer VA. Screening for gestational diabetes mellitus. US Preventive Services Task Force Recommendation Statement. *Ann Intern Med.* 2014;160(6):414–420. [PMID: 24424622]

Screening for Birth Defects

All women should be offered the option of aneuploidy screening or diagnostic testing for fetal genetic disorders, regardless of maternal age. Genetic testing should be discussed early in the pregnancy so that first-trimester screening options remain available. Referral to a genetic counselor can be helpful for women at higher risk for genetic diseases and can help with counseling, choosing the right test, and interpreting the results.

Women with positive screening tests should be referred for diagnostic testing via amniocentesis (second trimester) or chorionic villous sampling (first semester).

First-Trimester Genetic Screening

Screening for aneuploidy in the first trimester involves both US testing for nuchal translucency (NT) and serum measurement of β-human chorionic gonadotropin (β-hCG) and pregnancy-associated plasma protein A (PAPP-A). NT is a fluid collection seen at the back of the neck. It is larger in babies with Down syndrome and is also present in several other structural anomalies such as congenital cardiac defects, diaphragmatic hernias, and abdominal wall defects. First-trimester testing has a sensitivity of 82–87% with a 5% false-positive rate.

Special training is required to perform NT screening. It is still not available in all parts of the country. Furthermore, NT measurements cannot always be made in the first trimester, depending on the position of the fetus. First-trimester screening does not include screening for neural tube defects, which is included in second-trimester screening. Patients with a normal first-trimester screen should have an α-fetoprotein test performed in the second trimester.

Second-Trimester Genetic Screening

Serum testing for aneuploidy can be performed between 16 and 20 weeks' gestation in the form of the quadruple (quad) screen. The quad screen involves measuring levels of α-fetoprotein, intact β-hCG, inhibin A, and unconjugated estriol. Quad screening has an 81% sensitivity rate for Down syndrome.

Additional Genetic Screening Options

Combining first- and second-trimester screening tests will increase sensitivity for Down syndrome. In sequential screening, women are screened for Down syndrome in the first trimester. If the test indicates low risk, women can then obtain a second-trimester α-fetoprotein level, which is combined with the first-trimester results to calculate a final risk. Sequential screening increases sensitivity for detecting Down syndrome to 95% with a 5% false-positive rate.

Cell-free DNA screening is a newer option for genetic screening. Fetal DNA is released into the maternal circulation primarily from placental cells undergoing apoptosis and comprises approximately 7% of the total cell-free DNA in maternal blood. The test evaluates short segments of DNA to screen for a variety of conditions including trisomies, Rh status, fetal sex, and some paternally derived autosomal dominant genetic abnormalities. The positive detection rate for Down syndrome is 98%, with a 0.5% positive screening rate. Cell-free DNA testing does not provide information regarding the risks of neural tube defects. It should only be used as screening and is not considered a diagnostic test.

ACOG Committee on Practice Bulletins. ACOG Practice Bulletin no.163: screening for fetal aneuploidy. *Obstet Gynecol.* 2016;127(5):e123–e137. [PMID: 26938574]

ACOG Committee on Practice Bulletins. ACOG Practice Bulletin no. 162: prenatal diagnostic testing for genetic disorders. *Obstet Gynecol.* 2016;127(5):e108–e122. [PMID: 26938573]

Gill M, Quezada M, Revello R, et al. Analysis of cell-free DNA in maternal blood in screening for fetal aneuploidies: updated meta-analysis. *Ultrasound Obstet Gynecol.* 2015;45:249–266. [PMID: 25639627]

Malone F, Canick JA, Ball RH, et al. First- and Second-Trimester Evaluation of Risk (FASTER) Research Consortium. First-trimester or second-trimester screening, or both, for Down's syndrome. *N Engl J Med.* 2005;353(19):2001–2011. [PMID: 16282175]

PATIENT EDUCATION

Patient education is an integral part of prenatal care. Beginning with the initial prenatal visit, there are many important pregnancy-related topics to discuss with women. Many women and their partners also take an active role in learning all they can through books and the internet. It is helpful for providers to be able to recommend good, accurate resources for patients and their families. Many offices provide written and web-based content to augment what is taught during the visit. Topics covered during visits are focused on anticipatory guidance and vary by trimester.

First Trimester

During the first trimester and specifically at the initial visit, topics often involve an overview of the practice, dietary and nutritional counseling, patient safety, and lifestyle modifications. Women should receive information regarding the setup of the practice, after-hours phone numbers, members of the care team, and patient expectations. Because miscarriage is common, the warning signs and symptoms of impending pregnancy loss should be reviewed.

Dietary counseling includes recommendations on weight gain based on the woman's prepregnancy BMI. The Institute of Medicine recommendations for weight gain in pregnancy are a helpful clinical tool, but final recommendations should be individualized to the patient. Women should eat a well-balanced diet during pregnancy that is approximately 50% carbohydrates, 20% protein, and 30% fat. There is no benefit to protein supplementation. Women have an increased caloric requirement of approximately 150 calories during the first trimester, 300 calories during the second trimester, and 500 calories in the third trimester. However, the goal should be for healthy food choices and to avoid the idea of "eating for two." All women should take a prenatal vitamin daily, primarily for folic acid to prevent neural tube defects. Folic acid supplementation should be initiated prior to pregnancy, if possible, at a dose of 400 μg daily. This is the dose found in most prenatal vitamins. Women also have increased requirements for iron during pregnancy. In nonanemic patients, a prenatal vitamin should supply all the iron that they require (~15–30 mg elemental iron).

Dietary counseling should also focus on foods to avoid during pregnancy. Certain fish species contain high levels of mercury and should be avoided during pregnancy. These include shark, swordfish, and king mackerel. The US Food and Drug Administration recommends that ≤6 oz of solid white tuna be consumed weekly or ≤12 oz of canned light tuna. Other foods to avoid include unpasteurized dairy products such as unpasteurized cheeses, undercooked meats, and uncooked delicatessen meats, due to the risk for foodborne infections and illness. Caffeine should be limited to <300 mg daily (2–3 cups of coffee), although data on caffeine and adverse pregnancy outcomes are mixed.

Along with dietary hazards, women should also avoid exposure to infections such as influenza, varicella, parvovirus B19, cytomegalovirus, toxoplasmosis, and other infections associated with animals. Environmental and work exposures to toxic substances should be reviewed with the patient, including tobacco, alcohol, and illicit drug exposure and use. Most women can continue working right up to their due date, but those with very physically demanding jobs may have to stop working, especially if they are at risk for preterm labor. Intimate partner violence affects ≤20% of pregnant women, and abuse often worsens during pregnancy. All women should be asked about the safety of their home confidentially but directly. Providers should have a working knowledge of the community resources available in their area for victims of intimate partner violence.

Lifestyle changes associated with pregnancy are a common source of questions, especially regarding sexual activity, exercise, and travel. Most couples can continue normal sexual relations throughout pregnancy but will often have to adjust positions because of the gravid uterus. Sexual intercourse is contraindicated in placenta previa, cervical insufficiency, and preterm labor.

Mild to moderate exercise is safe during pregnancy for most women. Women who are inactive prior to pregnancy can be encouraged to engage in mild exercise to promote physical health and well-being. Low-impact activities such as swimming, water aerobics, and walking are good forms of exercise in pregnancy. Women who were physically active prior to pregnancy can maintain similar levels of exercise during pregnancy with some caveats; specifically, they should avoid activities that could increase the risk of falls and abdominal trauma, such as downhill skiing and horseback riding, and avoid activities that put heavy stress on the abdominal muscles such as pilates. As their center of gravity changes during pregnancy, runners should also be cautious to avoid falls. Maintaining adequate hydration and avoiding overheating are also important considerations. Exercise plans should be individualized based on a woman's prepregnancy fitness level.

Airline travel is safe for women with uncomplicated pregnancies up to 36 weeks' gestation. During the flight, women should wear seat belts when seated, maintain adequate hydration, and move around the cabin as much as possible to avoid venous thromboembolism. Car safety is especially important during pregnancy. Motor vehicle accidents are a leading cause of maternal morbidity and mortality and a common cause for placental abruption. Seat belts must be worn at all times. The lap belt should be worn low across the hips, under the uterus. The shoulder belt should go above the fundus and between the breasts. When taking long-distance car rides, it is important to make frequent stops.

Second & Third Trimesters

Patient education during subsequent visits involves reinforcement of previous recommendations, especially with regard to health and safety such as tobacco, alcohol, drug use, and domestic violence. Anticipatory guidance on the physiologic changes of pregnancy such as heartburn, leg swelling, and hemorrhoids should be covered. Signs and symptoms of preterm labor should be reviewed regularly along with warning signs and symptoms of preeclampsia. Fetal movement monitoring and "kick counts" should be reviewed. Up to 15% of women will call their physicians at some point during the third trimester because of perceived decreased fetal movement. Perform kick counts by having a woman eat something containing carbohydrates and then lie on her left side in a quiet room. With this technique, 10 movements over 2 hours is considered normal fetal movement.

Exclusive breastfeeding, as recommended by the WHO for the first 6 months of life, should be encouraged because of the many benefits to the mother and the baby. Women and their partners are often encouraged to sign up for childbirth classes if available. These classes allow for better understanding of the delivery hospital and the labor process and development of a birth plan. Options for labor anesthesia and analgesia should be discussed during the third trimester.

REFERRAL & MANAGEMENT OF HIGHER-RISK PATIENTS

When pregnant women develop conditions that require higher levels of monitoring and care, it is essential for family physicians to have a close working relationship with their obstetrical consultants. The American Academy of Family Physicians and the American College of Obstetricians and Gynecologists liaison committee has published recommendations for consultations between family physicians and obstetrician-gynecologists. Guidelines for consultation in the antepartum and peripartum period for women who develop high-risk conditions should be clearly established on the basis of local referral patterns and availability of obstetrician-gynecologists and maternal-fetal medicine specialists. All family physicians and obstetricians on the medical staff should agree to these guidelines for the best care of patients. Decisions regarding consultation or transfer of care should be delineated at the time of consultation as well as explained to the patient.

American Academy of Family Physicians, American College of Obstetricians and Gynecologists. Joint statement on cooperative practice and hospital privileges. https://www.aafp.org/about/policies/all/aafp-acog.html. Accessed June 29, 2018.

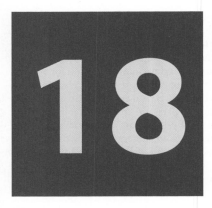

Contraception

Susan C. Brunsell, MD

General Considerations

According to the 2015–2017 National Survey of Family Growth (NSFG), changes in contraceptive method use among married, non-Hispanic white women have contributed to a significant decline in the proportion of unintended births among this group. Sixty-five percent of women of reproductive age are currently using contraception. Contraceptive use has been shown to increase with age; 37% of women age 15–19 compared to 74% of women age 40–49 are using contraceptive methods. Of women age 15–49, the most common methods of contraception are female sterilizations (18.6%), oral contraceptive pills (12.6%), and long-acting reversible contraceptives (10.3%). Use of long-acting reversible contraceptives has increased, whereas fewer women report that their partners are using condoms as their current most effective means of contraception. Addressing family planning and contraception is an important issue for providers of care to reproductive-age women. Because of the wide range of contraceptive options available, it is important that healthcare providers remain current with the recent advances concerning counseling, efficacy, safety, and side effects.

Curtis KM, Jatlaoui TC, Tepper NK, et al. U.S. selected practice recommendations for contraceptive use, 2016. *MMWR Recomm Rep*. 2016;65(4):1–66. [PMID: 27467319]
Curtis KM, Tepper NK, Jatlaoui TC, et al. U.S. medical eligibility criteria for contraceptive use, 2016. *MMWR Recomm Rep*. 2016;65(3):1–103. [PMID: 27467196]
Daniels K, Abma JC. *Current Contraceptive Status Among Women Aged 15-49: United States 2015-2017*. NCHS Data Brief, No 327. Hyattsville, MD: National Center for Health Statistics, 2018.

COMBINED ORAL CONTRACEPTIVES

According to the 2015–2017 NSFG, usage rate of the combined oral contraceptive (COC) pill has decreased to 12.6% for women between the ages of 15 and 44 from a rate of 28% in the 2006–2010 report. The availability of lower-dose COCs (<50 µg ethinyl estradiol) has provided many women a highly effective, safe, and tolerable method of contraception.

COCs suppress ovulation by diminishing the frequency of gonodotropin-releasing hormone pulses and halting the luteinizing hormone surge. They also alter the consistency of cervical mucus, affect the endometrial lining, and alter tubal transport. Most of the antiovulatory effects of COCs derive from the action of the progestin component. The estrogen doses are not sufficient to produce a consistent antiovulatory effect. The estrogenic component of COCs potentiates the action of the progestin and stabilizes the endometrium so that breakthrough bleeding is minimized. When administered correctly and consistently, they are >99% effective at preventing pregnancy. However, failure rates are as high as 9% during the first year of typical use. Noncompliance is the primary reason cited for the difference between these rates, frequently secondary to side effects such as abnormal bleeding and nausea. When appropriate contraceptive counseling is provided, women have higher rates of successful contraceptive use.

Hormonal Content

The estrogenic agent most commonly used in COCs is ethinyl estradiol, in doses ranging from 20 to 35 µg. It appears that decreasing the dose of estrogen to 20 µg reduces the frequency of estrogen-related side effects but increases the rate of breakthrough bleeding. In addition, there may be less margin for error with low-dose preparations such that missing pills may be more likely to result in breakthrough ovulation.

Each COC formulation will have at least one progestin agent included in the active ingredients. There are multiple progestin products that are used in separate COC formulations. Biphasic and triphasic oral contraceptives, which vary the dose of progestin over a 28-day cycle, were developed to decrease the incidence of progestin-related side effects and breakthrough bleeding. Although this was the intention, there is no convincing evidence that multiphasics indeed cause fewer adverse effects. As with estrogens, some progestins (norethindrone and levonorgestrel) are biologically active, whereas others are prodrugs that are activated by metabolism. Norethindrone acetate is converted to norethindrone, and norgestimate is metabolized into several active steroids, including levonorgestrel. Progestins that do not require hepatic transformation tend to have better bioavailability and a longer serum half-life. For example, levonorgestrel has a longer half-life than norethindrone. Norgestimate and desogestrel have lower androgenic potential than other progestins, which would be preferred for patients concerned about acne, oily skin, or hirsutism.

Drospirenone, a derivative of spironolactone, differs from other progestins because it has mild antimineralocorticoid activity. Contraceptive efficacy, metabolic profile, and cycle control are comparable to other COCs. Recent evidence has shown that the diuretic-like potential of drospirenone is generally safe, but because of its antimineralocorticoid effects and the potential for hyperkalemia, drospirenone should not be used in women with severe renal disease or hepatic dysfunction.

COCs are traditionally dosed cyclically, with 21 days of hormone and 7 days of placebo, during which a withdrawal bleed occurs. It is recommended to abstain from sexual intercourse or use a second method of contraceptive protection for 7 days after the inhiation of a COC. It is recommended to counsel the woman, man, or couple of appropriate strategies if a dose is missed.

To address the potential of escape ovulation in the lowest estrogen formulations (20 µg), many regimens reduce the number of hormone-free days to 2–4 days. Extended-cycle regimens or continuous hormonal regimens are safe and acceptable forms of contraception and may be more efficacious than cyclic regimens. Extended-cycle regimens result in fewer scheduled bleeding episodes; however, they also result in more unscheduled bleeding and/or spotting episodes during the first 3–6 months. Women who may particularly benefit from these regimens are those who have symptoms exacerbated by their menses. These include women who have seizure disorders, endometriosis, menstrual headaches, premenstrual dysphoric disorder, menorrhagia, or dysmenorrhea. There are several extended-cycle regimens approved by the US Food and Drug Administration (FDA; Seasonale, Seasonique, Amethyst); however, traditionally packaged COCs may also be prescribed as extended-cycle regimens. Women are advised to use the active pills and then start a new pack, ignoring the placebo pills. This regimen gives women the option of cycling as they desire, modifying the timing of individual periods on a month-by-month basis for personal reasons.

▶ Side Effects

Side effects may be due either to the estrogen component, the progestin component, or both. Side effects attributable to progestin include androgenic effects, such as hirsutism, male-pattern baldness, acne, and nausea. Switching to an agent with lower androgenic potential may decrease or resolve these problems. Estrogenic effects include nausea, breast tenderness, and fluid retention. Weight gain is commonly assumed to be a side effect of COCs; however, multiple studies have failed to confirm a significant effect. Weight gain can be managed by switching to a different formulation; however, appropriate diet and exercise should be emphasized.

Bleeding irregularities are the side effect most frequently cited as the reason for discontinuing COCs. Patients should be counseled that irregular bleeding/spotting is common in the first 3 months of COC use and will diminish with time. Spotting is also related to missed pills. Patients should be counseled regarding the importance of taking the pill daily. If the bleeding does not appear to be related to missed pills, the patient should be evaluated for other pathology such as infection, cervical disease, or pregnancy. If this evaluation is negative, the patient may be reassured. Another approach would be to change the pill formulation to increase the estrogen or progestin component. The doses can be tailored to the time in the cycle when the bleeding occurs. If the bleeding precedes the menses, consider a triphasic pill that increases the dose of estrogen (eg, Estrostep) or progestin (eg, Ortho Tri-Cyclen) sequentially through the cycle. If the bleeding follows the menses, consider Mircette, which has only 2 hormone-free days. Increase the estrogen and/or the progestin midcycle for midcycle bleeding (eg, Triphasil).

COCs may cause a small increase in blood pressure in some patients. The risk increases with age. The blood pressure usually returns to normal within 3 months if the COC is discontinued. Both estrogens and progestins are known to affect blood pressure. Therefore, switching to a lower estrogen formulation or a progestin-only pill may not resolve the problem. It is recommended to monitor the blood pressure prior to initiation of COCs and at every follow-up visit.

Combined oral contraceptives can be safely prescribed after a thorough medical history (including the use of tobacco products) and blood pressure documentation. Although a breast examination, Pap smear, and sexually transmitted disease (STD) screening may be indicated in a particular patient, these procedures are not required before a first prescription of COCs.

▶ Major Sequelae

The use of most oral contraceptives with <50 µg of estrogen approximately triples one's risk of venous thromboembolism (VTE). COCs containing third-generation progestogens (desogestrel but not norgestimate) or the progestin drospirenone have a greater risk of VTE (1.5- to 3.0-fold) over COCs containing levonorgestrel. Bias and confounding in these studies do not explain the consistent epidemiologic findings of increased risk. Evidence has shown that levo-norgestrel, norethisterone, and norgestimate have the lowest risk of VTE. Obesity, increasing age, and the factor V Leiden mutation are contributing risk factors. The best approach to identify women at higher risk of VTE before taking COCs is controversial. Universal screening for factor V Leiden is not cost effective. Furthermore, family history of VTE has unsatisfactory sensitivity and positive predictive value for identifying carriers of other common defects. Although the absolute risk of VTE remains low, women using COCs containing desogestrel and drospirenone should be counseled regarding potential increased risk. An FDA Advisory Committee has concluded that the benefits of COCs likely outweigh the risks in most women.

The risk of thrombotic or ischemic stroke among users of COCs appears to be relatively low. There is no evidence that the type of progestin influences risk or mortality associated with ischemic stroke. The risk of ischemic stroke does appear to be directly proportional to estrogen dose, but even with the newer low-estrogen preparations, there is still a slightly increased risk compared with nonusers. Hypertension and cigarette smoking interact with COC use to substantially increase the risk of ischemic stroke. The risk of hemorrhagic stroke in young women is low and is not increased by the use of COCs. History of migraine without focal neurologic signs is not a contraindication to hormonal contraception.

Current use of COCs is associated with an increased risk of acute myocardial infarction (AMI) among women with known cardiovascular risk factors (diabetes, cigarette smoking, hypertension) and among those who have not been effectively screened for risk factors, particularly for blood pressure. The risk for AMI does not increase with increasing duration of use or with past use of COCs.

Many epidemiologic studies have reported an increased risk of breast cancer among COC users. For current users of COCs, the relative risk of breast cancer compared with never-users is 1.24. This small risk persists for 10 years but essentially disappears after this time period. Although COC users have a modest increase in risk of breast cancer, the disease tends to be localized. The pattern of disappearance of risk after 10 years coupled with the tendency toward localized disease suggests that the overall effect may represent detection bias or perhaps a promotional effect.

▶ Contraindications

The CDC lists several contraindications for COC use, including age ≥35 years old and smoking ≥15 cigarettes per day, hypertension (systolic ≥160 mmHg or diastolic ≥100 mmHg), history of VTE, hypercoagulable mutations, history of ischemic cardiovascular disease, history of stroke, breast cancer, cirrhosis, and migraines with aura. Other methods of contraception are viable options for women with contraindications to COCs.

▶ Noncontraceptive Health Benefits

Most studies evaluating the relationship between COCs and ovarian cancer have shown a protective effect for oral contraceptives. There appears to be a 40–80% overall decrease in risk among users, with protection beginning 1 year after starting use, with a 10–12% decrease annually in risk for each year of use. Protection persists between 15 and 20 years after discontinuation. The mechanisms by which COCs may produce these protective effects include suppression of ovulation and the suppression of gonadotropins.

The use of COCs conveys protection against endometrial cancer as well. The reduction in risk of ≤50% begins 1 year after initiation and persists for ≤20 years after COCs are discontinued. The mechanism of action is likely reduction in the mitotic activity of endometrial cells because of progestational effects.

Numerous epidemiologic studies demonstrate that the use of COCs will reduce the risk of salpingitis by 50–80% compared with the risk to women not using contraception or who use a barrier method. The purported mechanisms for protection include progestin-induced thickening of the cervical mucus so that ascent of bacteria is inhibited and a decrease in menstrual flow resulting in less retrograde flow to the fallopian tubes. There is no protective effect against the acquisition of lower genital tract STDs. Other noncontraceptive benefits of COCs include decreased incidence of benign breast disease, relief from menstrual disorders (dysmenorrhea and menorrhagia), reduced risk of uterine leiomyomata, protection against ovarian cysts, reduction of acne, improvement in bone mineral density, and a reduced risk of colorectal cancer.

Maguire K. The state of hormonal contraception today: established and emerging noncontraceptive health benefits. *Am J Obstet Gynecol.* 2011;205(4 suppl):S4–S8. [PMID: 21961824]

Shulman LP. The state of hormonal contraception today: benefits and risks of hormonal contraceptives: combined estrogen and progestin contraceptives. *Am J Obstet Gynecol.* 2011;205(4 suppl): S9–S13. [PMID: 21961825]

Van Hylckma Vlieg A, Helmerhorst FM, Vanderboucke JP, Doggen CJ, Rosendaal FR. The venous thrombotic risk of oral contraceptives, effects of oestrogen dose and progestogen type: results of the MEGA case-control study. *Br Med J.* 2009;339:b2921. [PMID: 19679614]

TRANSDERMAL CONTRACEPTIVE SYSTEM

A transdermal contraceptive patch containing norelgestromin, the active metabolite of norgestimate, and ethinyl estradiol is marketed by Ortho-McNeil under the trade name Ortho-Evra. The system is designed to deliver 150 μg of norelgestromin and 20 μg of ethinyl estradiol daily directly to the peripheral circulation. The treatment regimen for each cycle is three consecutive 7-day patches (21 days) followed by 1 patch-free week so that withdrawal bleeding can occur. The patch can be applied to one of four sites on a woman's body: abdomen, buttocks, upper outer arm, or torso (excluding the breast).

Ortho-Evra's efficacy is comparable to that of COCs. Compliance with the patch is much higher than with COC, which may result in fewer pregnancies overall. However, pregnancy is more likely to occur in women weighing >198 lb. Breakthrough bleeding, spotting, and breast tenderness are slightly higher for Ortho-Evra than COCs in the first two cycles, but there is no difference in later cycles. Amenorrhea occurs in only 0.1% of patch users. Patch-site reactions occur in 2–3% of women.

Initiation of patch use is similar to initiation of COC use. Women apply the first patch on day 1 of their menstrual cycle. Another option is to apply the first patch on the Sunday after their menses begins. This becomes their patch change day. Subsequently, they change patches on the same day of the week. After three cycles, they have a patch-free week, during which they can expect their menses. A backup contraceptive should be used for the first 7 days of use.

The FDA requires labeling on the Ortho-Evra patch to warn healthcare providers and patients that this product exposes women to higher levels of estrogen than most birth control pills. Average concentration at steady state for ethinyl estradiol is approximately 60% higher in women using Ortho-Evra compared with women using an oral contraceptive containing 35 µg of ethinyl estradiol. In contrast, peak concentrations for ethinyl estradiol are approximately 25% lower in women using Ortho-Evra. In general, increased estrogen exposure may increase the risk of blood clots. The potential risks related to increased estrogen exposure with the patch should be balanced against the risk of pregnancy if patients have difficulty following the daily regimen associated with typical birth control pills.

Burkman RT. Transdermal hormonal contraception: benefits and risks. *Am J Obstet Gynecol.* 2007;197(2):134.e1–6. [PMID: 17689623]

INTRAVAGINAL RING SYSTEM

The NuvaRing vaginal contraceptive ring is a flexible, transparent ring made of ethylene vinylacetate copolymers, delivering an average of 120 µg of etonorgestrel and 15 µg of ethinyl estradiol per day. A woman inserts the NuvaRing herself, wears it for 3 weeks, and then removes and discards the device. After 1 ring-free week, during which withdrawal bleeding occurs, a new ring is inserted. Continuous use has been studied; results are similar to those observed with COCs. Rarely, NuvaRing can slip out of the vagina if it has not been inserted properly or while removing a tampon, moving the bowels, straining, or with severe constipation. If the NuvaRing has been out of the vagina for >3 hours, breakthrough ovulation may occur. Patients may be counseled to check the position of the NuvaRing before and after intercourse.

Peak serum concentrations of etonorgestrel and ethinyl estradiol occur about 1 week after insertion and are 60–70% lower than peak concentrations produced by standard COCs. The manufacturer recommends using backup birth control for the first 7 days of use if not switching from another hormonal contraceptive. NuvaRing prevents pregnancy by the same mechanism as COCs. Pregnancy rates for users of NuvaRing are between 1 and 2 per 100 woman-years of use.

The side effects of NuvaRing are similar to those of COC pills; the main adverse effect is disrupted bleeding. Breakthrough bleeding/spotting occurs in 2.6–11.7% of cycles, and absence of withdrawal bleeding occurs in 0.6–3.8% of cycles. Fewer than 1–2% of women experience discomfort or reported discomfort from their partners with NuvaRing. NuvaRing is associated with increased vaginal secretions, which is a result of both hormonal and mechanical effects. Although 23% of ring users reported vaginal discharge, the normal vaginal flora appears to be maintained. The ring is not associated with either adverse cytologic effects or bacteriologic colonization of the vaginal canal. The contraindications to NuvaRing are similar to those of COCs. In addition, the ring may not be an appropriate choice for women with conditions that render the vagina more susceptible to irritation or that increase the likelihood of ring expulsion, such as vaginal stenosis, cervical prolapse, cystocele, or rectocele.

The Annovera vaginal ring was approved in 2018 by the FDA as the first contraceptive with protection for up to 1 year. Annovera is a flexible silicone ring that is intended to be reused over 13 menstrual cycles. The ring delivers 150 µg of segesterone and 13 µg of ethinyl estradiol per day. The woman inserts the Annovera ring herself (similar to NuvaRing), wears it for 3 weeks, and then removes it for 1 week. The ring is washed and stored in a provided case, which does not require refrigeration. After 1 ring-free week, during which withdrawal bleeding occurs, the Annovera ring is reinserted. The increased ease of use with the need for yearly refill requirements could be favorable for certain patient populations.

The Annovera vaginal ring was originally studied in women age 18–40. Results showed a similar adverse effect profile compared to NuvaRing. The most common adverse effects included headache/migraine, nausea, vomiting, vaginal candidiasis, abdominal pain, and genitourinary tract infections. In clinical trials, 12% of patients appeared to have discontinued Annovera use due to adverse effects. The contraindications to Annovera are similar to those of COCs. The manufacturer recommends using backup birth control for the first 7 days of use if not switching from another hormonal contraceptive. Annovera prevents pregnancy by the same mechanism as COCs. Pregnancy rates for users of Annovera are between 2 and 4 per 100 woman-years with perfect use. Although there are only a few clinical studies, it appears that women will return to ovulation within 6 months of discontinuing Annovera. It is important to note that Annovera was not adequately studied for women >29 kg. The FDA is currently requesting postmarketing studies with concern for drug-drug interactions with CYP3A4 inhibitors, leading to decreased contraceptive efficacy, and Annovera's thromboembolic risk.

Bateson D, McNamee K, Briggs P. Newer non-oral hormonal contraception. *Br Med J.* 2013;346:f341. [PMID: 23412438]

Bitzer J, Simon JA. Current issues and available options in combined hormonal contraception. *Contraception.* 2011;84(4): 341–356. [PMID: 21920188]

Gemzell-Danielsson K, Sitruk-Ware R, Creinin MD, et al. Segesterone acetate/ethinyl estradiol 12-month contraceptive vaginal system safety evaluation. *Contraception.* 2019;99(6):323–328. [PMID: 30831102]

PROGESTIN-ONLY PILL

Progestin-only oral contraceptive pills (POPs), sometimes called the "minipill," are not widely used in the United States. Their use tends to be concentrated in select populations, notably breastfeeding women and those with contraindications to estrogen. Two formulations of POPs are available: one containing norgestrel and one containing norethindrone. POPs appear to prevent conception through several mechanisms, including suppression of ovulation, thickening of cervical mucus, alteration of the endometrium, and inhibition of tubal transport. Upon initiation of POPs, it is recommended to abstain from sexual intercourse or use a second method of contraception for 2 days. Efficacy of POPs requires consistent administration. The pills should be taken at the same time every day without interruption (no hormone-free week). If a pill is taken >3 hours late, a backup method of contraception should be used for the next 48 hours. No increase in the risk for thromboembolic events has been reported for POPs. The World Health Organization has deemed this contraceptive method acceptable for use in women with a history of venous thrombosis, pulmonary embolism, diabetes, obesity, or hypertension. Vascular disease is no longer considered a contraindication to use. The most common side effects of POPs are menstrual cycle disruption and breakthrough bleeding. Other common side effects include headache, breast tenderness, nausea, and dizziness. In general, POP use protects against ectopic pregnancy by lowering the chance of conception. If POP users do get pregnant, an average of 6–10% of pregnancies are extrauterine—higher than in women not using contraception. Therefore, POP users should be aware of the symptoms of ectopic pregnancy.

INJECTABLE CONTRACEPTIVES

Injectable long-acting contraception offers users convenient, safe, and reversible birth control as effective as surgical sterilization. Depot medroxyprogesterone acetate (DMPA) is a 3-month progestin-only formulation that can be administered by deep intramuscular injection (IM-DMPA) into the gluteus or deltoid muscle or subcutaneously (SC-DMPA). Patients using SC-DMPA can be taught to self-administer subcutaneously 4 times per year. Self-administration facilitates access to injectable contraception for many women, eliminating the need for an office visit. In addition to contraception, SC-DMPA is also indicated for the treatment of pain associated with endometriosis.

Studies have shown that DMPA acts primarily by inhibiting ovulation. With typical use, the failure rate of DMPA is 6 per 100 woman-years. Neither increasing weight nor use of concurrent medications has been noted to alter efficacy, apparently because of high circulating levels of progestin.

The first injection of DMPA can be administered at any time throughout the menstrual cycle or within 7 days of a first-trimester abortion. If a woman is postpartum and breastfeeding, then the drug should not be administered until at least 6 weeks postdelivery. When switching from COCs, the first injection may be given any time while the active pills are being taken or within 7 days of taking the last active pill. Repeat injections of DMPA should be administered every 3 months (13 weeks). Guidelines support early repeat injections but do not advise how soon a patient can receive her repeat injection of DMPA. If a patient presents at 15 weeks or later, it is recommended to exclude pregnancy before administering a repeat injection.

The use of DMPA has no permanent impact on fertility; however, return of fertility may be delayed after cessation of use. Fifty percent of women who discontinue DMPA to become pregnant will have conceived within 10 months of the last injection. In a small proportion of women, fertility is not reestablished until 18 months after the last injection.

Menstrual changes are the most common side effects reported by users of DMPA. After 1 year of use, approximately 75% of women receiving DMPA report amenorrhea, with the remainder reporting irregular bleeding or spotting. Some women, especially adolescents, view amenorrhea as a potential benefit of use. Women who voice concern over this side effect can be reassured that the amenorrhea is not harmful. Patients with persistent bleeding or spotting should be evaluated for genital tract neoplasia and infection as appropriate. If these are excluded and the symptoms are bothersome to the patient, a 1- to 3-month trial of low-dose estrogen can be considered or use of nonsteroidal anti-inflammatory drugs (NSAIDs) during days of bleeding (5–7 days). Early reinjection (eg, every 8–10 weeks) does not seem to decrease bleeding.

Other side effects attributed to DMPA include weight gain, mood swings, reduced libido, and headaches. Because of concerns regarding decreased bone mineral density (BMD) after prolonged use, the manufacturer no longer recommends use for >2 years. Reassuringly, results from several studies indicate almost complete recovery of BMD 2 years after discontinuation. Many clinicians recommend that users take supplemental calcium and vitamin D. DMPA may be used safely by smokers ≥35 years old and by other women at increased risk for arterial or venous events. Use of DMPA has not been associated with clinically significant alterations in hepatic function.

IMPLANTS

Implanon and Nexplanon are long-acting reversible contraceptives (LARCs) containing the progestin etonorgestrel, the active metabolite of desogestrel, and are approved for 3 years of use. Etonorgestrel has high progestational activity but weak androgenic activity. A single rod is inserted subdermally on the inside of the upper arm. Both LARCs release etonorgestrel at a rate of 60–70 µg per day initially, which decreases to 25–30 µg by the end of 3 years. Etonorgestrel levels are undetectable 1 week after removal. Nexplanon is bioequivalent to Implanon but has a preloaded applicator designed to reduce the risk of insertion errors. In addition, Nexplanon is radiopaque and can therefore be located by x-ray if necessary. Like other progestin-only contraceptives, the mechanism of action is by inhibition of ovulation and thickening of cervical mucus. The implants are effective, with a pregnancy rate of <1%. Implants are a favorable product for patients due to the ease of use and diminished risk of nonadherence leading to unplanned pregnancy. Irregular bleeding is the primary reason cited for discontinuation, accounting for 13–19% of discontinuations. Other adverse effects include headache, weight gain, acne, breast and abdominal pain, mood swings, depression, and decreased libido. The implants are not associated with decreased BMD or venous thromboembolic disease.

Timing of insertion depends on the patient's recent history. If she is not currently using contraception, insert during the menstrual cycle. If she is using COCs, insert during the pill-free week. If insertion occurs at other times, backup contraception is recommended for the first 7 days after insertion. Ovulation ordinarily returns to normal cycle within 10–14 days after removal of a LARC. Only healthcare providers who receive training from the manufacturer are allowed to order and insert the implant.

Mommers E. Nexplanon, a radiopaque etonorgestrel implant in combination with a next-generation applicator: 3-year results of a non-comparative multicenter trial. *Am J Obstet Gynecol.* 2012;207(5):388.e1–6. [PMID: 22939402]

INTRAUTERINE DEVICES

Currently there are five intrauterine devices (IUDs) marketed for use in the United States. IUDs are considered LARCs that can be used by women of all ages. The most common IUD used is the copper-T 380A (Paragard) made of polyethylene with fine-wire copper wrapped around the stem and copper in the sleeves of each horizontal arm. It is approved for 10 years of use. Two levonorgestrel-releasing IUDs (Mirena, Liletta) contain 52 mg of levonorgestrel. Mirena releases 20 µg of levonorgestrel per day and Liletta releases 18.6 µg of levonorgestrel per day. Kyleena contains 19.5 mg of levonorgestrel, releasing 15.7 µg of levonorgestrel per day. Lastly, Skyla contains 13.5 mg of levonorgestrel and releases 14 µg of levonorgestrel per day. Mirena, Liletta, and Kyleena are approved for 5 years of use, whereas Skyla is approved for 3 years of use. Although all four products have different amounts of levonorgestrel released per day and different approved durations, they all have similar efficacy rates. All four levonorgestrel-releasing IUDs are T-shaped with a polydimethylsiloxane sleeve frame. All IUDs are visible on x-ray.

The contraceptive action of IUDs is probably a result of a combination of factors. The IUD induces an inflammatory, foreign-body reaction within the uterus that causes prostaglandin release. This release results in altered uterine activity, inhibited tubal motility, and a direct toxic effect on sperm. The copper present in the copper-T enhances the contraceptive effects by inhibiting transport of ovum and sperm. IUDs containing a progestin produce a similar effect and, in addition, thicken cervical mucus and suppress ovulation. IUDs are not abortifacients; they prevent fertilization. The IUD is one of the most effective methods of reversible contraception available. Among women who use the IUD perfectly (checking strings regularly to detect expulsion), the probability of pregnancy in the first year of use is 0.8% for the copper-T and 0.2% for the levonorgestrel IUD. The progestational activity of the levonorgestrel IUD reduces menstrual blood loss and has been used to treat excessive uterine bleeding. The IUD may be inserted on any day of the month provided that the woman is not pregnant.

The main benefits of the IUD are a high level of effectiveness, lack of associated systemic metabolic effects, and provision of long-acting, reversible contraception. The most common reason cited for discontinuing the IUD is bleeding. Bleeding can be minimized with the use of a NSAID. However, if persistent or severe, the patient should be evaluated for infection or perforation. Patients can be reassured that the amount of bleeding and cramping usually decreases with time.

Expulsion occurs in 2–10% of women in the first year of use, with most expulsions occurring in the first 3 months. Nulliparity, abnormal amount of menstrual flow, and severe dysmenorrhea are risk factors for expulsion. In addition, the expulsion rate may be higher when the IUD is inserted at the time of the menses. Pregnancy may be the first sign of expulsion. Therefore, patients should be instructed to check for the IUD strings after each menstrual cycle. If a pregnancy does occur with an IUD in place, the IUD should be removed as soon as possible. In the presence of an IUD, 50–60% of pregnancies spontaneously abort. The risk drops to 20% when the

IUD is removed. Septic abortion is 26 times more common in women with an IUD. The copper-T IUD protects against ectopic pregnancy, whereas the progesterone IUD increases the risk of ectopic pregnancy almost twofold.

A common myth about IUDs is that they increase the risk of pelvic inflammatory disease (PID). However, it is now known that the risk of PID is highest in the first 20 days after insertion of an IUD and then returns to the baseline rate. The risk is eliminated if screening and treatment of sexually transmitted infections are done before insertion. Therefore, bacterial contamination associated with the insertion process is the likely cause of infection, not the IUD itself. IUD insertion should be delayed in a woman with active cervicitis. However, women with positive *Chlamydia* cultures after IUD insertion are unlikely to develop PID, even with retention of the IUD, if the infection is promptly treated. The levonorgestrel IUD may lower the risk of PID by thickening cervical mucus and thinning the endometrium. Routine antibiotic prophylaxis is not recommended before IUD insertion.

The incidental finding of *Actinomyces* on cervical cytology is more common in IUD users than in other women. If *Actinomyces* is detected on Pap smear and the patient has signs or symptoms of PID, the IUD should be removed immediately and the patient treated with doxycycline. If the patient is asymptomatic, antibiotic treatment is not recommended and the Pap smear is repeated in 1 year.

The following conditions are contraindications to insertion of an IUD: pregnancy; current or recent cervicitis, PID, or endometritis; uterine or cervical malignancy; undiagnosed vaginal or uterine bleeding; or an IUD already in place. Conditions commonly assumed to be contraindications but are *not* included are diabetes mellitus, valvular heart disease, history of ectopic pregnancy (except for the levonorgestrel IUD), nulliparity, treated cervical dysplasia, irregular menses, breastfeeding, corticosteroid use, age <25 years, and multiple sexual partners. Women with multiple sexual partners should be counseled to use condoms to reduce their risk of STD.

American College of Obstetricians and Gynecologists. Long-acting reversible contraception: implants and intrauterine devices. Practice Bulletin No. 186. *Obstet Gynecol.* 2017;130:e251–e269. [PMID: 29064972]

Ihongbe TO, Masho SW. Changes in the use of long-acting reversible contraceptive methods among U.S. nulliparous women: results from the 2006–2010, 2011–2013, and 2013–2015 National Survey of Family Growth. *J Womens Health.* 2018;27(3):245–252. [PMID: 29148890]

Winner B, Peipert JF, Zhao Q, et al. Effectiveness of long-acting reversible contraception. *N Engl J Med.* 2012;366(21):1998–2007. [PMID: 22621627]

BARRIER CONTRACEPTION

The percentage of women who used a method of contraception during their first premarital intercourse increased from 43% in the 1970s to 78% in 2006–2010. Most of this increase was due to an increase in use of the male condom at first premarital intercourse, from 22% in the 1970s to 68% in 2006–2010 (NSFG 2006–2010). Condoms are inexpensive, easy to use, and available without a prescription. Most commercially available condoms are manufactured from either latex or polyurethane. Although polyurethane and latex condoms offer similar protection against pregnancy, breakage and slippage rates appear to be higher with the polyurethane condom. Natural membrane condoms (made from sheep intestine) are also available; however, they do not offer the same degree of protection from STDs. Because couples vary widely in their ability to use condoms consistently and correctly, the failure rate also varies. The percentage of women experiencing an unintended pregnancy within the first year of use ranges from 2–5% with perfect use to 18–21% with typical use. Women relying on condoms for contraception and protection from STDs should be reminded that oil-based lubricants reduce the integrity of a latex condom and facilitate breakage. Because vaginal medications (eg, for yeast infections) often contain oil-based ingredients, they can damage latex condoms as well.

There are several vaginal barrier contraceptives available that are easy to use and effective. The contraceptive efficacy of all barrier methods depends on their consistent and correct use. The percentage of women experiencing an unintended pregnancy within the first year of typical use ranges from 15% to 32%.

The female condom is a soft, loose-fitting, latex sheath with two flexible rings at either end. One ring is inserted into the vagina and lies adjacent to the cervix. The other ring remains outside of the vagina, against the perineum. Sperm is captured within the condom. The sheath is coated on the inside with a silicone-based lubricant. It is available without a prescription and is intended for one-time use. Female and male condoms should not be used together because the two condoms can adhere to one another, causing slippage and displacement. With correct and consistent use, the female condom can decrease the transmission of STDs, including human immunodeficiency virus (HIV) and acquired immunodeficiency syndrome (AIDS).

The diaphragm is a dome-shaped latex rubber cup with a flexible rim. It is inserted, with a spermicide, into the vagina before intercourse. Once it is in position, the diaphragm provides contraceptive protection for 6 hours. If a longer interval has elapsed, insertion of additional spermicide is required. After intercourse, the diaphragm must be left in place for 6 hours, but no longer than 24 hours. Use of the diaphragm has been associated with an increase risk of urinary tract infections (UTIs). Spermicide exposure is an important risk factor for UTIs (due to alterations in vaginal flora), although mechanical factors in diaphragm use also may contribute to the risk of UTI. Use of the diaphragm requires an appointment with a healthcare provider for education, fitting, and a prescription. Oil-based vaginal products should not be used with the latex diaphragm.

The cervical cap is a cup-shaped silicone device that fits around the cervix. The device can be placed anytime before intercourse, with spermicide, and can be left in place for ≤48 hours. The advantages of the cervical cap over the diaphragm are that it can be left in place longer and it is more comfortable. Like the diaphragm, the cap is manufactured in different sizes and must be fitted by a clinician. The cap needs to be placed directly over the cervix to be effective, so it should not be used if a woman finds the placement to be difficult or uncomfortable.

The contraceptive sponge is a small, pillow-shaped polyurethane sponge containing a spermicide. The sponge protects for ≥12–24 hours, regardless of how many times intercourse occurs. After intercourse, the sponge must be left in place for ≥6 hours before it is removed and discarded. The sponge comes in one universal size and does not require a prescription.

Spermicides are an integral component of several of the barrier contraceptives. Nonoxynol-9, the active chemical agent in spermicides available in the United States, is a surfactant that destroys the sperm cell membrane. It is available in various formulations, including gel, foam, cream, film, suppository, or tablet. Spermicide use may lower the chance of infection with a bacterial STD by as much as 25%. However, women at high risk for acquiring HIV should not use products containing nonoxynol-9. Some studies have shown that it causes vaginal lesions, which could then be entry points for HIV.

FERTILITY AWARENESS–BASED METHODS

According to the NSFG 2015–2017 report, 1.5% of couples reported using a form of fertility awareness–based contraception. This method is generally called the "symptom-based method" or "naturally family planning." The concept of fertility awareness–based methods is to track the woman's menstrual cycle to estimate timing of ovulation during each menstrual cycle. Monitoring cervical mucus, body temperature, and length of the woman's menstrual cycle in days is a key component to the various fertility awareness–based methods. When all three components are monitored together, it is considered the symptothermal method. Using all three methods together has been shown to be more effective than using any one method alone.

The calendar method requires the couple to track the average number of days the woman's menstrual cycle lasts. The ovulation method and Billings method are fertility awareness-based methods that require the couple to track the woman's cervical mucus to determine ovulation and fertility of the woman. The temperature method requires the couple to track the woman's daily body temperature to estimate ovulation and fertility during her menstrual cycle. Basal or rectal thermometers are recommended when recording body temperature for the most accurate reporting. Couples that elect to use a fertility awareness–based method should frequently consult their doctor or counselor to decrease risk of unintended pregnancy.

With typical use, the fertility awareness–based methods have a failure rate of 24 per 100 person-years. Although perfect use is challenging to achieve due to many external factors, studies have shown the method to be >99% effective when perfect use is achieved. Women who take lithium, tricyclic antidepressants, anxiolytics, certain antibiotics, and certain anti-inflammatory medications should not use the fertility awareness–based method due to the alteration of cycle regularity and signs of fertility. Additional contraindications include irregular menses, postabortion, <6 weeks postpartum and breastfeeding, and <4 weeks postpartum and not breastfeeding.

EMERGENCY CONTRACEPTION

As many as half of the unintended pregnancies in the United States result from condom failure, missed birth control pills, or incorrect or inconsistent use of barrier contraception. Optimal use of emergency contraception could reduce unintended pregnancy in the United States by as much as 50%. Emergency contraceptions, available as COCs, POPs, and the copper IUD, are safe and effective. When taken as directed, emergency contraceptive pills (ECPs) can reduce the risk of pregnancy by 75–89% after a single act of unprotected intercourse, whereas a copper IUD inserted within 5 days of intercourse can reduce the risk by 99%.

Emergency contraception is appropriate when no contraception was used or when intercourse was unprotected as a result of contraceptive accidents (eg, condom slippage). Because pill regimens involve only limited exposure to hormones, ECPs are safe. They have not been shown to increase the risk of VTE, stroke, myocardial infarction, or other cardiovascular events. In addition, ECPs will not disrupt an implanted pregnancy and will not cause birth defects. ECPs work primarily by inhibiting ovulation, with some effects on sperm motility and thickening of cervical mucus. Unfortunately, ECPs do not protect against STDs. Of note, women who use hormonal ECP and have a body mass index (BMI) ≥30 kg/m² are at a three times greater risk of pregnancy than women with a BMI ≤25 kg/m².

The use of COCs for emergency contraception is frequently referred to as the *Yuzpe method*. Commercially available COCs containing ethinyl estradiol and levonorgestrel or norgestrel can be used as emergency contraception. Each of two doses separated by 12 hours must contain ≥100 µg ethinyl estradiol plus 0.5 mg levonorgestrel or 1.0 mg norgestrel (eg, four white Lo/Ovral pills per dose). When used correctly, the Yuzpe method decreases expected pregnancies by 75%. More specifically, 8 of every 100 women who have unprotected intercourse once during the second or third week of their cycles will become pregnant; however, 2 of 100 will become pregnant if the Yuzpe method is used. The most common adverse effects are nausea (50%) and vomiting (20%). Antiemetics taken 30–60 minutes before each dose help minimize these symptoms. Other side effects include delayed or early menstrual bleeding. Some women also experience heavier menses.

The most common progestin-only method of emergency contraception consists of 1.5 mg of levonorgestrel taken in one or two doses (Plan B One-Step or Next Choice). The progestin-only regimen is more effective than the Yuzpe method, preventing ≥85% of expected pregnancies. In addition, nausea occurs in <25% of patients, and vomiting is reduced to approximately 5% in women on the progestin-only regimen. Treatment is effective when initiated ≤5 days after unprotected intercourse, and a single 1.5-mg dose is as effective as two 0.75-mg doses 12 hours apart. Once hormonal contraceptive is resumed, it is recommended to use a second method of contraception for 7 days. Instruct women to complete a pregnancy test if they do not have withdrawal bleed within 3 weeks of emergency contraception use. Progestin-only emergency contraception is available without a prescription to women age ≥17 years.

Ulipristal (Ella), a progesterone receptor modulator, was approved by the FDA as a one-dose emergency contraception in 2010. It is effective when taken ≤5 days after unprotected intercourse. Ulipristal has been shown to be more effective than the progestin-only method of emergency contraception during days 3–5 after unprotected intercourse. Its mechanism of action is delay or inhibition of ovulation. Ulipristal requires that a prescription be dispensed. Advise patients to not resume their regular hormonal contraceptive for 5 days after ulipristal use. Once resumed, it is recommended to use a second method of contraception for 7 days. Instruct women to complete a pregnancy test if they do not have withdrawal bleed within 3 weeks of ulipristal use.

To prevent pregnancy, a copper-containing IUD can be inserted ≤5 days after unprotected intercourse. The IUD is highly effective and can be used for long-term contraception. An IUD is not recommended for anyone at risk for STDs or ectopic pregnancy or if long-term contraception is not desired. The IUD is the most effective method of emergency contraception, with failure rates of <1%.

Screening patients for ECP use is based on the time of unprotected intercourse and the date of the last normal menstrual period. There are no preexisting disease contraindications, and inadvertent use in pregnancy has not been linked to birth defects. Neither a pregnancy test nor a pelvic examination is required, although it may be done for other reasons (eg, screening for STDs). If EC use with a copper IUD is ineffective at preventing pregnancy, remove the IUD immediately and rule out an ectopic pregnancy. In contrast, IUD insertion for emergency contraception is an office-based procedure that requires appropriate counseling and screening as for any patient desiring an IUD for contraception.

Counseling regarding the availability of emergency contraception can occur any time that contraception or family planning issues are discussed. It is especially appropriate if the patient is relying on barrier methods or does not have a regular form of contraception. The counseling can be reinforced when patients present with contraceptive mishaps. Information that should be discussed includes the definition of emergency contraception, indications for use, mechanism of action, lack of protection against STDs, instructions on use, and follow-up plans including ongoing contraception.

American Academy of Pediatrics, Committee on Adolescence. Emergency contraception. *Pediatrics.* 2012;130(6):1174–1182. [PMID: 23184108]
Prine L. Emergency contraception, myths and facts. *Obstet Gynecol Clinics North Am.* 2007;34:127–136. [PMID: 17472869]

SPECIAL POPULATIONS

▶ Adolescents

Adolescent pregnancy continues to be a serious public health problem in the United States. Almost 1 in 10 adolescent females becomes pregnant each year, with 74–95% described as unintended. Improved contraceptive practices have contributed to an almost 40% decrease in the teen pregnancy rate. The general approach to adolescent contraception should focus on keeping the clinician-patient encounter interactive. Several suggestions include avoiding "yes/no" questions, keeping clinician speaking time short and focused, and avoiding the word "should."

Abstinence deserves emphasis, especially in young teenagers. Counseling should focus not on "just say no," but rather "know how to say no." Oral contraceptives (COCs) and condoms are the most common contraceptive methods chosen by teens. These methods should be promoted simultaneously as an approach to pregnancy and STD prevention. COC use is associated with health benefits that are especially important during adolescence including treatment for acne and menstrual cycle irregularity, decreased risk of PID and functional ovarian cysts, and decreased dysmenorrhea. The main concern that adolescents have regarding COCs is the development of side effects, especially weight gain. They can be reassured that many studies have proven that COCs do not cause weight gain. Another issue that may contribute to the reluctance of adolescents to seek contraception is fear of a pelvic examination. Contrary to popular belief, a pelvic examination is not necessary when contraception is prescribed, especially if it will delay the sexually active teens' access to needed pregnancy prevention. Adolescents should be counseled regarding missed pills and given anticipatory guidance about breakthrough bleeding and amenorrhea. Adolescents miss on average up to three pills per month, and the risk of contraceptive failure is twice as high among teenagers as it is among women age >30 years. These data underscore the potential benefits of offering adolescents long-acting reversible contraception (injectables, implants, and IUDs) to reduce unintended pregnancy in this high-risk group.

In some respects, DMPA (Depo-Provera) is an ideal contraceptive for adolescents. The dosing schedule allows flexibility and minimal maintenance, and the failure rate is extremely low. However, concerns regarding bone loss in long-term users have prompted the recommendation that use not exceed 2 years. Although available data on adolescents are scant, they indicate that this group may be especially vulnerable to BMD loss. It is not known whether bone loss before achieving peak bone density is recoverable or to what extent the loss impacts the future risk of fracture. In addition, adolescents are likely to demonstrate other risk behaviors for bone loss, including early sexual activity, smoking, alcohol use, and poor diet choices. Until the results of larger studies are available, definitive recommendations in teenagers cannot be made.

The etonorgestrel implant has many advantages for the teen who desires contraception: ease of use, discreet, improvement of acne, reduction of dysmenorrhea, and outstanding efficacy. Despite common misperceptions, implants are not associated with increased risk of VTE or decreased BMD. Unfortunately, despite its ease of use, high efficacy, and safety, many young women choose to discontinue this method early because of problems with unpredictable irregular bleeding.

Vaginal barrier contraceptives are not ideal choices for several reasons. Many adolescents are not prepared to deal so intimately with their own bodies and do not wish to prepare so carefully for each episode of intercourse. However, they can be an effective method for highly motivated, educated adolescents.

A discussion of emergency contraception should be part of contraceptive counseling for all adolescents. To increase the availability of emergency contraception, teens may be provided with a replaceable supply of emergency contraception pills to keep at home. Several studies in adolescents have shown that direct access to emergency contraception increases its rate of use but does not result in repetitive use. Although concern for improper use persists, women who are provided education on the method use the method correctly, and incorrect use does not pose a health risk beyond unintended pregnancy.

Breastfeeding Women

The lactational amenorrhea method is a highly effective, temporary method of contraception. However, to maintain effective protection against pregnancy, another method must be used as soon as menstruation resumes, the frequency or duration of breastfeeds is reduced, bottle-feeding or regular food supplements are introduced, or the baby reaches 6 months of age. Other good contraceptive options for lactating women include barrier methods, progestin-only methods, or an IUD. Some experts recommend that breastfeeding women delay using progestin-only contraception until 6 weeks postpartum. This recommendation is based on a theoretical concern that early neonatal exposure to exogenous steroids should be avoided if possible. The combined pill is not a good option for lactating women because estrogen decreases breast milk supply.

Perimenopausal Women

Women age >40 years have the second highest proportion of unintended pregnancies, exceeded only by girls age 13–14 years old. Although women still need effective contraception during perimenopause, issues including bone loss, menstrual irregularity, and vasomotor instability also need to be addressed. Oral contraceptives offer many benefits for healthy, nonsmoking perimenopausal women. They have been found to decrease the risk of postmenopausal hip fracture, regularize menses in women with dysfunctional uterine bleeding, and decrease vasomotor symptoms.

For perimenopausal women with cardiovascular risk factors, progestin-only methods may be preferred, including POPs, levonorgestrel (or copper) IUDs, contraceptive implants, and DMPA. Barrier methods or sterilization may also be appropriate in select women. Control of dysfunctional uterine bleeding can be obtained with injectable progestogens or the levonorgestrel IUD. Low-dose estrogen can be added to these methods if estrogen replacement is desired and appropriate.

Physiologically, menopause is the permanent cessation of menstruation as a consequence of termination of ovarian follicular activity. Determining the exact onset of menopause in a woman using hormonal contraception can be challenging. Many clinicians measure the level of follicle-stimulating hormone (FSH) during the pill-free interval to diagnose menopause. However, because suppression of ovulation can vary from month to month, a single FSH value is unreliable. In addition, in women using COCs, FSH levels can be suppressed even on the seventh pill-free day. Given that most women do not become menopausal until after age 50 and considering the limited utility of FSH testing, one approach to managing this transition avoids FSH testing entirely. Women continue to use their COCs until age 50–52, at which time they can discontinue use or transition to hormone replacement therapy.

Cornet A. Current challenges in contraception in adolescents and young women. *Curr Opin Obstet Gynecol.* 2013;25(suppl 1): S1–S10. [PMID: 23370330]

Hartmen LB, Monasterio E, Hwang L. Adolescent contraception: review and guidance for pediatric clinicians. *Curr Probl Pediatr Adolesc Health Care.* 2012;42(9):221–263. [PMID: 22959636]

Adult Sexual Dysfunction

Charles W. Mackett, III, MD, MMM

ESSENTIALS OF DIAGNOSIS

▶ Disturbance in one or more aspects of the sexual response cycle.

▶ Cause is often multifactorial, associated with medical conditions, therapies, and lifestyle.

▶ General Considerations

Sexual dysfunction is a disturbance in one or more of the aspects of the sexual response cycle. It is a common problem that can result from communication difficulties, misunderstandings, and side effects of medical or surgical treatment, as well as underlying health problems. Because sexual difficulties often occur as a response to stress, fatigue, or interpersonal difficulties, addressing sexual health requires an expanded view of sexuality that emphasizes the importance of understanding individuals within the context of their lives and defining sexual health across physical, intellectual, emotional, interpersonal, environmental, cultural, and spiritual aspects of their lives and their sexual orientation. Sexual dysfunction is extremely common. A survey of young to middle-aged adults found that 31% of men and 43% of women in the general population reported some type and degree of sexual dysfunction. The prevalence is even higher in clinical populations.

Recognition of sexual dysfunction is important. It may be the initial manifestation of significant underlying disease or provide a marker for disease progression and severity. It should be a consideration when managing a number of chronic medical conditions.

Sexual dysfunction is positively correlated with low relationship satisfaction and general happiness. Despite this, only 10% of affected men and 20% of affected women seek medical care for their sexual difficulties. The key to identification

of sexual function disorders is to inquire about their presence. A discussion of sexual health can be initiated in various ways. Educational material or self-administered screening forms convey the message that sexual health is an important topic that is discussed in the clinician's office. Table 19–1 lists several questionnaires that can be incorporated into self-administered patient surveys for office practices.

Sexual history can be included as part of the social history, as part of the review of systems under genitourinary systems, or in whatever manner seems most appropriate to the clinician. There are many other opportunities to bring a discussion of sexual health into the clinical encounter, as outlined in Table 19–2. Clinician anxiety may be reduced by asking the patient for permission prior to taking the sexual history.

Once the history confirms the existence of sexual difficulties, obtain as clear a description as possible of the following elements: the aspect of the sexual response cycle most involved, the onset, the progression, and any associated medical problems. Asking patients what they believe to be the cause can help the clinician identify possible etiologies. Asking patients what they have tried to do to resolve the problems and clarifying the patient's expectations for resolution can help facilitate an appropriate therapeutic approach. Involving the partner in diagnosis and subsequent management can be very valuable.

Sexual dysfunction is associated with many factors, conditions, therapies, and lifestyle choices (Table 19–3). In some instances, the underlying medical condition may be the cause of the sexual dysfunction (eg, arterial vascular disease causing erectile dysfunction). In other instances, the sexual dysfunction contributes to the associated condition (eg, erectile dysfunction leads to loss of self-esteem and depression). Sexual difficulties can begin with one aspect of the sexual response cycle and subsequently affect other aspects (eg, arousal difficulties causing depression, which can then negatively affect sexual interest).

Table 19–1. Sexual health screening questionnaires.

Sexual Health Inventory for Men (SHIM)
International Index of Erectile Function (IIEF)
World Health Organization (WHO) Intensity Score
Androgen Deficiency in the Aging Male (ADAM)
Female Sexual Function Index (FSFI)
Sexual Energy Scale
Brief Index of Sexual Function Inventory (BISF-W)
Changes in Sexual Functioning Questionnaire (CSFQ)

Nusbaum MR, Hamilton CD. The proactive sexual health inquiry. *Am Fam Physician.* 2002;66:1705. [PMID: 12449269]

DISORDERS OF DESIRE

▶ General Considerations

Difficulties with sexual desire are the most common sexual concern. Over 33% of women and 16% of men in the general population report an extended period of lack of sexual interest. Other investigators have reported prevalence rates as high as 87% in specific populations. Women who were younger, separated, nonwhite, less educated, and of lower socioeconomic status reported the highest rates. Men from the same demographics as well as increasing age reported the highest rates.

Table 19–2. Sexual health inquiry.

Review of systems or social history.
What sexual concerns do you have?
Has there been any change in your (or partner's) sexual desire or frequency of sexual activity?
Are you satisfied with your (or partner's) present sexual functioning?
Is there anything about your sexual activity (as individuals or as a couple) that you (or your partner) would like to change?
Counseling about healthy lifestyle (smoking or alcohol cessation, exercise program, weight reduction).
Discussing effectiveness and side effects of medications.
Inquire before and after medical event or procedures likely to impact sexual function (myocardial infarction, prostate surgery).
Inquire when there is an imminent or recent lifecycle change such as pregnancy, new baby, teenager, children leaving the home, retirement, menopause, "discovery" of past abuse.

Data from Nusbaum MRH. *Sexual Health.* Leawood, KS: American Academy of Family Physicians; 2001; Nusbaum MR, Hamilton C. The proactive sexual health inquiry: key to effective sexual health care. *Am Fam Physician.* 2002;66:1705–1712; Nusbaum M, Rosenfeld J. *Sexual Health Across the Lifecycle: A Practical Guide for Clinicians.* Cambridge, UK: Cambridge University Press; 2004.

Table 19–3. Factors associated with sexual dysfunction.

Aging
Chronic disease
Diabetes mellitus
Heart disease
Hypertension
Lipid disorders
Renal failure
Vascular disease
Endocrine abnormalities
Hypogonadism
Hyperprolactinemia
Hypo-/hyperthyroidism
Lifestyle
Cigarette smoking
Chronic alcohol abuse
Neurogenic causes
Spinal cord injury
Multiple sclerosis
Herniated disk
Penile injury/disease
Peyronie plaques
Priapism
Pharmacologic agents
Psychological issues
Depression
Anxiety
Social stresses
Trauma/injury
Pelvic trauma/surgery
Pelvic radiation

▶ Classification

Decrease in sexual desire can be related to decrease or loss of interest in or an aversion to sexual interaction with self or others. It can be primary or secondary, generalized, or situational in occurrence. Sexual aversion is characterized by persistent or extreme aversion to, and avoidance of, sexual activity. Separating these issues can be difficult. For example, a patient who has experienced sexual trauma may have difficulties with subsequent partners and ultimately develop an aversion to sexual activity.

A common situation in clinical practice is when partners differ in their level of sexual desire. Although most couples negotiate a workable solution, it may cause relationship dissatisfaction. It can also be a marker for extrarelationship affairs or domestic violence.

▶ Pathogenesis

Changes in or a loss of sexual desire can be the result of biological, psychological, social, or interpersonal factors. Numerous medical conditions directly or indirectly affect

Table 19–4. Common medical conditions that may affect sexual desire.

Pituitary/hypothalamic
 Infiltrative diseases/tumors
Endocrine
 Testosterone deficiency
  Castration, adrenal disease, age-related bilateral salpingo-oophorectomy, adrenal disease
 Thyroid deficiency
 Endocrine-secreting tumors
 Cushing syndrome
 Adrenal insufficiency
Psychiatric
 Depression and stress
 Substance abuse
Neurologic
 Degenerative diseases/trauma of the central nervous system
Urologic/gynecologic (indirect cause)
 Peyronie plaques, phimosis
 Gynecologic pain syndromes
Renal
 End-stage renal disease, renal dialysis
Conditions that cause chronic pain, fatigue, malaise
 Arthritis, cancer, chronic pulmonary or hepatic disease

Table 19–5. Drugs most commonly associated with sexual dysfunction.

Drug Class	Negative Effect on Sexual Response Cycle
Antihypertensives	Arousal difficulties
Diuretics Thiazides Spironolactone	Arousal and desire
Sympatholytics Central agents (methyldopa, clonidine)	Arousal and desire
Peripheral agents (reserpine)	Arousal and desire
α-Blockers	Arousal and orgasm
β-Blockers (particularly nonselective agents)	Arousal and desire
Psychiatric medications Antipsychotics	Multiple phases of sexual function

Antidepressants
  Tricyclic antidepressants
  MAO inhibitors
	Arousal and desire

SSRIs	Multiple phases of sexual function
Anxiolytics	Arousal and orgasm
Benzodiazepines	Arousal difficulties
Antiandrogenic agents Digoxin	Arousal and desire
H$_2$ receptor blockers	Arousal and desire
Others Alcohol (long-term, heavy use)	Arousal and desire
Ketoconazole	Arousal and desire
Niacin	Arousal and desire
Phenobarbital	Arousal and desire
Phenytoin	Arousal and desire

MAO, monoamine oxidase; SSRI, selective serotonin reuptake inhibitor.

sexual desire (Table 19–4). Illnesses and medications that decrease relative androgen levels, increase the level of sex hormone–binding globulin, or interfere with endocrine and neurotransmitter functioning can negatively affect desire. In both men and women, sexual desire is linked to levels of androgens, testosterone, and dehydroepiandrosterone (DHEA). In men, testosterone levels begin to decline in the fifth decade and continue to do so steadily throughout later life. For both genders, DHEA levels begin to decline in the 30s, decrease steadily thereafter, and are quite low by age 60.

Decreased sexual desire is a common manifestation of some psychiatric conditions, particularly affective disorders. Several medications can negatively affect desire and the sexual response cycle (Table 19–5). The agents most commonly associated with these changes are psychoactive drugs, particularly antidepressants, and medications with antiandrogen effects. Many psychosocial issues affect sexual desire. Factors as widely varied as religious beliefs, primary sexual interest in individuals outside the main relationship, specific sexual phobias or aversions, fear of pregnancy, lack of attraction to partner, and poor sexual skills in the partner can all diminish sexual desire.

▶ Clinical Findings

A. Symptoms and Signs

Evaluation of decreased sexual desire should include a detailed sexual problem history, which may clarify difficulties with sexual desire, identify predisposing conditions, and help establish a therapeutic plan. In addition to loss of desire, a diminished sense of well-being, depression, lethargy, osteoporosis, loss of muscle mass, and erectile dysfunction are other manifestations of androgen deficiency.

Physical examination should be directed toward the identification of unrecognized conditions such as endocrine abnormalities (eg, hypogonadism, hypothyroidism).

B. Laboratory Findings

Assessment of hormone status may be helpful. In men, assess androgen status. In women, assess both androgens and estrogen status.

Assessment of the total plasma testosterone level, obtained in the morning, is the most readily available study. In most men, levels below 300 ng/dL are symptomatic of hypogonadism; however, 200 ng/dL might be a more appropriate cutoff for diagnosis in older men. Free testosterone more accurately reflects bioavailable androgens. Levels <50 pg/mL suggest hypogonadism. If low testosterone is confirmed, further endocrine assessment and imaging are indicated to determine the specific underlying etiology.

▶ Treatment

Treatment is directed at the underlying etiology and consists of both nonspecific and specific therapy. Educating couples about the impact of extraneous influences—fatigue, preoccupation with childrearing, work-related stress, and interpersonal conflict—can improve awareness of these issues. Encouraging couples to set time aside for themselves, to schedule "dates," can be very effective. Educating partners about gender generalities and encouraging communication about sexual desires can be helpful. The quality of the relationship appears to be a critical component in women's sexual response cycle. Filbanserin, a multifunctional serotonin agonist antagonist, is approved by the US Food and Drug Administration (FDA) in low doses for sexual desire disorder in premenopausal women; however, it may cause severe hypotension and must be used with caution with alcohol.

An emotionally and physically satisfying relationship enhances sexual desire and arousal and has a positive feedback on the quality of the relationship. The importance of allowing time for sexual relations, incorporating the senses, understanding what is pleasing to one's partner, and incorporating seduction cannot be overemphasized.

The impact of potentially reversible medical conditions or medications on sexual desire should be addressed. Treating organic etiologies such as depression, hypothyroidism, hyperprolactinemia, and androgen deficiency can often restore sexual interest.

When medications affect desire, treatment approaches can include lowering the dosage, suggesting drug holidays, discontinuing potentially offensive medications, or switching to a different agent. Where continuation of therapy is indicated, adding specific agents to address the sexual manifestations can be useful. Hormone supplementation may be considered.

A. Androgen Replacement

The goal of replacement therapy is to raise the level to the lowest physiologic range that promotes satisfactory response (Table 19–6). Oral testosterone is not recommended due to the prominent first-pass phenomenon and the potential for significant liver toxicity. Intramuscular injections result in dramatic fluctuations in blood levels. Topical preparations offer the advantage of consistent levels in the normal range. Local skin reactions are common with patches. Topical gels tend to have fewer skin side effects.

Table 19–6. Androgen therapy: agents, routes, and dosages.

Route/Agent	Dosage for Women	Dosage for Men (mg/d)
Oral[a]		
Methyltestosterone	10 mg: ¼–½ tablet daily or 10 mg Monday, Wednesday, Friday	10–50
Fluoxymesterone	2 mg: ½ tablet daily or 1 tablet every other day	5–20
Estratest and Estratest HS	Either 1.25 or 0.625 mg	
Dehydroepiandrosterone	25–75 mg 3 times weekly to daily[a]	
Buccal		
Methyltestosterone[c]	5–25 mg daily USP tablet, 0.25 mg[b]	5–25
Sublingual		
Methyltestosterone	0.25 mg[b]	
Testosterone micronized USP tablet		
Transdermal		
Testosterone patch	2.5–5.0 mg applied every day or every other day	4–6
Topical testosterone	1% vaginal cream daily to clitoris and labia	5–10 (Androderm)
Testosterone micronized	1–2% gel daily to clitoris and labia[b]	
Intramuscular		
Testosterone enanthate	200 mg/mL: 0.25–0.5 mL every 3–5 weeks	50–400 mg every 2–4 weeks
Testosterone propionate	100 mg/mL: 0.25–0.5 mL every 3–4 weeks	25–50 mg 2–3 times weekly

[a]Oral methyltestosterone, aside from the combination Estratest, should be used only short term due to the risk of hepatotoxicity.
[b]Must be compounded by a pharmacist.
[c]Guay A. Advances in the management of androgen deficiency in women. *Med Aspects Hum Sex.* 2001;1:32–38.
Data from Nusbaum M, Rosenfeld J. *Sexual Health Across the Lifecycle: A Practical Guide for Clinicians.* Cambridge, UK: Cambridge University Press; 2004.

A diagnosis of androgen insufficiency is appropriate only in women who are adequately estrogenized, whose free testosterone is at or below the lowest quartile of the normal range for the reproductive age (20–40 years), and who present with clinical symptoms.

Androgen supplementation can be helpful for desire and arousal difficulties in both men and women (strength of recommendation: B). Dehydroepiandrosterone sulfate (DHEAS) is available over the counter and is dosed at 25–75 mg/d on the basis of response. Transdermal testosterone can be compounded as 1–2% cream, gel, or lotion that can be applied to the labial and clitoral area. Oral methyltestosterone, available as esterified estrogen/methyltestosterone for women, has been used safely for years. Oral administration of methyltestosterone is a less preferred route, given erratic absorption and concerns about liver effects.

Exogenous estrogens and progestins lower physiologically available androgens and can contribute to decreased sexual interest. Addition of androgens, methyltestosterone, or DHEAS can offset this negative impact. If no benefit occurs from this change, the physician should reassess the quality of the sexual relationship and also consider discontinuing the exogenous hormones. All oral contraceptive agents lower bioavailable androgen levels as a result of high sex hormone–binding globulin levels. Changing to oral contraceptive pills with greater androgen activity, such as those containing norgestrel, levonorgestrel, and norethindrone acetate, may be an effective change (Table 19–7).

B. Contraindications and Risk of Testosterone Therapy

Because testosterone treatment may stimulate tumor growth in androgen-, estrogen-, or progesterone-dependent cancers, it is contraindicated in men with prostate cancer and in men and women with a history of breast cancer. Although it is known that testosterone accelerates the clinical course of prostate cancer, there is no conclusive evidence that testosterone therapy increases the incidence of prostate cancer.

Certain patient populations such as the elderly and patients who have a first-degree relative with prostate cancer

Table 19–7. Relative androgenicity of progestational components of oral contraceptive agents.

Least
Norethindrone (0.4–0.5 mg)[a]
Norgestimate (0.18–0.25 mg)
Desogestrel (0.15 mg)
Ethynodiol diacetate (1.0 mg)
Medium/neutral
Norethindrone (0.5–1.0 mg)[a]
Greatest
Levonorgestrel (0.1–0.15 mg)
Norgestrel (0.075–0.5 mg)
Norethindrone acetate (1.0–1.5 mg)

[a]Norethindrone (0.35 mg) without estrogen, in progestin-only oral contraceptive pills, has medium relative androgenicity.
Data from Nusbaum MRH. *Sexual Health.* American Academy of Family Physicians; 2001 and Burham T, Short R: *Drug Facts and Comparisons.* Philadelphia, PA: Mosby; 2001.

may be at increased risk. Preexisting sleep apnea and hyperviscosity, including deep venous thrombosis or pulmonary embolism, are relative contraindications to testosterone use. Serious hepatic and lipid changes have been associated with the use of oral preparations. Benign prostatic hypertrophy, lipid changes, gynecomastia, sleep apnea, and increased oiliness of skin or acne are other reported side effects.

If androgen therapy is initiated for both men and women, close follow-up is recommended to assess androgen levels, lipid profile, hematocrit levels, and liver function. Periodic assessment of the prostate-specific antigen level may be considered. Until more data regarding long-term use are available, it is probably most prudent to check androgen, hematocrit, liver, and lipid levels every 3–6 months.

Faubion SS, Rullo JE. Sexual dysfunction in women: a practical approach. *Am Fam Physician.* 2015;92(4):281–288. [PMID: 26280233]
Petering RC, Brooks NA. Testosterone therapy: review of clinical applications. *Am Fam Physician.* 2017;96(7):441–449. [PMID: 29094914]

DISORDERS OF EXCITEMENT & AROUSAL

▶ General Considerations

Arousal disorders affect 18.8% of women and 5% of men in the general population. Prevalence of arousal difficulties is much higher in patient populations with coexisting illnesses such as depression, diabetes, and heart disease. Abuse also has a negative effect on arousal and sexual health.

▶ Pathogenesis

Arousal difficulties most likely result from a mix of organic and psychogenic etiologies. Organic causes include vascular, neurogenic, and hormonal etiologies. Vascular arterial or inflow problems are by far the most common. Regardless of the primary etiology, a psychological component frequently coexists. Optimal function requires an intact nervous system and responsive arterial vasculature. Sexual stimulation results in nitric oxide release, which initiates a cascade of events leading to a dramatic increase in blood flow to the penis, vagina, and clitoris. Nitric oxide causes an increase in the production of cyclic guanosine monophosphate (cGMP). As cGMP concentrations rise, vascular smooth muscle relaxes, allowing increased arterial blood flow. The cGMP buildup is countered by the enzyme phosphodiesterase type 5 (PDE5).

Inhibiting the action of PDE5 results in higher levels of cGMP, causing increased and sustained vasodilation. Arousal disorders appear to increase with age, but chronic illnesses and therapeutic intervention are more likely the root cause. Lifestyle factors such as tobacco, alcohol, exercise, and diet also contribute.

▶ Clinical Findings

A. Symptoms and Signs

The first step in assessment is to ensure that arousal is the primary problem. Some men may complain of erectile difficulties but, on detailed questioning, may lack desire or may have premature ejaculation. Detailed information about the onset, duration, progression, severity, and association with medical conditions, medications, and psychosocial factors will enable the provider to identify if the patient's problem has a primarily organic or psychogenic etiology.

Physical examination should be focused and directed by the history. The clinician should assess overall health, including lifestyle topics such as exercise, tobacco use, and alcohol use. Screening for manifestations of affective, cardiovascular, neurologic, or hormonal etiology should be performed.

B. Laboratory Findings

If not previously done, a lipid profile and fasting blood glucose may identify unrecognized systemic disease that can predispose to vascular disease. Measurement of androgen levels (including DHEA) should be performed if androgen supplementation is being considered.

▶ Treatment

Chronic medical conditions should be treated to reverse or slow their progression. Medications contributing to arousal problems (eg, antihypertensive agents) should be replaced with other agents, if possible, or reduced in dosage. Potentially reversible causes should be addressed.

Glucose control, moderating alcohol consumption, exercise (strength of recommendation: B), and smoking cessation (strength of recommendation: A) are important lifestyle changes necessary to maintain healthy sexual response. Nitric oxide appears to be androgen sensitive, so correction of androgen levels may be necessary before PDE5 inhibitors will be successful. Sexual lubricants such as Astroglide, Replens, and K-Y jelly can add lubrication and enhance sensuality.

A. Oral Agents

Sildenafil, vardenafil, tadalafil, and avanafil are PDE5 inhibitors and are the first-line treatment for male erectile dysfunction (strength of recommendation: A). Inhibitors do not result in spontaneous erection and require erotic or physical stimulation to be effective. PDE5 inhibitors are contraindicated in patients who take organic nitrates of any type. Nitrates are nitric oxide donors. The concomitant use of a PDE5 inhibitor and a nitrate can result in profound hypotension. PDE5 inhibitors are also contraindicated in patients with recent cardiovascular events or who are clinically hypotensive.

The side effects of PDE5 inhibitors are related to the presence of PDE5 in other parts of the body and cross-reactivity with other PDE enzyme subtypes. A transient disturbance in color vision, characterized typically by a greenish-blue hue, is due to a slight cross-reactivity with PDE5 isoenzyme in the retina. Because of this cross-reactivity, PDE5 inhibitors should not be used in patients with retinitis pigmentosa. Side effects tend to be mild and transient and include headache, flushing, dyspepsia, and rhinitis.

PDE5 inhibitors are not approved by the FDA for use in women, and their role in treating female arousal difficulties remains controversial. Studies of genital stimulation devices and topical warming gels have shown these adjuncts to be beneficial to sexual functioning.

B. Vacuum Constriction Devices

These devices are effective for most causes of erectile dysfunction, are noninvasive, and are a relatively inexpensive treatment option. The device consists of a cylinder, vacuum pump, and constriction band. The flaccid penis is placed in the cylinder. Pressing the cylinder against the skin of the perineum forms an airtight seal. Negative pressure from the pump draws blood into the penis, resulting in increased firmness. When sufficient blood has entered the erectile bodies, a constriction band is placed around the base of the penis, preventing the escape of blood. Following intercourse, the band is removed. Side effects include penile pain, bruising, numbness, and impaired ejaculation.

C. Intracavernosal Injection

With this method, synthetic formulations of prostaglandin E_1 (alprostadil alone or in combination with other vasoactive agents) are injected directly into the corpus cavernosum. This results in spontaneous erection. Intracavernosal injection is effective in producing erection in most patients with erectile dysfunction, including some who failed to respond to oral therapy.

D. Penile Prosthesis

In patients not responding to other therapies, a permanent penile prosthesis has proven to be safe and effective in many patients. Current models have a 7- to 10-year life expectancy or longer. Overall patient satisfaction is excellent.

▶ Sexual Pain Syndromes

Sexual pain syndromes can negatively affect arousal. Sexual pain syndromes occur in 14% of women and 3% of men in the general population, and >70% of samples of female patients. Peyronie plaques or other penile deformity, priapism, and lower urinary tract symptoms can be etiologic in male sexual pain syndrome. For women, vaginitis, vestibulitis, pelvic pathology, vaginismus, and inadequate vaginal lubrication may cause sexual pain. Sexual pain syndromes negatively affect desire, arousal, and thus orgasm.

Nusbaum MRH, Gamble G, Skinner B, et al. The high prevalence of sexual concerns among women seeking routine gynecological care. *J Fam Pract.* 2000;49:229–232. [PMID: 1073548]

Rew KT, Heidelbaugh JJ. Erectile dysfunction. *Am Fam Physician.* 2016;94(10);820–827. [PMID: 27929275]

DISORDERS OF EJACULATION & ORGASM

Premature ejaculation affects 29% of men in the general population, and orgasm difficulties affect 8% of men and 24% of women. Over 80% of women in patient populations report difficulties with orgasm.

Premature ejaculation results from a shortened plateau phase. In addition to heightened sensitivity to erotic stimulation and, often, learned behavior from rushed sexual encounters, organic etiology is also likely. The ejaculatory reflex involves a complex interplay between central serotonergic and other neurons. Premature ejaculation is speculated to be a dysfunction of serotonergic receptors.

Although premature ejaculation tends to improve with age by the natural lengthening of the plateau phase, it persists for many men. Like erectile dysfunction, premature ejaculation is often associated with shame and depression. Orgasmic difficulties can feed back negatively on arousal and then desire. Difficulty achieving orgasm affects a greater number of women than men and typically results from a prolonged arousal phase caused by inadequate stimulation. Medications can also interfere. Selective serotonin reuptake inhibitors (SSRIs) raise the threshold for orgasm, which makes them highly effective treatment options for men with premature ejaculation, but highly problematic for both genders who have difficulty achieving orgasm. Medications that lower the threshold for orgasm can be very problematic for men with premature ejaculation but can be very effective for treating problems with orgasm. These include cyproheptadine, bupropion, and possibly PDE5 inhibitors, which can be helpful for men with delayed ejaculation. Psychotropic agents and alcohol often delay ejaculation. Medications for treating sexual side effects of psychotropic agents or for women having difficulty with orgasm are also useful for treating delayed ejaculation (Table 19–8).

Retrograde ejaculation is caused by abnormal function of the internal sphincter of the urethra and can result from anatomic disruption (eg, transurethral prostatectomy), sympathetic nervous system disruptions (eg, damage from surgery), lymph node invasion, or diabetes. Retrograde ejaculation can result from interference with the sphincter function from medications such as antipsychotics, antidepressants, and antihypertensive agents as well as alcohol use. Dextroamphetamine, ephedrine, phenylpropanolamine, and pseudoephedrine are potentially effective in treating retrograde ejaculation.

Table 19–8. Antidotes for psychotropic-induced sexual dysfunction.

Drug	Dosage
Yohimbine	5.4–16.2 mg, 2–4 hours prior to sexual activity
Bupropion	100 mg as needed or 75 mg 3 times a day
Amantadine	100–400 mg as needed or daily
Cyproheptadine	2–16 mg a few hours before sexual activity
Methylphenidate	5–25 mg as needed
Dextroamphetamine	5 mg sublingually 1 hour prior to sex
Nefazodone	150 mg 1 hour prior to sex
Sildenafil	50–100 mg as needed

Data from Nusbaum MRH: *Sexual Health*. American Academy of Family Physicians; 2001 and Maurice W: *Sexual Medicine in Primary Care.* Philadelphia, PA: Mosby; 1999.

Evaluation should include a history of sexual problems, medications, and quality of the relationship. Treatment approaches include discontinuing, decreasing the dosage of, or drug holidays from offending medications. Small studies have shown a benefit from rescue agents that can be added as standing (or as needed) medications (see Table 19–8). SSRIs are the treatment of choice for premature ejaculation. It is helpful if women become familiar with the type of stimulation they require for orgasm and communicate that to their partners. An excellent reference for patients is the book by Nagowski (2015).

The resolution phase is typically not problematic for either gender, but misunderstandings of age-related changes can occur. Men, and their partners, need to understand that with increasing age the refractory period to sexual stimulation lengthens, sometimes up to 24 hours. Men may require more direct penile stimulation for sexual response as they age.

McMahon CG, Abdo C, Incrocci L, et al. Disorders of orgasm and ejaculation in men. *J Sex Med.* 2004;1(1)58–65. [PMID: 16422984]

Nagwoski E. *Come as You Are: The Surprising New Science That Will Transform Your Sex Life.* New York, NY: Simon & Schuster; 2015.

SEXUAL ACTIVITY & CARDIOVASCULAR RISK

Sexual activity and intercourse are associated with physiologic changes in heart rate and blood pressure. A patient's ability to meet the physiologic demands related to sexual activity should be assessed, particularly if the patient is not accustomed to the level of activity associated with sex or may be at increased risk for a cardiovascular event. Typical sexual intercourse is associated with an oxygen expenditure of 3–4 metabolic equivalents (METS), whereas vigorous sexual intercourse can expend 5–6 METS. Patients unaccustomed to the level of exercise associated with sexual activity and who have risk factors for cardiovascular events should be considered for cardiovascular screening. Men with erectile dysfunction are at significantly increased risk for cardiovascular, cerebrovascular, and peripheral vascular disease.

Jackson G, Rosen RC, Kloner RA, et al. The second Princeton consensus on sexual dysfunction and cardiac risk: new guidelines for sexual medicine. *J Sex Med.* 2006;3(1)28–36. [PMID: 11556163]

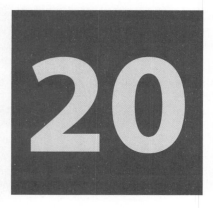

Acute Coronary Syndrome

Stephen A. Wilson, MD, MPH, FAAFP
Suzan Skef, MD, MS
Victoria McCurry, MD
Jacqueline S. Weaver-Agostoni, DO, MPH

▶ General Considerations

Acute coronary syndrome (ACS) encompasses unstable angina, ST-segment elevation myocardial infarction (STEMI), and non–ST-segment elevation myocardial infarction (NSTEMI). It is the symptomatic cardiac end product of cardiovascular disease (CVD) resulting in reversible or irreversible cardiac injury and even death.

▶ Diagnosis

The diagnosis of ACS requires two of the following: ischemic symptoms, diagnostic electrocardiogram (ECG) changes, or elevated serum marker of cardiac injury.

A. Symptoms

By themselves, signs and symptoms are not enough to diagnose or rule out ACS, but they start the investigatory cascade. Having known risk factors for coronary artery disease (CAD) (Table 20–1) or prior ACS increases the likelihood of ACS. Up to one-third of people with CAD progress to ACS with chest pain. Although chest pain is the predominant symptom of ACS, it is not always present. Symptoms include the following:

- Chest pain
  - Classic: substernal pain that occurs with exertion and alleviates with rest (in a person with a history of CAD, this is called "typical" or "stable" angina)
  - Dull, heavy pressure in or on the chest
  - Sensation of a heavy object on the chest
  - Initiated by stress, exercise, large meals, sex, or any activity that increases the body's demand on the heart for blood
  - Lasting >20 minutes
  - Change in quality or quantity over the preceding 24 hours
  - Radiating to the back, neck, jaw, left arm or shoulder, or both arms
  - Accompanied by feeling clammy or sweaty
  - Associated with sensation of dry mouth (women)
  - Not affected by inspiration
  - Not reproducible with chest palpation
  - Similar to a prior myocardial infarction (MI)
  - Left arm pain without chest pain
- Right-sided chest pain, occasionally
  - More common in African American patients
- Pain high in the abdomen or chest, nausea, and back pain; can occur in anyone but are more common in women
- Extreme fatigue or edema after exercise
- Indigestion or dyspepsia
- Shortness of breath
  - This can be the only sign in the elderly
  - More common in black than white patients
  - More common in women than men
- Levine's sign—chest discomfort described as a clenched fist over the sternum (the patient will clench his/her fist and rest it on or hover it over his/her sternum)
- Angor animi—great fear of impending doom/death
- Nausea, lightheadedness, or dizziness
- Less commonly
  - Mild, burning chest discomfort
  - Sharp chest pain
  - Pain that radiates to the right arm or back
  - A sudden urge to defecate in conjunction with chest pain

Chest pain that is present for days, is pleuritic, is positional, or radiates to the lower extremities or above the mandible is less likely to be cardiac in origin.

Table 20–1. Risk factors for coronary artery disease (CAD).

Nonmodifiable/Uncontrollable
Male sex
Age: men ≥45 years old
     women ≥55 years old or postmenopausal
Positive family history of CAD

Modifiable with Demonstrated Morbidity and Mortality Benefits

Hypertension	Overweight and obesity
Diabetes mellitus	Abdominal obesity
Dyslipidemia	Physical inactivity
HDL <35 mg/dL	Smoking tobacco
LDL >130 mg/dL	Low fruit and vegetable intake
Left ventricle hypertrophy	Excessive alcohol intake[a]

Potentially Modifiable but without Demonstrated Mortality and Morbidity Effects

Obstructive sleep apnea	Elevated uric acid
Depression	Lipoprotein(a)
Hypertriglyceridemia	Fibrinogen
Hyperhomocysteinemia	Elevated high-sensitivity C-reactive protein
Hyperreninemia	Stress

[a]>2 drinks per day in men, >1 drink per day in women and lighter-weight persons; 1 drink = 0.5 oz (15 mL) of ethanol: 12 oz beer, 5 oz wine, or 1.5 oz 80-proof whiskey.
HDL, high-density lipoprotein; LDL, low-density lipoprotein.

B. Physical Findings

Examination findings that increase the suspicion that symptoms are from ACS include hypotension, diaphoresis, and systolic heart failure indicated by a new S_3 gallop, new or worsening mitral valve regurgitation, pulmonary edema, and jugular venous distention. However, most patients with ACS have normal physical exams.

Chest pain reproducible with palpation is significantly less likely to be ACS.

C. Diagnostic Testing

Anyone suspected of having ACS should be evaluated with a 12-lead ECG and the serum cardiac biomarker troponin. CPK-MB is no longer used.

Notable ECG findings are as follows:

- ST-T segment (>1-mm elevation or depression) and T-wave (inversion) changes suggest ischemia.

- Q wave suggests accomplished infarction.

- ST elevation is absent in unstable angina and non–ST-segment elevation ACS.

- New bundle branch block or sustained ventricular tachycardia could indicate an evolving ACS event, particularly in setting of chest pain or elevated troponin.

Accurate ECG interpretation is essential for diagnosis, risk stratification, and guiding the treatment plan. Many findings are nonspecific, and the preexisting presence of bundle branch block, interventricular conduction delay, or Wolff-Parkinson-White syndrome reduces the diagnostic reliability of an ECG in patients with chest pain. If there is a recent ECG for comparison, the presence of a new bundle branch block or interventricular conduction delay raises the suspicion of ACS.

A normal ECG does *not* exclude ACS. Up to 25–50% of people with angina or silent ischemia have a normal ECG; 10% of ACS is subsequently diagnosed with a MI after an initial normal ECG.

The validated risk scoring tools used to predict ACS—HEART (history, ECG, age, risk factors, and troponin) and Thrombolysis in Myocardial Infarction (TIMI)—both include assessment of initial troponin (Tables 20–2 and 20–3).

Cardiac biomarkers are blood tests that indicate myocardial damage. Troponins T and I are preferred because of their high sensitivity and specificity for myocardial injury. Troponin I is most preferred because troponin T is more likely to be elevated by renal disease, polymyositis, or dermatomyositis. Newer highly sensitive troponin I assays have a 97–99% negative predictive value depending on the chosen cutoff value, as early as 3 hours after the onset of symptoms. However, the specificity is lower, resulting in a trade-off: fewer false negatives afford earlier diagnosis at the cost of more false positives. The potential impact of this will be discussed in the treatment section of this chapter. Troponin may remain elevated for 7–10 days and can therefore help identify prior recent infarctions.

When initial ECG and cardiac markers are normal, they should be repeated within 6–12 hours of symptom onset. If they are normal a second time, exercise or pharmacologic cardiac stress testing should be done to evaluate for inducible ischemia. Exercise stress testing (EST) is preferred, but stress testing with chemicals (dobutamine, dipyridamole, or adenosine) can be used to simulate the cardiac effects of exercise in those unable to exercise enough to produce a test adequate for interpretation. EST is done with ECGs for lower CAD risk, younger patients.

EST is the main test for evaluating those with suspected angina or heart disease (Table 20–4). Interpretation of the test is based on the occurrence of signs of stress-induced impairment of myocardial contraction, including ECG changes (Table 20–5) and/or symptoms and signs of angina or echocardiography changes

Adding *radionuclide myocardial perfusion imaging* to EST can improve sensitivity, specificity, and accuracy, especially in patients with a nondiagnostic exercise test or limited exercise ability. *Acute rest myocardial perfusion imaging* is very similar but is performed during or shortly after resolution of angina symptoms that were not induced by a stress test. Radionuclide EST can be advantageous in

Table 20–2. HEART (history, ECG, age, risk factors, troponin) score.

HEART risk factors	Answer choices (points)
History	Highly suspicious (+2) Moderately suspicious (+1) Slightly suspicious (0)
ECG	Significant ST depression (+2) Nonspecific repolarization disturbance (+1) Normal (0)
Age	≥65 years (+2) 45–65 years (+1) <45 years (0)
Risk factors (hypercholesterolemia, hypertension, diabetes, smoking, obesity [BMI >30], family history)	>3 risk factors or atherosclerosis history (+2) 1 or 2 risk factors are present (+1) No risk factors (0)
Troponin (protein complex involved in cardiac muscle contraction)	3 times higher than normal or more (2) 1–3 times higher than normal (1) Less than normal limit (0)

Interpreting HEART score.

HEART Score	MACE[a] Risk	Death	Recommendation
0–3	Low (1–2%)	0.05%	Discharge is an option, possible outpatient stress testing
4–6	Intermediate (12–17%)	1.3%	Clinical observation, further risk assessment, and investigation
7–10	High (50–65%)	2.8%	Observation, evaluation for early invasive treatment

[a]Major adverse cardiac events (MACE): group of cardiovascular conditions with sudden occurrence and resulting in high mortality and morbidity. It includes cardiac death, nonfatal myocardial infarction, and target lesion revascularization.
BMI, body mass index; ECG, electrocardiogram.

women because EST is less accurate in women compared to men. Radionuclide EST is preferred in instances of complete left bundle branch block, ventricular pacemaker, Wolf-Parkinson-White or other similar preexcitation syndromes, resting ECG has >1 millimeter of ST-segment depression, history of angina, prior cardiac revascularization, and inability to exercise enough to render a normal EST useful, which may also warrant additional use of medications to mimic exercise.

Chest radiography is used to assess for non-ACS causes of chest pain (eg, aortic dissection, pneumothorax, pulmonary embolus, pneumonia, rib fracture). This should be considered in the initial ACS workup.

Echocardiography can be used to determine left ventricle ejection fraction, assess cardiac valve function, and detect regional wall motion abnormalities that correspond to areas of myocardial damage. Its high sensitivity and low specificity make it most useful to exclude ACS if the study is normal. It can also be used as an adjunct to stress testing. Since

stress-induced impairment of myocardial contraction precedes ECG changes and angina, *stress echocardiography*, done and interpreted by experienced clinicians, can be superior to EST. It is also the preferred test for older, diabetic patients, those with a history of CAD, and those with a history of abnormal resting ECGs, as ECGs in these patients are more likely to have false-positive findings or to be uninterpretable.

Cardiac magnetic resonance imaging is not routinely used for initial care of ACS but is most often used in patients with multivessel disease or after a massive ACS event to assess myocardial viability.

Infrequently used in the past, *coronary computed tomography angiography* to detect the presence of CAD or stenosis has been recently identified as having excellent positive (91–93%) and negative (95–100%) predictive value for cardiac disease, allowing for confident assessment for CAD and the potential for early diagnosis and management of risk factors. Use of this modality depends on local radiographic and radiologist capabilities.

Table 20–3. Thrombolysis in Myocardial Infarction (TIMI) score.

1 point for each
- Age ≥65
- Aspirin use in the last 7 days (patient experiences chest pain despite aspirin use in past 7 days)
- At least 2 angina episodes within the past 24 hours
- ST changes of at least 0.5 mm in contiguous leads
- Elevated serum cardiac biomarkers
- Known coronary artery disease (CAD) (coronary stenosis ≥50%)
- At least 3 risk factors for CAD, such as:
  - Hypertension ≥140/90 mmHg or on antihypertensives
  - Current cigarette smoker
  - Low high-density lipoprotein cholesterol (<40 mg/dL)
  - Diabetes mellitus
  - Family history of premature CAD
    - Male first-degree relative or father younger than 55
    - Female first-degree relative or mother younger than 65

Score Interpretation
% risk at 14 days for all-cause mortality, new or recurrent myocardial infarction, or severe recurrent ischemia requiring urgent revascularization

0–1 = 4.7% risk
2 = 8.3% risk
3 = 13.2% risk
4 = 19.9% risk
5 = 26.2% risk
6–7 = at least 40.9% risk

Table 20–4. Exercise stress testing.

Indications	Contraindications
Confirm suspected angina	Cardiac failure
Evaluation of extent of myocardial ischemia and prognosis	Any febrile illness
Risk stratification after myocardial infarction	Left ventricular outflow tract obstruction or hypertrophic cardiomyopathy
Detection of exercise-induced symptoms (e.g., arrhythmias or syncope)	Severe aortic or mitral stenosis
• Evaluation of outcome of interventions (e.g., PCI or CABG)	Uncontrolled hypertension
• Assessment of cardiac transplant	Pulmonary hypertension
• Rehabilitation and patient motivation	Recent myocardial infarction
	Severe tachyarrhythmias
	Dissecting aortic aneurysm
	Left mainstem stenosis or equivalent
	Complete heart block

CABG, coronary artery bypass grafting; PCI, percutaneous coronary intervention.
Reproduced with permission from Grech ED: Pathophysiology and investigation of coronary artery disease. *Br Med J.* 2003;May10; 326(7397):1027–1030.

Table 20–5. Main end points for abnormal exercise electrocardiogram.

Target heart rate achieved (>85% of maximum predicted heart rate)
ST segment depression >1 mm (downsloping or planar depression of greater predictive value than upsloping depression)
Slow ST recovery to normal (>5 minutes)
Decrease in systolic blood pressure >20 mmHg
Increase in diastolic blood pressure >15 mmHg
Progressive ST segment elevation or depression
ST segment depression >3 mm without pain
Arrhythmias (atrial fibrillation, ventricular tachycardia)

Features Indicative of a Strongly Positive Exercise Test
Exercise limited by angina to <6 minutes of Bruce protocol
Failure of systolic blood pressure to increase >10 mmHg, or fall with evidence of ischemia
Widespread marked ST segment depression >3 mm
Prolonged recovery time of ST changes (>6 minutes)
Development of ventricular tachycardia
ST elevation in absence of prior myocardial infarction

Reproduced with permission from Grech ED: Pathophysiology and investigation of coronary artery disease. *Br Med J.* 2003;May10; 326(7397):1027–1030.

Coronary angiography is the gold standard. Main indications are listed in Table 20–6. Risks include death (1 in 1400), stroke (1 in 1000), coronary artery dissection (1 in 1000), arterial access complications (1 in 500), and minor risks such as arrhythmia; 10–30% of angiography studies are normal.

Table 20–6. Main indications for coronary angiography.

Uncertain diagnosis of angina (coronary artery disease cannot be excluded by noninvasive testing)
Assessment of feasibility and appropriateness of various forms of treatment (percutaneous intervention, bypass surgery, medical)
Class I or U stable angina with positive stress test or class III or W angina without positive stress test
Unstable angina or non-Q-wave myocardial infarction (medium- and high-risk patients)
Angina not controlled by drug treatment
Acute myocardial infarction—especially cardiogenic shock, ineligibility for thrombolytic treatment, failed thrombolytic reperfusion, re-infarction, or positive stress test
Life threatening ventricular arrhythmia
Angina after bypass surgery or percutaneous intervention
Before valve surgery or corrective heart surgery to assess occult coronary artery disease

Reproduced with permission from Grech ED: Pathophysiology and investigation of coronary artery disease. *Br Med J.* 2003;May10; 326(7397):1027–1030.

Boeddinghaus J, Nestelberger T, Twerenbold R, et al. Direct comparison of 4 very early rule-out strategies for acute myocardial infarction using high-sensitivity cardiac troponin I. *Circulation* 2017;135:1597–1611. [PMID: 28283497]

Neumann JT, Sörensen NA, Schwemer T, et al. Diagnosis of myocardial infarction using a high-sensitivity troponin I 1-hour algorithm. *JAMA Cardiol.* 2016;1(4):397–404. [PMID: 27438315]

▶ Pathogenesis & Epidemiology

CVD includes all diseases of the heart and vascular system (eg, stroke and hypertension). CAD, synonymous with coronary heart disease (CHD), affects the coronary arteries by diminishing their ability to be a conduit for carrying oxygenated blood to the heart.

A. Atherosclerosis Progression

Atherosclerotic disease is the thickening and hardening (loss of elasticity) of the arterial wall due to the accumulations of lipids, macrophages, T lymphocytes, smooth muscle cells, extracellular matrix, calcium, and necrotic debris. Figures 20–1 to 20–3 grossly depict the multifactorial and complex depository, inflammatory, and reactive processes that collaborate to occlude coronary arteries.

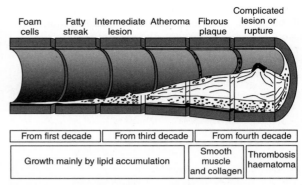

▲ **Figure 20–1. Atheromatous plaque progression.** (Reproduced with permission from Grech ED: Pathophysiology and investigation of coronary artery disease. *Br Med J.* 2003;May10;326(7397):1027–1030.)

B. Genetic Predisposition

Traditional risk factors for CAD include high low-density lipoprotein (LDL) cholesterol, low high-density lipoprotein (HDL) cholesterol, hypertension, family history of CAD, diabetes, smoking, menopause for women, and age >45 for men.

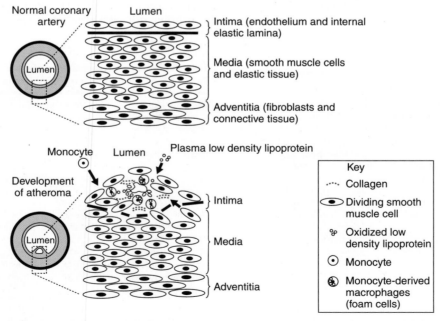

▲ **Figure 20–2. Mechanism of plaque development.** (Reproduced with permission from Grech ED: Pathophysiology and investigation of coronary artery disease. *Br Med J.* 2003;May10;326(7397):1027–1030.)

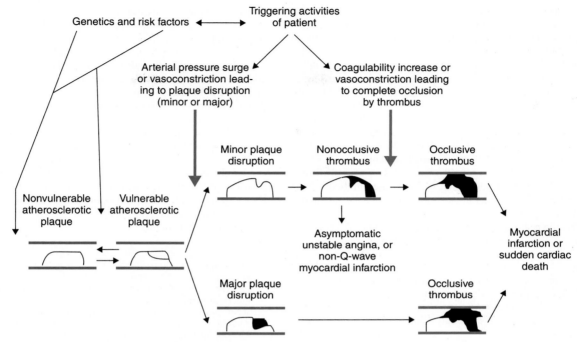

▲ **Figure 20–3.** Mechanism of coronary artery thrombosis. Hypothetical methods of possible trigger for coronary thrombosis: (1) physical or mental stress leads to hemodynamic changes leads to plaque rupture, (2) activities causing an increase in coagulability, and (3) stimuli leading to vasoconstriction. The role of coronary thrombosis in unstable angina, myocardial infarction, and sudden cardiac death has been well described. (Reproduced with permission from Muller JE, Abela GS, Nesto RW, et al: Triggers, acute risk factors and vulnerable plaques: the lexicon of a new frontier. *J Am Coll Cardiol.* 1994 Mar 1;23(3):809–813.)

Some inherited risk factors (eg, dyslipidemia and propensity for diabetes mellitus) are modifiable; others (eg, age and sex) are not. Genes affect the development and progression of disease and its response to risk factor modification and lifestyle decisions; nature (genetics) meets nurture (environment), and they responsively interrelate (Table 20–7). Obesity is an excellent example of the dynamics of the interplay between genetics and environment.

▶ Prevention: Primary, Secondary, & Tertiary

The cascade of events of CHD that lead to ACS can be interrupted, delayed, or treated. *Primary prevention* tries to prevent disease before it develops, namely, prevent or delay development of risk factors (eg, prevent the onset of smoking, obesity, diabetes, or hypertension). *Secondary prevention* attempts to prevent disease progression by identifying and treating risk factors or preclinical, asymptomatic disease (eg, treat hypertension or nicotine addiction *before* the occurrence of ACS). *Tertiary prevention* is treatment of established disease to restore and maintain highest function, minimize negative disease effects, and prevent complications, that is, help recover from and prevent recurrence of ACS (eg, treatment of hypertension and lowering LDL target from 100 mg/dL to 70 mg/dL after the occurrence of ACS).

Table 20–7. Genetic and environmental influences on congestive heart disease predisposition.

Gene-Environment Interaction	Favorable Genes	Unfavorable Genes
Favorable environment	Low risk	Moderate risk
Unfavorable environment	Moderate risk	High risk

Reproduced with permission from Scheuner MT. Genetic predisposition to coronary artery disease. *Curr Opin Cardiol.* 2001;July;16(4): 251–260.

Primary prevention of ACS should begin in childhood by preventing tobacco use, eating a diet rich in fruits and vegetable and low in saturated fats, exercising regularly for 20–30 minutes 5 times a week, and maintaining a body mass index of 18–28 kg/m². Compared to waiting to initiate secondary and tertiary strategies, these primary prevention strategies yield a larger impact on decreasing lifetime risk of death from ACS and years of productive life lost to ACS.

Secondary and tertiary preventions involve increasingly aggressive management of those who have known risk factors for or have experienced ACS (Figure 20–4 and Table 20–8). Although the association between cholesterol and ACS death is weaker in those age >65 years, HMG-CoA (3-hydroxy-3-methyl-glutaryl–coenzyme A) reductase inhibitor drugs (statins) still positively impact morbidity and mortality in this demographic. This may be due to their effects that go beyond their lipid-lowering effect, including pleiotropic effects such as anti-inflammation and endothelial stabilizing effects.

Some once-touted therapies have been found to be ineffective. Because of a lack of effect and potential harm, estrogen with or without progestin *hormone replacement therapy* should not be used as primary, secondary, or tertiary prevention of CAD. *Antibiotics* and the *antioxidants folate, vitamin C, and vitamin E* do not improve ACS morbidity and mortality.

▶ Cardiac Rehabilitation

Cardiac rehabilitation, an example of tertiary prevention, is a multidisciplinary attempt to prevent future ACS by focusing on three areas: exercise, risk factor modification, and psychosocial intervention. Optimal medical management is part of this process. Patient adherence to the plan is integral to long-term success.

Exercise-based rehabilitation programs reduce both all-cause and cardiac mortality in patients with a history of MI, surgical intervention (percutaneous coronary intervention [PCI], coronary artery bypass graft [CABG]), or stable CAD.

Risk factor modification addresses the content of Figure 20–4 and Table 20–8; involves dietician-guided nutritional training; and emphasizes smoking cessation via counseling, drug therapy (bupropion, varenicline), nicotine replacement, and formal cessation programs.

Psychosocial intervention emphasizes the identification and management of the psychological and social effects that can follow ACS. These effects can include depression, anxiety, family issues, and job-related problems. Depression has been linked to worse mortality in patients with CHD. Psychosocial intervention alone does not affect total or cardiac mortality, but does decrease depression and anxiety, which may impact quality of life.

American College of Cardiology. ASCVD Risk Estimator Plus. http://tools.acc.org/ascvd-risk-estimator-plus/#!/calculate/estimate/. Accessed November 11, 2019.

Arnett DK, Blumenthal RS, Albert MA, et al. 2019 ACC/AHA guideline on the primary prevention of cardiovascular disease: a report of the American College of Cardiology/American Heart Association Task Force on Clinical Practice Guidelines. *J Am Coll Cardiol.* 2019;74(10):1376–1414. [PMID: 30894319]

Balady GJ, Williams MA, Ades PA, et al. Core components of cardiac rehabilitation/secondary prevention programs: 2007 update: a scientific statement from the American Heart Association Exercise, Cardiac Rehabilitation, and Prevention Committee, the Council on Clinical Cardiology; the Councils on Cardiovascular Nursing, Epidemiology and Prevention, and Nutrition, Physical Activity, and Metabolism; and the American Association of Cardiovascular and Pulmonary Rehabilitation. *Circulation.* 2007;115:2675–2682. [PMID: 17513578]

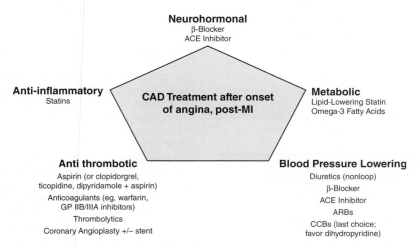

▲ **Figure 20–4.** Tertiary prevention for coronary artery disease (CAD). ACE, angiotensin-converting enzyme; ARB, angiotensin receptor blocker; CCB, calcium channel blocker; GP, glycoprotein; MI, myocardial infarction.

Table 20–8. Approach to comprehensive risk reduction for patients with coronary artery disease (CAD).

Risk Intervention	Recommendations			
Smoking: *Goal*: complete cessation	Strongly encourage patient and family to stop smoking. The greatest modifiable risk factor for ACS is tobacco smoking. Provide counseling, nicotine replacement, bupropion, varenicline, and formal cessation programs as appropriate.			

Lipids:
Primary goal
  LDL <100 mg/dL
Secondary goals
  HDL >35 mg/dL
  TG <200 mg/dL
	AHA Step II Diet (30% fat, <200 mg/d cholesterol)
	Assess fasting lipid profile
	  • In post-MI patients, lipid profile may take 4–6 weeks to stabilize
	Add drug therapy according to the following table:			

	LDL <100 mg/dL	LDL 100–130 mg/dL	LDL >130 mg/dL	HDL <35 mg/dL
	Use statin in all patients with CAD; if post-MI, target LDL <70 mg/dL	Use statin in all patients with CAD; dosing based on risk	Use statin in all patients with CAD; dosing based on risk	Emphasize weight management and physical activity Emphasize smoking cessation
	Statins as first-line suggested drug therapy			If needed to achieve LDL goals, consider statin, fibrate, fish oil
	TG <200 mg/dL	TG 200–400 mg/dL	TG >400 mg/dL	
	Statin Resin Omega-3 fatty acids (fish oil)	Statin Omega-3 fatty acids (fish oil)	Consider combined drug therapy (statin, resin, fish oil)	
	If LDL goal not achieved, consider combination therapy			
Physical activity: Minimum goal: 150 minutes per week of moderate exercise	Assess risk, preferably with exercise test, to guide prescription Encourage minimum of 150 minutes of moderate-intensity activity weekly (walking, jogging, cycling, or other aerobic activity) supplemented by an increase in daily lifestyle activities (eg, walking breaks at work, using stairs, gardening, household work) 75 minutes of vigorous aerobic activity weekly is also an option if preferred, tolerated, and achievable Maximum exercise benefit reached at about 300 minutes weekly Add moderate- to high-intensity muscle-strengthening activity (eg, resistance or weights) on at least 2 days per week; advise medically supervised programs for moderate- to high-risk patients			
Weight management Ideal BMI: 18.5–25 kg/m²	Start intensive diet and appropriate physical activity intervention, as outlined above, in patients >120% of ideal weight for height Particularly emphasize need for weight loss in patients with hypertension, elevated TG, or elevated glucose levels Desirable waist-to-hip ratio for men, <0.9; for middle-aged and elderly women, <0.8			
Antiplatelet agents/ anticoagulants	Start aspirin 80–325 mg/d, if not contraindicated Manage warfarin to international normalized ratio of 2–3 for post-MI patients not able to take or who failed aspirin, then consider ticlopidine, clopidogrel, or dipyridamole plus aspirin			
ACE inhibitors after MI	Start after MI in stable patients, within 24 hours in patients with anterior MI, CHF, renal insufficiency, EF <40% (LV dysfunction) Maximize dose as tolerated indefinitely Use to manage blood pressure or symptoms in all other patients			
β-Blockers	After MI, as tolerated			
Estrogens	No role More evidence of harm than help			
Blood pressure Goal: ≤*140*/90 mmHg	Initiate lifestyle modification: tobacco cessation, weight control, physical activity, and alcohol moderation in all patients with blood pressure >140 mmHg systolic or ≥90 mmHg diastolic Add blood pressure medication, individualize to other patient requirements and characteristics (eg, age, race, need for drugs with specific benefits) if blood pressure is ≥140 mmHg systolic or ≥90 mmHg diastolic in 3 months if initial blood pressure is >160 mmHg systolic or ≥100 mmHg diastolic Based on risk factors, some patients' target blood pressure should be <130/80 mmHg			

ACE, angiotensin-converting enzyme; ACS, acute coronary syndrome; AHA, American Heart Association; BMI, body mass index; CHF, congestive heart failure; EF, ejection fraction; HDL, high-density lipoprotein; LDL, low-density lipoprotein; LV, left ventricular; MI, myocardial infarction; TG, triglycerides.

Data from Smith SC Jr, Blair SN, Bonow RO, et al. AHA/ACC guidelines for preventing heart attack and death in patients with atherosclerotic cardiovascular disease. *J Am Coll Cardiol*. 2001 Nov 1;38(5):1581–1583.

James PA, Oparil S, Carter BL, et al. 2014 evidence-based guideline for the management of high blood pressure in adults: report from the panel members appointed to the Eight Joint National Committee (JNC 8). *JAMA*. 2014;311:507–520. [PMID: 24352797]

National Heart, Lung, and Blood Institute. Seventh Report of the Joint National Committee on Prevention, Detection, Evaluation and Treatment of High Blood Pressure (JNC7). https://www.nhlbi.nih.gov/files/docs/guidelines/jnc7full.pdf. Accessed November 11, 2019.

Smith SC Jr, Benjamin EJ, Bonow RO, et al. AHA/ACCF secondary prevention and risk reduction therapy for patients with coronary and other atherosclerotic vascular disease: 2011 update. A guideline from the American Heart Association and American College of Cardiology Foundation. *Circulation*. 2011;124:2458–2473. [PMID: 22052934]

Differential Diagnosis of ACS Signs & Symptoms

These are listed as follows:

- Anemia
- Aortic aneurysm
- Aortic dissection
- Cardiac tamponade
- Cardiac valve rupture
- Cardiomyopathy
- Cholecystitis
- Costochondritis
- Coronary artery anomaly or aneurysm
- Diaphragramatic irritation/inflammation due to
  - Hepatitis
  - Infection
  - Mass effect from nearby cancer
  - Pancreatitis
  - Pulmonary edema/effusion
- Drug use (eg, cocaine)
- Duodenal ulcer
- Esophageal spasm
- Esophagitis
- Gastritis
- Generalized anxiety disorder
- Gastroesophageal reflux disease
- Hiatal hernia
- High-altitude exposure
- Hyperthyroidism
- Panic attack
- Peptic ulcer disease

- Pericardial effusion
- Pericarditis
- Pleurisy/pleuritis
- Pneumothorax
- Prinzmetal angina (coronary vasospasm)—more common in women
- Pulmonary embolus
- Pulmonary hypertension
- Radiculopathy
- Shoulder arthropathy
- Stress reactional anxiety
- Supraventricular tachycardia
- Vasculitis

ACS Complications

There are five major complications:

1. Death
2. MI
3. Hospitalization
4. Cardiac dysfunction:
   - Angina/ischemia: Lifestyle and activity options are diminished because the heart is unable to supply the oxygenated blood the body needs to fulfill its demand because the coronary arteries are unable to supply the heart muscle.
   - Arrhythmia: Poor blood supply or irreversible damage to the heart muscle can predispose patients to significant heart rhythm disturbances.
   - Heart failure: Irreversible damage to heart muscle can lead to decreased pump function of the heart.
5. Stroke

There is one important formula to keep in mind for management of ACS:

Treatment: time = tissue!

ACS causes MI in three ways:

1. Atheromatous plaque buildup increases until the artery is totally occluded.
2. An atheromatous plaque ruptures or tears, leading to occlusions via inflammatory response and thrombus formation as platelets adhere to the site to seal off the plaque.
3. Superimposition of thrombus on a disrupted atherosclerotic plaque.

The *goal of treatment* is to save cardiac muscle by reducing myocardial oxygen demand and/or increasing oxygen supply.

All patients with ACS should be hospitalized, be medically stabilized, and receive further cardiac evaluation to determine STEMI versus NSTEMI versus unstable angina and then receive treatment appropriate to the diagnosis. Immediate PCI can be beneficial for STEMI but can be safely delayed in low-risk NSTEMI. All ACS patients should receive medical management, which begins with the mnemonic **HOBANACS**:

Heparin (low-molecular-weight heparin → fewer MIs and deaths)

Oxygen

Beta-blocker (β-blocker; if hemodynamically stable: metoprolol, timolol, propranolol, or carvedilol if decreased ejection fraction)

Aspirin (initially 160–325 mg each day, then 70–162 mg daily indefinitely)

Nitroglycerin (for pain; stop if hypotension occurs)

ACE inhibitor (angiotensin-converting enzyme inhibitor; within the first 24 hours if anterior location infarct, heart failure, or ejection fraction of ≤40%, unless contraindicated)

Clopidogrel (up to 1 year; not within 5 days of CABG)

Statins (high-dose HMG-CoA reductase inhibitors; goal LDL <70 mg/dL)

Morphine may be added for pain and anxiety relief. It also provides some afterload reduction.

Anticoagulation with *heparin* starts with low-molecular-weight heparin if PCI is not planned. Unfractionated heparin should be used if creatinine clearance is <60 mL/min or if early PCI or CABG is planned within 24 hours. Fondaparinux is as effective as enoxaparin with less major bleeding and lower long-term mortality.

β-Blockers decrease the workload on the heart by slowing it down and decreasing blood pressure. The goal should be <130/85 mmHg or <130/80 mmHg if diabetes or chronic kidney disease is present; optimal blood pressure for some may be 120/80 mmHg.

Aspirin (ASA) should be continued indefinitely. Once ACS is stabilized, a dose of 81 mg/d should suffice. If ASA is not tolerated, clopidogrel should be used. If there is a history of gastrointestinal bleeding and either ASA or clopidogrel is used, drugs to decrease the risk of recurrent gastrointestinal bleeding (eg, proton pump inhibitors) should be given.

Clopidogrel requires a loading dose (300–600 mg) followed by the daily maintenance dose (75 mg). If there is no plan for PCI, it should be added to aspirin and anticoagulant therapy as soon as possible after admission. If PCI is likely, it can be added before the procedure. Duration of treatment should be for at least 3 months and ideally up to 1 year. Ticagrelor (180 mg load, then 90 mg twice daily) compared to clopidogrel resulted in lower all-cause

mortality, vascular mortality, and MI rate without increase in major bleeding or stroke. Prasugrel (5–10 mg daily) compared to clopidogrel has not shown lower risk of death from cardiovascular causes, MI, or stroke, and bleeding risks are similar.

Platelet glycoprotein IIB/IIIA (GP IIB/IIIA) receptor inhibitors are beneficial for ACS patients undergoing revascularization: 100 STEMIs need to be treated to prevent one MI or death, but for every one prevention, there is one major bleeding complication. Caution and dose adjustment are necessary when using in the elderly and those with chronic kidney disease. *Reperfusion–PCI, CABG, and medications* can also be used. If cardiac tissue is to survive, blood flow must be restored. STEMI (active infarction) requires medical thrombolysis or emergent angioplasty to achieve this. Primary PCI is the recommended method of reperfusion. If PCI or CABG cannot be initiated within 120 minutes, then thrombolytic, fibrinolytic agents should be started within 30–60 minutes. When medical therapy is used because PCI/CABG cannot be initiated within 120 minutes, if blood flow is still not restored, then proceed to PCI/CABG as soon as possible without a "cooling-off" period. A cooling-off period (ie, delaying PCI or CABG because of failed medical thrombolysis) increases mortality without decreasing bleeding complications.

Although there is a modest decrease in recurrent ischemia, *early PCI* within 24 hours of symptom onset for lower-risk NSTEMI patients does not decrease mortality compared to *late PCI* within 36 hours. Higher-risk patients (ST >1-mm depression, T-wave inversion, impaired renal function, hemodynamically unstable, TIMI score >4, GRACE [Global Registry of Acute Coronary Events] score >140, presence of heart failure) with NSTEMI benefit from early PCI within 24 hours. There is no difference in NSTEMI mortality with PCI in 70 minutes compared to 21 hours in higher-risk patients (TIMI score >4).

The 2-year risk of death or recurrent MI is the same for PCI and CABG, but approximately 5% of patients who receive CABG have less angina.

Post-MI care should center around tertiary care (see cardiac rehabilitation, illustrated in Figure 20–4 and Table 20–8). Optimal blood pressure is closer to 115/75 mmHg, since in 40- to 70-year-olds, each increment of 20 mmHg in systolic blood pressure or 10 mmHg in diastolic blood pressure doubles the risk of CVD across the entire blood pressure range from 115/75 mmHg to 185/115 mmHg.

Cyclooxygenase-2 (COX-2) nonsteroidal anti-inflammatory drugs and naproxen should be avoided because they increase risk for ACS.

For some individuals, using warfarin (goal international normalized ratio [INR], 2.0–3.0) together with aspirin or warfarin alone (goal INR, 3.0–4.0) results in a better all-cause mortality than taking aspirin alone. It reduces the risk of MI and stroke but increases the risk of major bleeding.

Fihn SD, Blankenship JC, Alexander KP, et al. 2014 ACC/AHA/ AATS/PCNA/SCAI/STS focused update of the guideline for the diagnosis and management of patients with stable ischemic heart disease. A report of the American College of Cardiology/ American Heart Association Task Force on Practice Guidelines, and the American Association for Thoracic Surgery, Preventive Cardiovascular Nurses Association, Society for Cardiovascular Angiography and Interventions, and Society of Thoracic Surgeons. *J Am Coll Cardiol.* 2014;64(18):1929–1949. [PMID: 25077860]

GRACE: Global Registry of Acute Coronary Events calculator. http://www.outcomes-umassmed.org/grace/. Accessed November 11, 2019.

TIMI: Thrombolysis In Myocardial Infarction calculators. http://www.mdcalc.com/timi-risk-score-for-uanstemi. Accessed November 11, 2019.

CULTURAL CONSIDERATIONS

Cultural issues can affect the diagnosis, treatment, and outcome of ACS. Some clinical symptoms are more common in certain patient populations (see prior symptoms list). Overall, atypical symptoms are more prevalent in women and elderly patients. Symptoms may include jaw and neck pain, dyspnea, fatigue, dry mouth, palpitations, indigestion, cough, and nausea and emesis. Perhaps because atypical symptoms occur more frequently in women and older adults, they tend to experience delaying diagnosis, less aggressive treatment, and increased rates of in-hospital mortality.

Other notable differences exist between patient populations that relate to diagnosis and treatment of cardiac disease. Both men and women with ACS respond to early invasive treatment. Women tend to have a more severe first ACS, are less likely to receive thrombolysis, and are at greater risk for death and hospital readmission at 6 months. Patients with symptoms of acute MI are less often hospitalized if they are nonwhite or have a normal or nondiagnostic ECG. Patients experiencing ACS who are women <55 years of age, are nonwhite, have shortness of breath as their chief complaint, or have a normal or indeterminate ECG are less often hospitalized, thus increasing their morality. After ACS, women are more likely than men to experience depression and hence its ramifications.

Patients are more likely to adhere to treatment plans that they can afford. This should be considered when deciding which medication to prescribe and which diets and exercise plans to recommend. Emphasize free and low-cost exercise options; remember that some diet approaches are less expensive than others.

For patients 75 years of age or older, treatment considerations should be patient-specific and made in the context of overall health status.

PROGNOSIS

Approximately 60% of MI deaths occur within the first hour of symptom onset. Prognosis following a survived MI without subsequent intervention carries a mortality rate of 10% the first year and 5% each additional year. Reperfusion strategies and medications (eg, aspirin, statins, and β-blockers) have improved 30-day mortality (~3–6%). Sudden death, more common in patients with a lower ejection fraction, following ACS occurs in 1.4% of patients during the first month and decreases to 0.14% per month after 2 years.

The type of MI affects prognosis. STEMI often has a higher mortality than NSTEMI, even when aggressively treated. Patients experiencing STEMI who receive timely revascularization, within 2 hours of symptom onset, have a mortality of 3–8%, compared to 2–4% mortality in those experiencing NSTEMI.

When either troponin T or I level is normal at 2, 4, and 6 hours after the onset of chest pain in patients with a normal ECG, the 30-day risk of cardiac death and nonfatal acute MI is nearly zero.

Normal troponin T levels at 10–12 hours after symptom onset in patients with chest pain and a normal ECG indicate a low risk of adverse events for the next 12 months. Newer high-sensitivity cardiac troponin assays result in higher analytical sensitivity, which allows for more rapid rule out of ACS within 1–2 hours of symptom onset. Even slight elevations in cardiac troponin levels in patients with unstable angina and NSTEMI help identify high-risk patients who may benefit the most from early invasive treatment.

Website-accessible scoring systems (eg, HEART and TIMI) can help risk-stratify patients with chest pain and aid prognosis given a range of different circumstances by analyzing individual patient characteristics and test results. Prognostic tools are valuable when educating patients about possible outcomes and when discussing and deciding on treatment options.

Boeddinghaus J, Nestelberger T, Twerenbold R, et al. Direct comparison of 4 very early rule-out strategies for acute myocardial infarction using high-sensitivity cardiac troponin I. *Circulation.* 2017;135:1597–1611. [PMID: 28283497]

HEART Score for Major Cardiac Events. https://www.mdcalc.com/ heart-score-major-cardiac-events. Accessed November 11, 2019.

Jneid H, Addison D, Bhatt DL, et al. 2017 AHA/ACC clinical performance and quality measures for adults with ST-elevation and non–ST-elevation myocardial infarction: a report of the American College of Cardiology/American Heart Association Task Force on Performance Measures. *J Am Coll Cardiol.* 2017;70(16):2048–2090. [PMID: 28943066]

The HEART Score. www.heartscore.nl/score. Accessed November 11, 2019.

TIMI Risk Score for UA/NSTEMI. http://www.mdcalc.com/ timi-risk-score-for-uanstemi. Accessed November 11, 2019.

Websites for Information on ACS & CVD

American Academy of Family Physicians. http://www.aafp.org and http://familydoctor.org

American College of Cardiology. http://www.acc.org

American Heart Association. http://www.americanheart.org

ASCVD Risk Estimator Plus. http://tools.acc.org/ascvd-risk-estimator-plus/#!/calculate/estimate/

Centers for Disease Control and Prevention. http://www.cdc.gov

Family Practice Notebook. http://fpnotebook.com/CV/index.htm

Mayo Clinic. http://www.mayoclinic.com

Medline Plus. http://www.medlineplus.gov

Medtronic. http://www.medtronic.corn/cad

Merck Manual: Overview of Acute Coronary Syndrome (ACS). https://www.merckmanuals.com/professional/cardiovascular-disorders/coronary-artery-disease/overview-of-acute-coronary-syndromes-acs?query=ACS

National Institutes of Health–health topics. http://health.nih.gov/

The HEART Score. www.heartscore.nl/score

TIMI Risk Score. https://www.mdcalc.com/timi-risk-score-ua-nstemi

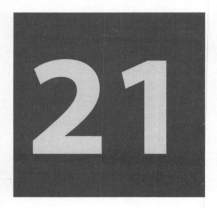

Heart Failure

Michael King, MD, MPH, FAAFP
Angelina Rodriguez, MD, FAAFP
Yelena Tarasenko, DO
Tiffany Simon, DO, MS
Billy R. Davis, DO

ESSENTIALS OF DIAGNOSIS

► Left ventricular dysfunction by echocardiography.

► Dyspnea on exertion and fatigue are common, but paroxysmal nocturnal dyspnea, orthopnea, and peripheral edema are more diagnostic.

► Unintentional weight loss, intractable volume overload, and signs of inadequate perfusion (eg, hypotension and narrowed pulse pressure) may represent advanced heart failure.

► Third (S_3) heart sound, displaced cardiac apex, jugular venous distension, hepatojugular reflux, rales, murmur.

► Any electrocardiographic (ECG) abnormality, radiographic evidence of pulmonary venous congestion, cardiomegaly, or pleural effusion.

► Elevated B-type natriuretic peptide (BNP) or N-terminal pro-BNP levels.

General Considerations

According to the 2016 statistical update from the American Heart Association (AHA) and the Centers for Disease Control and Prevention, approximately 5.7 million adults in the United States are diagnosed with heart failure. This correlates to 1.77% of the overall population, with men having a higher incidence than women, and this incidence increases with age. The age-adjusted incidence of heart failure has declined by only 11% per decade in men and by 17% per decade in women over a 40-year observation period, despite improved treatments for ischemic heart disease, hypertension, and valvular heart disease. These advances in treatment during the four-decade period of observation did not translate into significant improvements in overall survival after onset of heart failure. The delineation of heart failure has changed in recent decades as well, with a lower prevalence of left ventricular systolic dysfunction (LVSD) or heart failure with reduced ejection fraction (HFrEF) and an increased occurrence of heart failure with preserved ejection fraction (HFpEF). In patients with clinical symptoms of heart failure, moderate or severe isolated diastolic dysfunction appears to be as common as systolic dysfunction, and systolic dysfunction appears to increase with the severity of diastolic dysfunction.

Pathogenesis

As defined by the AHA and the American College of Cardiology (ACC), heart failure is "a complex clinical syndrome that can result from any structural or functional cardiac disorder that impairs the ability of the ventricle to fill with or eject blood." As cardiac output decreases in response to the stresses placed on the myocardium (Table 21–1), activation of the sympathetic nervous and renin-angiotensin-aldosterone system occurs. These neurohormonal adaptations help increase blood pressure for tissue perfusion and also increase blood volume to enhance preload, stroke volume, and cardiac output. These compensatory mechanisms, which increase afterload, also lead to further myocardial deterioration and worsening myocardial contractility.

Causes of Cardiac Failure

The First National Health and Nutrition Examination Survey (NHANES I) found coronary artery disease (CAD), diabetes mellitus, hypertension, cigarette smoking, valvular heart disease, and obesity to be significant risk factors for heart failure in the United States. It is estimated that 60–70% of patients who have systolic heart failure have CAD as the underlying etiology. CAD is a substantial predictor of developing symptomatic heart failure with LVSD compared to asymptomatic LVSD. Heart failure is twice as common in

Table 21–1. Causes of heart failure.

Most common causes
Coronary artery disease
Diabetes
Hypertension
Idiopathic cardiomyopathy
Valvular heart disease

Less common causes
Arrhythmias (tachycardia, atrial fibrillation/flutter, bradycardia, heart block)
Collagen vascular disease (systemic lupus erythematosus, scleroderma)
Endocrine/metabolic disorders (thyroid disease, pheochromocytoma, other genetic disorders)
Hypertrophic cardiomyopathy
Myocarditis (including human immunodeficiency virus)
Pericarditis
Postpartum cardiomyopathy
Restrictive cardiomyopathies (amyloidosis, hemochromatosis, sarcoidosis, other genetic disorders)
    Stress-induced cardiomyopathy/takotsubo cardiomyopathy
    Toxic cardiomyopathy (alcohol, cocaine, heavy metals, chemotherapy, radiation)

Data from King M, Kingery J, Casey B. Diagnosis and evaluation of heart failure. *Am Fam Physician*. 2012 Jun 15;85(12):1161–1168 and Institute for Clinical Systems Improvement (ICSI). *Heart Failure in Adults*. Bloomington, MN: Institute for Clinical Systems Improvement (ICSI); 2011.

diabetic patients and is one of the most significant factors for developing heart failure in women. This is likely due to the direct effect of diabetes in developing cardiomyopathy as well as the effects of CAD risk and progression. There are racial differences as well with CAD being a more common cause in whites where hypertension is a more common cause in African Americans. Decreased physical activity and lower cardiorespiratory fitness also remain as major precipitants in the development of heart failure. There is a higher risk for heart failure in those with lower socioeconomic status, possibly due to limited access to higher quality care, resulting in decreased adherence to treatment of modifiable risk factors such as hypertension, diabetes mellitus, and CAD.

Conrad N, Judge A, Tran J, et al. Temporal trends and patterns in heart failure incidence: a population-based study of 4 million individuals. *Lancet*. 2018; 391:572–580. [PMID: 29174292]

Nayor M, Vasan RS. Preventing heart failure: the role of physical activity. *Curr Opin Cardiol*. 2015;30:543–550. [PMID: 26154074]

Vasan RS, Xanthakis V, Lyass A, et al. Epidemiology of left ventricular systolic dysfunction and heart failure in the Framingham study: an echocardiographic study over 3 decades. *JACC Cardiovasc Imaging*. 2018;11:1–11. [PMID: 28917679]

▶ **Classification & Prevention**

The most important component to classifying heart failure is whether left ventricular ejection fraction (LVEF) is preserved or reduced (<50%). A reduced LVEF in heart failure is a powerful predictor of mortality. The ACC and AHA classified heart failure into stages, emphasizing the progressive nature of the clinical syndrome. These stages more clearly define appropriate therapy at each level that can reduce morbidity and mortality and delay the onset of clinically evident disease (Table 21–2).

Patients in ACC/AHA stages A and B do not have clinical symptomatic heart failure but are at risk for developing heart failure. Stage A includes those at risk but not manifesting structural heart disease. Early identification and aggressive treatment of modifiable risk factors remain the best prevention for heart failure. Lifestyle modification, pharmacologic therapy, and counseling can improve or correct conditions such as CAD, hypertension, diabetes mellitus, hyperlipidemia, obesity, tobacco abuse, and alcohol or illicit substance abuse. Stage B represents patients who are asymptomatic but have structural heart disease or LVSD. Stage C comprises the majority of patients with heart failure who have past or current symptoms and associated underlying structural heart disease, including LVSD. Stage D includes refractory patients with heart failure who may need advanced and specialized treatment strategies.

The NYHA classification gauges the severity of symptoms for patients with stage C and D heart failure. The NYHA classification is a more subjective assessment that can change frequently, secondary to treatment response, but it is a well-established predictor of mortality.

▶ **Clinical Findings**

A high index of suspicion is necessary to diagnose the syndrome of heart failure early in its clinical presentation because of nonspecific signs and symptoms. Patients are often elderly with comorbidity, symptoms may be mild, and routine clinical assessment lacks specificity. A prompt diagnosis allows for early treatment with therapies proven to delay the progression of heart failure and improve quality of life. Evaluation is directed at confirming the presence of heart failure, determining cause, identifying comorbid illness, establishing severity, and guiding response to therapy. Heart failure is a clinical diagnosis for which no single symptom, examination, or test can establish the presence or absence with certainty.

Yancy CW, Jessup M, Bozkurt B, et al. 2013 ACCF/AHA guideline for the management of heart failure: a report of the American College of Cardiology/American Heart Association Task Force on Practice Guidelines. *Circulation*. 2013;128:e240–327. [PMID: 28461007]

A. Symptoms and Signs

The most common manifestation of symptomatic heart failure is dyspnea, but many conditions present with these

Table 21–2. Progression of heart failure and recommended evidence-based therapies.

	Progression of Heart Failure				
	At Risk for Heart Failure		**Heart Failure**		
NYHA classification	Not applicable	Class I: asymptomatic	Class II: symptoms with significant exertion	Class III: symptoms on minor exertion	Class IV: symptoms at rest
ACC/AHA stage	Stage A: high risk	Stage B: asymptomatic with cardiac structural abnormalities (MI, remodeling, reduced EF, valvular disease)	Stage C: cardiac structural abnormalities (reduced EF) and symptomatic or history of heart failure		Stage D: refractory end-stage heart failure
Treatments: beneficial, effective, recommended	*Goals:* disease management: Hypertension[a] Lipid disorders[a] Diabetes mellitus[c] Thyroid disease[c] Secondary prevention of atherosclerotic vascular disease[c] Behavior change[c] Smoking cessation Regular exercise Avoidance of alcohol and illicit drug use	*Goals:* stage A measures *Drugs* (in appropriate patients): ACEI[a] or ARB[a] β-blockers (history of MI[a]; no MI[c])	*Goals:* stage A/B measures, dietary sodium restriction[c] *Drugs/devices:* Routine use: Diuretics[c] (fluid retention) ACEI[a] or ARB[a] or ARNI[b] β-Blockers[a] In selected patients: ARB[a] or ARNI[b] Aldosterone antagonists[a] Hydralazine or nitrates[b] Implantable cardioverter defibrillator[a]		*Goals:* stage A, B, and C measures Meticulous fluid retention control[b] Decision regarding appropriate level of care and referral to heart failure program *Options:* End-of-life care or hospice[c] Extraordinary measures: heart transplantation[c]
Treatments: reasonably beneficial, probably recommended	*Drugs* (in appropriate patients): ACEI[a] or ARB[c] (in patients with vascular disease or diabetes mellitus)	–	*Drugs/devices (in selected patients):* Cardiac resynchronization therapy[b] I Ivabradine[b]		*Options:* Extraordinary measures: permanent mechanical support[b]

[a]SORT A (consistent, good-quality, patient-oriented evidence).
[b]SORT B (inconsistent or limited-quality, patient-oriented evidence).
[c]SORT C (consensus, disease-oriented evidence).
ACC/AHA, American College of Cardiology/American Heart Association; ACEI, angiotensin-converting enzyme inhibitor; ARB, angiotensin receptor blocker; ARNI, angiotensin receptor-neprilysin inhibitor; EF, ejection fraction; MI, myocardial infarction; NYHA, New York Heart Association; SORT, Strength of Recommendation Taxonomy.
Data from Yancy CW, Jessup M, Bozkurt B, et al. 2017 ACC/AHA/HFSA focused update of the 2013 ACCF/AHA guideline for the management of heart failure: a report of the American College of Cardiology/American Heart Association Task Force on Clinical Practice Guidelines and the Heart Failure Society of America. *Circulation.* 2017 Aug 8;136(6):e137–e161 and Yancy CW, Jessup M, Bozkurt B, et al. 2013 ACCF/AHA guideline for the management of heart failure: a report of the American College of Cardiology Foundation/American Heart Association Task Force on Practice Guidelines. *Circulation.* 2013 Oct 15;128(16):e240–e327.

symptoms. Limited exercise tolerance and fluid retention may eventually lead to pulmonary congestion and peripheral edema. Neither of these symptoms necessarily dominates the clinical picture at the same time. The absence of dyspnea on exertion is helpful to rule out the diagnosis of heart failure with a sensitivity of 84%. Other symptoms that are helpful in diagnosing heart failure include orthopnea, paroxysmal nocturnal dyspnea (PND), and peripheral edema. PND has the highest specificity (84%) of any symptom for heart failure. It is important to remember that no single clinical symptom has been shown to be both sensitive and specific. A substantial portion of the population has asymptomatic LVSD, and the history alone is insufficient to make the diagnosis of heart failure. However, a detailed history and review of symptoms remain the best approach in identifying the cause of heart failure and assessing response to therapy.

B. Physical Examination

The clinical examination is helpful to assess the degree of reduced cardiac output, cardiac filling, volume overload, and ventricular enlargement. It can also provide clues to noncardiac causes of dyspnea. A third heart sound, S_3 (ventricular filling gallop), on examination is specific for increased left ventricular end-diastolic pressure and decreased LVEF. It has the best specificity of any exam finding for heart failure (99%). Thus, a third audible sound along with a displaced cardiac apex are both very predictive and effectively rule in a diagnosis of LVSD. Volume overload from heart failure can present with many signs on examination. Jugular venous distention and a hepatojugular reflex can be present and are moderately effective in diagnosing heart failure. Other signs such as pulmonary rales (crackles), a murmur, and peripheral edema have a smaller but helpful role in diagnosing heart failure.

Additional exam findings can assist in determining causes of heart failure or assessing for other differential diagnoses. Cardiac murmurs may be an indication of primary valvular disease. Asymmetric rales or rhonchi on the pulmonary examination may suggest pneumonia or chronic obstructive pulmonary disease (COPD). Dullness to percussion or auscultation of the lungs could indicate pleural effusion. Examination of the thyroid can exclude thyromegaly or goiter, which could cause abnormal thyroid function precipitating heart failure. Hepatomegaly can indicate passive hepatic congestion.

C. Laboratory Findings

Objective tests can aid in confirmation of heart failure by assessing the differential diagnosis and excluding other possible causes for the signs and symptoms. A complete blood count can rule out anemia as a cause of high-output failure. Electrolyte (including magnesium and calcium) analysis may reveal deficiencies that are commonplace with treatment and can render the patient prone to arrhythmias. Hyponatremia is a poor prognostic sign indicating significant activation of the renin-aldosterone-angiotensin system. Abnormalities on liver tests can indicate hepatic congestion. Thyroid function tests can detect hyper- or hypothyroidism. Fasting lipid profile, fasting glucose, and hemoglobin A1c level can reveal comorbid conditions that may need to be better controlled. Iron studies can detect iron deficiency or overload. If the patient is malnourished or an alcoholic and presents with high-output failure, thiamine testing is indicated to rule out deficiency related to beriberi. Further testing to determine any other etiologic factors of heart failure should be based on historical findings.

1. B-type natriuretic peptide—B-type natriuretic peptide (BNP) and N-terminal pro-BNP levels can be effectively used to evaluate patients presenting with dyspnea for heart failure. BNP is a cardiac neurohormone secreted from the ventricles and, to some extent, the atrial myocardium in response to stretching and increased wall tension from volume and pressure overload. Circulating BNP levels are increased in patients with heart failure and have a rapid turnover; thus, they vary as volume status changes. Factors to consider when interpreting BNP levels are that they increase with age, are higher in women and African American individuals, and can be elevated in renal failure. Overall, BNP appears to have better reliability than N-terminal pro-BNP, especially in older populations. Although no BNP threshold indicates the presence or absence of heart failure with 100% certainty, multiple systematic reviews have shown that normal or low BNP (<100 pg/mL) or N-terminal BNP (<300 pg/mL) levels can effectively rule out a heart failure diagnosis. The average BNP and N-terminal pro-BNP levels for diagnosing heart failure in one review were 95 pg/mL and 642 pg/mL, respectively. Elevated BNP levels can assist in diagnosing heart failure, but the effect of this diagnostic tool is small at these cutoffs. As the levels increase, the specificity and likelihood of heart failure increase, as does the ability to differentiate between a pulmonary and cardiac cause of dyspnea (Table 21–3).

Certain studies have also shown that higher BNP levels (>200 pg/mL) or N-terminal pro-BNP levels (>5180 pg/mL) during acute heart failure are a strong predictor of mortality and cardiovascular admission events during the following 2–3 months. Some evidence also suggests that a 30–50%

Table 21–3. Factors influencing B-type natriuretic peptide (BNP) levels.

Factors That Cause Elevated BNP (>100 pg/mL)	Factors That Lower BNP in the Setting of Heart Failure
Heart failure	Acute pulmonary edema
Advanced age	Stable NYHA class I disease with low ejection fraction
Renal failure[a]	Acute mitral regurgitation
Acute coronary syndromes	Mitral stenosis
Lung disease with cor pulmonale	Atrial myxoma
Acute large pulmonary embolism	
High-output cardiac states	

[a]Adjusted levels are based on glomerular filtration rate (GFR). GFR 60–89 mL/min: no adjustment in the 100 pg/mL threshold (see text). GFR 30–59 mL/min: BNP >201. GFR 15–29 mL/min: BNP >225. GFR <15 mL/min: unknown utility of BNP levels.
NYHA, New York Heart Association
Data from Wang CS, FitzGerald JM, Schulzer M, et al. Does this dyspneic patient in the emergency department have congestive heart failure? *JAMA.* 2005 Oct 19;294(15):1944–1956.

reduction in BNP at hospital discharge led to improved survival and less frequent rehospitalization. Similarly, studies suggest that having improved outpatient BNP targets showed improvements in decompensations, hospitalizations, and mortality.

2. Electrocardiography (ECG)—The ECG helps identify possible causes of heart failure. Signs of ischemic heart disease, acute or previous myocardial infarction (MI), left ventricular hypertrophy, left bundle branch block, or atrial fibrillation can be identified and lead to further cardiac evaluation and treatment options. A left bundle branch block with heart failure is a poor prognostic sign, with an increased 1-year mortality rate from any cause, including sudden death. In terms of diagnostic value, a normal ECG (or only minor abnormalities) has a small effect on ruling out systolic heart failure. Similarly, the presence of atrial fibrillation, new T-wave changes, or any abnormality has a small effect on the diagnostic probability of heart failure being present.

Balion C, Santaguida PL, Hill S, et al. Testing for BNP and NT-proBNP in the diagnosis and prognosis of heart failure. *Evid Rep Technol Assess.* 2006(142):1–147. [PMID: 17764210]

Chen W-C, Tran KD, Maisel AS. Biomarkers in heart failure. *Heart.* 2010;96(4):314–320. [PMID: 20194212]

Ewald B, Ewald D, Thakkinstian A, et al. Meta-analysis of B type natriuretic peptide and N-terminal pro B natriuretic peptide in the diagnosis of clinical heart failure and population screening for left ventricular dysfunction. *Intern Med J.* 2008;38:101–113. [PMID: 18290826]

Madhok V, Falk G, Rogers A, et al. The accuracy of symptoms, signs and diagnostic tests in the diagnosis of left ventricular dysfunction in primary care: a diagnostic accuracy systematic review. *BMC Fam Pract.* 2008;9:56. [PMID: 2569936]

D. Imaging Studies

1. Chest radiography—The chest radiograph can provide valuable clues in patients presenting with acute dyspnea, especially to identify pulmonary causes such as pneumonia, COPD, pneumothorax, or a mass. The presence of venous congestion and interstitial edema is more conclusive and effective in diagnosing heart failure (specificity of 96% and 97%, respectively). Findings such as cardiomegaly and a pleural effusion are suggestive of heart failure but only slightly increase the likelihood of the diagnosis in dyspneic patients. Likewise, the absence of cardiomegaly or venous congestion only slightly decreases the probability of a diagnosis of heart failure.

2. Cardiac Doppler echocardiography—Echocardiography with Doppler imaging is the most important component in evaluation of suspected heart failure (Table 21–4). It identifies systolic dysfunction through assessment of LVEF. Diastolic dysfunction can also be determined by assessing for elevated left atrial pressures as well as impaired left ventricular relaxation and decreased compliance.

Table 21–4. Echocardiographic parameters useful in the diagnosis of heart failure.

Parameter	Information Provided
Left ventricular function (ejection fraction)	Normal value: ≥55–60% Abnormal value: <50% Significant systolic dysfunction value: ≤35–40%
Diastolic function	Elevated left atrial pressures Decreased left ventricular compliance Impaired left ventricular relaxation
Pulmonary artery pressure	Normal value: ≤30–35 mmHg

Data from Yancy CW, Jessup M, Bozkurt B, et al. 2017 ACC/AHA/HFSA focused update of the 2013 ACCF/AHA guideline for the management of heart failure: a report of the American College of Cardiology/American Heart Association Task Force on Clinical Practice Guidelines and the Heart Failure Society of America. *Circulation.* 2017 Aug 8;136(6):e137–e161 and Vitarelli A, Tiukinhoy S, Di Luzio S, et al. The role of echocardiography in the diagnosis and management of heart failure. *Heart Fail Rev.* 2003 Apr;8(2):181–189.

Echocardiographic findings can also help differentiate among the various causes of heart failure, including ischemic heart disease (wall motion abnormalities), valvular heart disease, or various cardiomyopathies such as dilated (idiopathic), hypertrophic, restrictive, or hypertensive cardiomyopathy (left ventricular hypertrophy). Other potential reversible etiologies of heart failure are pericardial disorders such as effusion or tamponade.

The routine reevaluation with echocardiography of clinically stable patients in whom no change in management is contemplated is not recommended. If the echocardiography results are inadequate or the body habitus of the patient makes it impractical, transesophageal echocardiography, radionuclide ventriculography, or cardiac catherization ventriculogram can be performed to assess LVEF.

3. Cardiac catheterization—Coronary angiography is recommended for patients with new-onset heart failure of uncertain etiology, despite the absence of anginal symptoms or negative findings on exercise stress testing. Coronary angiography should be strongly considered for patients with LVSD and a strong suspicion of ischemic myocardium based on noninvasive testing (echocardiography or nuclear imaging).

As stated, heart failure remains a clinical diagnosis for which no single finding can establish its presence or absence with certainty. Criteria such as the Framingham and Boston criteria have been developed that use history, examination, and chest radiography to better determine a clinical diagnosis of heart failure. Ultimately, using a combination of history, examination, laboratory analysis (including BNP testing), chest radiography, and ECG provides the best information in suspected cases while proceeding to evaluate left ventricular function by echocardiography.

King M, Kingery J, Casey B. Diagnosis and evaluation of heart failure. *Am Fam Physician.* 2012;85(12):1161–1168. [PMID: 22962896]

Wang CS, FitzGerald JM, Schulzer M, et al. Does this dyspneic patient in the emergency department have congestive heart failure? *JAMA.* 2005;294:1944–1956. [PMID: 16234501]

▶ Differential Diagnosis

Because heart failure is estimated to be present in only approximately 30% of patients with dyspnea in the primary care setting, clinicians need to consider differential diagnoses for dyspnea such as asthma, COPD, infection, interstitial lung disease, pulmonary embolism, anemia, thyrotoxicosis, carbon monoxide poisoning, arrhythmia, anginal equivalent (CAD), valvular heart disease, cardiac shunt, obstructive sleep apnea, and severe obesity causing hypoventilation syndrome. The prevalence of COPD ranges from 20% to 30% in patients with heart failure.

▶ Treatment

Most evidence-based treatment strategies have focused on patients with systolic rather than diastolic heart failure; hence, stage-specific outpatient management of patients with chronic systolic heart failure (LVSD) is the focus of the discussion that follows. Although stages A–D of the ACC/AHA heart failure classification represent progressive cardiac risk and dysfunction, the treatment strategies recommended at earlier stages are applicable to and recommended for later stages (see Table 21–2).

A. Systolic Heart Failure

1. High risk for systolic heart failure (stage A)—Individuals with conditions and behaviors that place them at high risk for heart failure but who do not have structurally abnormal hearts are classified as ACC/AHA stage A and should be treated with therapies that can delay progression of cardiac dysfunction and development of heart failure. Optimizing hypertension treatment based on the current national guidelines, such as the Eighth Report of the Joint National Committee on Detection, Evaluation, and Treatment of High Blood Pressure (JNC 8) and recommendations by the ACC/AHA, can reduce new-onset heart failure by 50%. The use of hydroxymethylglutaryl–coenzyme A (HMG-CoA) reductase inhibitors or statin therapy in CAD patients based on current hyperlipidemia guidelines (the updated Adult Treatment Panel III [ATP III]) can also reduce the incidence of heart failure by 20% (Strength of Recommendation Taxonomy [SORT]: A).

Evidence-based disease management strategies for diabetes mellitus, atherosclerotic vascular disease, and thyroid disease, as well as patient avoidance of tobacco, alcohol, cocaine, amphetamines, and other illicit drugs that can be cardiotoxic, are also important components of early risk modification for prevention of heart failure. In diabetic patients, both angiotensin-converting enzyme inhibitors (ACEIs) and angiotensin receptor blockers (ARBs; specifically losartan and irbesartan) have been shown to reduce new-onset heart failure compared with placebo. In CAD or atherosclerotic vascular disease patients without heart failure, reviews of the EUROPA (European Trial on Reduction of Cardiac Events with Perindopril in Stable Coronary Artery Disease) and HOPE (Heart Outcomes Prevention Evaluation) results show a 23% reduction in heart failure with ACEI therapy, as well as reduced mortality, MIs, and cardiac arrest.

ALLHAT Officers and Coordinators for the ALLHAT Collaborative Research Group. Major outcomes in high-risk hypertensive patients randomized to angiotensin-converting enzyme inhibitor or calcium channel blocker vs. diuretic: the Anti-hypertensive and Lipid-Lowering Treatment to Prevent Heart Attack Trial (ALLHAT). *JAMA.* 2002;288:2981. [PMID: 12479763]

Baker DW. Prevention of heart failure. *J Card Fail.* 2002;8:333. [PMID: 12411985]

Yancy CW, Jessup M, Bozkurt B, et al. 2013 ACCF/AHA guideline for the management of heart failure: a report of the American College of Cardiology/American Heart Association Task Force on Practice Guidelines. *Circulation.* 2013;128:e240–327. [PMID: 23741058]

2. Asymptomatic with cardiac structural abnormalities or remodeling (stage B)—Patients who do not have clinical symptoms of heart failure but who have a structurally abnormal heart, such as a previous MI, evidence of left ventricular remodeling (left ventricular hypertrophy or low ejection fraction), or valvular disease, are at a substantial risk of developing symptomatic heart failure. Prevention of further progression in these at-risk patients is the goal, and appropriate therapies are dependent on the patient's cardiac condition.

In patients with any history of MI, regardless of ejection fraction, ACEIs and β-blockers are the mainstay of therapy (SORT: A). Both therapies have been demonstrated in randomized controlled trials to cause a significant reduction in cardiovascular death and symptomatic heart failure. These therapies are vital in post-MI patients, as is evidence-based management of an ST-segment elevation MI and chronic stable angina, to help further achieve reduction in heart failure morbidity and mortality.

In asymptomatic patients who have not had an MI but have a reduced LVEF (nonischemic cardiomyopathy), clinical trials reported an overall 37% reduction in symptomatic heart failure when treated with ACEI therapy (SORT: A). The SOLVD (Studies of Left Ventricular Dysfunction) trial and a 12-year follow-up study confirmed the long-term benefit of ACEIs regarding the onset of symptomatic heart failure and mortality. A substudy of the SOLVD trial showed how enalapril attenuates progressive increases in left ventricular dilation and hypertrophy, thus inhibiting left ventricular remodeling. Despite a lack of evidence from randomized controlled trials, the ACC/AHA guidelines recommend β-blockers in patients with stage B heart failure, given the significant survival benefit that these agents provide in worsening stages of heart failure. The RACE (Ramipril Cardioprotective Evaluation) trial provided a clue as to why ACEIs are advantageous over β-blockers for nonischemic cardiomyopathy by demonstrating that ramipril is more effective than the β-blocker atenolol in reversing left ventricular hypertrophy in hypertensive patients.

There is no clear outcome evidence for the use of ARBs in asymptomatic patients with reduced LVEF. ARB therapy is, however, a guideline-recommended alternative in ACEI-intolerant patients. VALIANT (Valsartan in Acute Myocardial Infarction) was one trial that showed that the ARB valsartan was as effective as but not superior to captopril, an ACEI, in reducing cardiovascular morbidity and mortality in post-MI patients with heart failure or a reduced LVEF. The combination of both therapies was no better than captopril alone.

Agabiti-Rosei E, Ambrosioni E, Dal Palù C, et al. ACE inhibitor ramipril is more effective than the beta-blocker atenolol in reducing left ventricular mass in hypertension. Results of the RACE (ramipril cardioprotective evaluation) study on behalf of the RACE study group. *J Hypertens.* 1995;13:1325–1334. [PMID: 8984131]

Flather MD, Yusuf S, Køber L, et al. Long-term ACE-inhibitor therapy in patients with heart failure or left-ventricular dysfunction: a systematic overview of data from individual patients. ACE-Inhibitor Myocardial Infarction Collaborative Group. *Lancet.* 2000;355:1575–1581. [PMID: 10821360]

3. Symptomatic systolic heart failure (stage C)—Patients with structural heart disease and a clinical diagnosis of symptomatic heart failure compose ACC/AHA stage C. This stage encompasses NYHA classes II, III, and IV, excluding patients who develop refractory end-stage heart failure (see Table 21–2). In patients with symptomatic heart failure and left ventricular dysfunction, neurohormonal activation creates deleterious effects on the heart, leading to pulmonary and peripheral edema, persistent increased afterload, pathologic cardiac remodeling, and a progressive decline in cardiac function. The overall goals in this stage are to improve the patient's symptoms, slow or reverse the deterioration of cardiac functioning, and reduce the patient's long-term morbidity and mortality.

Accurate assessment of the cause and severity of heart failure; the incorporation of previous stage A and B treatment recommendations; and correction of any cardiovascular, systemic, and behavioral factors (Table 21–5) are important to achieve control in patients with symptomatic heart failure.

Table 21–5. Factors contributing to worsening heart failure.

Cardiovascular factors
Ischemia or infarction
New-onset or uncontrolled atrial fibrillation
Uncontrolled hypertension
Unrecognized or worsened valvular disease

Systemic factors
Anemia
Fluid retention from drugs (chemotherapy, COX-1 and -2 inhibitors, licorice, glitazones, glucocorticoids, androgens, estrogens)
Infection
Pregnancy
Pulmonary causes (pulmonary embolism, cor pulmonale, pulmonary hypertension)
Renal causes (renal failure, nephrotic syndrome, glomerulonephritis)
Sleep apnea
Thyroid dysfunction
Uncontrolled diabetes mellitus

Patient-related factors
Fluid overload (sodium intake, water intake, medication compliance)
Alcohol use
Substance abuse

Data from Basow DS: UpToDate. Waltham, MA, 2013 and King M, Kingery J, Casey B. Diagnosis and evaluation of heart failure. *Am Fam Physician.* 2012 Jun 15;85(12):1161–1168.

Moderate dietary sodium restriction of <2400 mg/d and daily weight measurement further enhance volume control and allow for lower and safer doses of diuretic therapies. Exercise training is beneficial and should be encouraged to prevent physical deconditioning, which can contribute to exercise intolerance in patients with heart failure.

Patients with symptomatic heart failure should be routinely managed with a standard therapy of an ACEI (or ARB if intolerant), a β-blocker, and a diuretic (see Table 21–2). Aldosterone receptor agonists have been shown to reduce hospitalizations when used in those with preserved ejection fraction ≥45% and elevated BNP or heart failure admission within 1 year, along with other criteria discussed later. Additional pharmacologic management should be guided by the need for further symptom control versus the desire to enhance survival and long-term prognosis. A stepwise approach to therapy and recommendations for newer medications are presented in Table 21–6 and expanded on later.

A. ACE INHIBITORS—ACEIs are prescribed to all patients with symptomatic heart failure unless contraindicated and have proven benefit in alleviating heart failure symptoms, reducing hospitalization, and reducing morbidity and mortality (SORT: A). Current ACC/AHA guidelines recommend that all patients with LVSD be started on low-dose ACEI

Table 21–6. Pharmacologic steps in symptomatic heart failure.[a]

Pharmacotherapy	Indications and Considerations
Standard therapy	
Loop diuretic	Titrate accordingly for fluid control and symptom relief (dyspnea, edema)
Angiotensin-converting enzyme inhibitor (ACEI)[b]	Initiate at low dose, titrating to target, during or after optimization of diuretic therapy for survival benefit
β-Blocker	Initiate at low dose once stable on ACEI, ARB, or ARNI for survival benefit
	May initiate before achieving ACEI, ARB, or ARNI target doses and should be titrated to target doses unless symptoms become limiting
Additional therapies[c]	
Angiotensin II receptor blocker (ARB)	ARB: Used in ACEI-intolerant patients, as above, for survival benefit
	May be effective for persistent symptoms and survival (NYHA class II–IV)
Angiotensin receptor-neprilysin inhibitor (ARNI)	ARNI: shown to reduce cardiovascular death or HF hospitalization by 20%
Aldosterone antagonist	For worsening symptoms and survival in moderately severe to severe heart failure (NYHA class III with decompensations)
Ivabradine	Inhibits the I$_f$ current in the sinoatrial node, providing heart rate reduction. Shown to reduce cardiovascular death and HF hospitalization
Hydralazine plus isosorbide dinitrate	Effective for persistent symptoms and survival, particularly in African Americans

[a]Assessment of clinical response and tolerability should guide decision making and allow for variations.
[b]ARBs are recommended in patients who are intolerant to ACEIs.
[c]Decisions about whether to use additional therapy are guided by the need for symptom control versus mortality benefit.
HF, heart failure; NYHA, New York Heart Association.
Data from Basow DS: UpToDate. Waltham, MA, 2013 and Yancy CW, Jessup M, Bozkurt B, et al. 2017 ACC/AHA/HFSA focused update of the 2013 ACCF/AHA guideline for the Management of Heart Failure: a report of the American College of Cardiology/American Heart Association task force on clinical practice guidelines and the Heart Failure Society of America. *Circulation.* 2017 Aug 8;136(6):e137–e161.

therapy to avoid side effects and be slowly titrated to a maintenance or target dose (Table 21–7). ACEI titration should be adjusted every 2 weeks with monitoring of renal function, potassium, and blood pressure. For ACEIs as a class, there does not appear to be any difference in agents in terms of effectiveness at improving heart failure outcomes. Patients with NYHA class II and III symptoms who can tolerate an ACEI and ARB should transition to an angiotensin receptor-neprilysin inhibitor (ARNI) to further reduce morbidity and mortality.

B. Angiotensin II receptor blockers—Certain ARBs (see Table 21–7) have been shown in clinical trials to be nearly as effective as, but not consistently as effective and not superior to, ACEIs as first-line therapy for symptomatic heart failure (SORT: A). The use of ARBs is recommended in ACEI-intolerant patients. A recent systematic review that analyzed the benefit of ARBs in heart failure showed reduction in mortality compared to placebo. Drug withdrawals due to adverse effect were also significantly less common with the ARBs compared to the ACEIs. There is no improvement in morbidity and mortality by adding an ARB to current ACEI therapy, and combination therapy is not recommended.

C. β-Blockers—In patients with NYHA class II, III, and stable class IV heart failure, the β-blockers bisoprolol, metoprolol succinate (sustained release), and carvedilol have been shown to improve mortality, reduce hospitalizations, and improve event-free survival (SORT: A). These benefits are in addition to ACEI therapy and support the use of β-blockers as part of standard therapy in these patients.

β-Blocker therapy should be initiated near the onset of a diagnosis of LVSD and mild heart failure symptoms, given the added benefit on survival and disease progression. Data from the CIBIS III trial suggest that initiating ACEI titration and β-blocker titration first are both safe and effective, although titrating ACEI therapy to a target dose is often better tolerated and will not exacerbate heart failure in the short term. Starting doses should be very low, given their effectiveness (see Table 21–7), but doubled at regular intervals, every 2–3 weeks as tolerated, toward target doses to achieve heart rate reductions. Longer time periods may be indicated for hemodynamically instable or frail patients.

β-Blocker therapy should be titrated to the maximal dose tolerated (see Table 21–7), based on the evidence and studied doses of therapy. The MERIT-HF trial also supported lower than maximal doses as effective when those doses successfully decrease the patient's heart rate. The clinical difference

Table 21–7. Medications used in treatment of symptomatic heart failure in patients with reduced left ventricular ejection fraction.

Drug Therapy	Initial Daily Dose	Target or Maximum Daily Dose
Angiotensin-converting enzyme inhibitors		
Captopril	6.25 mg three times daily	50 mg three times daily
Enalapril	2.5 mg twice daily	10–20 mg twice daily
Fosinopril	5–10 mg once daily	40 mg once daily
Lisinopril	2.5–5 mg once daily	20–40 mg once daily
Perindopril	2 mg once daily	8–16 mg once daily
Quinapril	5 mg twice daily	20 mg twice daily
Ramipril	1.25–2.5 mg once daily	10 mg once daily
Trandolapril	1 mg once daily	4 mg once daily
Angiotensin II receptor blockers		
Candesartan	4–8 mg once daily	32 mg once daily
Losartan	25–50 mg once daily	50–150 mg once daily
Valsartan	20–40 mg twice daily	160 mg twice daily
β-Blockers		
Bisoprolol	1.25 mg once daily	10 mg once daily
Carvedilol	3.125 mg twice daily	50 mg twice daily
Carvedilol CR	10 mg once daily	80 mg once daily
Metoprolol succinate, extended release (CR/XL)	12.5–25 mg once daily	200 mg once daily
Loop diuretics		
Bumetanide	0.5–1.0 mg/dose	10 mg/d
Furosemide	20–40 mg/dose	600 mg/d
Torsemide	5–10 mg/dose	200 mg/d
Aldosterone antagonists		
Eplerenone	25 mg once daily	50 mg once daily
Spironolactone	12.5–25 mg once daily	25 mg once or twice daily
Other medication		
Hydralazine plus isosorbide dinitrate	37.5 mg/20 mg three times daily	75 mg/40 mg three times daily
	20–50 mg/20–30 mg three times daily	100 mg/40 mg three times daily
Ivabradine	5 mg BID	7.5 mg BID
Sacubitril/valsartan	24/26 mg or 49/51 mg BID	97/103 mg BID

Data from Yancy CW, Jessup M, Bozkurt B, et al: 2017 ACC/AHA/HFSA Focused Update of the 2013 ACCF/AHA Guideline for the Management of Heart Failure: A Report of the American College of Cardiology/American Heart Association Task Force on Clinical Practice Guidelines and the Heart Failure Society of America. *Circulation.* 2017 Aug 8;136(6):e137–e161.

among the β-blockers used for heart failure may be the effects on blood pressure. Patients with lower blood pressures initially are less likely to tolerate carvedilol due to its vasodilator properties. A recent systematic review and meta-analysis suggests that the benefits may be a class effect with no superior agent over other agents. Limited data are available on the direct comparison of carvedilol and sustained-release metoprolol for treatment of heart failure.

Traditionally, the negative inotropic effects of β-blockers were considered harmful in heart failure, but this impact is outweighed by the beneficial effect of inhibiting sympathetic nervous system activation. Current evidence suggests that these beneficial effects may not necessarily be equivalent

among proven β-blockers. The COMET (Carvedilol or Metoprolol European Trial) findings showed that carvedilol (an α_1-, β_1-, and β_2-receptor inhibitor) is more effective than twice-daily dosed immediate-release metoprolol tartrate (a highly specific β_1-receptor inhibitor) in reducing heart failure mortality (40% vs 34%, respectively). Previous trials had investigated metoprolol succinate (sustained-release, once-daily dosing), but the COMET trial showed a mortality reduction even with metoprolol tartrate, a very cost-effective alternative.

β-Blockers may cause a 4- to 10-week increase in symptoms before improvement is noted; therefore, therapy should be initiated when patients have no or minimal evidence of fluid retention. Patients should be instructed to weigh themselves daily and report any increase in weight >1 kg lasting >2 days. Other adverse effects of β-blockers include the worsening of heart failure, including bradycardia, hypotension, hypoperfusion, and exacerbation of peripheral vascular disease. Contraindications include second- or third-degree heart block, a P-R interval of >0.24 seconds, severe COPD, or a history of asthma. Race or gender differences in efficacy of β-blocker therapy have not been noted.

D. DIURETICS—Patients with heart failure who present with common congestive symptoms (pulmonary, elevated jugular venous pressure, and peripheral edema) are given a diuretic and asked to adhere to a low-sodium diet to manage fluid retention and achieve and maintain a euvolemic state. Diuretic therapy is specifically aimed at treating the compensatory volume expansion driven by renal tubular sodium retention and activation of the renin-angiotensin-aldosterone system.

Oral loop diuretics are the first choice in diuretics because they increase sodium excretion by 20–25% and substantially enhance free water clearance. Furosemide is most commonly used, but patients may respond better to bumetanide or torsemide because of superior, more predictable absorptions and longer durations of action. To minimize the risk of over- or underdiuresis, the diuretic response should guide the dosage of loop diuretics (see Table 21–7), with dose increases until a response is achieved. Frequency of dosing is guided by the time needed to maintain active diuresis and sustained volume and weight control. If reaching a high dose of a loop diuretic, consider changing to a different diuretic or adding thiazide in addition to the loop diuretic. Thiazide diuretics should not be used as solitary treatment, as they increase sodium excretion by only 5–10% and tend to decrease free water clearance overall.

Symptom improvement with diuretics occurs within hours to days, as compared with weeks to months for other heart failure therapies. For long-term clinical stability, diuretics alone are not sufficient, and exacerbations can be greatly reduced when diuretics are combined with ACEI and β-blocker therapies.

E. HYDRALAZINE AND NITRATES—The combination of hydralazine and isosorbide dinitrate (H-I) is a reasonable treatment in patients, particularly African Americans, who have persistent heart failure symptoms with standard therapy (SORT: B). In V-HeFT I (Vasodilator Heart Failure Trial), the mortality of African American patients receiving H-I combination therapy was reduced, but the mortality of white patients did not differ from that of the placebo group. In V-HeFT II, a reduction in mortality with the H-I combination was seen only in white patients who had been receiving enalapril therapy. No effect on hospitalization was found in either trial.

The A-HeFT (African-American Heart Failure Trial) findings further supported the benefit of a fixed-dose H-I combination (see Table 21–7) by showing a reduction in mortality and heart failure hospitalization rates as well as improved quality-of-life scores in patients with moderate to severe heart failure (NYHA class III or IV) who self-identified as African American. The H-I combination was in addition to standard therapies that included ACEIs or ARBs, β-blockers, and spironolactone.

F. ALDOSTERONE ANTAGONISTS—For selected patients with moderately severe to severe symptoms who are difficult to control (NYHA class II with reduced ejection fraction of <30%, class III or class IV with reduced ejection fraction of <35%), additional treatment options include the aldosterone antagonists spironolactone and eplerenone (see Table 21–7) to improve mortality and reduce hospitalizations (SORT: A).

The addition of aldosterone antagonist therapy can cause life-threatening hyperkalemia in patients with heart failure, who are often already at risk because of reduced left ventricular function and associated renal insufficiency. Current guidelines recommend careful monitoring to ensure that creatinine is <2.5 mg/dL in men or <2.0 mg/dL in women and that potassium is maintained below 5.0 mEq/L (levels >5.5 mEq/L should trigger discontinuation or dose reduction). The ACC/AHA recommends that potassium and creatinine should be checked 2 days after starting an aldosterone antagonist, again at 1 week, and 1 month. Subsequent testing can occur monthly and increased slowly to every 3 months if stable. Higher doses of aldosterone antagonists and ACEI therapy should also raise concern for possible hyperkalemia, and the use of nonsteroidal anti-inflammatory drugs (NSAIDs), cyclooxygenase-2 (COX-2) inhibitors, and potassium supplements should be avoided if possible. If the clinical situation does not allow for proper monitoring, the risk of hyperkalemia may outweigh the benefit of aldosterone antagonist therapy.

G. NOVEL THERAPIES—The ACC/AHA focused update of the management of heart failure guidelines included several novel medications, the first approved ARNI valsartan/sacubitril and the sinoatrial node modulator ivabradine. An ARNI is a combination of an ARB and a neprilysin inhibitor, which results in increased natriuretic peptides, bradykinin, and adrenomedullin. Valsartan/sacubitril was found to be superior to enalapril in the PARADIGM-HF (Prospective Comparison of ARNI with ACEI to Determine Impact on Global Mortality and Morbidity in Heart Failure) trial, reducing heart failure hospitalization and cardiac death by 20%. Based on these new clinical trial data, it is recommended that patients with NYHA class II–III HFrEF who are able to tolerate an ACEI or an ARB should be transitioned to an ARNI (SORT: B). A history of angioedema is a contraindication for the use of an ARNI, with an increased risk seen in smokers and African Americans. A 36-hour waiting period is required between stopping an ACEI and starting an ARNI, and vice versa, due to breakdown of bradykinin, which may increase the risk of angioedema. Adverse effects of ARNIs include hypotension, hyperkalemia, and impaired renal function. After initiation of treatment, renal function and potassium should be checked in 1–2 weeks, then monthly for 3 months, and subsequently every 3 months. It is important to take into consideration that BNP levels of patients taking an ARNI will be elevated and N-terminal pro-BNP levels may be decreased. Ivabradine reduces the heart rate by selectively inhibiting the sinoatrial node and prolonging the slow depolarization phase. The use of ivabradine demonstrated decreased heart failure hospitalization and cardiac death in one trial. However, only 25% of patients studied were on optimal doses of β-blockers. Ivabradine can be a useful adjunct treatment in patients already on optimal β-blocker therapy in sinus rhythm with NYHA class II–IV heart failure with LVEF <35% and a resting heart rate >70 bpm.

H. Adverse therapies—The AHA issued a comprehensive statement discussing drugs that can either cause or exacerbate heart failure. NSAIDs can exacerbate heart failure through peripheral vasoconstriction and by interfering with the renal effects of diuretics and the unloading effects of ACEIs, resulting in sodium and water retention. Multiple observational studies have demonstrated increased risk for heart failure in patients taking NSAIDs, and as a result, the ACC/AHA guidelines discourage their use when possible. Calcium channel blockers offer no morbidity or mortality benefit in heart failure and should generally be avoided. The nondihydropyridine calcium channel blockers diltiazem and verapamil can worsen heart failure due to negative inotropic effects. The dihydropyridine calcium channel blocker nifedipine has been found to worsen heart failure in several small trials. Amlodipine has also been found to increase peripheral and pulmonary edema. Class I and III antiarrhythmic drugs (except amiodarone and dofetilide) have an adverse impact on heart failure and survival because of their negative inotropic activity and proarrhythmic effects. Phosphodiesterase inhibitors (cilostazol, sildenafil, vardenafil, and tadalafil) can cause hypotension and are potentially hazardous in patients with heart failure. Thiazolidinediones and metformin, both used in treatment of diabetes, can be detrimental in patients with heart failure because they increase the risk of excessive fluid retention and lactic acidosis, respectively. The dipeptidyl peptidase-4 enzyme (DPP-4) inhibitors saxagliptin and sitagliptin have been found to be associated with a higher likelihood of heart failure hospitalizations due to an unknown mechanism. Although there is a slightly elevated risk of thromboembolic events in patients with heart failure, anticoagulation is only indicated in the presence of a prior history of such event or atrial fibrillation or flutter. Aspirin can decrease the effectiveness of ACEIs and should only be used for proper indications.

I. Implantable devices—Nearly one-third of all heart failure deaths occur as a result of sudden cardiac death. The ACC/AHA recommendations include the use of implantable cardioverter-defibrillators (ICDs) for primary prevention of sudden cardiac death in patients with symptomatic heart failure and a reduced LVEF and for secondary prevention in patients with a history of cardiac arrest, ventricular fibrillation, or hemodynamically unstable ventricular tachycardia. ICDs are recommended for patients with NYHA class II or III heart failure, a LVEF of <35%, and a reasonable 1-year survival with no recent MI (SORT: A). A 3-month period of guideline-directed medical therapy followed by reevaluation of LVEF is recommended in patients newly diagnosed with heart failure to reassess the need for ICD implantation. Multiple trials have demonstrated a 31% decrease in all-cause mortality in patients with an ICD in comparison to medical therapy alone. The wearable cardioverter-defibrillator is another alternative for temporary prevention of sudden cardiac death in patients with LVEF <35% who are ineligible for an ICD, including patients awaiting heart transplant and patients with MI within 40 days, revascularization within 90 days, and newly diagnosed nonischemic cardiomyopathy. In patients with NYHA class IV heart failure awaiting heart transplantation, multiple observational studies have demonstrated benefit of an ICD.

As heart failure progresses, ventricular dyssynchrony, loss of coordinated contraction defined by a QRS duration of >120 milliseconds in patients with an LVEF <35%, and NYHA class III or IV heart failure can also occur. Clinical trials have shown that cardiac resynchronization therapy (CRT) with biventricular pacing can improve quality of life, functional class, exercise capacity, exercise distance, LVEF, and survival in these patients. The COMPANION (Comparison of Medical Therapy, Pacing, and Defibrillation in Heart Failure) trial demonstrated that patients with optimized pharmacologic therapy combined with CRT with defibrillation had a 36% decrease in all-cause mortality. Patients who meet criteria for CRT and an ICD should receive a combined device, unless contraindicated.

Al-Khatib SM, Stevenson WG, Ackerman MJ, et al. 2017 AHA/ACC/HRS guideline for management of patients with ventricular arrhythmias and the prevention of sudden cardiac death. *Heart Rhythm*. 2018 Oct;15(10):e190–e252. [PMID: 29097320]

Chatterjee S, Biondi-Zoccai G, Abbate A, et al. Benefits of beta blockers in patients with heart failure and reduced ejection fraction: network meta-analysis. *Br Med J*. 2013;346:f55. [PMID: 23325883]

Heran BS, Musini VM, Bassett K, Taylor RS, Wright JM. Angiotensin receptor blocker for heart failure. *Cochrane Database Syst Rev*. 2012;4:CD003040. [PMID: 23325883]

Jong P, Yusuf S, Rousseau MF, et al. Effect of enalapril on 12-year survival and life expectancy in patients with left ventricular systolic dysfunction: a follow-up study. *Lancet*. 2003;361: 1843–1848. [PMID: 12788569].

McMurray J, Packer M, Desai A, et al. Angiotensin-neprilysin inhibition versus enalapril in heart failure. *N Engl J Med*. 2014;371(11): 993–1004. [PMID: 25176015]

Page R, O'Bryant C, Cheng D, et al. Drugs that may cause or exacerbate heart failure. American Heart Association. *Circulation*. 2016;134(6):e32–e69. [PMID: 27400984]

Yancy CW, Jessup M, Bozkurt B, et al. 2013 ACCF/AHA guideline for the management of heart failure: a report of the American College of Cardiology Foundation/American Heart Association Task Force on Practice Guidelines. *Circulation*. 2013;128: e240–327. [PMID: 23741058]

Yancy CW, Jessup M, Bozkurt B, et al. 2017 ACC/AHA/HFSA focused update of the 2013 ACCF/AHA guideline for the management of heart failure: a report of the American College of Cardiology/American Heart Association Task Force on Clinical Practice Guidelines and the Heart Failure Society of America. *Circulation*. 2017;136:e137–e161. [PMID: 28455343]

4. Refractory end-stage heart failure (stage D)—Despite optimal medical therapy, some patients deteriorate or do not improve and experience symptoms at rest (NYHA class IV). These patients can have rapid recurrence of symptoms, leading to frequent hospitalizations and a significant or permanent reduction in their activities of daily living. Before classifying patients as being refractory or having end-stage heart failure, providers should verify an accurate diagnosis, identify and treat contributing conditions that could be hindering improvement, and maximize medical therapy.

Control of fluid retention to improve symptoms is paramount in this stage, and referral to a program with expertise in refractory heart failure or referral for cardiac transplantation should be considered. Other specialized treatment strategies, such as mechanical circulatory support, continuous intravenous positive inotropic therapy, and other surgical management, can be considered, but there is limited evidence in terms of morbidity and mortality to support the value of these therapies. Careful discussion of the prognosis and options for end-of-life care should also be initiated with patients and their families. In this scenario, patients with ICDs should receive information about the option to inactivate defibrillation.

B. Diastolic Heart Failure

Clinically, diastolic heart failure is as prevalent as LVSD, and the presentation of diastolic heart failure is indistinguishable from LVSD. Nearly 40–50% of patients with symptomatic heart failure experience diastolic failure. Patients with diastolic heart failure are more likely to be women, older, and have hypertension, atrial fibrillation, and left ventricular hypertrophy, but no history of CAD. Diastolic heart failure remains a diagnosis of exclusion in which a thorough differential of heart failure needs to be considered. Compared to systolic heart failure, the treatment of diastolic heart failure lacks validated evidence-based therapies. Management focuses on controlling systolic and diastolic blood pressure, ventricular rate, and volume status and reducing myocardial ischemia, because these entities are known to exert effects on ventricular relaxation. Diuretics are used to control symptoms of pulmonary congestion and peripheral edema, but care must be taken to avoid overdiuresis, which can cause decreased volume status and preload, manifesting as worsening heart failure.

King M, Kingery J, Casey B. Diagnosis and evaluation of heart failure. *Am Fam Physician*. 2012;85(12):1161–1168. [PMID: 22962896]

Yancy CW, Jessup M, Bozkurt B, et al. 2013 ACCF/AHA guideline for the management of heart failure: a report of the American College of Cardiology Foundation/American Heart Association Task Force on Practice Guidelines. *Circulation*. 2013;128:e240–e327. [PMID: 23741058]

▶ **Prognosis**

Despite favorable trends in survival and advances in treatment of heart failure and associated comorbidities, prognosis is poor, thus indicating the importance of appropriate diagnosis and treatment. Following diagnosis, survival is 90% at 1 month but declines to 78% at 1 year and only 58% at 5 years. Mortality increases in patients both with and without symptomatic heart failure as systolic function declines. There is also no difference in survival between diastolic and systolic heart failure.

Websites

American College of Cardiology clinical guidelines. https://www.acc.org/guidelines

American Heart Association (AHA). http://www.americanheart.org

AHA health topics. https://www.heart.org/en/health-topics

National Heart, Lung, and Blood Institute patient information. https://www.nhlbi.nih.gov/health-topics/heart-failure

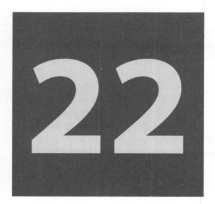

Dyslipidemias

Brian V. Reamy, MD

▶ Serum cholesterol values greater than ideal for the prevention of atherosclerotic cardiovascular disease (ASCVD).

▶ Patients with clinical ASCVD or low-density lipoprotein (LDL) cholesterol ≥190 mg/dL, diabetic patients age 40–75, or those with an elevated 10-year risk for ASCVD require treatment.

▶ General Considerations

The Framingham Heart Study firmly established an epidemiologic link between elevated serum cholesterol and an increased risk of morbidity and mortality from ASCVD. Although the benefits of lowering cholesterol were assumed for many years, not until 2001 had enough evidence accumulated to show unequivocal benefits from using lifestyle and pharmacologic therapy to lower serum cholesterol. Evidence in support of using statin agents is particularly strong and has revolutionized the treatment of dyslipidemias.

The efficacy of lipid reduction for the *secondary prevention* of ASCVD (reducing further disease-related morbidity in those with manifest disease) is supported by multiple trials and is appropriate in all patients with ASCVD. The efficacy of *primary prevention* (reducing the risk of disease occurrence in those without overt cardiovascular disease) is now supported by growing evidence that has been reviewed by the Cochrane Collaboration and led to 2016 guidelines for primary prevention from the US Preventive Services Task Force (USPSTF). The USPSTF now endorses the use of statins in adults age 40–75 years with a calculated 10-year risk of 10% or greater.

The American College of Cardiology (ACC) and American Heart Association (AHA) released new integrated guidelines for cardiovascular disease reduction in 2013. These guidelines emphasize aggressive treatment of dyslipidemias and other cardiovascular risk factors with lifestyle interventions and targeted use of statin medications, with the intensity of treatment titrated to the patients risk status. These guidelines form the foundation for the approach to the treatment of dyslipidemias.

▶ Pathogenesis

Serum cholesterol is carried by three major lipoproteins: high-density lipoprotein (HDL), LDL, and very-low-density lipoprotein (VLDL). All clinical laboratories can measure the total cholesterol, total triglycerides (TG), and the HDL fraction, and most can now directly measure the LDL fraction.

The triglyceride fraction and, to a lesser extent, the HDL level vary considerably depending on the fasting status of the patient. The ACC/AHA guidelines recommend that fasting measurements of total cholesterol, triglycerides, HDL cholesterol, and LDL cholesterol be used to guide management decisions unless a direct measure of LDL cholesterol is available.

Different populations have different median cholesterol values. For example, Asian populations tend to have total cholesterol values 20–30% lower than those of populations living in Europe or the United States. It is important to recognize that unlike a serum sodium electrolyte value, there is no normal cholesterol value. Instead, there are cholesterol values that predict higher morbidity and mortality from ASCVD if left untreated and lower cholesterol values that correlate with less likelihood of cardiovascular disease.

Atherosclerosis is an inflammatory disease in which cells and mediators participate at every stage of atherogenesis from the earliest fatty streak to the most advanced fibrous lesion. Elevated glucose, increased blood pressure, and inhaled cigarette by-products can trigger inflammation. However, one of the key factors triggering this inflammation is oxidized LDL.

When LDL is taken up by macrophages, it triggers the release of inflammatory mediators, which can lead to thickening and/or rupture of plaque lining the arterial walls. Ruptured or unstable plaques are responsible for clinical events such as myocardial infarction and stroke. Lipid lowering, whether by diet or medication, can therefore be regarded as an anti-inflammatory and plaque-stabilizing therapy.

► Clinical Findings

A. Symptoms and Signs

Most dyslipidemia patients have no signs or symptoms of the disease, which is usually detected by routine laboratory screening in an asymptomatic individual. Rarely, patients with familial forms of hyperlipidemia may present with yellow xanthomas on the skin or in tendon bodies, especially the patellar tendon, Achilles tendon, and the extensor tendons of the hands.

A few associated conditions can cause a secondary hyperlipidemia (Table 22–1). These conditions should be considered before lipid-lowering therapy is begun or when the response to therapy is much less than predicted. In particular, poorly controlled diabetes and untreated hypothyroidism can lead to an elevation of serum lipids resistant to pharmacologic treatment.

B. Screening

The USPSTF 2016 evidence summary found no direct evidence for the benefits or harms of screening young adults age 21–39 years and stated that the potential effects of screening must be extrapolated from studies in older adults.

Table 22–1. Secondary causes of lipid abnormalities.

I. Hypercholesterolemia
Hypothyroidism
Nephrotic syndrome
Obstructive liver disease
Acute intermittent porphyria
Diabetes mellitus
Chronic renal insufficiency
Cushing disease
Drugs (oral contraceptives, diuretics)
II. Hypertriglyceridemia
Diabetes mellitus
Alcohol use
Obesity
Chronic renal insufficiency
Drugs (estrogens, isotretinoin)
III. Hypocholesterolemia
Malignancy
Hyperthyroidism
Cirrhosis

In contrast, the 2013 ACC/AHA guidelines recommend the use of a global cardiovascular risk assessment in adults between the ages of 20 and 79 years who are free of overt cardiovascular disease. They also state that it is reasonable to reassess 10-year and lifetime risk for cardiovascular disease every 4–6 years. Screening children and adolescents is controversial. Integrated guidelines released by the National Heart, Lung, and Blood Institute in 2011 recommended universal screening of all 9- to 11-year-olds and gave this a grade B recommendation. Expert opinion recommends screening children from 2–8 years of age with significant family histories of hypercholesterolemia and premature ASCVD.

► Treatment

The 2013 ACC/AHA treatment guidelines are as rooted in evidence as possible and begin with an assessment of global risk for cardiovascular disease in 10 years and over the lifetime through the use of the Pooled Cohort Risk Equation calculator found at www.cvriskcalculator.com. No risk calculation is required for those with overt ASCVD. The ACC/AHA calculator is the only tool with full external validation and includes the risks attributable to different ethnicities. Of note, no risk calculator is completely accurate, and each requires an individualized application to the patient being evaluated. Improvements to risk assessment are an active area of research.

A. Lifestyle Optimization

After the calculation of risk, all patients should be instructed in lifestyle optimization to include: no tobacco use, maintaining a body mass index <25 kg/m^2, engaging in 150 minutes of moderate aerobic exercise per week, and optimizing the diet by following recommended guidelines such as the AHA Healthy Heart Diet or a Mediterranean-style diet.

B. Pharmacologic Treatment

Statins are recommended in four risk groups: those with known ASCVD, patients with an LDL cholesterol ≥190 mg/dL, patients 40–75 years of age with diabetes, and those with a 10-year risk for disease >5–7.5%. In selected patients, additional factors may be considered to decide on the need for medications, including family history of premature ASCVD, an abnormal coronary artery calcium score, a high-sensitivity C-reactive protein of ≥2 mg/L, comorbidities, the chance for drug-drug interactions, and age >75 years. Patients with known ASCVD or LDL ≥190 mg/dL and diabetics with a 10-year risk >7.5% should be treated with a high-intensity statin. Other patients at risk should be prescribed a moderate-intensity statin (Table 22–2). A flowchart that includes recommended intensity of statin treatment can be found in the ACC/AHA guidelines.

The addition of ezetimibe to a statin may also aid in secondary prevention. Niacin and fibrates both reduce TG and

Table 22–2. High-intensity and moderate-intensity statin medications and dosing.

Medication	Dose for High Intensity	Dose for Moderate Intensity
Atorvastatin	40–80 mg/d	10–20 mg/d
Rosuvastatin	20–40 mg/d	5–10 mg/d
Simvastatin	Do not use 80 mg/d (FDA black box warning)	20–40 mg/d
Pravastatin	Not possible	40–80 mg/d
Lovastatin	Not possible	40 mg/d

FDA, US Food and Drug Administration.

LDL and raise HDL cholesterol, but have not been shown to reduce cardiovascular risk and are no longer recommended. There is also no definitive evidence to support the use of fish oil supplements for the prevention of cardiovascular disease. The PCSK9 inhibitors, alirocumab and evolocumab, are the newest and highest potency class of medications for the reduction of LDL cholesterol. They are indicated for use when maximum-dose statins do not lower LDL cholesterol sufficiently or when a patient has an intolerance to statins. The addition of one of these medications to a statin can lower LDL an additional 50–60%.

Patients should be reevaluated at 12 weeks with lipid levels and a focused medical history to assess compliance with medication and lifestyle changes. Subsequently, at least annual visits are advised to assure sufficient reduction in LDL cholesterol and to assess medication compliance and continued implementation of lifestyle changes. Although most patients' LDL cholesterol levels respond fairly predictably to the use of statins, there are some who are resistant or overly sensitive, and this can only be assessed and corrected with repeat lipid assessments and patient reevaluation.

C. Complementary and Alternative Therapies

Several complementary or alternative therapies are employed for cholesterol reduction, but the evidence supporting their use is variable. Several are harmless, and some could lead to significant side effects. Oat bran (½ cup/d) is a soluble fiber that can reduce total cholesterol by 5 mg/dL and TG by 5%. Fish oil (1 g daily of unsaturated omega-3 fatty acids) can reduce triglycerides by ≤30% and raise HDL slightly with long-term use.

Garlic has few side effects, but several trials have shown that it changes lipids minimally. Soy can reduce LDL by ≤15%, with an intake of 25 g/d. This amount is unlikely to be achieved in a Western-style diet. Went yeast (*Monascus purpureus*) is the natural source for statin agents. As such,

it is effective at lowering lipid values, but carries the same side effect profile as statins. Red wine can raise HDL; however, in amounts of >2 glasses per day, red wine will raise TG and potentially cause hepatic damage and other deleterious health effects. Several other supplements such as ginseng, chromium, and myrrh all have putative cholesterol-lowering effects but little patient-oriented clinical outcome evidence.

D. Treatment of Special Groups

The treatment of dyslipidemias in special groups presents problems because fewer trial data are available.

1. Women—Several statin trials included women, although they accounted for only 15–20% of the total enrolled patient population. Subset analysis and meta-analysis reveal that statins reduced coronary events by a similar proportion in women as in men.

2. Elderly—Given that ASCVD is more common in the elderly, it is expected that the benefits of cholesterol lowering would extend to this subgroup. Because of the increased frequency of ASCVD events in this population, the number needed to treat is reduced from approximately 35:1 in patients age 40–55 years to just 4:1 in patients age 65–75 years. The 2002 Prospective Study of Pravastatin in the Elderly at Risk (PROSPER) study and several others have confirmed the benefits of lipid lowering with statins for the primary and secondary prevention of ASCVD in patients age 65–84 years. However, subanalysis of older patients in the ALLHAT trial raised questions as to the efficacy of statin treatment in the elderly.

3. Children—There are accumulating studies showing the safety of statins in adolescents. However, given concerns of interrupting cholesterol synthesis in the growing body, therapy is usually confined to the very high risk. Lifestyle interventions are safe and can have a profound impact on the long-term health of the child. Cholesterol levels should not be checked in children age <2 years.

E. Indications for Referral

Patients who do not respond to combination therapy or have untoward side effects following therapy should be considered for specialty consultation. Combinations of multiple agents or lipid plasmapheresis may sometimes be required.

Anonymous. Statins for the primary prevention of cardiovascular disease. *Cochrane Database Syst Rev.* 2013;1:CD004816. [PMID: 23440795]

National Heart, Lung, and Blood Institute. Integrated guidelines for cardiovascular health and risk reduction in children and adolescents: summary report. https://www.nhlbi.nih.gov/node/80308. Accessed November 11, 2019.

Oldways. Mediterranean diet. http://oldwayspt.org/traditional-diets/mediterranean-diet. Accessed November 11, 2019.

Stone NJ, Robinson JG, Lichtenstein AH, et al. 2013 ACC/AHA guideline on the treatment of blood cholesterol to reduce atherosclerotic cardiovascular risk in adults: a report of the ACC/AHA task force on practice guidelines. *Circulation*. 2014;129(suppl2):S1–S45. [PMID: 24222016]

US Preventive Services Task Force, Bibbins-Domingo K, Grossman DC, et al. Statin use for the primary prevention of cardiovascular disease in adults: US Preventive Services Task Force Recommendation Statement. *JAMA*. 2016;316(19):1997–2007. [PMID: 27838723]

Van Horn L, Carson JA, Appel LJ, et al. Recommended dietary pattern to achieve adherence to the American Heart Association/American College of Cardiology (AHA/ACC) Guidelines: a scientific statement from the American Heart Association. *Circulation*. 2016;134(22):e505–e529. [PMID: 27789558]

Websites

American Heart Association. https://www.heart.org (best peer-reviewed source for diet, exercise, and lifestyle information for physicians and patients)

American Heart Association. https://www.heart.org/en/healthy-living (advice for patients on lifestyle)

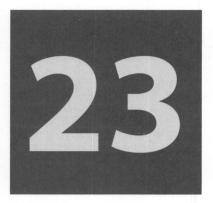

Urinary Tract Infections

Joe E. Kingery, DO, MBA, FACOFP

Urinary tract infections (UTIs) are among the most common bacterial infections encountered in medicine. Accurately estimating incidence is difficult because UTIs are not reportable, but they are estimated to result in 10.5 million office visits and 2–3 million emergency department visits per year in the United States.

A *UTI* is defined by urologists as any infection involving the urothelium, which includes urethral, bladder, prostate, and kidney infections. Some of these are diseases that have been clearly characterized (eg, cystitis and pyelonephritis), whereas others (eg, urethral and prostate infections) are not as well understood or described.

The terms *simple UTI* and *uncomplicated UTI* are often used to refer to cystitis. In this chapter, *UTI* is used to refer to any infection of the urinary tract, and *cystitis* is used to specify a bladder infection. The generic term *complicated UTI* is often used to refer to cystitis occurring in a person with preexisting metabolic, immunologic, or urologic abnormalities, including kidney stones, diabetes, and acquired immunodeficiency syndrome (AIDS), or caused by multidrug-resistant organisms.

Asymptomatic bacteriuria, uncomplicated cystitis, complicated cystitis, two urethral syndromes, four prostatitis syndromes, and pyelonephritis are discussed in this chapter. Although separated into different diagnoses, differentiating among syndromes and deciding treatment is left to the clinician's discretion.

Antibiotic resistance is a topic that has been left mostly to the reader. General recommendations about specific antibiotics are inappropriate, given that antibiotic resistance differs from location to location. It is the responsibility of individual physicians to be familiar with local antibiotic resistances and to determine the best first-line therapies for their practice. Always keep in mind that antibiotic use breeds resistance, and try to keep first-line drugs as simple and narrow spectrum as possible.

Drekonja DM, Johnson JR. Urinary tract infections. *Prim Care*. 2008:35:345–367; vii. [PMID: 18486719]

Flores-Mireles AL, Walker JN, Caparon M, Hultgren SJ. Urinary tract infections: epidemiology, mechanisms of infection and treatment options. *Nat Rev Microbiol*. 2015;13(5):269–284. [PMID: 25853778]

ASYMPTOMATIC BACTERIURIA

 ESSENTIALS OF DIAGNOSIS

▶ Asymptomatic patient.

▶ Urine culture with more than 10^5 colony-forming units (CFUs); bacteria in spun urine; or urine dipstick analysis positive for leukocytes, nitrites, or both.

General Considerations

Asymptomatic bacteriuria is defined separately for men, women, and the type of specimen. For women, clean-catch voided specimens on two separate occasions must contain $>10^5$ CFU/mL of the same bacterial strain, or one catheterized specimen must contain $>10^2$ CFU/mL of bacteria. For men, a single clean-catch specimen with $>10^5$ CFU/mL of bacteria or one catheterized specimen with $>10^2$ CFU/mL of bacteria suffices for the diagnosis. By definition, the patient must be asymptomatic, that is, should not be experiencing dysuria, suprapubic pain, fever, urgency, frequency, or incontinence. Screening for bacteriuria does not need to be done in young, healthy, nonpregnant women; elderly healthy or institutionalized men or women; diabetic women; persons with spinal cord injury; or catheterized patients while the catheter remains in place. Studies show, except in the case of pregnancy, that the presence of asymptomatic bacteriuria is not harmful in adult populations and treatment of asymptomatic bacteriuria does not improve outcomes. Pregnant women are now the only group that should be routinely screened and treated for asymptomatic bacteriuria. There are multiple guidelines recommending screening of this group of patients. Screening should occur between 12 and 16 weeks' gestation. The incidence is approximately 5–10% of pregnant women. There are numerous studies showing an association between asymptomatic bacteriuria and premature birth, low birth weight, and a high incidence of pyelonephritis. In the United States, screening is usually done by urine culture because dipstick screening can miss patients without pyuria or with unusual organisms.

► Treatment

Treatment should be guided by local rates of resistance, keeping in mind safety of the antibiotic in pregnancy. The usual first-line treatment in the absence of significant resistance or penicillin allergy is a 7-day course of amoxicillin. Nitrofurantoin or a cephalosporin is suggested for penicillin-allergic pregnant patients, again for 7 days.

Avelluto GD, Bryman PN. Asymptomatic bacteriuria vs. symptomatic urinary tract infection: identification and treatment challenges in geriatric care. *Urol Nursing.* 2018;38(3):129–135, 143. [No PMID]

Guinto V, De Guia B, Festin MR, et al. Different antibiotic regimens for treating asymptomatic bacteriuria in pregnancy. *Cochrane Database Syst Rev.* 2010;9:CD007855. [PMID: 20824868]

Lin K, Fajardo K. Screening for asymptomatic bacteriuria in adults: evidence for the U.S. Preventive Services Task Force reaffirmation recommendation statement. *Ann Intern Med.* 2008;149:W20–W24. [PMID: 18591632]

Widmer M, Lopez I, Gülmezoglu AM, et al. Duration of treatment for asymptomatic bacteriuria during pregnancy. *Cochrane Database Syst Rev.* 2011;11:CD000491. [PMID: 22161364]

UNCOMPLICATED BACTERIAL CYSTITIS

ESSENTIALS OF DIAGNOSIS

► Dysuria.

► Frequency, urgency, or both.

► Urine dipstick analysis positive for nitrites or leukocyte esterase.

► Positive urine culture (>10^4 organisms).

► No fever or flank pain.

► General Considerations

Acute, uncomplicated cystitis is most common in women. Approximately one-third of all women have experienced at least one episode of cystitis by the age of 24 years, and nearly half will experience at least one episode during their lifetime. Young women's risk factors include sexual activity, use of spermicidal condoms or diaphragm, and genetic factors such as blood type or maternal history of recurrent cystitis. Healthy, noninstitutionalized older women can also experience recurrent cystitis. Risk factors among these women include changes in the perineal epithelium and vaginal microflora after menopause, incontinence, diabetes, and history of cystitis before menopause.

Although men can also suffer from cystitis, it is rare (annual incidence: <0.01% of men age 21–50 years) in men age <35 years who have normal urinary anatomy. Urethritis from sexually transmitted pathogens should always be considered in this age group, and prostatitis should always be ruled out in the older age group by a rectal examination. Any cystitis in a man is complicated, due to the presence of the prostate gland, and should be treated for 10–14 days to prevent a persistent prostatic infection.

► Prevention

A. Young Women

Considering the frequency and morbidity of cystitis among young women, it is hardly surprising that the lay press and medical literature contain a host of ideas about how to prevent recurrent cystitis. These range from the suggestion that cotton underwear is "healthier" to wiping habits, voiding habits, and choice of beverage. Unfortunately, the vast majority of these preventive measures do not hold up to scientific study (Table 23–1).

Recent studies have shown no effect of front-to-back wiping, precoital voiding, tampon use, underwear fabric choice, or use of noncotton hose or tights. Behaviors that do appear to have an impact on frequency of cystitis in young women include sexual activity (four or more episodes per month in

Table 23–1. UTI risk in young women.

Factors with No Evidence of Effect on Cystitis	Factors with Evidence of Effect on Cystitis	
	Promote	Prevent
Precoital voiding	Spermicide[a]	Cranberry juice
Underwear fabric	Diaphragm[a]	Prophylactic antibiotics
Wiping pattern	Cervical cap[a]	
Douching	Sexual activity	
Hot tub use	Genetic predisposition	
	Delayed postcoital voiding[a]	

[a]Data from Drekonja DM, Johnson JR: Urinary tract infections. *Prim Care* 2008: Jun;35(2):345–367.

one study), delayed postcoital voiding, use of spermicidal condoms (several studies), use of unlubricated condoms (one study), use of diaphragms or cervical caps, and intake of cranberry juice.

It can be concluded from Table 23–1 that a few behaviorally oriented strategies can be offered to young women who suffer from recurrent cystitis. Recommending a change in contraception to oral contraceptive pills, intrauterine devices, or nonspermicidal, lubricated condoms may be helpful.

Cranberry juice and cranberry extract have long been proposed as a possible way to prevent UTIs. Cranberries supposedly contain a substance that changes the surface properties of *Escherichia coli* and prevents it from adhering to the bladder wall. An updated *Cochrane Review* showed that although some small studies demonstrated a small benefit for women with recurrent UTIs, there was no statistically significant differences when a much larger study was included. Thus, although cranberry juice is likely benign, the evidence suggests it does not prevent UTIs.

Probiotics that contain *Lactobacillus* are likely effective in decreasing recurrent UTIs in women. They may be particularly useful for women with a history of recurrent, complicated UTIs or who have had prolonged use of antibiotics. Probiotics do not cause antibiotic resistance and may offer other health benefits as they tend to recolonize the vaginal area with lactobacilli.

Prophylactic antibiotics, either low-dose daily antibiotics or postcoital antibiotics, remain the mainstay of prevention of recurrent UTIs for young women and can reduce recurrence rates by ≤95%.

B. Postmenopausal Women

Risk factors for cystitis in older women include urologic factors such as incontinence, cystocele, and postvoid residual; hormonal factors resulting in a lack of protective *Lactobacillus* colonization; and a prior history of cystitis. For the previously mentioned risk factors, the most easily administered effective prevention is estrogen.

There are many possible ways to administer estrogen. These include traditional oral hormone replacement therapy, which is still considered indicated (after thorough discussion with the patient of risks and benefits) for menopausal symptoms, vaginal estrogen rings, or vaginal creams.

The only form of estrogen that has been proven to decrease recurrent UTIs in postmenopausal women is vaginal. The usual side effects of estrogen can be seen with vaginal use as well as oral. These include breast tenderness, vaginal bleeding, vaginal discharge, and vaginal irritation. Contraindications (as with oral estrogens) include a history of endometrial carcinoma, breast carcinoma, thromboembolic disorders, and liver disease. Patients' functional abilities and cultural preferences should be considered before prescribing vaginal applications.

C. Young Men

The only studies focusing on prevention of UTI in young men have investigated infant circumcision; because the risk of UTI is so low in normal men, these studies are prohibitively expensive. In boys with recurrent UTI or high-grade ureteral reflux, the numbers needed to treat (NNTs) are 11 and 4, respectively. The complication rate of circumcision is 2–10%, with adverse sequelae ranging from minor transient bleeding (common) to amputation of the penis (extremely rare). It does appear to decrease the chance of UTI in boys and men. The risk of UTI in normal boys hovers around 1% in the first 10 years of life, given that the NNT for circumcision is 111. In 2012, the American Academy of Pediatrics found that the scientific evidence of newborn male circumcision benefits outweighed the risks. Additionally, in 2014, the Centers for Disease Control and Prevention released a draft policy stating that male circumcision was an important public health measure. This was based on several factors, one of which was decreasing UTIs in men.

D. Future Trends in Prevention

Several investigations are ongoing in finding ways to prevent recurrent UTIs, given the high prevalence and health burden that they impose. Vaginal vaccines are working their way through clinical trials and are not yet commercially available; whether they will prove to be more efficacious than prophylactic antibiotics is yet to be determined. Currently, a sublingual bacterial vaccine is also in development. This also looks promising, but needs more research.

▶ Clinical Findings

A. Symptoms and Signs

Symptoms include dysuria, ideally felt more internally than externally, and of sudden onset; suprapubic pain; cloudy, smelly urine; frequency; and urgency.

Physical examination in the afebrile, otherwise healthy patient with a classic history is done essentially to rule out other diagnoses and to ensure that red flags are not present. The examination might range from checking a temperature and percussing the costovertebral angles to a full pelvic examination, depending on where the history leads. There are no pathognomonic signs on physical examination for cystitis.

B. Laboratory Findings

Laboratory studies include dipstick test of urine, urinalysis, and urine culture. In some cases, laboratory tests are not required to diagnose cystitis with high accuracy; however, they should probably be omitted only in settings where follow-up can be easily arranged in case of failure of treatment, which would, of course, indicate further workup.

1. Urine dipstick testing—Dipstick findings are positive for leukocyte esterase or nitrite, or both. Several references now support treatment of simple, uncomplicated UTIs in the young, nonpregnant woman on the grounds of clinical history alone, if that history leads to high suspicion for cystitis (and low suspicion of sexually transmitted disease). In a meta-analysis, a woman who presented with dysuria and frequency, no risk factors for complicated infection, and no vaginal discharge had a 90% probability of UTI. For women with an equivocal clinical history, urine dipstick analysis may suffice to reassign the women to high or low suspicion and treat or not treat accordingly.

2. Urinalysis—Urinalysis will be positive for white blood cells (WBCs), with few or no epithelial cells. It should be noted, however, that urinalysis is more expensive than dipstick analysis and only minimally more accurate.

3. Urine culture—The gold standard of diagnosis is a culture growth of 100,000 (10^5) organisms in a midstream clean-catch sample. However, some patients have classic clinical cases of UTI and only 100 (10^2) organisms on culture.

Few laboratories are equipped to detect anything fewer than 10^4 organisms. Culture is strongly suggested if a relapsing UTI or pyelonephritis is suspected to ensure sensitivities and eradication. Any patient who has risk factors for a complicated UTI or whose symptoms do not respond to initial treatment should have a urine culture and sensitivity done.

C. Imaging Studies

Imaging studies are seldom required for patients with simple uncomplicated UTIs.

D. Special Tests

These tests are generally required only for failures of treatment, symptoms suggesting a diagnosis other than cystitis, or complicated cystitis (see section on complicated cystitis, later).

▶ **Differential Diagnosis**

See Table 23–2.

Table 23–2. Red flag symptoms and differential diagnoses.

If Patient Has	Consider
Fever	Urosepsis, pyelonephritis, pelvic inflammatory disease (PID)
Vaginal discharge	Sexually transmitted disease (STD), PID
External burning pain	Vulvovaginitis, especially candidal vaginitis
Costovertebral angle tenderness	Pyelonephritis
Nausea/vomiting	Pyelonephritis, urosepsis, inability to tolerate oral medications
Recent urinary tract infection (UTI; <2 weeks)	Incompletely treated, resistant pathogen; urologic abnormality, including stones and unusual anatomy; interstitial cystitis
Dyspareunia	STD, PID, psychogenic causes
Recent trauma or instrumentation	Complicated UTI
Pregnancy	Antibiotic choice, treatment duration
Severe, colicky flank pain	UTI complicated by stones; preexisting or struvite stone caused by urea-splitting bacteria
Joint pains, sterile urine	Spondyloarthropathy (eg, Reiter or Behçet syndrome)
History of childhood infections, urologic surgery	Abnormal anatomy
History of kidney stones	Complicated UTI; bacterial persistence in stones
Diabetes	Complicated UTI
Immunosuppression	Complicated UTI

Complications

There are virtually no complications from repeated uncomplicated cystitis if it is recognized and treated. Delay in treatment may lead to ascending infection and pyelonephritis. In the case of infection with urea-splitting bacteria, "infection stones" of struvite with bacteria trapped in the interstices may be formed. These stones lead to persistent bacteriuria and must be completely removed to clear the infection. *Proteus mirabilis*, *Staphylococcus saprophyticus*, and *Klebsiella* bacteria can all split urea and lead to stones.

Treatment

A. Acute Cystitis

There is ample evidence from randomized clinical trials to support the superiority of 3-day antibiotic therapy to 1-day treatment and, equivalently, of therapy for longer periods of time, with the exception of nitrofurantoin. This is true for treatment of older, noninstitutionalized women as well. Trimethoprim-sulfamethoxazole (TMP-SMX), in the absence of allergies to sulfa and local resistance rates of >10–20%, should be considered first-line therapy and taken for 3 days. Risk factors for TMP-SMX resistance include recent antibiotic exposure, recent hospitalization, diabetes mellitus, three or more UTIs in the past year, and possibly use of oral contraceptive pills or estrogen replacement therapy. For patients who are allergic to sulfa drugs, a 5- to 7-day course of nitrofurantoin or a 3-day course of a fluoroquinolone (eg, ciprofloxacin) can be used. However, because of concern regarding fluoroquinolone resistance and frequency of cystitis, they should be used sparingly. β-Lactam antibiotics are not as effective as other classes of drugs against urinary pathogens and should not be used as first-line agents except in pregnant patients.

B. Acute Cystitis in the Pregnant Woman

Treatment with amoxicillin, a cephalosporin, nitrofurantoin, or another pregnancy-safe antibiotic for 7 days remains the standard. Asymptomatic bacteriuria, if found on cultures, is treated in pregnant women with the same antibiotics (see section on asymptomatic bacteriuria, earlier). Urine culture should be done after treatment to confirm eradication of bacteriuria.

C. Prophylaxis for Recurrent Cystitis

Low-dose, prophylactic antibiotics have been shown to decrease recurrences by ≤95%. Most recommendations suggest starting prophylaxis after a patient has had more than three documented UTIs in 1 year. Prophylactic antibiotics are usually administered for 6 months to 1 year but can be given for longer periods of time. Antibiotics can be taken daily at bedtime or used postcoitally by women whose infections are associated with intercourse (Table 23–3). Unfortunately,

Table 23–3. Prophylactic antibiotics for recurrent urinary tract infection in women.

Regimen	Drug and Dose
Daily	Trimethoprim, 100 mg every day
	Trimethoprim-sulfamethoxazole, 80 mg/400 mg every day
	Nitrofurantoin, 50 mg every day[a]
	Nitrofurantoin macrocrystals, 100 mg every day
	Cranberry juice, 8 oz 3 times a day
	Cranberry tablets, 1:30 twice a day
Postcoital	One dose of any of the above antibiotics after coitus

[a]Preferred if patient could become pregnant. Trimethoprim should be avoided in the first trimester.

prophylaxis does not change the propensity of these women for recurrent UTIs; when prophylaxis is stopped, approximately 60% of women develop a UTI within 3–4 months. Prophylaxis should not start until cultures have shown no growth after treatment, to rule out bacterial persistence.

Prognosis

Long-term prognosis in terms of kidney function is excellent; prognosis of arresting recurrent cystitis without permanent prophylaxis is not as good. New preventive treatments are currently being explored, and it is hoped that these will prove beneficial.

Chisholm AH. Probiotics in preventing recurrent urinary tract infections in women: a literature review. *Urol Nurs.* 2015;35(1):18–21, 29. [PMID: 26298938]

Drekonja DM, Johnson JR. Urinary tract infections. *Prim Care.* 2008:35:345–367, vii. [PMID: 18486719]

Gupta K, Larissa G, Trautner B. Urinary tract infection. *Ann Intern Med.* 2017;167(7):ITC49–ITC64. [PMID: 28973215]

Jepson RG, Craig JC. Cranberries for preventing urinary tract infections. *Cochrane Database Syst Rev.* 2012;1:CD001321. [PMID: 18253990]

Lorenzo-Gomez MF, Padilla-Fernández B, García-Criado FJ, et al. Evaluation of a therapeutic vaccine for the prevention of recurrent urinary tract infections versus prophylactic treatment with antibiotics. *Int Urogynecol J.* 2013;24(1):127–134. [PMID: 22806485]

Michels TC. Dysuria: evaluation and differential diagnosis in adults. *Am Fam Physician.* 2015;92(9):778–786. [PMID: 26554471]

Morris BJ, Krieger JN, Klausner JD. CDC's male circumcision recommendations represent a key public health measure. *Glob Health Sci Pract.* 2017;5(1):15–27. [PMID: 28351877]

Nicolle LE. Short-term therapy for urinary tract infection: success and failure. *Int J Antimicrob Agents.* 2008;31(suppl 1):S40–S45. [PMID: 18023152]

Perrotta C, Aznar M, Mejia R, et al. Oestrogens for preventing recurrent urinary tract infection in postmenopausal women. *Cochrane Database Syst Rev.* 2008;2:CD005131. [PMID: 18425910]

COMPLICATED CYSTITIS & SPECIAL POPULATIONS

ESSENTIALS OF DIAGNOSIS

► Any cystitis not resolved after 3 days of appropriate antibiotic treatment.

► Any cystitis in a special population, such as a diabetic patient, a man, a patient with an abnormal urinary tract, or a patient with ureteral stones.

► Any cystitis involving multidrug-resistant bacteria.

General Considerations

The infections listed above warrant further workup by a physician or referral to a urologist. These infections should all be cultured to ensure that the antibiotics used are appropriate and that the organisms are sensitive to the chosen antibiotic. Risk factors for complicated UTIs include male sex, postmenopause, pregnancy, diabetes mellitus, immunocompromised state, history of recurrent UTIs, indwelling catheter, neurogenic bladder, and urolithiasis, among others.

Clinical Findings

Special tests should include ultrasound and/or computed tomography (CT) to evaluate for stones, intravenous pyelogram (IVP) to evaluate anatomy and stones, and cystoscopy and biopsy to rule out interstitial cystitis, cancer, or unusual pathogens.

Treatment

Patients with complicated UTIs should be treated with long-course (≥10–14 days), appropriate antibiotics. Initial empiric treatment should be broad spectrum and can be penicillins, β-lactams, cephalosporins, fluoroquinolones, or carbapenems. Single-dose or 3-day regimens are not appropriate for this group of patients.

ACUTE URETHRAL SYNDROME

ESSENTIALS OF DIAGNOSIS

► Dysuria.

► Frequency and urgency.

► No vaginal discharge.

► Urine dipstick analysis may be negative or positive.

► Negative culture.

General Considerations

Acute urethral syndrome is a term used by some to describe a young, healthy, sexually active woman who complains of recent-onset symptoms of cystitis but does not meet strict guidelines for diagnosis of cystitis (growth of ≤10^4 or 10^5 organisms on culture). Some authors now feel that even 100 CFUs found on culture of a dysuric woman represent a true UTI. Because most laboratories are equipped to detect only ≥10^4 organisms, these are patients in usual practice found to have "negative" cultures. They may have positive or negative urine dipstick analysis and positive or negative spun urine for bacteria, although bacteria and WBCs in the urine are more convincing for cystitis than a completely negative workup.

Clinical Findings

Testing depends on the physician's assessment of the patient. In patients at low risk of acquiring a sexually transmitted disease (STD), no testing might be appropriate or maybe only after failure of empirical treatment for cystitis. In patients at higher risk of acquiring an STD, *Chlamydia* testing, by cervical swab, urine polymerase chain reaction (PCR), or ligase chain reaction (LCR), might be appropriate.

Differential Diagnosis

This syndrome is not well defined. It is usually taken to represent an early cystitis, but it can also be an STD (*Chlamydia trachomatis* has been noted in women with the previously described symptoms).

Treatment

There is some evidence that the acute urethral syndrome will respond to antibiotics commonly used in the treatment of UTIs. Because the prevalence of *C trachomatis* was found to be high in at least one study of women with these symptoms, use of antibiotics effective against STDs or *Chlamydia* testing for patients who do not respond completely to a course of antibiotics is highly recommended.

Leibovici L. Trimethoprim reduced dysuria in women with symptoms of urinary tract infection but negative urine dipstick test results. *Evid Based Med.* 2006;11:19. [PMID: 17213061]

Michels TC. Dysuria: evaluation and differential diagnosis in adults. *Am Fam Physician.* 2015;92(9):778–786. [PMID: 26554471]

Richards D, Toop L, Chambers S, et al. Response to antibiotics of women with symptoms of urinary tract infection but negative dipstick urine test results: double blind randomized controlled trial. *Br Med J.* 2005;331:143. [PMID: 15972728]

Sabith A, Leslie SW. Complicated urinary tract infections. *StatPearls.* 2018. https://www.ncbi.nlm.nih.gov/books/NBK436013/ [PMID: 28613784]

URETHRITIS

ESSENTIALS OF DIAGNOSIS

▶ Pain or irritation on urination.
▶ No frequency or urgency.
▶ Discharge from the urethra (predominantly males).
▶ Vaginal discharge possible.

▶ General Considerations

Isolated urethritis in men or women is almost always an STD, most often caused by *C trachomatis*. This syndrome is differentiated from acute urethral syndrome by the time course of symptoms; symptoms that have a gradual onset or persist without evolution into classic cystitis symptoms, including suprapubic symptoms such as pain, urgency, or frequency, are more indicative of urethritis than of acute urethral syndrome.

▶ Clinical Findings

It can be very difficult to differentiate a symptomatic chlamydial infection from bacterial cystitis with coliform organisms, and testing for both may be required. The advent of *Chlamydia* urine PCR or LCR tests makes ruling out *Chlamydia* much easier than in the past, as the same urine sample can be sent for both tests.

▶ Treatment

See Chapter 14 for current diagnosis and treatment of STDs such as *Chlamydia*.

ACUTE BACTERIAL PROSTATITIS

ESSENTIALS OF DIAGNOSIS

▶ Dysuria, frequency, urgency.
▶ Tender prostate.
▶ Leukocyte esterase or nitrite on urine dipstick analysis.
▶ Positive urine culture.

▶ General Considerations

Prostatitis is a very common disease among men, with a prevalence and incidence among men ranging between 11% and 16%. Approximately 35–50% of men are reported to be affected by symptoms of prostatitis during their lifetime. It is estimated that 2 million office visits per year occur for prostatitis (1% of all primary care office visits), so it is useful for the primary care practitioner to be able to evaluate men for symptoms of prostatitis.

Previously, prostatitis was simply described as "acute," "chronic," or "nonbacterial." In 1995, the National Institutes of Health (NIH) revised the categorization of prostatitis, and the disease is now differentiated into four categories, as follows:

• Category I: acute bacterial prostatitis
• Category II: chronic bacterial prostatitis
• Category IIIA: inflammatory chronic pelvic pain syndrome
• Category IIIB: noninflammatory chronic pelvic pain syndrome
• Category IV: asymptomatic inflammatory prostatitis

Category IV is a diagnosis made incidentally, while working up other symptoms, and is not considered severe enough to require treatment. Discussion of category I, or acute bacterial prostatitis, follows. The other categories are discussed separately in this chapter.

Acute bacterial prostatitis is different from other types of prostatitis in that it is a well-defined entity with a relatively clear-cut etiology, diagnosis, and treatment. Acute bacterial prostatitis is caused by typical uropathogens and responds well to antibiotic treatment.

▶ Prevention

There is no evidence for interventions that will prevent spontaneous prostatitis.

▶ Clinical Findings

Symptoms and signs include dysuria, frequency, and urgency; low back, perineal, penile, or rectal pain; or tense or "boggy" tender prostate. Fever and chills may be present.

Laboratory findings include a urine dipstick analysis that is positive for leukocyte esterase or nitrites, or both, and urine culture that is positive for a single uropathogen. Imaging studies are rarely performed for acute uncomplicated prostatitis.

Prostatic massage is not generally performed in patients with acute bacterial prostatitis because it may lead to acute bacteremia.

▶ Differential Diagnosis

Abnormal anatomy may include urethral strictures, polyps, diverticula, redundancies, or valves anywhere in the system from the penis to the kidneys (Table 23–4).

Table 23–4. Differential diagnosis of dysuria in men.

If Patient Has	Consider
Acute, colicky flank pain or history of kidney stones	Kidney stone; complicated cystitis
Costovertebral angle tenderness, fevers	Pyelonephritis
Urethral discharge	Sexually transmitted disease
Diabetes/immunosuppression	Complicated cystitis, unusual pathogens
Testicular pain	Torsion; epididymo-orchitis
Joint pains	Spondyloarthropathy (ie, Reiter or Behçet syndrome)
History of childhood UTI or urologic surgery	Abnormal anatomy; complicated cystitis
Recurrent symptoms after treatment	Abnormal anatomy; abscess; stone; chronic prostatitis; resistant organism; inadequate length of treatment; Munchausen syndrome; somatization disorder

Complications

Complications of acute bacterial prostatitis may include ascending infection, infection-related stones, abscess, fistula, cysts, and acute urinary retention. In the case of acute urinary retention precipitated by prostatitis, a suprapubic catheter rather than a Foley catheter should be placed to avoid damage to the prostate.

Treatment

Treatment is determined by the severity of illness as well as local resistance rates. In cases of very ill patients, broad-spectrum parenteral antibiotics should be initiated. Typically, a penicillin or penicillin derivative and an aminoglycoside can be used. As the illness is treated, the patient can be transitioned to oral therapy with either a quinolone or TMP-SMX for at least 3–4 weeks. Less ill patients can be started on oral therapy with a quinolone, TMP-SMX, or doxycycline. Ciprofloxacin is currently recommended as first-line therapy and should be taken for 28 days. TMP-SMX and doxycycline are considered second-line therapy. The duration of treatment for these drugs is also 28 days. An α-blocker can be considered for mild urinary retention. A urinary catheter should be considered for more severe retention.

Prognosis

The prognosis is very good for patients with acute uncomplicated bacterial prostatitis.

Murphy AB, Macejko A, Taylor A, et al. Chronic prostatitis: management strategies. *Drugs.* 2009;69:71–84. [PMID: 19192937]

Rees J, Abrahams M, Doble A, Cooper A. Diagnosis and treatment of chronic bacterial prostatitis and chronic prostatitis/chronic pelvic syndrome: a consensus guideline. *BJU Int.* 2015;116: 509–525. [PMID: 25711488]

CHRONIC BACTERIAL PROSTATITIS

 ESSENTIALS OF DIAGNOSIS

▶ Dysuria, frequency, urgency.

▶ Symptoms lasting >3 months.

▶ Urine dipstick analysis positive for leukocyte esterase or nitrites, or both.

▶ Pyuria on microscopy.

▶ Positive four-glass or two-glass test for prostatic origin.

General Consideration

Chronic bacterial prostatitis, or NIH category II prostatitis, is quite rare, and consequently, very few studies have examined it. Bacterial disease represents only a small percentage of the cases of chronic prostatitis. It has been estimated that both acute and chronic bacterial prostatitis cases constitute only 5–10% of all prostatitis diagnoses, and of the bacterial cases, the vast majority are acute.

Prevention

Early and sufficient treatment of acute bacterial prostatitis is considered by some authors to prevent chronic prostatitis.

► Clinical Findings

A. Symptoms and Signs

Symptoms and signs include dysuria, frequency, and urgency; prostatic tenderness on examination; low back pain; and perineal, penile, or rectal pain. Symptoms are usually present for more than 3 months.

B. Laboratory and Imaging Findings

A urine dipstick analysis will be positive for leukocyte esterase or nitrites, or both. Additionally, a four- or two-glass test (discussed in the following sections) will be positive for prostatic origin. A transrectal prostatic ultrasound should be performed if an abscess or a stone is suspected.

C. Special Tests

1. Four-glass test—Not used by the majority of practitioners, this is a localization test for chronic prostatitis. The patient should not have been on antibiotics for a month, should not have ejaculated for 2 days, and needs a reasonably full bladder. Signs and symptoms of urethritis or cystitis should have been worked up previously and treated. To perform the test, the patient first cleans himself and carefully retracts the foreskin, then urinates the first 5–10 mL into a sterile container (VB_1). He then urinates 100–200 mL into the toilet, and a second 10- to 20-mL sample into a sterile container (VB_2). Prostatic massage is then done, milking secretions from the periphery to the center, and any expressed prostatic secretions are caught in a third sterile container. The patient then cleans himself again, and urinates a final 10–20 mL sample into a fourth container (VB_3).

All urine samples are examined microscopically and cultured. Expressed prostatic secretions are wet-mounted, examined, and cultured. The test is positive for prostatic localization if WBCs per high-power field (HPF) and colony counts in VB_3 are ≥10 times greater than in VB_1 or VB_2, or if there are 10 polymorphonuclear leukocytes/HPF in the wet mount. If there is a significant colony count in both VB_2 and VB_3, the patient should be treated for 3 days with nitrofurantoin, which does not penetrate the prostate, and the test should be repeated.

2. Two-glass test—A verified modification of the four-glass test, this test requires an initial clean-catch urine sample, prostatic massage, and a postmassage urine sample. It is functionally equivalent to the VB_2 and VB_3 portions of the four-glass test and more often used in clinical practice.

► Differential Diagnosis

See Table 23–4.

► Complications

Complications of chronic bacterial prostatitis may include ascending infection, infection-related stones, abscess, fistula, cysts, and acute urinary retention.

► Treatment

Antibiotic treatment with quinolones has shown the best results. Therapy is with an oral quinolone for at least 4–6 weeks. TMP-SMX for 1–3 months can also be considered. α-Blockers may provide some benefit to treatment as well.

► Prognosis

The prognosis for treatment of chronic bacterial prostatitis is not known. A clear differentiation of which patients will or will not respond to antibiotics has not been obtained.

Nickel JC, Xiang J. Clinical significance of nontraditional bacterial uropathogens in the management of chronic prostatitis. *J Urol.* 2008;179:1391–1395. [PMID: 18289570]

Weidner W, Wagenlehner FM, Marconi M, et al. Acute bacterial prostatitis and chronic prostatitis/chronic pelvic pain syndrome: andrological implications. *Andrologia.* 2008;40: 105–112. [PMID: 18336460]

CHRONIC ABACTERIAL PROSTATITIS/CHRONIC PELVIC PAIN SYNDROME

 ESSENTIALS OF DIAGNOSIS

Not very well characterized; most suggestive symptoms include the following:

► Perineal pain.

► Lower abdominal pain.

► Penile, especially penile tip, pain.

► Testicular pain.

► Ejaculatory discomfort or pain.

► STDs and UTI ruled out.

► General Considerations

Chronic abacterial prostatitis was renamed by the NIH in 1995. It is now called *chronic pelvic pain syndrome* and can be further subclassified into inflammatory, meaning with inflammatory cells isolated in tests, or noninflammatory. This change was made in an attempt to recognize that the pain syndrome that physicians have been referring to as "chronic abacterial prostatitis" or even "prostatodynia" in the absence of inflammatory cells on examination has never been proved to originate in the prostate.

The NIH further divided chronic prostatitis/chronic pelvic pain syndrome (CP/CPPS) into two categories: inflammatory (IIIA) and noninflammatory (IIIB). In category IIIA prostatitis, leukocytes are found in semen, in expressed prostatic secretions, or in a post–prostatic massage urine sample. In category IIIB prostatitis, no leukocytes are found in secretions. Recent evidence suggests cytokines may play a role in diagnosis in the future. Current research efforts include the Chronic Prostatitis Clinical Research Network, founded in 1997 by the NIH to investigate the chronic pelvic pain syndrome. Their work is ongoing and not definitive at this time.

The etiology of chronic prostatitis remains unknown. Current theories include infection with unusual or fastidious organisms, lower urinary tract obstruction or dysfunctional voiding, intraprostatic ductal reflux and subsequent chemical irritation with urea from urine forced into the gland, immunologic or autoimmune processes, or neuromuscular causes, such as reflex sympathetic dystrophy. Although none of these theories has been proved, continued research, it is hoped, will increase our understanding of this problem.

▶ Prevention

Trials of preventive measures for chronic prostatitis or chronic pelvic pain syndrome are lacking, and risk factors for prostatitis or chronic pelvic pain have not been investigated.

▶ Clinical Findings

A. Symptoms and Signs

Symptoms include dysuria, frequency, urgency, other irritative voiding symptoms, and pain in the perineal area for >3 of the past 6 months.

B. Laboratory Findings

Laboratory testing shows no evidence of current cystitis or demonstrable bacterial infection. Patients with inflammatory-type chronic pelvic pain syndrome have leukocytes in expressed prostatic secretions or post–prostatic massage urine.

C. Special Tests

If the patient has hematuria, urine cytology should be performed. The two-glass test (first part of a clean-catch urine sample in one bottle; prostatic massage milking from periphery to center; second urine sample into a sterile container) has been shown to be as reliable as the more complicated four-glass test (discussed earlier) at distinguishing chronic bacterial prostatitis and inflammatory and noninflammatory prostatitis.

▶ Differential Diagnosis

See Table 23–4.

▶ Treatment

There is no clear-cut prescription for the treatment of chronic prostatitis of either the inflammatory or noninflammatory type. This treatment discussion therefore groups inflammatory and noninflammatory prostatitis into one entity for discussion.

Although CP/CPPS does not have a bacterial etiology, antimicrobials do improve symptoms in ≤50% of patients. Patients with a shorter duration of symptoms are more likely to respond. The antimicrobials used most include fluoroquinolones and TMP-SMX for 4–6 weeks. α-Blockers such as tamsulosin, terazosin, and doxazosin have shown some improvement in patients as well. Once again, the sooner treatment is started, the better are the outcomes. At least 6 weeks of therapy are needed with α-blockers. A combination of antimicrobial and α-blocker shows slight improvement over monotherapy. Despite high use by providers, nonsteroidal anti-inflammatory drugs (NSAIDs) have shown only minimal effects. To prevent unwanted adverse effects, NSAIDs should only be used for short-term treatment. Unless the patient has concomitant benign prostatic hyperplasia, 5α-reductase inhibitors (eg, finasteride) have also demonstrated only minimal effects. Due to concern for dependency, opioids for pain management should be avoided. However; if the pain is considered to be neuropathic in origin, treatment with a gabapentinoid (gabapentin or pregabalin), a tricyclic antidepressant, or a serotonin-norepinephrine reuptake inhibitor may be used.

There are several other modalities of treatment that need further review: (1) transurethral microwave thermotherapy, (2) cooled transurethral microwave thermotherapy, (3) transurethral needle ablation, (4) botulinum toxin A injections, (5) transurethral resection of the prostate, (6) electromagnetic therapy, and (7) electroacupuncture and application of capsaicin on the perineal area. Although none of these have been studied extensively, modalities 2 and 6 show promising results.

Table 23–5 reviews the controlled trials that have shown possible efficacy of treatments.

▶ Prognosis

The prognosis for chronic prostatitis and chronic pelvic pain syndrome category III is not good. Prognosis appears to be worse for patients with previous episodes or more severe pain.

Kastner C. Update on minimally invasive therapy for chronic prostatitis/chronic pelvic pain syndrome. *Curr Urol Rep.* 2008;9: 333–338. [PMID: 18765134]

Table 23–5. Effective therapies for chronic abacterial prostatitis/chronic pelvic pain syndrome.

Therapy	Dose	Comments
Fluoroquinolone	Levofloxacin 500 mg every day Ciprofloxacin 500 mg twice a day	Although no infectious etiology in this disease, studies suggest that ~50% of patients can improve if treated early; treatment is for 6 weeks; currently considered a first-line therapy
α-Blockers	Tamsulosin 0.4 mg every day[a] Doxasozin 4 mg every day 1 mg every day for 4 days 2 mg every day for 10 days 5 mg every day for 12 weeks	All considered first-line therapy; well tolerated; can be combined with fluoroquinolone for improved benefits Needs to be taken for ≥6 weeks[b–d] Studies have used ≥3 months of therapy[d]
Finasteride	5 mg every day	Minimal benefit; not first-line therapy; mostly useful only if concomitant benign prostatic hyperplasia; need to take for >1 year[b,c]
Pentosan polysulfate	100 mg 3 times a day for 6 months	Minimal improvement, with no statistical significance[b]
Thermotherapy		Still experimental, but some promising results[d]

[a]Ye ZQ, Lan RZ, Yang WM, et al. Tamsulosin treatment of chronic non-bacterial prostatitis. *J Intern Med Res.* 2008:36:244–252. [PMID: 18380933]
[b]Murphy M, Macejko A, Taylor A, et al. Chronic prostatitis: management strategies. *Drugs.* 2009;69:71–84. [PMID: 19192937]
[c]Nickel JC. Treatment of chronic prostatitis/chronic pelvic pain syndrome. *Int J Antimicrob Agents.* 2008;31(suppl 1):S112–S116. [PMID: 17954024]
[d]Kastner C. Update on minimally invasive therapy for chronic prostatitis/chronic pelvic pain syndrome. *Curr Urol Rep.* 2008;9:333–338. [PMID: 18765134]

Murphy AB, Macejko A, Taylor A, et al. Chronic prostatitis: management strategies. *Drugs.* 2009;69:71–84. [PMID: 19192937]

Nickel JC, Alexander RB, Anderson R, et al. Category III chronic prostatitis/chronic pelvic pain syndrome: insights from the National Institutes of Health Chronic Prostatitis Collaborative Research Network studies. *Curr Urol Rep.* 2008;9:320–327. [PMID: 18765132]

Rees J, Abrahams M, Doble A, Cooper A. Diagnosis and treatment of chronic bacterial prostatitis and chronic prostatitis/chronic pelvic syndrome: a consensus guideline. *BJU Int.* 2015;116:509–525. [PMID: 25711488]

Ye ZQ, Lan RZ, Yang WM, et al. Tamsulosin treatment of chronic non-bacterial prostatitis. *J Int Med Res.* 2008;36:244–252. [PMID: 18380933]

PYELONEPHRITIS

 ESSENTIALS OF DIAGNOSIS

▶ Fever.

▶ Chills.

▶ Flank pain.

▶ More than 100,000 CFUs on urine culture.

General Considerations

Pyelonephritis is an infection of the kidney parenchyma. It has been estimated to result in >100,000 hospitalizations per year. Information on outpatient visits is not readily available, but because many cases are now managed on an outpatient basis, it is likely to be seen by most primary care providers. Pyelonephritis usually results from upward spread of cystitis but can also result from hematogenous seeding of the kidney from another infectious source. The infection can be complicated by stones or renal scarring if untreated but usually resolves without sequelae in young, healthy people if treated promptly.

The most common bacteria involved are the same organisms that cause uncomplicated cystitis: *E coli, S saprophyticus, Klebsiella* species, and occasionally *Enterobacter*. As with simple cystitis, women with genetic predispositions are more commonly affected than other women.

Prevention

There are no recent studies on prevention of pyelonephritis. Prompt treatment of cystitis may prevent some cases of pyelonephritis, but this has not been demonstrated.

Clinical Findings

Symptoms and signs include fever, chills, malaise, dysuria, and flank pain. Nausea and vomiting may also occur.

Laboratory findings include a urine dipstick analysis that is positive for leukocyte esterase or nitrites and urine culture showing >100,000 CFUs.

Imaging studies are seldom required unless the patient is diabetic or there is suspicion that stones are complicating the infection, in which case a CT scan is the test of choice.

Differential Diagnosis

See Table 23–6.

Complications

Diabetic patients can experience emphysematous pyelonephritis. It is a severe necrotizing renal infection characterized by gas production within the renal parenchyma. This is diagnosed by CT scan or other imaging study showing gas in the renal collecting system or around the kidney. In a diabetic patient with emphysematous pyelonephritis, the definitive treatment is percutaneous drainage. If there is extensive, diffuse gas, nephrectomy is advised, as the mortality rate in diabetics approaches 75%. This condition rarely occurs in non-diabetic patients and is often related to obstruction. In some of these cases, relief of the obstruction and antibiotics may suffice.

Stones can complicate pyelonephritis by causing a partial or complete obstruction. These stones can be spontaneous or "infection" stones of struvite, caused by urea-splitting organisms. Stones complicating pyelonephritis must be removed before the infection can completely resolve.

People with a history of childhood pyelonephritis can experience renal scarring and recurrent infections. These scars are unusual in healthy adults with pyelonephritis. Young men with pyelonephritis should be investigated for a cause.

Table 23–6. Differential diagnosis of pyelonephritis.

If Patient Has	Consider
Negative urine dipstick or culture	Pelvic inflammatory disease; stone obstructing ureter; lower lobe pneumonia; herpes zoster
Guarding/rebound	Acute cholecystitis; acute appendicitis; perforated viscus
Recurrent infection	Kidney stone, spontaneous or infection-related; anatomic abnormality; resistant organism; inadequate treatment
Diabetes	Emphysematous pyelonephritis
History of childhood infections, urologic surgery	Abnormal anatomy
History of kidney stones	Pyelonephritis complicated by stones

Patients who do not respond to 48 hours of appropriate antibiotics should be worked up for occult complicating factors or other diagnoses.

Treatment

The best drugs for treatment of pyelonephritis are bactericidal, with a broad spectrum to cover gram-positive and gram-negative bacteria, and concentrate well in urine and renal tissues. Fluoroquinolones and TMP-SMX are highly efficacious as they do attain high concentrations within the urine and renal tissue both. In contrast, nitrofurantoin and oral fosfomycin only attain adequate concentrations in the urine; they do not concentrate in the renal tissue. Aminoglycosides; aminopenicillins such as amoxicillin with clavulanic acid, ticarcillin, or piperacillin; cephalosporins; and, in extreme cases, imipenem, are all also appropriate. Cure rates have been shown to be >90% with a 5-to-7-day course of a fluoroquinolone or aminoglycoside. This cure rate has also been seen with a 14-day course of TMP-SMX. As always, it is important to be aware of local resistance patterns of bacteria and adjust therapy appropriately based on that or on culture and sensitivity reports once those are available from the lab.

Patients experiencing severe nausea and vomiting who are unable to tolerate oral agents may need to be hospitalized for parenteral therapy. Patients with severe illness, suspected bacteremia, or sepsis should also be admitted.

Prognosis

Prognosis after an acute episode of uncomplicated pyelonephritis in a previously healthy adult is excellent.

Colgan R, Williams M, Johnson JR. Diagnosis and treatment of acute pyelonephritis in women. *Am Fam Physician.* 2011;84:519–526. [PMID: 21888302]

Johnson JR, Russo TA. Acute pyelonephritis in adults. *N Engl J Med.* 2018;378:48–59. [PMID: 29562155]

Sandberg T, Skoog G, Hermansson AB, et al. Ciprofloxacin for 7 days versus 14 days in women with acute pyelonephritis: a randomized, open-label and double-blind, placebo-controlled, non-inferiority trial. *Lancet.* 2012;380:484–490. [PMID: 22726802]

Arthritis: Osteoarthritis, Gout, & Rheumatoid Arthritis

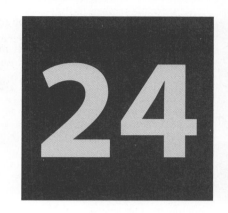

Bruce E. Johnson, MD

Arthritis is a complaint and a disease afflicting many patients and accounting for >10% of appointments to a generalist practice. Arthritis is multifaceted and can be categorized in several different fashions. For simplicity, this chapter focuses on conditions affecting the anatomic joint composed of cartilage, synovium, and bone. Other discussions would include localized disorders of the periarticular region (eg, tendonitis and bursitis) and systemic disorders that have arthritic manifestations (eg, vasculitides, polymyalgia rheumatica, and fibromyalgia). The chapter discusses three prototypical types of arthritis: osteoarthritis, as an example of a cartilage disorder; gout, as an example of both a crystal-induced arthritis and an acute arthritis; and rheumatoid arthritis, as an example of an immune-mediated, systemic disease and a chronic deforming arthritis.

OSTEOARTHRITIS

ESSENTIALS OF DIAGNOSIS

▶ Degenerative changes in the knee, hip, shoulder, spine, or virtually any other joint.

▶ Pain with movement that improves with rest.

▶ Joint deformity and mechanical alteration.

▶ Sclerosis, thickening, spur formation, warmth, and effusion in the joints.

▶ General Considerations

Arthritis is among the oldest identified conditions in humans. Anthropologists examining skeletal remains from antiquity deduce levels of physical activity and work by searching for the presence of the degenerative changes of osteoarthritis (OA). OA is more prevalent among people in occupations characterized by steady, physically demanding activity such as farming, construction, certain sports, and production-line work. Obesity is a significant risk factor for OA, especially of the knee. Heredity and gender play a role in a person's likelihood of developing OA, regardless of work or recreational activity.

▶ Pathogenesis

It is increasingly accepted that most OA results, at least in part, from altered mechanics within the joint. Certain metabolic conditions such as hemochromatosis and Gaucher disease involve a genetic defect in collagen/cartilage. Altered mechanics may occur from minor gait abnormalities or major traumas that, over a lifetime, result in repeated stress and damage to cartilage. Repeated trauma may result in microfracture of cartilage, with incomplete healing due to continuation of the altered mechanics. Disruption of the otherwise smooth cartilage surface allows differential pressure on remaining cartilage, as well as stress on the underlying bone. Debris from fractured cartilage acts as a foreign body, causing low-level inflammation within the synovial fluid. Indeed, increasing evidence suggests that inflammation, from damaged cartilage or even as a primary activity, is involved in most OA, and actions taken to reduce inflammation are increasingly used to alter the path to joint damage. These multiple influences combine to alter intrinsic efforts at cartilage repair, leading to progressive cartilage destruction and bony joint change. Current thinking suggests that the process is not immutable, but any intervention would have to be made while the joint is still asymptomatic—an unlikely occurrence.

▶ Prevention

It is difficult to advise patients on measures to prevent OA. Obese persons should lose weight, but few occupational or recreational precautions can be expected to alter the natural history of OA. Altered mechanics may be an important precipitating cause of arthritis, but recognizing minor changes, especially within the currently accepted range of normal, makes diagnosis and preventive steps unrealistic.

Berenbaum F, Wallace IJ, Lieberman DE, et al. Modern-day environmental factors in the pathogenesis of osteoarthritis. *Nat Rev Rheumatol.* 2018;14(11):674–681. [PMID: 30209413]
Brandt KD, Dieppe P, Radin E. Etiopathogenesis of osteoarthritis. *Med Clin North Am.* 2009;93:1–24. [PMID: 19059018]

▶ Clinical Findings

A. Symptoms and Signs

Symptomatic OA represents the culmination of damage to cartilage, usually over many years. OA typically progresses from symptomatic pain to physical findings to loss of function, but actually any of these can be first to present. OA can occur at any joint, but the most commonly involved joints are the knee, hip, thumb (carpometacarpal), ankle, foot, and spine. The strongly inherited (primarily females) spur formations at the distal interphalangeal joins (Heberden nodes) and proximal interphalangeal joints (Bouchard nodes) are often mistakenly referred to as OA. In fact, the swelling and deformity are more an abnormality of bone itself rather than the joint. Indeed, pain or disability is actually rather uncommon in what otherwise appear to be significantly altered joints (Figure 24–1).

Cartilage has no pain fibers, so the pain of OA arises from other tissues, most significantly bone itself. Osteoarthritic pain is typically associated with movement, meaning that at rest the patient may be relatively asymptomatic. Patient's awareness that at rest the joint is less painful can be maladaptive, especially at weight-bearing such as knees, hips, and ankles. A protective role played by surrounding muscle

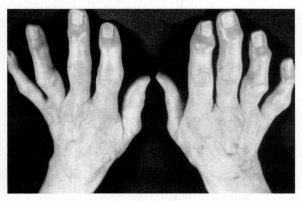

▲ **Figure 24–1.** Heberden nodes (distal interphalangeal joint) noted on all fingers and Bouchard nodes (proximal interphalangeal joint) noted on most fingers.

of both a normal and arthritic joint is that of a shock absorber. Well-maintained muscle can actually reduce mechanical stress on cartilage and bone. However, if a patient learns to favor the involved joint, disuse of supporting muscle groups may result in relative muscle weakness. Such weakness may decrease the shock-absorber effect, hastening joint damage. This mechanism also may lead to the complaint that a joint "gives way," resulting in dropped items (if at the wrist) or falls (if at the knee). In joints with mild OA, pain and instability may counterintuitively improve with exercise or activity.

Advanced OA is characterized by bony destruction and alteration of joint architecture. Secondary spur formation with deformity, instability, or restricted motion is a common finding. Fingers, wrists, knees, and ankles appear abnormal and asymmetric. Warmth and effusion are seen in joints with advanced OA. At this stage, pain may be exacerbated by any movement, weight-bearing, or otherwise.

B. Laboratory Findings

There are few laboratory studies of relevance to the diagnosis of OA. Rarely, the erythrocyte sedimentation rate (ESR) will be raised, but only if an inflammatory effusion is present (and even then, an elevated ESR or C-reactive protein is more likely to be misleading than helpful). If an effusion is present, arthrocentesis can be helpful in ruling out other conditions (see discussion of laboratory findings in gout, later).

Osteoarthritis can be secondary to other conditions, and these diseases have their own laboratory evaluation. Examples include OA secondary to hemochromatosis (elevated iron and ferritin, liver enzyme abnormalities), Wilson disease (elevated copper), acromegaly (elevated growth hormone), and Paget disease (elevated alkaline phosphatase).

C. Imaging Studies

Radiographs are seldom helpful in early stages of OA because changes in cartilage are difficult to see in plain film radiographs. Plain films of joints afflicted with advanced OA show changes of sclerosis, thickening, spur formation (enlargement of some aspects of bone), loss of cartilage with narrowing of the joint space, and malalignment (Figure 24–2). Such radiographic changes typically occur late in the disease process. Patients may complain of significant pain despite a relatively normal appearance of the joint on plain films. Conversely, considerable radiographic damage may be seen with only modest symptoms. In addition, plain-film radiography does not provide useful information about cartilage, tendons, ligaments, or any soft tissue. Such findings may be crucial to explaining a patient complaint, especially if there is loss of function.

To see cartilage, ligaments, and tendons, magnetic resonance imaging (MRI) is important and, in many instances, essential. MRI can detect abnormalities of the meniscus or ligaments of the knee; cartilage or femoral head deterioration

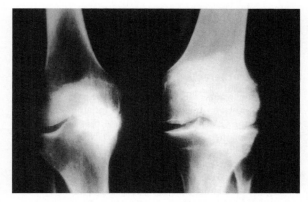

▲ **Figure 24–2.** Osteoarthritis of the knees showing loss of joint space with marked reactive sclerosis and probable malalignment.

at the hip; misalignment at the elbow; rupture of muscle and fascia at the shoulder; and a host of other abnormalities. Any of these findings may be incorrectly diagnosed as OA before MRI scanning.

Computed tomography (CT) and ultrasonography have lesser, more specialized uses. CT, especially with contrast, can detect structural abnormalities of large joints such as the knee or shoulder. Ultrasonography is an inexpensive means of detecting joint or periarticular fluid or unusual collections of fluid such as a popliteal (Baker) cyst at the knee.

▶ Differential Diagnosis

In practice, it should not be difficult to differentiate among the three prototypical arthritides discussed in this chapter. Table 24–1 suggests some key differential findings.

A common source of confusion and misdiagnosis occurs when a bursitis-tendinitis syndrome mimics the pain of OA.

A common example is anserine bursitis. This bursitis, located medially at the tibial plateau, presents in a fashion similar to OA of the knee, but can be differentiated by a few simple questions and directed physical findings.

▶ Treatment

Typically, the early development of OA is silent. When pain occurs, and pain is almost always the presenting complaint, the osteoarthritic process has already likely progressed to joint damage. Cartilage is damaged, bone reaction occurs, and debris mixes with synovial fluid. Consequently, when a diagnosis of OA is established, goals of therapy become control of pain, restoration of function, and reduction of disease progression. Although control of the patient's complaints is possible, and long periods of few or no symptoms may ensue, the patient permanently carries a diagnosis of OA.

Treatment of OA involves multiple modalities and is inadequate if only a prescription for anti-inflammatory drugs is written. Patient education, assessment for physical therapy and devices, and consideration of intra-articular injections are additional measures in the total management of the patient.

Hochberg MC, Altman RD, April KT, et al. American College of Rheumatology 2012 recommendations for the use of nonpharmacologic and pharmacologic therapies for osteoarthritis of the hand, hip and knee. *Arthritis Care Res.* 2012;64(4):465–474. [PMID: 22563589]

A. Patient Education

Patient education is a crucial step. Patients must be made aware of the role they play in successful therapy. Many resources are available to assist the provider in patient education. Patient education pamphlets are widely available from government organizations, physician organizations (eg, American College of Rheumatology, American Academy

Table 24–1. Essentials of diagnosis.

	Osteoarthritis	Gout	Rheumatoid Arthritis
Key presenting symptoms	Pauciarticular; pain with movement, improving with rest; site of old injury (sport, trauma); obesity; occupation	Monoarticular; abrupt onset; pain at rest and movement; precipitating event (meal, physical stress); family history	Polyarticular; gradual, symmetric involvement; morning stiffness; hands and feet initially involved more than large joints; fatigue, poorly restorative sleep
Key physical findings	Infrequent warmth, effusion; crepitus; enlargement/spur formation; malalignment	Podagra; swelling, warmth; exquisite pain with movement; single joint (exceptions: plantar fascia, lumbar spine); tophi	Symmetric swelling, tenderness; MCP, MTP, wrist, ankle usually before larger, proximal joints; rheumatoid nodules
Key laboratory, x-ray findings	Few characteristic (early); loss of joint space, spur formation, malalignment (late)	Synovial fluid with uric acid crystals; elevated serum uric acid; 24-hour urine uric acid	Elevated ESR/CRP; rheumatoid factor; anemia of chronic disease; early erosions on x-ray, osteopenia at involved joints

CRP, C-reactive protein; ESR, erythrocyte sedimentation rate; MCP, metacarpophalangeal; MTP, metatarsophalangeal.

of Family Physicians), insurance companies, pharmaceutical companies, or patient advocacy groups (eg, the Arthritis Foundation). Many communities have self-help or support groups that are rich sources of information, advice, and encouragement.

One of the most effective long-term measures to both improve symptoms and slow progression of disease is weight loss. Less weight carried by the hip, knee, ankle, or foot reduces stress on the involved arthritic joint, decreases the destructive processes, and probably slows progression of disease. Unfortunately, because of the pain and occasional limited mobility of OA, exercise—an almost required component of weight loss regimens—is less likely to be utilized. On the other hand, exercise is a crucial modality that should not be overlooked. Evaluation for appropriate exercise focuses on two issues: overall fitness and correction of any joint-specific disuse atrophy. One must be flexible in the choice of exercise. Swimming is an excellent exercise that limits stress on the lower extremities. Many older persons are reluctant to learn to swim anew, yet they may be amenable to water aerobic exercises. These exercises encourage calorie expenditure, flexibility, and both upper and lower muscle strengthening in a supportive atmosphere. Stationary bicycle exercise is also accessible to most people, is easy to learn, and may be acceptable to those with arthritis of the hip, ankle, or foot. Advice from an occupational or recreational therapist can be most helpful.

Connelly AE, Tucker AJ, Kott LS, et al. Modifiable lifestyle factors are associated with lower pain levels in adults with knee osteoarthritis. *Pain Res Manag*. 2015;20(5):241–248. [PMID: 26125195]

B. Physical Therapy and Assistive Devices

The pain of OA can result in muscular disuse. The best example is quadriceps weakness resulting from OA of the knee. The patient who favors the involved joint loses quadriceps strength. This has two repercussions—both cushioning (shock absorption) and stabilization are lost. The latter is usually the cause of the knee "giving way." Sudden buckling at the knee, often when descending stairs, is rarely due to the destruction of cartilage or bone but rather to inadequate strength in the quadriceps to handle the load required at the joint. Physical therapy with quadriceps strengthening is highly efficacious, resulting in improved mobility, increased patient confidence, and reduction in pain.

The physical therapist or physiatrist should also be consulted for advice regarding assistive devices. Advanced OA of lower extremity joints may cause instability and fear of falls that can be addressed by canes of various types. Altered posture or joint malalignment can be corrected by orthotics, which has the advantage, when used early, of slowing progression of OA. Braces can protect the truly unstable joint and permit continued ambulation.

Fransen M, McConnell S. Land-based exercise for osteoarthritis of the knee: a metaanalysis of randomized controlled trials. *J Rheumatol*. 2009;36:1109–1117. [PMID: 19447940]

C. Pharmacotherapy

The patient wants relief from pain. Despite the widespread promotion of nonsteroidal anti-inflammatory drugs (NSAIDs) for OA, there is no evidence that NSAIDs alter the course of the disease. Nevertheless, NSAIDs are used for their analgesic, rather than disease-modifying effects. Although effective as analgesics, NSAIDs have significant side effects and are not necessarily first-line drugs.

Begin with adequate doses of acetaminophen. Acetaminophen should be prescribed in large doses, 3–4 g/d, and continued at this level until pain control is attained. Once pain is controlled, dosage can be reduced if possible. Maintenance of adequate blood levels is essential, and because acetaminophen has a relatively short half-life, frequent dosing is necessary (3 or 4 times a day). High doses of acetaminophen are generally well tolerated, although caution is important in patients with liver disease or in whom alcohol ingestion is heavy.

Some patients find relief with medications delievered as gels or creams. There are a couple NSAIDs and capsaicin products that are formulated this way, although compounding pharmacies may assist in delivering other products. Gels or creams tend to be more effective in small joints (fingers, wrist, ankle) than larger joints, although it is occasionally surprising how benefit can be seen even in large, deeper joints such as the hip or shoulder. One distinct advantage to gels or creams is relatively consistent lack of gastrointestinal upset. Unfortunately, this treatment rarely gives long-lasting relief.

Two main classes of NSAIDs are available, differentiated largely by half-life. NSAIDs with shorter half-lives (eg, diclofenac, ibuprofen) need more frequent dosing than longer-acting agents (eg, naproxen, meloxicam). Several NSAIDs are available in generic or over-the-counter (OTC) form, which reduces cost. Despite differing pharmacology, there is little difference in efficacy, so a choice of medication should be based on individual patient issues such as dosing intervals, tolerance, toxicity, and cost. As with acetaminophen, adequate doses must be used for maximal effectiveness. For example, ibuprofen at doses of ≤800 mg 3 or 4 times a day should be maintained (if tolerated) before concluding that a different agent is necessary. Examples of NSAID dosing are given in Table 24–2.

Occasionally patients find help with pain management by use of medications originally developed for psychiatric conditions. The more common medications used in this manner include duloxetine (Cymbaltra), escitalopram (Lexapro), and citalopram (Celexa). It is unclear how these medications help with arthritic pain management since patients are

Table 24–2. Selected nonsteroidal anti-inflammatory drugs with usual and maximal doses.

Drug	Frequency of Administration	Usual Daily Dose (mg/d)	Maximal Dose (mg/d)
Oxaprozin (eg, Daypro)	Every day	1200	1800
Piroxicam (eg, Feldene)	Every day	10–20	20
Nabumetone (eg, Relafen)	1–2 times a day	1000–2000	2000
Sulindac (eg, Clinoril)	Twice a day	300–400	400
Naproxen (eg, Naprosyn)	Twice a day	500–1000	1500
Diclofenac (eg, Voltaren)	2–4 times a day	100–150	200
Ibuprofen (eg, Motrin)	3–4 times a day	600–1800	2400
Etodolac (eg, Lodine)	3–4 times a day	600–1200	1200
Ketoprofen (eg, Orudis)	3–4 times a day	150–300	300

infrequently diagnosed with depression, anxiety, or bipolar disorders. However, the use of such agents should at least be considered before proceeding to some other medications or more invasive treatments.

Because such a major thrust of OA management is pain control, one must acknowledge the role played by narcotics. Narcotics should be confined to the patient with severe disease incompletely controlled by nonpharmacologic and nonnarcotic analgesics and in whom joint replacement is not indicated. The narcotic medication should be additive to all other measures; for instance, full-dose acetaminophen or NSAIDs should be continued. The patient must be reminded of the fluctuating nature of OA symptoms and not expect complete elimination of pain. Once narcotics are started (in any patient for any cause), most generalist practices institute monitoring measures such as a "drug contract" or referral to a specialist pain management clinic.

Zhang W, Moskowitz RW, Nuki G, et al. OARSI recommendations for the management of hip and knee arthritis, Part II: OARSI evidence-based, expert consensus guidelines. *Osteoarthr Cartilage.* 2008;16:137–162. [PMID: 18279766]

D. Intra-articular Injections

Hyaluronic acid (hyaluronan) is a constituent of both cartilage and synovial fluid. Injection of hyaluronic acid, usually in a series of several weekly intra-articular insertions, is purported to provide improvement in symptomatic OA for ≤6 months. It is unknown why hyaluronic acid helps; there is no evidence that hyaluronic acid is incorporated into cartilage, and it apparently does not slow the progression of OA. It is expensive, and the injection process is painful. Use of these agents (Synvisc, Artzal) is limited to patients who have failed other forms of OA therapy.

Intra-articular injection of corticosteroids has been both under- and overutilized in the past. There is little question that steroid injection rapidly reduces inflammation and eases symptoms. The best use is one in which the patient has an exacerbation of pain accompanied by signs of inflammation (warmth, effusion). The knee is most commonly implicated and is most easily approached. Most authorities recommend no more than two injections during one episode and limiting injections to no more than two or three episodes per year. Benefits of injection are often shorter in duration than similar injection for tendinitis or bursitis, but the symptomatic improvement buys time to reestablish therapy with oral agents, physical exercise, and assistive devices.

New therapeutic investigation and translational studies hold some promise for actual cartilage modification of damaged joints. Therapies involving strontium ranelate, platelet-rich plasma injections, and mesenchymal stem cells are currently in stages of development and may truly alter the otherwise somewhat relentless progression of this disease.

Reginster JY, Badurski J, Bellamy N, et al. Efficacy and safety of strontium ranelate in the treatment of knee osteoarthritis: results of a double-blind, randomized placebo-controlled trial. *Ann Rheum Dis.* 2013;72:179–186. [PMID: 23117245]
Two new intra-articular injections for knee osteoarthritis. *JAMA.* 2018;320(21):2262–2263. [PMID: 30512097]

E. Surgery

At one time, orthopedic surgeons performed arthroscopic surgery on osteoarthritic knees in an effort to remove accumulated debris and to polish or débride frayed cartilage. However, a clinical trial using a sham-procedure methodology demonstrated that benefit from this practice could be explained by the placebo effect. Numbers of these procedures have reduced rather significantly, although there still remain some indications for performing this operation.

Joint replacement is a well-established option for treatment of OA, especially of the knee and hip. Pain is reduced or eliminated altogether. Mobility is improved, although infrequently to premorbid levels. Expenditures for total joint replacement have been increasing dramatically as the Baby Boomer generation reaches the age at which OA of large joints is more common. Indications for joint replacement (which also apply to other joints, including shoulder, elbow, and fingers) include pain poorly controlled with maximal therapy, malalignment, and decreased mobility. Improvement in pain relief and quality of life should be realized in approximately 90% of patients undergoing the procedure. Because complications of both the surgery and rehabilitation are increased by obesity, few orthopedic surgeons will consider hip or knee replacement without at least an attempt by the obese patient to lose weight. Patients need to be in adequate medical condition to undergo the operation and even more so to endure the often lengthy rehabilitation process. Some surgeons refer patients for "prehabilitation" or physical training prior to the operation. Counseling of patients should include the fact that there often is a 4- to 6-month recovery period involving intensive rehabilitation.

Kirkley A, Birmingham TB, Litchfield RB, et al. A randomized trial of arthroscopic surgery for osteoarthritis of the knee. *N Engl J Med.* 2008:359(11):1097–1107. [PMID: 18784099]

Moseley JB, O'Malley K, Petersen NJ, et al. A controlled trial of arthroscopic surgery for osteoarthritis of the knee. *N Engl J Med.* 2002;347:81. [PMID: 12110735]

F. Complementary and Alternative Therapies

Glucosamine, capsaicin, bee venom, acupuncture, and a host of other products have been promoted as alternative therapies for OA. Glucosamine and chondroitin sulfate are components of glycosaminoglycans, which make up cartilage; although some advocates might suggest otherwise, there is no evidence that orally ingested glucosamine or chondroitin sulfate is actually incorporated into cartilage. Studies suggest these agents are superior to placebo in symptomatic relief of mild OA. The onset of action is delayed, sometimes by weeks, but the effect may be prolonged after treatment is stopped. Glucosamine–chondroitin sulfate combinations are available over the counter and are generally well tolerated by patients.

Capsaicin, a topically applied extract of the chili pepper, relieves pain by depletion of substance P, a neuropeptide involved in pain sensation. Capsaicin is suggested for tendinitis or bursitis but may be tried for OA of superficial joints such as the fingers. The cream should be applied 3 or 4 times a day for ≥2 weeks before reaching any conclusion regarding benefit.

Bee venom is promoted in complementary medicine circles. A mechanism for action in OA is unclear. Although anecdotal reports are available, comparison studies to other established treatments are difficult to find. Various vitamins (D, K) and minerals have been recommended for treatment of OA but are supported, if at all, by only poorly controlled studies.

Acupuncture can be useful in managing pain and improving function. There are more comparisons between acupuncture and conventional treatment for OA of the back and knee than for other joints. Generally, acupuncture is equivalent to oral treatments for mild symptoms at these two sites.

▶ Prognosis

Investigations into restoring and rebuilding damaged cartilage continue, but consistent positive results are elusive. Prevention, or at least delay of development, of OA is the major impact physicians can have on the population. However, these efforts involve activities that are themselves challenging to accomplish, such as weight control or avoidance of joint stress from jobs and recreational activities. Much of the current, and anticipated, management of OA will continue to be pain control, appropriate exercise for joint protection, orthotics and braces/devices, and surgery.

GOUT

 ESSENTIALS OF DIAGNOSIS

- ▶ Podagra (intense inflammation of the first metatarsophalangeal joint).
- ▶ Inflammation of the overlying skin.
- ▶ Pain at rest and intense pain with movement.
- ▶ Swelling, warmth, redness, and effusion.
- ▶ Tophi (in long-established disease).
- ▶ Elevated serum uric acid level.

▶ General Considerations

Gout, first described by Hippocrates in the fourth century BCE, has a colorful history, characterized as a disease of excesses, primarily gluttony. An association with diet is germane, as gout has a lower incidence in countries in which obesity is uncommon and the diet is relatively devoid of alcohol and reliance on meat and abdominal organs (liver, spleen). Gout is strongly hereditary as well, affecting as many as 25% of the men in some families.

▶ Prevention

Despite the previously noted associations, it is difficult with any assurance to advise patients on measures to prevent gout.

Even thin vegetarians develop gout, although at a markedly lower rate than obese, alcohol-drinking men. Gout has multiple etiologies, and no consistent preventive steps are available to patients.

▶ Clinical Findings

A. Symptoms and Signs

Gout classically presents as an acute monoarthritis, perhaps best described by Thomas Sydenham in the seventeenth century. Podagra—abrupt, intense inflammation of the first metatarsophalangeal joint—remains the most common presentation (Figure 24–3). The first attack often occurs overnight, with intense pain awakening the patient. Any pressure, even a bed sheet on the toe, increases the agony. Walking is difficult. The overlying skin can be intensely inflamed. On questioning, an exacerbating event may be elicited. Common stories include an excess of alcohol, a heavy meal of abdominal organs, or a recent physiologic stress such as surgery or serious medical disease. Alcohol alters renal excretion of uric acid, allowing rapid buildup of serum uric acid levels. Foods such as liver, sweetbread, anchovies, sardines, asparagus, salmon, and legumes contain relatively large quantities of purines that, when broken down, become uric acid.

Acute gout is not limited to the great toe; any joint may be affected, although lower extremity joints are more common.

The typical abrupt, single-joint presentation may be overlooked (Table 24–3). Hence, given any acute monoarthritis, one should certainly search for both inflammatory and noninflammatory clues that would be suggestive of a diagnosis other than gout.

Table 24–3. Inflammatory and noninflammatory causes of monoarthritis.

Inflammatory	Noninflammatory
Crystal-induced gout	Fracture or meniscal tear or
Pseudogout (calcium pyrophosphate	other
deposition disease)	trauma
Apatite (and others)	Osteoarthritis
Infectious	Tumors
Bacteria	Osteochondroma
Fungi	Osteoid osteoma
Lyme disease or other spirochetes	Pigmented villonodular
Tuberculosis and other mycobacteria	synovitis
Viruses (eg, HIV, hepatitis B)	Precancerous growths
Systemic diseases	Osteonecrosis
Psoriatic or other spondyloarthropathies	Hemarthrosis
Reactive (eg, inflammatory bowel,	Cancers
Reiter syndrome)	
Systemic lupus erythematosus	

Reproduced with permission from Klipper JH: *Primer on the Rheumatic Diseases*, 11th ed. Atlanta, GA: Arthritis Foundation; 1997.

Gout in joints other than the great toe is actually not uncommon in older women and in men who have already had several previous attacks of podagra (gout of the great toe). A not uncommon presentation of gout in an older woman may initially be mistaken for plantar fasciitis. Gout of the ankle with inflammation and even a positive Homans sign can be mistaken for phlebitis.

Untreated, attacks of gout spontaneously resolve, with the involved joint becoming progressively less symptomatic over 8–10 days. Longstanding, untreated gout with consistent elevated uric acid can result in the development of extra-articular manifestations. Tophi are deposits of urate crystals and are classically found as nodules in the ear helix or elsewhere; atypically placed tophi (eg, Heberden nodes, heart valves) serve as the source of colorful medical anecdotes. Chronic, untreated gout is a contributor to renal insufficiency (especially in association with heavy metal lead exposure).

Physiologic stress is a common precipitating factor for an acute attack. Monoarthritis within days of a surgical procedure raises concern of infection (which it should!) but is just as likely due to crystal-induced gout or pseudogout. In some circumstances, prophylaxis in a person with known gout can prevent these attacks.

Approximately 10% of kidney stones include uric acid. A person with nephrolithiasis due to uric acid stones need not have attacks of gout, but patients with gout are at increased risk of developing uric acid stones. A prior history of nephrolithiasis is an important factor in choosing therapy in the patient with gout.

Gout is largely a disease of men, with a male-to-female ratio of 9:1. The first attack of podagra typically occurs in

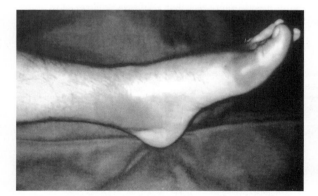

▲ **Figure 24–3.** Classic podagra involving the first metatarsophalangeal joint. In this photo, the ankle is also involved and the intense erythema could be mistaken for cellulitis.

men in their 30s or 40s. One attack need not necessarily predict future attacks. In fact, some 20% of men who have a first attack of gout never have a second episode. In addition, even after a second attack of gout, about 5% do not progress to recurrent attacks. Hence, although a correct diagnosis should be made, it may not be necessary to institute long-term therapy after a first of second episode of acute monarthritis due to gout.

Premenopausal women rarely have gout; indeed, confirmed gout in a young woman might raise the question of an inborn error of metabolism. Diagnosis of gout in postmenopausal women is infrequent, less so because it does not occur than because it is unsuspected. Gout is also more likely to have an atypical presentation in joints other than the great toe in women. A high index of suspicion must be practiced.

B. Laboratory Findings

The fundamental abnormality in gout is excess uric acid. In most first attacks of gout, serum uric acid is elevated. In longstanding disease, the uric acid value may be within the normal range, yet symptoms still occur. It is important to note, however, that mild hyperuricemia has a rather high prevalence in the general population. Indeed, fewer than 25% of persons with elevated uric acid will ever have gout.

During acute attacks of gout, the white blood cell count may be slightly elevated and ESR increased, reflecting acute inflammation. Gout is not uncommon in chronic kidney disease, and measurement of blood urea nitrogen and creatinine is recommended following a first gout attack.

Gout usually results from either inappropriately low renal excretion of uric acid (implicated in 90% of patients) or abnormally high endogenous production of uric acid. Collecting a 24-hour urine sample for the evaluation of uric acid and creatinine clearance can be useful in therapy (discussed as follows).

A strong recommendation must be made to attempt arthrocentesis of the joint in suspected acute gout. First episodes of gout present as an acute monoarthritis, for which the differential diagnosis is noted in Table 24–3. It is extremely important to rule out infectious arthritis because this condition could lead to sepsis as well as possible permanent damage to the joint. Synovial fluid analysis should distinguish between infection and the crystal conditions, gout and pseudogout. This may be somewhat difficult on the basis of clinical presentation alone. However, excess white blood cells (plus bacteria if seen on stain) or crystals should lead to a diagnosis. The presence of negatively birefringent needle-shaped crystals is diagnostic of gout and confirms the correct diagnosis. Features of synovial fluid in selected disease settings are highlighted in Table 24–4.

C. Imaging Studies

Radiographs are not needed for the diagnosis of gout. Other means of diagnosing gout (eg, arthrocentesis) are more useful. Characteristic erosions occur with longstanding gout but are rarely seen in first attacks.

▶ Differential Diagnosis

The first attack of gout must be distinguished from an acute monoarthritis. A review of Tables 24–1 and 24–3 is relevant.

▶ Treatment

The inflammation of acute gout is effectively managed with anti-inflammatory medications. Once recognized, most cases of gout can be controlled within days, occasionally within hours. Remaining as a challenge is the decision regarding long-term treatment.

Standard therapy for acute gout is a short course of NSAIDs at adequate levels. As one of the first NSAIDs developed, indomethacin (50 mg 3 or 4 times a day) is occasionally assumed to be somehow unique in the treatment of gout. In fact, all NSAIDs are probably equally effective, although many practitioners feel that response is faster with short-acting agents such as naproxen (375–500 mg 3 times a day) or ibuprofen (800 mg 3 or 4 times a day). Pain often decreases

Table 24–4. Synovial fluid analysis in selected rheumatic diseases.

Disease	Fluid	WBC Count (in Fluid)	Differential	Glucose	Crystals
Gout	Clear/cloudy	10–100,000	>50% PMNs	Normal	Needle-shaped, negative birefringence
Pseudogout	Clear/cloudy	10–100,000	>50% PMNs	Normal	Rhomboid-shaped, positive birefringence
Infectious	Cloudy	>50,000	Often >95% PMNs	Decreased	None[a]
Osteoarthritis	Clear	2–10,000	<50% PMNs	Normal	None[a]
Rheumatoid arthritis	Clear	10–50,000	>50% PMNs	Normal or decreased	None[a]

[a]Debris in synovial fluid may be misleading on plain microscopy, but only crystals respond to polarizing light.
PMNs, polymorphonuclear leukocytes; WBC, white blood cells.

on the first day, with treatment indicated for not much more than 3–5 days.

A classic medication for acute gout is colchicine. Typically given orally, the instructions to the patient can sound bizarre. The drug is prescribed every 1–2 hours "until relief of pain or uncontrollable diarrhea." Most attacks actually respond to the first two or three pills, with a maximum of six pills in 24 hours as a prudent upper limit. Most patients develop diarrhea well before the sixth pill. Colchicine is then dosed 3 times daily and, as with NSAIDs, is seldom needed after 3–5 days. Around 2009, using a feature in US Food and Drug Administration (FDA) law, colchicine actually received new medication status and was allowed to be patented. This permitted the pharmaceutical company to charge prices as much as 50 times the previous cost. By 2016, the FDA persuaded the company to allow a generic version of colchicine to be marketed, resulting (once again) in more affordable medication for an acute episode of gout.

On occasion, corticosteroids are used in acute gout. Oral prednisone (eg, ≥60 mg), methylprednisolone or triamcinolone (eg, 40–80 mg) intramuscularly, or intra-articular agents can be used. Indications include intense overlying skin involvement (mimicking cellulitis), polyarticular presentation of gout, and contraindication to NSAID or colchicine therapy. Intra-articular steroid use may be considered for ankle or knee gout, if infection is ruled out.

Decisions regarding long-term treatment of gout must factor in the individual's history of attacks. The first attack, especially in young men with a clear precipitating event (eg, an alcohol binge), may not be followed by a second attack for years, even decades. As stated earlier, as many as 20% of men will never have a second gouty attack. Data from the Framingham longitudinal study suggest that intervals of ≤12 years are common between first and second attacks. This is not always the case for young women with gout (who tend to have a uric acid metabolic abnormality) or for either men or women who have polyarticular gout. But for many young men, a reasonable recommendation after a first episode is to watch expectantly but not necessarily to treat with uric acid–lowering drugs.

The physician and patient may even decide to withhold prophylactic medication after a second attack, but when episodes of gout become more frequent than one or two a year, both physician and patient are usually ready to consider long-term medication. The primary medications used at this point are probenecid and the xanthine oxidase inhibitors allopurinol and febuxostat. Probenecid is a uric acid tubular reuptake inhibitor that results in increased excretion of uric acid in the urine. Allopurinol and febuxostat inhibit the uric acid synthesis pathway, blocking the step at which xanthine is converted to uric acid. Xanthine is much more soluble than uric acid and is not implicated in acute arthritis, nephrolithiasis, or renal insufficiency.

Until recently, guidelines recommended obtaining 24-hour uric acid excretion levels. The patient found to have low excretion of uric acid (<600 mg/d) and normal renal function was often prescribed probenecid. Probenecid loses effectiveness when the creatinine clearance falls below 50 mL/min, so alternative therapy was necessary in patients with chronic kidney disease. If the patient had uric acid nephrolithiasis, probenecid was contraindicated to avoid increased delivery of uric acid to the stone-forming region.

Recent guidelines from the American College of Rheumatology have modified this approach. These guidelines now suggest that initial therapy can begin with a xanthine oxidase inhibitor, obviating the need to measure 24-hour uric acid excretion. The guidelines recommend treating to a serum uric acid level of ≤6 g/dL. If this goal cannot be reached with xanthine oxidase inhibitors alone (an infrequent occurrence), probenecid might then be added. This newer modification recognizes that both allopurinol and febuxostat are well tolerated with infrequent toxic side effects. An important difference, though, is that allopurinol is usually dosed lower in chronic kidney disease because of the potential for adverse effects, whereas febuxostat does not seem to have such dosing requirements. Interestingly, a relatively recent (2016) American College of Physicians guideline on treatment of gout reinforced the treat-to-symptoms approach more typically used by physicians—that is, to treat several attacks of gout with anti-inflammatory agents such as NSAIDs or colchicine with no chronic medication until there have been several attacks, which then warrant long-term treatment with either a uric acid excretion agent or a xanthine oxidase inhibitor.

Recently, the FDA has issued a "black box" warning for both allopurinol and febuxostat. The warning is regarding possible cardiovascular adverse events with the use of either agent. The likelihood of any adverse event is felt to be low but is an issue that should be considered when choosing one of these agents for long-term therapy.

White WB, Saag KG, Becker MA, et al. Cardiovascular safety of febuxostat and allopurinol in patients with gout. *N Engl J Med.* 2018;378(13):1200–1210. [PMID: 29527974]

Xanthine oxidase inhibitors are especially indicated for treatment of tophaceous gout and for uric acid nephrolithiasis. These agents also are drugs of choice for those with uric acid metabolic abnormalities (often young women) and polyarticular gout. Caution must be used, however, when starting any uric acid–lowering drug for the first time. Rapid lowering of the serum uric acid causes instability of uric acid crystals within the synovial fluid and can actually precipitate an attack of gout. Consequently, prior establishment of either NSAID or colchicine therapy is recommended to obviate this complication.

Patients are occasionally seen who have been prescribed long-term therapy with colchicine. There is some conceptual attraction to this choice. Between attacks of gout (the "intercritical period"), examination of synovial fluid continues to show uric acid crystals. Using colchicine to prevent the spiral to inflammation seems to make sense. But this choice is deceptive. Colchicine does nothing to lower uric acid levels. Long-term use allows deposition of uric acid into destructive tophi or contributes to renal disease and kidney stones. Colchicine can be an effective prophylactic agent, however, if started prior to a surgical procedure in a patient with known gout who is not using allopurinol or probenecid. However, use of this drug as a solo agent can result in significant complications.

▶ Prognosis

Gouty attacks can be both effectively treated and prevented. A clear diagnosis is important, and arthrocentesis is essential. Management is relatively straightforward, and no patient should have to endure tophi or repeated acute attacks.

Kanna D, Fitzgerald JD, Khanna PP, et al. American College of Rheumatology guidelines for management of gout. Part 1: systemic nonpharmacologic and pharmacologic therapeutic approaches to hyperuricemia. *Arthritis Care Res.* 2012;64: 1431–1446. [PMID: 23024028]

Kanna D, Khanna PP, Fitzgerald JD, et al. American College of Rheumatology guidelines for management of gout. Part 2: therapy and anti-inflammatory prophylaxis of acute gouty arthritis. *Arthritis Care Res.* 2012;64:1447–1461. [PMID: 23024029]

Qaseem A, Harris RP, Forciea MA, et al. Management of acute and recurrent gout: A clinical practice guideline from the American College of Physicians. *Ann Intern Med.* 2017; 166(1):58–68. [PMID: 27802508]

RHEUMATOID ARTHRITIS

ESSENTIALS OF DIAGNOSIS

▶ Arthritis of three or more joint areas.

▶ Arthritis in hands, feet, or both (bilateral joint involvement).

▶ Morning stiffness.

▶ Fatigue.

▶ Swelling, tenderness, warmth, and loss of function.

▶ Rheumatoid nodules.

▶ Elevated ESR and C-reactive protein.

▶ Positive test for rheumatoid factor.

▶ General Considerations

Bony changes consistent with rheumatoid arthritis (RA) have been found in the body of a Native American who lived 3000 years ago. Differentiation of RA from other types of arthritis is more recent, delineated only in the late

nineteenth century. RA is more frequently seen in women, with the ratio of premenopausal women to age-matched men approximately 4:1; after the age of menopause, the ratio of incident RA is closer to 1:1.

▶ Pathogenesis

Although the etiology of RA is not known, the pathophysiology has been elucidated to a remarkable degree in recent decades. Important knowledge of all inflammatory processes has come from studies in RA. Early in the disease process, the synovium of joints is targeted by T cells (this is the feature that leads to the "autoimmune" moniker). Release of interleukins, lymphokines, cytokines, tissue necrosis factor, and other messengers attracts additional inflammatory cells to the synovium. Intense inflammation ensues, experienced by the patient as pain, warmth, swelling, and loss of function. Reactive cells move to the inflammatory synovium, attempting to repair damaged tissue. Without treatment, this intense reaction develops into the pathologic tissue called *pannus*, an exuberant growth of tissue engulfing the joint space and causing destruction itself. Cartilage becomes swept into the pathologic process, resulting in breakdown, deterioration, and eventual destruction. Periarticular bone responds to inflammation with resorption, seen as erosions on radiographs. All these changes clearly are maladaptive and responsible for deformity and disability.

▶ Prevention

Because the etiology of RA is not fully elucidated, it is difficult to counsel patients on measures that might prevent the arthritis. Besides, because it is not even clear that there is a hereditary component to the disease, there rarely are occasions when the physician would be approached about steps that might be taken to prevent it. There is some suggestion that RA may be more common in smokers, but clearly there are stronger reasons to advise patients to stop smoking than bringing up the somewhat remote possibility of developing RA.

▶ Clinical Findings

A. Symptoms and Signs

RA is a systemic disease always involving joints but with inflammatory responses that include fatigue, rash, nodules, and even clinical depression as joints become increasingly stiff and inflamed. Most, but by no means all, of the initial symptoms are in the joints. There is inflammation, so the presence of swelling, warmth, and loss of function is imperative to the diagnosis. Joints of the hands (Figure 24–4) and feet are typically affected first, although larger joints can be involved at any time. The disease is classically symmetric with symptoms present bilaterally in hands, feet, or both. This mirroring is almost unique to RA; systemic lupus erythematosus, which is often confused with RA in its early stages, is not so consistently symmetric.

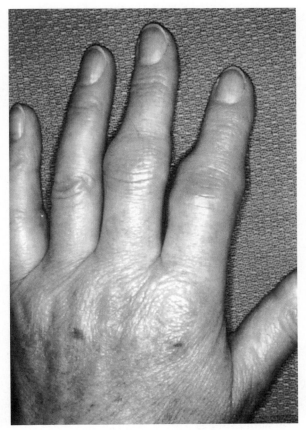

▲ **Figure 24–4.** Swelling of the proximal interphalangeal joints of the second and third fingers in rheumatoid arthritis. Symmetric swelling might be expected on the other hand.

Fingers and wrists are stiff and sore in the mornings, requiring heat, rubbing, and movement to be functional ("morning stiffness"). Stiffness after prolonged lack of movement ("gelling") is seen in many joint disorders, but the morning stiffness of RA is prolonged and characteristic enough that queries regarding this symptom are quite helpful as one works toward a diagnosis.

The patient often reports fatigue out of proportion to lack of sleep. Daytime naps are almost unavoidable, yet are not fully restorative. Anorexia, weight loss, or even low-grade fever can be present. Along with musculoskeletal complaints, these somatic concerns may lead to mistaken diagnoses of fibromyalgia or even depression.

RA can eventually involve almost any joint in the body. Selected important manifestations of RA in specific joints are listed in Table 24–5. Because the hand and wrist are so commonly affected by RA, the complications listed for these sites

Table 24–5. Manifestations of rheumatoid arthritis in specific joints.

Joint	Complication
Hand	Ulnar deviation (hand points toward ulnar side), swan neck deformity (extension of PIP joint), Boutonniere deformity (flexion at DIP)
Wrist	Swelling causing carpal tunnel syndrome
Elbow	Swelling causing compressive neuropathy Deformity preventing complete extension, loss of power
Shoulder	"Frozen shoulder" (loss of abduction, nighttime pain)
Neck	Subluxation of C_1-C_2 joint with danger of dislocation and spinal cord compression ("hangman's injury")
Foot	"Cockup" deformity and/or subluxation at MTP
Knee	Effusion leading to Baker cyst (evagination of synovial lining and fluid into popliteal space)

DIP, distal interphalangeal; MTP, metatarsophalangeal; PIP, proximal interphalangeal.

are so likely seen in long-standing disease as to be almost pathognomonic. The cause of any one manifestation may be unique to a particular joint and the surrounding periarticular structure. Common features include inflammation-induced stretching of tendons and ligaments resulting in joint laxity, subconscious restriction of movement resulting in "frozen" joints, and consequences of inflammatory synovitis with cartilage destruction and periarticular bone erosion. An objective sign of destruction includes the high-pitched, "crunchy" sound of crepitus.

Extra-articular manifestations of RA can be seen at any stage of disease. Most common are rheumatoid nodules, found at some point in ≤50% of all patients with RA. These occur almost anywhere in the body, especially along pressure points (the typical olecranon site), along tendons, or in bursae. Vasculitis is an uncommon initial presentation of RA. Dry eyes and mouth are seen in the RA-associated sicca syndrome. Dyspnea, cough, or even chest pain may signal respiratory interstitial disease. Cardiac, gastrointestinal, and renal involvement in RA is not common. Peripheral nervous system symptoms are seen as compression neuropathies (eg, carpal or tarsal tunnel syndrome) and reflect not so much direct attack on nerves, but rather primarily as consequences of squeezing compression as nerves are forced into passages narrowed by nearby inflammation.

B. Laboratory Findings

In contrast to OA, the laboratory findings in RA can be significant and helpful. A normocytic anemia is common in active RA. This anemia is almost always the so-called anemia of chronic disease. The white blood cell count is normal or even slightly elevated; an exception is the rare Felty syndrome (leukopenia and splenomegaly in a patient with known RA).

RA does not typically affect electrolytes and renal function. There is no pathophysiologic reason why transaminases, bilirubin, alkaline phosphatase, or other liver, pancreatic, or bone enzymes should be altered. Similarly, calcium, magnesium, and phosphate values should be unchanged. Most hormone measurements are normal, particularly thyroid and the adrenal axis. Any chronic inflammatory disease may alter the menstrual cycle, but measurement of luteinizing hormone and follicle-stimulating hormone is of little help.

An elevated ESR is almost ubiquitous in RA; this is not surprising since RA is clearly a strong, chronic inflammatory state. However, there are more than a few conditions in which the measured ESR might be altered because of other physiologic states. For instance, the ESR, even in a patient with active RA, might be inappropriately "normal" if there also are red blood cell changes such as sickle cell or microcytosis, or blood protein abnormalities such as hyperviscosity or polycythemia. For these reasons, rheumatologists often also measure the C-reactive protein (CRP), another measure of inflammation. The CRP is not affected by many of the conditions that can interfere with measurement of the ESR. An elevated CRP, just as the ESR, is indicative of an inflammatory state (though is not specific for RA).

The test most associated with RA is the rheumatoid factor (RF) blood test. RF is actually a family of antibodies, the most common of which is an immunoglobulin M (IgM) antibody directed against the Fc (fragment, crystallizable) portion of immunoglobulin G (IgG). There is no question this antibody is frequently present in RA, with RF-negative RA accounting for only approximately 5% of all patients with RA. The problem lies with the low specificity of the test. Surveys demonstrate that in a young population, 3–5% of "normal" individuals have a high RF titer (positive test), whereas in an older cohort, the prevalence of positive RF reaches 25%. With the national prevalence of RA only 1%, it is clear that many people with an elevated RF titer do not have RA. In fact, a false-positive RF titer is a common reason for incorrect referral of patients to rheumatologists. Some of the conditions that are associated with a positive RF test are listed in Table 24–6.

Another frequent test useful for diagnosis of RA in the early stages is the anticyclic citrullinated peptide (anti-CCP; also called *anticitrullinated protein/peptide antibody* [ACPA]). This test is positive in most patients with RA and may precede the onset of clinically diagnosed RA by months or even years. When combined with the RF test, this test will confirm the diagnosis even in confusing settings.

Table 24–6. Conditions associated with a positive rheumatoid factor test.

Normal aging
Chronic bacterial infections
Subacute bacterial endocarditis
Tuberculosis
Lyme disease
Others
Viral disease
Cytomegalovirus
Epstein-Barr virus
Hepatitis B
Chronic inflammatory diseases
Sarcoidosis
Periodontal disease
Chronic liver disease (especially viral)
Sjögren syndrome
Systemic lupus erythematosus
Mixed cryoglobulinemia

Nishimura K, Sugiyama D, Kogata Y, et al. Meta-analysis: diagnostic accuracy of anti-cyclic citrullinated peptide antibody and rheumatoid factor for rheumatoid arthritis. *Ann Intern Med.* 2007;146:797–808. [PMID: 17548411]

Suarez-Almazor ME, Gonzalez-Lopez L, Gamez-Nava JI, et al. Utilization and predictive value of laboratory tests in patients referred to rheumatologists by primary care physicians. *J Rheumatol.* 1998;25:1980–1985. [PMID: 9779854]

C. Imaging Studies

Radiographs are no longer needed for the initial diagnosis of RA. Other means of diagnosing RA are more useful. Nonetheless, RA is a disease of synovial tissue, and, because the synovium lies on and attaches to bone, inflammation can cause changes on plain film radiography. Small erosions, or lucencies, on the lateral portions of phalanges are early indications of significant inflammation and should prompt immediate suppressive treatment.

Computed tomography and/or MRI have limited but useful supporting roles. An undesired complication of treatment of RA, aseptic necrosis (eg, of the femoral head), has a characteristic appearance on MRI. Although MRI can be used to differentiate the synovitis of RA from infection (eg, septic arthritis, osteomyelitis), positive cultures are much more important to eventual diagnosis and treatment.

► Differential Diagnosis

In practice, it should not be difficult to differentiate among the three prototypical arthritides discussed in this chapter (see Table 24–1). Relatively new (2010) criteria developed by subspecialty organizations give valuable guidelines to

Table 24–7. 1987 American College of Rheumatology diagnostic criteria for rheumatoid arthritis.

The diagnosis of rheumatoid arthritis is confirmed if the patient has had at least four of the seven following criteria, with criteria 1–6 present for ≥6 weeks:
1. Morning stiffness (≥1 hour)
2. Arthritis of three or more joint areas (areas are right or left of proximal interphalangeal joints, metacarpophalangeal, wrist, elbow, knee, ankle, and metatarsophalangeal)
3. Arthritis of hand joints (proximal interphalangeal joints or metacarpophalangeal joints)
4. Symmetric arthritis, by area
5. Subcutaneous rheumatoid nodules
6. Positive test for rheumatoid factor
7. Radiographic changes (hand and wrist radiography showing erosion of joints or unequivocal demineralization around joints)

Adapted with permission from Arnett FC, Edworthy SM, Bloch DA, et al: The American Rheumatism Association 1987 revised criteria for the classification of rheumatoid arthritis. *Arthritis Rheum* 1988; Mar;31(3):315–324.

making an accurate diagnosis of RA (Table 24–7). Because treatment started early is generally successful, rheumatologists promote early referral—treating a new diagnosis of RA almost as a "medical emergency."

Moreland LW, Bridges SL Jr. Early rheumatoid arthritis: a medical emergency? *Am J Med.* 2001;111:498. [PMID: 11690579]

Neil VP, Machold KP, Eberl G, et al. Benefit of very early referral and very early therapy with disease-modifying anti-rheumatic drugs in patients with early rheumatoid arthritis. *Rheumatology.* 2004;43:906–914. [PMID: 15113999]

▶ Complications

Serious extra-articular manifestations of RA are not infrequent. Some of these are life-threatening and require sophisticated management by physicians experienced in dealing with these crises. The responsibility often remains with the primary care physician to recognize these conditions and refer the patient appropriately. Table 24–8 lists several of these complications with a brief description of the clinical presentation.

▶ Treatment

Therapy of RA has changed from managing inflammation to specific measures directed against the fundamental sources of the inflammation. In more recent decades, treatment of RA has undergone perhaps the most wholesale shift of any of the rheumatologic conditions. Therapy is now directed at fundamental processes and begins with aggressive,

Table 24–8. Extra-articular manifestations of rheumatoid arthritis (RA).

Complication	Brief Comments
Rheumatoid nodules	Found over pressure points, classically olecranon; typically fade with disease-modifying antirheumatic drug (DMARD) therapy; also may be found in internal organs; if causing disability, may attempt intralesional steroids, or surgery
Popliteal cyst	Usually asymptomatic unless ruptures, then mimics calf thrombophlebitis; ultrasonography (and high index of suspicion) useful
Anemia	Usually "chronic disease" and, despite low measured iron, does not respond to oral iron therapy; improves with control of inflammatory disease
Scleritis/episcleritis	Inflammatory lesion of conjunctiva; more prolonged, intense, and uncomfortable than "simple" conjunctivitis; requires ophthalmologic management
Pulmonary disease	Ranges from simple pleuritis and pleural effusion (noted for low glucose) to severe bronchiolitis, interstitial fibrosis, nodulosis, and pulmonary vasculitis; may require high-dose steroid therapy once diagnosis established by bronchoscopy or even open-lung biopsy
Sjögren syndrome	Often occurring with RA, includes sicca syndrome with thickened respiratory secretions, dysphagia, vaginal atrophy, hyperglobulinemia, and distal renal tubule defects; treatment of sicca syndrome possible with muscarinic receptor agonists; other manifestations more difficult
Felty syndrome	Constellation of RA, leukopenia, splenomegaly, and often anemia, thrombocytopenia; control underlying RA with DMARDs; may need granulocyte colony-stimulating factor, especially if infectious complications are frequent
Rheumatoid vasculitis	Spectrum from digital arteritis (with hemorrhage) to cutaneous ulceration to mononeuritis multiplex to severe, life-threatening multisystem arteritis involving heart, gastrointestinal tract, and other organs; resembles polyarteritis nodosum

potentially toxic disease-modifying drugs. The outlook can be hopeful, with preservation of joints, activity, and lifestyle a realistic goal. RA need no longer be the "deforming arthritis" by which it was known just a short time ago.

Kremers HM, Nicola P, Crowson CS, et al. Therapeutic strategies in rheumatoid arthritis over a 40-year period. *J Rheumatol.* 2004;31:2366–2373. [PMID: 15570636]

A. Assessment of Prognostic Factors

One of the early steps in treating RA is to assess prognostic factors in the individual patient. Poor prognosis leads to the decision to start aggressive treatment earlier. Some prognostic features are demographic, such as female sex, age >50 years, low socioeconomic status, and a first-degree relative with RA. Clinical features associated with poor prognosis include a large number of affected joints, especially involvement of the flexor tendons of the wrist, with persistence of swelling at the fingers; rheumatoid nodules; high ESR or C-reactive protein and high titers of RF; presence of erosions on radiographs; and evidence of functional disability. Formal functional testing and disease activity questionnaires are frequently employed, not only in establishing stage of disease but also at interval visits. In practice, though, most rheumatologists urge their generalist colleagues to refer patients identified with new-onset RA early. Despite certain prognostic factors noted earlier, most patients are indicated for, and respond to, early therapeutic intervention.

Anderson J, Caplan L, Yazdany J, et al. Rheumatoid arthritis disease activity measures: American College of Rheumatology recommendations for use in clinical practice. *Arthritis Care Res.* 2012;64:640–647. [PMID: 22473918]

B. Patient Education

Therapy begins with patient education, and again, there are multiple sources of information from support and advocacy groups, professional organizations, government sources, and pharmaceutical companies. Patients should learn about the natural history of RA and the therapies available to interrupt the course. They should learn about joint protection and the likelihood that at least some activities need to be modified or discontinued. RA, especially before disease modification is established, is a fatiguing disorder. Patients should realize that rest is as important as appropriate types of activity. Of vital importance is the patient's acknowledgment that drug regimens about to be started are complex but that compliance is critical to successful outcomes. The patient should frankly be told that the drugs are toxic and may have adverse effects.

C. Pharmacotherapy

1. Pain relief—Pain in RA is caused by inflammation, and establishment of effective anti-inflammatory drugs is the first goal of RA intervention. This is a step often expected of generalist physicians if there is likely to be delay in referral of the newly diagnosed RA patient to the rheumatologist. NSAIDs, at doses recommended earlier (see Table 24–2), give the patient early relief. NSAIDs continue to be used throughout the course of treatment; it is not uncommon to switch from one to another as effectiveness falters. It should be noted, though, that NSAIDs will not alter the course of the disease, and the patient should not be deluded into thinking that early pain relief substitutes for comprehensive treatment.

However, the effective management of RA should limit uncontrolled pain. Indeed, the goal of RA management is to find treatments that will alter the otherwise progressive course of disease and that will also alter and control joint pain. Indeed, the goal of any RA management is to find therapies that will limit pain. Consequently, both generalist and specialist physicians to the patient with RA should continuously seek treatment modifications rather than settle for a degree of uncontrolled pain that might prompt use of narcotics.

2. Complementary and alternative medicine—If the patient is reluctant to start drugs, fish oil supplementation may provide symptomatic relief. But the same caution mentioned earlier for pain relief applies to complementary and alternative therapies—these products do not alter the natural history of RA. Even with some degree of pain relief and anti-inflammatory efficacy, these products are no substitute for effective treatment.

Nevertheless, physicians regularly are asked for recommendations of alternative treatments. Both omega-3 and omega-6 fatty acids in fish oil modulate synthesis of highly inflammatory prostaglandin E_2 and leukotriene E_4. The fish oil chosen must contain high concentrations of the relevant fatty acids. A large number of capsules need to be taken, and palatability, diarrhea, and halitosis are frequent adverse effects. γ-Linolenic acid interrupts the pathway of arachidonic acid, another component of the inflammatory cascades. Extracted from the oils of plant seeds such as linseed, sunflower seed, and flaxseed, γ-linolenic acid demonstrates some efficacy in short-term studies using large doses of the extract.

3. Anti-inflammatory medications—RA is an inflammatory disease, and all treatments are directed, in one way or another, to the reduction or elimination of the inflammatory process. Patients with RA will be taking one form of anti-inflammatory medication throughout the course of the disease.

As noted earlier, NSAIDs are almost continuously recommended, even with other effective treatments established.

It is common to switch from one drug to another as efficacy wanes. It is important to modify use of NSAIDs if well-identified effects are noted. Gastrointestinal upset, even gastrointestinal bleeding, is common; this may be ameliorated as well by use of H_2-blockers such as ranitidine or proton pump inhibitors such as omeprazole. NSAID use should be modified, if not discontinued, in advancing stages of chronic kidney disease.

Steroids are widely used in RA. Relatively high-dose oral or parenteral use of steroids can reduce inflammation in the early stages of RA or at times of RA flare. Certain manifestations of RA, such as vasculitis or pulmonary involvement, will require steroids for more prolonged periods of time. The use of steroids for intra-articular injection into symptomatic joints can enhance systemic anti-inflammatory medications. The well-known complications of high-dose steroids require that these be used only for short periods of time if at all possible

Sulfasalazine has been noted to have some efficacy as an anti-inflammatory in RA; initially, this was found when patients with RA were also being treated for another inflammatory condition (eg, inflammatory bowel disease). Another antibiotic, minocycline, may have similar anti-inflammatory effects. It is evident that the mechanism is not through some bacterial/viral effect but likely through inhibition of metalloproteinase metabolism.

4. Disease-modifying antirheumatic drugs (DMARDs)— These agents are almost always the first line of intensive therapy for patients newly diagnosed with RA. Fortunately, a large number of patients can be maintained in disease remission with use of medications in this category. Depending on the classification used to describe RA therapy, there may be a limited number of DMARD agents available, or some of these may be used in combination with agents described under anti-inflammatories earlier. Nonetheless, almost all patients with RA will be prescribed agents in this class at some time during their therapy.

The prototypical DMARD agent is methotrexate. Methotrexate is effective at decreasing inflammation, lowering ESR, slowing bony erosions, and reducing destructive pannus. Methotrexate is generally given in weekly doses with beneficial results seen as early as 4–6 weeks. Treatment can be continued for years. Toxicity includes liver and hematologic changes, and regular monitoring is essential. Other adverse effects are not infrequent and may require modification of dose. For most patients, there will be regular modification of the dose in an attempt to find the lowest effective dose.

Azathioprine and cyclosporine are occasionally used as DMARDs, although rarely concurrently with methotrexate. Complications from these drugs are well recognized, and patient counseling should be extensive before use. One use for these agents appears to be during therapy for complications such as vasculitis. Another antibiotic, the antimalarial

drug hydroxychloroquine, is often given in conjunction with methotrexate. There is a rare, but unfortunate, adverse effect to the retina seen with use of hydroxychloroquine that requires periodic ophthalmologic visits. Leflunomide blocks protein synthesis by lymphocytes and has been shown to be almost as effective as methotrexate. However, its half-life is almost 2 weeks, and liver toxicity is not infrequent. In addition, leflunomide has been associated with birth defects, making effective contraception mandatory when used in women of reproductive age.

5. Tissue necrosis factor (TNF) inhibitors—TNF is a messenger that attracts other inflammatory cells to a site. TNF is also involved in production of interferon and interleukins. Blockade of these TNF effects diminishes the inflammatory response, both decreasing patient symptoms and slowing disease progression. Etanercept, infliximab, and adalimumab are examples of frequently used TNF inhibitors in treatment of RA. Other TNF inhibitors are available and occasionally used in very specific circumstances. These drugs require subcutaneous or intravenous injection, as often as every other week. Yet, they are relatively well tolerated, and any hematologic toxicity responds to discontinuation. Although TNF inhibitors carry FDA indication for moderate to severe RA, they are often given with methotrexate or even as single agents.

A serious consideration relates to the role of TNF inhibitors in host defenses. In particular, patients on TNF inhibitors who have tuberculosis often have rapid extrapulmonary spread and poor response to treatment. Consequently, assurance of the absence of tuberculosis, either by the purified protein derivative test or even the blood-based test QuantiFERON, is indicated.

6. Interleukin (IL) inhibitors—IL inhibitors have found increasing use in RA, typically in conjunction with other modalities. IL-6 inhibitor (tocilizumab) and IL-1 inhibitor (anakinra) block different steps in both immune response and acute-phase response. Both inhibitors can be used with methotrexate for added disease-modifying activity. Side effects are not uncommon, ranging from local injection inflammation to leukopenia, liver enzyme abnormalities, and even alterations in lipids. In addition, interleukin inhibitors should not be used with TNF inhibitors because infectious complications are increased.

7. T-cell blockade—Continuing the effort to block parts of the immune and/or inflammatory response, the T-cell blocker abatacept functions by arresting activation of naïve T cells. When used in conjunction with other DMARDs, there can be a moderate improvement in response criteria in a significant number of patients. This agent does carry an increased risk of infection. In addition, perhaps because of suppressed immune surveillance, there is concern for increased risk of neoplasia.

8. B-cell depletion—The biologic agent rituximab is widely used in treatment of B-cell lymphoma and has also been demonstrated to have efficacy in RA similar to that of abatacept. Rituximab works by blocking a signaling molecule from mature B cells, resulting in the depletion of B cells. Reduction of B cells reduces the inflammatory response in the synovium of the patient with RA. This agent, along with abatacept, may be used in patients with a poor response to TNF inhibitors. Other "biologics" are being developed or introduced for therapy of RA. The choice of one agent over another is very often related as much to the rheumatologist preference and experience as to medical studies showing increased efficacy.

9. Drug administration and precautions—Although many of the anti-inflammatory and DMARD medications can be taken orally, most of the TNF inhibitors, the IL inhibitors, and the T- and B-cell blockers must be given either by injection (subcutaneous) or intravenous infusion. Since the frequency of administration, even once stabilized, ranges from weekly to monthly, it is clear that the patient will have frequent office visits to the rheumatologist. Unfortunately, local or systemic reaction to these agents is frequent and may require coadministration of other drugs (often steroids) to ameliorate the reactions.

As noted earlier, a frequent concern in use of biologics is increased infection. Patients are routinely tested for subclinical tuberculosis infection and are strongly advised to remain up to date with immunizations. Specific immunizations to be considered should include pneumococcal (both 23 and 13 strains), human papillomavirus, hepatitis B, and herpes zoster. The yearly influenza vaccine should be strongly considered. Most vaccines can be given even while the patient is receiving DMARDS; current evidence suggests that even the herpes zoster vaccine is effective if given to a patient receiving biologic agents. A concern also alluded to earlier is the possibility of increased occurrence of neoplasm. Since the purpose of most of these products is to suppress the immune/inflammatory response, the very real concern is that neoplasia surveillance mechanisms are also suppressed. To date, although tumors have been reported during use of these agents, there does not seem to be a significant increase in incidence.

Singh JA, Furst DE, Bharat A, et al. 2012 Update of the 2008 American College of Rheumatology recommendations for the use of disease-modifying antirheumatic drugs and biologic agents in the treatment of rheumatoid arthritis. *Arthritis Care Res.* 2012;64:625–639. [PMID: 22473917]

Singh JA, Saag KG, Bridges SL Jr, et al. 2015 American College of Rheumatology guideline for the treatment of rheumatoid arthritis. *Arthritis Care Res.* 2016;68:1–25. [PMID: 26545825]

Smolen JS, Landewé R, Bijlsma J, et al. EULAR recommendations for the management of rheumatoid arthritis with synthetic and biological disease-modifying antirheumatic drugs. *Ann Rheum Dis.* 2010;69:964–977. [PMID: 28264816]

D. Surgery

Joint instability and resultant disability are often due to a combination of joint destruction, a primary effect of synovial inflammation, and tendon or ligament laxity, a secondary effect or "innocent bystander." The innocent bystander effect notes that these connective tissues are stretched, weakened, or malaligned as a result of inflammation of the joints over which they cross, but not the result of a direct attack on the tendon or ligament itself. Nonetheless, at some point, joint destruction and connective tissue laxity combine to produce useless, and frequently painful, joints. At this point, the surgeon has much to offer. Joint stabilization, connective tissue reinsertion, and joint replacement of both small (interphalangeal) and large (hip, knee) joints provide return of function and reduction of pain. The timing of surgery is still an art and is most effective when close collaboration exists between the treating physician and surgeon.

▶ Prognosis

Morbidity and mortality are increased in patients with RA over age-matched persons without RA. Correlated with active disease, there is a well-described increase in stroke and myocardial infarction. These manifestations may be due to a hypercoagulable state induced by the autoimmune process and circulating antibodies. There are suggestions that the increased rate of stroke and myocardial infarction may be reduced by effective DMARD therapy. Even so, it is recommended that appropriate cardiovascular interventions be considered (eg, aspirin, lipid management). Even under conscientious treatment, complications from infection, pulmonary and renal disease, and gastrointestinal bleeding occur at rates higher than those in the general population. Many of the latter complications are related as much to the drugs used to control the disease as to the disease itself.

Aletaha D, Smolen JS. Diagnosis and management of rheumatoid arthritis. *JAMA.* 2018;320(13);1360–1372. [PMID: 30285183]

Myasoedova E, Gabriel SE. Cardiovascular disease in rheumatoid arthritis: a step forward. *Curr Opin Rheumatol.* 2010;22:342–347. [PMID: 20164773]

Websites

American Academy of Family Physicians (Family doctor–designed for patient information more than the academy website). www.familydoctor.org

American College of Physicians (for physicians; little of relevance for patients—nothing on OA, gout, or RA readily found—and much that requires sign-in by members). www.acponline.org

American College of Rheumatology (a section for patients, "Patient Resources," with appropriately written information is available without sign-in). www.rheumatology.org

Arthritis Foundation (user-friendly information for patients, written without medical jargon, somewhat superficial, strong community support). www.arthritis.org

National Center for Complementary and Alternative Medicine (National Institutes of Health [NIH]) (for physicians and patients; easy to use; comprehensive; balanced information on conventional and alternative treatments). www.nccam.nih.gov

National Guideline Clearinghouse (for physicians; functions as a search engine for guidelines on subject desired; links to publications, some of which require sign-in; comprehensive and international). www.guideline.gov

National Institute of Arthritis and Musculoskeletal and Skin Diseases (NIH) (for physicians and sophisticated patients; relatively easy to use; comprehensive, though technical, information). www.niams.nih.gov

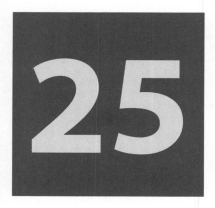

Low Back Pain in Primary Care: An Evidence-Based Approach

Charles W. Webb, DO, FAAFP, FAMSSM, CAQSM

Francis G. O'Connor, MD, MPH

▶ General Considerations

Low back pain (LBP)—discomfort, tension, or stiffness below the costal margin and above the inferior gluteal folds—is one of the most common conditions encountered in primary care as an acute self-limited problem, second only to the common cold. LBP has an annual incidence of 5% and a lifetime prevalence of 60–90%. It is the leading cause of disability in the United States for adults age <45 years, is responsible for one-third of workers' compensation costs, and accounts for direct and indirect costs of nearly $90 billion per year. At any given time, 1% of the US population is chronically disabled and another 1% temporarily disabled as a result of back pain. Numerous studies report a favorable natural history for acute and subacute LBP, with <90% of patients regaining function within 6–12 weeks with or without physician intervention. Recent evidence suggests that about one in five acute LBP patients will have persistent back pain resulting in limitations in activity at 1 year. Approximately 85% of back pain has no readily identifiable cause, and up to one-third of all patients will develop chronic LBP. This chapter reviews a detailed evidence-based approach to the assessment, diagnosis, and management of the adult patient with acute, subacute, and chronic LBP.

Casazza BA. Diagnosis and treatment of acute low back pain. *Am Fam Physician*. 2012;85(4):343–350. [PMID: 22335313]

Dagenais S, Caro J, Haldeman S. A systematic review of low back pain cost of illness studies in the United States and internationally. *Spine J*. 2008;8:8–20. [PMID: 18164449]

Fourney DR, Andersson G, Arnold PM, et al. Chronic low back pain. *Spine*. 2011;36:S1–S9. [PMID: 21952181]

Herndon CM, Zoberi KS, Gardner BJ. Common questions about chronic low back pain. Am Fam Physician. 2015;91(10): 708-714. [PMID: 25978200].

Stochkendahl MJ, Kjaer P, Hartvigsen J, et al. National Clinical Guidelines for non-surgical treatment of patients with recent onset low back pain or lumbar radiculopathy. *Eur Spine J*. 2018;27(1):60–75. [PMID: 28429142]

▶ Prevention

LBP is a heavy medical and financial burden to not only the patients who are experiencing the ailment but also society. The US Preventive Services Task Force produced a recommendation statement on primary care interventions to prevent LBP in adults stating that, currently, there is insufficient evidence to support or rebuke the routine use of exercise to prevent LBP. However, regular physical activity has been shown to be beneficial in the treatment and limitation of recurrent episodes of chronic LBP. Lumbar supports (back belts) and shoe inserts (orthotics) have not been found to be effective in the prevention of LBP. Worksite interventions, including education on lifting techniques, have been shown to have some short-term effects, such as decreasing lost time from work for patients with back pain.

Risk factor modifications may be the only way to truly prevent LBP. These risk factors can be classified as individual, psychosocial, occupational, and anatomic. Table 25–1 lists the prominent risk factors for LBP.

Casazza BA. Diagnosis and treatment of acute low back pain. *Am Fam Physician*. 2012;85(4):343–350. [PMID: 22335313]

Dagenais S, Caro J, Haldeman S. A systematic review of low back pain cost of illness studies in the United States and internationally. *Spine J*. 2008;8:8–20. [PMID: 18164449]

Herndon CM, Zoberi KS, Gardner BJ. Common questions about chronic low back pain. *Am Fam Physician*. 2015;91(10): 708–714. [PMID: 25978200].

Lillios S, Young J. The effects of core and lower extremity strengthening on pregnancy-related low back and pelvic girdle pain: a systematic review. *J Womens Health Phys Ther*. 2012;36(3): 116–124. [No PMID]

Stochkendahl MJ, Kjaer P, Hartvigsen J, et al. National Clinical Guidelines for non-surgical treatment of patients with recent onset low back pain or lumbar radiculopathy. *Eur Spine J*. 2018; 27(1):60–75. [PMID: 28429142]

Table 25–1. Risk factors associated with low back pain.

Unchangeable Risk Factors			
Individual		**Anatomic**	
Increasing age Birth defects of the spine High birth weight		Degenerative disk disease	
Male gender		Osteoarthritis	
Family history		Synovial cyst formation	
Previous back injury		Lumbosacral transitional vertebra	
Pregnancy		Schmorl nodes	
History of spine surgery		Annular disruption	
High birth weight		Spondylolysis Spondylolisthesis History of birth defects (eg, spina bifida)	
Modifiable Risk Factors			
Individual	**Psychosocial**	**Occupational**	**Others**
Sedentary lifestyle	Stress	Unemployment	Poor pain tolerance
Smoking	Depression	Perceived inadequate income	History of recurrent back pain
Overweight or obese	Decreased cognition	Monotonous tasks	Presence of sciatic
Poor posture and biomechanics	Somatization	Long periods of sitting or standing	Corticosteroid use
Education level	Fear/avoidance behaviors	Heavy lifting	Chronic illness that causes chronic cough (eg, chronic obstructive pulmonary disease)
Poor general health	History of anxiety	Repetitive twisting, bending, squatting, pushing, pulling	Participation in strenuous or contact sports
	Neurotic personality disorder	Constant vibration Lack of recognition at work Poor job satisfaction Poor relations with employer, supervisor, and coworkers Low job control High pressure on time Unavailability of light duty Belief that job is dangerous for the lower back	

▶ Clinical Findings

The key elements in the correct diagnosis and management of the issues surrounding the causes of LBP include an evaluation for serious health problems, screening for red and yellow flags (Tables 25–2 and 25–3), symptom control for acute and subacute LBP, and follow-up evaluation of patients whose condition worsens or fails to improve. The first step is the accurate and timely identification of clinical conditions for which LBP is a symptom.

A. Symptoms and Signs

A careful medical history and physical examination are critical in determining the presence of a more serious condition in the patient presenting with LBP. On examining

Table 25–2. Red flags and appropriate actions.

Condition	Red Flag	Action
Cancer	History of cancer Unexplained weight loss Age ≥50 years Failure to improve with therapy Pain ≥4–6 weeks; night/rest pain	If malignant disease of the spine is suspected, imaging is indicated, and CBC and ESR should be considered Identification of possible primary malignancy should be investigated, eg, PSA, mammogram, UPEP/SPEP/IPEP
Infection	Fever History of intravenous drug use Recent bacterial infection: UTI, skin, pneumonia Immunocompromised states (steroid, organ transplants, diabetes, HIV) Rest pain	If infection in the spine is suspected, MRI, CBC, ESR, and/or UA are indicated
Cauda equina syndrome	Urinary retention or incontinence Saddle anesthesia Anosphincter tone decrease/fecal incontinence Bilateral lower extremity weakness/numbness or progressive neurologic deficit	Request immediate surgical consultation
Fracture	Use of corticosteroids Age ≥70 or history of osteoporosis; recent significant trauma	Appropriate imaging and surgical consultation
Acute abdominal aneurysm	Abdominal pulsating mass Other atherosclerotic vascular disease; rest/night pain; age ≥ 60 years	Appropriate imaging (ultrasound) and surgical consultation
Significant herniated nucleus pulposus (HNP)	Major muscle weakness (drop foot) (abnormal gait with lack of heel to toe ambulation)	Appropriate imaging and surgical consultation

CBC, complete blood count; ESR, erythrocyte sedimentation rate; HIV, human immunodeficiency virus; IPEP, immunoprotein electrophoresis; MRI, magnetic resonance imaging; PSA, prostate-specific antigen; SPEP, serum protein electrophoresis; UA, urinalysis; UPEP, urine protein electrophoresis; UTI, urinary tract infection.

the patient, the primary care provider must look for "red and yellow flags" that indicate the presence of a significant medical or psychological condition. If any red flags are identified, patients requiring emergent or urgent care should be given immediate consultation or referral to the appropriate specialist. Nonemergent patients with red flags should be scheduled for the appropriate diagnostic test to determine whether they have a condition that requires a referral. If any yellow flags are identified, this signifies the presence of psychological distress and strongly correlates to chronicity and poor patient outcomes in both pain control and disability. When yellow flags are identified early, an interdisciplinary approach should be considered.

1. History—The history should focus on the location of the pain, the mechanism of injury (to ascertain what the patient was doing when he/she first noticed the pain, whether it was insidious or whether there was a specific trauma or inciting activity), the character (mechanical, radicular, claudicant, or nonspecific), and duration of the pain (acute, <6 weeks; subacute, between 6 and 12 weeks; or chronic, >12 weeks).

The provider must identify neurologic symptoms (bowel/bladder symptoms, weakness in the extremities, saddle anesthesia) suggestive of cauda equina syndrome (CES; a true neurosurgical emergency). The functional status of the patient should be noted, as should any exacerbating or ameliorating factors. The presence of fever, weight loss, and night pain is particularly concerning because these could indicate a more serious disease, such as an underlying malignancy. The social history should include information about drug use/abuse, intravenous (IV) drug use, tobacco use, any physical demands at work, and the presence of psychosocial stressors. Past medical and surgical history should also be obtained, particularly a history of previous spinal surgery or immunosuppression (history of cancer, steroid use, human immunodeficiency virus [HIV]). A thorough history enables the primary care provider to identify any red and/or yellow flags that require a more extensive workup to rule out a potentially serious and disabling disease processes.

2. Physical examination—The physical examination supplements the information obtained in the history by helping

Table 25–3. Yellow flags in low back pain.

Attitudes and Beliefs	Comorbid Conditions

Fear/avoidance
Fear of movement, use of
   excessive rest
Catastrophizing
Excessive focus on pain
Feeling out of control
Passivity toward rehabilitation
	Lack of or decreased sleep
	History of other disabling injuries
	   or conditions
	Lack of financial incentive to return
	   to work
	Pending litigation
	Overprotective family

Affective factors
Poor work history
Poor compliance with rehabilitation
Withdrawal from activities (activities
   of daily living, social)
History of substance abuse
   (self-medicating)
Depression
Anxiety
Irritability
History of psychological or
   physical abuse
History of irregular or episodic
   physical activity
Conflicting diagnosis from different
   providers
Multiple medical providers
	Waddell signs
	Pain with axial loading of spine
	Superficial tenderness to palpation
	   (light touch)
	Overreaction (pain out of proportion
	   to physical findings)
	Straight leg raise test improves
	   with distraction
	Regional weakness

to identify underlying serious medical conditions or possible serious neurologic compromise. The primary elements of the physical examination are inspection, palpation, observation (including range-of-motion testing), and a specialized neuromuscular evaluation. The examination should start with an evaluation of the spinal curvature and lumbar range of motion, specifically noting the amount of pain-free movement. Palpation should include the paraspinal muscles, the spinous processes, the sacroiliac joints, the piriformis muscles, and the position of the pelvic bones. Because the lumbar spine is kinetically linked to the pelvis (particularly the sacroiliac area), pain from the pelvis is often referred to the lumbar spine. Hip flexors and hamstring flexibility should also be assessed as a potential cause for the pain. The Waddell signs, which describe five physical signs (tenderness, simulation, distraction, regional numbness, and overreaction), are clinically useful in the identification of patients who have physical findings without a specific anatomic cause that would benefit from surgical intervention. If three or more of these tests are positive, psychological overlay might be present, and this should be assessed with the yellow flags described earlier.

3. Neurologic evaluation—The neurologic evaluation should include Achilles (S_1) and patellar tendon (L_2–L_4) reflex testing, ankle and great toe dorsiflexion (L_4–L_5), and

plantarflexion (S_1) strength, as well as the location of sensory complaints (dermatomes involved). Light touch testing for sensation in the medial (L_4), dorsal (L_5), and lateral (S_1) aspects of the foot should also be performed. In patients presenting with acute LBP and no specific limb complaints, a more elaborate neurologic examination is seldom necessary. A seated and supine straight leg raise test evaluates for nerve root impingement. This abbreviated neurologic evaluation of the lower extremity allows detection of clinically significant nerve root compromise at the L_4–L_5 or L_5–S_1 levels. These two sites represent >90% of all significant radiculopathy secondary to lumbar disk herniation. Because this abbreviated examination may fail to diagnose some of the less common causes of LBP, any patient who has not improved in 4–6 weeks should return for further evaluation.

4. Risk stratification—All patients with acute LBP should be risk-stratified with an initial assessment attempting to identify red flags: responses or findings in the history and physical examination that indicate a potentially serious underlying condition, such as a fracture, tumor, infections, abdominal aneurysm, or CES that can lead to considerable patient morbidity and/or mortality. These clinical clues (red flags) include a history of major trauma, minor trauma in patients >50 years old, persistent fever, history of cancer, metabolic disorder, major muscle weakness, bladder or bowel dysfunction, saddle anesthesia, decreased sphincter tone, and unrelenting night pain. Red flags risk-stratify the patient to an increased risk and should prompt an earlier clinical action, such as imaging or laboratory workup. See Table 25–2 for a listing of red flags and their related conditions.

Psychosocial factors also significantly affect pain and function in LBP patients. These psychosocial factors are known as "yellow flags" and are better predictors of treatment outcomes than physical factors in some patients. These yellow flags are listed in Table 25–3.

Casazza BA. Diagnosis and treatment of acute low back pain. *Am Fam Physician*. 2012;85(4):343–350. [PMID: 22335313]

Chapman R, Norvell C, Hermsmeyer T, et al. Evaluating common outcomes for measuring treatment success for chronic low back pain. *Spine*. 2011;36:S54–S68. [PMID: 21952190]

Fisher CG, Vaccaro AR, Mulpuri K, et al. Evidence-based recommendations for spine surgery. *Spine*. 2012;37(1):E3–E9. [PMID: 22751143]

Fourney DR, Andersson G, Arnold PM, et al. Chronic low back pain. *Spine*. 2011;36:S1–S9. [PMID: 21952181]

Herndon CM, Zoberi KS, Gardner BJ. Common questions about chronic low back pain. *Am Fam Physician*. 2015;91(10):708–714. [PMID: 25978200].

Sembrano JN, Reiley MA, Polly DW, et al. Diagnosis and treatment of sacroiliac joint pain. *Curr Orthop Pract*. 2011;22(4):344–350. [No PMID]

Waddell G, McCulloch JA, Kummel E, et al. Nonorganic physical signs in low back pain. *Spine*. 1980;5(2):117–125. [PMID: 6446157]

B. Imaging Studies

Diagnostic imaging is rarely indicated in the acute setting of LBP. Even though some studies have indicated greater patient satisfaction with lumbar radiography, the evidence demonstrates that it may not lead to greater improvement in outcomes. After the first 4–6 weeks of symptoms, the majority of patients will have regained function. However, if the patient is still limited by back symptoms, diagnostic imaging should be considered to look for conditions that present as LBP. Patients for whom diagnostic imaging should be considered include children, patients age >50 years with new-onset back pain, trauma patients, or patients for whom back pain fails to improve despite appropriate conservative treatment. Imaging studies must always be interpreted carefully since disk degeneration and protrusion have been noted in 20–25% of asymptomatic individuals. Therefore, abnormal findings on diagnostic imaging may or may not represent the reason for the patient's pain.

Plain films remain the most widely available modality for imaging the lumbar spine and are rarely useful in evaluating or guiding treatment of adults with acute LBP in the absence of red flags. Plain lumbar x-rays are helpful in detecting spinal fractures and evaluating tumor and/or infection. Anteroposterior and lateral views allow assessment of lumbar alignment, the intervertebral disk space, and bone density and a limited evaluation of the soft tissue. Oblique views should be used only when spondylolysis is suspected as they double the radiation exposure and add only minimal information. Sacroiliac views are used to evaluate ankylosing spondylitis and, again, should be used only when this is suspected.

When the history or physical examination suggests an anatomic abnormality as a cause for the back pain with neurologic deficits, four imaging studies are commonly used: (1) plain myelography, (2) computed tomography (CT) scan, (3) magnetic resonance imaging (MRI) scan, and (4) CT myelography. These four tests are used in similar clinical situations and provide similar information. The objective of these studies is to define a medically or surgically remediable anatomic condition. These tests are not done routinely and should be used only for patients who present with certain clinical findings, such as persistent radicular symptoms and clinically detectable nerve root compressive symptoms and signs (radiculopathy) severe enough to consider surgical intervention (major muscle weakness, progressive motor deficit, intractable pain, and persistent radicular pain beyond 6 weeks). For a listing of these and other special tests and tier indications and recommendations, see Table 25–4.

Diagnostic imaging plays a central role in diagnosing spinal infections. Plain films should be obtained but are often helpful only in the advanced stages of the infection. MRI is the imaging modality of choice in evaluating spinal infection. When infection is identified or suspected, a spinal surgeon should be consulted immediately.

Table 25–4. Special tests and indications/recommendations.

Special Test	Indications/Recommendations
Plain x-ray	Not recommended for routine evaluation of acute LBP unless red flags present Recommended for ruling out fractures Obliques are only recommended when findings are suggestive of spondylolisthesis or spondylolysis
Electrophysiologic tests (EMG and SPEP)	Questionable nerve root dysfunction with leg symptoms ≥6 weeks Not recommended if radiculopathy is obvious
MRI or CT myelography	Back-related leg symptoms and clinically detectable nerve root compromise History of neurogenic claudication suspicious for spinal stenosis Findings suggesting CES, fracture, infection, tumor
ESR	Suspected tumors, infection, inflammatory conditions, metabolic disorders
CBC	Suspected tumors, myelogenous conditions, infections
UA	Suspected UTI, pyelonephritis, myeloma
IPEP	Suspected multiple myeloma
Chemistry profile to include TSH, calcium, and alkaline phosphatase	Suspected electrolyte disorders, thyroid dysfunction, metabolic dysfunction
Bone scan	Suspected occult pars interarticularis fracture or metastatic disease Contraindicated in pregnant patient

CBC, complete blood count; CES, cauda equina syndrome; CT, computed tomography; EMG, electromyelogram; ESR, erythrocyte sedimentation rate; IPEP, immunoprotein electrophoresis; LBP, low back pain; MRI, magnetic resonance imaging; SPEP, serum protein electrophoresis; TSH, thyroid-stimulating hormone; UA, urinalysis; UTI, urinary tract infection.

Casazza BA. Diagnosis and treatment of acute low back pain. *Am Fam Physician.* 2012;85(4):343–350. [PMID: 22335313]

Chapman R, Norvell C, Hermsmeyer T, et al. Evaluating common outcomes for measuring treatment success for chronic low back pain. *Spine.* 2011;36:S54–S68. [PMID: 21952190]

Fisher CG, Vaccaro AR, Mulpuri K, et al. Evidence-based recommendations for spine surgery. *Spine.* 2012;37(1):E3–E9. [PMID: 22751143]

Fourney DR, Andersson G, Arnold PM, et al. Chronic low back pain. *Spine.* 2011;36:S1–S9. [PMID: 21952181]

Qaseem A, Wilt TJ, McLean RM, Forciea MA. Noninvasive treatments for acute, subacute, and chronic low back pain: a clinical practice guideline from the American College of Physicians. *Ann Intern Med.* 2017;166(7):514–530. [PMID: 28192789]

Sembrano JN, Reiley MA, Polly DW, et al. Diagnosis and treatment of sacroiliac joint pain. *Curr Orthop Pract.* 2011;22(4):344–350. [No PMID]

Stochkendahl MJ, Kjaer P, Hartvigsen J, et al. National Clinical Guidelines for non-surgical treatment of patients with recent onset low back pain or lumbar radiculopathy. *Eur Spine J.* 2018;27(1):60–75. [PMID: 28429142]

C. Laboratory Testing

Laboratory testing should be reserved for patients who seem to have conditions masquerading as simple LBP such as cancer or infection (Table 25–5). Laboratory tests that are recommended in evaluating patients with a suspicious history for cancer include a complete blood count with differential and an erythrocyte sedimentation rate (ESR). An ESR of >50 mm/h is suggestive of malignancy, infection, or inflammatory disease. Blood urea nitrogen, creatinine, and urinalysis are helpful for identifying underlying renal or urinary tract disease. Serum calcium, phosphorus, and alkaline phosphatase should be checked in patients with osteopenia, osteolytic vertebral lesions, or vertebral body collapse. If prostate carcinoma is suspected, prostate-specific antigen and acid phosphatase levels should be checked. If multiple myeloma is suspected, a serum immunoelectrophoresis can help guide treatment.

Historical red flags such as IV drug abuse and immunocompromise, as well as fever, should raise concern for an underlying infection. An elevated white blood cell count is a clue to an underlying infection, but can be within normal limits even in acute infection. The ESR and C-reactive protein can be used to monitor the efficacy of treatment of spinal infections. Urinalysis and urine culture should be obtained because urinary tract infection often precedes spinal infection. Blood cultures should be obtained as well. Although they are usually negative, positive cultures identify the infecting organism and provide antibiotic sensitivity to guide treatment.

Table 25–5. Differential diagnosis of lower back pain.

System	Conditions	System	Conditions
Vascular	Expanding aortic aneurysm	Psychogenic	Affective disorder
Gastrointestinal	Pancreatitis		Conversion disorder
	Peptic ulcers		Somatization disorder
	Cholecystitis		Malingering
	Colonic cancer	Infection	Osteomyelitis
Genitourinary	Endometriosis		Epidural/paraspinal abscess
	Tubal pregnancy		Disk space infection
	Kidney stones		Pyogenic sacroiliitis
	Prostatitis		Varicella-zoster
	Chronic pelvic inflammatory disease	Neoplastic	Skeletal metastases
	Perinephric abscess		Spinal cord tumors
	Pyelonephritis		Leukemia
Endocrinologic/metabolic	Osteoporosis		Lymphoma
	Osteomalacia		Retroperitoneal tumors
	Hyperparathyroidism		Primary lumbosacral tumors
	Paget disease		Benign
	Acromegaly		Metastatic
	Cushing disease	Miscellaneous	Sarcoidosis
	Ochronosis		Subacute endocarditis
Hematologic	Hemoglobinopathy		Retroperitoneal fibrosis
	Myelofibrosis		Herpes zoster
	Mastocytosis		Fat herniation of lumbar space
Rheumatologic/ inflammatory	Spondyloarthropathies		Spinal stenosis
	Ankylosing spondylitis	Musculoskeletal	Piriformis syndrome
	Reiter syndrome		Osteoarthritis of the hip
	Psoriatic arthritis		Spondylolysis
	Enteropathic arthritis		Sacroiliac joint dysfunction
	Beçhet syndrome		Traumatic fracture
	Familial Mediterranean fever		Trochanteric bursitis
	Whipple disease		
	Diffuse idiopathic skeletal hyperostosis		

Casazza BA. Diagnosis and treatment of acute low back pain. *Am Fam Physician*. 2012;85(4):343–350. [PMID: 22335313]

Fourney DR, Andersson G, Arnold PM, et al. Chronic low back pain. *Spine*. 2011;36:S1–S9. [PMID: 21952181]

Herndon CM, Zoberi KS, Gardner BJ. Common questions about chronic low back pain. *Am Fam Physician*. 2015;91(10): 708–714. [PMID: 25978200]

▶ Differential Diagnosis

After potential red flags have been ruled out, the differential diagnosis for LBP remains extensive. Table 25–5 presents a list of conditions that can present as simple LBP.

▶ Treatment

If the patient has no red flags and the history and physical examination do not suggest an underlying cause, the diagnosis of mechanical LBP can be made, and treatment may be initiated. The patient should be reassured with a discussion of the natural history of mechanical LBP, and treatment should then focus on pain control and improving individual function. Methods of symptom control should focus on providing comfort and keeping the patient as active as possible while awaiting spontaneous recovery. Evidence for the most common treatments currently used in the primary care setting is presented as follows. Depending on the patient, this treatment may include activity modification, bed rest (of short duration), conservative medications, progressive range of motion and exercise, manipulative treatment, and patient education. This line of treatment should be used for 4–6 weeks before ordering an additional diagnostic test unless the history and physical examination identify a more concerning diagnosis.

A. Patient Education

Patient education is the cornerstone of effective treatment of LBP. Patients who present to the primary care clinic with acute LBP should be educated about expectations for recovery and the potential recurrence of symptoms. Management of patients' expectations of therapy and educating patients about the management goals is an effective way to decrease apprehension and promote a quick recovery. Management goals focus on decreasing pain and improving overall function of the patient. Patients should be informed of safe and reasonable activity modifications and be given information on how to limit the recurrence of low back problems through proper lifting techniques, treatment of obesity, and tobacco cessation. If medications are used, patients should be given information on their use and the potential side effects. Patients should be instructed to follow-up in 1–3 weeks if they fail to improve with conservative treatment, develop bowel or bladder dysfunction, or experience worsening neurologic function.

B. Activity Modification

Patients with acute LBP may be more comfortable if they are able to temporarily limit or avoid specific activities that are known to increase mechanical stress on the spine. Prolonged unsupported sitting and heavy lifting, especially while bending or twisting, should be avoided. Activity recommendations for the employed patient with acute LBP should consider the patient's age and general health and the physical demands of the job.

C. Bed Rest

A gradual return to normal activities is more effective than prolonged bed rest for the treatment of LBP. Bed rest for >4 days may lead to debilitating muscle atrophy and increased stiffness and therefore is not recommended. Most patients with acute or subacute LBP will not require bed rest. For patients with severe initial symptoms, however, limited bed rest for 2–4 days remains an option.

D. Medications

Oral medications (acetaminophen, nonsteroidal anti-inflammatory drugs [NSAIDs], muscle relaxants, and opioids) and injection treatments are available for the treatment of LBP. Most patients with chronic LBP will self-medicate with an over-the-counter (OTC) pain reliever (acetaminophen and ibuprofen). In addition, most patients are prescribed at least one medication to control pain and improve function. Currently, there is good evidence supporting the use of NSAIDs and skeletal muscle relaxants for the management of acute LBP, but these agents are less effective when used as monotherapy. NSAIDs have both anti-inflammatory and analgesic properties and are widely used for all types of LBP. However, they can cause gastrointestinal, renal, and hepatic side effects and have been linked to increased risk of cardiovascular events. Therefore, all of these medications should be used with caution and at the lowest possible dose for the shortest duration. There is no clinical difference in efficacy between selective and nonselective cyclooxygenase (COX) inhibitors. Because opioids are only slightly more effective in relieving low back symptoms than other analgesics (aspirin, acetaminophen) and because of their potential for other complications (dependence), opioid analgesics, if used, should be used only over a time-limited course. Oral corticosteroids are not recommended for the treatment of acute LBP.

There is limited evidence supporting the use of homeopathic and herbal remedies, such as devil's claw, willow bark, and capsicum, for the treatment of acute episodes of chronic LBP.

Injection therapy for the treatment of low back symptoms includes acute pain management; trigger point; ligamentous, sclerosant, and facet joint; and epidural injections. Injections are an invasive treatment option that exposes patients to potentially serious complications. No conclusive studies have proved the efficacy of trigger point, sclerosant, ligamentous, or facet joint injections in the treatment of acute LBP. However, epidural and facet joint injections may benefit patients who fail conservative treatment as a means of avoiding surgery. A series of one to three epidural steroid injections may be beneficial for patients who have radiculopathy that has not improved after 4–6 weeks of conservative therapy.

E. Spinal Manipulation

There is some evidence supporting the use of manipulative therapy in the treatment of acute LBP. Spinal manipulation techniques attempt to restore joint and soft tissue range of motion. Impaired motion of synovial joints has a detrimental effect on joint cartilage and vertebral disk metabolism, leading to degenerative spinal changes. Manipulation is useful early after symptom onset for patients who have LBP without radiculopathy. A 2011 Cochran Review found that spinal manipulation, when compared to all other therapies for chronic LBP, resulted in a statistically significant improvement of patients' pain level at both 1 and 6 months. If the patient's physical findings suggest progressive or severe neurologic deficit, aggressive manipulation should be postponed pending an appropriate diagnostic assessment.

F. Physical Agents and Modalities

Physical agents include ice and moist heat treatments. There is good evidence to support the use of superficial heat for muscle relaxation and analgesia. The evidence supporting cryotherapy is limited at best.

Transcutaneous electrical nerve stimulation (TENS) is thought to modify pain perception by counterstimulation of the nervous system. However, in a Cochran Review of the evidence, including four high-quality randomized controlled trials, TENS was no more effective than placebo. Currently, there is insufficient evidence on the efficacy of TENS to recommend its routine use.

Shoe insoles (or inserts) can vary from OTC foam or rubber inserts to custom orthotics. These devices aim to reduce back pain due to leg length discrepancies or abnormal foot mechanics. There is limited evidence that shoe orthotics (either OTC or custom-made) may provide short-term benefit for patients with mild back pain, although there is no evidence supporting their long-term use or their use in prevention of back pain. The role of leg length discrepancies in LBP has not been established, and differences of <2 cm are unlikely to produce symptoms.

Lumbar support devices for low back problems include corsets, support belts, various types of braces, and molded jackets, and back rests for chairs and car seats. Lumbar corsets and support belts may be beneficial in preventing LBP and time lost from work for individuals whose jobs require frequent lifting; however, the evidence is lacking. There is

some recent evidence that lumbar belts in the setting of subacute LBP can increase functional status and decrease both pain and medication use. Lumbar corsets have not been shown to be beneficial in the treatment of LBP.

A randomized controlled trial found that mattresses of medium firmness are beneficial in reducing pain symptoms and disability in patients with chronic LBP.

Acupuncture and other dry needling techniques have not been found to be beneficial for treating acute or subacute LBP patients. However, recent evidence does suggest that traditional Chinese medical acupuncture and therapeutic massage are beneficial in the treatment of chronic LBP. Acupuncture, when added to conventional therapies, improves function, sleep, and pain better than conventional therapy alone and decreases medication use.

G. Exercise

Therapeutic exercises should be started early to control pain, avoid deconditioning, and restore function. Intensive therapeutic exercise can help decrease pain and improve function in patients with chronic LBP. No single treatment or exercise program has proved effective for all patients with LBP. Poor endurance and abnormal firing of the hip muscles have been noted in patients with both acute and chronic LBP. Various studies have shown that the occurrence of LBP may be reduced by strengthening the back, legs, and abdomen (core muscle groups) and by improving muscular stabilization. Initial exercises should focus on strengthening and stabilizing the spine and stretching the hip flexors. Lower extremity muscle tightness is common with LBP and must be corrected to allow normal range of motion of the lumbar spine.

There is moderate evidence that yoga, compared to non-exercise controls, results in small to moderate improvements in back related function at 3 and 6 months. Yoga improves functional disability, pain intensity, and depression in patients with chronic LBP. It was found to be a cost-effective treatment by reducing office visits as well as medication use, with improved function at 3 and 6 months after intervention.

H. Behavioral Therapy

Multitudinous factors play a role in the patient's return to function and decreasing pain. Psychological stressors (yellow flags) have emerged as the strongest single baseline predictor of 4-year outcomes exceeding pain intensity. Fear/avoidance beliefs also have a strong influence on recovery. These factors highlight the importance of exercise as a management tool for LBP. Exercise reduces fear/avoidance behavior and facilitates function despite ongoing pain. Graded behavior intervention reinforces the fact that pain does not necessarily mean harm. A patient may still have pain but be able to function and thereby improve his or her prognosis over time. Cognitive intervention and exercise programs have demonstrated similar results for improving disability as lumbar fusion in patients with chronic back pain and disk degeneration.

I. Reevaluation

For patients with LBP whose condition worsens during the time of symptom control, reevaluation and consultation or referral to specialty care are recommended. Patients with LBP should always be reevaluated as indicated after 1–3 weeks to assess progress. This can be accomplished with either a follow-up phone call or an office visit. This empowers patients to take the initiative in their disease course. Patients must be advised to follow up sooner if their condition worsens. Any worsening of neurologic symptoms warrants a complete reevaluation.

Conservative treatment is warranted for 4–6 weeks from the initial evaluation. This follow-up visit is also the appropriate time to consider a work-related ergonomic evaluation. As the patient improves, there should be a gradual return to normal activity and a weaning of the medications.

J. Referral

Any patient who has LBP for >6 weeks despite an adequate course of conservative therapy should be reexamined in the office. A comprehensive reevaluation, including a psychosocial assessment and physical examination, should be performed. During follow-up visits, questions should be directed at identifying any detriments in the patient's condition, including new neurologic symptoms, increased pain, or increased medication use. If such problems are found, the patient should be reevaluated for other health problems, consultation, and/or imaging modalities.

For patients with pain that radiates below the knee, especially with a positive tension sign, the anatomy should be evaluated with an imaging study. If there are abnormal findings, then consultation with a neurosurgeon or spine surgeon is appropriate. If, however, the imaging study does not reveal anatomic pathology, then a nonsurgical back specialist may be necessary to help manage the patient. Table 25–6 lists these specialists and indications for their referral. Table 25–7 further identifies useful websites that can assist the provider in identifying resources for management and indications for referral.

If there are no abnormal findings on a comprehensive reassessment, including selected diagnostic tests, it is crucial to start patients on a program that will enable them to resume their usual activities. Management of the patient without structural pathology should be directed toward a physical conditioning program designed with exercise to progressively build activity tolerance and overcome individual limitations. This may include referral to behavior modification specialists, activity-specific educators, or an organized multidisciplinary back rehabilitation program.

Table 25–6. Surgical back specialists.

Specialist	Indications
Physiatrist/physical medicine and rehabilitation	Chronic back pain >6 weeks Chronic sciatica >6 weeks Chronic pain syndrome Recurrent back pain
Neurology	Chronic sciatica for >6 weeks Atypical chronic leg pain (negative straight leg raise) New or progressive neuromotor deficit
Occupational medicine	Difficult workers' compensation situations Disability/impairment ratings Return-to-work issues
Rheumatology	Rule out inflammatory arthropathy Rule out fibrositis/fibromyalgia Rule out metabolic bone disease (eg, osteoporosis)
Primary care sports medicine specialist	Chronic back pain for >6 weeks; chronic sciatica for >6 weeks Recurrent back pain

Table 25–7. Helpful websites.

Address	Information
https://www.ahrq.gov/patients-consumers/index.html	Agency for Healthcare Research and Quality
http://orthoinfo.aaos.org	American Academy of Orthopedic Surgeons information page
https://www.uspreventiveservices-taskforce.org/	US Preventative Services Task Force
http://www.medinfo.co.uk/conditions/lowbackpain.html	European Clinical Practice Guideline on the Treatment of Low Back Pain, including the pediatric population
http://www.chirobase.org/07Strategy/AHCPR/ahcprclinician.html	Quick reference to the US Agency for Health Care Policy and Research (1994) practice guideline
http://familydoctor.org/	FamilyDoctor.org, patient education handouts
https://www.fda.gov/drugs/postmarket-drug-safety-information-patients-and-providers/nonsteroidal-anti-inflammatory-drugs-nsaids	US Food and Drug Administration; analysis and recommendations for nonsteroidal anti-inflammatory drugs and cardiovascular risk

Casazza BA. Diagnosis and treatment of acute low back pain. *Am Fam Physician.* 2012;85(4):343–350. [PMID: 22335313]

Chang DG, Holt JA, Sklar M, Groessl EJ. Yoga as a treatment for chronic low back pain: a systematic review of the literature. *J Orthop Rheumatol.* 2016;3(1):1–8. [PMID: 27231715]

Chapman R, Norvell C, Hermsmeyer T, et al. Evaluating common outcomes for measuring treatment success for chronic low back pain. *Spine.* 2011;36:S54–S68. [PMID: 21952190]

Chuang LH, Soares MO, Tilbrook H, et al. A pragmatic multi-centered randomized controlled trial of yoga for chronic low back pain: economic evaluation. *Spine.* 2012;37(18):1593–1601. [PMID: 22433499]

Deckers K, Smedt KD, Mitchell B, et al. New therapy for refractory chronic mechanical low back pain-restorative neurostimulation to activate the lumbar multifidus: one year results of a prospective multicenter clinical trial. *Neuromodulation.* 2018;21(1): 48–55. [PMID: 29244235]

Herndon CM, Zoberi KS, Gardner BJ. Common questions about chronic low back pain. *Am Fam Physician.* 2015;91(10): 708–714. [PMID: 25978200]

Knezevic NN, Mandalia S, Raasch J, et al. Treatment of chronic low back pain- new approaches on the horizon. *J Pain Res.* 2017;10:1111–1123. [PMID: 28546769]

Koes BW, Backes D, Bindels PJE. Pharmacotherapy for chronic non-specific low back pain: current and future options. *Expert Opin Pharmacother.* 2018;19(6):537–545. [PMID: 29578822]

Lin HT, Hung WC, Hung JL, et al. Effects of pilates on patients with chronic non-specific low back pain: a systematic review. *J Phys Ther Sci.* 2016;28(10):2961–2969. [PMID: 27821970]

Qaseem A, Wilt TJ, McLean RM, Forciea MA. Noninvasive treatments for acute, subacute, and chronic low back pain: a clinical practice guideline from the American College of Physicians. *Ann Intern Med.* 2017;166(7):514–530. [PMID: 28192789]

Ruddock JK, Sallis H, Ness A, Perry RE. Spinal manipulation vs sham manipulation for nonspecific low back pain: a systematic review and meta-analysis. *J Chiropr Med.* 2016;15(3):165–183. [PMID: 27660593]

Russo M, Deckers K, Eldabe S, et al. Muscle control and non-specific chronic low back pain. *Neuromodulation.* 2018;21(1):1–9. [PMID: 29230905]

Sitthipornvorakul E, Klinsophon T, Sihawong R, et al. The effects of walking intervention in patients with chronic low back pain: a meta-analysis of randomized controlled trials. *Musculoskelet Sci Pract.* 2018;34:38–46. [PMID: 29257996]

Standaert C. Comparative effectiveness of exercise, acupuncture, and spinal manipulation for low back pain. *Spine.* 2011;36: S120–S130. [PMID: 21952184]

Stochkendahl MJ, Kjaer P, Hartvigsen J, et al. National Clinical Guidelines for non-surgical treatment of patients with recent onset low back pain or lumbar radiculopathy. *Eur Spine J.* 2018;27(1):60–75. [PMID: 28429142]

Tavee JO, Levin KH. Low back pain. lifelong learning in neurology. *Continuum.* 2017;23(2):467–486. [PMID: 28375914]

Thomas KJ, MacPherson H, Thorpe L, et al. Randomized controlled trial of a short course of traditional acupuncture compared with usual care for persistent non-specific low back pain. *Br Med J.* 2006;333:623–626. [PMID: 16980316]

White AP. Pharmacologic management of chronic low back pain: synthesis of the evidence. *Spine.* 2011;36:S131–S143. [PMID: 21952185]

▶ Prognosis

The long-term course of LBP is variable. Fortunately, it does not develop into a chronic disabling condition for the majority of patients. One recent review discovered that one in five patients report persistent LBP after an acute episode 12 months after initial onset of symptoms. However, 90% of patients will regain function with decreasing pain after 6 weeks, despite physician intervention.

Chapman R, Norvell C, Hermsmeyer T, et al. Evaluating common outcomes for measuring treatment success for chronic low back pain. *Spine.* 2011;36:S54–S68. [PMID: 21952190]

Fourney DR, Andersson G, Arnold PM, et al. Chronic low back pain. *Spine.* 2011;36:S1–S9. [PMID: 21952181]

Wirth B, Ehrler M, Humphreys BK. First episode of acute low back pain: an exploratory cluster analysis approach for early detection of unfavorable recovery. *Disabil Rehabil.* 2017;39(25): 2559–2565. [PMID: 27758141]

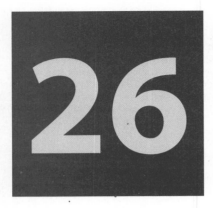

Neck Pain

Stephanie Singh, DO

Garry W. K. Ho, MD, FACSM, FAMSSM, FAAFP, RMSK, CIC

Thomas M. Howard, MD, FACSM, RMSK

General Considerations

Neck pain is a common clinical problem experienced by nearly two-thirds of people. Neck pain can be quite disabling, in some countries accounting for nearly as much disability as low back pain. Neck pain is also similar to low back pain in that the etiology is poorly understood and the clinical diagnoses can be vague. Compared to low back pain, however, neck pain has received limited study. The few available randomized controlled studies lack consistency in study design. This chapter reviews the epidemiology and anatomy of neck pain and provides an evidence-based guide for the evaluation, diagnosis, and management of this challenging disorder.

Neck pain is most prevalent in middle-aged adults; however, prevalence tends to vary with differing definitions and differing survey methodologies of neck pain. Worldwide prevalence of neck pain has been reported at 4.9% and ranked fourth in terms of disability. One study found that the 1-year prevalence in adults ranged from 16.7% (youngest) to 75.1% (oldest). Almost 85% of neck pain may be attributed to chronic stress and strains or acute or repetitive injuries associated with poor posture, anxiety, depression, and occupational or sporting risks. The acceleration-deceleration of a whiplash injury may result in cervical sprains or strains, which, in turn, are common causes of neck pain. Radicular neck pain occurs later in life, with an estimated incidence of 10% among 25- to 29-year-olds, rising to 25–40% in those age >45 years.

Occupational neck pain is ubiquitous and not limited to any particular work setting. Predictors for occupational neck pain include prolonged static positioning, other work-related psychosocial factors, and perceived general tension. Predictors of occupational neck pain include prolonged sitting at work (>95% of the workday), especially with the neck forward-flexed ≥20° for >70% of the work time. A neck angle of 30° forward flexion increases the weight of the head on the cervical spine to 40 pounds, and an angle of 60° increases the weight of the head to 60 pounds. Over time, the increased weight of the head on the cervical spine can cause disruption in the neck muscles and functionality.

More recently, the adolescent population has seen an increasing number of primary physician visits for neck pain. Neck pain was reported in up to 20% of adolescents, and screen time was found to be a major contributing factor. In one study, exercise and physical activity were found to be protective among adolescents in this group.

Fejer R, Kyvik KO, Hartvigsen J. The prevalence of neck pain in the world population: a systematic critical review of the literature. *Eur Spine J.* 2006;15:834. [PMID: 15999284]

Hoy D, March L, Woolf A, et al. The global burden of neck pain: estimates from the global burden of disease 2010. *Ann Rheum Dis.* 2014;73:1309–1315. [PMID: 24482302]

Myrtveit SM, Sivertsen B, Skogen JC, et al. Adolescent neck and shoulder pain: the association with depression, physical activity, screen-based activities, and use of health care services. *J Adolesc Health.* 2014;55:366–372. [PMID: 24746679]

Pathogenesis & Functional Anatomy

The cervical spine is a highly mobile column that supports the 6- to 8-lb head, provides protection for the cervical spinal cord, and consists of 7 vertebrae intercalated by 5 intervertebral disks; 14 facet joints (zygapophyseal joints or Z-joints); 12 joints of Luschka (uncovertebral joints); and 14 paired anterior, lateral, and posterior muscles. The vertebrae can be viewed as three major groups: the atlas (C_1), the axis (C_2), and the others (C_3–C_7). C_1 is a ring-shaped vertebra with two lateral masses articulating with the occiput and C_2. The C_2 consists of a large vertebral body (the largest in the cervical spine) with the anterior odontoid process (dens) articulating with C_1. This odontoid process has a precarious blood supply, placing it at risk for nonunion when fractured. The atlantooccipital articulation accounts for 50% of the flexion and extension neck range of motion (RoM), and the C_1–C_2 joints account for 50% of the rotational RoM of the neck. The remaining cervical vertebrae consists of an anterior body with a posterior projecting ring of the transverse and spinous processes that form the vertebral foramen for the spinal cord, as well as provide attachment sites for ligaments and muscles, which, in turn, can become sprained or strained. The most prominent palpable spinous processes are C_2 and C_7 (vertebral prominens). The joints of Luschka and the facet joints can be involved in degenerative and inflammatory processes. The most important ligaments are the anterior and posterior longitudinal ligaments along the vertebral bodies, the ligamentum nuchae along the spinous process, and the ligamentum flavum along the anterior surfaces of the laminae. The weaker posterior longitudinal ligaments stabilize the intervertebral disks posteriorly and are often damaged in disk herniation. Ligamentum flavum hypertrophy may contribute to spinal stenosis or nerve root impingement.

Eight cervical nerve roots exit posterolaterally through neuroforamina, each emerging above the vertebra of its number (ie, the C_6 root arises between C_5 and C_6), with C_8 exiting between C_7 and T_1. The cervical cord also directly gives rise to nerves that innervate the neck, upper extremity, and diaphragm. Each intervertebral disk consists of a gelatinous center (nucleus pulposus) surrounded by a tougher, multilayered annulus fibrosis. Degenerative or acute disk injury may lead to herniation to the nucleus pulposus, which, in turn, can impinge on nearby cervical nerve roots, contributing to radiculopathy.

The musculature of the cervical spine includes flexors, extensors, lateral flexors, and rotators. Major flexors include the sternocleidomastoid, scalenes, and prevertebrals. Extensors include the posterior paravertebral muscles (splenius, semispinalis, capitis) and trapezius. Lateral flexors include the sternocleidomastoid, scalenes, and interspinous (between the transverse processes) muscles, and the rotators include the sternocleidomastoid and the interspinous muscles. Of particular recent interest are the roles that the deep cervical flexors (longus coli, longus capitis) and deep cervical extensors (rectus capitis posterior major and minor, obliquus capitis superior and inferior) play in chronic neck pain. The ability of the cervical spine to absorb and diffuse the energy from acute trauma is related to its lordotic curvature, the paraspinal muscles, and intervertebral disks. At 30° of forward flexion, the cervical spine is straight and most vulnerable to axial load–type injuries. The paraspinal muscles can be strained and become spastic. Occasionally, so-called trigger points—hyperirritable myo-nodules and taut muscle fiber bands—may develop. The combined motion of all the preceding structures gives a significant RoM to the neck, allowing the head to scan the environment with the eyes and ears. Flexion and extension are centered at C_5–C_6 and C_6–C_7, respectively; hence, degeneration and injury often occur at these levels.

The mechanism of injury of the cervical spine can be classified in multiple ways: acute injuries—including a fall, blow to the head, or the whiplash injury—or chronic repetitive injury—associated with recreational or occupational activities or degenerative processes. Other classifications include the direction of the stress or force generating the injury: flexion, extension-hyperextension, axial load, lateral flexion, or rotation. Most chronic neck pain is associated with poor posture and ergonomics, anxiety or depression, neck strain, or occupational and sports-related injuries.

▶ **Prevention**

Prevention strategies for high-risk groups have been employed for both neck and lower back pain. A review of 27 investigations into educational efforts, exercises, ergonomics, and risk factor modification found sufficient evidence for only strengthening exercises as an effective prevention strategy. A more recent randomized controlled trial showed that specific resistance and all-around exercise programs were more effective than general health counseling in preventing occupation-related neck pain. Accordingly, early intervention and counseling may still prove beneficial for the adolescent population as functional habits are formed during this time. The shift in earlier use of technologies (eg, computers, cell phones, tablets) that contribute to occupational neck pain has recently become a new area of study. As more links are made to earlier exposure, the emphasis will focus on prevention.

Anderson LL, Jørgensen MB, Blangsted AK, et al. A randomized controlled intervention trial to relieve and prevent neck/shoulder pain. *Med Sci Sports Exerc.* 2008;40(6):983–990. [PMID: 18461010]

▶ **Clinical Findings**

A. Symptoms and Signs

In the evaluation of cervical spine problems, it is critical to obtain a thorough history, ascertaining the mechanism of injury. In many cases, the mechanism of injury may identify the injury or guide the physical examination. A survey of prior injuries or problems with the cervical spine (eg, a history of prior surgery or degenerative arthritis) is helpful. Radicular or radiating symptoms in the upper extremity should be identified, including radiating pain, motor weakness, numbness, or paraesthesias of the extremities. Determining both the apparent origin and source of radiating symptoms is important. Occasionally, a myofascial trigger point may exhibit referral pain patterns mimicking those of radiculopathy and often plays a role in chronic neck pain. Conversely, musculoskeletal neck pain can refer to the head playing a large role in cervicogenic headaches. The examiner should ask about any symptoms related to possible upper motor neuron pathology, including bowel or bladder dysfunction or gait disturbance.

Additional information should include the duration and course of symptoms, aggravating and alleviating motions or activities, and attempted prior treatments. Comorbid diseases such as inflammatory spondyloarthropathies, cardiac disease, or gastrointestinal problems should be identified, as well as a history of tobacco or alcohol abuse. Current occupational and recreational activities and requirements should be identified, as they may contribute to the underlying problem and identify the desired end point for recovery and return to activity.

B. Cervical Spine Examination

The cervical spine is examined in an organized and systematic way that includes adequate exposure of the neck, upper back, and shoulders for observation; palpation of bony and soft tissues; evaluation of RoM; tests for cervical radiculopathy (Spurling test, Lhermitte sign); upper extremity motor and sensory examination; and evaluation for upper motor neuron symptoms.

1. Observation—Observation should begin as the patient walks into the examination room, looking for the presence or absence of normal fluid motion of the neck and arm swing with walking. After exposure, the examiner may note the posture (look for a poor head-forward, rounded-shoulder posture contributing to chronic cervical muscular strain), shoulder position (looking for elevation from muscle spasm), evidence of atrophy, and any head tilt or rotation.

2. Palpation—Palpation of major bony prominences and the soft tissues should be performed. The spinous processes and the facet joints (~1 cm lateral and deep to the spinous process) should be gently palpated, noting (more than expected) tenderness. Palpation of the prevertebral and paravertebral muscles may reveal hypertonicity and pain. Common sites for trigger points include the levator scapulae (off the superior, medial margin of the scapula), upper trapezius, rhomboids, and upper paraspinals near the occiput. Palpation of trigger points may elicit tenderness, referred pain (which may mimic radicular symptoms), or a local twitch response.

3. Range of motion—Active RoM should be tested first with judicious use of passive motion as pain permits. Normal RoM includes extension of 70° (chin pointed straight up to the ceiling), flexion of 60° (chin on chest, or within 3 cm of chest), lateral flexion of approximately 45° (ear to shoulder), and rotation of approximately 80° (looking right and left). RoM should be tested in each of these planes and for both left and right sides, recording findings in degrees from the neutral position or as a percentage of the expected norm.

4. Spurling test—This test assesses for nerve root irritation, which can be related to spondylotic compression, discogenic

compression, or the stinger-burner syndrome (a compression or stretch injury of the brachial plexus, commonly seen in sports injuries). To perform the Spurling test, the examiner extends, side-bends, and partially rotates the patient's head toward the side being tested. An axial load is then gently applied to the top of the head. A positive test is indicated by radiation of pain, generally into the posterior shoulder or arm on the ipsilateral side.

5. Lhermitte sign—The Lhermitte sign may also be used to test for cervical radiculopathy. Forward flexion of the neck that causes paraesthesias down the spine or extremities suggests cervical radiculopathy, spondylosis, myelopathy, or multiple sclerosis. Manual cervical distraction may reduce neck and limb symptoms in cervical radiculopathy.

6. Upper extremity motor examination—This includes manual muscle testing and deep tendon reflexes (DTRs; Table 26–1). A useful mnemonic to keep the upper extremity motor findings in order is *blocker > beggar > kisser > grabber > Spock* (Figure 26–1). The examiner systematically checks arm abduction (blocking position) for deltoid function, then resisted elbow flexion and extension (biceps and triceps), wrist extension and flexion, grip, and finger abduction (spread fingers). DTRs should be checked for the biceps (C_5), triceps (C_7), and brachioradialis (C_6). Sensory testing should focus on the dermatomes for the cervical roots, with focus on the lateral deltoid area (C_5), dorsal first web space (C_6), dorsal middle finger (C_7), small finger (C_8), and inner arm (T_1). Testing for thoracic outlet syndrome can be accomplished with the Adson test and Roo test. In the Adson test, the patient's neck is extended, with the head rotated toward the affected side and lungs in deep inspiration, while the examiner palpates the ipsilateral radial pulse. Decrease in the amplitude of the radial pulse with this maneuver is a positive test. The Roo test (also called the *elevated arm stress test*) is performed with both the patient's arms (shoulders) in an abducted and externally rotated position (90° each) and the elbow flexed to 90°. The patient then opens and closes both hands for 3 minutes. Inability to continue this maneuver for 3 minutes due to reproduction of symptoms suggests thoracic outlet syndrome. Reasonably low false-positive rates make the Roo test the preferred test.

7. Upper motor neuron symptoms—Upper motor neuron findings can be demonstrated by a Hoffman sign; with the third finger extended, a quick flexion-flick of the third distal interphalangeal joint is applied; an abnormal flexion reflex in the thumb or other fingers is a positive test (positive Hoffman sign). Lower extremity testing for upper motor neuron findings should be performed, including DTRs (looking for hyperreflexia), assessment for ankle clonus, and testing for the Babinski reflex. The Babinski reflex may be elicited by firmly stroking the sole (plantar surface) of the foot. The reflex is present if the great toe dorsiflexes and

Table 26–1. Upper extremity motor and sensory innervations.

Spinal Level	Motor	Reflex	Sensory	Peripheral Nerve
C_5	Deltoid (shoulder abduction) Biceps	Biceps	Lateral shoulder	Axillary
C_6	Biceps (elbow flexion) Wrist extensors	Brachioradialis	Lateral forearm Dorsal first web space	Musculocutaneous Radial
C_7	Triceps (elbow extension) Wrist flexion Finger extension	Triceps	Dorsal middle finger	Median
C_8	Finger flexors Thumb flexion/opposition	None	Ring finger Small finger Medial forearm	Ulnar Medial antebrachial cutaneous
T_1	Hand intrinsics (finger abduction/adduction)	None	Medial arm axilla	Medial brachial cutaneous

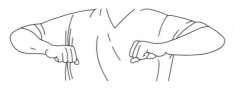

C₅: Blocker
    Arm abduction
    Elbow flexion

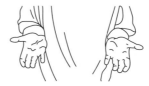

C₆: Beggar
    Elbow flexion
    Wrist extension

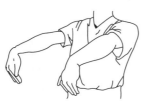

C₇: Kisser
    Elbow extension
    Wrist flexion
    Finger extension

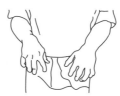

C₈: Grabber
    Finger flexion

T₁: Spock
    Finger abduction

▲ **Figure 26–1.** Upper extremity motor evaluation.

the other toes fan out (abduct). This is normal in younger children, but abnormal after the age of 2 years.

C. Laboratory Findings

In cases with upper extremity weakness not improving with therapy, electromyography (EMG) and nerve conduction studies (NCSs) may be considered in evaluating upper extremity neurologic disorders and to help distinguish between peripheral (including brachial plexus) and nerve root injuries. EMG and NCS also distinguish between stable and active denervating and recovery processes. Testing may not be diagnostic until 3–4 weeks after an acute nerve injury, so this study should not be ordered in the acute setting. Routine follow-up EMG and NCS in patients with whiplash injuries may not contribute useful information to clinical and imaging findings. Other laboratory studies—including complete blood count, sedimentation rate, rheumatoid factor, and others—should be reserved for the evaluation of spondyloarthropathies and play little role in the evaluation of most cases of isolated neck pain.

D. Imaging Studies

Potential imaging studies of the cervical spine can include plain radiographs, magnetic resonance imaging (MRI), computed tomography (CT), bone scan, and myelography. Bone scan does not significantly contribute to the evaluation of neck pain in most acute or chronic settings. Plain films include the basic three-view series (anteroposterior, lateral, open mouth), oblique, and lateral flexion-extension views. Indications for the use of imaging studies in the evaluation of neck pain can be divided into recommendations for acute (traumatic) or chronic neck pain.

In the acute trauma situation, the three-view radiograph is the basic study of choice, when CT is not available. CT or lateral flexion and extension views can be used to further evaluate nondiagnostic radiographs or cases of high clinical suspicion for injury. Cervical fractures may be ruled out on a clinical basis if the patient does not complain of neck pain when asked; does not have a history of loss of consciousness; does not have mental status change from trauma, drugs, or alcohol; does not have symptoms referable to the neck (paralysis or sensory change—present or resolved); does not have midline cervical tenderness to palpation; and does not have other distracting painful injuries. The American College of Radiology (ACR) appropriateness criteria for imaging of suspected cervical spine trauma recommend that thin-section CT, and not plain radiography, be the screening study of choice, and once a decision is made to scan the patient, the entire spine should be examined owing to the high incidence of noncontiguous multiple injuries. If CT scanning is not readily available, those with cervical tenderness should have, at a minimum, the basic three-view plain-film series. Patients who have upper or lower extremity paraesthesias (or other neurologic findings), are unconscious at the time of evaluation, have distracting injuries, or are in an altered mental state (due to alcohol or drugs) should undergo a CT scan of the cervical spine; MRI of the cervical spine may be considered, depending on the CT findings or in cases where myelopathy is suspected. Patients with neck pain and clinical findings suggestive of ligamentous injury, with normal radiographic and CT findings, may be considered for MRI of the cervical spine.

The ACR appropriateness criteria for imaging of chronic neck pain concluded that there are no existing evidence-based guidelines for the radiologic evaluation of the patient with chronic neck pain. The initial imaging study should be the three-view series. The most common findings include a loss of lordosis (straight cervical spine) or disk space narrowing with degenerative change at the C_5–C_6 and C_4–C_5 levels. When patients have chronic neck pain after hyperextension or flexion injury with normal radiographs and persistent pain or evidence of neurologic injury, lateral flexion-extension views should be considered to rule out instability. Abnormal findings include >3.5-mm horizontal displacement or >11° of rotational difference to that of the adjacent vertebrae on resting or flexion-extension lateral radiographs. Oblique radiographs may be helpful to look for bony encroachment of the neuroforamina in the evaluation of radicular neck pain. MRI should be performed on all patients who have chronic neck pain with neurologic signs or symptoms. If there is a contraindication to MRI (ie, pacemaker, nonavailability, claustrophobia, or interfering hardware in the neck), CT myelography is recommended.

American College of Radiology (ACR), Expert Panel on Musculoskeletal Imaging. *Chronic Neck Pain in ACR Appropriateness Criteria.* Reston, VA: ACR; 2010:1–9.
American College of Radiology (ACR), Expert Panel on Musculoskeletal Imaging. *Suspected Spine Trauma in ACR Appropriateness Criteria.* Reston, VA: ACR; 2012:1–20.

▶ Differential Diagnosis

See Table 26–2.

▶ Treatment

Multiple treatment options are available, although there is limited evidence-based support for the efficacy of most of these. Early management focuses on proper initial evaluation, use of analgesics, early return to motion, and judicious use of physical modalities. Acupuncture and manual therapy may help reduce pain early. Chronic neck pain can be related to psychosocial factors at home and in the workplace and may be tied to litigation in whiplash-type injuries. Specialty consultation beyond physical therapy is rarely needed.

Table 26–2. Differential diagnosis of neck pain.

Acute Injury	Noninflammatory Disease	Inflammatory Disease	Infectious Causes	Neoplasm	Referred Pain
Cervical sprain, strain, spasm, whiplash	Cervical osteoarthritis (spondylosis)	Rheumatoid arthritis	Meningitis	Primary	Temporomandibular joint
Cervical tendonitis, tendinosis	Discogenic neck pain	Spondyloarthropathies	Osteomyelitis	Myeloma	Cardiac
Cervical instability	Cervical spinal stenosis	Juvenile rheumatoid arthritis	Infectious discitis	Cord tumor	Diaphragmatic irritation
Fractures	Cervical myelopathy	Ankylosing spondylitis		Metastatic	Gastrointestinal
Vertebral body	Myofascial pain				Gastric ulcer
Teardrop	Trigger points				Gall bladder
Burst	Fibromyalgia				Pancreas
Chance	Reflex sympathetic dystrophy/ complex regional pain syndrome				Thoracic outlet syndrome
Compression					Shoulder disorders
Spinous process					Brachial plexus injuries
Transverse process	Migraines (or variants)				Occipital neuralgia
Facet	Torticollis				Peripheral nerve injury
Odontoid (C_2)					
Hangman (C_2)					
Jefferson (C_1)					
Stinger or burner					

A. Initial Care

Initial management includes avoidance of aggravating factors at work or with recreational activities, as well as pain management, recognizing that most pain is self-limiting. Management should focus on early return to motion, isometric strengthening, and modification of occupational or recreational aggravating factors with return to activity with ergonomic precautions.

Absolute rest, including cervical collars, should be limited to a very short period of time (ie, <1–2 days). Early motion should be encouraged as soon as severe pain allows. Early mobilization after whiplash injury is associated with a better prognosis. Proprioceptive neuromuscular facilitation or muscle energy techniques may be employed in a structured physical therapy program or home program with the goal to improve motion. In one study, mobilizing physical therapy showed significant improvement in cervical motion at 8 weeks. As one example of muscle energy, patients move their heads in a direction to the point of pain. Next, they attempt to move in the opposite direction against the resistance of their own hands on the chin for a count of 5, contracting the rehabilitating muscle throughout the entire maneuver. Then they attempt to further move in the original direction of pain, usually with improved motion. This should be done in the six major RoM directions. Patients should focus on proper posture (neck centered and back over the shoulders) and gentle stretching of the neck for RoM. Each position should be held for 15–20 seconds.

B. Pain Management

Pain management may take the form of ice, medications, physical modalities, or manual therapy techniques.

Application of ice (15 minutes every 2 hours) is effective for acute pain after injury or for postactivity pain during the recovery process. Medications used in the management of acute and chronic neck pain include salicylates (aspirin), nonsteroidal anti-inflammatory drugs (NSAIDs; ibuprofen, naproxen, indomethacin, diclofenac, celecoxib), acetaminophen (500–1000 mg 4 times daily), muscle relaxants (diazepam, methocarbamol, cyclobenzaprine), narcotic medications (acetaminophen with codeine, acetaminophen with oxycodone, acetaminophen with hydrocodone, meperidine), and systemic corticosteroids. NSAIDs and muscle relaxants are most commonly prescribed for acute pain; however, selecting which medications to prescribe should be made on a case-by-case basis, taking into account individual risks and comorbidities. Due to recent concerns regarding opioid overprescribing, opioids for pain management should be carefully reserved for patients who fail first- and second-line treatments. For acute radicular symptoms, a short course of systemic corticosteroids may be considered to reduce inflammation associated with a herniated nucleus pulposus. Although there is no literature to support the use of ice or systemic steroids, anecdotal evidence suggests that they may be helpful in the acute setting.

For chronic neck pain (eg, lasting >30 days), tricyclic antidepressants (TCAs; nortriptyline, amitriptyline), selective norepinephrine reuptake inhibitors (SNRIs; venlafaxine, duloxetine), or selective serotonin reuptake inhibitors (SSRIs; fluoxetine, sertraline) at bedtime may be used for chronic pain management and management of sleep disturbance that often accompanies chronic pain of any source. Side effects of TCAs include excessive drowsiness, dry mouth, urinary retention, and potential cardiac conduction problems. Side effects of SNRIs and SSRIs include insomnia, drowsiness, dry mouth, nausea, headache, and anorexia. Any combination of SSRIs, SNRIs, and TCAs may result in increased serum levels of the TCA and toxicity. Randomized controlled studies support the use of simple analgesics and NSAIDs in the management of acute pain but do not support the other treatment options.

C. Physical Modalities

Multiple physical modalities are available for pain management and to improve RoM, although there is little evidence of their effectiveness and few well-designed randomized controlled studies that support their use in management of acute or chronic neck pain. These modalities include the application of heat, cold, ultrasound, cervical traction, acupuncture, and electrical stimulation (including transcutaneous electrical nerve stimulation). However, evidence supporting the use of electrotherapy in neck disorders is limited and conflicting. Cervical traction can be effective for relief of spasm or in the management of radicular pain and may be performed in a controlled setting at physical therapy or with the use of home traction units. Typical sessions in physical therapy are 2–3 days per week for 30 minutes per session. A typical home cervical traction regimen would start at 10 lb of longitudinal traction and increase by 5 lb every 1–2 days until a goal of 20–30 lb is reached. Home traction is used on a daily or alternate-day basis.

D. Acupuncture, Acupressure, and Needling

Acupuncture can be effective in the treatment of neck pain, although literature supporting its effectiveness beyond five treatment sessions for acute neck pain or 4 weeks of treatment for chronic neck pain is limited. A home program of ischemic pressure (acupressure) with stretching can also be effective in the management of myofascial neck pain and trigger points. Although much of the evidence on trigger point injections has been conflicting, systematic reviews have reported that trigger point injections may be useful in relieving trigger point–related pain in chronic conditions lasting >3 months. Outcomes were not significantly different with regard to the injectant used, including dry needling. Intramuscular injections of botulinum toxin type A have been found to be no more efficacious than saline. However, the injection of a local anesthetic does seem to decrease discomfort related to the needling process.

E. Manual Therapy

Manual therapy (eg, osteopathic and chiropractic manipulation or manual therapy techniques applied by a physical therapist) is commonly used in the management of chronic neck and lower back pain. Osteopathic manipulative techniques (OMT) can be part of a beneficial treatment strategy both initially after injury and in chronic neck pain. Early focus is aimed at relieving somatic dysfunction through both direct (eg, high velocity–low amplitude, muscle energy) and indirect (eg, muscle energy, strain-counterstrain, balanced ligamentous tension) techniques. These techniques engage agonist and antagonist muscle groups as well as fascial planes to relieve dysfunction and pain and increase mobility in the neck. Early manipulation therapies should be combined with an exercise program and patient-directed treatment. For acute neck injuries, there is some evidence supporting the use of manual techniques involving passive neck motion aimed at restoring normal spinal RoM and function, excluding spinal manipulations. A study on the use of manual therapy in the treatment of neck and low back pain showed an average improvement of 53.8% in acute pain and 48.4% in chronic pain with 12 treatments over a 4-week period. A case report of a patient with persistent neck and arm pain—after failed cervical disk surgery with resolution after a program of manual therapy and rehabilitative exercises—further supports the use of manual therapy in the management of both myofascial and radicular neck pain. However, caution should be exercised, because one study reported that 30% of patients undergoing spinal manipulation had adverse effects, especially in those with severe neck pain or severe headache prior to treatment.

F. Therapeutic Exercise

There is some evidence to support the effectiveness of active RoM exercises for acute mechanical neck disorders. As patients recover, a program of strengthening should be instituted. Simple isometric exercises focusing on resisted forward flexion, extension, and right and left lateral flexion will improve pain and strength, contributing to recovery and long-term resistance to further injury. Attention to posture and an ergonomic survey are also important and can help in customizing a complete therapeutic exercise program for both treatment and prevention of neck pain. There is evidence to support the use of yoga in relieving chronic nonspecific neck pain.

G. Referral

Specialty referral may be considered at multiple points in the recovery process to aid in diagnosis or treatment of acute or chronic neck pain. OMT and physical therapy may be used early in the process to incorporate physical modalities and initiate a strengthening program. *Physical medicine and rehabilitation* (PM&R) involvement may be considered for co-management of chronic pain of any source and to obtain EMGs. The input of a neurologist may be considered to obtain EMGs or for consultation in patients with confusing neurologic conditions. Neurosurgery or orthopedic-spinal surgery should be considered for patients requiring operative management. Early referral should be considered for severe muscle weakness, fractures, and evidence of myelopathy (upper motor neuron signs). Success rates for surgery have been reported to be as high as 80–90% for radicular pain and 60–70% for myelopathy. There is insufficient evidence to compare conservative treatment with surgical management of patients who have neck pain and radiculopathy, and a recent systematic review found low-quality evidence that showed no overall differences between conservative and surgical management. For patients who have chronic radiating pain despite 9–12 weeks of conservative management, referral for chronic pain management at an anesthesiology, neurology, PM&R, or other pain management clinic should be considered for co-management or consideration of epidural steroid injections (ESI), facet joint injections, or medial branch nerve procedures. Randomized controlled studies provide some evidence to support the use of ESI in chronic neck pain.

Cramer H, Lauche R, Hohmann C, et al. Randomized-controlled trial comparing yoga and home-based exercise for chronic neck pain. *Clin J Pain*. 2013;29(3):216–223. [PMID: 23249655]

Manchikanti L, Cash KA, Pampati V, Malla Y. Cervical epidural injections in chronic fluoroscopic cervical epidural injections in chronic axial or disc-related neck pain without disc herniation, facet joint pain, or radiculitis. *J Pain Res*. 2012;5:227–236. [PMID: 22826642]

Nadler S. Nonpharmacologic management of pain. *J Am Osteopath Assoc*. 2014;104:S6–S12. [PMID: 15602035]

Scott NA, Guo B, Barton PM, Gerwin RD. Trigger point injections for chronic non-malignant musculoskeletal pain: a systematic review. *Pain Med*. 2009;10(1):54–69. [PMID: 18992040]

Van Middelkoop M, Rubinstein SM, Ostelo R, et al. Surgery versus conservative care for neck pain: a systematic review. *Eur Spine J*. 2013:22:87–95. [PMID: 20949289]

▶ Prognosis

Neck pain usually resolves in days to weeks, but like low back pain, it can become recurrent. High initial pain intensity is an important predictor of delayed functional recovery. The single best estimation of handicap due to whiplash injury was return of normal cervical RoM. Up to 40% of patients with whiplash injuries report symptoms for ≤15 years after injury. These patients have a 3 times higher risk of neck pain in the next 7 years. A Swedish study showed that 55% of an exposed group and 29% of a control group had residual symptoms up to 17 years after injury. The incidence of chronic standing neck pain is approximately 10%, and approximately 5% of people will experience severe disability. Patients who experience these symptoms for at least 6 months have a <50% chance of recovering even with aggressive therapy. Predictors of chronic neck pain include a prior history of neck pain or injury, motor vehicle collision, age of >60 years, female gender, number of children, poor self-assessed health, poor socioeconomic and psychological status (eg, excessive concerns about symptoms, unrealistic expectations of treatment, and psychosocial concerns), and history of low back pain.

Palmlöf L, Skillgate E, Alfredsson L, et al. Does income matter for troublesome neck pain? A population-based study on risk and prognosis. *J Epidemiol Community Health*. 2012;66:1063–1070. [PMID: 22412154]

Websites

The following are useful websites for patient education on topics such as home rehabilitation and correction of occupational and postural risk factors:

American Academy of Family Physicians. Neck pain. https://familydoctor.org/symptom/neck-pain/

Nicholas Institute of Sports Medicine and Athletic Trauma. https://nismat.org/wp-content/uploads/2019/03/ue_exercises.pdf

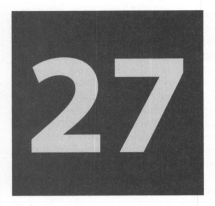

Cancer Screening in Women[1]

Nicole Powell-Dunford, MD, MPH, FAAFP, FAsMA

Katie L. Westerfield, DO, IBCLC, FAAFP

Abigail K. Vargo, MD, MPH

BREAST CANCER

ESSENTIALS OF DIAGNOSIS

- ▶ Lobular or ductal carcinoma in situ is localized breast cancers.
- ▶ Invasive breast cancer extends beyond the ducts and lobules and may present as a palpable mass.
- ▶ Inflammatory breast cancers can be mistaken for skin infection.
- ▶ Guidelines for early detection have evolved significantly.

General Considerations

Breast cancer is the second most common cancer in women after skin cancer. *BRCA1* and *BRCA2* tumor suppressor genes confer strong risk. Other risk factors include earlier age of menarche, later age of menopause, nulliparity, and late age of first birth, all reflecting higher total number of ovarian cycles. Obesity, alcohol use, older age, decreased physical activity, and other genetic and environmental factors have been linked to breast cancer. Recent studies challenge hormone replacement therapy (HRT) as a risk for breast cancer. Prenatal exposure to diethylstilbestrol (DES) has also been linked to increased risk for breast cancer.

Prevention

Women positive for the heritable *BCRA* mutation may benefit from the prophylactic selective estrogen receptor modulator tamoxifen and prophylactic total mastectomy. Women whose family history is associated with an increased risk for *BRCA* mutation be referred for genetic counseling and evaluation for *BRCA* testing (Table 27–1). Neither routine *BRCA* testing nor prophylactic medication is recommended for the general population. Smoking is a risk factor for cancer development, and cessation should be recommended in all current smokers.

Clinical Findings

Breast cancer most commonly presents as a painless, irregularly bordered mass. Other presentations may include local swelling, dimpling, breast pain, nipple discharge, and other breast or nipple changes. Advanced clinical presentations may include pain and/or fracture from bony metastasis.

Differential Diagnosis

A. Clinically Evident Mass

A concerning breast mass can be further evaluated through diagnostic mammography, ultrasound with or without fine-needle aspiration, and/or ductal lavage and/or ductogram. Genetic and hormonal receptor testing further differentiates breast cancers.

B. Preclinical Detection

Screening guidelines for normal- and high-risk women have evolved considerably, balancing benefits of early detection against the anxiety, financial loss, and morbidity of false-positive screening. Table 27–2 outlines recommendations of several organizations.

Complications

Metastatic spread is often to lungs, liver, and bone.

---

[1]The views and information presented are those of the authors and do not represent the official position of the US Army Medical Department Center and School Health Readiness Center of Excellence, the US Army Training and Doctrine Command, or the Departments of Army, Department of Defense, or US Government.

Table 27–1. Indications for genetic referral for *BRCA* testing.

A first-degree relative with breast cancer before age 40
Two or more relatives with breast or ovarian cancer at any age
Three or more relatives with breast, ovarian, or colon cancer at any age

Data from Smith RA, Saslow D, Sawyer KA, et al: American Cancer Society guidelines for breast cancer screening: update 2003, CA. *Cancer J Clin.* 2003 May–Jun;53(3):141–169.

▶ **Treatment**

Treatment may include surgery, radiotherapy, chemotherapy, hormone therapy, and/or targeted therapy depending on the stage at diagnosis. Staging is based on the size and location of the primary tumor, the spread of cancer to nearby lymph nodes or other parts of the body, tumor grade, and biomarker presence. The TNM (tumor, node, metastasis) system, the grading system, and the biomarker status determine the clinical prognostic breast cancer stage (Table 27–3).

The pathologic prognostic stage is used when surgery is the first treatment and uses the TNM system, grading system, biomarker status, and laboratory evaluation of removed breast and lymph node tissues during surgery. Breast conservation therapy, consisting of lumpectomy and radiation therapy, is standard treatment for early-stage cancer and is not associated with increased 20-year mortality compared to mastectomy. Hormonal therapy is often given for 5 years to prevent relapse in early-stage breast cancer. Invasive cancer is usually treated with both surgery and adjuvant systemic therapy. Determination of progesterone receptor, estrogen receptor, and human epidermal growth factor receptor 2 (HER2) status is important because there are drugs that can block these receptors. Targeted therapy involves the use of drugs or other substances such as monoclonal antibodies to identify and attack specific cancer cells. Treatment guidelines differ for men and pregnant women. Treatment strategies also differ based on pre- or postmenopausal status. The National Comprehensive Cancer Network updates detailed treatment guidelines for each population and breast cancer stage regularly. Second opinions are valuable. The National

Table 27–2. Breast cancer screening.

2012 Screening Recommendations	AAFP	ACOG	ACS	USPSTF	Other Guidance
Breast self-examination (BSE)	Recommend against	May be part of breast self-awareness	20+: BSE is optional; educate on benefits/ limitations	Insufficient evidence	USPSTF, AAFP, ACS, and ACOG encourage breast self-awareness and/or early reporting of breast changes
Clinical breast examination	Insufficient evidence	40+: annual 20–39: every 1–3 years	40+: annual 20–39: every 1–3 years	Insufficient evidence	Use of fingerpads of the middle three fingers, overlapping dime-sized circular motions, and sequential application of light, medium, and deep levels of pressure recommended
Mammography	40–49: individualize 50–74: biennial screening 75+: insufficient evidence	40+: offer annual 75+: individualize	40 through age of good health: offer annual	<50: individualize 50–74: biennial screening 75+: evidence lacking	Breast density influences ability to detect
Magnetic resonance imaging (MRI)	Consider in high risk	Not for normal-risk screen	Not for normal-risk screen	Insufficient evidence for normal-risk screen	MRI may afford very high sensitivity in detecting small masses but is expensive, associated with intravenous contrast risks, does not detect all breast cancers that mammography can, and is not widely available with guided biopsy
High-risk women	Refer high-risk women by family history for genetic counseling and *BRCA* testing	Early enhanced screen	Annual mammogram + MRI for high-risk women 30+	Early enhanced screen	High risk considered to be *BRCA* positive ± ≥20% risk on a valid prediction model

AAFP, American Academy of Family Physicians; ACOG, American College of Obstetricians and Gynecologists; ACS, American Cancer Society; USPSTF, US Preventive Services Task Force.

Table 27–3. Stages of breast cancer.

Stage 0 (carcinoma in situ)	Ductal carcinoma in situ (noninvasive, may progress) Lobular carcinoma in situ (seldom invasive, but breast cancer risk) Paget disease of nipple
Stage IA	Tumor ≤2 cm; no lymph nodes (LN) involved Microscopic invasion possible but does not exceed 1 mm
Stage IB	No tumor; LN cancer >0.2 mm but ≤2 mm Tumor ≤2 cm; LN cancer >0.2 mm but ≤2 mm
Stage IIA	No tumor; 1–3 axillary/sternal LN >2 mm Tumor ≤2 cm; 1–3 axillary/sternal LN >2 mm Tumor is >2 cm but <5 cm; no LN involved
Stage IIB	Tumor >2 cm but ≤5 cm; LN (>0.2 mm but ≤2 mm) Tumor >2 cm but ≤5 cm; 1–3 axillary/sternal LN Tumor >5 cm; no LN involved
Stage IIIA	No tumor or any size; 4–9 axillary/sternal LNs Tumor >5 cm; LN > 0.2 mm and ≤2 mm Tumor >5 cm; 1–3 axillary/sternal LN
Stage IIIB	No tumor or tumor of any size has spread to the chest wall and/or to the skin of the breast, causing swelling or an ulcer, with up to 9 axillary/sternal LNs May be inflammatory breast cancer
Stage IIIC	No tumor or tumor of any size; ≥10 axillary/sternal LNs; or LNs above or below the collarbone May be inflammatory breast cancer
Stage IV	The cancer has spread to other parts of the body, most often the bones, lungs, liver, or brain

Cancer Institute can help enroll patients who wish to participate in ongoing clinical trials.

▶ Prognosis

The 5-year survival rate for Surveillance, Epidemiology, and End Results (SEER) localized stage breast cancer is 99%. The 5-year survival rates for SEER regional stage and distant stage are 85% and 27%, respectively. Combined, all breast cancer SEER stages have a 5-year survival rate of 90%. HER2 oncogene expression is associated with higher risk for relapse and shorter survival. HER2 expression, hormonal receptors, biomarkers, and tumor gene signature are being used to predict disease outcome, recurrence risk, and/or response to specific medications.

American Academy of Family Physicians. Clinical Preventive Service Recommendation: breast cancer, breast self-exam. https://www.aafp.org/patient-care/clinical-recommendations/all/breast-cancer-self-bse.html. Accessed April 9, 2019.

Blichert-Toft M, Nielsen M, During M, et al. Long-term results of breast conserving surgery vs. mastectomy for early stage invasive breast cancer: 20-year follow-up of the Danish randomized DBCG-82TM protocol. Acta Oncol. 2008;47:672–681. [PMID: 18465335]

Committee on Practice Bulletins—Gynecology. Practice Bulletin no. 179: breast cancer risk assessment and screening in average-risk women. Ostet Gynecol. 2017;130(1):e1–e16. [PMID: 28644335]

Committee on Practice Bulletins–Gynecology, Committee on Genetics, Society of Gynecologic Oncology. Practice Bulletin no. 182: hereditary breast and ovarian cancer syndrome. Obstet Gynecol. 2017;130(3):e110–e126. [PMID: 28832484]

Hoover RN, Hyer M, Pfeiffer RM, et al. Adverse health outcomes in women exposed in utero to diethylstilbestrol. N Engl J Med. 2011;65(14):1304–1314. [PMID: 21991952]

National Cancer Institute. Breast Cancer Treatment (Adult) (PDQ®)–Patient Version. https://www.cancer.gov/types/breast/patient/adult/breast-treatment-pdq. Accessed April 9, 2019.

National Cancer Institute, Surveillance, Epidemiology, and End Results Program. Cancer stat facts: female breast cancer. https://seer.cancer.gov/statfacts/html/breast.html. Accessed April 9, 2019.

National Comprehensive Cancer Network. NCCN Guidelines Breast Cancer version 1. 2013. http://www.nccn.org/professionals/physician_gls/pdf/breast.pdf. Accessed April 9, 2019.

Oeffinger KC, Fontham ETH, Etzioni R et al. Breast cancer screening for women at average risk. 2015 guideline update from the American Cancer Society. JAMA. 2015;2314(15):1599–1614. [PMID: 26501536]

Saslow D, Hannan J, Osuch J, et al. Clinical breast examination: practical recommendations for optimizing performance and reporting. CA Cancer J Clin. 2004;54(6):327–344. [PMID: 15537576]

Shapiro S, Farmer R, Stevenson J, et al. Does hormone replacement therapy (HRT) cause breast cancer? An application of causal principles to three studies. J Fam Plann Reprod Health Care. 2013;39(2):80–88. [PMID: 23493592]

Tria TM. Breast cancer screening update. Am Fam Physician. 2013;87(4):274–278. [PMID: 23418799]

US Preventative Service Task Force. Breast cancer: screening. https://www.uspreventiveservicestaskforce.org/Page/Document/UpdateSummaryFinal/breast-cancer-screening1. Accessed April 9, 2019.

Weigel MT, Dowsett M. Current and emerging biomarkers in breast cancer: prognosis and prediction. Endocr Relat Cancer. 2010;17:245–253. [PMID: 20647302]

CERVICAL CANCER

ESSENTIALS OF DIAGNOSIS

▶ Cervical cancer often develops at the transition zone, making Pap smear screening useful in early diagnosis.

▶ Human papillomavirus (HPV) infections induce squamous cell and adenomatous cervical cancer. Cervical cancers of other histology are rare.

▶ Frequent spontaneous regression of HPV in young women has resulted in evolved screening guidelines.

General Considerations

Although largely preventable, cervical cancer is the third most common gynecologic cancer in the United States and the third leading cause of gynecologic death. HPV infections cause the overwhelming majority of cervical cancer cases. Prenatal exposure to DES also increases risk for cervical cancer. Factors such as smoking, long-term oral contraceptive pill (OCP) use, immunosuppression, sexual activity patterns, and parity influence either HPV acquisition or natural history of disease progression.

Pathogenesis

HPV, especially high-risk types 16 and 18, triggers dysplastic changes.

Prevention

The Centers for Disease Control and Prevention Advisory Committee on Immunization Practices recommend the use of a two-dose schedule of HPV immunization for girls and boys who initiate the vaccination series at age 9 through 14 years. Three doses remain recommended for persons who initiate the vaccination series at age 15 through 26 years and for immunocompromised persons. Although immunization is safe and highly effective, adolescents in the United States remain underimmunized for HPV. As with any immunization, fainting may occur. Abstinence, monogamy, and use of barrier devices may reduce oncogenic viral transmission. Abstinence-only education programs may not reduce behaviors associated with HPV transmission. Smoking, family history of cervical cancer, high-risk sexual activity, personal history of vulvar/vaginal cancer, current use of OCPs, and immune suppression are other risk factors for cervical cancer.

Clinical Findings

Signs and symptoms often include heavy or irregular menstrual bleeding and/or postcoital bleeding. Advanced disease may manifest with pelvic or lower back pain.

Differential Diagnosis

A. Clinically Evident Disease

Abnormal vaginal bleeding/discharge and pelvic pain are initially evaluated through speculum and clinical pelvic examination in conjunction with infectious disease testing with or without colposcopy and focused biopsy, which may differentiate benign cysts, cervical infection/inflammation, and other noncancerous conditions from cervical cancer. Metastatic cancer can be further delineated through computed tomography (CT) and/or magnetic resonance imaging (MRI) with or without positron emission tomography and serologic studies.

B. Preclinical Detection

Screening has dramatically lowered mortality rates. Precancerous cervical changes are identified through cytology. HPV testing guides further management of cytology results. Colposcopy examination and focused biopsy are used to evaluate significant initial screening abnormalities. A biopsy result of cervical intraepithelial neoplasia (CIN) I is often associated with spontaneous disease remission in younger populations; CIN II and CIN III are precursors to invasive cancer, which entail closer follow-up. Certain diagnostic procedures such as biopsy and the loop electrosurgical excision procedure (LEEP) may be simultaneously diagnostic and therapeutic. Comprehensive guidelines, which include colposcopy follow-up recommendations, are regularly updated and published electronically by the American Society for Colposcopy and Cervical Pathology.

For low-risk women, the 2018 US Preventive Services Task Force (USPSTF) guidelines recommend screening for cervical cancer every 3 years with cervical cytology alone in women age 21–29 years. For women age 30–65 years, the USPSTF recommends screening every 3 years with cervical cytology alone, every 5 years with high-risk HPV (hrHPV) testing alone, or every 5 years with hrHPV testing in combination with cytology (cotesting). The USPSTF recommends against screening for cervical cancer in women younger than 21 years of age. Women older than 65 years who have had adequate prior screening and are not otherwise at high risk for cervical cancer should be discontinued from screening. Likewise, women who have had a hysterectomy with removal of the cervix and do not have a history of a high-grade precancerous lesion (ie, CIN II or III) or cervical cancer should be discontinued from screening. Women with human immunodeficiency virus (HIV) positivity, organ transplant, or forms of immunosuppression should be screened more frequently than low-risk women. The American Cancer Society recommends that women with a history of maternal DES exposure receive four-quadrant Pap smear testing in order to sample cells from all quadrants of the vaginal wall, because DES-related cancers include vaginal cancers. Iodine staining may be used to highlight areas of adenosis, with further colposcopic evaluation as indicated.

Complications

Bladder, bowel, and other pelvic organs may be locally invaded. Metastatic spread to the liver, lung, bones, and other distant organs may occur.

Treatment

LEEP and/or cone biopsy can be both diagnostic and therapeutic for dysplasia. Cervical cancer is treated with surgery, brachytherapy, radiotherapy, and/or a chemotherapy regimen that includes cisplatin. Patients with recurrent disease may be candidates for further cycles of standard treatments, palliative care, or clinical trials.

Prognosis

Short-term disease-free survival is significantly shortened in women presenting with abnormal bleeding and/or pain compared to women identified through screening. The vast majority of invasive cancers identified through Pap smear screening are limited to nonmetastatic disease, with significantly increased rates of disease-free survival.

American Cancer Society. DES exposure: questions and answers. https://www.cancer.org/cancer/cancer-causes/medical-treatments/des-exposure.html. Accessed July 25, 2019.

American Society for Colposcopy and Cervical Pathology. ASCCP guidelines. Last updated May 2018. http://www.asccp.org/asccp-guidelines. Accessed 14 March 2019.

Appleby P, Beral V, Berrington de González A, et al. International collaboration of epidemiological studies of cervical cancer, cervical cancer and hormonal contraceptives: collaborative reanalysis of individual data for 16,573 women with cervical cancer and 35,509 women without cervical cancer from 24 epidemiological studies. *Lancet*. 2007;370(9599):1609–1620. [PMID: 17993361]

Brady M, Byington C, Davies H, et al. HPV vaccine recommendations; American Academy of Pediatrics Policy Statement. *Pediatrics*. 2012;1(3):602–605. [PMID: 22371460]

Centers for Disease Control and Prevention. Human papillomavirus (HPV) vaccination & cancer prevention. https://www.cdc.gov/vaccines/vpd/hpv/index.html. Accessed March 14, 2019.

De Sanjose S, Quint WG, Alemany L, et al. Human papillomavirus genotype attribution in invasive cervical cancer: a retrospective cross-sectional worldwide study. *Lancet Oncol*. 2010;11(11):1048–1056. [PMID: 20952254]

Hemminki K, Chen B. Familial risks for cervical tumors in full and half siblings: etiologic apportioning. *Cancer Epidemiol Biomarkers Prevent*. 2006;15(7):1413. [PMID: 16835346]

Hoover RN, Hyer M, Pfeiffer RM, et al. Adverse health outcomes in women exposed in utero to diethylstilbestrol. *N Engl J Med*. 2011;365(14):1304–1314. [PMID: 21991952]

Huh WK, Ault KA, Chelmow D, et al. Use of primary high-risk human papillomavirus testing for cervical cancer screening: interim clinical guidance. *Gynecol Oncol*. 2015;136(2):178–182. [PMID: 25579107]

Massad I, Einstein M, Huh W, et al. 2012 updated consensus guidelines for the management of abnormal cervical cancer screening tests and cancer precursors. *J Low Genit Tract Dis*. 2013;17(5 suppl 1):s1–s27. [PMID: 23635684]

Meites E, Kempe A, Markowitz L. Use of a 2-dose schedule for human papillomavirus vaccination: updated recommendations of the advisory committee on immunization practices. *MMWR Morb Mortal Wkly Rep*. 2016;65(49);1405–1408. [PMID: 27977643]

Moyer VA. Screening for cervical cancer: US Preventive Services Task Force recommendation statement. *Ann Intern Med*. 2012;156(12):880–891. [PMID: 22711081]

National Institute of Health. Human papillomavirus disease. https://aidsinfo.nih.gov/guidelines/html/4/adult-and-adolescent-opportunistic-infection/343/hpv. Accessed July 25, 2019.

Rerucha CM, Caro RJ, Wheeler V. Cervical cancer screening. *Am Fam Physician*. 2018;97(7):441–448. [PMID: 29671553]

Saslow D, Solomon D, Lawson HW, et al. American Cancer Society, American Society for Colposcopy and Cervical Pathology, and American Society for Clinical Pathology screening guidelines for the prevention and early detection of cervical cancer. *Cancer J Clin*. 2012;62(3):147–172. [PMID: 22431528]

Siegel RL, Miller KD, Jemal A. Cancer statistics, 2018. *Cancer J Clin*. 2018;68(1):7–30. [PMID: 29313949]

US Preventative Service Task Force. Cervical cancer: screening. https://www.uspreventiveservicestaskforce.org/Page/Document/UpdateSummaryFinal/cervical-cancer-screening2. Accessed July 24, 2019.

Vesikari T, Brodszki N. A randomized, double-blind, phase iii study of the immunogenicity and safety of a 9-valent human papillomavirus l1 virus-like particle vaccine (v503) versus Gardasil® in 9-15-year-old girls. *Pediatr Infect Dis J*. 2015;34(9):992–998. [PMID: 26090572]

Walker TY, Elam-Evans LD. National, regional, state, and selected local area vaccination coverage among adolescents aged 13-17 years–United States, 2016. *MMWR Morb Mortal Wkly Rep*. 2017;66(33):874–882. [PMID: 28837546]

OVARIAN CANCER

 ESSENTIALS OF DIAGNOSIS

▶ Epithelial cell cancers represent the vast majority of ovarian cancers, usually affecting older women and having a poor prognosis.

▶ Germ cell cancer, carcinosarcoma, and borderline epithelial cell and sex chord stromal cancers are rarer forms of ovarian cancer that affect younger women and have a better prognosis.

▶ Fallopian tube and primary peritoneal cancers are currently managed in a fashion similar to that for ovarian cancer.

▶ A gynecologic oncologist should manage ovarian cancer.

General Considerations

Epithelial ovarian cancer is the leading cause of gynecologic cancer death in the United States. Risk generally increases with age. Risk is reduced in women with early childbearing, multiple pregnancies, breastfeeding, tubal ligation or hysterectomy, and/or OCP use, but is increased in women with early menarche, late menopause, endometriosis, infertility, or nulliparity and in women who delivered a first child at age ≥35 years.

HRT has been associated with increased risk for the two most common types of ovarian cancer: serous and endometrioid. It is unlikely that in vitro fertilization is associated with increased risk for ovarian cancer.

Women with family history of ovarian cancer are at higher risk, especially if *BRCA* positive. Women with a history of breast, uterine, or colon cancer, as well as women of Eastern European (Ashkenazi) Jewish descent, also have higher than average risk.

Clinical Findings

Symptoms that are significantly associated with ovarian cancer are pelvic/abdominal pain, increased abdominal size/bloating, and feeling full (easily satiated) when these symptoms are present for <1 year and have occurred >12 days per month. Early symptoms are often missed because of their nonspecific nature. Advanced cancer may present with acute symptoms of metastatic bowel obstruction or pleural effusion.

Prevention

The USPSTF found adequate evidence that screening for ovarian cancer does not reduce ovarian cancer mortality. The USPSTF found adequate evidence that the harms from screening for ovarian cancer are at least moderate and may be substantial in some cases and include unnecessary surgery for women who do not have cancer. This recommendation applies to asymptomatic women who are not known to have a high-risk hereditary cancer syndrome. Prophylactic surgery and/or enhanced cancer screening in conjunction with genetic counseling may be beneficial in *BRCA*-positive women.

Differential Diagnosis

Ovarian cancer must be differentiated from other causes of abdominal mass and/or distension such as noncancerous ovarian conditions, gastrointestinal disease, lymphoma, and uterine or pancreatic cancers. Ultrasound with or without CT is used to further delineate the undiagnosed pelvic mass. Fine-needle aspiration of an ovarian mass should be avoided to prevent malignant seeding of the peritoneal cavity. Tumor markers and chest imaging are often obtained in the patient with a mass suspicious for ovarian cancer. Preclinical detection through CA-125 or other biomarker screening and/or ultrasound screening of asymptomatic women is not recommended.

Treatment

Select young women with very-early-stage ovarian cancer may be candidates for fertility-sparing surgery. Most cancers are treated with total abdominal hysterectomy and bilateral salpingo-oophorectomy in conjunction with staging laparotomy. Intraperitoneal therapy, debulking with cytoreduction surgery, and chemotherapy are used to treat advanced disease. Early trials show a survival benefit for *BRCA*-positive women with advanced epithelial ovarian cancer who are treated with poly(adenosine diphosphate-ribose) polymerase (PARP) inhibitors. Radiation therapy is used for palliative symptom control.

Complications

Complication of ovarian cancer include locally invasive disease and metastatic spread to the peritoneum, liver, and lungs.

Prognosis

Because most cancers are high grade at the time of diagnosis, less than half of women with ovarian cancer are cured. However, survival is very good for the small group of women diagnosed with isolated local disease, nonepithelial tumors, or borderline epithelial tumors.

Beral V, Gaitskell K, Hermon C, et al. Menopausal hormone use and ovarian cancer risk: individual participant meta-analysis of 52 epidemiological studies. *Lancet.* 2015;385(9980):1835–1842. [PMID: 25684585]

Centers for Disease Control and Prevention. What are the risk factors for ovarian cancer? https://www.cdc.gov/cancer/ovarian/basic_info/risk_factors.htm. Accessed March 27, 2019.

Ebell MH, Culp MB, Radke TJ. A systematic review of symptoms for the diagnosis of ovarian cancer. *Am J Prev Med.* 2016;50(3):384–394. [PMID: 26541098]

Ledermann JA, Raja FA, Fotopoulou C, et al. Newly diagnosed and relapsed epithelial ovarian carcinoma: ESMO Clinical Practice Guidelines for diagnosis, treatment and follow-up. *Ann Oncol.* 2013;24.S6:vi24–32. [PMID: 24078660]

Moore K, Colombo N, Scambia G, et al. Maintenance olaparib in patients with newly diagnosed advanced ovarian cancer. *N Engl J Med.* 2018;379(26):2495. [PMID: 30345884]

Siristatidis C, Sergentanis TN, Kanavidis P, et al. Controlled ovarian hyperstimulation for IVF: impact on ovarian, endometrial and cervical cancer: a systematic review and meta-analysis. *Hum Reprod.* 2013;19(2):105–123. [PMID: 23255514]

US Preventive Services Task Force. Ovarian cancer: screening. https://www.uspreventiveservicestaskforce.org/Page/Document/RecommendationStatementFinal/ovarian-cancer-screening1. Accessed April 2, 2019.

UTERINE CANCER

 ESSENTIALS OF DIAGNOSIS

▶ Cancers of the uterus include endometrial cancer and uterine sarcoma.

▶ Incidence increases with age.

▶ Commonly presents with abnormal vaginal bleeding or discharge.

General Considerations

Endometrial cancer is the most common gynecologic cancer in the United States; uterine sarcoma represents 5% of all uterine cancers. Uterine cancer is more common in older women and typically presents with abnormal vaginal bleeding. Postmenopausal estrogen therapy, infertility/nulliparity, obesity, and diabetes are risk factors. Tamoxifen and estrogen-secreting ovarian cancers increase risk. Women with hereditary nonpolyposis colon cancer (HNPCC) syndrome have an increased risk of endometrial cancer. A family history of uterine, colon, or ovarian cancer; a personal history of breast or ovarian cancer; and a history of pelvic radiation therapy also increase risk. Reduced number of lifetime menstrual cycles, pregnancy, OCP use, regular physical activity, maintaining a healthy weight, and the use of nonhormonal intrauterine devices reduce the risk of endometrial cancer. Endometrial hyperplasia may progress to endometrial cancer.

Clinical Findings

Abnormal vaginal bleeding is the earliest sign of endometrial cancer, with advanced cancer potentially presenting as pelvic pain and/or mass.

Prevention

The American Cancer Society recommends educating women about risks and symptoms of endometrial cancer beginning at menopause. Total hysterectomy is preventive but not indicated in low-risk women. Hysterectomy in conjunction with genetic counseling is considered for women with select hereditary syndromes. There are no medications accepted for the prevention of uterine cancer.

Differential Diagnosis

A. Clinically Evident Disease

Abnormal vaginal bleeding may be caused by benign tumors such as polyps, benign hyperplasia, fibroids, infection, or other gynecologic malignancy; endometrial biopsy is diagnostic. A negative office biopsy with clinical suspicion should be followed up by a dilation and curettage with or without hysteroscopy. Imaging can define extrauterine disease.

B. Preclinical Diagnosis

The American Cancer Society recommends offering annual endometrial biopsy beginning at age 35 to women with history of infertility, obesity, failure of ovulation, abnormal uterine bleeding, or use of estrogen therapy or tamoxifen. Women at high risk of endometrial cancer due to known or suspected HNPCC-associated genetic mutations should be routinely screened with endometrial biopsy beginning at age 35.

Complications

Local invasion and metastatic spread to the bone, liver, lungs, peritoneum, and vagina can occur.

Treatment

In premenopausal women with low-grade disease, ovary-sparing surgery is acceptable. Radiation therapy may afford symptom control and delay disease progression in inoperable patients. Postoperative symptoms of estrogen withdrawal may be treated with estrogen replacement, which does not increase risk of relapse. Detailed current treatment guidelines are available through the National Comprehensive Cancer Network.

Prognosis

Because of early presentation with abnormal bleeding, 75% of women diagnosed with endometrial cancer are diagnosed with noninvasive disease and have a good prognosis.

American Cancer Society. Can endometrial cancer be found early? https://www.cancer.org/cancer/endometrial-cancer/detection-diagnosis-staging/detection.html. Accessed April 10, 2019.

George SM, Ballard R, Shikany JM, et al. A prospective analysis of diet quality and endometrial cancer among 84,415 postmenopausal women in the Women's Health Initiative. *Ann Epidemiol.* 2015;25(10):788–93. [PMID: 26260777]

Henley SJ, Miller JW, Dowling NF, et al. Uterine cancer incidence and mortality—United States, 1999–2016. *MMWR Morb Mortal Wkly Rep.* 2018;67(48):1333. [PMID: 30521505]

Luo J, Chlebowski RT, Hendryx M, et al. Intentional weight loss and endometrial cancer risk. *J Clin Oncol.* 2017;35(11):1189. [PMID: 28165909]

National Comprehensive Cancer Network. NCCN guidelines: uterine neoplasms version 2.2013. http://www.nccn.org/professionals/physician_gls/pdf/uterine.pdf. Accessed March 20, 2013.

US Preventive Services Task Force. Final recommendation statement: ovarian cancer: screening. https://www.uspreventiveservicestaskforce.org/Page/Document/RecommendationStatementFinal/ovarian-cancer-screening1. Accessed July 28, 2019.

Respiratory Problems

Anja Dabelić, MD, FAAFP

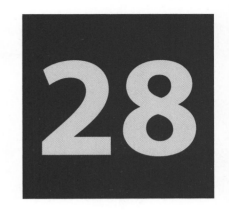

Respiratory infections and chronic lung diseases are among the most common reasons why patients consult primary care physicians. Most respiratory problems encountered by primary care physicians are acute, with the majority comprising respiratory infections, exacerbations of asthma, chronic obstructive pulmonary diseases (COPDs), and pulmonary embolism (PE).

UPPER RESPIRATORY TRACT INFECTIONS

COMMON COLDS/UPPER RESPIRATORY TRACT INFECTIONS

ESSENTIALS OF DIAGNOSIS

▶ Sore throat, congestion, low-grade fever, mild myalgias, and fatigue.

▶ Symptoms lasting for 12–14 days.

▶ General Considerations

Although colds are mild, self-limiting, and short in duration, they are a leading cause of sickness in industrial and school absenteeism. Each year, colds account for 170 million days of restricted activity, 23 million days of school absence, and 18 million days of work absence.

Most colds are caused by viruses. Rhinoviruses are the most common type of virus and are found in slightly more than half of all patients. Coronaviruses are the second most common cause. Rarely (0.05% of all cases) can bacteria be cultured from individuals with cold symptoms. It is not clear whether these bacteria cause the cold, are secondary infectious agents, or are simply colonizers. Bacterial pathogens

that have been identified include *Chlamydia pneumoniae, Haemophilus influenzae, Streptococcus pneumoniae,* and *Mycoplasma pneumoniae.*

▶ Prevention

The mechanisms of transmission suggest that colds can be spread through contact with inanimate surfaces, but the primary transmission appears to be via hand-to-hand contact. The beneficial effects of removing viruses from the hands are supported by observations that absences of children have been reduced through the use of antiseptic hand wipes throughout the day at school or daycare.

▶ Clinical Findings

Colds generally last 12–14 days. Reassurance and education of patients reduce misconceptions that symptoms lasting >1 week are abnormal. When the symptoms of congestion persist longer than 2 weeks, other causes of chronic congestion should be considered (Table 28–1).

Symptoms of colds include sore throat, congestion, low-grade fever, and mild myalgias and fatigue. In general, early in the development of a cold, the discharge is clear. As more inflammation develops, the discharge takes on some coloration. A yellow, green, or brown-tinted nasal discharge is an indicator of inflammation, not secondary bacterial infection. Discolored nasal discharge raises the likelihood of sinusitis, but only if other predictors of sinusitis are present. Therefore, education of patients and reassurance are needed, and not reflexive antibiotic prescriptions, which some patients ultimately desire.

▶ Complications

Primary complications from upper respiratory tract infection are otitis media and sinusitis. These complications develop from obstruction of the eustachian tube or sinus ostia from

Table 28–1. Differential diagnosis for congestion and rhinorrhea.

Common cold
Sinusitis
   Viral
   Allergic
   Bacterial
   Fungal
Seasonal allergic rhinitis
Vasomotor rhinitis
Rhinitis secondary to α-agonist withdrawal
Drug-induced rhinitis (eg, cocaine)
Nasal foreign body

nasal passage edema. Although treatment of these infections with antibiotics is common, the vast majority of infections clear without antibiotic therapy.

One misconception is that using antibiotics during the acute phase of a cold can prevent these complications. Evidence shows that taking antibiotics during a cold does not reduce the incidence of sinusitis or otitis media. Nor do antibiotics give a faster recovery than placebos.

▶ Differential Diagnosis

The differential diagnosis of colds includes complications of the cold such as sinusitis or otitis media, acute bronchitis, and noninfectious rhinitis. Influenza shares many of the symptoms of a common cold, but generally patients have a much higher fever, myalgias, and more intense fatigue.

▶ Treatment

Despite the widespread recognition that viruses cause common colds, several studies have shown that patients with the common cold who are seen in physicians' offices are often treated with antibiotics. The prescribing of antibiotics for colds occurs more often in adults than children. Although this practice appears to have declined in adults, the use of broad-spectrum antibiotics for colds is still common in children. The need to reduce the use of antibiotics for viral conditions has important ramifications on communitywide drug resistance; in areas in which prescribing antibiotics for respiratory infections has been curtailed, reversals in antibiotic drug resistance have been observed.

Currently, the most effective treatment is symptom reduction with over-the-counter (OTC) decongestants, the most popular of which include pseudoephedrine hydrochloride and topically applied vasoconstrictors. These agents produce short-term symptomatic relief. However, patients must be warned to use topical agents for a limited duration because prolonged use is associated with rebound edema of the nasal mucosa (rhinitis medicamentosa).

Several OTC medications contain a mix of decongestants, cough suppressants, and pain relievers. Again, the use of these preparations will not cure the common cold but will provide symptomatic reduction and relief.

Antihistamines, with a few exceptions, have not been shown to provide effective treatment. Zinc gluconate lozenges are available without a prescription, but a meta-analysis of 15 previous studies on zinc concluded that zinc lozenges were not effective in reducing the duration of cold symptoms.

Some herbal remedies are useful for treatment of the common cold. Echinacea, also known as the "American coneflower," has been purported to reduce the duration of the common cold by stimulating the immune system; however, evidence for its efficacy is mixed. Echinacea should be used for only 2–3 weeks to avoid liver damage and other possible side effects that have been reported during long-term use of this herb. Ephedra, also known as *ma huang*, has decongestant properties that make it similar to pseudoephedrine. Ephedra is more likely than pseudoephedrine to cause increased blood pressure tachyarrhythmia. This is especially true if used in conjunction with caffeine.

Linde K, Barrett B, Wölkart K, et al. Echinacea for preventing and treating the common cold. *Cochrane Database Syst Rev.* 2006;(2):CD000530. [PMID: 16437427]

Mainous AG 3rd, Hueston WJ, Davis MP, et al. Trends in antimicrobial prescribing for bronchitis and upper respiratory infections among adults and children. *Am J Public Health.* 2003;93:1910–1914. [PMID: 14600065]

SINUSITIS

ESSENTIALS OF DIAGNOSIS

▶ "Double-sickening" phenomenon.

▶ Maxillary toothache and purulent rhinorrhea.

▶ Poor response to decongestants.

▶ History of discolored nasal discharge.

▶ Facial pain/pressure/fullness; increasing pain with bending forward.

▶ Nasal congestion.

▶ General Considerations

Sinusitis is most often a complication of an upper respiratory viral infection, so the incidence peaks in the winter cold season. Medical conditions that may increase the risk for sinusitis include cystic fibrosis, asthma, immunosuppression, and allergic rhinitis. Cigarette smoking may also increase the risk of bacterial sinusitis during a cold because of reduced mucociliary clearance.

Most cases of acute sinusitis are caused by viral infection. The inflammation associated with viral infection clears without additional therapy. Bacterial superinfection of upper respiratory infections (URIs) is rare and occurs in only 0.5–1% of colds. Fungal sinusitis is very rare and usually occurs in immunosuppressed individuals or those with diabetes mellitus.

Clinical Findings

Acute sinusitis has considerable overlap in its constellation of signs and symptoms with URIs. One-half to two-thirds of patients with sinus symptoms seen in primary care are unlikely to have sinusitis. URIs are often precursors of sinusitis, and at some point, symptoms from each condition may overlap. Sinus inflammation from a URI without bacterial infection is also common.

The signs and symptoms that increase the likelihood that the patient has acute sinusitis are a "double-sickening" phenomenon (whereby the patient seems to improve following the URI and then deteriorates), maxillary toothache, purulent nasal discharge, poor response to decongestants, and a history of discolored nasal discharge. In addition, on examination, patients will have tenderness to palpation of their sinuses and worsening pain with bending forward.

Treatment

Nonsevere symptoms, such as mild pain and afebrile state of <7 days' duration should be treated with supportive care. Treatment would include analgesics, decongestants, and saline nasal irrigation. Narrow-spectrum antibiotics should be reserved for patients with no improvement in 7 days or worsening symptoms. No radiologic imaging is required. A rare complication of sinusitis to be aware of is orbital and/or intracranial bony involvement. If symptoms fail to improve with therapy course, consider referral to an otorhinolaryngologist. The effectiveness of antibiotics is unclear. Amoxicillin/clavulanate acid (ACA) is preferred over amoxicillin alone in treatment of children and adults, provided the patient is not allergic to the components. High doses of ACA at 90 mg/kg daily in twice-a-day dosing is recommended for regions with >10% endemic rate of sinusitis, severe infection, children who attend daycare, a child <2 years old, an adult age >65 years, a recently hospitalized patient, any recent antibiotic use, or an immunocompromised patient. There are increasing rates of resistance to macrolides and sulfamethoxazole/trimethoprim, and these should not be used for empiric therapy. Alternatives in case of allergy to ACA would be doxycycline or levofloxacin/moxifloxacin. Treatment should be for 5–7 days for adults and 10–14 days for children on antibiotics for sinusitis.

American Academy of Pediatrics. Subcommittee on Management of Sinusitis and Committee on Quality Improvement: clinical practice guideline: management of sinusitis. *Pediatrics.* 2001;108:798. [PMID: 11533355]

Aring AM, Chan MM. Acute rhinosinusitis in adults. *Am Acad Fam Physicians.* 2011;83(9):1057–1063. [PMID: 21534518]

Chow AW, Benninger MS, Brook I, et al. IDSA clinical practice guideline for acute bacterial rhinosinusitis in children and adults. *Clin Infect Dis.* 2012;54(8):e72–e112. [PMID: 22438350]

Williams JW Jr, Aguilar C, Cornell J, et al. Antibiotics for acute maxillary sinusitis. *Cochrane Database Syst Rev.* 2000;2:CD000243. [PMID: 12804392]

INFLUENZA (ADULTS)

ESSENTIALS OF DIAGNOSIS

- ► High fever.
- ► Extreme fatigue.
- ► Myalgias.

Diagnosis, treatment, and prevention of influenza in children are reviewed extensively in Chapter 5.

General Considerations

Although most cases of the flu are mild and usually resolve without medical treatment within 2 weeks, some will develop complications. Currently, three types of viruses causing influenza have been identified in the United States: A, B, and C. Seasonal epidemics from influenza types A and B are seen every winter. Type C influenza usually causes a mild respiratory illness and is not responsible for epidemics. If a new strain emerges and infects a population, an influenza pandemic can result.

Influenza A is identified by two proteins on the virus surface: a hemagglutinin (H) and a neuraminidase (N). These proteins result in 16 different H subtypes and 9 different N subtypes. The A form of influenza can be further divided into strains. The two subtypes of influenza A found in humans currently are A(H1N1) and A(H3N2). In 2009, an influenza pandemic occurred when a very different strain of influenza A(N1H1) developed in humans. Influenza B is broken down by different strain, but not by subtypes.

Prevention

Vaccination is the most effective prevention against influenza. The seasonal flu vaccination is a trivalent vaccine, with each component selected to protect against one of the three main groups of influenza viruses circulating in humans. The influenza viruses in the seasonal flu vaccine are selected each year from surveillance-based forecasts about which viruses are most likely to cause illness in the upcoming season. The World Health Organization (WHO) recommends specific vaccine viruses for inclusion, but each country decides independently which strains should be included. The US Food and Drug Administration (FDA) determines which vaccine viruses will be used in US-licensed vaccines. Influenza vaccinations require annual dosing for adults and children age >1 year. Therefore, the influenza vaccine does not cover all strains of the influenza virus, and patients who have received their annual vaccination can still develop influenza; this is an important education point for all patients. A complete listing of who should be immunized can be found on the Centers for Disease Control and Prevention's (CDC) Advisory Committee on Immunization Practices (ACIP) website and others.

The spread of influenza is from person to person by sneezing or coughing. Therefore, everyday care to stay healthy can help prevent contracting the flu and/or spreading the flu to others. Simple steps, such as covering nose and mouth when sneezing or coughing with a tissue; avoiding touching mouth, nose, and eyes if sick; washing hands frequently with soap or germicide solution; and staying home if sick to avoid others, may help prevent the spread of influenza. Additionally, if a patient has been exposed to influenza by another, influenza antiviral prescription drugs can be used as chemoprophylaxis of influenza.

▶ Clinical Findings

The flu can last from 3 days to 2 weeks. Mild cases may be assumed to have the common cold and receive no medical treatment. Symptoms include high fever, extreme fatigue, and myalgias. Other symptoms associated with the flu include sore throat, rhinorrhea, cough, headache, and chills. Some people experience nausea, vomiting, and diarrhea. The diagnosis is most commonly clinical, but there are laboratory confirmation tests available, such as rapid influenza diagnostic tests (RIDTs), viral cultures, immunofluorescence, and reverse transcription polymerase chain reaction. Clinicians should realize that a negative RIDT result does not exclude a diagnosis of influenza, because sensitivities are 40–70%. When there is a clinical suspicion of influenza and antiviral treatment is indicated, the treatment should be started without waiting for results of additional influenza testing.

▶ Complications

Complications can lead to hospitalization and even death. These complications include, but are not limited to, otitis media, sinusitis, acute bronchitis, and pneumonia. Exacerbations of chronic illnesses such as asthma, congestive heart failure, and chronic obstructive lung disease are further complications of the flu.

▶ Differential Diagnosis

One must consider other viruses, such as the common cold viruses, which have many of the same symptoms in less severity.

Table 28–2. High-risk populations for flu-related complications.

Children <5 years of age
Adults >64 years of age
Pregnant women
Heart disease (heart failure, coronary artery disease, congenital heart disease, and others)
Asthma
Neurologic disorders (cerebral palsy, intellectual disability, developmental delay, spinal cord injury, epilepsy, muscular dystrophy, stroke, and others)
Kidney diseases
Liver diseases
Blood disorders (sickle cell disease and others)
Chronic lung disease (chronic obstructive pulmonary disease, cystic fibrosis, and others)
Endocrine diseases (diabetes mellitus and others)
Metabolic disorders
Immune deficiencies (people with cancer, HIV or AIDS, chronic steroid use, and others)
Younger than 19 years on chronic aspirin therapy

▶ Treatment

People who develop flu symptoms should seek medical treatment as soon as possible, especially those in the high-risk group, as shown in Table 28–2. If treatment with antivirals is begun within 48 hours of the first signs or symptoms of illness, the patient gets the greatest benefit. These benefits include shortening the illness by at least 24 hours, preventing serious complications, and decreasing the likelihood of spreading the disease to others. Treatment with oseltamivir or zanamivir is effective against all forms of human influenza, including A(H1N1)/(H3N2), 2009 A(H1N1), and B. Two older medications, amantadine and rimantadine, remain susceptible to influenza A but not to B. The CDC recommends the use of oseltamivir or zanamivir at this time, due to the emergence of the new strain of A(N1H1). Treatment guidelines differ for age groups and high-risk groups. Therefore, it is important when considering treatment options to refer to the *Physician's Desk Reference* to ensure that appropriate treatment is given. Symptomatic treatment can be given with an antipyretic for the fever and an anti-inflammatory for pain and myalgias.

Centers for Disease Control and Prevention (CDC). 2009 H1N1 flu. http://www.cdc.gov/h1n1flu/. Accessed February 12, 2010.

Centers for Disease Control and Prevention (CDC). Antiviral agents for the treatment and chemoprophylaxis of influenza. Recommendations of the Advisory Committee on Immunization Practices (ACIP). www.cdc.gov/mmwr/pdf/rr/rr6601.pdf. Accessed January 21, 2011.

Centers for Disease Control and Prevention (CDC). People at high risk of developing flu-related complications. http://www.cdc.gov/about/disease/high_risk.html. Accessed November 1, 2012.

Centers for Disease Control and Prevention (CDC). Types of influenza viruses. http://www.cdc.gov/FLU/about/viruses/types .htm. Accessed March 22, 2012.

Centers for Disease Control and Prevention (CDC), Advisory Committee on Immunization Practices (ACIP). Recommended Adult Immunization Schedule—United States 2011. http://www .cdc.gov/vaccines/pubs/ACIP-list.htm. Accessed January 28, 2011.

▼ LOWER RESPIRATORY TRACT INFECTIONS

ACUTE BRONCHITIS

ESSENTIALS OF DIAGNOSIS

► Cough lasting >3 weeks.
► Fever, constitutional symptoms, and a productive cough.

▶ General Considerations

Viral infection is the primary cause of most episodes of acute bronchitis. A wide variety of viruses have been shown to cause acute bronchitis, including influenza, rhinovirus, adenovirus, coronavirus, parainfluenza, and respiratory syncytial virus. Nonviral pathogens, including *M pneumoniae* and *Chlamydophila pneumoniae* (Taiwan acute respiratory agent [TWAR]), have also been identified as causes.

The etiologic role of bacteria such as *H influenzae* and *S pneumoniae* in acute bronchitis is unclear because these bacteria are common upper respiratory tract flora. Sputum cultures for acute bronchitis are therefore difficult to evaluate because it is unclear whether the sputum has been contaminated by pathogens colonizing the nasopharynx.

▶ Clinical Findings

Patients with acute bronchitis may have a cough for a significant time. Although the duration of the condition is variable, one study showed that 50% of patients had a cough for >3 weeks and 25% for >4 weeks. Other causes of chronic cough are shown in Table 28–3.

Both acute bronchitis and pneumonia can present with fever, constitutional symptoms, and a productive cough. Although patients with pneumonia often have rales, this finding is neither sensitive nor specific for the illness. When pneumonia is suspected because of the presence of a high fever, constitutional symptoms, severe dyspnea, and certain physical findings or risk factors, a chest radiograph should be obtained to confirm the diagnosis.

Table 28–3. Causes of chronic cough.

Pulmonary causes
Infectious
 Postobstructive pneumonia
 Tuberculosis
 Pneumocystis jiroveci (formerly, *Pneumocystis carinii*)
 Bronchiectasis
 Lung abscess
Noninfectious
 Asthma
 Chronic bronchitis
 Allergic aspergillosis
 Bronchogenic neoplasms
 Sarcoidosis
 Pulmonary fibrosis
 Chemical or smoke inhalation
Cardiovascular causes
Congestive heart failure/pulmonary edema
Enlargement of left atrium
Gastrointestinal tract
Reflux esophagitis
Other causes
Medications, especially angiotensin-converting enzyme (ACE) inhibitors
Psychogenic cough
Foreign-body aspiration

▶ Differential Diagnosis

Asthma and allergic bronchospastic disorders can mimic the productive cough of acute bronchitis. When obstructive symptoms are not obvious, mild asthma may be diagnosed as acute bronchitis. Further, because respiratory infections can trigger bronchospasm in asthma, patients with asthma that occurs only in the presence of respiratory infections resemble patients with acute bronchitis.

Finally, nonpulmonary causes of cough should enter the differential diagnosis. In older patients, congestive heart failure may cause cough, shortness of breath, and wheezing. Reflux esophagitis with chronic aspiration can cause bronchial inflammation with cough and wheezing. Bronchogenic tumors may produce a cough and obstructive symptoms.

▶ Treatment

Clinical trials of the effectiveness of antibiotics in treating acute bronchitis have had mixed results. Meta-analyses indicated that the benefits of antibiotics in a general population are marginal and should be weighed against the impact of excessive use of antibiotics on the development of antibiotic resistance as well as complications of developing *Clostridium difficile*.

Data from clinical trials suggest that bronchodilators may provide effective symptomatic relief to patients with acute bronchitis. Treatment with bronchodilators demonstrated significant relief of symptoms, including faster resolution of cough and return to work. The effect of albuterol in a population of patients with undifferentiated cough was evaluated, and no beneficial effect was found. Because various conditions present with cough, there may have been some misclassification in generalizing this finding to acute bronchitis.

Albert RH. Diagnosis and treatment of acute bronchitis. *Am Fam Physician.* 2010;82(11):1345–1350. [PMID: 21121518]

Bent S, Saint S, Vittinghoff E, et al. Antibiotics in acute bronchitis: a meta-analysis. *Am J Med.* 1999;107:62. [PMID: 10403354]

Braman SS. Chronic cough due to acute bronchitis. *Chest.* 2006;129(1 suppl):95S–103S. [PMID: 16428698]

Smucny JJ, Becker LA, Glazier RH, et al. Are antibiotics effective treatment for acute bronchitis? A meta-analysis. *J Fam Pract.* 1998;47:453. [PMID: 9866671]

COMMUNITY-ACQUIRED PNEUMONIA

 ESSENTIALS OF DIAGNOSIS

▶ Fever and cough (productive or nonproductive).

▶ Tachypnea.

▶ Rales or crackles.

▶ Positive chest radiograph.

▶ General Considerations

Pneumonia is the cause of >10 million visits to physicians annually, accounts for 3% of all hospitalizations, and is the eighth leading cause of death in the United States, per the American Lung Association. A variety of factors, including increasing age, increase the risk of pneumonia. Among the elderly, institutionalization and debilitation further increase the risk for acquiring pneumonia. Patients age ≥55 years, smokers, and patients with chronic respiratory diseases are more likely to require hospitalization for pneumonia. Those with congestive heart failure, cerebrovascular diseases, cancer, diabetes mellitus, and poor nutritional status are more likely to die. Thus, age and comorbidities are important factors to consider when deciding whether to hospitalize a patient with pneumonia. These risk factors are summarized in Table 28–4.

▶ Prevention

Pneumococcal pneumonia may be prevented through immunization with multivalent pneumococcal vaccine. There are currently two pneumococcal vaccines. The pneumococcal conjugate vaccine, PCV13, is currently recommended for all children age <5 years and adults age ≥19 years with certain medical conditions. The other is a 23-valent pneumococcal polysaccharide vaccine (PPSV23) and is indicated for all adults age >65 years and children age ≥2 years with high risk for disease (ie, diabetes mellitus, chronic pulmonary, or cardiac disease, without a spleen, or with immunocompromise). The PPSV23 is also recommended for adults age 19–64 years who smoke cigarettes or have asthma. Additionally, anyone who lives in a long-term care facility should be vaccinated. The CDC recommends immunization of all patients with the following medical conditions: immunosuppressed patients, including those with human immunodeficiency virus (HIV) infection; alcoholism; cirrhosis; chronic renal failure; nephrotic syndrome; functional or anatomic asplenia (eg, sickle cell disease or splenectomy); cochlear implants; cerebrospinal fluid leaks; or multiple myeloma.

In addition to initial vaccination, clinicians should advise patients that the duration of protection is uncertain. Those at particularly high risk of mortality from pneumococcal pneumonia, such as patients with chronic pulmonary disease, lacking a spleen, or with chronic renal disease or nephrotic disease, functional or anatomic asplenia, or immunocompromising conditions, should receive a one-time revaccination after 5 years from their first vaccination. For patients age >65 years, a one-time revaccination is also recommended if their last vaccination was earlier than 5 years ago or if they were <65 years old when they received their first vaccination.

Table 28–4. Risk factors associated with mortality in community-acquired pneumonia.

Category	Characteristics	Mortality	Location of Care
Very low risk	Age <60, no comorbidities	<1%	Outpatient
Low risk	Age >60, but healthy Age <60, mild comorbidity	3%	80% can be cared for as outpatient (depending on comorbidity)
Moderate risk	Age >60 with comorbidity	13–25%	Hospitalization
High risk	Serious compromise present on presentation (eg, hypotension, respiratory distress) regardless of age	50%	Intensive care unit

Clinical Findings

The most common presenting complaints for patients with pneumonia are fever and a cough that may be either productive or nonproductive. As an example, in one study, 80% of patients with pneumonia had a fever. Other symptoms that may be suggestive of pneumonia include dyspnea and pleuritic chest pain. However, none of these symptoms is specific for pneumonia.

Symptoms of pneumonia may be nonspecific in older patients. Elderly individuals who suffer a general decline in their function, become confused or have worsening dementia, or experience more frequent falls should increase suspicion of infection. Elderly patients who have preexisting cognitive impairment or depend on someone else for support of their daily activities are at highest risk for not exhibiting typical symptoms of pneumonia.

The most consistent sign of pneumonia is tachypnea. In one study of elderly patients, tachypnea was observed to be present 3–4 days before the appearance of other physical findings of pneumonia. Rales or crackles are often considered the hallmark of pneumonia, but these may be heard in only 75–80% of patients. Other signs of pneumonia such as dullness to percussion or egophony, which are usually believed to be indicative of consolidation, occur in less than a third of patients with pneumonia.

Chest radiography is the standard for diagnosing pneumonia. In rare cases, the chest x-ray may be falsely negative. This generally occurs in patients exhibiting profound dehydration, early pneumonia (first 24 hours), infection with *Pneumocystis*, and severe neutropenia.

Microbiological testing for pneumonia is not very useful in relatively healthy patients with nonsevere pneumonia. Blood and sputum cultures are most likely to be beneficial in patients with risk factors for unusual organisms or who are very ill.

Differential Diagnosis

Other conditions such as postobstructive pneumonitis, pulmonary infarction from an embolism, radiation pneumonitis, and interstitial edema from congestive heart failure all may produce infiltrates that are indistinguishable from an infectious process.

Treatment

With the emergence of other pathogens causing pneumonia and the development of resistance to penicillin and other drugs in *S pneumoniae*, treatment decisions have become more complex. The 2007 update to the Infectious Disease Society of America (ISDA) and American Thoracic Society (ATS) guidelines for the treatment of community-acquired pneumonia differ depending on the health and age of patients (ie, those age ≥65 years), whether they have recently been treated with an antibiotic, and whether they are at risk for an

Table 28–5. Recommendations for empiric treatment of community-acquired pneumonia.

Treatment of patients not requiring hospitalization
No comorbidities or comorbidities but no recent antibiotic use: respiratory fluoroquinolone,[a] macrolide plus high-dose amoxicillin, or macrolide plus amoxicillin-clavulanic acid
With comorbidities and recent antibiotic use: respiratory fluoroquinolone, macrolide plus β-lactam (second- or third-generation cephalosporin or lactam-lactamase inhibitor)
Treatment of hospitalized patients not critically ill
β-Lactam with or without a macrolide or respiratory fluoroquinolone
Treatment of critically-ill hospitalized patients
Pseudomonas not suspected: β-lactam with or without a macrolide or respiratory fluoroquinolone
Pseudomonas possible: antipseudomonal cephalosporin plus ciprofloxacin or antipseudomonal cephalosporin plus aminoglycoside plus respiratory fluoroquinolone
Other situations
Suspected aspiration: clindamycin or a β-lactam with β-lactamase inhibitor
Influenza superinfection: respiratory fluoroquinolone or β-lactam (second- or third-generation cephalosporin or lactam-lactamase inhibitor)

[a]Includes levofloxacin, sparfloxacin, and grepafloxacin.

aspiration pneumonia or influenza superinfection (Table 28–5). For patients with no serious comorbidities, the ISDA/ATS recommends a respiratory quinolone or an advanced macrolide plus high-dose amoxicillin (or ACA) as first-line therapy. If an antibiotic has been used recently, then either a respiratory quinolone or an advanced macrolide plus a second- or third-generation cephalosporin is a recommended option. If aspiration is suspected, the ISDA/ATS guidelines include a choice of ACA or clindamycin as initial treatment.

Suitable empiric antimicrobial regimens for inpatient pneumonia include an intravenous β-lactam antibiotic, such as cefuroxime, ceftriaxone sodium, or cefotaxime sodium, or a combination of ampicillin sodium and sulbactam sodium plus a macrolide. New fluoroquinolones with improved activity against *S pneumoniae* can also be used to treat adults with community-acquired pneumonia. Vancomycin hydrochloride is not routinely indicated for the treatment of community-acquired pneumonia or pneumonia caused by drug-resistant *S pneumoniae*.

Centers for Disease Control and Prevention (CDC). Recommended adult immunization schedule United States 2010. http://www.cdc.gov/vaccines/pubs/ACIP-list.htm. Accessed February 9, 2010.

Centers for Disease Control and Prevention (CDC). Vaccine Information Sheet (VIS) PCV13. www.cdc.gov/vaccines/hcp/vis/vis-statements/pcv13.html. Accessed February 27, 2013.

Centers for Disease Control and Prevention (CDC). Vaccine Information Sheet (VIS) PPSV23. www.cdc.gov/vaccines/hcp/vis/vis-statements/ppv.html. Accessed October 6, 2009.

Ebell MH. Outpatient vs. inpatient treatment of community-acquired pneumonia. *Am Fam Physician.* 2006;73:1425. [PMID: 16669565]

Mandell LA, Bartlett JG, Dowell SF, et al. Infectious Diseases Society of America: update of practice guidelines for the management of community-acquired pneumonia in immunocompetent adults. *Clin Infect Dis.* 2003;37:1405–1433. [PMID: 14614663]

Ramanujam P, Rathlev NK. Blood cultures do not change management in hospitalized patients with community-acquired pneumonia. *Acad Emerg Med.* 2006;13:740. [PMID: 16766742]

▼ NONINFECTIOUS RESPIRATORY PROBLEMS

ASTHMA

ESSENTIALS OF DIAGNOSIS

▶ Recurrent wheezing, shortness of breath, or cough.

▶ Histories of allergies in children.

▶ Increase in airway secretions.

▶ Airway constriction, obstruction, or both.

▶ Bronchospasm documented on spirometry.

▶ Dyspnea.

▶ General Considerations

Asthma is one of the most common illnesses in childhood. Risk factors for the development of asthma include living in poverty and being in a nonwhite racial group. Part of the difference in asthma rates noted among different races may be related to increased exposure to allergens and other irritants such as air pollution, cigarette smoke, dust mites, and cockroaches in less affluent families, but racial differences persist even after adjusting for socioeconomic status.

Allergy is an important factor in asthma development in children but does not appear to be as significant a factor in adults. Although as many as 80% of children with asthma also are atopic, 70% of adults age <30 years and fewer than half of all adults age ≥30 years have any evidence of allergy. Therefore, although an allergic component should be sought in adults, it is less commonly found than in children with asthma.

▶ Clinical Findings

In most cases, the diagnosis of asthma is based on symptoms of recurrent wheezing, shortness of breath, or cough. Children with recurrent cases of "bronchitis" who experience nighttime cough or have difficulty with exercise tolerance should be suspected of having asthma. An additional history of allergies is useful, because 80% of childhood asthma is associated with atopy.

Formal spirometry testing can usually be accomplished in children as young as 5 years of age and can confirm the diagnosis of asthma. Both the forced expiratory volume in 1 second (FEV_1) and FEV_1 to forced vital capacity (FVC) ratio are useful in documenting obstruction to airway flow. Further confirmation is provided by improvement of the FEV_1 by ≥12% following the use of a short-acting bronchodilator. For a valid test, though, children should avoid using a long-acting β-agonist in the previous 24 hours or a short-acting β-agonist in the previous 6 hours.

In some patients with asthma, spirometry may be normal. When there is a high index of suspicion that asthma may still be present, provocative testing with methacholine may be necessary to make the diagnosis.

It is useful to stratify patients with asthma by the severity of their illness. The severity of asthma is based on the frequency, intensity, and duration of baseline symptoms; level of airflow obstruction; and the extent to which asthma interferes with daily activities. Stages of severity range from severe persistent (step 4), in which symptoms are chronic and limit activity, to mild intermittent (step 1), in which symptoms are present no more than twice a week and pulmonary function studies are normal between exacerbations (Table 28–6). Patients are classified as to severity on the basis of their worst symptom and frequency, regardless of whether they met all or the majority of the criteria in any category.

▶ Treatment

The approach to managing asthma relies on acute management of exacerbations, treatment of chronic airway inflammation, monitoring of respiratory function, and control of the factors that precipitate wheezing episodes. For all of these, patient and family education is vital.

Treatment of persistent asthma requires daily medication to prevent long-term airway remodeling. Mild, intermittent asthma may require therapy only during wheezing episodes. Guidelines for the management of asthma are based on the child's age (≤6 years) and are stratified by severity of illness. Guidelines for older children, adults, and younger children are provided in Table 28–7.

The treatment of exacerbations of asthma relies on fast-acting bronchodilators to produce rapid changes in airway resistance along with management of the late-phase changes that occur several hours after the initial symptoms are manifested. The failure to recognize the late-phase component of an acute exacerbation may lead to a rebound of symptoms several hours after the patient has left the office or emergency department. Corticosteroids are the mainstay for preventing the late-phase response.

For patients with persistent symptoms (step 2 and higher), chronic therapy is required. The management of persistent asthma may include long-acting bronchodilators to control intermittent symptoms and nighttime cough, but also should

Table 28–6. Classification of asthma severity.

Step	Symptoms	Nighttime Symptoms	Lung Function
Step 4 Severe persistent	Continual symptoms Limited physical activity Frequent exacerbations	Frequent	Forced expiratory volume in 1 second (FEV_1) or peak expiratory flow (PEF) ≤60% predicted PEF variability >30%
Step 3 Moderate persistent	Daily symptoms Daily use of inhaled short-acting β_2-agonist Exacerbations affect activity Exacerbations ≥2 times a week; may last days	>1 time a week	FEV_1 or PEF >60–<80% predicted PEF variability >30%
Step 2 Mild persistent	Symptoms >2 times a week but <1 time a day Exacerbations may affect activity	>2 times a month	FEV_1 or PEF ≥80% predicted PEF variability 20–30%
Step 1 Mild intermittent	Symptoms <2 times a week Asymptomatic and normal PEF between exacerbations Exacerbations are brief; variable intensity	≤2 times a month	FEV_1 or PEF ≥80% predicted PEF variability <20%

provide chronic anti-inflammatory therapy to prevent long-term remodeling. Both inhaled steroids and nonsteroidal anti-inflammatory medications (ie, cromoglycates) can provide anti-inflammatory therapy. When symptoms are recurrent or large doses of anti-inflammatory agents are required, treatment with a leukotriene inhibitor can provide additional anti-inflammatory therapy and may allow a reduction in the dose of other anti-inflammatory agents such as steroids.

When drugs are selected for the treatment of asthma, the potential side effects of each agent need to be weighed against the potential benefits. For children, chronic use of inhaled steroids has been associated with a small decrease in total height attained. Although the difference in height attainment is small, it might be preferable to use nonsteroidal anti-inflammatory agents such as cromolyn and nedocromil in children.

In addition to pharmacologic management, patients with asthma should avoid known and possible airway irritants. These include cigarette smoke (including second-hand inhalation of smoke), environmental pollutants, suspected or known allergens, and cold air. Children who have difficulty participating in sports may benefit from the use of a short-acting β-agonist such as albuterol before participating in exertion to prevent wheezing or cough.

The monitoring of pulmonary function is an important component of asthma management for all patients with persistent disease. Children and adults should be provided with a peak-flow meter and instructed on how to use the device reliably. The use of a peak-flow meter can detect subtle changes in respiratory function that may not cause symptoms for several days. To use a peak-flow meter, patients must establish a "personal best," which represents the best reading that they can obtain when they are as asymptomatic as possible. Daily or periodic recordings of peak flows are compared with this personal best to gauge the current pulmonary function. Readings between 80% and 100% of the personal best indicate that the patient is doing well. Peak flows between 50% and 80% of an individual's personal best are cause for concern even if symptoms are mild. Patients should be instructed beforehand how to respond in these instances. If a repeat of the peak flow later in the day after appropriate measures have been taken does not show improvement, patients should seek further medical attention. Patients should be told that severe decreases in peak flow to <50% are cause for immediate medical attention.

For patients with allergic symptoms, the use of immunotherapy should be considered. However, although immunotherapy usually results in improvements in symptoms of allergic rhinitis, it seldom improves asthma symptoms.

Namazy JA, Schatz JM. Current guidelines for the management of asthma during pregnancy. *Immunol Allergy Clin North Am.* 2006;26:93. [PMID: 16443415]

Siwik JP, Nowak RM, Zoratti EM. The evaluation and management of acute, severe asthma. *Med Clin North Am.* 2002;86:1049. [PMID: 12428545]

CHRONIC OBSTRUCTIVE PULMONARY DISEASE

 ESSENTIALS OF DIAGNOSIS

▶ Productive cough featuring sputum production for ≥3 months for 2 consecutive years.

▶ Chronic dyspnea.

▶ FEV_1 >80% predicted.

Table 28–7. Asthma drug therapy based on severity.

Step	Ages 6 Years Through Adulthood	
	Daily Medications	**Quick Relief**
Step 4 Severe persistent	Choose all needed High-dose inhaled corticosteroid Long-acting bronchodilator A leukotriene modifier Oral corticosteroid	Short-acting bronchodilator Daily or increasing use of short-acting inhaled β_2-agonist indicates need for additional long-term control therapy
Step 3 Moderate persistent	Usually need two Either low- or medium-dose inhaled corticosteroid Long-acting bronchodilator	Short-acting bronchodilator Daily or increasing use of short-acting inhaled β_2-agonist indicates need for additional long-term control therapy
Step 2 Mild persistent	Choose one Low-dose inhaled corticosteroid cromolyn Sustained-release theophylline (to serum concentration of 5–15 µg/mL) A leukotriene modifier	Short-acting bronchodilator Daily or increasing use of short-acting inhaled β_2-agonist indicates need for additional long-term control therapy
Step 1 Intermittent	No daily medication needed	Short-acting bronchodilator Use of short-acting inhaled β_2-agonist >2 times per week indicates need for additional long-term control therapy
	Step Down	**Step Up**
	Review treatment every 1–6 months; a gradual step-wise reduction in treatment may be possible	If control is not maintained, consider step up; first, review patient medication technique, adherence, and environmental control (avoidance of allergens and/or other factors that contribute to asthma severity)
Step	**Daily Anti-inflammatory Medications**	**Quick Relief**
Step 4 Severe persistent	High-dose inhaled corticosteroid with spacer/holding chamber and facemask and, if needed, add systemic corticosteroids 2 mg/kg per day and reduce to lowest daily or alternate-day dose that stabilizes symptoms	Short-acting bronchodilator as needed for symptoms By nebulizer or metered-dose inhaler (MDI) with spacer/holding chamber and facemask or oral β_2-agonist Daily or increasing use of short-acting inhaled β_2-agonist indicates need for additional long-term control therapy
Step 3 Moderate persistent	Either medium-dose inhaled corticosteroid with spacer/holding chamber and facemask or low- to medium-dose inhaled corticosteroid and long-acting bronchodilator (theophylline)	Short-acting bronchodilator as needed for symptoms By nebulizer or MDI with spacer/holding chamber and facemask or oral β_2-agonist Daily or increasing use of short-acting inhaled β_2-agonist indicates need for additional long-term control therapy
Step 2 Mild	Young children usually begin with a trial of cromolyn or low-dose inhaled corticosteroid with spacer/holding chamber and facemask	Short-acting bronchodilator as needed for symptoms By nebulizer or MDI with spacer/holding chamber and facemask or oral β_2-agonist Daily or increasing use of short-acting inhaled β_2-agonist indicates need for additional long-term control therapy
Step 1 Intermittent	No daily medication	Short-acting bronchodilator as needed for symptoms <2 times a week By nebulizer or MDI with spacer/holding chamber and facemask or oral β_2-agonist Two times weekly or increasing use of short-acting inhaled β_2-agonist indicates need for additional long-term control therapy
	Step Down	**Step Up**
	Review treatment every 1–6 months; a gradual step-wise reduction in treatment may be possible	If control is not maintained, consider step up; first, review patient medication technique, adherence, and environmental control (avoidance of allergens and/or other factors that contribute to asthma severity)

General Considerations

Chronic airway disease is the second leading cause of disability in the United States after coronary artery disease. It is also fourth in the list of leading causes of death in the United States. Consistently more women died secondary to COPD than men. Symptoms of chronic bronchitis first develop when patients are between 30 and 40 years of age and become increasingly common as patients reach their 50s and 60s. The development of chronic bronchitis is associated with heavier cigarette use; those smoking over 25 cigarettes per day have a risk of chronic bronchitis that is 30 times higher than that for nonsmokers. Although chronic bronchitis affects both genders and all socioeconomic strata, it is more commonly observed in men and in those of lower socioeconomic classes. It is presumed that these populations may be at higher risk due to higher consumption of cigarettes observed in these groups.

In addition to smoking, air pollution may affect the development and exacerbation of symptoms in patients with chronic bronchitis. Patients with COPDs who live in industrialized areas with heavy levels of particulate air pollution may be at increased risk of recurrent disease and death.

Only 10–15% of smokers will develop COPD, so other factors must also play a role in the progression from acute to chronic lung damage. The development of chronic bronchitis is assumed to include both a predisposition to inflammatory damage and exposure to the proper stimuli that cause inflammation, such as cigarette smoke or pollutants. Genetic factors, prolonged heavy exposure to other inflammatory mediators such as environmental pollutants, preexisting lung impairment from other inflammatory processes such as recurrent infection or childhood passive smoke exposure, and other mechanisms may all predispose individuals to the development of chronic bronchitis from smoking.

α_1-Antitrypsin deficiency is a rare genetic abnormality that causes panlobular emphysema in adults and is responsible for approximately 2–3% of cases of COPD. This trait is inherited in an autosomal recessive pattern. Nonsmokers with this genetic defect develop emphysema at young ages. Those with this trait who smoke develop progressive emphysema at very early ages. Emphysema related to α_1-antitrypsin deficiency rarely shows up below age 25 and rarely in nonsmokers.

Clinical Findings

COPD includes both chronic bronchitis and emphysema, and these two often coexist. Chronic bronchitis is characterized by a productive cough featuring sputum production for ≥3 months for 2 consecutive years. Emphysema causes chronic dyspnea due to destruction of lung tissue, resulting in enlargement of airspace and reduced compliance. In most cases, chronic bronchitis and emphysema can be differentiated according to whether the predominant symptom is a chronic cough or dyspnea. In contrast to asthma, changes in COPD are relatively fixed and only partially reversible with bronchodilator use.

When suspected clinically, COPD can be confirmed with chest radiography and spirometry. Although chest radiographic findings occur much later in the course of the disease than alterations in pulmonary function testing, a chest x-ray may be useful in patients suspected of having COPD because it can detect several other clinical conditions often found in these patients.

Spirometry is generally used to diagnose COPD because it can detect small changes in lung function and is easy to quantify. Changes in the FEV_1 and the FVC can provide an estimate of the degree of airway obstruction in these patients. Symptoms of COPD usually develop when FEV_1 falls below 80% of the predicted rate. In addition, a peak expiratory flow rate of <350 L/min in adults is a sign that COPD is likely to be present.

Spirometry also is useful in gauging the severity of COPD. Decreases in FEV_1 on serial testing are associated with increased mortality rates (ie, patients with a faster decline in FEV_1 have a higher rate of death). The major risk factor associated with an accelerated rate of decline of FEV_1 is continued cigarette smoking. Smoking cessation in patients with early COPD improves lung function initially and slows the annual loss of FEV_1. Once FEV_1 falls below 1 L, 5-year survival is approximately 50%.

The US Preventive Services Task Force (USPSTF) has recommended against the use of spirometry to screen asymptomatic adult patients for COPD, which carries a D recommendation.

Treatment

A. Nonpharmacologic Therapy

The first step in treating the patient with chronic bronchitis or COPD is to promote a healthy lifestyle. Regular exercise and weight control should be started and smoking stopped to maximize the patient's therapeutic options.

Smoking cessation is the first and most important treatment option in the management of chronic bronchitis or COPD. Several interventions to assist patients in smoking cessation are available. These include behavioral modification techniques as well as pharmacotherapy (see the next section). A combination of behavioral and pharmacologic approaches such as nicotine replacement appears to yield the best results. Even minimal counseling from the provider improves the effectiveness of the nicotine patch.

Once patients have stopped smoking, those who are hypoxemic with a Pao_2 (partial pressure of oxygen in arterial blood) of ≤55 mmHg or an O_2 saturation of ≤88% while sleeping should receive supplemental oxygen. Along with smoking cessation, home oxygen is the only therapy shown to reduce mortality in COPD. Continuous long-term oxygen therapy (LTOT) should be considered in patients with stable chronic pulmonary disease with Pao_2 of <55 mmHg on room air, at rest, and awake. The presence of polycythemia, pulmonary hypertension, right heart failure, or hypercapnia (Pao_2 >45 mmHg) is also an indication for use of continuous LTOT.

Exercise and pulmonary rehabilitation may also be beneficial as adjunct therapies for patients whose symptoms are not adequately controlled with appropriate pharmacotherapy. Exercise and pulmonary rehabilitation are most useful for patients who are restricted in their activities and have decreased quality of life.

B. Pharmacotherapy

1. Smoking cessation pharmacotherapy—Multiple medications are available to assist with smoking cessation. Nicotine can be substituted 1 mg (1 cigarette) per milligram with the use of the patch, gum, or inhaler to help with symptoms of nicotine withdrawal. Patches and gum are both available over the counter as well as by prescription. Some evidence suggests that use of the patch and gum simultaneously enhances quit rates, but use of both is not approved by the US Food and Drug Administration. Although all these products state that patients must not smoke while using nicotine replacement because of early case reports of myocardial infarction, more recent studies show that smoking is relatively safe when using nicotine replacement and may help reduce smoking before a patient actually quits. However, even at best, the cessation rate is only ~20–30% at 1 year.

Bupropion also is approved for smoking cessation as an adjunct to behavior modification. The main effect of bupropion is to reduce symptoms of nicotine withdrawal. Bupropion should be instituted for 2 weeks before the quitting target date. Then a nicotine substitute can be used in combination to maximize alleviation of symptoms of nicotine withdrawal. Because many patients with chronic bronchitis are already taking multiple medications, potential drug interactions and adverse effects must be considered before instituting therapy with bupropion.

A third agent to assist in smoking cessation is varenicline tartrate. Varenicline is a selective nicotine receptor partial agonist. The drug stimulates nicotine receptors to produce a nicotine replacement–type effect but also blocks the receptors from additional exogenous nicotine stimulation. Use of varenicline has been reported to achieve quit rates of 40% at 12 weeks and continuous quit rates of ~22% after 1 year, which was significantly more than either bupropion or nicotine replacement alone. Adverse effects of varenicline occur in 20–30% of patients and include nausea, insomnia, headache, and abnormal dreams but necessitated discontinuation of the drug in 2–3% of patients in clinical trials.

2. Bronchodilators—An anticholinergic agent such as ipratropium bromide is the drug of choice for patients with persistent symptoms of chronic bronchitis. Anticholinergic agents such as ipratropium bromide or tiotropium have fewer side effects and a better response than intermittent β-agonists. Although both of these agents have a delayed onset of action compared with short-acting β-agonists, the beneficial effects are prolonged. Ipratropium requires dosing several times a day; in contrast, tiotropium can be used once a day.

For patients with mild to moderately severe symptoms, intermittent use of a β-agonist inhaler such as albuterol is sometimes beneficial even without significant changes in their FEV_1. Adverse effects of β-agonist agents include tachycardia, nervousness, and tremor. Short-acting β-agonists may not last through the night; when nighttime symptoms develop, long-acting β-agonists such as salmeterol may be more useful. Levalbuterol, the active agent of racemic albuterol, has recently been studied and appears to have greater efficacy than albuterol with fewer side effects.

Combination inhalers of ipratropium bromide and albuterol have also been used in the treatment of patients with chronic bronchitis but have demonstrated only minimal changes in outcomes compared with single agents.

3. Antibiotics—Patients with acute exacerbations of chronic bronchitis pose a more difficult therapeutic dilemma. Many of these exacerbations are probably due to viral infections. However, a meta-analysis of studies using a wide range of antibiotics (ampicillin, sulfamethoxazole-trimethoprim, and tetracyclines) demonstrated some benefit from empiric use of antibiotics for exacerbations of chronic bronchitis.

4. Other agents—As symptoms increase, addition of inhaled β-agonists, theophylline, and corticosteroids may provide symptomatic relief of symptoms of chronic bronchitis. In a multicenter randomized placebo-controlled trial, patients who used inhaled fluticasone had improved peak expiratory flows, FEV_1, FVC, and midexpiratory flow. At the end of treatment, patients also showed increased exercise tolerance compared with the placebo group. Corticosteroids at a therapeutic dose of 60 mg/d for 5 days have been shown to provide some symptomatic relief for severe exacerbations.

Mucolytics have not been shown to be beneficial. Iodinated glycerol has not been shown to improve any objective outcome measurements.

Newer agents such as aerosolized surfactant also have been used to treat stable chronic bronchitis. A prospective randomized controlled trial showed a minimal but statistically significant improvement in spirometry and sputum clearance. However, the cost of such a treatment regimen is high and may not add any advantage to the underlying treatment.

For the treatment of cough, agents that may be of benefit for patients with chronic bronchitis include ipratropium bromide, guaimesal, dextromethorphan, and viminol.

Anabolic steroids have recently been used for patients who have severe malnutrition and in those in whom weight loss is a concern. These agents show some beneficial effects.

American Lung Association. Chronic obstructive pulmonary disease (COPD) fact sheet. http://www.lungusa.org/lung-disease/copd/resources/facts-figures/COPD-Fact-Sheet.html. Accessed May 2014.

Armstrong C. ACP updates guideline on diagnosis and management of stable COPD. *Am Fam Physician*. 2012;85(2):204–205. [PMID: 22335223]

Bach PB, Brown C, Gelfand SE, et al. American College of Physicians—American Society of Internal Medicine; American College of Chest Physicians: management of acute exacerbations of chronic obstructive pulmonary disease: a summary and appraisal of published evidence. *Ann Intern Med*. 2001;134:600. [PMID: 11281745]

Snow V, Lascher S, Mottur-Pilson C, et al. Joint Expert Panel on Chronic Obstructive Pulmonary Disease of the American College of Chest Physicians and the American College of Physicians—American Society of Internal Medicine: evidence base for management of acute exacerbations of chronic obstructive pulmonary disease. *Ann Intern Med*. 2001;134:595. [PMID: 11281744]

Stephens MB, Yew KS. Diagnosis of chronic obstructive pulmonary disease. *Am Fam Physician*. 2008;78(1):87–92. [PMID: 18649615]

US Preventive Screening Task Force (USPSTF). Screening for chronic obstructive pulmonary disease using spirometry. http://www.ahrq.gov/clinic/uspstf08/copd/copdrs.htm. Accessed March 2008.

EMBOLIC DISEASE

ESSENTIALS OF DIAGNOSIS

▶ Dyspnea.

▶ Hypoxia.

▶ Pleuritic pain.

General Considerations

Pulmonary embolism (PE) usually results from the mobilization of blood clots from thromboses in the lower extremities or pelvis. However, embolization of other materials, including air, fat, and amniotic fluid, also can obstruct the pulmonary vasculature. The symptoms of PE range from mild, intermittent shortness of breath or pleuritic chest pain to complete circulatory collapse and death.

The most common source of embolism is the disruption of thrombi formed in the deep veins. Mortality in untreated cases is 30% but can be reduced to 2% with prompt recognition and appropriate management. Recurrent PE carries a very high mortality in the range of 45–50%.

Strong risk factors for PE are leg or hip fracture, major general surgery, knee or hip replacement, spinal cord injury, and major trauma. Other risk factors include venous stasis, trauma, abnormalities in the deep veins, and hypercoagulable states. Hypercoagulability occurs with some cancers as well as with inherited conditions such as factor V Leiden

mutation, which results in resistance to the anticoagulant effects of protein C. Other congenital hypercoagulation disorders include protein C deficiency, protein S deficiency, and antithrombin III deficiency.

Hypercoagulation states also exist with the use of certain medications. Use of estrogens either as part of hormone replacement therapy or for contraception increases the risk by a factor of 3. The effects of these drugs are compounded in patients with factor V Leiden mutation. Pregnancy and postpartum states increase the risk of PE.

In addition, smoking appears to be an independent risk factor for deep vein thrombosis (DVT) and PE. The presence of more than two of these risk factors places the patient at a synergistic increased risk for the development of venous thromboembolism.

Prevention

Because PEs usually arise from lower extremity thromboses, prophylactic anticoagulation can be used to reduce the incidence of these thrombi in high-risk individuals. Both low-molecular-weight heparin products and unfractionated heparin are effective in preventing DVT. Selection of the agent and the dose is based on the risk. The decision to initiate VTE prophylaxis should be based on the patient's individual risk of thromboembolism and bleeding and the balance of benefits versus harms. Risk factors for thromboembolism are inherited (eg, factor V Leiden mutation, prothrombin gene mutation, protein S or C deficiency, antithrombin deficiency) or are acquired (eg, surgery, cancer, immobilization, trauma, presence of a central venous catheter, pregnancy, medication use, congestive heart failure, chronic renal disease, antiphospholipid antibody syndrome, obesity, smoking, older age, history of thromboembolism). Although there are many tools for assessing thromboembolism risk, there is insufficient evidence to recommend one over the others. General evidence regarding risk factors also may be used to make decisions about the need for prophylaxis.

Heparin or a related drug can increase the risk of bleeding, especially in older patients; women; patients with diabetes mellitus, hypertension, cancer, alcoholism, liver disease, severe chronic kidney disease, peptic ulcer disease, anemia, poor treatment adherence, previous stroke or intracerebral hemorrhage, bleeding lesions, or bleeding disorder; and patients taking certain concomitant medications.

Prophylaxis with heparin has been shown to significantly reduce PEs in hospitalized patients, although bleeding events were increased. In most patients, the clinical benefit of decreased PEs outweighs the risk of bleeding. Evidence is insufficient to conclude that these risks and benefits differ in patients with stroke, although prevention of recurrent stroke may be an added benefit in these patients.

The optimal duration of heparin therapy is unclear. The benefits and risks are not significantly different between low-molecular-weight heparin and unfractionated heparin, and fondaparinux (Arixtra) has not been directly compared with heparin. The choice of medication should be based on ease of use, adverse effect profile, and cost.

Use of graduated compression stockings was not shown to be effective in preventing VTE or reducing mortality and can cause clinically important damage to the skin. Intermittent pneumatic compression may be a reasonable option if heparin is contraindicated, because evidence suggests that it is beneficial in patients undergoing surgery. However, the therapy has not been sufficiently evaluated as a standalone intervention in other patients.

In addition to preventing initial thrombi, the PE can be reduced through the use of a venacaval filter in patients with known thrombi and contraindications to long-term anticoagulation. The long-term impact of intravenacaval (IVC) filters has not been studied extensively. One study showed a complication rate, such as thrombi trapped in the filter or the filter tilting, malpositioning, or migrating, in nearly 50% of those who survived 3 years. However, given the high mortality rates from recurrent PE, the complication rates from long-term IVC filter insertion appear to be a worthwhile trade-off in high-risk patients.

▶ Clinical Findings

Patients with PEs usually exhibit dyspnea and hypoxia and often have pleuritic chest pain. However, other than hypoxia, most routine studies including chest radiographs may be normal. The clinical assessment of the patient should include the criteria in the Wells score looking at signs and symptoms consistent with DVT, different diagnosis less likely, a heart rate of >100 bpm, previous PE or DVT, surgery within the past 4 weeks or immobilization, current malignancy, and presence of hemoptysis. Scores placed patients in either a low, intermediate, or high probability of having a PE. The Christopher study (modified Wells study) further divided the scoring into PE likely or unlikely. Suspicious signs of embolism on a chest radiograph include a wedge-shaped infiltrate resulting from lobar infarction, new pleural effusion, or both. Confirmation of a PE is based on either demonstrating obstruction of vascular flow through pulmonary angiography, finding a mismatch of perfusion and ventilation, or visualization of a clot on spiral (helical) computed tomography (CT) scanning. Although pulmonary angiography is considered the gold standard, because of its invasiveness, spiral CT and ventilation-perfusion scan are usually employed to make the diagnosis. Of the noninvasive tests available, spiral CT has the best sensitivity for detecting pulmonary artery thrombi (95–100%), although it is not as useful in identifying subsegmental emboli.

D-dimer testing has been evaluated as a serum marker for PE or DVT. The presence of D-dimer is not specific for thrombotic disease because D-dimer also rises in other conditions such as recent surgery, congestive heart failure, myocardial infarction, and pneumonia. Although the presence of D-dimer is not useful in diagnosing thrombosis or embolism, the negative predictive value of the absence of D-dimer is very high (97–99%), so this test can be useful in ruling out embolism. Clinically predictive rules, such as the modified Wells, can be used together with the D-dimer test to identify those in the "PE unlikely" group who would not require further study. On the basis of these two tools, clinical assessment and laboratory test, those that fall into the "PE likely" category can be further evaluated with CT angiography or spiral CT.

▶ Treatment

Options for management of patients with an acute PE include anticoagulation to prevent further embolism from occurring, clot lysis with thrombolytic agents, or surgical removal of the clot.

Patients without life-threatening embolism can be managed with acute anticoagulation with heparin followed by long-term maintenance on warfarin. Heparin may be administered as either unfractionated heparin or low-molecular-weight heparin. Unfractionated heparin is generally administered intravenously with the dosage rate titrated to produce a suitable anticoagulation state. The use of a weight-based nomogram for loading and maintenance dosing can improve the time to achieve adequate anticoagulation and reduce the risks of bleeding. The drawbacks of unfractionated heparin include the need for hospitalization to monitor coagulation status and administer the intravenous drug plus the possibility of thrombocytopenia associated with the use of this agent. Should bleeding occur as a complication of treatment with unfractionated heparin, stopping the heparin is the first step to stop further anticoagulation. If bleeding continues after stopping the heparin, protamine can be given to reverse the anticoagulation.

In contrast, low-molecular-weight heparin can be administered as a daily intramuscular dose without titration or frequent anticoagulation monitoring. As a result, low-molecular-weight heparin therapy usually can be provided in the patient's home.

To achieve long-term anticoagulation, warfarin should be started promptly at a dose of 5 mg/d. Starting with a higher dose of warfarin does not appear to achieve oral anticoagulation any faster or reduce the total number of days when heparin is needed. Heparin can be discontinued when a prothrombin time indicates that the international normalized ratio (INR) has reached 2.0–3.0. Should excessive anticoagulation resulting from administering warfarin and bleeding occur, vitamin K can be given to reverse the effect of warfarin.

The duration of anticoagulation for PE depends on whether the precipitating event is known and reversible or whether the cause is unknown. In situations in which the thrombosis and embolism are the result of an acute event such as an injury or surgery, treatment for 6 months is recommended. If the risk factor associated with the embolic event is not reversible, such as cancer or coagulation disorder, then lifetime anticoagulation is advisable. When a risk factor or event causing the embolism is not known, so-called idiopathic embolism, treatment with anticoagulants for 6 months is indicated.

The use of thrombolytic agents for PE is usually reserved for patients with extensive embolism who show hemodynamic instability. Thrombolytic agents available for use in this situation include urokinase, streptokinase, tissue plasminogen activator (tPA), and reteplase. Embolectomy is rarely performed and is reserved for patients in whom embolism is rapidly diagnosed and a very large embolism is suspected that completely occludes the pulmonary arteries. In most situations, this is treated as a "last ditch" effort to save the patient.

Geerts WH, Pineo GF, Heit JA, et al. Prevention of venous thromboembolism: the Seventh ACCP Conference on Antithrombotic and Thrombolytic Therapy. *Chest.* 2004;126:338S–400S. [PMID: 15383478]

Gopinath A, Thomas R. *Pulmonary Embolism: Gildea of Cleveland Clinic Center for Continuing Education.* 2010. http://www.clevelanclinicmeded.com/medicalpubs/diseasemanagement/pulmonary/pulmonary-embolism/.

Piazza G, Goldhaber SZ. Acute pulmonary embolism. Part I: epidemiology and diagnosis. *Circulation.* 2006;114:e28. [PMID: 16831989]

Piazza G, Goldhaber SZ. Acute pulmonary embolism. Part II: treatment and prophylaxis. *Circulation.* 2006;114:e42. [PMID: 16847156]

Qaseem A, Chou R, Humphrey LL, et al. Venous thromboembolism prophylaxis in hospitalized patients: a clinical practice guideline from the American College of Physicians. *Ann Intern Med.* 2011;155(9):625–632. [PMID: 22041951]

Takagi H, Umemoto T. An algorithm for managing suspected pulmonary embolism. *JAMA.* 2006;295:2603. [PMID: 16772621]

29

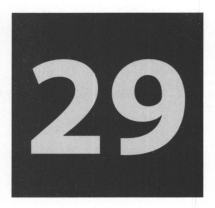

Evaluation & Management of Headache

Scott A. Harper, MD
Jennifer E. Roper, MD
Rachel K. F. Woodruff, MD, MPH
C. Randall Clinch, DO, MS

ESSENTIALS OF DIAGNOSIS

- Migraine.
  - Headache lasting 4–72 hours.
  - Unilateral onset, often spreading bilaterally.
  - Pulsating quality and moderate or severe intensity of pain.
  - Aggravated by or inhibiting physical activity.
  - Nausea and/or photophobia and phonophobia.
  - May present with an aura.
- Cluster headache.
  - Strictly unilateral orbital, supraorbital, or temporal pain lasting 15–180 minutes.
  - Explosive, excruciating pain.
  - One attack every other day to eight attacks per day.
- Tension-type headache.
  - Pressing or tightening (nonpulsating) pain.
  - Bilateral band-like distribution of pain.
  - Not aggravated by routine physical activity.

General Considerations

Headache is among the most common pain syndromes, consistently ranking as the fourth or fifth leading reason to present to an emergency department (ED) and accounting for approximately 3% of all ED visits. Population-based studies reveal that approximately 15% of all US adults report having had a migraine or severe headache in the last 3 months, with a female-to-male ratio of approximately 2.4:1. Regarding tension-type headache, the prevalence among both genders is 31.2–38.3% for episodic and 2.2% for chronic tension-type headache. Cluster headache has a prevalence of about 0.1% of the US population, with a male-to-female ratio of approximately 3:1. Although headache disorders such as migraine, tension-type, and cluster headaches are most frequently encountered, the main task before the primary care provider is to determine whether the patient has a potentially life-threatening headache disorder and, if not, to provide appropriate management to limit disability from headache.

A distinction between primary headaches (ie, benign, recurrent headaches having no organic disease as their cause) and secondary headaches (ie, those caused by an underlying, organic disease) is practical in primary care. Over 90% of patients presenting to primary care providers have a primary headache disorder. These disorders include migraine (with and without aura), tension-type headache, and cluster headache. Secondary headache disorders constitute the minority of presentations; however, given that their underlying etiology may range from sinusitis to subarachnoid hemorrhage, these headache disorders often present the greatest diagnostic challenge to the practicing clinician. The International Headache Society provides a detailed classification of primary and secondary headache disorders on their website (https://www.ichd-3.org/).

Burch R, Rizzoli P, Loder E. The prevalence and impact of migraine and severe headache in the United States: figures and trends from government health studies. *Headache.* 2018;58(4): 496–505. [PMID: 29527677]

Headache Classification Committee of the International Headache Society (IHS). The International Classification of Headache Disorders, 3rd edition. *Cephalalgia.* 2018;38:1–211. [PMID: 29368949]

Hoffmann J, May A. Diagnosis, pathophysiology, and management of cluster headache. *Lancet Neurol.* 2018;17:75–83. [PMID: 29174963]

Kaniecki RG. Tension-type headache. *Continuum.* 2012;18: 823–834. [PMID: 22868544]

Table 29–1. Questions to ask when obtaining a headache history.

H:	How severe is your headache on a scale of 1–10 (1 = minimal pain, 10 = severe pain)? How did this headache start (gradually, suddenly, other)? How long have you had this headache?
E:	Ever had headaches before? Ever had a headache this bad before (first or worst headache)? Ever have headaches just like this one in the past?
A:	Any other symptoms noted before or during your headache? Any symptoms right now?
D:	Describe the quality of your pain (throbbing, stabbing, dull, other). Describe the location of your pain. Describe where your pain radiates. Describe any other medical problems you may have. Describe your use of medications (prescription and over-the-counter products). Describe any history of recent trauma or any medical or dental procedures.

► Clinical Findings

A. Symptoms and Signs

1. History—The majority of patients presenting with headache have a normal neurologic and general physical examination; for this reason, the headache history is of utmost importance (Table 29–1). A key issue in the headache history is identifying patients presenting with "red flags"—diagnostic alarms that prompt greater concern for the presence of a secondary headache disorder and a greater potential need for additional laboratory evaluation and/or neuroimaging (Table 29–2). The mnemonic SNOOP can be an aid in identifying red flags in the history of a patient with headache. SNOOP stands for **s**ystemic symptoms, conditions, or illness; **n**eurologic signs or symptoms; **o**nset (eg, sudden, trauma-related); **o**lder age of onset (ie, age ≥50 years); and **p**attern of change in a previous headache condition.

The onset of primary headache disorders is usually between 20 and 40 years of age; however, they may occur at any age. Patients without a history of headaches who present with a new-onset headache outside this age range should be considered at higher risk for a secondary headache disorder. Additional testing or neuroimaging in these patients or those complaining of their "first or worst" headache should be seriously considered. Temporal (giant cell) arteritis should be a consideration in any patient age ≥50 years with a new complaint of head, facial, or scalp pain, diplopia, or jaw claudication.

Symptoms suggesting a recurring, transient neurologic event, typically lasting 30–60 minutes and preceding headache onset, strongly suggest the presence of an aura and an associated migraine headache disorder. Migraine without aura, the most common form of migraine (formerly called common migraine), may present with unilateral pain in the head (cephalalgia) with subsequent generalization of pain to the entire head. Bilateral cephalalgia is present in a small percentage of migraineurs at the onset of their headache.

Table 29–2. Red flags in the evaluation of acute headaches in adults.

Red Flag	Potential Etiologies	Possible Evaluation
Headache beginning after 50 years of age	Temporal arteritis, tumor/mass	Erythrocyte sedimentation rate, MRI with and without contrast
Headache of sudden onset	Subarachnoid hemorrhage, pituitary hemorrhage, expansion or hemorrhage of arteriovenous malformation (AVM)	CT without contrast (to assess for acute bleed), lumbar puncture if CT is negative
Headaches increasing in frequency and severity	Expansion of AVM or mass, subdural hematoma, medication overuse	MRI with and without contrast versus CT with contrast, urine drug screen
New-onset headache in immunocompromised patient (eg, HIV, cancer)	Meningitis, brain abscess, metastatic disease	MRI with and without contrast, lumbar puncture if neuroimaging is negative
Headache with signs of systemic illness (eg, fever, stiff neck, rash)	Meningitis, encephalitis, Lyme disease, systemic infection, collagen vascular disease	MRI with and without contrast, lumbar puncture, serology
Focal neurologic signs or symptoms (other than typical aura)	Mass/tumor, AVM, ischemic/hemorrhagic stroke, collagen vascular disease	MRI with and without contrast versus CT, serologic evaluation for collagen vascular disease evaluation
Papilledema	Mass/tumor, benign intracranial hypertension, meningitis	MRI with and without contrast versus CT, lumbar puncture
Posttraumatic headache	Intracranial hemorrhage, subdural hematoma, epidural hematoma, posttraumatic headache	CT without contrast versus MRI with and without contrast of brain, skull, and, possibly, cervical spine

CT, computed tomography; HIV, human immunodeficiency virus; MRI, magnetic resonance imaging.

Nausea accompanying a migraine may be debilitating and warrant specific treatment. A three-question screening tool, ID-Migraine, can assist primary care providers in making a diagnosis of migraine. If the screen is positive for two or more of the items, the sensitivity and specificity for migraine diagnosis are 82% and 75%, respectively.

Cluster headaches, most common among the trigeminal autonomic cephalalgia category, are strictly unilateral in location and are typically described as an explosive, deep, excruciating pain. Cluster headaches have a greater prevalence in men and are associated with ipsilateral autonomic signs and symptoms including lacrimation, conjunctival injection, ptosis, miosis, eyelid edema, nasal congestion and/or rhinorrhea, and forehead or facial sweating.

Tension-type headaches, the most prevalent form of primary headache disorder, often present with pericranial muscle tenderness and a description of a bilateral band-like distribution of the pain.

Patients with chronic medical conditions have a greater possibility of having an organic cause of their headache (see Table 29-2). Patients with cancer or human immunodeficiency virus (HIV) infection may present with central nervous system (CNS) metastases, lymphoma, toxoplasmosis, or meningitis as the etiology of their headache. Patients with hypertension in the range consistent with a hypertensive crisis (with diastolic pressures >110 mmHg) may present with headache; otherwise, headache is not typically a symptom related to hypertension. Elevated blood pressure has actually been demonstrated to be associated with a lower incidence of nonmigrainous headache in a large prospective study. Numerous medications have headache as a reported adverse effect, and medication overuse headache (formerly drug-induced headache) may occur following frequent use of analgesics or any antiheadache medication, including the triptans (eg, sumatriptan). The duration and severity of withdrawal headache following discontinuation of the medication vary with the medication itself, typically lasting from 2 to 10 days. Medical or dental procedures (eg, lumbar punctures, rhinoscopy, tooth extraction) may be associated with postprocedure headaches. Any history of head trauma or loss of consciousness should prompt concern for an intracranial hemorrhage in addition to a postconcussive disorder.

2. Physical examination—Physical examination is performed to attempt to identify a secondary, organic cause for the patient's headache. Additionally, any red flags identified during the headache history (see Table 29-2) warrant special attention on exam. A general physical examination should be performed, including vital signs; general appearance; and examinations of the head, eyes (including a funduscopic examination), ears, nose, throat, teeth, neck, and cardiovascular regions. Palpation of the head, face, and neck should also be a priority.

A detailed neurologic examination should be performed and the findings well documented. Assessment includes mental status testing; level of consciousness; pupillary responses; gait; coordination and cerebellar function; motor strength; sensory, deep tendon, and pathologic reflex testing; and cranial nerve tests. The presence or absence of meningeal irritation should be sought. Examinations such as evaluation for Kernig and Brudzinski signs should be documented; both signs may be absent, however, even in the presence of subarachnoid hemorrhage.

B. Laboratory Findings and Imaging Studies

Additional laboratory investigations should be driven by the history and any red flags that have been identified (see Table 29-2). The routine use of electroencephalography is not warranted in the evaluation of the patient with headache.

The rate of significant intracranial abnormalities (eg, acute cerebral infarct, neoplastic disease, hydrocephalus, or vascular abnormalities such as aneurysm or arteriovenous malformation) among patients with headache and a normal neurologic exam is <1%; as such, the routine use of neuroimaging is not cost effective. The American College of Radiology has published detailed recommendations about the appropriateness of neuroimaging for a wide variety of headache disorders.

In the setting of a severe, acute headache, computed tomography (CT) scanning without contrast medium followed, if negative, by lumbar puncture and cerebrospinal fluid (CSF) analysis is the preferred approach to attempt to diagnose subarachnoid hemorrhage. Xanthochromia, a yellow discoloration detectable on spectrophotometry, may aid in diagnosis if the CT scan and CSF analysis are normal but suspicion of subarachnoid hemorrhage remains high. Xanthochromia is present within 2 hours and may persist for up to 2 weeks following a subarachnoid hemorrhage. A validation study of the Ottawa Subarachnoid Hemorrhage Rule revealed a negative predictive value of 100% for a subarachnoid hemorrhage when the rule was applied against a cohort of patients presenting to the centers previously used during the derivation of the rule. Additional study may reveal that the application of this rule allows for the identification of patients who do not need additional investigation to rule out subarachnoid hemorrhage.

In addition to CSF analysis, lumbar puncture is useful for documenting abnormalities of CSF pressure in the setting of headache. Headaches are associated with low CSF pressure (<90 mmH$_2$O as measured by a manometer) and elevated CSF pressure (>200–250 mmH$_2$O). Headaches related to CSF hypotension include those caused by posttraumatic leakage of CSF (ie, after lumbar puncture or CNS trauma). Headaches related to CSF hypertension include those associated with idiopathic intracranial hypertension and CNS space-occupying lesions (ie, tumor, infection, mass, hemorrhage).

Table 29–3. Choosing Wisely Campaign recommendations about evaluation and management options in patients with headaches.

Organization	Recommendation
American Academy of Neurology	Don't perform electroencephalography (EEG) for headaches.
American Academy of Neurology	Don't use opioid or butalbital treatment for migraine except as a last resort.
American College of Emergency Physicians	Avoid computed tomography (CT) of the head in asymptomatic adult patients in the emergency department with syncope, insignificant trauma, and a normal neurologic evaluation.
American Headache Society	Don't perform neuroimaging studies in patients with stable headaches that meet criteria for migraine.
American Headache Society	Don't perform CT imaging for headache when magnetic resonance imaging (MRI) is available, except in emergency settings.
American Headache Society	Don't recommend surgical deactivation of migraine trigger points outside of a clinical trial.
American Headache Society	Don't prescribe opioid or butalbital-containing medications as first-line treatment for recurrent headache disorders.
American Headache Society	Don't recommend prolonged or frequent use of over-the-counter (OTC) pain medications for headache.
American College of Radiology	Don't do imaging for uncomplicated headache.

The Choosing Wisely Campaign provides several evidence-based recommendations from national organizations including the American Academy of Neurology, the American College of Emergency Physicians, the American Headache Society, and the American College of Radiology related to the evaluation and management of patients with headache (Table 29–3).

Buttgereit F, Dejaco C, Matteson EL, Dasgupta B. Polymyalgia rheumatica and giant cell arteritis: a systematic review. *JAMA.* 2016;315:2442–2458. [PMID: 27299619]

Choosing Wisely Recommendations. Five things patients and providers should question. http://www.choosingwisely.org/wp-content/uploads/2015/01/Choosing-Wisely-Recommendations.pdf. Accessed November 9, 2019.

Dodick DW. Diagnosing headache: Clinical clues and clinical rules. https://pdfs.semanticscholar.org/8f11/dd601f346b88c83cd353e1331d812a82ee39.pdf. Accessed November 9, 2019.

Douglas AC, Wippold FJ, Broderick DF, et al. ACR appropriateness criteria headache. *J Am Coll Radiol.* 2014;11:657–667. [PMID: 24933450]

Hagen K, Stovner LJ, Vatten L, Holmen J, Zwart J-A, Bovim G. Blood pressure and risk of headache: a prospective study of 22 685 adults in Norway. *J Neurol Neurosurg Psychiatry.* 2002;72: 463–466. [PMID: 11909904]

Jay GW, Barkin RL. Primary headache disorders part I: migraine and the trigeminal autonomic cephalalgias. *Dis Mon.* 2017;63: 308–338. [PMID: 28886860]

Jay GW, Barkin RL. Primary headache disorders part 2: tension-type headache and medication overuse headache. *Dis Mon.* 2017;63:342–367. [PMID: 28886861]

Katsarava Z, Fritsche G, Muessig M, Diener HC, Limmroth V. Clinical features of withdrawal headache following overuse of triptans and other headache drugs. *Neurology.* 2001;57(9): 1694–1698. [PMID: 11706113]

Katz M. The cost-effective evaluation of uncomplicated headache. *Med Clin North Am.* 2016;100:1009–1017. [PMID: 27542421]

Lipton RB. Risk factors for and management of medication-overuse headache. *Continuum (Minneap Minn).* 2015;21(4 Headache): 1118–1131. [PMID: 26252595]

Mehndiratta M, Nayak R, Garg H, Kumar M, Pandey S. Appraisal of Kernig's and Brudzinski's sign in meningitis. *Ann Indian Acad Neurol.* 2012;15:287–288. [PMID: 23349594]

Peng K-P, Wang S-J. Migraine diagnosis: screening items, instruments, and scales. *Acta Anaesthesiol Taiwan.* 2012;50:69–73. [PMID: 22769861]

▶ Differential Diagnosis

In addition to migraine, tension-type, and cluster headaches, a differential diagnosis for acute headaches in adults is presented in Table 29–2.

▶ Treatment

Treatment of headache is best individualized with respect to a thorough history, physical examination, and the interpretation of appropriate ancillary testing. Secondary headaches require accurate diagnosis and therapy directed at the underlying etiology. Nonpharmacologic measures and cognitive behavioral therapy (CBT) are worth consideration in most patients with primary headache disorders. CBT may have a prophylactic effect in migraine similar to propranolol (ie, an approximate 50% reduction). Cluster headache, chronic tension-type headache, and medication overuse headache respond poorly to CBT as monotherapy. The evidence for a benefit of acupuncture in the preventive treatment of migraine and the acute and preventive treatment of tension-type headache now reveals it to be an effective option. A systematic review of six randomized controlled trials of manual therapies in chronic headache revealed a positive effect of massage and physiotherapy in the treatment of chronic tension-type headache.

Coeytaux RR, Befus D. Role of acupuncture in the treatment or prevention of migraine, tension-type headache, or chronic headache disorders. *Headache*. 2016;56:1238–1240. [PMID: 27411557]

Perry JJ, Sivilotti MLA, Sutherland J, et al. Validation of the Ottawa Subarachnoid Hemorrhage Rule in patients with acute headache. *CMAJ*. 2017;189:E1379–E1385. [PMID: 29133539]

UK National External Quality Assessment Scheme for Immunochemistry Working Group. National guidelines for analysis of cerebrospinal fluid for bilirubin in suspected subarachnoid haemorrhage. *Ann Clin Biochem*. 2003;40:481–488. [PMID: 14503985]

A. Migraine

The following are general management guidelines for treatment of migraine patients:

- Educate migraine sufferers about their condition and its treatment and encourage them to participate in their own management.

- Use migraine-specific agents (eg, triptans) in patients with more severe migraine and in those whose headaches respond poorly to nonsteroidal anti-inflammatory drugs (NSAIDs) or combination analgesics such as aspirin plus acetaminophen plus caffeine.

- Select a nonoral route of administration for patients whose migraines present early with nausea or vomiting as a significant component of the symptom complex.

- Consider a self-administered rescue medication for patients with severe migraine who do not respond well to (or fail) other treatments.

- Guard against medication overuse headache by educating patients and using prophylactic medications in patients with frequent headaches (>10 headaches per month).

Pharmacologic treatment options are numerous in the management of migraine headache. See Table 29–4 for a summary of medication options. Due to side effects, rebound, and overuse concerns, narcotic medications are not first-line treatment for acute migraine headaches, although they may be effective.

In the emergency setting where parenteral medications are available, see Table 29–4 for evidence-based treatment options. Parenteral dexamethasone should be offered to patients to reduce the risk of having a moderate or severe migraine headache at 24–72 hours after ED evaluation. The optimal dose is not known, but three large randomized controlled trials used doses of 10, 20, and 24 mg. Greater occipital nerve (GON) block is a minimally invasive procedure used when medication has been ineffective for acute migraine. GON block has been shown to be effective in reducing headache severity and number of headache days and lowering medication use, but it did not affect duration of migraine headache.

The goal of therapy in migraine prophylaxis is a reduction in the severity and frequency of headache by ≥50%. Selection of prophylactic medications should be guided by patient characteristics and expected side effects. There is good evidence for amitriptyline, atenolol, flunarizine, fluoxetine, metoprolol, pizotifen, propranolol, timolol, topiramate, and valproate to reduce episodic migraine frequency and severity. Preventive medications are recommended for at least 3–6 months, with better pain control and decreased frequency when used for a longer duration. Frovatriptan is most effective for preventing menstrual migraine when taken twice daily perimenstrually. In a Cochrane review of 22 randomized controlled trials, acupuncture was shown to be superior to prophylactic medication for episodic migraine suppression at 3 months (standardized mean difference, –0.25 [confidence interval, –0.39 to –0.10]) but was not superior at 6 months. Acupuncture was superior to usual care and sham acupuncture at both 3 months and 6 months. One small review of physical therapy interventions showed a decrease in migraine intensity and frequency, but further studies are needed. Noninvasive neurostimulation may be another adjunct for migraine patients with unsatisfactory outcomes with medication prophylaxis, although more studies are needed. The US Food and Drug Administration (FDA) has approved transcutaneous supraorbital nerve stimulation for migraine prevention and transcranial magnetic stimulation to treat migraine with aura. OnabotulinumtoxinA is the only agent FDA approved to prevent chronic migraine (ie, 15+ headaches per month, at least 8 of which have migraine features). It is ineffective for episodic migraine (ie, <15 headaches per month).

B. Tension-Type Headache

Initial medical therapy of episodic tension-type headache often includes aspirin, acetaminophen, or NSAIDs. Avoidance of habituating, caffeine-containing. over-the-counter or prescription drugs as well as butalbital-, codeine-, or ergotamine-containing preparations (including combination products) is recommended given the significant risk of developing drug dependence or medication overuse headache.

Similar general management principles for treatment of migraine headaches can be applied to the treatment of chronic tension-type headaches. A systematic review of tricyclic antidepressants (TCAs) and tetracyclic antidepressants revealed TCAs were superior to placebo in reducing headache frequency and the consumption of analgesic medications; TCAs were more effective than selective serotonin reuptake inhibitors. Tetracyclic antidepressants were found to be no better than placebo for chronic tension-type headache. A Cochrane systematic review suggests that acupuncture reduces both frequency and severity of headaches compared to routine care and sham acupuncture and should be considered for treatment and prophylaxis of tension-type headaches. OnabotulinumtoxinA use is not associated with an improvement in the frequency of either chronic or episodic tension-type headaches.

Table 29–4. Evidence for pharmacologic treatment of migraine headache.

Level of Evidence	Acute Migraine Treatment	Acute Migraine Treatment in ED	Prophylactic Migraine Treatment	Intermittent Menstrual Migraine Treatment
Level A: Established as effective	Acetaminophen DHE nasal or inhaled NSAIDS: Aspirin, diclofenac, ibuprofen, naproxen Butorphanol nasal Triptans: Almotriptan, eletriptan, frovatriptan, naratriptan, rizatriptan, sumatriptan (PO, nasal), zolmitriptan Acetaminophen/aspirin/caffeine Sumatriptan/naproxen	None	Divalproex/sodium valproate Metoprolol *Petasites* (butterbur) Propranolol Timolol Topiramate	Frovatriptan
Level B: Probably effective	Antiemetics: Chlorpromazine IV, droperidol IV, metoclopramide IV, prochlorperazine IV/IM Ergots: DHE IV/IM/SC, ergotamine/caffeine NSAIDS: Flurbiprofen, ketoprofen, ketorolac IV/IM $MgSO_4$ IV Isometheptene Codeine/acetaminophen Tramadol/acetaminophen	Metoclopramide IV Prochlorperazine IV Sumatriptan SC	Amitriptyline Fenoprofen Feverfew Histamine Ibuprofen Ketoprofen Magnesium Naproxen/naproxen sodium Riboflavin Venlafaxine Atenolol	Naratriptan Zolmitriptan
Level C: Possibly effective	Valproate IV Ergotamine NSAID: Phenazone Opioids: Butorphanol IM, codeine, meperidine IM, methadone IM, tramadol IV Steroid: Dexamethasone IV	Acetaminophen IV Acetylsalicylic acid IV Chlorpromazine IV Dexketoprofen IV Dipyrone IV Droperidol IV Haloperidol IV Ketorolac IV Valproate IV	Candesartan Carbamazepine Clonidine Guanfacine Lisinopril Nebivolol Pindolol Flurbiprofen Mefenamic acid Coenzyme Q10 Cyproheptadine	Estrogen
Level U: Conflicting or inadequate evidence	Celecoxib Lidocaine IV Hydrocortisone IV	Dexamethasone IV Dihydroergotamine IV Ergotamine IV Ketamine IV Lysine clonixinate IV Magnesium IV (may benefit if aura) Meperidine IV Nalbuphine IV Propofol IV Promethazine IV Tramadol IV Trimethobenzamide IM	Acenocoumarol Acetazolamide Aspirin Bisoprolol Coumadin Cyclandelate Fluoxetine Fluvoxamine Gabapentin Hyperbaric oxygen Indomethacin Nicardipine Nifedipine Nimodipine Omega-3 Picotamide Protriptyline Verapamil	

(Continued)

Table 29–4. Evidence for pharmacologic treatment of migraine headache. (*Continued*)

Level of Evidence	Acute Migraine Treatment	Acute Migraine Treatment in ED	Prophylactic Migraine Treatment	Intermittent Menstrual Migraine Treatment
Levels B and C Negative: Probably or possibly ineffective	Octreotide SC Chlorpromazine IM Granisetron IV Ketorolac tromethamine nasal Acetaminophen IV	Diphenhydramine IV Hydromorphone IV Lidocaine IV Morphine IV Octreotide IV	Acebutolol Clomipramine Clonazepam Lamotrigine Montelukast Nabumetone Oxcarbazepine Telmisartan	

DHE, dihydroergotamine; IM, intramuscular; IV, intravenous; MgSO$_4$, magnesium sulfate; NSAID, nonsteroidal anti-inflammatory drug; PO, oral; SC, subcutaneous.

Jackson JL, Cogbill E, Santana-Davila R, et al. A comparative effectiveness meta-analysis of drugs for the prophylaxis of migraine headache. *PloS One.* 2015;10:e0130733. [PMID: 26172390]

Linde K, Allais G, Brinkhaus B, et al. Acupuncture for the prevention of episodic migraine. *Cochrane Database Syst Rev.* 2016;6:CD001218. [PMID: 27351677]

Luedtke K, Allers A, Schulte LH, May A. Efficacy of interventions used by physiotherapists for patients with headache and migraine-systematic review and meta-analysis. *Cephalalgia.* 2016;36:474–492. [PMID: 26229071]

Marmura MJ, Silberstein SD, Schwedt TJ. The acute treatment of migraine in adults: the american headache society evidence assessment of migraine pharmacotherapies. *Headache.* 2015;55:3–20. [PMID: 25600718]

Orr SL, Friedman BW, Christie S, et al. Management of adults with acute migraine in the emergency department: the American Headache Society evidence assessment of parenteral pharmacotherapies. *Headache.* 2016;56:911–940. [PMID: 27300483]

Schwedt TJ, Vargas B. Neurostimulation for treatment of migraine and cluster headache. *Pain Med.* 2015;16:1827–1834. [PMID: 26177612]

Silberstein SD, Holland S, Freitag F, Dodick DW, Argoff C, Ashman E. Evidence-based guideline update: pharmacologic treatment for episodic migraine prevention in adults: report of the Quality Standards Subcommittee of the American Academy of Neurology and the American Headache Society. *Neurology.* 2012;78:1337–1345. [PMID: 22529202]

Simpson DM, Hallett M, Ashman EJ, et al. Practice guideline update summary: botulinum neurotoxin for the treatment of blepharospasm, cervical dystonia, adult spasticity, and headache. *Neurology.* 2016;86:1818–1826. [PMID: 27164716]

Tang Y, Kang J, Zhang Y, Zhang X. Influence of greater occipital nerve block on pain severity in migraine patients: a systematic review and meta-analysis. *Am J Emerg Med.* 2017;35:1750–1754. [PMID: 28844531]

C. Cluster Headache

Acute management of cluster headache includes the use of sumatriptan in its subcutaneous (FDA-approved indication), intranasal, or oral forms (the latter two are less effective due to their slower onset of action); intranasal zolmitriptan; inhalation of 100% oxygen at 12 L/min for 15 minutes via nonrebreather facemask; and intranasal lidocaine. Subcutaneous octreotide may also be effective for abortive treatment. Verapamil (target dose of 360 mg/d; monitor for heart block) and lithium (target dose of 900 mg/d) have been demonstrated to reduce attack frequency. Other agents, including divalproex sodium, gabapentin, lithium, melatonin (possibly), topiramate (possibly), methysergide, baclofen, and TCAs, have been used in cluster headache, but the preventive benefits are not well established. Because of side effects related to chronic use, methysergide and prednisone should be used with caution. When prednisone or prednisolone is used, standard dosing is 1 mg/kg (maximum, 60 mg) daily for 5 days, which is subsequently reduced by 10 mg every 3 days. This regimen often reduces the frequency of cluster headaches; another preventive agent should be started at the same time. There is increasing evidence supporting the use of OnabotulinumtoxinA, neurostimulation, and occipital nerve blocks, particularly for refractory cluster headaches.

Cohen AS, Burns B, Goadsby PJ. High-flow oxygen for treatment of cluster headache: a randomized trial. *JAMA.* 2009;302:2451–2457. [PMID: 19996400]

Francis GJ, Becker WJ, Pringsheim TM. Acute and preventive pharmacologic treatment of cluster headache. *Neurology.* 2010;75:463–473. [PMID: 20679639]

Gaul C, Roguski J, Dresler T, et al. Efficacy and safety of a single occipital nerve blockade in episodic and chronic cluster headache: a prospective observational study. *Cephalalgia.* 2017.37:873–880. [PMID: 27313215]

Lampl C, Rudolph M, Brautigam E. OnabotulinumtoxinA in the treatment of refractory chronic cluster headache. *J Headache Pain.* 2018;19:45. [PMID: 29915913]

May A, Leone M, Afra J, et al. EFNS guidelines on the treatment of cluster headache and other trigeminal-autonomic cephalalgias. *Eur J Neurol.* 2006;13:1066–1077. [PMID: 16987158]

D. Referral

Referral to a headache specialist should be considered for patients whose findings are difficult to classify into a primary or secondary headache disorder. Additionally, referral is often warranted in cases of daily or intractable headache, drug rebound, habituation, or medication overuse headache, or in any scenario in which the primary care provider feels uncomfortable in making a diagnosis or offering appropriate treatment. Patients who request referral, who do not respond to treatment, or whose condition continues to worsen should be considered for referral.

Chaibi A, Russell MB. Manual therapies for primary chronic headaches: a systematic review of randomized controlled trials. *J Headache Pain.* 2014;15:67. [PMID: 25278005]

Coeytaux RR, Befus D. Role of acupuncture in the treatment or prevention of migraine, tension-type headache, or chronic headache disorders. *Headache.* 2016;56:1238–1240. [PMID: 27411557]

Derry S, Wiffen PJ, Moore RA. Aspirin for acute treatment of episodic tension-type headache in adults. *Cochrane Database Syst Rev.* 2017;1:CD011888. [PMID: 28084009]

Derry S, Wiffen PJ, Moore RA, Bendtsen L. Ibuprofen for acute treatment of episodic tension-type headache in adults. *Cochrane Database Syst Rev.* 2015;7:CD011474. [PMID: 26230487]

Perry JJ, Sivilotti MLA, Sutherland J, et al. Validation of the Ottawa Subarachnoid Hemorrhage Rule in patients with acute headache. *CMAJ.* 2017;189:E1379–E1385. [PMID: 29133539]

UK National External Quality Assessment Scheme for Immunochemistry Working Group. National guidelines for analysis of cerebrospinal fluid for bilirubin in suspected subarachnoid haemorrhage. *Ann Clin Biochem.* 2003;40:481–488. [PMID: 14503985]

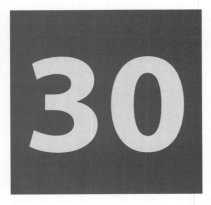

Osteoporosis

Jeannette E. South-Paul, MD, DHL (Hon), FAAFP

Mehret Birru Talabi, MD, PhD

General Considerations

Osteoporosis is a public health problem affecting >40 million people, one-third of postmenopausal women, and a substantial portion of the elderly in the United States and almost as many in Europe and Japan. An additional 54% of postmenopausal women have low bone density measured at the hip, spine, or wrist. Osteoporosis results in approximately 1,500,000 fractures annually in women in the United States alone and is a significant cause of fractures in men as well. The overall incidence of hip fracture in the United States increased from 1986 to 1995 and then steadily declined from 1995 to 2012, but it has now plateaued at higher levels than predicted for the years 2013 to 2015. At least 90% of all hip and spine fractures among elderly women are a consequence of osteoporosis. The direct expenditures for osteoporotic fractures have increased during the past decade from $5 billion to almost $15 billion per year. The number of women experiencing osteoporotic fractures annually exceeds the number diagnosed with heart attack, stroke, and breast cancer combined. Thus, family physicians and other primary care clinicians (1) will frequently care for patients with subclinical osteoporosis, (2) should recognize the implications of those who present with osteoporosis-related fractures, and (3) must determine when to implement prevention for younger people.

Osteoporotic fractures are more common in whites and Asians than in African Americans and Hispanics and are more common in women than in men. The female-to-male fracture ratios are reported to be 7:1 for vertebral fractures, 1.5:1 for distal forearm fractures, and 2:1 for hip fractures. Approximately 30% of hip fractures in persons age ≥65 years occur in men. Osteoporosis-related fractures in older men are associated with lower femoral neck bone mineral density (BMD), quadriceps weakness, higher body sway, lower body weight, and decreased stature. Little is known regarding the influence of ethnicity on bone turnover as a possible cause of the variance in bone density and fracture rates among different ethnic groups. Significant differences in bone turnover in premenopausal and early perimenopausal women can be documented. The bone turnover differences do not appear to parallel the patterns of BMD. Other factors, such as differences in bone accretion, are likely responsible for much of the ethnic variation in adult BMD. Estimates of numbers needed to screen to prevent one hip fracture over 5 years (from data from the Fracture Intervention Trial of bisphosphonate use in postmenopausal women age 54–81 years) are 1667, 1000, and 556 for postmenopausal women age 55–59 years, 60–64 years, and 65–69 years, respectively. These findings, as well as the absence of data on the benefits of osteoporosis treatment beginning between ages 50 and 59, suggest that early screening is not an evidence-based rationale.

Cauley JA. Screening for osteoporosis. *JAMA.* 2018;319(24):2483–2485. [PMID: 29946707]

Finkelstein JS, Sowers M, Greendale GA, et al. Ethnic variation in bone turnover in pre- and early perimenopausal women: effects of anthropometric and lifestyle factors. *J Clin Endocrinol Metab.* 2002;87:3051–3056. [PMID: 12107200]

Gourlay ML. Osteoporosis screening: 2 steps may be too much for women younger than 65 years. *JAMA Int Med.* 2018;178(9):1159–1160. [PMID: 29946684]

Watts NB, Bilezikian JP, Camacho PM, et al. American Association of Clinical Endocrinologists Medical Guidelines for Clinical Practice for the diagnosis and treatment of postmenopausal osteoporosis. *Endocr Pract.* 2010;16(Suppl 3):1–37. [PMID: 21224201]

Pathogenesis

Osteoporosis is characterized by microarchitectural deterioration of bone tissue that leads to decreased bone mass and bone fragility. The major processes responsible for osteoporosis are accelerated bone loss during the perimenopausal period (mid-50s to the sixth decade) in women and the seventh decade in men and beyond and, to a lesser extent, poor

Table 30–1. Risk factors for osteoporosis.

Lifestyle and patient-centric factors that contribute independently to risk for osteoporosis	Myeloma and some malignancies
Age	Chronic renal disease
Previous fragility fracture	Chronic liver disease
Maternal history of hip fracture	Chronic obstructive pulmonary disease
Current smoking	Chronic inflammatory disease
Alcohol intake ≥ 3 drinks/day	Rheumatoid arthritis
Falls	Ankylosing spondylitis
Sedentary lifestyle	HIV/AIDS
Major depression	Immobility
Chronic factors that contribute to risk for osteoporosis due to effects on bone mineral density	Drugs
	Aromatase inhibitors
Anorexia	Androgen deprivation therapy
Body mass index ≤ 19	Chemotherapy and immunosuppression
Collagen metabolism disorders	Glucocorticoids
Ehlers Danlos syndrome	Tamoxifen
Marfan syndrome	Gonadotropin-release hormones
Osteogenesis imperfecta	Heparin
Malabsorption	Lithium
Celiac disease	Medroxyprogesterone acetate (Depo Provera)
Cystic fibrosis	Proton-pump inhibitors
Crohn's disease	Selective serotonin uptake inhibitors
Gastric bypass or resection	Thiazolinediones
Endocrine disease	Barbituates
Acromegaly	Antiepileptic drugs (phenobarbital, phenytoin, primidone, valproate, carbamazepine)
Type 1 and 2 diabetes	Vitamin D deficiency
Growth hormone deficiency	Hemophilia
Hypercortisolism	Systemic mastocytosis
Hyperthyroidism	Thalassemia
Hyperparathyroidism	Porphyria
Hypogonadism (untreated)	

Data from Poole KE, Compston JE: Osteoporosis and its management, *BMJ*. 2006 Dec 16;333(7581):1251–1256.

bone mass acquisition during adolescence. Both processes are regulated by genetic and environmental factors. Reduced bone mass, in turn, is the result of varying combinations of hormone deficiencies, inadequate nutrition, decreased physical activity, comorbidity, and the effects of drugs used to treat various medical conditions.

The term *primary osteoporosis* is now used less frequently than in the past and signifies deterioration of bone mass not associated with other chronic illness, usually related to increasing age and decreasing gonadal function. Therefore, early menopause or premenopausal estrogen deficiency states may hasten its development. Prolonged periods of inadequate calcium intake, a sedentary lifestyle, and tobacco and alcohol abuse also contribute to primary osteoporosis.

Secondary osteoporosis results from chronic conditions that contribute significantly to accelerated bone loss. These include endogenous and exogenous thyroxine excess,

hyperparathyroidism, cancer, gastrointestinal diseases, medications, renal failure, and connective tissue diseases. Secondary forms of osteoporosis are listed in Table 30–1. If secondary osteoporosis is suspected, appropriate diagnostic workup may identify a different management course.

Camacho PM, Petak SM, Binkley N, et al. American Association of Clinical Endocrinologists and American College of Endocrinology clinical practice guidelines for the diagnosis and treatment of postmenopausal osteoporosis–2016. *Endocr Pract.* 2016;22(Suppl 4):1–42. [PMID: 27662240]

Kelman A, Lane NE. The management of secondary osteoporosis. *Best Pract Res Clin Rheumatol.* 2005;19(6):1021–1037. [PMID: 16301195]

Kok C, Sambrook PN. Secondary osteoporosis in patients with osteoporotic fracture. *Best Pract Res Clin Rheumatol.* 2009;23:769–779. [PMID: 19945688]

▶ Prevention

A. Nutrition

Bone mineralization is dependent on adequate nutritional status in childhood and adolescence. Therefore, measures to prevent osteoporosis should begin with increasing the milk intake of adolescents to improve bone mineralization as well as other nutrients essential for bone health. A balance between calcium and protein intake and other calorie sources is needed. Substituting phosphorus-laden soft drinks for calcium-rich dairy products and juices compromises calcium uptake by bone and promotes decreased bone mass.

The nutritional impact of eating disorders results in low body mass and bone loss. The body weight history of women with anorexia nervosa predicts the presence of osteoporosis as well as the likelihood of recovery. The BMD of these patients does not increase to a normal range, even several years after recovery from the disorder, and all persons with a history of an eating disorder remain at high risk for osteoporosis in the future.

Major demands for calcium are placed on the mother by the fetus during pregnancy and lactation. The axial spine and hip show losses of BMD during the first 6 months of lactation, but this bone mineral loss appears to be completely restored 6–12 months after weaning.

B. Lifestyle

Sedentary lifestyle or immobility (confinement to bed or a wheelchair) increases the incidence of osteoporosis. Low body weight and cigarette smoking negatively influence bone mass. Excessive alcohol consumption has been shown to depress osteoblast function and, thus, to decrease bone formation. Those at risk for low BMD should avoid drugs that negatively affect BMD (see Table 30–1).

C. Behavioral Measures

Behavioral measures that decrease the risk of bone loss include eliminating tobacco use and excessive consumption of alcohol and caffeine. A balanced diet with adequate calcium and vitamin D intake and a regular exercise program (see next section) retard bone loss. Medications, such as glucocorticoids, that decrease bone mass should be avoided if possible. The importance of maintaining estrogen levels in women should be emphasized. Measurement of bone density should be considered in the patient who presents with risk factors, but additional evidence is needed before instituting preventive measures.

D. Exercise

Regular physical exercise can reduce the risk of osteoporosis and delay the physiologic decrease of BMD. Short- and long-term exercise training (measured up to 12 months; eg, walking, jogging, stair climbing) in healthy, sedentary, postmenopausal women results in improved bone mineral content. Bone mineral content increases >5% above baseline after short-term, weight-bearing exercise training. With reduced weight-bearing exercise, bone mass reverts to baseline levels. Similar increases in BMD have been seen in women who participate in strength training. In the elderly, progressive strength training has been demonstrated to be a safe and effective form of exercise that reduces risk factors for falling and may also enhance BMD.

Estrogen deficiency results in diminished bone density in younger women as well as in older women. Athletes who exercise much more intensely and consistently than the average person usually have above-average bone mass. However, the positive effect of exercise on the bones of young women is dependent on normal levels of endogenous estrogen. The low-estrogen state of exercise-induced amenorrhea outweighs the positive effects of exercise and results in diminished bone density. When mechanical stress or gravitational force on the skeleton is removed, as in bed rest, space flight, immobilization of limbs, or paralysis, bone loss is rapid and extensive. Weight-bearing exercise can significantly increase the BMD of menopausal women. Furthermore, weight-bearing exercise and estrogen replacement therapy have independent and additive effects on the BMD of the limb, spine, and Ward triangle (hip).

There have been no randomized prospective studies systematically comparing the effect of various activities on bone mass. Recommended activities include walking and jogging, weight training, aerobics, stair climbing, field sports, racquet sports, court sports, and dancing. Swimming is of questionable value to bone density (because it is not a weight-bearing activity), and there are no data on cycling, skating, or skiing. It should be kept in mind that any increase in physical activity may have a positive effect on bone mass for women who have been very sedentary. To be beneficial, the duration of exercise should be between 30 and 60 minutes and the frequency should be 3–4 times per week.

Cadogan J, Eastell R, Jones N, et al. Milk intake and bone mineral acquisition in adolescent girls: randomised, controlled intervention trial. *Br Med J.* 1997;315:1255. [PMID: 9390050]

Ernst E. Exercise for female osteoporosis. A systematic review of randomised clinical trials. *Sports Med.* 1998;25:359. [PMID: 9680658]

Rantalainen T, Nikander R, Heinonen A, et al. Differential effects of exercise on tibial shaft marrow density in young female athletes. *J Clin Endocrinol Metab.* 2013;98(5):2037–2044. [PMID: 23616150]

▶ Clinical Findings

A. Symptoms and Signs

The history and physical examination are neither sensitive enough nor sufficient for diagnosing primary osteoporosis. However, they are important in screening for secondary forms of osteoporosis and directing the evaluation. The goals of the evaluation should be to (1) establish the diagnosis of osteoporosis by assessing bone mass, (2) determine fracture risk, and (3) determine whether intervention is needed. A medical history provides valuable clues to the presence of chronic conditions, behaviors, physical fitness, and the use of long-term medications that could influence bone density. Those already affected by complications of osteoporosis may complain of upper or midthoracic back pain associated with activity, aggravated by long periods of sitting or standing, and easily relieved by rest in a recumbent position. The history should also assess the likelihood of fracture. Other indicators of increased fracture risk are low bone density, a propensity to fall, taller stature, and the presence of prior fractures. See Table 30–2.

The physical examination should be thorough for the same reasons. For example, lid lag and enlargement or nodularity of the thyroid suggest hyperthyroidism. Moon facies, thin skin, and a "buffalo hump" (dorsocervical fat pad) suggest hypercortisolism. Cachexia mandates screening for an eating disorder or cancer. A pelvic examination is one aspect of the total evaluation of hormonal status in women and a necessary part of the physical examination in women. Osteoporotic fractures are a late physical manifestation. Common fracture sites are the vertebrae, forearm, femoral neck, and proximal humerus. The presence of a "dowager hump" in elderly patients suggests multiple vertebral fractures and decreased bone volume.

The US Preventive Services Task Force (USPSTF) evaluated the accuracy of clinical risk assessment tools to identify risk of osteoporosis. the USPSTF focused on their accuracy to identify osteoporosis because all the treatment studies evaluated by the USPSTF enrolled patients based on bone measurement testing, specifically BMD measured by central dual-energy x-ray absorptiometry (DXA). Many of the clinical risk assessment tools can also be used to calculate risk of future fractures. Several tools developed to help determine which postmenopausal women younger than age 65 years should be screened with bone density testing are as follows: the Simple Calculated Osteoporosis Risk Estimation (SCORE; Merck); the Osteoporosis Risk Assessment Instrument (ORAI); the Osteoporosis Index of Risk (OSIRIS); and the Osteoporosis Self-Assessment Tool (OST). These tools seem to perform similarly and are moderately accurate at predicting osteoporosis. The Fracture Risk Assessment (FRAX) tool (University of Sheffield), which assesses a person's 10-year risk of fracture, is also a commonly used tool. The FRAX does not require previous DXA results to estimate fracture risk and uses primary data from nine large patient cohorts in North America, Europe, Asia, and Australia. BMD measurements are most valuable in postmenopausal women under 65 years of age who have a 10-year FRAX risk of major osteoporotic fracture greater than that of a 65-year-old white woman without major risk factors. This tool estimates the 10-year, patient-specific absolute risk of hip or major osteoporotic fracture (hip, spine, shoulder, or wrist), taking into account death from all causes and death hazards (eg, smoking). The tool may be used alone employing individual clinical risk factors, with or without BMD, and is easily accessed online.

Table 30–2. Assessment for osteoporosis and fracture risk in postmenopausal women.

Medical history and physical examination to identify:
• Prior nontraumatic fracture (other than fingers, toes, and skull) after age 50
• Clinical risk factors for osteoporosis
• Age >65
• Low body weight (<57.6 kg or 127 lb)
• Family history of osteoporosis or fractures
• Smoking
• Early menopause
• Excessive alcohol intake (>3 drinks daily)
• Secondary osteoporosis
• Height loss or kyphosis
• Risk factors for falling
• Patient's reliability, understanding, and willingness to accept interventions
Lateral spine imaging with standard x-ray or vertebral fracture assessment in patients with unexplained height loss, self-reported but undocumented prior spine fractures, or glucocorticoid therapy equivalent to >5 mg prednisone daily for 3 months or more
Bone mineral density measurements in those at increased risk for osteoporosis and fractures and willing to consider pharmacologic treatment if low bone mass is documented:
• All women >65 years of age
• Younger postmenopausal women
• With a history of fracture(s) without major trauma
• Starting or taking long-term systemic glucocorticoid therapy
• With radiographic osteopenia
• With clinical risk factors for osteoporosis (low body weight, cigarette smoking, family history of spine or hip fractures, early menopause, or secondary osteoporosis)
In women who are candidates for pharmacologic therapy, laboratory evaluation to identify coexisting conditions that may contribute to bone loss and/or interfere with therapy

Reproduced with permission from Camacho PM, Petak SM, Binkley N, et al: American Association of Clinical Endocrinologists and American College of Endocrinology Clinical Practice Guidelines for the Diagnosis and Treatment of Postmenopausal Osteoporosis–2016. *Endocr Pract.* 2016 Sep 2;22(Suppl 4):1–42.

Kanis JA, McCloskey EV, Johansson H, et al. European guidance for the diagnosis and management of osteoporosis in postmenopausal women. *Osteoporos Int.* 2008;19:399–428. [PMID: 18266020]

Kanis JA, Johnell O, Oden A, et al. FRAX and the assessment of fracture probability in men and women from the UK. *Osteoporos Int.* 2008;19:385–397. [PMID: 18292978]

US Preventive Services Task Force. Curry SJ, Krist AH, et al. Screening for osteoporosis to prevent fractures: US Preventive Services Task Force Recommendation Statement. *JAMA.* 2018;319(24):2521–2531. [PMID: 29946735]

Watts NB, Ettinger B, LeBoff MS. FRAX facts. *J Bone Miner Res.* 2009;24:975–979. [PMID: 19364271]

B. Laboratory Findings

Basic chemical analysis of serum is indicated when the history suggests other clinical conditions may be influencing bone density. Secondary causes of osteoporosis may include endocrinopathies, vitamin deficiency, liver disease, and malignancy. The following se tests provide clues tocertain serious illnesses that may otherwise have gone undetected and that, if treated, could result in resolution or modification of the bone loss.

Endocrinopathies: Hypogonadism among men may be diagnosed by low testosterone levels; among women, low estrogen levels, and high gonadotropin levels (LH and FSH) may be diagnostic. Hyperthyroidism may be assessed by low TSH and elevated T4. Hyperparathyroidism may be assessed through increased PTH, serum calcium levels, and 1,25OH vitamin D levels. Cushing syndrome may be diagnosed through elevated 24-hour urine free cortisol excretion levels, and overnight dexamethasone suppression test.

Vitamin Deficiency: Vitamin D deficiency is a major risk factor for osteoporosis, and may be detected by low 25 (OH) vitamin D levels.

Malignancy: Multiple myeloma is a malignancy that often manifests with "punched-out" lesions of the bone; while a rare cause of osteoporosis, it is important to detect. Laboratory tests including abnormal serum and urine protein electrophoresis, increased sedimentation rate, anemia, hypercalcemia, and decreased parathyroid hormone, may be used to diagnose this malignancy.

The utility of serum or urine tests to diagnose osteoporosis is less clear. Specific biochemical markers (human osteocalcin, bone alkaline phosphatase, immunoassays for pyridinoline crosslinks, and type 1 collagen–related peptides in urine) that reflect the overall rate of bone formation and bone resorption are now available. These markers are primarily of research interest and are not recommended as part of the basic workup for osteoporosis. They suffer from substantial biological variability and diurnal variation and do not differentiate causes of altered bone metabolism. For example, measures of bone turnover increase and remain elevated after menopause but do not necessarily provide information that can direct management.

C. Imaging Studies

Plain radiographs are not sensitive enough to diagnose osteoporosis until total bone density has decreased by 50%, but bone densitometry is useful for measuring bone density and monitoring the course of therapy. Single- or dual-photon absorptiometry has been used in the past but provides poorer resolution, less accurate analysis, and more radiation exposure than x-ray absorptiometry. The most widely used techniques for assessing BMD are DXA and quantitative computed tomography (CT). These methods have errors in precision of 0.5–2%. Quantitative CT is most sensitive but results in substantially greater radiation exposure than DXA. For this reason, DXA is the diagnostic measure of choice. Vertebral fracture assessment is now available through imaging completed with the DXA assessment and provides more accurate assessment of the patient's bone density.

Smaller, less expensive systems for assessing the peripheral skeleton are also available. These include DXA scans of the distal forearm and the middle phalanx of the nondominant hand and a variety of devices for performing quantitative ultrasound (QUS) measurements on bone. Prospective studies using QUS of the heel have predicted hip fracture and all nonvertebral fractures nearly as well as DXA at the femoral neck. Both of these methods provide information regarding fracture risk and predict hip fracture better than DXA at the lumbar spine. Clinical trials of pharmacologic agents have used DXA rather than QUS, so it is unclear whether the results of these trials can be generalized to patients identified by QUS to have high risk of fracture.

Bone densitometry reports provide a T score (the number of standard deviations above or below the mean BMD for sex and race matched to young controls) or Z score (comparing the patient with a population adjusted for age as well as for sex and race). The BMD result enables the classification of patients into three categories: normal, osteopenic, and osteoporotic. Normal patients receive no further therapy; osteopenic patients are counseled, treated, and followed so that no further bone loss develops; osteoporotic patients receive active therapy aimed at increasing bone density and decreasing fracture risk. Osteoporosis is indicated by a T score of >2.5 standard deviations below the sex-adjusted mean for normal young adults at peak bone mass. Z scores are of little value to the practicing clinician.

There is little evidence from controlled trials that women who receive bone density screening have better outcomes (improved bone density or fewer falls) than women who are not screened. The USPSTF suggests that the primary argument for screening is that postmenopausal women with low bone density are at increased risk for subsequent fractures of the hip, vertebrae, and wrist and that interventions can slow the decline in bone density after menopause. The presence of multiple risk factors (eg, age ≥80 years, poor health, limited physical activity, poor vision, prior postmenopausal fracture, psychotropic drug use) seems to be a stronger predictor of hip fracture than low bone density. The patient who is not symptomatic but may have one or two risk factors can benefit from BMD screening.

Davison KS, Kendler DL, Ammann P, et al. Assessing fracture risk and effects of osteoporosis drugs: bone mineral density and beyond. *Am J Med.* 2009;122:992–997. [PMID: 19854322]

Lewiecki EM, Watts NB, McClung MR, et al; International Society for Clinical Densitometry. Official positions of the international society for clinical densitometry. *J Clin Endocrinol Metab.* 2004;89(8):3651–3655. [PMID: 15292281]

US Preventive Services Task Force. Curry SJ, Krist AH, et al. Screening for osteoporosis to prevent fractures: US Preventive Services Task Force Recommendation Statement. *JAMA*. 2018;319(24):2521–2531. [PMID: 29946735]

▶ Differential Diagnosis & Screening

The approach to the patient is governed by the presentation. The greatest challenge for clinicians is to identify which asymptomatic patients would benefit from screening for osteoporosis, rather than determining a treatment regimen for those with known disease (see Table 30–2). All women and girls should be counseled about appropriate calcium intake and physical activity. Assessment of osteoporosis risk is also important when following a patient for a chronic disease known to cause secondary osteoporosis (see Table 30–1). Preventive measures are always the first step in therapy.

Should there be a suspicion of osteoporosis in a man or evidence of a pathologic fracture in a man or a woman, assessment of risk via medical history and determination of BMD should be completed. BMD measurement and laboratory evaluation are necessary to document the extent of bone loss and to rule out secondary causes of osteoporosis. Should there be clinical evidence of a particular condition, the evaluation can focus on the suspected condition when the basic laboratory work has been completed.

Recognizing the variety of conditions conferring risk of osteoporosis, the National Osteoporosis Foundation makes the following recommendations to physicians:

Universal recommendations:

- Counsel on the risk of osteoporosis and related fractures.
- Advise on a diet rich in fruits and vegetables and that includes adequate amounts of total calcium intake (1000 mg/d for men age 50–70 years; 1200 mg/d for women age ≥51 years and men ≥71 years).
- Advise on vitamin D intake (800–1000 IU/d), including supplements if necessary for individuals age ≥50 years.
- Recommend regular weight-bearing and muscle-strengthening exercise to improve agility, strength, posture, and balance and reduce the risk of falls and fractures.
- Assess risk factors for falls (e.g., neurologic disorders, hearing or vision impairment, medication side effects, weakness, home and environmental safety factors) and offer appropriate modifications (eg, home safety assessment, balance training exercises, correction of vitamin D insufficiency, avoidance of certain medications, and bifocals use when appropriate).
- Advise on cessation of tobacco smoking and avoidance of excessive alcohol intake.
- Measure height annually, preferably with a wall-mounted stadiometer.

Diagnostic assessment:

- BMD testing should be performed.
  - In women age ≥65 years and men age ≥70 years, recommend BMD testing.
  - In postmenopausal women and men age 50–69 years, recommend BMD testing based on risk factor profile.
- Recommend BMD testing and vertebral imaging to those who have had a fracture to determine degree of disease severity.
- BMD testing should be performed at DXA facilities using accepted quality assurance measures.
- Vertebral imaging should be performed.
  - In all women age ≥70 years and all men age ≥80 years.
  - In women age 65–69 and men age 75–79 years if BMD T score is ≤1.5.
  - In postmenopausal women age 50–64 and men age 50–69 years with specific risk factors:
    - Low trauma fracture
    - Historical height loss of ≥1.5 inches (4 cm)
    - Prospective height loss of ≥0.8 inch (2 cm)
    - Recent or ongoing long-term glucocorticoid treatment
- Check for causes of secondary osteoporosis.

When monitoring patients who have the diagnosis of osteoporosis, perform BMD testing 1–2 years after initiating therapy to reduce fracture risk and every 2 years thereafter. In certain clinical situations, more frequent testing may be indicated. Likewise, the interval for repeat screening may be longer if the initial T score is in the normal or upper low bone mass range or the patient is without major risk factors.

Cosman F, de Beur SJ, LeBoff MS, et al. Clinician's guide to prevention and treatment of osteoporosis. https://my.nof.org/file/bonesource/Clinicians-Guide.pdf. Accessed December 9, 2018.

▶ Treatment

Decisions to intervene when osteoporosis is diagnosed are designed to prevent early or continuing bone loss, a belief that there can be an immediate impact on the patient's well-being, and a willingness to comply with the patient's desires. Bone densitometry can assist in the decision-making process if the patient's age confers risk, there are no manifestations of disease, and the decision point is prevention rather than treatment. BMD measurements can also assist in therapy when there are relative contraindications to a specific agent, and demonstrating efficacy could encourage continuation of therapy. Medicare currently reimburses costs of bone densitometry if they have the conditions outlined above under vertebral imaging recommendations. The decision to intervene with pharmacologic therapy involves clinical judgment based on a global assessment, rather than BMD measurement alone.

The USPSTF has reviewed the evidence on drug therapies for the primary prevention of osteoporotic fractures and found that drug therapies are effective. The vast majority of the studies were done exclusively in women; only two were conducted in men. Currently approved therapeutic agents for the prevention and treatment of osteoporosis work by inhibiting or decreasing bone resorption or stimulating new bone formation.

A. Bisphosphonates

Bisphosphonates are antiresorptive agents and effective for preventing bone loss associated with estrogen deficiency, glucocorticoid treatment, and immobilization. Antiresorptive agents improve the quality of bone by preserving trabecular architecture. They may increase bone strength by methods other than by increasing BMD. All bisphosphonates act similarly on bone in binding permanently to mineralized bone surfaces and inhibiting osteoclastic activity. Thus, less bone is degraded during the remodeling cycle. First-, second-, and third-generation bisphosphonates are now available (alendronate, risedronate, etidronate, ibandronate, and zoledronic acid). Bisphosphonates were studied most frequently by the USPSTF. Because food and liquids can reduce the absorption of bisphosphonates, they should be given with a glass of plain water 30 minutes before the first meal or beverage of the day. Patients should not lie down for at least 30 minutes to lessen the chance of esophageal irritation. In addition, patients should consider taking supplemental calcium and vitamin D if their dietary intake is inadequate. Bisphosphonates are of comparable efficacy to hormone replacement therapy in preventing bone loss and have a demonstrated positive effect on symptomatic and asymptomatic vertebral fracture rate as well as on nonvertebral fracture rate (forearm and hip). More than 4 years of treatment would be needed in women with low bone density (T score $\geq$ −2.0), but without preexisting fractures, to substantially reduce the risk of clinical fracture. Based on pooled analyses, studies of bisphosphonates showed no increased risk of discontinuation adverse effects, serious adverse events, or upper gastrointestinal events.

Concerns have been raised regarding osteonecrosis of the jaw and atypical femoral fractures. The USPSTF reviewed multiple trials as well as a systematic review that did not meet inclusion criteria (because it included populations with a previous fracture) and found a higher incidence of osteonecrosis of the jaw with intravenous bisphosphonate use and with longer use. No studies that met inclusion criteria in the most recent review reported on atypical fractures of the femur, although some studies and systematic reviews that did not meet inclusion criteria (because of wrong study population, study design, or intervention comparator) reported an increase in atypical femur fractures with bisphosphonate use.

In clinical trials, alendronate was generally well tolerated and no significant clinical or biological adverse experiences were observed. Alendronate appears to be effective at doses of 5 mg daily in preventing osteoporosis induced by long-term glucocorticoid therapy. In placebo-controlled studies of men and women (age 17–83) who were receiving glucocorticoid therapy, femoral neck bone density and the bone density of the trochanter and total body increased significantly in patients treated with alendronate. Alendronate appears to be a safe, well-tolerated, and lower-cost agent for the osteoporosis and is a good first-line treatment. Some small-scale studies suggest an additional benefit of adding alendronate to hormone replacement therapy, and ongoing studies should provide additional information. However, all of the bisphosphonates accumulate over time in bone, and further research is needed to determine their long-term impact as well as their potential for use in premenopausal women and men.

Risedronate is a pyridinyl bisphosphonate approved as treatment for several metabolic bone diseases in 2000. In doses of 5 mg daily, risedronate reduces the incidence of vertebral fractures in women with two or more fractures by rapidly increasing BMD at sites of cortical and trabecular bone. The 2.5-mg dose was found to be ineffective in a large trial of postmenopausal women with osteoporosis, but the 5-mg group showed a 41% reduction in risk of new vertebral fractures and a 39% reduction in incidence of nonvertebral fractures after 3 years of treatment. Risedronate has also been shown to significantly reduce the risk of hip fracture in older women with osteoporosis. Bisphosphonates should be prescribed for 3–4 years in women with osteoporosis and low bone density.

Ibandronate is also approved by the US Food and Drug Administration (FDA) for the treatment and prevention of osteoporosis in postmenopausal women. Over a 3-year period, ibandronate was shown to decrease the incidence of new vertebral fractures by 52% and to increase BMD at the spine by 5%. It can be administered daily or once a month.

Zoledronic acid was approved by the FDA in 2011 and is prescribed as a single annual intramuscular dose of 5 mg. Femoral neck BMD increased by 3.7% above placebo 3 years after a single dose of zoledronic acid. Clinical fracture rates were reduced by 32% in patients receiving single infusions and 34% in those receiving three infusions over a 3-year period. There is no general agreement regarding how long to wait before repeating the injection.

Compston J, Bowring C, Cooper A, et al. Diagnosis and management of osteoporosis in postmenopausal women and older men in the UK: National Osteoporosis Guideline Group (NOGG) update 2013. *Maturitas*. 2013;75(4):392–396. [PMID: 23810490]

Reid IR, Black DM, Eastell R, et al. Reduction in the risk of clinical fractures after a single dose of zoledronic acid 5 milligrams. *J Clin Endocrinol Metab*. 2013;98(2):557–563. [PMID: 23293335]

Whitaker M, Guo J, Kehoe T, et al. Bisphosphonates for osteoporosis—where do we go from here? *N Engl J Med*. 2012; 366:2048–2051. [PMID: 22571168]

US Preventive Services Task Force. Curry SJ, Krist AH, et al. Screening for osteoporosis to prevent fractures: US Preventive Services Task Force Recommendation Statement. *JAMA*. 2018;319(24):2521–2531. [PMID: 29946735]

B. Selective Estrogen Receptor Modulators

Raloxifene was the first drug to be studied from a class of drugs termed selective estrogen receptor modulators and has a mixed agonist-antagonist action on estrogen receptors: specifically, estrogen agonist effects on bone and antagonist effects on breast and endometrium. It blocks estrogen in a manner similar to tamoxifen, while also binding and stimulating other tissue receptors to act like estrogen. Raloxifene inhibits trabecular and vertebral bone loss in a manner similar, but not identical, to estrogen (ie, by blocking the activity of cytokines that stimulate bone resorption). Raloxifene therapy results in decreased serum total and low-density lipoprotein (LDL) cholesterol without any beneficial effects on serum total high-density lipoprotein (HDL) cholesterol or triglycerides. Side effects associated with raloxifene are vaginitis and hot flashes. Investigators in the Multiple Outcomes of Raloxifene (MORE) trial of >7000 postmenopausal, osteoporotic women over 3 years showed a decreased risk of breast cancer in those already at low risk for the disease. Pooled analyses showed no increased risk of discontinuation due to adverse events or increased risk of leg cramps, although there was a nonsignificant trend for increased risk of deep vein thrombosis as well as an increased risk of hot flashes. A third-generation selective estrogen receptor modulator combined with estrogen, bazedoxifene, has had FDA approval since 2013 and is designed to preserve bone density and decrease biochemical markers. As with other selective estrogen receptor modulators, the rate of deep venous thrombosis is higher than what is seen with placebo, but it has favorable endometrial and breast safety profiles. A summary of guidelines for dosing the pharmacologic agents is given in Table 30–3.

Christiansen C, Chesnut CH, Adachi JD, et al. Safety of bazedoxifene in a randomized, double-blind, placebo- and active-controlled phase 3 study of postmenopausal women with osteoporosis. *BMC Musculoskelet Disord.* 2010;11:130. [PMID: 20569451]

C. Denosumab

Denosumab, a fully human, monoclonal antibody that inhibits RANKL, a key modulator of osteoclast formation, function, and survival, was approved by the FDA in 2012. The FREEDOM study of 7808 postmenopausal women with osteoporosis compared 60 mg of denosumab with placebo given every 6 months for 36 months. DXA and quantitative CT scans were used for monitoring. Denosumab significantly increased BMD and did not appear to delay fracture healing. A recent longitudinal study of femoral neck T scores did not demonstrate measurable improvement after approximately 1 year of treatment in a diverse group of community-dwelling patients except in those receiving intravenous bisphosphonates or denosumab. Denosumab use warrants caution in the presence of hypocalcemia; serious side effects include skin infections (cellulitis and erysipelas), osteonecrosis of the jaw, and suppression of bone turnover, which could include atypical femoral fracture after long-term use. An observational study of patients who had used denosumab for 8 years found that 1 year after denosumab discontinuation, BMD decreased by 6.7% in the lumbar spine and 6.6% in the hip, after gains of 16.8% and 6.2% from baseline; thus, the effects of denosumab on BMD may be time limited.

Berry SD, Dufour AB, Travison TG, et al. Changes in bone mineral density (BMD): a longitudinal study of osteoporosis patients in the real-world setting. *Arch Osteoporos.* 2018;13(1):124. [PMID: 30421141]

McClung MR, Wagman RB, Wang A, Lewiecki EM. Observations following discontinuation of long-term denosumab therapy. *Osteoporos Int.* 2017;28:1723–1732. [PMID: 28144701]

D. Estrogen

Adequate estrogen levels remain the single most important therapy for maintaining adequate bone density in women. Prior to 2003, estrogen replacement therapy was considered for all women with decreased bone density, absent contraindications. However, in July 2002, the Women's Health Initiative randomized controlled primary prevention trial was stopped at a mean of 5.2 years of follow-up by the Data and Safety Monitoring Board because the test statistic for invasive breast cancer exceeded the stopping boundary for the adverse effects of estrogen and progesterone versus placebo. Estimated hazard ratios were excessive for coronary heart disease, breast cancer, and strokes, but were <1.0 for colorectal cancer, endometrial cancer, and hip fracture. Therefore, careful risk assessment is needed for each patient to determine whether the improvement of risk for hip fracture (0.66) balances the risk for cardiovascular and breast disease.

Current estrogen users who started estrogen therapy at menopause had the highest BMD levels, which were significantly higher than those of women who never used estrogen therapy or past users who started at menopause (with a duration of use of ≥10 years). BMD was similar for women using unopposed estrogen or estrogen plus progestin and for current smokers or nonsmokers. Current users who started estrogen within 5 years of menopause had a decreased risk of hip, wrist, and all nonspinal fractures compared with those who never used estrogen. Long-term users who initiated therapy 5 years after menopause had no significant reduction in risk for all nonspinal fractures, despite an average duration of use of 16 years. Therefore, early initiation of estrogen with respect to menopause may be more important than the total duration of use. Estrogen initiated early in the menopausal period and continued into late life appears to be associated with the highest bone density.

As more and more women use estrogen therapy, there has been increasing concern regarding its impact on breast

Table 30–3. Medications for treating osteoporosis.

Treatment	Dosing	Effects on bone	Licensed indication	Comments
Alendronate (Fosamax, Binosto)	Treatment: 70 mg PO weekly or 5 mg or 10 PO mg once daily Prevention: 35 mg PO weekly or 5 mg PO daily	Antiresorptive	Postmenopausal osteoporosis; glucocorticoid-induced osteoporosis; male osteoporosis	Contraindications: Esophageal abnormalities, hypocalcemia Use with caution if GFR<30 mL/min Use with caution if patient is unable to sit or stand upright for 30 minutes or more after administration Major adverse effects: Gastrointestinal or esophageal irritation; atypical femur fractures; osteonecrosis of jaw
Risedronate (Actonel, Atelvia)	Treatment or prevention: 5 mg PO daily or 35 mg PO weekly, or 150 mg PO monthly Treatment with delayed release: 35 mg PO weekly	Antiresorptive	Postmenopausal osteoporosis; glucocorticoid-induced osteoporosis	Contraindications and major adverse effects are the same as Alendronate.
Zolendronic acid (Reclast)	Treatment: 5 mg intravenous infusion annually Prevention: 5 mg intravenous infusion every 2 years	Antiresorptive	Postmenopausal osteoporosis, hypercalcemia of malignancy and bony metastatic disease	Contraindications: Hypocalcemia Major adverse effects: Atypical femur fractures; osteonecrosis of jaw
Denosumab (Prolia)	Treatment: 60 mg subcutaneous every 6 months	Antiresorptive RANK-L inhibitor	Postmenopausal osteoporosis	Contraindications: Hypocalcemia, pregnancy
Ibandronate (Boniva)	Treatment: 150 mg oral monthly Prevention: 150 mg oral monthly	Antiresorptive Bisphosphonate		

Other Therapies

Treatment	Dosing	Effects on bone	Licensed indication	Comments
Teriparatide (Forteo)	Treatment: 20 micrograms subcutaneously daily for up to 2 years	Anabolic Recombinant human parathyroid hormone	Postmenopausal osteoporosis	Major adverse effects: Orthostatic hypotension Increased risk of osteosarcoma May exacerbate urolithiasis Avoid in patients with Paget's disease of the bone or with high alkaline phosphatase of unclear etiology
Raloxifene (Evista)	Treatment: 60 mg PO daily	Antiresorptive Selective estrogen agonist/antagonist	Postmenopausal osteoporosis	Contraindications: Current or historical venous thromboembolism, pregnancy, breastfeeding Increased risk of death among women with known cardiovascular disease FDA approved for risk reduction of invasive breast cancer for postmenopausal women with osteoporosis and for postmenopausal women without osteoporosis who are at increased risk for invasive breast cancer
Calcitonin	Treatment: 200 units (1 spray) in one nostril daily 100 units intramuscularly or subcutaneously daily	Antiresorptive	Postmenopausal osteoporosis Paget's disease of the bone Hypercalcemia	Use among postmenopausal women who cannot tolerate or use other treatments. Major adverse effects: Rhinitis and epistaxis. Unclear association with malignancy.

cancer risk. The relation between the use of hormones and the risk of breast cancer in postmenopausal women was assessed in a follow-up survey of participants in the Nurses' Health Study in 1992. The risk of breast cancer was significantly increased among women who were currently using estrogen alone or estrogen plus progestin, as compared with postmenopausal women who had never used hormones. Women currently taking hormones who had used such therapy for 5–9 years had an adjusted relative risk (RR) of breast cancer of 1.46, as did those currently using hormones who had done so for a total of 10 or more years (RR, 1.46). The addition of progestins to estrogen therapy does not reduce the risk of breast cancer among postmenopausal women.

The only randomized trial of estrogen-progesterone therapy describes secondary prevention of coronary heart disease in postmenopausal women (Heart and Estrogen/ Progestin Replacement Study [HERS]) and included only women who had a prior history of cardiovascular disease. Women received either estrogen alone or estrogen plus progesterone. There was an excessive number of deaths from coronary heart disease and a threefold excess risk of venous thrombosis during the first year of the trial in women on estrogen and a small risk of stroke in women on estrogen and progesterone. Recommendations at the conclusion of the trial included not starting women who already have clinical cardiovascular disease on estrogen and progesterone therapy (ie, secondary prevention).

E. Calcium and Vitamin D

Calcium supplementation produces small beneficial effects on bone mass throughout postmenopausal life and may reduce fracture rates by more than the change in BMD would predict—possibly as much as 50%. Postmenopausal women receiving supplemental calcium over a 3-year period in a placebo-controlled, randomized clinical trial had stable total body calcium and BMD in the lumbar spine, femoral neck, and trochanter compared with the placebo group.

Vitamin D increases calcium absorption in the gastrointestinal tract, so that more calcium is available in the circulation and is subsequently reabsorbed in the renal proximal tubules. There is now evidence of significant reductions in nonvertebral fracture rates from physiologic replacement of vitamin D in the elderly. Vitamin D supplementation is important in those of all ages with limited exposure to sunlight. Dietary calcium augmentation should be recommended to maintain lifetime calcium levels and to help prevent early postmenopausal bone loss. Adults should ingest 1200 mg of elemental calcium per day for optimal bone health. Teenagers, pregnant or lactating women, women age >50 years taking estrogen replacement therapy, and everyone age >65 years should ingest 1500 mg of elemental calcium per day for optimal bone health. If this cannot be achieved by diet alone, calcium supplementation is recommended. Calcium preparations should be compared relative to elemental calcium content. Therefore, attention to which form the patient is ingesting is important.

F. Calcitonin

Calcitonin, a hormone directly inhibiting osteoclastic bone resorption, is an alternative for patients with established osteoporosis in whom estrogen replacement therapy is not recommended. A unique characteristic of calcitonin is that it produces an analgesic effect with respect to bone pain and, thus, is often prescribed for patients who have suffered an acute osteoporotic fracture. The American College of Rheumatology recommends treatment until the pain is controlled, followed by tapering of medication over 4-6 weeks. Calcitonin decreases further bone loss at vertebral and femoral sites in patients with documented osteoporosis but has a questionable effect on fracture frequency. Calcitonin has been shown to prevent trabecular bone loss during the first few years of menopause, but it is unclear whether it has any impact on cortical bone. Calcitonin is also thought to be effective in decreasing the fracture rate of vertebrae and peripheral bones.

For reasons that are poorly understood, the increase in BMD associated with administration of calcitonin may be transient, or there may be the development of resistance. Therefore, calcitonin should be prescribed more acutely and other medications used for chronic management. Calcitonin can be provided in two forms. Nasal congestion and rhinitis are the most significant side effects of the nasal form. The injectable formulation has gastrointestinal side effects and is less convenient than the nasal preparation. The increase in bone density observed by this therapy is significantly less than that achieved by bisphosphonates or estrogen and may be limited to the spine, but it still has recognized value in reducing risk of fracture.

The FDA is currently reviewing prescribing recommendations for calcitonin and new guidelines are forthcoming in the near future.

https://link.springer.com/article/10.1007/s00198-014-2794-2#Sec30.

G. Teriparatide

Teriparatide (Forteo), or recombinant parathyroid hormone, is FDA approved for the treatment of osteoporosis in perimenopausal women who are at high risk for fracture. Teriparatide also has FDA labeling for increasing bone mass in men with primary or hypogonadal osteoporosis who are at high risk for fracture. Unlike antiresorptive agents, teriparatide stimulates new bone formation. There are some concerns regarding extended use of teriparatide because of the long-term effects on multiple organ systems (ie, significant hepatotoxicity, reduced HDL, and elevated LDL cholesterol).

Teriparatide is the first approved agent for the treatment of osteoporosis that stimulates new bone formation.

It is administered once a day by injection (20 µg/d) in the thigh or abdomen. Patients treated with 20 µg/d of teriparatide, along with calcium and vitamin D supplementation, had statistically significant increases in BMD at the spine and hip when compared with patients receiving only calcium and vitamin D supplementation. Clinical trials also demonstrated that teriparatide reduced the risk of vertebral and nonvertebral fractures in postmenopausal women. The effects of teriparatide on fracture risk have not been studied in men. However, in a small prospective cohort of teriparatide users, females appeared to have greater loss in BMD than did men after teriparatide discontinuation.

Of note, osteosarcoma developed in animals in early studies, and the possibility that humans treated with teriparatide may face an increased risk of developing this cancer cannot be ruled out. This safety issue is highlighted in a black box warning in the drug label for health professionals and explained in a brochure for patients. Children and adolescents with growing bones and patients with Paget disease of the bone have a higher risk for developing osteosarcoma and should not be treated with this agent. Because the effects of long-term treatment with teriparatide are not known, therapy for >2 years is not recommended.

Adami S. Denosumab treatment in postmenopausal women with osteoporosis does not interfere with fracture-healing: results from the FREEDOM trial. *J Bone Joint Surg Am.* 2012;94: 2113–2119. [PMID: 23097066]

Leder BZ, Neer RM, Wyland JJ, Lee HW, Burnett-Bowie S, Finkelstein JS. Effects of teriparatide treatment and discontinuation in postmenopausal women and eugonadal men with osteoporosis. *J Clin Enocrinol Metab.* 2009;94(8):2915–2921. [PMID: 19435827]

Simon JA, Recknor C, Moffett AH, et al. Impact of denosumab on the peripheral skeleton of postmenopausal women with osteoporosis. *Menopause.* 2013;20(2):130–137. [PMID: 23010883]

The European Medicines Agency. The European Medicines Agency recommends limiting long term use of calcitonin medicines. http://www.ema.europa.eu/ema/index.jsp?cur/pages/medicines/human/public_health_alerts/2012/07/human_pha_detail_000065.jsp&mid=wc0b01ac058001d126. Accessed October 17, 2012.

H. Complementary and Alternative Therapies

Nutraceuticals are now being used more frequently by patients to promote bone health. There is a paucity of data confirming the benefit of these products, but likewise no evidence of harm. The most common nutraceuticals used for bone health are phytoestrogens (isoflavones, lignins, and coumestans), vitamin A, the B vitamins (B_2 [folate] and B_{12}), vitamin K, magnesium, and omega-3 fatty acids. Evidence from animal studies suggests a beneficial effect of phytoestrogens on bone, but long-term human studies are lacking. Epidemiologic evidence that Asian women have a lower fracture rate than white women, even though the bone density of

Asian women is less than that of African American women, promotes consideration of the impact of nutrition. It is possible that high soy intake contributes to improved bone quality in Asian women. A comparison study of a soy protein and high isoflavone diet versus a milk protein diet or medium isoflavone and soy protein diet demonstrated that only those receiving the higher isoflavone preparation were protected against trabecular (vertebral) bone loss.

A topical form of natural progesterone derived from diosgenin in either soybeans or Mexican wild yam has been promoted as a treatment for osteoporosis, hot flashes, and premenstrual syndrome and as a prophylactic against breast cancer. However, eating or applying wild yam extract or diosgenin does not produce increased progesterone levels in humans because humans cannot convert diosgenin to progesterone.

All patients should be encouraged to maintain a bone-healthy diet. This includes reducing soft drink and sodium consumption, eating potassium-rich foods, encouraging iron and folate supplementation in adolescent females and women of childbearing age, vitamin B_{12} supplementation in persons age ≥50 years, and vitamin D supplementation in the elderly, in dark-skinned people, and in those with low ultraviolet B exposure.

Nieves J. Nutraceuticals: effects on bone metabolism. Talk presented at 8th International Symposium on Osteoporosis Meeting, Washington, DC, April 1–5, 2009.

Weaver C. Nutrition and osteoporosis. Talk presented at 8th International Symposium on Osteoporosis Meeting. Washington, DC, April 1–5, 2009.

I. Glucocorticoid-Induced Osteoporosis

Glucocorticoids are widely used in the treatment of many chronic diseases, particularly asthma, chronic lung disease, and inflammatory and rheumatologic disorders, and in those who have undergone organ transplantation. The risk that oral steroid therapy poses to BMD, among other side effects, has been known for some time. The FRAX score attempts to adjust for steroid exposure of 3 months or greater at a daily dose of 5 mg or more; however, FRAX likely underestimates the probability of fracture if the prednisone dose is >7.5 mg daily and overestimates the probability of fracture if the prednisone dose is <2.5 mg daily.

Clinicians have eagerly substituted inhaled steroids in an endeavor to protect the patient from unwanted negative steroid effects. Recent evaluations of the effects of inhaled glucocorticoids on bone density in premenopausal women demonstrated a dose-related decline in bone density at both the total hip and the trochanter. Women with asthma were enrolled and were divided into three groups: those using no inhaled steroids, those using four to eight puffs per day, and those using more than eight puffs per day at 100 µg per puff. No dose-related effect was noted at the femoral neck or the spine. Serum and urinary markers of bone turnover or adrenal function did not predict the degree of bone loss. To achieve the best possible outcome for the patient, given the potentially devastating effects of systemic steroids, therapy to combat the steroids should begin as soon as the steroids are begun.

American College of Rheumatology recommendations are to initiate bisphosphonate use in glucocorticoid-induced osteoporosis and to initiate therapy if (1) the glucocorticoid use will equal or exceed 3 months, (2) the patient has a T score of < −1, or (3) the patient is receiving long-term glucocorticoid therapy and has had fractures on or cannot tolerate hormone replacement therapy. For individuals <40 years old, the Z score is preferred to the T score; Z scores compare a patient's bone density to the average bone density of others of the same age and gender. Bisphosphonate treatment may be considered for Z scores < −3 at the hip or spine.

J. Children

Bisphosphonates are rarely prescribed to children except for specific pediatric subgroups. For example, bisphosphonates are a mainstay of therapy for children with skeletal fragility, including osteogenesis imperfecta and idiopathic juvenile osteoporosis, or inflammatory bone conditions (eg, chronic recurrent multifocal osteomyelitis). Long-term effects of oral bisphosphonates have not been shown to impair the skeletal development of children, but studies on this subject are limited.

It may be challenging to assess a child's probability of fracture, as the FRAX is generally not used for patients <40 years old. Therefore, bisphosphonates are rarely used for fracture prophylaxis, even among children at high risk of secondary osteoporosis (eg, cerebral palsy, inflammatory conditions). Calcium and vitamin D supplementation are generally recommended. However, bisphosphonates may be used among children with confirmed osteoporotic fractures. The American College of Rheumatology recommends that children who have experienced an osteoporotic fracture and who remain on glucocorticoids at a dose >0.1 mg/kg/d use an oral bisphosphonate, or intravenous bisphosphonate if oral bisphosphonate is not tolerated, in combination with calcium and vitamin D supplementation.

Buckley L, Guyatt G, Fink H, et al. 2017 American College of Rheumatology Guideline for the prevention and treatment of glucocorticoid-induced osteoporosis. *Arthritis Care Res (Hoboken).* 2017;69(8):1095–1110. [PMID: 28585410]

Israel E, Banerjee TR, Fitzmaurice GM, et al. Effects of inhaled glucocorticoids on bone density in premenopausal women. *N Engl J Med.* 2001;345:941–947. [PMID: 11575285]

Leib ES, Saag KG, Geusens PP, Binkley N, McCLoskey EV, Hans DB; FRAX Position Development Conference Members. Official positions for FRAX clinical regarding glucocorticoids: the impact of the use of glucocorticoids on the estimate by FRAX of the 10 year risk of fracture from the Joint Official Positions Development Conference of the International Society for Clinical Densitometry and International Osteoporosis Foundation on FRAX. *J Clin Densitom.* 2011;14(4):212–219. [PMID: 21810527]

Rossouw JE, Anderson GL, Prentice RL, et al. Risks and benefits of estrogen plus progestin in healthy postmenopausal women: principal results from the Women's Health Initiative randomized controlled trial. *JAMA.* 2002;288:321–333. [PMID: 12117397]

Saag KG, Emkey R, Schnitzer TJ, et al. Alendronate for the prevention and treatment of glucocorticoid-induced osteoporosis: glucocorticoid-Induced Osteoporosis Intervention Study Group. *N Engl J Med.* 1998;339:292–299. [PMID: 9682041]

Simm PJ, Biggin A, Zacharin MR, et al. Consensus guidelines on the use of bisphosphonate therapy in children and adolescents. *J Paediatr Child Health.* 2018;54(3):223–233. [PMID: 29504223]

▶ Summary Recommendations

Summary recommendations for postmenopausal women and men age ≥50 years are to (1) counsel on the risk of osteoporosis and fractures, (2) check for secondary causes, (3) advise on adequate calcium and vitamin D, (4) recommend regular exercise, and (5) advise on avoidance of tobacco and alcohol intake. In women age ≥65 years and men age ≥70 years, recommend BMD testing. In postmenopausal women between the ages of 50 and 69, recommend BMD testing based on the risk factor profile. Furthermore, when a patient has already experienced a fracture, recommend BMD to determine the severity of the disease.

Websites

Food and Drug Administration: Approved Drug Products: http://www.accessdata.fda.gov/scripts/cder/drugsatfda
National Osteoporosis Foundation: http:/www.nof.org

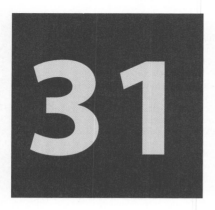

Abdominal Complaints

Cindy M. Barter, MD, MPH, IBCLC, CTTS, FAAFP

Laura Dunne, MD, CAQSM, FAAFP

Carla Jardim, MD, FAAP

► General Considerations

Abdominal pain is a common presenting complaint in both the emergency department and office. It accounts for up to 10% of emergency department visits and is one of the top 10 reasons for presenting to a primary care office. Because of the wide differential diagnoses, accurate diagnosis can be difficult. This usually can be achieved through a detailed history and thorough physical examination. Although most complaints of abdominal pain are related to benign conditions, it is important to identify the patients with severe or life-threatening conditions. A thoughtful and logical approach to the use of diagnostic testing is necessary. Follow-up, continuity, and patient-centered care are important components to the treatment both acute and chronic abdominal pain regardless of etiology.

► Clinical Findings

A. History

ESSENTIALS OF DIAGNOSIS

► Acuity, onset, and duration of symptoms.

► Quality, location, and radiation of pain.

► Associated symptoms.

History is the most important component of evaluating abdominal pain. Effective communication is necessary for a thorough, accurate history. Adequate time should be allowed for an open-ended history using the method "engage, empathize, educate, enlist."

1. Onset—Determining the onset of pain can help determine the cause of abdominal pain as well as the need for emergent

referral. Abdominal pain is categorized as acute, subacute, or chronic. Symptoms lasting >3 months are considered chronic. Acute pain is often associated with peritoneal irritation, such as seen with appendicitis and abdominal organ rupture, and may require emergency management and consultation with a surgeon. Many patients present to the office with a more gradual onset of their abdominal pain (Table 31–1).

2. Quality of pain—A patient's description of the quality of their pain provides important clues to etiology. Pain can be sharp, stabbing, burning, dull, gnawing, colicky, crampy, gassy, focal, migrating, or radiating. Pain described as pressure, such as "an elephant sitting on me," suggests cardiac ischemia. Focal symptoms help determine both the location and diagnosis.

3. Location—Location and radiation of pain are important clues to etiology. The abdomen is separated into four quadrants—right upper (RUQ), left upper (LUQ), right lower (RLQ), and left lower (LLQ)—or as midepigastric or suprapubic. Some causes of abdominal pain have classic patterns of location and radiation. Pain may be referred. For example, lower esophageal pain may be experienced higher in the chest and confused with pain from cardiac conditions.

4. Frequency and timing—Frequency and pattern of pain are particularly useful in identifying the causes of chronic pain. Symptoms may be associated with eating, types of food, defecation, body position, or movement. Peritoneal irritation may be eased by lack of movement. Visceral pain may trigger a patient to move more to try to find a more comfortable position. Pain caused by colonic pathology may be relieved by defecation.

5. Other diagnostic clues and symptoms—Physicians should determine whether associated symptoms are present such as nausea, vomiting, diarrhea, constipation, melena,

Table 31–1. Common causes of abdominal pain by location.

Localized
  Midepigastric
    Dyspepsia
    GERD
    Pancreatitis
    PUD
  RUQ
    Gallbladder diseases
    Hepatitis
    Hepatomegaly
  RLQ
    Appendicitis
    Crohn disease
    GYN-related diseases
      Ruptured ovarian cyst
      Ectopic pregnancy
      PID
      Pregnancy
    Meckel diverticulitis
  LUQ
    MI
    Pneumonia
    Sickle cell crisis
    Lymphoma
    Splenomegaly—EBV
    Gastritis
  LLQ
    Diverticulitis
    Bowel obstruction
    Ischemic colitis
    Ulcerative colitis
    Urinary calculi
  Suprapubic
    Cystitis
    Prostatitis
    Urinary retention
Generalized
  Abdominal wall pain—multiple causes
  Celiac disease
  Constipation
  Chronic diarrhea
  IBS
  Gastroenteritis/infectious diarrhea
  Mesenteric lymphadenitis
  Perforated colon
  Ruptured aortic aneurysm
  Trauma

EBV, Epstein-Barr virus; GERD, gastroesophageal reflux disease; GYN, gynecologic; IBS, irritable bowel syndrome; LLQ, left lower quadrant; LUQ, left upper quadrant; MI, myocardial infarction; PID, pelvic inflammatory disease; PUD, peptic ulcer disease; RLQ, right lower quadrant; RUQ, right upper quadrant.

mucus, or hematochezia. Fever and chills suggest an infectious etiology. Feculent emesis correlates with a bowel obstruction. The presence of melena or blood in the stool should prompt evaluation for gastrointestinal (GI) bleeding. A patient's age may be a factor in both cause and perception of pain. The elderly may not present with classic symptoms of serious conditions and instead complain of vague or mild pain. There is a 10–20% reduction in pain perception for each decade of age over 60 years. Emotional stress can trigger symptoms from functional bowel disease. Organic diseases also may be exacerbated by emotional stress.

Past medical history provides important clues to the etiology of pain. Previous abdominal surgery increases the risk for bowel obstruction secondary to adhesions, strangulation, or hernia. Patients with cardiovascular diseases are at greater risk for GI ischemia and bowel infarction. Tobacco, alcohol, or medications such as nonsteroidal anti-inflammatory drugs (NSAIDs) are associated with an increased incidence of gastroesophageal reflux disease (GERD) and peptic ulcer disease (PUD). Alcohol abuse is a common cause of pancreatitis. Multiparity, obesity, and diabetes mellitus increase the risk of gallbladder disease. Tubal ligation or pelvic inflammatory disease (PID) history indicate a greater risk for an ectopic pregnancy.

Medication history should include the use of prescription and over-the-counter (OTC) medications and herbal supplements. Aspirin and other platelet aggregation inhibitors, steroids and NSAIDs, and antidepressants increase the risk of GI bleeding. Antibiotics can cause abdominal cramping, nausea, and diarrhea.

B. Physical Examination

ESSENTIALS OF DIAGNOSIS

► Inspect, auscultate, palpate, and percuss abdomen.
► Palpate for tenderness and rebound tenderness.
► Assess bowel sounds

1. Inspection—Examine the patient in the supine position with knees slightly bent. Inspect for distention, discoloration, scars, and striae. Distention suggests ascites, obstruction, or other masses. Discoloration from bruising associated with hemoperitoneum is found in the central portion of the abdomen, especially following abdominal trauma. The location of scars helps to clarify and confirm the past history. Striae suggest rapid growth of the abdomen. New striae or those related to endocrine abnormalities tend to be purplish or dark pink. Striae may appear as darkening of the skin in darker-skinned persons. The abdomen should be inspected for hernias with the patient in an upright position.

2. Auscultation—Auscultation is performed prior to palpation. Bowel sounds may be normal, hypoactive, hyperactive, or high-pitched. Hypoactive or hyperactive bowel sounds can be present with partial bowel obstruction, or ileus. Bruits over the aorta, renal arteries, and femoral arteries suggest stenosis or aneurysms. Gentle palpation while auscultating decreases the likelihood that a patient will guard, embellish, or magnify symptoms.

3. Palpation—Palpation of the abdomen begins with light touch away from the area of greatest pain. Assess for rigidity, tenderness, masses, and organ size. Increased rigidity may indicate an acute abdomen and need for emergent intervention. A Murphy sign is the sudden cessation of a patient's inspiratory effort during deep palpation of the RUQ and suggests acute cholecystitis.

Pain from visceral organs may radiate because of shared nerve innervation. Pain from pancreatitis often radiates to the back. Abdominal pain radiating to the left shoulder (Kehr sign) indicates splenic rupture, renal calculi, or ectopic pregnancy. Radiation of pain may be caused by inflammation of surrounding tissues.

The iliopsoas muscle test, performed by having the patient flex the right hip while lying supine and applying pressure to the leg, can be used to evaluate the deep muscles of the abdomen. Inflammation of the psoas muscle may indicate inflammation of nearby structures as seen with appendicitis or retroperitoneal dissection.

Rebound tenderness indicates peritoneal irritation and can occur with GI perforation or non-GI sources such as a ruptured ovarian cyst and PID. Peritoneal irritation is often associated with guarding. Voluntary guarding occurs when a patient anticipates the pain. Patients who close their eyes as the examiner approaches ("closed-eye sign") are more likely to have underlying psychosocial factors contributing to pain. Involuntary guarding is caused by flexion of the abdominal wall muscle as the body attempts to protect internal organs. The Carnett test, performed by having the patient flex the abdominal wall as the point of greatest tenderness is palpated, may help differentiate visceral pain from abdominal wall or psychogenic pain. Pain that is less severe with palpation of the flexed abdomen wall has a higher probability of being visceral than pain from abdominal wall pathology or nonorganic causes.

Two approaches may help examine a ticklish patient: use of a stethoscope for light palpation by curling fingers past the edge of the stethoscope to create a less sensitive touch; and placement of hands over the patient's hand to palpate.

Evaluate liver and spleen by having the patient take a deep breath and exhale while palpating the organ's border. The normal liver span at the midclavicular line is 6–12 cm depending on the height and gender of the patient. Assessing the mid-sternal liver size can be helpful. The normal span is 4–8 cm. A span of >8 cm is considered enlarged. The tip of the spleen may not be palpable.

Examine for masses that may be seen with colon cancer, kidney abnormalities, and non-GI tumors. A palpated mass should be examined for location, size, shape, consistency, pulsations, mobility, and movement with respiration.

4. Percussion—Percussion can help determine the size of organs and other abdominal pathology. A change in the character of the sound indicates a solid organ. The examiner should percuss both liver edges. The upper border usually sits at the fifth to seventh intercostal space. Inferior displacement suggests emphysema or other pulmonary diseases. The span of the spleen is evaluated in the left mid-axillary line and usually extends from the sixth to the tenth ribs. The scratch test is another form of percussion. It is performed by placing the stethoscope over the liver and gently scratching the surface of the skin beginning above the upper border of the liver and progressing to below the lower border of the liver. The quality of the sound changes as the examiner's scratch travels from the lung field to liver and abdomen. Changes in sound help identify the liver borders.

Increased tympany should be present over the stomach in the area of the left lower border of the rib cage and left epigastrium because of the gastric air bubble. Increased tympany throughout the rest of the abdomen suggests dilation or perforation of the bowel. Dullness can be stationary, as with solid masses, or shifting, as with mobile fluid. Shifting dullness generally is present with significant ascites.

5. Pelvic exam—A pelvic examination may be indicated in female patients with abdominal pain.

C. Laboratory Findings

ESSENTIALS OF DIAGNOSIS

▶ Complete blood cell count, electrolytes, blood urea nitrogen, creatinine, and glucose are useful in most patients.

▶ All women of childbearing age should have a pregnancy test.

▶ Consider iron studies for adults age >50 years.

Testing should include complete blood cell count (CBC), electrolytes, blood urea nitrogen (BUN), creatinine, and glucose. Alkaline phosphatase and liver function tests can be helpful. Normal hemoglobin and hematocrit in the setting of acute rapid blood loss can be misleading and should be rechecked after the patient is fluid-resuscitated. Anemia, especially in those age >50 years, should prompt iron studies, including ferritin level. Hypothyroidism in the elderly may present with vague abdominal pain, so a thyroid-stimulating hormone level may be helpful.

RUQ pain should be evaluated with bilirubin, lipase, amylase, trypsin, and liver function tests. Hepatitis panels may be useful. Amylase is elevated in pancreatitis and many other abdominal problems. Therefore, lipase and trypsin levels are more specific for pancreatitis.

Stool studies may be indicated when the patient presents with abdominal pain and diarrhea. Stool testing should be done for dehydration, blood in the stool, and immunocompromised patients. Stool white blood cell (WBC) count, hemoccult testing, ova and parasite, culture for enteric pathogens, and *Clostridium difficile* toxin level are indicated for chronic or bloody diarrhea. Erythrocyte sedimentation rate (ESR) and C-reactive protein (CRP) should be checked if inflammatory bowel disease is suspected, especially if WBCs are found in stool. Intermittent symptoms suggesting celiac disease may warrant laboratory tests for antiendomysial antibody.

Women of childbearing age should have a pregnancy test regardless of history of tubal ligation. Patients with lower abdominal pain may need a urinalysis (UA), although other intraabdominal problems can cause changes in UA similar to urinary tract infection. Consider vaginal testing for sexually transmitted infections, including gonorrhea and *Chlamydia*. Cardiac studies should be considered for at-risk patients. Studies including magnesium, calcium, and vitamin D levels may be indicated for nonspecific complaints.

D. Imaging Studies

ESSENTIALS OF DIAGNOSIS

▸ A computed tomography (CT) scan is the test of choice for acute abdominal pain.

▸ An ultrasound is the test of choice for RUQ pain.

▸ Colonoscopy should be considered for abdominal pain in all patients age >50 years.

Plain films of the abdomen are low-cost, widely available, and safe initial diagnostic tests. Upright and lateral decubitus films of the abdomen can show dilated small bowel loops (suggestive of obstruction), free air (perforated organ), mass (tumor or other obstructing cause), or stones (biliary or renal). Small bowel follow-through may show ulcer or mass. Barium enema can be useful for evaluation of constipation.

CT of the abdomen and pelvis is the test of choice for many acute and nonacute causes of abdominal pain. Protocols for specific problems limit radiation exposure while providing accurate information. Spiral CT for appendicitis and renal calculus has been shown to be fast, safe, effective, and cost effective. Other problems well visualized by CT scan include diverticulitis, bowel obstruction, pancreatitis, abdominal aortic aneurysm, pneumoperitoneum, soft tissue tumors, and radiopaque renal and biliary stones.

Ultrasonography is the most reliable imaging study for the biliary system and pelvic organs and the test of choice for most RUQ pain; in addition, it can identify hernias. The lack of contrast material and radiation makes it useful for pregnant patients. Children may tolerate ultrasound better than CT scan because the exam time is shorter and there is less need to remain completely still. The accuracy of ultrasound is more operator dependent and is limited by obesity.

Direct visualization of the GI tract is often needed for chronic pain. Upper endoscopy is used for evaluation of dyspepsia, ulcers, and other upper gastric abnormalities. This imaging modality allows for visualization, biopsy of mucosal lesions, and treatment of bleeding. Colonoscopy or sigmoidoscopy is indicated for most patients age >50 years or with other risk factors for cancer. Direct visualization of the colonic mucosa can help in diagnosis of diverticulosis, cancer, diarrhea, and inflammatory bowel disease.

Other modalities available for imaging of the abdomen include magnetic resonance imaging (MRI). Imaging modalities for urinary system problems are discussed elsewhere.

DYSPEPSIA

▸ General Considerations

The term *dyspepsia* was first used in the early 18th century to describe a person's ill humor, indigestion, or disgruntlement. The term now describes a set of symptoms encompassing different diseases and the etiologies associated with them. Chronic or recurrent discomfort centered in the upper abdomen commonly describes dyspepsia and can be associated with heartburn, belching, bloating, nausea, or vomiting. Common etiologies include PUD and GERD. Rare causes include gastric and pancreatic cancers. No specific etiology is found for >50% of patients presenting with epigastric pain. Dyspepsia is reported to affect 20% of the world's adult population, accounts for 2–3% of all visits to primary care providers, and costs the US healthcare system >$18 billion per year. It is more common in women, smokers, and patients taking NSAIDs. Dyspepsia may have a significant effect on the quality of life.

Nonulcer dyspepsia or *functional dyspepsia* applies to patients with symptoms lasting >3 months without a clear etiology. Other infrequent etiologies include gastric, esophageal, and pancreatic cancer; biliary tract disease; gastroparesis; pancreatitis; carbohydrate malabsorption; medication-induced symptoms; hepatoma; intestinal parasites; non-GI diseases such as sarcoidosis, diabetes, thyroid, and parathyroid conditions; and metabolic disturbances such as hypercalcemia and hyperkalemia. Studies have shown that symptoms and degree of symptoms do not correlate with findings on endoscopy.

Dyspepsia is caused by PUD in 15–25% and GERD in 5–15% of cases. Abdominal exam may be unremarkable unless an ulcer perforates, causing signs of peritonitis. Treatment for dyspepsia depends on the etiology and is discussed in sections on PUD, GERD, and nonulcer dyspepsia.

Moayyedi PM, Lacy BE, Andrews CN, et al. Management of dyspepsia. *Am J Gastroenterol.* 2017;112(7):988–1013. [PMID: 28631728]
Stanghellini V, Chan FK, Hasler WL, et al. Gastroduodenal disorders. *Gastroenterology.* 2016;150:1380–1392. [PMID: 27147122]

Peptic Ulcer Disease

▶ General Considerations

The four major causes of ulcers are *Helicobacter pylori*–induced ulcers, NSAIDs, acid hypersecretory conditions, and idiopathic ulcers. Clear evidence supports eradication of *H pylori* in patients with documented ulcers. Since the early 1990s, the association of *H pylori* with peptic ulcers has decreased from 90% to as low as 15–20% in some countries. This decrease is related to increased treatment of *H pylori* infections, which are commonly associated with low income, low educational levels, and overcrowded living conditions. African Americans and Hispanics have about a one-third higher rate of infection than white Americans. In the United States, 40% of adults are infected with *H pylori* by the age of 50, compared with only 5% of children age 6–12 years. In developing countries, children commonly are infected at a younger age, and there is a higher incidence of infection in the entire population.

▶ Pathogenesis

In the past, infection with *H pylori* was the leading cause of peptic ulcers, and NSAID use was second. Now NSAID use and idiopathic ulcers are the most common causes. In the United States, one in seven individuals uses NSAIDs. Of long-term NSAID users undergoing upper endoscopy, 5–20% are found to have an ulcer. Compared with nonusers, NSAID users have a four times higher risk of complications of PUD. Risk factors for developing ulcers due to NSAID use are a personal history of ulcer, age >65 years, current steroid use, use of anticoagulants, history of cardiovascular disease, and impairment of another major organ. NSAIDs are prescribed to nearly 40% of all persons age >65 years. Elderly patients treated with a course of NSAIDs have a 1–8% chance of being hospitalized within the first year of therapy for GI complications. Patients who are *H pylori* positive and take NSAIDs have a higher risk of complications. The disease is uncommon in patients without *H pylori* infection and who do not take NSAIDs or aspirin.

▶ Prevention

Eradication of *H pylori* infection before starting a course of treatment with NSAIDs reduces the risk of developing an ulcer early in the treatment, particularly with duodenal ulcers. Treatment with a proton pump inhibitor (PPI) is standard for secondary prevention of gastroduodenal ulcers.

▶ Clinical Findings

Factors suggesting PUD include gnawing pain with the sensation of hunger, prior personal or family history of ulcers, tobacco use, and a report of melena. The most accurate diagnostic test is esophagogastroduodenoscopy (EGD). It allows both visualization and biopsy of an ulcer as well as testing for *H pylori*. Good evidence supports a "test and treat" approach. The most cost-effective noninvasive test is the monoclonal stool antigen test, although there have not been any large, randomized, controlled trials using the stool antigen test. Breath urea testing is noninvasive but more expensive. Serology testing is used mainly for research or surveillance but may be indicated for actively bleeding ulcers, complicating performance of an EGD.

▶ Complications

Elderly patients (age ≥80 years) with ulcers who take aspirin or have *H pylori* infection have a much higher incidence of complications. A hypersecretory condition, such as Zollinger-Ellison syndrome, caused by a gastrin-producing tumor should be suspected in patients with multiple ulcers. The incidence of GI bleeding from the upper GI tract has decreased. This may be related to the increased treatment of *H pylori*.

▶ Treatment

Treatment of PUD requires initial eradication of *H pylori* if present, reducing or discontinuing NSAID use, and treatment with a PPI. The recommended standard first-line therapy is a quadruple therapy for 14 days (PPI, a bismuth salt, tetracycline, and metronidazole; or PPI, clarithromycin, amoxicillin, and metronidazole) depending on local resistance. Refer to the Centers for Disease Control and Prevention (CDC) and local guidelines since antibiotic resistance is increasing. Treatment of *H pylori* facilitates healing of ulcers and decreases rate of recurrence in the first year from 75% to 10%. Increased effectiveness of medical treatment for PUD has decreased the need for surgical intervention. Surgery, when performed, is commonly laparoscopic. A vaccine for *H pylori* is currently being developed.

Chan FK, Kyaw M, Tanigawa T, et al. Similar efficacy of proton-pump inhibitors vs H2-receptor antagonists in reducing risk of upper gastrointestinal bleeding or ulcers in high-risk users of low-dose aspirin. *Gastroenterology.* 2017;152:105–10.e1. [PMID: 27641510]
El-Serag HB, Kao JY, Kanwal F, et al. Houston consensus conference on testing for *Helicobacter pylori* infection in the United States. *Clin Gastroenterol Hepatol.* 2018;16(7):992–1002. [PMID: 29559361]

Lanas A, Chan FKL. Peptic ulcer disease. *Lancet*. 2017;390(10094): 613–624. [PMID: 28242110]

Malfertheiner P, Megraud F, O'Morain CA, et al. Management of *Helicobacter pylori* infection—the Maastricht V/Florence Consensus Report. *Gut*. 2017;66:6–30. [PMID: 27707777]

Nyssen OP, McNicholl AG, Megraud F, et al. Sequential versus standard triple first-line therapy for *Helicobacter pylori* eradication. *Cochrane Database Syst Rev*. 2016;6:CD009034. [PMID: 27351542]

Gastroesophageal Reflux Disease

▶ Clinical Findings

Heartburn is the single most common symptom of GERD. Ten percent of the US population experiences heartburn at least once a day, and almost 50% experiences symptoms once a month. Other common symptoms include regurgitation, belching, and dysphagia. GERD can be associated with extraesophageal symptoms and conditions. Pulmonary conditions include asthma, chronic bronchitis, aspiration pneumonia, sleep apnea, atelectasis, and interstitial pulmonary fibrosis. Ear, nose, and throat manifestations of GERD include chronic cough, sore throat, hoarseness, halitosis, enamel erosion, subglottic stenosis, vocal cord inflammation, granuloma, and, possibly, cancer. Noncardiac chest pain, chronic hiccups, and nausea may be associated with GERD. Changes in body position such as lying down or bending forward may exacerbate symptoms of GERD.

The esophagus has three mechanisms in place to prevent mucosal injury. The lower esophageal sphincter (LES) creates a barrier to acid reflux. Peristalsis, gravity, and saliva provide acid clearance mechanisms. Epithelial cells provide resistance.

Diagnosis is based on the medical history and response to treatment with H_2-receptor antagonists, prokinetic agents, or PPIs. Symptomatic improvement following treatment can indicate GERD. Diagnosis may be suggested by use of symptom questionnaires, catheter and wireless pH-metry, and impedance–pH monitoring. Upper endoscopy fails to reveal 36–50% of patients diagnosed via esophageal pH monitoring. Patients with typical symptoms and response to PPIs do not need further evaluation. Endoscopy should be performed if alarming symptoms are present, such as bleeding, weight loss, dysphagia, or persistence of symptoms after treatment with a PPI, especially in elderly patients. Complications of GERD include Barrett esophagus, esophageal strictures, ulceration, hemorrhage, and rarely, perforation. Barrett esophagus is found in 8–20% of patients who undergo upper endoscopy for GERD.

▶ Treatment

Lifestyle modifications with the greatest impact on reducing symptoms of GERD include weight loss in overweight and obese patients, cessation of smoking, moderation of alcohol consumption, and reduction of dietary fat intake. Limiting foods that decrease LES pressure (chocolate), stimulate acid secretion (coffee, tea, and cola beverages), or produce symptoms by their acidity (orange or tomato juice) may be helpful. Elevating the head of the bed by 6 inches, avoiding bedtime snacks, and reducing meal size, particularly in the evening, may help ameliorate symptoms.

Medication treatment options decrease acid or help with other defense mechanisms. Commonly used OTC medications include antacids, simethicone, and H_2-blockers. Prescription medications include prescription-strength H_2-blockers, PPIs, prokinetic agents, bethanechol, and sucralfate. Agents that irritate the mucosa (eg, aspirin and NSAIDs) should be avoided. Other agents to avoid include α-adrenergic antagonists, anticholinergics, β-adrenergic agonists, calcium channel blockers, diazepam, narcotics, progesterone, and theophylline.

If a patient's symptoms resolve or significantly improve with treatment, no further evaluation is needed. If the symptoms do not improve with an 8-week course of PPIs, endoscopy is indicated. Extensive use of PPIs without monitoring and reassessment is concerning and increases the risk of adverse effects (vitamin B_{12} deficiency, hypomagnesemia, pneumonia, *Clostridium difficile* infection, diarrhea, headache, and fractures). Patients with Barrett esophagus need close monitoring because of a 50- to 100-fold increased risk of developing esophageal cancer.

Boghossian TA, Rashid FJ, Thompson W, et al. Deprescribing versus continuation of chronic proton pump inhibitor use in adults. *Cochrane Database Syst Rev*. 2017;3:CD011969. [PMID: 28301676]

Sandhu DS, Fass R. Current trends in the management of gastroesophageal reflux disease. *Gut Liver*. 2018;12(1):7–16. [PMID: 28427116]

Nonulcer Dyspepsia

ESSENTIALS OF DIAGNOSIS

▶ Persistent or recurrent dyspepsia present for the past 3 months; onset at least 6 months prior to diagnosis, without evidence of organic disease.

▶ Diagnosis made by excluding other causes of dyspepsia.

▶ No diagnostic gold standard; consider EGD to rule out other causes if no response to PPIs and "test and treat" for *H pylori*.

▶ General Considerations

Nonulcer dyspepsia, also called *idiopathic* or *functional dyspepsia*, is defined as persistent or recurrent dyspepsia without evidence of organic disease present for 3 months with onset >6 months prior to diagnosis, not relieved by defecation, and not associated with the onset of change in stool frequency or form. Nonulcer dyspepsia is divided into at least two distinct subgroups: postprandial distress syndrome, which features postprandial fullness and early satiety; and epigastric pain syndrome, which features more constant and less meal-related symptoms.

Nonerosive reflux disease (NERD) is defined as having typical symptoms of GERD but absence of visible esophageal mucosal injury when EGD is performed. Nonulcer dyspepsia and NERD may represent different aspects of the same disease entity.

▶ Pathogenesis

The pathophysiology of nonulcer dyspepsia is not entirely clear and is probably multifactorial. Suggested causes include changes in gastric physiology, nociception, motor dysfunction, central nervous system (CNS) dysfunction, and psychological and environmental factors. *H pylori* and its effects on nonulcer dyspepsia are not completely understood. Individuals with nonulcer dyspepsia and *H pylori* should be treated because a significant percentage have improvement in symptoms.

▶ Clinical Findings

Nonulcer dyspepsia is diagnosed by excluding other causes of dyspepsia. Endoscopy is negative with nonulcer dyspepsia and NERD. A therapeutic trial of PPIs and/or "test and treat" for *H pylori* are common practices supported in the literature. Cost-effectiveness data indicate that testing and treating patients for *H pylori* decreases the number of EGDs performed by about one-third.

▶ Treatment

Management of nonulcer dyspepsia is multifactorial. Early diagnosis and explanation of the relevant physiology are helpful to patients. Physicians should avoid excessive investigation, although patients with previous diagnosis of nonulcer dyspepsia should be investigated whenever alarm symptoms are present or a new objective symptom arises. Alarm symptoms are highlighted by the mnemonic **VBAD:** **v**omiting, evidence of **b**leeding or anemia, presence of **a**bdominal mass or weight loss, and **d**ysphagia. The prevalence of *H pylori* in the community may factor into the decision to "test and treat" or perform other investigations. Physicians should determine why the patient with chronic symptoms presented at this particular time.

Psychosocial factors exacerbate symptoms. Physicians should address these issues and offer counseling. Postevaluation reassurance is a mainstay of management. Patients should be told to avoid foods or substances that exacerbate symptoms (NSAIDs, alcohol, tobacco, and certain foods). Not all patients want or need prescription medications and may prefer to explore other treatment options. Eating six small meals per day may alleviate symptoms of bloating or postprandial fullness.

Numerous medications have been used in studies of nonulcer dyspepsia. Results are confounded by different study definitions of the disorder and the lack of differentiation of symptom types. Medications include antacids, H_2-blockers, PPIs, bismuth, and sucralfate. PPIs appear to benefit ulcer-like dyspepsia but not dysmotility like dyspepsia. Prokinetic agents such as metoclopramide have been poorly studied. Cisapride, which was taken off the market, showed a twofold decrease in symptoms compared to placebo. Domperidone has been shown to be superior to placebo and does not cross the blood-brain barrier to cause CNS side effects but is not available in the United States. Peppermint and caraway oils produced similar results when compared to cisapride. Motilin agonists such as erythromycin increase the rate of gastric emptying. Visceral analgesics such as fedotozine reduce gastric hypersensitivity. Buspirone and 5-HT_1 agonists such as sumatriptan have shown promise. Antispasmodics such as dicyclomine have not been shown to be more effective than placebo in patients with dyspepsia. Antinausea agents such as ondansetron and prochlorperazine have been shown to modestly improve symptoms. Prochlorperazine had more side effects. Antihistamines such as dimenhydrinate and cyclizine decrease gastric dysrhythmias. Promethazine has been used to treat mild nausea. Tricyclic antidepressants have been the most extensively studied antidepressant treatment of functional dyspepsia. Selective serotonin reuptake inhibitors have shown promising results with other functional bowel diseases (eg, irritable bowel syndrome [IBS]).

Other treatment approaches include acupuncture, acupressure, and gastric electrical stimulation. No randomized, double-blind, controlled trials have been performed to evaluate their effectiveness. Follow-up appointments are important to assess patient function and response to treatment.

Drossman DA. Functional gastrointestinal disorders: history, pathophysiology, clinical features and Rome IV. *Gastroenterology*. 2016;19:S0016-5085(16)00223-7. [PMID: 27144617]

Pinto-Sanchez MI, Yuan Y, Hassan A, Bercik P, Moayyedi P. Proton pump inhibitors for functional dyspepsia. *Cochrane Database Syst Rev*. 2017;11:CD011194. [PMID: 29161458]

DISEASES OF THE GALLBLADDER & PANCREAS

The four main causes of abdominal pain related to the gallbladder and pancreas are biliary colic, gallstones, cholecystitis, and pancreatitis. Gallbladder-related pain usually is located in the midepigastric region with radiation to the right shoulder, right scapula, right clavicular area, or back. Pancreatitis often produces pain throughout the entire upper abdomen with frequent radiation to the back. See Chapter 33 for a detailed discussion of these and other diseases of the biliary tract and pancreas.

IRRITABLE BOWEL SYNDROME

▶ General Considerations

Estimates indicate that symptoms consistent with a diagnosis of IBS are present in 3–20% of adults in the Western world. Although IBS occurs worldwide, cultural and social factors affect its presentation. Women in Western countries have a higher incidence of IBS and are more likely to consult a physician. In India and Sri Lanka, men have a higher incidence. IBS symptoms are common in South Africans who live in urban zones and unusual in people who live in rural areas. In the United States, prevalence is similar in blacks and whites. Some studies show lower prevalence in Hispanics from Texas and Asians from California.

Up to 50% of individuals with symptoms consistent with IBS do not seek physician care. Many who seek care had a major life event such as a death in the family or loss of job before presenting. Primary care providers see more of these patients than GI specialists.

▶ Pathogenesis

Physiologic changes contributing to symptoms of IBS have not been elucidated. Many theories exist, including disturbance in motility, postinfectious changes, altered perception either locally in the GI tract or in the CNS, visceral hypersensitivity, mucosal inflammation, autonomic nerve dysfunction, and psychological disturbance. More recently, altered gut immune activation, intestinal permeability, and intestinal and colonic microbiome have been proposed as possible contributing mechanisms. A study using positron emission tomography (PET) examined the activity of the brain when GI symptoms were induced. Patients with IBS did not activate the anterior cingulate cortex associated with opiate binding but activated the prefrontal cortex associated with hypervigilance and anxiety. Studies to determine whether patients with IBS have a lower threshold of pain with colonic distention are inconclusive. Studies have not clarified whether symptoms of IBS are a normal perception of an abnormal function or an abnormal perception of a normal function.

▶ Clinical Findings

A. Symptoms and Signs

IBS is a functional bowel disorder, without identified organic cause, in which abdominal discomfort or pain is associated with defecation or change in bowel habits and with features of disordered defecation. Diagnostic criteria developed by the Rome Consensus Committee for IBS are presence of symptoms at least 3 days per month for the past 3 months with onset at least 6 months prior to diagnosis of abdominal discomfort or pain characterized by two of the following three features: (1) relieved with defecation, (2) onset associated with a change in frequency of stool, and (3) onset associated with change in form or appearance of the stool.

The Bristol Stool Form Scale describes seven types of stool forms. Other symptoms supporting the diagnosis of IBS include abnormal stool frequency (more than three per day or fewer than three per week), abnormal stool form (lumpy/hard or loose/watery), abnormal stool passage (straining, urgency, or feeling of incomplete evacuation), passage of mucus, and sensation of bloating or feeling of abdominal distention. Stool form has been demonstrated to reflect GI transit time. Using the Bristol Stool Form Scale and frequency of bowel movements is more precise and useful than using the imprecise terms *diarrhea* and *constipation*, since these terms have different meanings to different patients. Patients may complain of feeling constipated because of a feeling of incomplete evacuation despite having just passed soft or watery stool.

B. History

Patient history is the single most useful tool in diagnosing IBS. Continuity of care and a well-established rapport contribute significantly to obtaining accurate and complete history. A positive physician-patient interaction, psychosocial history, precipitating factors, and discussion of diagnosis and treatment with patients result in fewer return visits for IBS and lower utilization of healthcare resources. Chronic or recurrent abdominal pain indicates a need to assess quality of life. In a study of undergraduate students with IBS, quality-of-life scores similar to those of patients with congestive heart failure indicated the significant impact of IBS symptoms. As noted earlier, stressful life events often precede onset of symptoms of IBS. Although stressful life events may not be the cause of IBS, they may factor into the decision by patients to seek care. The decision of women with IBS symptoms to seek care has been shown to have a significant and positive correlation between daily stress levels and daily symptoms.

A history of abuse should be sought in patients with chronic abdominal pain. A study at a tertiary care gastroenterology clinic revealed that 60% of the overall study population reported a history of physical or sexual abuse. All were women. Self-reported history of abuse was highest for those with functional bowel disease (≤84%) and lowest for those with organic bowel disease, such as ulcerative colitis (38%). Treatment success can be affected by exploring a patient's psychosocial stressors. Physicians should assess for abuse when considering referral to a gastroenterologist. Family physicians are uniquely positioned to assess and address issues associated with abuse.

Patients with IBS have not been demonstrated to have a higher incidence of psychiatric diagnosis such as depression, anxiety, somatization, stress, lack of social support, or abnormal illness behavior compared with other patients presenting with abdominal pain of organic origin. However, patients presenting with abdominal pain do have more psychosocial concerns than control subjects without abdominal pain. Psychosocial factors have not been shown to help in differentiating between organic and functional abdominal disease but do help in understanding some health-seeking behaviors.

Signs or symptoms of an anatomic disease should be absent. These include fever, GI bleeding, unintentional weight loss, anemia, and abdominal mass. Laxative use should be assessed because laxatives may cause IBS-like symptoms. Patients with IBS may have had surgery, particularly appendectomy, hysterectomy, or ovarian surgery. The most common discharge diagnosis for patients hospitalized for abdominal pain is "nonspecific abdominal pain." A study of patients discharged with this diagnosis showed that 37% of women and 19% of men met the criteria for IBS 1–2 years after discharge. Of these patients, 70% had prior attacks of abdominal pain. Only 6% of charts listed IBS in the differential diagnosis on the initial admission. Of patients presenting with acute pain of <1 week's duration, 50% had symptoms of IBS at time of admission. Assessing for diagnostic criteria of IBS symptoms may reduce length of hospitalization, extent of testing, and cost of treatment for patients presenting with acute abdominal pain who do not need immediate surgical intervention.

C. Physical Examination

Physical examination is often unremarkable except for abdominal tenderness and an increased likelihood of abdominal scars.

D. Special Tests

No specific testing is required for diagnosis of IBS, although normal CBC and ESR may be reassuring. Patients with criteria for colon cancer screening should be examined by flexible sigmoidoscopy or colonoscopy with random colon biopsies to evaluate for microscopic colitis. Other studies may include *C difficile* toxin if the patient has recently taken antibiotics, testing for giardiasis in endemic areas, and evaluation for lactose intolerance. A meta-analysis found a fourfold increased likelihood of biopsy-proven celiac disease in patients with IBS symptoms, so tissue transglutaminase antibodies (tTG-IgA) should be tested to evaluate for celiac disease. CRP or fecal calprotectin can be used to evaluate for inflammatory bowel disease.

▶ Treatment

A. Therapeutic Relationship

A therapeutic relationship is critical to the effective management of IBS. The therapeutic relationship is achieved by a nondirective, patient-centered, nonjudgmental history, eliciting the patient's understanding of the illness and his or her concerns, identifying and responding realistically to the patient's expectation for improvement, setting consistent limits, and involving the patient in the treatment approach. The most effective treatment option is explanation and reassurance. A confident diagnosis based on previously outlined clinical criteria helps convey the lack of association with a higher risk of other diseases such as cancer and chronic nature of symptoms. Patients' reasons for seeking care and possible contributing psychosocial issues should be assessed. Counseling regarding psychosocial stressors may not resolve all the symptoms of IBS, but may help patients cope better with symptoms.

B. Diet and Exercise

Many different dietary approaches have been tried. Patients in whom gas-forming vegetables, lactose, caffeine, or alcohol exacerbate symptoms should be counseled to minimize exposure. There is more recent evidence that short-chain, poorly absorbed, highly fermentable carbohydrates, known as FODMAPs (fermentable oligosaccharides, disaccharides, monosaccharides, and polyols), increase IBS symptoms and that lower intake of FODMAPs has improved symptoms; however, the evidence is not of high quality, so it is difficult to recommend a low-FODMAP diet for patients with IBS symptoms. Dietary fiber has been shown to improve symptoms of constipation, hard stools, and straining, particularly if 30 g of soluble fiber is consumed each day. Patients often need to gradually increase the amount of fiber to improve adherence, as a sudden increase can increase symptoms of bloating and gas. The most common reason for failure of a high-fiber diet is insufficient dose. Fiber is safe and inexpensive and should be routinely recommended, particularly to patients for whom constipation is a predominant symptom. Nondietary bulking agents have not been found to be more effective than placebo. Probiotics have been found to provide global improvement in IBS symptoms and abdominal pain. The exact mechanism contributing to the improvement in symptoms is not completely understood and can vary between strains and dose used. There is insufficient evidence to recommend the use of one particular strain or dose. Patients should be encouraged to consume probiotic-rich fermented foods such as yogurt, kefir, miso, tempeh, and sauerkraut. Increased physical activity has shown improvement in severity of IBS symptoms and significantly lower likelihood of worsening of symptoms. Given the multiple benefits of increased physical activity, it should be routinely recommended.

C. Complementary and Alternative Therapies

A meta-analysis of five double-blind, placebo-controlled randomized trials of peppermint oil given as a mono-preparation in a dosage range of 0.2–0.4 mL suggested a significant (P <.001) positive effect compared with placebo. Randomized controlled trials of Chinese herbal medicine indicated that both a standardized herbal formulation (Tong Xie Yao Fang is a commonly used formula) as well as individualized Chinese herbal medicine treatment improved symptoms of IBS compared with placebo. Padma Lax, a Tibetan herbal digestive formula, has been used and studied in Europe and has shown global improvement in symptoms. Acupuncture has been shown to be more beneficial than some antispasmodic medications. Moxibustion has been shown to be helpful compared to placebo treatments.

D. Psychological Therapies

Various psychological therapies have been studied in randomized controlled trials comparing control therapy and a physician's "usual management." Psychological therapies studied include hypnotherapy, relaxation training, multicomponent psychological therapy, dynamic psychotherapy, cognitive behavioral therapy (CBT), stress management, and self-administered CBT. Dramatic improvements in a high proportion of patients with poorly controlled IBS symptoms were seen for both individual and group hypnotherapy. Therapeutic audiotapes are an easy, low-cost alternative but may be somewhat inferior to hypnotherapy. Psychotherapy effectiveness relies on the relationship between therapist and patient, making it difficult to study in randomized, controlled trials. The quality of the data is not as strong as that for pharmacotherapy, but the number needed to treat with psychological therapies to prevent IBS symptom persistence for one patient is four. The number needed to treat with antidepressants to prevent persistent symptoms also is four. Patients with IBS are more likely to have coexisting mood disorders and anxiety. Psychological interventions should be considered.

E. Pharmacotherapy

A meta-analysis that concluded that smooth muscle relaxants and anticholinergics were better than placebo has been criticized for methodologic inadequacies. Common GI complaints and the drugs most frequently used to treat them are as follows:

Constipation: Psyllium, methylcellulose, calcium polycarbophil, lactulose, 70% sorbitol, and polyethylene glycol (PEG) solution. A partial 5-HT$_4$ agonist (tegaserod) was removed from the market secondary to cardiovascular side effects. Lubiprostone is a chloride channel activator that stimulates intestinal fluid secretion, and linaclotide is a guanylate cyclase-C agonist that works to increase intestinal chloride secretions.

Diarrhea: Loperamide, cholestyramine. Alosetron for female patients with diarrhea-predominant IBS symptoms was removed from the market secondary to risk of ischemic colitis and severe constipation but is now available again with warnings.

Gas, bloating, or flatus: Aimethicone, α-galactosidase (Beano), probiotic, antibiotics. Rifaximin is expensive and not recommended for long-term treatment.

Abdominal pain: Anticholinergics and antispasmodics (dicyclomine, hyoscine, cimetropium, and pinaverium).

Chronic pain: Tricyclic antidepressants, selective serotonin reuptake inhibitors.

A positive therapeutic relationship and regular visits to a family physician can prevent a continual and costly quest by patients for a "miracle" cure.

Chey WD, Kurlander J, Eswaran S. Irritable bowel syndrome: a clinical review. *JAMA.* 2015;313(9):949–958. [PMID: 25734736]

Dionne J, Ford AC, Yuan Y, et al. A systematic review and meta-analysis evaluating the efficacy of a gluten-free diet and a low FODMAPs diet in treating symptoms of irritable bowel syndrome. *Am J Gastroenterol.* 2018;113:1290–1300. [PMID: 30046155]

Ford AC, Lacy BE, Harris LA, et al. Effect of antidepressants and psychological therapies in irritable bowel syndrome: systematic review and meta-analysis. *Am J Gastroenterol. Am J Gastroenterol.* 2019;114(1):21–39. [PMID: 30177784]

Lewis SJ, Heaton KW. Stool Form Scale as a useful guide to intestinal transit time. *Scand J Gastroenterol.* 1997;32:920. [PMID: 9299672]

CELIAC DISEASE

 ESSENTIALS OF DIAGNOSIS

► Abdominal pain due to autoimmune destruction of mucosa.

► Testing for immunoglobulin (Ig) A endomysial antibodies and IgA tissue transglutaminase.

► Confirm with small bowel biopsy.

► Confirm with resolution of symptoms on gluten-free diet.

General Considerations

Celiac disease is an immune-mediated small intestine enteropathy triggered by the exposure to gluten proteins found in wheat, rye, and barley. It is reported to affect between 0.3% and 2% of Western populations. It is commonly associated with other autoimmune conditions and has a genetic predisposition. Repeated exposure to gluten causes destruction of the small bowel mucosa, infiltration of mucosa with lymphatic T cells, and enlargement of crypts. Although many affected individuals are asymptomatic, patients may present with classic signs and symptoms of malabsorption as well as abdominal pain. Diagnosis of celiac disease and avoidance of gluten can resolve symptoms, improve quality of life, and reduce the risk of GI and lymphoproliferative cancers. Currently, there is insufficient evidence to recommend screening for celiac disease in asymptomatic persons.

▶ Clinical Findings

Symptoms of clinical disease (or celiac sprue) include abdominal pain, diarrhea, weight loss, and failure to thrive. Signs of malabsorption may include short stature, skin problems, osteoporosis, excessive flatulence, neurologic dysfunction, liver enzyme abnormalities, and iron deficiency anemia. Severe deficiency of vitamin D, vitamin K, and iron may be present. Psychological comorbidities such as anxiety and depression are not uncommonly seen.

▶ Diagnosis

Testing for serum IgA endomysial antibodies and IgA tissue transglutaminase (tTG) antibodies should be performed while a patient consumes a diet containing gluten. The accuracy of testing is higher in patients at increased risk such as those with iron deficiency anemia, other autoimmune disorders, or positive family history. Positive results need confirmation with endoscopic small bowel biopsy in four locations. Testing for IgA deficiency may be helpful if clinical suspicion remains high despite negative endoscopy.

▶ Treatment

The treatment for celiac disease is a strict lifelong gluten-free diet. To help achieve this, patients should be referred to a knowledgeable nutritionist as well as for psychological support. Symptoms and nutritional deficiencies usually improve significantly by 3 months. Strict adherence to a gluten-free diet may help decrease the risk of GI cancers.

Chou R, Bougatsos C2, Blazina I, et al. Screening for celiac disease: evidence report and systematic review for the US Preventive Services Task Force. *JAMA*. 2017;317(12):1258–1268. [PMID: 28350935]

Leonard MM, Sapone A, Catassi C, et al. Celiac disease and non-celiac gluten sensitivity: a review. *JAMA*. 2017;318(7):647–656. [PMID: 28810029].

Ludvigsson JF, Card T, Ciclitira PJ, et al. Support for patients with celiac disease: a literature review. *United European Gastroenterol J*. 2015;3(2):146–159. [PMID: 25922674]

Talley NJ, Walker MM. Celiac disease and nonceliac gluten or wheat sensitivity: the risks and benefits of diagnosis. *JAMA Intern Med*. 2017;177(5):615–616. [PMID: 28350893]

Zingone F, Swift GL, Card TR, et al. Psychological morbidity of celiac disease: a review of the literature. *United European Gastroenterol J*. 2015;3(2):136–145. [PMID: 25922673]

CONSTIPATION

ESSENTIALS OF DIAGNOSIS

▶ Best treated with lifestyle modification.

▶ Laboratory studies and imaging rarely needed.

▶ Caution if red flags present, including bleeding or weight loss.

▶ General Considerations

Constipation is common in the United States. It affects all ages and populations. About 16% of adults have symptoms of constipation. Symptoms are more common in women and people over the age of 60. Symptoms of constipation may include abdominal pain. Causes of constipation often can be identified and addressed without laboratory studies or imaging studies.

▶ History

History includes infrequent stooling (<3 times per week), straining in >25% of attempts, need for maneuvers to help facilitate defecation such as digital evacuation, support of pelvic floor, or rare loose stools without use of laxatives. Diet, especially fiber intake; prescription and OTC medication and supplement use; activity level; and other medical conditions should be reviewed. Further evaluation for underlying disorders should be explored if warning signs ("red flags") are present. Red flags include bleeding, anemia, change in stool caliper, unintended weight loss of ≥10 lb, and abnormal findings on exam.

▶ Physical Examination

Examination should include abdominal and rectal exams. The rectal exam should evaluate anal wink, integrity and strength of the anal sphincter, presence of impacted stool, pain with palpation, presence of fissures or hemorrhoids, and the presence of blood.

▶ Diagnostic Studies

Laboratory or imaging studies are occasionally needed. Endoscopy should be performed in patients age >50 years without prior colon cancer screening; patients with evidence of bleeding, rectal prolapse, or change in stool caliper; and patients with weight loss. Simple radiologic studies can demonstrate the presence of large amounts of stool in the rectum and large bowel. Laboratory testing includes CBC, complete metabolic panel, and screening for hypothyroidism. A vitamin D level may be useful if toxicity is suspected.

Defecography and colon transit testing may be helpful to confirm slow transit of stool. Pelvic floor dysfunction testing, including radiography, anal manometry, and electromyography, should be reserved for patients not responsive to initial treatment attempts.

Treatment

The most effective initial treatment for constipation is lifestyle modification. Modifications include increased physical activity, dietary fiber, and fluid intake. Medications known to cause constipation should be adjusted or eliminated if possible. Biofeedback techniques and physical therapy may be used for pelvic floor dysfunction. Secondary treatment includes consistent intake of osmotic agents such as magnesium hydroxide or lactulose.

Polyethylene glycol (Miralax) should be tried if lifestyle modification is not successful Other laxatives have shown variable effectiveness in clinical trials. These include senna, bisacodyl, methylcellulose, docusate, psyllium, and other bulking agents. Studies on probiotics and prebiotics show mixed results. Most studies were done in patients with constipation-dominant IBS rather than isolated constipation. The use of some probiotics seems to improve transit time and stool consistency. Stimulants such as 5-HT$_4$ agonists should be reserved for patients after further evaluation from a GI specialist.

Nelson AD, Camilleri M, Chirapongsathorn S, et al. Comparison of efficacy of pharmacological treatments for chronic idiopathic constipation: a systematic review and network meta-analysis. *Gut.* 2017;66(9):1611–1622. [PMID: 27287486]
Stern T, Davis AM. Evaluation and treatment of patients with constipation. *JAMA.* 2016;315(2):192–193. [PMID: 26757468]
Wald A. Constipation: advances in diagnosis and treatment. *JAMA.* 2016;315(2):185–191. [PMID: 26757467]
National Institute of Diabetes and Digestive and Kidney Diseases. Constipation. https://www.niddk.nih.gov/health-information/digestive-diseases/constipation. Accessed November 10, 2019.

APPENDICITIS

 ESSENTIALS OF DIAGNOSIS

► History of periumbilical pain migrating to RLQ with anorexia, nausea, and vomiting is often diagnostic.

► CT scan is test of choice for most suspected cases that need confirmation.

► Urgent surgical consult is needed.

► Left shift of elevated WBC count to 7000–19,000/mm^3 is helpful in diagnosis.

General Considerations

Appendicitis occurs in >290,000 people per year in the United States alone. Appendicitis occurs in people of any age and is most common in later childhood through young adulthood. The presentation of appendicitis in young children and the elderly is often atypical. There is no race or gender predilection. Diagnosis in female patients can be more difficult, although males are more likely to have a perforated appendix.

Pathogenesis

The appendix is a long diverticulum extending from the cecum. Appendicitis results when the lumen is occluded. Proliferation of lymphoid tissue, associated with viral infections, Epstein-Barr virus, upper respiratory infection, or gastroenteritis, is the most common cause of obstruction and appendicitis in young adults. Other causes of occlusion include tumors, foreign bodies, fecaliths, parasites, and complications of Crohn disease.

Clinical Findings

A. Symptoms and Signs

History is the most important component of diagnosis. The presence of the following historical indicators should be elicited: abdominal pain, usually RLQ pain often preceded by periumbilical pain (~100%); anorexia (~100%); nausea (90%), with vomiting (75%); progression of abdominal pain from periumbilical to RLQ (50%); and classic progression from vague abdominal pain to anorexia, nausea, vomiting, RLQ pain, and low-grade fever (50%).

B. Physical Examination

Careful abdominal examination with inspection, palpation, and percussion often identifies the cause of abdominal pain. Peritoneal signs, including rigidity, rebound tenderness, and guarding, and a low-grade fever (38°C [100.4°F]) are characteristic findings. Findings of RLQ pain with palpation, rebound pain, psoas sign, obturator sign, and Rovsing sign all are highly suggestive of appendicitis. Guarding, rigidity, and pain with cough or motion also support the diagnosis. Decreased bowel sounds, no palpable mass, and no organomegaly generally are found. The size and location of the appendix vary, so pain may occur at a remote distance from the classic McBurney point.

Acetaminophen, NSAID, and opioid use has been shown to help manage pain during evaluation of patients with suspected appendicitis without risk of missed diagnosis or delay of treatment.

C. Laboratory Findings

Many laboratory studies are performed routinely on patients with abdominal pain. Few, if any, are truly helpful and can be misleading. Studies suggest the WBC count is seldom helpful diagnostically, although if the WBC count is <7000/mm³, appendicitis is unlikely. A WBC count of >19,000/mm³ is associated with an 80% probability of appendicitis. The presence of neutrophilia makes the diagnosis of appendicitis more likely but is not diagnostic. Increased WBCs with neutrophilia generally is accompanied by increased CRP levels. The presence of all three is not diagnostic, but the absence of all three rules out appendicitis.

Routine use of a chemistry examination is helpful to determine the level of dehydration. UA commonly shows leukocytosis and increased red blood cells and thus may be misleading. All women of childbearing age should have a pregnancy test. Urine markers of acute pediatric appendicitis may help improve diagnostic accuracy in children. Recent introduction of the APPY-1 lab test panel has been very helpful, with 98% accuracy in the pediatric population that increases to 99% when used with ultrasound evaluation.

D. Imaging Studies

Imaging studies can delay treatment, increase cost, and increase radiation exposure. When the diagnosis is clear from the history and physical, rapid surgical consult should be obtained prior to imaging studies. Studies are helpful in less clear cases and may decrease rate of removal of normal appendices. Current rate of negative pathology is ~1%. Ultrasound evaluation is the current diagnostic test of choice. Ultrasound is fast, has no radiation exposure, allows for visualization of some gynecologic issues more clearly, and is better for children and pregnant patients. CT scan is useful in more complex cases where the differential may be more broad. Complete abdominal radiographs can be misleading, are not diagnostic in most cases, delay other testing, and add additional radiation exposure. Focused spiral CT without contrast can be performed in less than an hour and is very sensitive and specific for appendicitis. Use of contrast may be helpful in certain cases, especially in patients who are thin or older and those with unclear etiology.

▶ Treatment

Treatment consists of surgical removal of inflamed appendix via laparotomy or laparoscopy. Laparotomy is faster, simpler, and less expensive and has a lower rate of complications. Laparoscopy allows visualization of other possible causes of pain. Recent advances in surgical technology have shown other benefits of laparoscopic procedures: faster recovery, shorter hospital stay, and decreased postoperative pain. Choice of surgical options should be made on an individual basis and based on surgical experience and opinion at time of surgery. A few small studies suggest that treatment with antibiotics and observation can result in temporary resolution of symptoms but generally result in high recurrence rates. This may be an option for medically unstable patients or where surgery is not readily available. Use of antibiotics may result in faster recovery in surgical cases.

Benabbas R, Hanna M, Shah J, at al. Diagnostic accuracy of history, physical examination, laboratory tests, and point-of-care ultrasound for pediatric acute appendicitis in the emergency department: a systematic review and meta-analysis. *Acad Emerg Med.* 2017;24(5):523–551. [PMID: 28214369]

Depinet H, von Allmen D, Towbin A, et al. Risk stratification to decrease unnecessary diagnostic imaging for acute appendicitis. *Pediatrics.* 2016;138(3): e20154031. [PMID: 27553220]

Di Saveio, Sibilio A, Giorgini E, et al. The NOTA Study (Non Operative Treatment for Acute Appendicitis): prospective study on the efficacy and safety of antibiotics (amoxicillin and clavulanic acid) for treating patients with right lower quadrant abdominal pain and long-term follow-up of conservatively treated suspected appendicitis. *Ann Surg* 2014;260(1):109–117. [PMID: 24646528]

Huang L, Yin Y, Yang L, et al. Comparison of antibiotic therapy and appendectomy for acute uncomplicated appendicitis in children: a meta-analysis. *JAMA Pediatr.* 2017;171(5):426–434. [PMID: 28346589]

Salminen P, Paajanen H, Rautio T, et al. Antibiotic therapy vs appendectomy for treatment of uncomplicated acute appendicitis: the APPAC randomized clinical trial. *JAMA.* 2015; 313(23):2340–2348. [PMID: 26080338]

Snyder MJ, Guthrie M, Cagle S. Acute appendicitis: efficient diagnosis and management. *Am Fam Physician.* 2018;98(1):25–33. [PMID: 30215950]

INFLAMMATORY BOWEL DISEASE

 ESSENTIALS OF DIAGNOSIS

▶ Inflammatory bowel disease should be considered in patients with abdominal pain associated with blood in stool or elevated sedimentation rate.

▶ CT scan remains helpful; colonoscopy is essential only after control of acute attack.

▶ Current medical management is changing rapidly.

▶ General Considerations

Inflammatory bowel disease (IBD) is a broad category encompassing several disease subtypes. The most common are ulcerative colitis (UC) and Crohn disease (CD). Other inflammatory bowel conditions, including acute infectious colitis and gastroenteritis, are addressed elsewhere. Genetic advances have shown specific genetic loci associated with 20–40 times higher prevalence of both UC and CD. Prevalence of CD is much higher in whites with higher education and lower physical activity level, especially those of Jewish descent. Onset of IBD is most commonly seen at ages 15–30 years. Susceptibility is increased with smoking, higher antibiotic use, and low physical activity, and decreased by exposure to animals (pets and farm animals). All of these factors seem to influence the microflora of the gut, thus influencing an inappropriate inflammatory response to normal intestinal microbiology.

Environmental factors may make IBD more prevalent in people who work indoors and less prevalent in manual laborers who work outdoors. There is a 20–50% increase in the prevalence of IBD in first-degree relatives and a 50- to 100-fold increase in the offspring of patients with IBD. Risk factors, including work environment and diet, differ among subtypes of IBD. Smoking appears to decrease the risk of UC but increases risk and severity of CD. Patients with IBD have a higher incidence of ankylosing spondylosis, cholangitis, and psoriasis.

▶ Pathogenesis

Increased knowledge of genetic susceptibility has increased the understanding of pathogenesis. Environmental factors seem to allow for altered immunologic responses to normal intestinal flora and destruction within the mucosa of the GI tract. CD appears to be related to altered macrophage function. UC is more likely related to a pathologic inflammatory response to normal intestinal microflora. Changes within the microflora, combined with the immune response, result in altered mucosal barriers, luminal antigens, and macrophage function.

▶ Clinical Findings

A. Symptoms and Signs

IBDs can present with abdominal pain, bleeding (usually rectal), diarrhea (often nocturnal), abdominal cramping, weight loss (>5% body weight in 3 months), and anemia. Abdominal pain is more common in patients with CD, which can present anywhere from mouth to anus (skip lesions). RLQ pain is present in most patients with CD, reflecting involvement of the terminal ileum in 85% of cases. CD can affect the entire bowel wall, resulting in more destructive lesions causing fistula, bowel obstruction, and extraintestinal lesions. CD can be associated with liver, skin, joint, and ocular lesions. In contrast, UC presents with perirectal pain and bloody diarrhea due to the disease process being focal to the rectum and sometimes colon with only the mucosa involved.

B. Physical Examination

Physical examination findings are not specific. Evaluation of the rectum for evidence of fissures, ulceration, or abscess can be helpful. Fullness or a palpable mass suggests abscess. Examination often reveals nonspecific generalized tenderness, with focal findings dependent on extent and activity of disease. Skin examination may be useful. CD is associated with erythema nodosum and aphthous stomatitis. UC is

associated with pyoderma gangrenosa. Growth retardation and delayed sexual maturation can occur from the disease process and medications used to treat disease.

C. Laboratory Findings

Recommended laboratory tests include ESR; CRP; CBC; liver function tests (LFTs); albumin and prealbumin; electrolytes; stool studies; vitamin B_{12}, folate, and vitamin D levels; and pregnancy test. ESR is elevated in 80% of patients with CD and 40% of patients with UC. Elevated CRP is present in 95% of symptomatic patients with CD. Anemia from iron deficiency and blood loss is common. Leukocytosis with increased eosinophilia is noted often. Liver involvement in patients with CD (eg, sclerosing cholangitis, autoimmune hepatitis, and cirrhosis) may affect LFTs. Albumin and prealbumin are indicators of malnutrition from malabsorption. Stool studies rule out infectious etiologies of colitis. Fecal calprotectin is very useful in diagnosis and rule out of CD and nearly 100% specific in pediatric patients. Perinuclear antineutrophil antibody (pANCA) titer is useful to differentiate between CD and UC. pANCA is present in ~6% of patients with CD and 70% of patients with UC. *Saccharomyces cerevisiae* (anti–*S cerevisiae* antibodies [ASCA]) is found in ~50% of individuals with CD and correlates closely with involvement of small bowel, stenosing lesions, and perforation. Stool studies for *C difficile* and ova and parasites as well as culture and lactoferrin can help with management.

D. Imaging Studies

Endoscopy is the most accurate diagnostic test and allows for direct visualization of mucosa and biopsy. It is not recommended in acute active disease because of the risk of perforation. Histologic variances help differentiate CD from UC. Visualization of skip lesions, cobblestoning, and strictures suggests CD. Colonoscopy with ileoscopy, capsule endoscopy, CT scan, and small bowel follow-through help evaluate all areas of disease. Capsule endoscopy, when combined with other testing, improves sensitivity to >90% and improves specificity. Capsule endoscopy is contraindicated in patients with known or suspected stricture. MRI and ultrasound help identify extraintestinal areas and complications of disease. Plain films are most helpful in identifying toxic megacolon and the "thumbprinting" sign (seen with bowel wall edema) and may identify strictures, skip lesions, and perforation. The classic string sign is seen on barium enema. Abdominal CT is helpful in identifying abscess, fistula, bowel wall thickening, and fat striation.

▶ Treatment

Management of IBD includes medical therapy, nutritional support, psychological support, and surveillance for cancer. Familial and genetic counseling is important to help family members cope with exacerbations of the disease and because of the strong pattern of inheritance.

Many medical treatment options are available for treatment of IBD, including steroids, immune modulator, and biologics. Prednisone is the most commonly used medicine in the acute setting until remission is achieved. Long-term steroid use has many risks and should be avoided by the addition or substitution of other treatment options. Rapid advances in medical treatment with immune modulators and biologics such as monoclonal antibodies are occurring. The best options should be reevaluated with the most updated recommendations as many treatments have been shown to be useful only in combination or at certain times of treatment and show a higher level of infection and cancer despite being more well tolerated than other treatment options. Probiotics and omega-3 supplements have no current evidence supporting use.

Antibiotics, including metronidazole and ciprofloxacin, are widely used and have anti-inflammatory as well as anti-infectious properties. Methotrexate use can enable the practitioner to wean the patient from steroids but may cause bone marrow suppression, leukopenia, hepatic fibrosis, and pneumonitis.

Patients with severe disease require hospital admission for bowel rest, parenteral nutritional support, and corticosteroids. Increased use of immunomodulators has allowed for less use of systemic steroids.

Nutritional therapy is helpful to maintain remission and decrease likelihood of nutritional deficiency due to malabsorption, especially in children. Research suggests that the use of fecal bacteriotherapy, helminthic therapy, and other biologics may have a role in treatment by altering the bacterial flora of the gut.

Surgical therapy is often required. Approximately 85% of patients with persistent elevation of CRP and frequent liquid stools require total colectomy. Strictures and abscess formation may necessitate surgical excision of small segments of bowel or strictureplasty. Surgery is performed for intractable bleeding, abscess, or fistula formation. Patients with limited resection have fewer stools and better anorectal function.

Risk of adenocarcinoma is increased in patients with chronic colon disease. Risk of cancer development in UC is equivalent to CD with colon involvement. Biannual colonoscopy and biopsy are recommended for disease present for ≥10 years. Risk of other cancers, such as adenocarcinoma of the jejunum and ileum (when involved), lymphoma, and squamous cell carcinoma of the vulva and rectum, is increased in CD.

Ananthakrishnon AN. Epidemiology and risk factors for IBD. *Nat Rev Gasteenterol Hepitol.* 2015;12(4):205–217. [PMID: 25732745]

Centers for Disease Control and Prevention. Inflammatory bowel disease. www.cdc.gov/ibd/. Accessed December 18, 2018.

Dignas AU, Gasche C, Bettenworth D, et al. European Crohn's and Colitis Organization: European consensus on the diagnosis and management of iron deficiency anemia in inflammatory bowel diseases. *J Crohns Colitis.* 2015;9(3):211–222. [PMID: 25518052]

Lichtenstein GR, Loftus EV, Isaacs KL, et al. ACG clinical guideline: management of Crohn's disease in adults. *Am J Gastroenterol.* 2018;113(40):481–517. [PMID: 29610508]

Veauthier B, Hornecker JR. Crohn's disease: diagnosis and management. *Am Fam Physician.* 2018;98(1):661–669. [PMID: 30485038]

DIVERTICULITIS

ESSENTIALS OF DIAGNOSIS

▶ More than 3 days of abdominal pain with low-grade fever.

▶ Commonly left-sided pain (right-sided pain more common in people of Asian descent).

▶ CT scan is test of choice.

▶ Early antibiotic treatment, bowel rest, hydration.

▶ General Considerations

Diverticulitis occurs in 10–25% of patients with diverticulosis. In the 20th century, the incidence of diverticulosis increased as fiber intake decreased. In addition to insufficient fiber, age is the single greatest risk factor. Typically, diverticulosis is seen in patients age ≥60 years, is uncommon before age 40, and is present in 50% of people age >90 years. Patients of Western European descent have increased prevalence of left-sided diverticula. Patients of Asian descent have increased prevalence of right-sided diverticula.

▶ Pathogenesis

The pathology of diverticulitis is directly related to the anatomy of the bowel wall. True diverticula consist of outpouching of all three layers of the wall: mucosa, submucosa, and muscular layer. Meckel diverticulum also contains gastric or pancreatic tissue due to being an outpouching of intestine derived from the fetal yolk stalk. Most cases of diverticulitis involve pseudodiverticula with herniation of the mucosa and submucosa through the muscular layer. Diverticula tend to form in rows between mesenteric and lateral teniae. The area of penetration of the vasa recta has the greatest muscular weakness and is therefore the most common site of herniation.

Lack of dietary fiber contributes to the development of diverticula. As fiber content of the stool decreases, colonic pressure increases and transit time decreases. As we age, increased cross-fibers within the collagen and elastin render the bowel wall less compliant, resulting in high pressure in the colon and essentially blowing out areas of weakness in the colon wall. Previous recommendations to avoid seeds, nuts, and corn were based on the misconception that these foods caused aggravation of diverticulitis. Recent studies do not support avoiding these foods and suggest that higher intake of corn and nuts could help decrease the incidence of diverticulitis, at least in men.

Colonic pressure and the ability of the structures of the wall to contain that pressure are the underlying factors that cause diverticula to form or become problematic. Genetics affect the tensile strength of the wall, as does age. The use of aspirin and NSAIDs affect the structure and integrity of the bowel wall. Obesity increases risk. Higher levels of exercises are associated with higher gut motility and with lower rates of diverticular disease.

Diverticulitis occurs when infection is associated with one or more of these diverticula. Micro- or macroperforations of diverticula may occur, resulting in bowel contents contacting the peritoneum and infecting the pericolonic fat, mesentery, and associated organs. This can localize and result in the development of an abscess, peritonitis, or fistula. A fistula can form between the colon and an abdominal organ. A colovesical fistula, connecting the colon and urinary bladder, is most common.

▶ Clinical Findings

A. Symptoms and Signs

LLQ pain occurs in 93–100% of patients. Pain may be right-sided, especially in patients of Asian descent. A duration of ≥3 days of RLQ pain is suggestive of diverticulitis rather than appendicitis. Patients commonly have nausea, vomiting, constipation, or diarrhea. Dysuria and urinary frequency may be present. Complicated diverticulitis, as with a colovesical fistula, can present with recurrent urinary tract infections. In macroperforation, diffuse abdominal pain is present.

B. Physical Examination

Abnormal vital signs, including tachycardia and temperature of ≥38.1°C (≥100.7°F), give supporting evidence for the diagnosis of diverticulitis. Fever is present in most patients. Examination should include complete abdominal examination. Signs suggestive of diverticulitis include tender LLQ or less frequently RLQ tenderness, signs of peritoneal irritation such as guarding or tenderness to percussion, and occasional presence of a tender mass, suggesting the presence of an abscess. Rectal examination may demonstrate rectal tenderness or mass.

C. Laboratory Findings

Patients suspected of having diverticulitis should undergo a CBC and UA. The WBC count is increased in more than two-thirds of patients, with a high prevalence of polymorphonuclear leukocytes. Anemia may be noted if there is associated diverticular bleeding. UA can show evidence of inflammation if there is irritation of the peritoneum surrounding the bladder or evidence of infection if a fistula is present. Other useful testing includes pregnancy test, CRP, and fecal occult blood testing.

D. Imaging Studies

Flat and upright abdominal films, or CT of the abdomen and pelvis if the diagnosis is unclear, should be obtained. Abdominal films can show evidence of free air, ileus, or mass. CT scan shows a thickened colonic wall and allows insertion of percutaneous drainage if an abscess is present, allowing for delay in surgical intervention. Similar findings can be seen on ultrasound, but CT best confirms diverticulitis by revealing the presence and location of an abscess and allowing for identification of other pathologic processes such as cancer, CD, and appendicitis. Ureteral obstruction, fistula, or air in the bladder can be seen. Colonoscopy should be done 6–8 weeks after resolution of diverticulitis to evaluate for concomitant cancerous lesions, and if IBD is suspected, in at-risk patients, or if cancer screening is otherwise indicated.

▶ Treatment

Treatment depends on severity of disease and the health of the patient. Outpatient treatment includes clear liquid diet and rest. Use of oral broad-spectrum antibiotics can be considered, although research does not show clear benefit with the use of antibiotics. Current recommendations include broad-spectrum antibiotics for gram-negative rods as well as anerobic bacteria. Medications such as morphine increase colonic pressure and should be avoided. Meperidine is the best choice for pain control because it decreases colonic pressure. Steroids and NSAIDs should be avoided because of the increased risk of GI bleeding and perforation. Mesalamine and *Lactobacillus casei* are effective to prevent recurrence.

Patients with signs and symptoms of inflammation, such as fever and leukocytosis, require hospitalization. Treatment includes complete bowel rest, intravenous fluids, and intravenous broad-spectrum antibiotics. A nasogastric tube is not needed unless there is significant ileus or obstruction. Most patients improve in 48–72 hours, at which time they can resume their regular diet, receive oral antibiotics, and be discharged home with close follow-up. A high-fiber diet is recommended for all patients after recovery. Surgical resection is recommended for perforation or uncontrolled bleeding.

Surgery is seldom recommended after a first attack, given a recurrence rate of 20–30%. However, this rate increases with each subsequent attack, as does the risk of associated morbidity. Therefore, surgery should be considered after the second or third attack. Surgical intervention can be considered with a first attack for immunocompromised patients because of their increased risk of morbidity and mortality. Surgical intervention is done on a case-by-case basis for complicated diverticulitis. Allowing decreased inflammation of the bowel wall prior to resection and anastomosis by use of percutaneous drainage and antibiotic treatment improves outcome. Morbidity and mortality rates are improved when primary anastomosis can be performed, rather than a two-stage approach with colostomy. Patients age <40 years at the first attack have an increased lifelong risk due to the increased life expectancy, although risk with each attack is not increased. These cases are determined on an individual basis based on frequency and severity of attacks.

Bolkenstein HE, van de Wall BJM, Consten ECJ, et al. Risk factors for complicated diverticulitis: systematic review and meta-analysis. *Int J Colorectal Dis.* 2017;32(10):1375–1383. [PMID: 28799055]

Dahl C, Crichton M, Jenkins J, et al. Evidence for dietary fibre modification in the recovery and prevention of reoccurrence of acute, uncomplicated diverticulitis: a systematic literature review. *Nutrients.* 2018;10(2):E137. [PMID: 29382074]

O'Leary DP, Lynch N, Clancy C, et al. International, expert-based, consensus statement regarding the management of acute diverticulitis. *JAMA Surg.* 2015;150(9):899–904. [PMID: 26176318]

Wilkins T, Embry K, George R. Diagnosis and management of acute diverticulitis. *Am Fam Physician.* 2013;87(9):612–620. [PMID: 23668524].

ABDOMINAL WALL PAIN

There are many presentations of abdominal wall pain because of the multiple different causes of abdominal wall pain. Causes include hernias, herpes zoster, neuromas, hematomas of the abdominal wall or rectus sheath, desmoid tumor, endometriosis, myofascial tears, intraabdominal adhesions, neuropathies, slipping rib syndrome, and general myofascial pain. Examination findings suggesting abdominal wall pain include lack of evidence for an intraabdominal process; pain unrelated to meals or bowel function; pain related to posture; a trigger point; and a positive Carnett sign. When examining the area of pain, the clinician has the patient flex the abdominal muscles while palpating the area. Pain with this maneuver is considered a positive sign and suggests abdominal wall rather than visceral pain.

Hernias

Types of hernias include inguinal, femoral, umbilical, epigastric, spigelian, and Richter hernias. Hernias are more commonly identified by exam rather than history. History can be confusing with herniation of bowel wall or omentum. Bowel herniation causes visceral pain and obstruction. Omentum herniation causes visceral pain without signs of obstruction. A history of prior surgery, especially laparoscopic surgery, increases the likelihood of a hernia.

Men more typically develop inguinal hernias. Women tend to develop femoral hernias. Umbilical and epigastric hernias are more common in obese or gravid patients. Spigelian hernias, a hernia along the border of the arcuate ligament, is most common in athletes.

Richter hernia is defined by the pathology rather than the location of the hernia. The side of the bowel wall herniates, rather than the entire bowel segment. Often the hernia produces a slight bulge that may be confused with adenopathy or fat. Because this type of hernia results in subtle findings, there often is a delay in diagnosis and a higher fatality rate. Richter hernia is generally found in women age >50 years, but the incidence is increasing in young men, due to the increased frequency of laparoscopic procedures. Because the instruments used for laparoscopy are so small, the abdominal wall defect remaining after surgery may allow only a portion of the bowel wall to herniate. The resultant tight hernia causes strangulation of the tissue passing through. Prior surgical sites must be examined. Erythema at these sites can be a sign of local infection, fistula formation, or an inflammatory process at the site of scarring.

Point-of-care ultrasound evaluation is the single best test to examine the abdominal wall. It allows for visualization of trigger point, nerve entrapment, and hernia. Ultrasound is also useful in diagnosis when combined with local injection of painful region. Ultrasound allows for injection with needle visualization to help avoid intra-abdominal penetration with needle. Although CT scans can identify hernias, hernias are often overlooked unless the radiologist is focused on thorough examination of the abdominal wall.

Hernias are best treated surgically. If surgery is contraindicated, hernias causing pain or posing risk of bowel obstruction can be treated with a truss or other restrictive garment. Nerve entrapment or other nerve disorders can be treated surgically as well as with focal treatment with ultrasound guidance without true surgical intervention.

Rectus Sheath Hematoma

Rectus sheath hematomas can be difficult to diagnose. They tend to occur more commonly in elderly or pregnant patients. The epigastric vessels are sheared, resulting in intramuscular bleeding. Shearing can occur from trauma or twisting motions. History is the most important factor in directing the clinician. A history of unilateral midabdominal pain, use of anticoagulants such as aspirin or warfarin, and abdominal trauma are all important risk factors. Pain is unilateral and worse when patients tense their abdominal muscles. There is often a palpable mass within the rectus sheath.

Coagulation studies and blood count are the most useful laboratory studies. Helpful imaging studies include CT, ultrasound, and MRI. Ultrasound is the cheapest and most useful study if the diagnosis is highly suspected. CT is more useful for identifying other possible causes. MRI sometimes helps if the diagnosis remains unclear. Treatment is generally expectant, but severe cases may warrant reversal of coagulation abnormalities, administration of fluids, or surgical evacuation and ligation or coagulation of vessels.

Herpes Zoster

Herpes zoster should be suspected when there is an abrupt onset of severe abdominal wall pain. Pain associated with zoster can precede the rash by >1 week, although more commonly by 2–4 days. Zoster occurs most frequently in patients age >50 years. Postherpetic neuralgia (PHN) causes persistent pain, especially in patients age >60 years. Thorough history and close follow-up are the best measures to establish the diagnosis. Varicella vaccine may help prevent zoster. Treatment of acute zoster with acyclovir, valacyclovir, or famciclovir in combination with a prednisone taper seems to decrease incidence and severity of PHN. Treatment of PHN has proved difficult. Many modalities have been tried with minor success, including analgesics, narcotics, nerve stimulation, antidepressants, capsaicin, biofeedback, and nerve blocks.

Other Causes of Abdominal Wall Pain

Surgical scars are the location of many causes of abdominal wall pain. Hernias and endometriosis can occur at these sites. Neuromas often form at the border of scars. Other unusual causes include desmoid tumors, myofascial tears, and intraabdominal adhesions. Desmoid tumors are dysplastic tumors of the connective tissue, tend to form in young adults, and can be identified only after surgical removal. Myofascial tears and intraabdominal adhesions occur most frequently in athletes.

▶ Treatment

Trigger points often reproduce abdominal wall pain. Finding this point can help both diagnosis and treatment. Trigger points are often found along the lateral border of the rectus abdominis muscle, where nerve roots become stretched, compressed, and irritated. Points are also found at areas of tight-fitting clothing or at insertion points of muscles. The Carnett sign, described earlier, is useful for diagnosis of trigger points. Relief of many causes of abdominal wall pain can be achieved by injection of lidocaine or its equivalent into the point of most tenderness. This treatment can be diagnostic and therapeutic. Insertion of the needle into the correct point elicits intense pain, which improves dramatically after injection. Areas requiring more than one injection can be injected with a small amount of steroids. Steroids should be avoided in areas near hernias or in fascia, as they can cause hernia formation. Dry needling has proved useful, but initial treatment may cause more pain. Patients with severe needle aversion may benefit from a therapeutic trial of a transcutaneous lidocaine patch. Pain clinics may help in more difficult cases.

Management of this type of pain can be difficult. Patient education and reassurance are important. Unnecessary further testing can be avoided by decreasing patients' concerns about the pain. Tricyclic antidepressants can be useful at low doses.

Koop H, Koprdova S, Schürmann C. Chronic abdominal wall pain. *Dtsch Arztebl Int.* 2016;113(4):51–57. [PMID: 26883414]

Shian B, Larson ST. Abdominal wall pain: clinical evaluation, differential diagnosis, and treatment. *Am Fam Physician.* 2018;98(7):429–436. [PMID: 30252418]

GYNECOLOGIC CAUSES OF ABDOMINAL PAIN

Gynecologic causes of abdominal pain can be separated into three categories: acute causes in nonpregnant patients, chronic problems in nonpregnant patients, and acute causes in pregnant patients. Acute causes include PID, adnexal torsion, ruptured ovarian cyst, hemorrhagic corpus luteum cyst, endometriosis, and tuboovarian abscess. Chronic causes in nonpregnant patients include dysmenorrhea, mittelschmerz, endometriosis, obstructive müllerian duct abnormalities, leiomyomas, cancer, and pelvic congestion syndrome. Causes in pregnant patients include ectopic pregnancy, retained products of conception, septic abortion, and ovarian torsion. Psychological factors greatly contribute to abdominal and pelvic pain. Patients can present with acute pain after a sexual assault.

A wide differential, careful history, and pregnancy test should be considered when evaluating women and girls with abdominal pain. History includes last menstrual period, detailed menstrual history, sexual history including possible assault, and family history. Physical examination includes careful abdominal, pelvic, and rectovaginal examinations. Laboratory evaluation is based on findings from the physical examination. LFTs can help identify Fitz-Hughes and Curtis syndromes, especially in the presence of RUQ pain.

PID occurs in 11% of US women of reproductive age, although it is rare in pregnancy. Numerous biological factors contribute to a higher incidence of PID in adolescents, including lower prevalence of protective chlamydial antibodies, more penetrable cervical mucus, and larger zones of cervical ectopy with more vulnerable columnar cells. Other risk factors increasing the likelihood of PID include early age at first sexual intercourse, higher number of lifetime partners, or a new partner within the past 30–60 days. Diagnosis of PID requires the presence of abdominal pain, adnexal pain, cervical motion tenderness, and at least one of the following: temperature of >38.3°C (>101°F), vaginal discharge, leukocytosis with a cell count of >10,500/mm³, positive cervical cultures, intracellular diplococci, or WBCs on vaginal smear. Treatment depends on whether the patient requires inpatient or outpatient treatment. Inpatient treatment is required for surgical emergencies, pregnancy, no response to outpatient therapy in 72 hours, nausea and vomiting, or immunodeficiency.

Endometriosis is found in 15–32% of women undergoing laparoscopic evaluation of abdominopelvic pain. The pain is generally cyclical but can present acutely with ruptured ovarian endometrioma. A retroverted, fixed uterus with ash spots on the cervix suggests endometriosis. Conservative treatment includes NSAIDs and oral contraceptive use.

Most gynecologic causes of abdominal pain can be evaluated by ultrasound. Laparoscopy may be needed and can be therapeutic as in ovarian torsion. CT may help delineate unclear ultrasound findings. Consultation with a gynecologist often is warranted.

Baines PA, Allen GM. Pelvic pain and menstrual related illness. *Emerg Med Clin North Am.* 2011;19:763. [PMID: 11554286]

Anemia

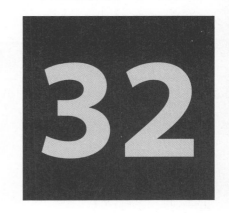

32

Alan K. David, MD

Anemia is defined as a reduced red blood cell (RBC) mass resulting in decreased oxygen-carrying capacity of the blood. Oxygen levels depend on the RBC mass, lung function, available erythropoietin (EPO), and the bone marrow. Some would define it as an abnormally low hematocrit/hemoglobin (H/H) level, but there are exceptions to this definition. Long-distance runners and pregnant women may have an increased plasma volume, diluting the H/H to abnormal or borderline low levels and suggesting a diagnosis of anemia when, in fact, the RBC mass and oxygen-carrying capacity of the blood are normal. Thus, the physiologic definition is most accurate. Anemia is the most frequent hematologic disorder seen by family physicians. Iron deficiency is the most common anemia seen in family medicine and the most common nutritional deficiency in the world. Children age 1–2 years (7%) and females age 12–48 years (8–16%) are the most commonly affected due to inadequate supply or increased requirement via blood loss, respectively. Anemia in men is most likely due to blood loss. Although in some instances elderly patients tend to have borderline low H/H levels, anemia in the elderly deserves evaluation instead of writing it off as an "anemia of aging."

PHYSIOLOGY

A normal RBC lasts 120 days, whereas white blood cells (WBCs) last several days but only spend 6 hours in the circulation. The normal myeloid-to-erythroid ratio of the bone marrow is 3:1, but in severe blood loss, this will be reversed so that erythroid precursors become the dominant form. The bone marrow can change and expand its production of any cell line under appropriate circumstances. In responding to anemia, the bone marrow can increase production of RBCs by 10%, and this response can be measured by the percentage of new RBCs called reticulocytes. These are new RBCs in which the RNA has not yet disintegrated. They can be counted using a supravital stain and reported as a percentage per 100 RBCs. In the face of acute blood loss or treatment of an anemia with iron, this percentage may or may not accurately reflect the expected bone marrow response. To correct for this, one must multiply the reticulocyte percentage on blood smear:

$$\% \times \frac{\text{actual hemoglobin}}{\text{normal hemoglobin}} = \text{corrected reticulocyte count}$$

A reticulocytosis of 10% after an acute bleed would seem to be an appropriate response, but if the hemoglobin dropped to 7.5 gms% (grams of Hgb/100 dl of blood) from a normal 15 gms%, the corrected response is:

$$10\% \times \frac{7.5}{15.0} = 5\%$$

This is still an effective response, but more accurately reflects bone marrow capacity in a particular patient.

Many laboratories report reticulocytes as an actual number such as $35–70 \times 10^3$. In this case, one can see if an appropriate response occurs relative to the degree of anemia if the actual count dramatically rises 3- to 10-fold. Reticulocyte measurement and correction can also provide significant insight into the cause of a given anemia. A marked reticulocytosis suggests acute RBC loss through bleeding or hemolysis or sudden replacement of something like iron or folic acid. Low reticulocyte numbers suggest a hypoproliferative situation such as nutrient deficiencies (eg, iron, vitamin B_{12}, folate), inadequate erythropoietin production, or marrow dysfunction from chemicals, medications, or invasion.

CLASSIFICATION OF ANEMIAS

A variety of classifications have been proposed in the literature to help organize the diagnosis and approach to anemia in a systematic fashion. These include RBC descriptive terms such as normocytic/microcytic/macrocytic or a kinetic

Table 32–1. Classification of anemias.

Hypoproliferative anemias
Aplastic anemia
Anemia of inflammation
Chronic renal insufficiency
Hypothyroidism
Mild iron deficiency

Maturation disorders
Megaloblastic anemias
Myelodysplasia
Severe iron deficiency
Thalassemia syndromes

Hemolytic-hemorrhagic anemia
Hereditary red blood cell defect
Autoimmune hemolysis
Drug- or chemical-induced hemolysis
Acute or chronic blood loss
Sickle cell anemia
Microangiopathic anemias
Paroxysmal nocturnal hemoglobinuria
Glucose-6-phosphate dehydrogenase deficiency

system of classification of decreased production versus red cell loss through bleeding or hemolysis. The system used here is more expansive and physiologic based, connecting the categories to bone marrow responsiveness or lack thereof. Table 32–1 depicts this classification scheme.

Hypoproliferative anemias are caused by three mechanisms of bone marrow impairment: marrow damage, inflammation, or inadequate EPO production. Examples of marrow damage are aplastic anemia/marrow aplasia characterized by a low reticulocyte index, elevated EPO, and a hypocellular bone marrow. Inflammation most commonly seen in the anemia of inflammation involves altered iron balance, decreased EPO, and decreased iron absorption, resulting in a picture similar to iron deficiency, but it does not respond to iron supplementation. Inadequate EPO production is seen most commonly in chronic renal insufficiency. Hypometabolism seen in hypothyroidism can also cause reduction in EPO, leading to anemia.

Maturation disorders are different because there is elevated EPO production and erythroid marrow hyperplasia but a low level of reticulocytosis. Thus, red cell production is impaired by nuclear or cytoplasmic maturation deficits. Examples of nuclear maturation defects are folate/B_{12} deficiencies, severe iron deficiency, and myelodysplastic states (eg, primary bone marrow neoplasms). Cytoplasmic maturation defects involve the abnormal hemoglobinopathies such as thalassemia.

Hemolytic-hemorrhagic anemia can be classified as hemolysis involving extracorpuscular defects or intracorpuscular defects. Some extracorpuscular etiologies

are ABO incompatibility, autoimmune hemolytic anemia (AIHA), microangiopathic hemolysis, thrombotic thrombocytopenic purpura, malaria, or inflammation such as seen in collagen vascular disease. Some intravascular etiologies cause abnormal RBC shapes or forms that trigger hemolysis and destruction by the reticuloendothelial system (RES)—liver, spleen, and nodes—such as hereditary spherocytosis, paroxysmal nocturnal hemoglobinuria, glucose-6-phosphate dehydrogenase (G6PD) deficiency, and sickle cell disease.

CLINICAL FEATURES OF ANEMIA

Anemia is most often discovered by finding an abnormal H/H on a complete blood count or subtle signs on physical examination. As the level of anemia increases, physical findings and symptoms become more evident. Fatigue, increasing skin pallor seen in the conjunctiva or nail beds, unexplained tachycardia at rest or with minimal exertion, and increased dyspnea on exertion are all signs that might be caused by anemia. However, at mild levels of anemia (hemoglobin = 10.0–11.0 gm/dl), there may be only minimal symptoms or physical findings. In acute bleeding, the H/H may not accurately reflect the degree of loss until 48 hours later. Vascular symptoms may appear with 10–15% blood loss, whereas a 30% blood volume loss will result in severe vascular contraction and postural hypotension plus tachycardia. Volume losses >40% cause frank shock. A careful history of indolent blood loss in terms of increasing menstrual volumes/frequency, darkening of stools, or intermittent hematemesis is critical to achieving the correct diagnosis.

HYPOPROLIFERATIVE ANEMIAS: IRON-DEFICIENCY ANEMIA & ANEMIA OF INFLAMMATION

This section will focus on iron deficiency/iron-deficiency anemia and the anemia of inflammation because they are the most common disorders in the hypoproliferative group.

Iron deficiency and iron-deficiency anemia are part of a single continuum that involves a hypoproliferative mechanism early on and transitions into a maturation disorder as the disease progresses. Iron has multiple functions; it carries oxygen, catalyzes metabolic oxidative reactions, and aids in cellular growth and proliferation. Iron hemostasis is the balance between absorption and loss and is influenced by body stores and EPO levels. Women and men have about 40 mg iron/kg and 50 mg iron/kg, respectively. Plasma iron is transported by transferrin to developing RBCs in the marrow. It is recovered from senescent RBCs and attached to transferrin again. Ferritin functions as a storage molecule of iron atoms and is found in the cytoplasm of macrophages and hepatocytes in the RES system. Ferritin stores only a small amount of total iron but is a good indicator of total body iron.

Early iron deficiency causes a reduction in erythroid proliferation, whereas in severe iron deficiency, the marrow becomes stimulated by more EPO and thus has an appearance of hyperplasia but ineffective maturation. In both cases, there is low serum iron, low transferrin saturation, and very low ferritin levels. There is a steady progression toward a microcytic, hypochromic picture on blood smear. The predominant cause varies by age and gender. Children may not receive enough iron in their diet; women may lose more iron in their menstrual cycles than they take in; and men with iron deficiency should always be suspected of blood loss, especially in the gastrointestinal tract.

In contrast, the mechanisms of anemia of inflammation involve tumor necrosis factor and interferons that block iron absorption and release of iron from the RES to transferrin, resulting in low serum iron and low transferrin saturation along with a microcytic, hypochromic laboratory picture. However, ferritin levels are normal or elevated. Treating with iron is ineffective, and adding EPO may increase the number of RBCs, but they are less effective than normal RBCs in terms of oxygen-carrying capacity. Elevated ferritin levels may also be a result of inflammatory conditions such as infection, liver disease, or cancer because it is a proinflammatory marker like the erythrocyte sedimentation rate or C-reactive protein. Treatment of anemia of inflammation should be directed at discovering the cause of inflammation, focusing on reducing or eliminating the inflammatory process. When a cause cannot be found or remedied, high-dose EPO (30,000–40,000 units/wk subcutaneously) may be helpful (Strength of Recommendation [SOR]: C). Table 32–2 outlines the major differences in iron deficiency and anemia of inflammation.

Treatment of iron deficiency should be directed at discovering any source of iron loss and should supply iron to both correct the hemoglobin deficit and replace iron stores. Oral iron in the form of ferrous sulfate, 325 mg 2–3 times per day, is usually well tolerated. If not, ferrous fumarate or gluconate may be better tolerated. Three tablets per day will provide 150 mg of elemental iron. Reticulocytosis will occur in 1 week and subside after 2 weeks. Hemoglobin should begin to rise in 2 weeks. The H/H may return to normal in 6–8 weeks, but microcytosis will take 4 months to resolve. Iron is best taken on an empty stomach, although ascorbic acid may enhance absorption. If oral forms cannot be tolerated, then intravenous (IV) iron is preferred. Iron dextran provides large amounts of iron at one time but has side effects including anaphylaxis. Nondextran iron such as ferric carboxymaltose may be better tolerated and can be given safely over several minutes to hours in multiple applications. Serum ferritin will remain low until the anemia is resolved, but iron therapy should continue for 3–4 months longer until iron stores are corrected and the ferritin level returns to normal.

Note that most clinicians recommend screening pregnant women for iron-deficiency anemia and routine iron supplementation in pregnant women. The US Preventive Services Task Force (USPSTF) found that evidence for screening asymptomatic pregnant women for iron-deficiency anemia and use of iron supplementation in pregnant women is insufficient and the balance of harms and benefits cannot be determined.

The USPSTF found there is insufficient evidence to assess the balance of benefits and harms of screening for iron deficiency in young children based on systematic review. In contrast, the American Academy of Pediatrics recommends screening all infants for iron-deficiency anemia with a hemoglobin test at 1 year of age.

Auerbach M, Adamson JW. How we diagnose and treat iron deficiency anemia. *AM J Hemoatol.* 2016;91(1):31–38. [PMID: 26408108]

McDonagh MS, Blazina I, Dana T, et al. Screening and routine supplementation for iron deficiency anemia: a systematic review. *Pediatrics.* 2015;135(4):723–733. [PMID: 25825534]

Siu AL; US Preventive Services Task Force. Screening for iron deficiency anemia and iron supplementation in pregnant women to improve maternal health and birth outcomes: U.S. Preventive Services Task Force Recommendation Statement. *Ann Intern Med*, 2015;163(7):529–536. [PMID: 26344176]

Baker RD, Greer FR; Committee on Nutrition American Academy of Pediatrics. Diagnosis and prevention of iron deficiency and iron-deficiency anemia in infants and young children (0-3 years of age). *Pediatrics.* 2010;126(5):1040–1050. [PMID: 20923825]

Table 32–2. Major differences between iron deficiency and anemia of inflammation.

Iron Deficiency	Anemia of Inflammation
Low serum iron level	Low serum iron level
Elevated TIBC	TIBC normal or reduced
Transferrin saturation low (<15%)	Transferrin saturation low (15–20%)
Serum ferritin level low (<15 ng/mL)	Serum ferritin level normal or elevated
Microcytic, hypochromic RBCs	Normocytic to microcytic RBCs
RBC protoporphyrin level elevated	RBC protoporphyrin level elevated

RBCs, red blood cells; TIBC, total iron-binding capacity.

MATURATION DISORDERS

Maturation disorders include megaloblastic anemias, myelodysplasia, severe iron deficiency, and thalassemia. Because severe iron deficiency has been discussed previously, this section will focus on megaloblastic anemias and thalassemia.

MEGALOBLASTIC ANEMIAS

Anemias in this category are generally macrocytic, with mean corpuscular volumes (MCVs) >100 fL. This is caused by abnormal DNA replication and is often seen in conjunction with hypersegmented neutrophils. Vitamin B_{12} and/or folic acid deficiencies are often responsible for this picture, but antiviral medicines or medications such as hydroxyurea may cause a similar picture. EPO is found in sufficient quantities and the bone marrow has erythroid hyperplasia, but an adequate reticulocytosis matching the degree of anemia does not occur. Thus, production of RBCs is ineffective, hence the term *maturation disorder*.

Vitamin B_{12} deficiency is usually caused by inadequate absorption in patients with atrophic gastritis, bowel resections, or intestinal bypass because intrinsic factor produced by parietal cells in the stomach is required for vitamin B_{12} absorption, which occurs in the small intestine. Development of antibodies to intrinsic factor or parietal cells resulting in impairment of intrinsic factor production or effectiveness has been called pernicious anemia. The old Schilling test has been replaced by testing for parietal cell and intrinsic factor antibodies, increasing the ease and probability of making this diagnosis. Patients with vitamin B_{12} deficiency may also have neurologic symptoms including memory issues and neuropathy. Older patients with memory issues should be evaluated for vitamin B_{12} deficiency. B_{12} deficiency can be treated with vitamin B_{12} 1000 mg/d orally or 1000 mg intramuscularly once a day for 1 week, then once a week for 4 weeks, and then once a month as a maintenance dose.

Folate deficiency is most often caused by heavy alcohol consumption and poor diet. Folate levels can rise with one good meal or supplementation, but RBC folate levels are less likely to change transiently in these situations. Alcohol also inhibits the release of folic acid to tissues. Its relative absence may be due to both dietary insufficiency and impaired release. In a patient with severe megaloblastic anemia, folate deficiency, and neuropathy, treatment with folate alone may correct some of the macrocytosis and anemia, but the neuropathy associated with concomitant vitamin B_{12} deficiency will not resolve and, in fact, may worsen. Testing for both folate and vitamin B_{12} in macrocytic anemia is imperative. Sometimes, actual vitamin B_{12} deficiency will be seen in the face of a "normal" serum B_{12} level. Determination of homocysteine and methylmalonic acid levels may help distinguish between the two. Both are elevated in B_{12} deficiency, but in folate deficiency, homocysteine is the only one elevated. Anemia due to folate deficiency may be best treated by marked reduction or elimination of alcohol consumption, a balanced diet, and 1 mg of folic acid per day until macrocytosis is resolved, which usually takes a minimum of 4 months. Periodic reassessment is necessary due to often recurrent dietary and alcohol issues.

Liver dysfunction, hypothyroidism, heavy metal poisoning, anticancer drugs, and antiretroviral therapy such as zidovudine are may be causes of macrocytosis. Myelodysplastic syndromes are essentially bone marrow neoplasms produced by abnormal clones of RBC precursors. These syndromes do not respond to vitamin replacement and should be suspected in older adults with macrocytosis who do not have gastrointestinal issues, excessive alcohol consumption, or inadequate diets. Over time, myelodysplastic syndromes may progress to a frank neoplastic state, overtaking production of normal cellular elements in the bone marrow.

THALASSEMIA

Thalassemia is the result of gene deletion on chromosomes 11 and 16, resulting in a reduction of hemoglobin α chains, defining α-thalassemia. β-Thalassemia is caused by a reduction in β chains. These phenomena occur in many populations worldwide, especially in regions where malaria is endemic because the heterozygous forms provide some protection against malaria. In either form, excess α or β chains are produced and accumulate in the RBC, altering its shape, oxygen-carrying capacity, and maturation. Ineffective erythropoiesis occurs in the marrow in both types.

▶ β-Thalassemia

In β-thalassemia, β chains are not produced or are markedly reduced, resulting in misshapen, rigid RBCs that are unstable and fragment easily. The cells are microcytic and hypochromic and appear as target cells. The body compensates by making RBCs with HbA_2 or HbF. This can be diagnosed by hemoglobin electrophoresis. When a patient presents with an anemia characterized by an MCV <75 fL and an RBC count of >5 million cells/μL, there is an 85% chance that this is a thalassemia syndrome (SOR: C).

β-Thalassemia major (Cooley anemia) is the most severe form in which no β chains are synthesized. Severe anemia is noted by the age of 1 year, along with an enlarged spleen/liver, bone marrow expansion, and jaundice. The blood smear demonstrates hypochromic RBCs, nucleated RBCs, and α chains on supravital staining. Treatment consists of RBC transfusions every 3–6 weeks when the hemoglobin level drops to 9–10.5 g/dL. Hepatitis B vaccine should be given prior to the start of this therapy. This therapy reduces risks of skeletal deformities, cardiac dilatation, and extramedullary hematopoiesis. A major complication of repeated RBC transfusions is iron overload, which can be treated with iron-chelating agents (eg, deferoxamine [parenteral] or oral agents such as deferasirox). Hydroxyurea may be used to increase HbF levels, but it is not uniformly effective. These therapies greatly improve life expectancy, but patients develop endocrinopathies secondary to endocrine organ iron deposition and cardiac disease secondary to myocardial iron deposition, plus high output syndrome secondary to chronic anemia. Transplantation of allogenic stem cells from human leukocyte antigen–matched sibling donors or, in some cases, with cord blood can be curative. A worse prognosis occurs in patients with an enlarged liver or liver fibrosis.

β-Thalassemia Minor (Trait)

These patients are heterozygous for β-globin production and present with a mild anemia or, in some cases, no anemia. HbA$_2$ and HbF are compensatory hemoglobins, and patients with higher HbF levels are less severely affected. The clinical picture is one of hypochromic/microcytic RBCs, normal or elevated serum ferritin, and an RBC count of >5 million RBCs/μL. Periodic monitoring of the H/H and treatment with transfusion in case of a bleed may be all that are needed.

Thalassemia Intermedia

Patients with thalassemia intermedia have mixed levels of hemoglobin types but present with a low hemoglobin (in the range of 6–8 g/dL) and hepatosplenomegaly requiring periodic transfusions. Iron overload should be monitored and treated.

α-Thalassemia

There are no substitutes for the α-globin chains, but there are four α-globin genes versus two β-globin genes. As a result, there are multiple variations of α-globin chain loss depending on how many α-globin gene sites have been affected. Infants who are homozygous for α-thalassemia produce no α chains, and the alternative hemoglobins formed by other globin chains such as hemoglobin β are nonfunctional in terms of delivering oxygen to tissues. This results in severe hypoxia in utero, resulting in hydrops fetalis. Mothers experience greater risk of preeclampsia, high blood pressure, and antepartum hemorrhage in this situation.

Hemoglobin H disease, which is caused by deletion of three of the four α chain genes, presents with a variable level of anemia resulting from hemolysis of unstable RBCs. Hemolysis is increased by infection or oxidative stress. RBC transfusions may be required in these instances.

Heterozygous α-thalassemia involves deletion of two α chain genes, is common in Asian populations, and causes limited to no anemia. Hemoglobin Constant Spring (HbCS) is caused by an α-globin that contains 31 additional amino acids. Homozygotes have a more profound anemia than heterozygotes.

Individuals coming from families in which thalassemia is present can seek genetic counseling, which can provide prenatal counseling and risk factoring. The risk of infants being born with thalassemia major has decreased markedly in recent years.

HEMOLYTIC-HEMORRHAGIC ANEMIA

Hemolysis may be an indolent slow process or one that is acute and relatively rapid. One tends to think of hemolysis when an anemia is persistent with what appears to be an adequate bone marrow response and no evidence of blood loss. There are two major forms of hemolysis: intracorpuscular and extracorpuscular. Intracorpuscular causes are related to defects in the red cell membrane, metabolism, or structure of hemoglobin. Extracorpuscular etiologies involve structures, proteins, or agents that change the RBC and cause the red cells to be removed from the circulation. Table 32–3 lists major forms of each.

INTRACORPUSCULAR HEMOLYSIS

RBCs rupture intravascularly due to a variety of causes, listed in Table 32–3, and spill their contents into the plasma, where hemoglobin is bound by haptoglobin, the main hemoglobin-binding protein. Thus, hemoglobinuria and extremely low haptoglobin levels are measures of intravascular hemolysis. Causes of intravascular rupture include hereditary stomatocytosis, a genetically inherited red cell with excess membrane permeability to Na$^+$ and K$^+$; hereditary elliptocytosis, in which the RBC membrane is unstable and, under stress, assumes an elliptical shape leading to rupture; and hereditary spherocytosis, in which RBCs become microspheres instead of the normal biconcave RBC shape. This results in a failure to pass through the spleen, resulting red cell trapping and ultimately hemolysis. This occurs in approximately 1 in 2000 persons of northern European ancestry. The bone marrow tends to chronically increase RBC production so much so that up to 25% of patients with this diagnosis do not have evidence of anemia despite the ongoing low-grade hemolysis. Stress, such as infection, pregnancy, or hypoxic conditions, may increase the hemolysis, resulting in anemia, jaundice, and an enlarged spleen. Diagnosis may be made due to a mean corpuscular hemoglobin concentration >35 g/dL, a positive osmotic fragility test (sensitivity, 81%),

Table 32–3. Hemolytic anemias.

Intracorpuscular	Extracorpuscular
Hereditary elliptocytosis	Microangiopathic hemolysis
Hereditary spherocytosis	Autoimmune hemolysis
Paroxysmal nocturnal hemoglobinuria	Drug-induced hemolysis
Glucose-6-phophate dehydrogenase deficiency	External agents
Sickle cell disease	

reticulocytosis, jaundice, splenomegaly, and positive family history. Transfusions and folic acid, 1 mg/d, should be given when there is evidence of severe or ongoing hemolysis.

Paroxysmal Nocturnal Hemoglobinuria

Paroxysmal nocturnal hemoglobinuria is the result of a genetically derived membrane defect that prevents the RBC from defending itself against a complement-mediated attack. It should be considered in any patient with unexplained chronic or episodic hemolysis. It can lead to aplastic anemia and myelodysplastic syndromes. The diagnosis is made by special fluorescent antigen-antibody complement testing.

Prednisone is indicated in flare-ups of hemolysis. Transfusions should be devoid of complement (ie, leukocytic poor). Iron deficiency is often present and should be addressed. Newer monoclonal antibody preparations directed at complement decrease hemolysis and improve survival. Although approximately 15% of cases resolve spontaneously, monoclonal antibody treatments increase median survival by 10–15 years.

Glucose-6-Phosphate Dehydrogenase Deficiency

G6PD deficiency affects almost 500 million people worldwide and is most prevalent where malaria is endemic because it reduces the risk of severe malaria by about 50%. It is caused by a sex-linked genetic defect, making affected males heterozygotes and females either homozygous or heterozygous. G6PD deficiency means the RBC has less reducing power to prevent oxidation, which then allows hemoglobin to be degraded in the RBC as evidenced by Heinz bodies on peripheral smear. There are several subtypes with varying degrees of enzyme deficiency. Thus, there are varying degrees of resultant hemolytic anemia severity. Because the RBC mechanisms to protect oxidation from occurring too rapidly are deficient, stress such as low-oxygen situations, exposure to oxidant drugs, infection, or fava bean exposure causes hemoglobin breakdown. Heinz body formation and altered RBC morphology occur, which result in red cell rupture. Patients report jaundice, dark urine like cola, and back pain. Hemoglobin decreases in the next several days, whereas bilirubin, lactate dehydrogenase, and reticulocytes are elevated and haptoglobin is decreased. Treatment is focused on removing stressors such as certain foods, oxidative drugs, and exposure to low oxygen saturation environments. Severe cases may require transfusions and supplementation with iron, folate, and vitamin B_{12} when hemolysis seems to be repetitive.

Sickle Cell Disease

Sickle cell anemia is an inherited autosomal recessive condition in which glutamic acid in the sixth position on the β-globin chain is replaced by a valine (Glu6Val). This results in hemoglobin SS in the homozygous state. Sickle cell trait, or hemoglobin AS, is found in 8–10% of African Americans in the United States, and sickle cell anemia occurs in about 1 in 400, or about 70,000 individuals. The gene for HbS is prevalent in sub-Saharan Africa. Persons of Mediterranean descent and those from India or Saudi Arabia have varying but somewhat lower percentages of the carrier state for HbSS. Sickle cell anemia occurs worldwide but predominates in Mediterranean, Saudi Arabian, and Indian populations. This distribution appears to be associated with independent mutations in these regions. People with hemoglobin AS or SS are somewhat protected against malaria because their erythrocytes are resistant to invasion by malarial parasites. If the parasite infects the cell, the rate of sickling increases, causing the cell with the parasite to be removed from the circulation more rapidly.

The pathophysiology of the sickling process is related to the oxygenation of the molecule. When deoxygenated, HbSS tends to polymerize into long, tubelike fibrils. This results in an elongated, rigid cell subject to trapping in the microcirculation, resulting in vaso-occlusive crisis. Hypoxemia, acidosis, dehydration of the RBC, hyperosmolality of the renal medulla, and viral infections can play a role in triggering or accentuating the sickling process. Sickled RBCs are also more adhesive to endothelial cells, activate endothelial cells, and contribute to the interaction between neutrophils and activated endothelium in the microvasculature. When the conditions that cause sickling are corrected, the sickle cell may return to a more normal shape and function. However, some sickled RBCs are irreversibly changed, indicating that the membrane cytoskeleton has been damaged. Irreversibly sickled cells are generally removed in the sinusoidal RES networks, but approximately one-third may be hemolyzed intravascularly. Some degree of anemia has a protective effect in vaso-occlusive crises by helping reduce blood viscosity and deoxygenation, thereby reducing the likelihood of polymerization and sickling.

During vaso-occlusive crises, the microvascular capillaries, capillary bed, and veins become occluded. Contributing to this locally are low pH, prolonged capillary transit time, and infection. Increased numbers of sickled RBCs occlude the vessels, which leads to painful ischemia, infarction, and reduced organ function over time. Areas particularly affected include the portal circulation, in which oxygen tension is low; the kidney, in which the renal medulla is hyperosmolar and dehydrates RBCs; the lungs; and the brain. It is not clear why some patients have severe, frequent episodes and others do not. Avascular necrosis of the bone marrow is often the cause of severe pain. WBCs may have a role in vaso-occlusive crises. In circumstances where the WBC is ≥15,000/μL, the risk of death increases. When hydroxyurea is used to reduce the frequency and severity of sickle cell crises, it may be effective in part because it reduces the WBC count.

Clinically, symptoms occur in childhood with shortness of breath, reduced exercise tolerance, and tachycardia all related to anemia. The complete blood count shows elongated RBCs and the appearance of Howell-Jolly bodies (cytoplasmic remnants usually removed by the spleen) in the RBCs over time due to recurrent splenic infarcts after multiple vaso-occlusive episodes resulting in autosplenectomy. WBC and platelet counts may be elevated. Bone marrow testing reveals erythroid hyperplasia unless there is an aplastic crisis.

The diagnosis of sickle cell disease is easily made by finding sickled cells on the peripheral smear, preparing a sickle cell sample, or carrying out a screening hemoglobin electrophoresis, which will confirm the Hb type. For a sickle cell preparation, blood is mixed with 2% sodium metabisulfite, which produces sickling. The proportion of sickled cells is measured initially and then 1 hour later to make the diagnosis. The "gold standard" of diagnosis is Hb electrophoresis, which shows the relative amounts of Hb forms.

Patients may experience a myriad of complications, including bilirubin gallstones in 40–60% of patients, aseptic necrosis of the femoral head, pulmonary vascular occlusion leading to an acute chest syndrome, renal papillary necrosis, retinal hemorrhages, and skin breakdown over bony prominences. Infections are more likely to occur, including *Salmonella* from decreased complement activation and streptococcal sepsis and *Haemophilus* infections caused by encapsulated bacteria all usually rendered ineffective or removed by the spleen. Patients should be given Pneumovax (PCV13) as early as 6 weeks of age while *Haemophilous influenza* and Influenza vaccine should be initiated at 6 months of age. Pneumococcal polysaccharide vaccine (PPSV 23) should not be started till age 24 months as it is not effective before age 2 years. Prophylactic penicillin should be given to all children with sickle cell disease up to 5 years of age (SOR: C). Parvovirus infection can be devastating, leading to RBC aplasia. Vascular problems such as stroke are increased, with thrombotic stroke being more common in children and hemorrhage more common in adults.

Prevention should focus on good hydration, prevention of infection, and maintenance of a moderately low H/H to prevent occlusive crises. Acute crisis requires emergent hydration, rest, and pain reduction starting with nonsteroidal anti-inflammatory drugs (NSAIDs), acetaminophen, and then oral narcotics all the way to delivery by IV. Diphenhydramine and/or lorazepam may be helpful in reducing anxiety. Long-acting pain medications (MS Contin) may be needed until the crisis resolves. Supplemental oxygen in patients with a normal PaO_2 has not been proven to be beneficial (SOR: B). For prevention, all patients should receive folic acid and a multivitamin without iron.

Medications such as hydroxyurea increase the percentage of HbF and reduce the WBC count, thus shortening sickle crisis episodes. Given chronically and prophylactically (15 mg/kg/d), hydroxyurea results in fewer sickle cell occlusive episodes, reduced levels of pain, and reduction in hospital admissions. The complete blood cell count should be done every 2 weeks during chronic therapy. A decrease in the WBC count is a predictor of success, and chronic therapy decreases mortality by 40%. L-glutamine was approved in 2017 to reduce complications in children older than 5 years of age because of its antioxidant property. It is useful in patients who have a suboptimal response to hydroxyurea (SOR: A). Nitric oxide resulting in vasodilation may be useful in an acute crisis. In some cases of severe disease, sibling-donor allogenic bone marrow transplantation can result in a cure or conversion to sickle cell trait status, resulting in an 86% 5-year survival. Patients undergoing general anesthesia should have their HbA increased to 50% or more by preoperative RBC transfusions to reduce hypoxia, sickling, and sickle cell crises.

Sickle cell anemia should be viewed as a chronic disease that requires a team approach to be successful. Primary care physicians, nurses, social workers, pain experts, pharmacists, hematologists, and behavioral medicine may all be involved.

Niihara Y, Miller ST, Kanter J, et al. A phase 3 trial of l-glutamine in sickle cell disease. *N Engl J Med.* 2018;379(3):226–235. [PMID: 30021096]

▶ Sickle Cell Trait

Patients with sickle cell trait are heterozygous for the sickle gene and have a much lower likelihood of sickling than those who are homozygous. Most heterozygotes are asymptomatic throughout life. Patients with sickle cell trait, however, may develop complications if put into an extremely hypoxic environment such as high altitude, heat stroke, or dehydration, or if they develop pulmonary infections.

EXTRACORPUSCULAR HEMOLYTIC ANEMIAS

Changes can occur in RBCs from external agents such as heart valves, antibodies, toxins, drugs, or organ dysfunction.

▶ Macroangiopathic Hemolysis

Altered aortic valves, ventricular septal defects, arteriovenous shunts, vasculitis, thrombotic thrombocytopenic purpura, infections with sequelae such as hemolytic-uremic syndrome, and metastatic cancer may all cause shearing or stretching conditions on RBCs, leading to rupture or hemolysis. Some of the latter conditions produce disseminated intravascular coagulation (DIC) in which protein strands partially block blood vessel lumens, traumatizing RBCs as they attempt to pass through. The blood smear reveals fragmented RBCs such as schistocytes, helmet cells, and red cell fragments. In severe cases, platelet counts may drop and DIC may occur as a sequela instead of an inciting event, as noted earlier. Treatment of the resulting anemia is secondary to discovering the cause: a bad aortic valve may need replacement;

an infection may need antibiotics, or a vasculitis may require steroids. In chronic or severe cases, iron and folate may be low and replacement is required.

▶ Autoimmune Hemolytic Anemia

AIHA involves self-generated antibodies against antigens on the RBC cell or immunoglobulin (Ig) G complexes with complement that become attached to the RBC cell wall.

The Coombs test is useful because the *direct* Coombs detects immunoglobins already residing on the RBCs and is performed on the patient's RBCs, whereas the *indirect* Coombs detects the presence or absence of serum antibodies in the circulation with testing of the patient's serum instead of the patient's RBCs. RBCs attacked by IgG only are removed in the spleen, whereas RBCs clumped with IgG and complement are generally removed by Kupffer cells in the liver, which carry complement receptors. Some forms of AIHA are primary/idiopathic with cause unknown, whereas others are secondary to connective tissue disorders such as systemic lupus erythematosus, lymphomas, infections such as human immunodeficiency virus or hepatitis C, or inflammatory bowel disorders.

Patients present with varying degrees of anemia depending on whether the nature of the problem is acute or chronic. Most have a positive Coombs test and demonstrate macrocytosis-spherocytosis and RBC agglutination on the blood smear. Treatment focuses on decreasing the IgG antibody production and reduction of the RBC destruction process primarily through the use of large divided doses of prednisone (60–100 mg/d). Response to treatment can be seen by a reticulocytosis and rise in H/H levels. The Coombs test titer should be declining as well and can be a guide to reducing prednisone dosing. Although 20% of patients who respond will never have a recurrence, chronic steroid therapy implies a poorer prognosis. Splenectomy may cure some patients, but recurrence after splenectomy is fairly common. The monoclonal antibody to CD20, rituximab, is more effective than splenectomy. Recurrences may require use of immunosuppressive agents such as cyclosporine or azathioprine.

▶ Drug-Induced Immune Hemolysis

Two types of drug-induced hemolysis occur: hapten type or alteration of an RBC antigen. In the hapten type, a drug used in high doses such as from the penicillin or cephalosporin family may bind directly to the RBC cell wall. The body then produces an IgG antibody, leading to hemolysis in the RES. The direct Coombs test is positive in 20% of cases, and stopping the drug resolves the RBC-antigen complex formation, ending the hemolysis. Drugs such as levodopa, procainamide, and mefenamic acid are implicated. Diclofenac, an NSAID, can cause severe intracorpuscular and extracorpuscular hemolysis, leading to organ damage and disseminated intravascular coagulation.

Drug-induced autoimmune hemolysis will resolve once the offending agent is identified and stopped. Monitoring the patient for complications until stable may be necessary, along with monitoring until the H/H stabilizes and starts to rise.

SUMMARY

Anemia can be both a sign that something is wrong and a broad-based diagnosis by itself. Using a classification scheme based on the physiology of marrow responsiveness can be helpful in arriving at a diagnosis. The process of discovering the cause or diagnostic rationale for a given anemia is an interesting challenge and provides one with a sense of accomplishment, satisfying the dual agendas of helping a patient and mastery of interesting clinical problems.

Hepatobiliary Disorders

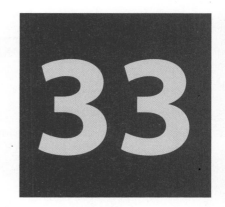

Samuel C. Matheny, MD, MPH, FAAFP
Kristin L. Long, MD, MPH, FACS
J. Scott Roth, MD, FACS

BILIARY DISEASES

Kristin Long, MD
J. Scott Roth, MD, FACS

GENERAL CONSIDERATIONS

Approximately 10–20% of the population has gallstones, making biliary pathology an increasing consideration in a patient with abdominal pain. Females are twice as likely to have gallstones. Gallstones are more frequently seen with increasing age and obesity and are more common in whites and Native Americans than African Americans. Most patients with cholelithiasis remain asymptomatic and never require surgery, but the sequelae of biliary disease remain significant: symptomatic cholelithiasis, gallstone pancreatitis, acute cholecystitis, chronic cholecystitis, choledocholithiasis, and ascending cholangitis. Understanding the basic pathophysiology of each of these conditions is essential to appropriately diagnose and treat patients with biliary disease.

A basic understanding of biliary diseases requires a vocabulary of terms used in describing them. Many have similar sounding names and can be confusing. A summary of the definitions can be found in Table 33–1. Although the treatment of most biliary diseases ultimately requires cholecystectomy, each condition must be evaluated and treated in a unique fashion.

OPERATIVE PROCEDURES & COMPLICATIONS

Laparoscopic Cholecystectomy

Laparoscopic cholecystectomy has replaced the open operation as the gold standard for removing the gallbladder. Many studies have documented an improved recovery time, decreased postoperative ileus, and decreased pain along with improved esthetics associated with laparoscopy.

Although associated with less morbidity, laparoscopic cholecystectomy does require pneumoperitoneum (insufflation of carbon dioxide gas into the abdomen) and may not be feasible in patients with other severe comorbid conditions (eg, the morbidly obese, those with severe congestive heart failure, advanced pulmonary disease, or uncontrolled coagulopathy). If operation is required, open cholecystectomy remains the only viable option for these patients.

Advanced Laparoscopic & Robotic Cholecystectomy

In carefully selected patients, both single-incision laparoscopic cholecystectomy and robotic cholecystectomy have been shown to be feasible and safe approaches in institutions with available technology. Although both techniques have been noted to have slightly longer operative times (mean difference of 18.5 minutes), a steep learning curve is observed and no increase in overall complication rates has been reported.

Postoperative Complications

The most feared complication of laparoscopic cholecystectomy is injury to the common bile duct. The reported incidence of bile duct injuries varies from 0% to 3% depending on the underlying pathology necessitating cholecystectomy. Minor biliary injuries include cystic duct leaks and biliary leaks from the hepatic parenchyma. These injuries may be managed with percutaneous drain placement or endoscopic retrograde cholangiopancreatography (ERCP) to facilitate drainage into the duodenum.

Major biliary injuries include clipping or transection of the common hepatic or common bile duct. When identified intraoperatively, these injuries are best managed with immediate repair, requiring open operation and a skilled surgeon. Those biliary injuries identified in the postoperative setting are best treated with externalization of the bile flow

Table 33–1. Basic definitions.

Term	Definition
Cholelithiasis	Presence of stones in the gallbladder
Cholecystitis	Inflammation of the gallbladder
Choledocholithiasis	Presence of gallstones in the common bile duct
Cholangitis	Inflammation (most commonly due to infection) of the bile ducts ascending into the liver
Cholecystectomy	Surgical removal of the gallbladder
Cholecystic	Relating to the gallbladder
Calculous	Related to the presence of gallstones
Acalculous	In absence of gallstones
ERCP	Endoscopic retrograde cholangiopancreatography

(percutaneous transhepatic biliary drainage) and a definitive repair at a later date, often 2–3 months following the initial injury. In most circumstances, a Roux-en-Y hepaticojejunostomy is required to reconstruct the biliary tree.

Patients who present with jaundice after elective cholecystectomy should be evaluated for retained common bile duct stones or a biliary injury. Presence of common bile duct dilatation on abdominal ultrasound should prompt immediate ERCP for both diagnosis and treatment. Patients undergoing elective cholecystectomy should be aware that ≤12% of those undergoing surgery may experience postcholecystectomy syndromes, including diarrhea (usually responsive to dietary measures), continued abdominal pain, or dyspepsia. Late sequelae of cholecystectomy can include bile duct strictures or recurrent bile duct stones. Patients suspected of these diagnoses should be promptly referred back to the operating surgeon.

Gurusamy KS, Davidson BR. Surgical treatment of gallstones. *Gastroenterol Clin North Am.* 2010;39(2):229–244. [PMID: 20478484]

Song T, Liao B, Cheng N. Single-incision versus conventional laparoscopic cholecystectomy: a systematic review of available data. *Surg Laparosc Endosc Percutan Tech.* 2012;22(4):190–196. [PMID: 22874697]

CHOLELITHIASIS

Asymptomatic Cholelithiasis

A landmark study from the University of Michigan followed the course of 123 faculty members identified as having asymptomatic gallstones during a routine health examination.

After >2 decades of follow-up, 14 (11%) patients went on to develop complications requiring surgery. Subsequent studies have not demonstrated a survival advantage with prophylactic cholecystectomy, and as a result, cholecystectomy for asymptomatic cholelithiasis is rarely indicated. Hemolytic conditions such as hereditary spherocytosis remain one indication to consider prophylactic cholecystectomy during other abdominal operations such as splenectomy.

Symptomatic Cholelithiasis

 ESSENTIALS OF DIAGNOSIS

▶ Episodic right upper quadrant (RUQ) pain.
▶ Ultrasound evidence of gallstones.

Unlike asymptomatic cholelithiasis, symptomatic cholelithiasis will generally necessitate operative intervention. The typical patient presentation will include RUQ abdominal pain, usually following a fatty meal and frequently associated with nausea (biliary colic). The pain can be severe and debilitating, and a trip to the emergency room is not an infrequent occurrence. Symptoms are related to transient obstruction of the gallbladder neck or infundibulum by stones or biliary sludge. As the gallbladder attempts to contract in response to cholecystokinin secretion, the obstructed cystic duct prevents the egress of bile from the gallbladder into the biliary system, resulting in acute RUQ pain. In addition to RUQ pain, the character of biliary colic is often described as a colicky or crampy pain that may radiate to the back or shoulder. The pain is generally postprandial in nature and typically resolves within 1–2 hours. Persistence of pain beyond this time should prompt the clinician to suspect acute cholecystitis or other disorders discussed later.

In most circumstances, there will be no abnormalities in the liver function tests or complete blood counts of patients with symptomatic cholelithiasis. An abdominal ultrasound will reveal the presence of cholelithiasis without gallbladder wall thickening or pericholecystic fluid. The treatment of symptomatic cholelithiasis remains elective cholecystectomy in patients suitable to undergo a general anesthetic. Following cholecystectomy, most patients (95%) with symptomatic cholelithiasis will have no further sequela of biliary diseases.

Chronic Cholecystitis

The term *chronic cholecystitis* is often used synonymously with *symptomatic cholelithiasis*. It may also be a result of multiple episodes of untreated acute cholecystitis. The gallbladder will become scarred from multiple episodes of inflammation. Pathologic examination will demonstrate

Rokitansky-Aschoff sinuses. The patient will usually describe multiple episodes of biliary colic. Ultrasound will demonstrate cholelithiasis and occasionally gallbladder wall thickening (from the scarring).

The treatment of chronic cholecystitis is cholecystectomy. Following cholecystectomy, most patients recover with no adverse effects.

Gracie WA, Ransohoff DF. The natural history of silent gallstones: the innocent gallstone is not a myth. N Engl J Med. 1982;307: 798–800. [PMID: 7110244]

Z'Graggen K, Wehrli H, Metzger A, et al. Complications of laparoscopic cholecystectomy in Switzerland. A prospective study of 10,174 patients. Swiss Association of Laparoscopic and Thoracoscopic Surgery. Surg Endosc. 1998;12:1301–1310. [PMID: 9788852]

ACUTE CHOLECYSTITIS

ESSENTIALS OF DIAGNOSIS

▶ Persistent severe RUQ pain (>4–6 hours).

▶ RUQ tenderness.

▶ Fever, leukocytosis.

▶ Ultrasound evidence of gallstones.

Acute cholecystitis is caused most commonly by obstruction of the cystic duct, resulting in localized edema and inflammation. Biliary cultures of most patients reveal bacteria. Women are 3 times more likely to develop acute cholecystitis than men. Over 90% of cases of acute cholecystitis are related to gallstones causing obstruction (calculous cholecystitis). The remaining cases are classified as acalculous cholecystitis, in which other comorbid conditions result in gallbladder wall ischemia or biliary stasis.

Acute cholecystitis is defined by the triad of RUQ pain, fever, and leukocytosis. Abdominal ultrasound will demonstrate gallbladder wall thickening (>3 mm) with pericholecystic fluid. Symptoms typically begin after a meal. The pain is similar to, but far more severe than, that of symptomatic cholelithiasis. In cases where acalculous cholecystitis is suspected or when ultrasound is inconclusive, radionucleotide scanning (ie, hepatobiliary iminodiacetic acid [HIDA]) may be used. Presence of radionucleotide in the extrahepatic biliary tree without filling the gallbladder is diagnostic of acute cholecystitis.

The treatment of acute cholecystitis is cholecystectomy. The timing of the operation is a controversial subject matter for general surgeons. Localized edema and subsequent scar formation after an episode of acute cholecystitis can make laparoscopic cholecystectomy difficult. Traditional teaching has been that cholecystectomy should be performed within 3 days of onset of symptoms—before myoepithelial changes can occur in the RUQ. The localized edema associated with acute cholecystitis aides with dissection of tissue planes and facilitates cholecystectomy. Compared to delayed cholecystectomy (after 7 days of symptoms), this approach is associated with a decreased conversion rate to open operation (2% vs 30%) and decreased recovery time (12 vs 28 days). Many patients present, however, outside the initial 72-hour window. Most current recommendations extend the period for safely performing laparoscopic cholecystectomy during acute cholecystitis to within 1 week of symptom onset. If outside of this 7-day window, many surgeons advocate a course of intravenous and (later) oral antibiotics with a plan to perform cholecystectomy in a delayed fashion at least 6 weeks later. This delay will allow the scarring in the RUQ to subside, allowing for safer and easier dissection during laparoscopy. If the patient has continued pain or recurrence of cholecystitis during this waiting period, laparoscopic cholecystectomy should be attempted immediately. The patient should be counseled on the high probability of conversion to an open operation. For patients who are not operative candidates, percutaneous tube cholecystostomy remains a viable option to drain the infected bile as a bridge to elective cholecystectomy when the patient has stabilized.

Untreated cholecystitis can lead to gallbladder ischemia, necrosis, or perforation, resulting in biliary leak or fistula formation to the surrounding structures. Those undergoing successful immediate cholecystectomy will generally have no further sequel of biliary disease. The potential for choledocholithiasis and common bile duct injury must be considered in patients presenting with jaundice after cholecystectomy.

Gurusamy K, Samraj K, Gluud C, Wilson E, Davidson BR. Meta-analysis of randomized controlled trials on the safety and effectiveness of early versus delayed laparoscopic cholecystectomy for acute cholecystitis. Br J Surg. 2010;97(2):141–150. [PMID: 20035546]

The Southern Surgeons Club. A prospective analysis of 1518 laparoscopic cholecystectomies. N Engl J Med. 1991;324:1073–1078. [PMID: 1826143]

Choledocholithiasis

Choledocholithiasis, or common bile duct stones, are present in ≤10% of patients undergoing cholecystectomy. The treatment is cholecystectomy with evaluation of the biliary tree and clearance of all stones within the ductal system. Choledocholithiasis should be suspected in any patient with biliary ductal dilatation seen on imaging, elevated bilirubin levels (conjugated), elevated alkaline phosphatase levels, or elevated amylase and lipase levels. Patients presenting with choledocholithiasis may develop symptoms related to obstruction of the bile duct, pancreatic duct, or both.

Gallstone Pancreatitis

ESSENTIALS OF DIAGNOSIS

- ▶ RUQ or epigastric pain.
- ▶ Elevated serum amylase and lipase.
- ▶ Ultrasound evidence of gallstones.

Gallstones small enough to pass through the biliary tree may enter the pancreatic duct and potentially obstruct at the level of the ampulla of Vater. These stones will then cause obstruction of the pancreatic ductal system, resulting in pancreatitis. Gallstones are associated with approximately 45–50% of all cases of pancreatitis in the United States.

Patients presenting with pancreatitis typically have varying degrees of abdominal pain, usually located in the epigastrium or RUQ. The pain may radiate to the back or shoulders. Nausea and vomiting are common. Laboratory studies will reveal elevation of lipase and (occasionally) amylase. If gallstones remain in the biliary tree, then liver transaminases and bilirubin may also be elevated. Although ultrasound is useful to confirm presence of gallstones, computed tomography (CT) scanning is useful in delineating the severity of pancreatitis.

The treatment of gallstone pancreatitis is eventual cholecystectomy. As the gallbladder is the source of the stones, cholecystectomy will prevent subsequent episodes of pancreatitis. Cholecystectomy should not be attempted until the resolution of pancreatitis. Treatment for pancreatitis involves bowel rest with intravenous hydration. Severe cases of pancreatitis may require intensive care unit admission with cardiovascular and respiratory support. Regardless of the patient's condition, cholecystectomy should be postponed until after the pancreatitis has resolved. It has been suggested that morbidity and mortality are improved if these patients undergo ERCP within 2 days of onset of symptoms. ERCP may be able to remove an impacted stone and thus allow for pancreatic decompression. This approach is generally considered in patients with moderate or severe pancreatitis.

The presence or absence of a persistent bile duct stone should be determined prior to proceeding with cholecystectomy. In most circumstances, normalization of serum lipase, amylase, and liver function tests (if originally elevated) occurs rapidly. In these circumstances, no imaging of the biliary tree is required because of the low probability of a persistent bile duct stone. However, patients with persistent abnormalities of their liver functions, amylase, or lipase should be evaluated for the presence of common bile duct stones. Biliary imaging may be obtained by means of intraoperative cholangiography at the time of cholecystectomy, perioperative ERCP, or magnetic resonance cholangiopancreatography (MRCP). MRCP is the least invasive modality but is only diagnostic. ERCP allows for both visualization and extraction of stones of diameter ≤1.5 cm. ERCP may be used to extract common bile duct stones either antecedent or subsequent to cholecystectomy. Common bile duct stones not amenable to endoscopic removal are removed operatively by performing a common bile duct exploration.

The overall long-term outcome of patients is related to the severity of the pancreatitis. Localized morbidity includes pancreatic necrosis, splenic vein thrombosis with gastric varices, hemorrhagic pancreatitis, and pancreatic abscess formation. Systemic morbidity can result in multisystem organ failure or even death.

Behrns KE, Ashley SW, Hunter JG, et al. Early ERCP for gallstone pancreatitis: for whom and when? *J Gastrointest Surg.* 2008;12:629–633. [PMID: 17846851]

Kaw M, Al-Antably Y, Kaw P. Management of gallstone pancreatitis: cholecystectomy, or ERCP and endoscopic sphincterotomy. *Gastroinest Endosc.* 2002;56:61–65. [PMID: 12085036]

Tse F, Yuan Y. Early routine endoscopic retrograde cholangiopancreatography strategy versus early conservative management strategy in acute gallstone pancreatitis. *Cochrane Database Syst Rev.* 2012;16:CD009779. [PMID: 22592743]

Cholangitis

ESSENTIALS OF DIAGNOSIS

- ▶ Persistent RUQ pain.
- ▶ Jaundice.
- ▶ Fever.
- ▶ Hypotension, mental status changes (acute suppurative cholangitis).

Cholangitis is defined as inflammation of the biliary system. It is most commonly caused by an impacted gallstone at the ampulla of Vater preventing bile drainage into the duodenum, although other etiologies such as extrinsic compression from an adjacent mass, inflammatory process, or a primary tumor of the ampulla, duodenum, or bile duct should also be considered. Cholangitis is considered a medical emergency.

Patients with cholangitis may present with Charcot's triad (fever, RUQ pain, and jaundice) or with Reynold's pentad (the addition of hypotension or mental status changes). Laboratory studies will show hyperbilirubinemia and leukocytosis. Ultrasound will likely show biliary ductal dilatation.

With clinical suspicion of cholangitis, patients should be immediately resuscitated and given broad-spectrum antibiotics. Biliary decompression should be urgently performed by ERCP. If ERCP fails to resolve the obstruction or is not available, percutaneous transhepatic cholangiography (PTC) with drainage may be performed. In the presence of stones, once biliary decompression has been performed, cholecystectomy should be performed electively following resolution of the cholangitis. In rare circumstances in which percutaneous or endoscopic biliary drainage is not possible, urgent cholecystectomy with common bile duct exploration should be performed.

The mortality associated with cholangitis varies widely and is related to the underlying etiology of the cholangitis. Cholangitis secondary to stones is associated with a low overall mortality provided the patient can be successfully supported through the infectious period. Cholangitis related to an underlying periampullary malignancy requires careful oncologic consideration prior to surgical intervention. This may require a more involved oncologic resection (eg, a pancreaticoduodenectomy or extrahepatic biliary resection) or palliative care depending on the extent of the malignancy. In the event of an unresectable periampullary tumor, a biliary bypass (hepaticojejunostomy) may be considered. Most periampullary cancers are associated with very poor 5-year survival even with complete extirpation of the tumor.

Lai EC, Mok FP, Tan ES, et al. Endoscopic biliary drainage for severe acute cholangitis. *N Engl J Med*. 1992;326:1582–1586. [PMID: 1584258]

Lee JG. Diagnosis and management of acute cholangitis. *Nat Rev Gastroenterol Hepatol*. 2009;6(9):533–541. [PMID: 19652653]

Sugiyama M, Atomi Y. Treatment of acute cholangitis due to choledocholithiasis in elderly and younger patients. *Arch Surg*. 1997;132:1129–1133. [PMID: 9336514]

Biliary Dyskinesia

A small group of patients will present with RUQ abdominal pain and symptoms that follow the pattern of biliary disease but will have essentially negative imaging for biliary pathology. One key factor in ascertaining whether the gallbladder is contributing to their pain would be to perform a HIDA scan with cholecystokinin (CCK) injection. Likewise, measurement of gallbladder ejection fraction (EF) during this scan can further identify patients with biliary pathology. EFs of <35% are considered pathophysiologic and warrant evaluation for cholecystectomy. Reproduction of pain with CCK injection is diagnostic for biliary dyskinesia, and these patients benefit from referral for cholecystectomy. Laparoscopic cholecystectomy has been reported to alleviate pain in ≤94% of patients with biliary dyskinesia. Patients with the highest success rate were those presenting with complaints of nausea or pain or with EF <15% by HIDA scan. Patients with vague abdominal complaints should be cautioned that laparoscopic cholecystectomy is not guaranteed to alleviate their symptoms, and the decision to proceed with surgical intervention should be made carefully on a case-by-case basis.

Bingener J, Sirinek KR, Schwesinger WH, et al. Laparoscopic cholecystectomy for biliary dyskinesia. *Surg Endosc*. 2004;18:802–806. [PMID: 15054652]

Yost F, Murayama K. Cholecystectomy is an effective treatment for biliary dyskinesia. *Am J Surg*. 1999;178(6):462–465. [PMID: 10670853]

BILIARY MALIGNANCIES

Gallbladder Polyps

Gallbladder polyps are present in ~5% of the population and are usually found incidentally during abdominal ultrasonography. The different types of polyps include cholesterolosis, adenomyomatosis, hyperplastic cholecystosis, and adenocarcinomatosis. The goal of surgical management is to identify which polyps are cancerous (adenocarcinoma) or at risk of developing cancer (adenomyomatosis) and select these patients for cholecystectomy.

Unfortunately, short of cholecystectomy, there is currently no way to distinguish among the different types of gallbladder polyps. With the relative safety of laparoscopic cholecystectomy, some advocate surgery immediately after discovering polyps. Patients who have polyps with gallstones or are age >50 years should be referred for cholecystectomy. Further imaging techniques, including endoscopic ultrasound (EUS), have been advocated for small polyps. Recent recommendations include removing polyps of diameter ≥6 mm because of an increased likelihood of malignancy. If cancer is present in the surgical specimen, the depth of invasion dictates the next course of therapy.

Gallahan WC, Conway JD. Diagnosis and management of gallbladder polyps. *Gastroenterol Clin North Am*. 2010;39(2):359–367. [PMID: 20478491]

Gallbladder Cancer

Patients with gallbladder cancer have presentations similar to those with symptomatic cholelithiasis or chronic cholecystitis. Presentation is often late, and with advanced disease, systemic complaints such as gradual weight loss and loss of appetite also appear. Since presentation is often assumed to be related to gallstone disease, ultrasound is usually the initial diagnostic modality used. Ultrasound findings of a mass >1 cm, calcified gallbladder wall, discontinuity of gallbladder wall layers, and loss of interface between the gallbladder wall and the liver should raise suspicion of gallbladder cancer. CT is useful in these circumstances to delineate anatomic structures for resectability, as well as evidence of metastatic disease.

The presence of paraaortic or peripancreatic lymphadenopathy is deemed unresectable disease. This can be confirmed with EUS with biopsies. Cancers that are limited to the mucosa or muscular layer of the gallbladder can be treated with cholecystectomy with negative margins alone. Tumors that invade the pericholecystic connective tissue require resection of the gallbladder fossa with en bloc cholecystectomy. Tumors that invade the liver require formal resection of the involved segments. Unfortunately, 15–50% of tumors that penetrate the muscular wall of the gallbladder have nodal disease that will render them unresectable. Gallbladder cancer may also be found incidentally in cholecystectomy specimens. If it is invasive, additional resection of involved hepatic margins will be necessary. The 5-year survival of early tumors (those confined to the muscular or mucosal layer) is excellent (90–100%). The survival for more advanced tumors is measured in terms of weeks or months.

Bartlett DL, Fong Y, Fortner JG, et al. Long-term results after resection for gallbladder cancer: implications for staging and management. *Ann Surg.* 1996;224:639–646. [PMID: 8916879]

Fong Y, Jarnagin W, Blumgart LH. Gallbladder cancer: comparison of patients presenting initially for definitive operation with those presenting after prior noncurative intervention. *Ann Surg.* 2000;232:557–569. [PMID: 10998654]

Choledochal Cyst

Classically, a choledochal cyst is described as a palpable RUQ mass in a young female with jaundice. Most choledochal cysts are described in Asian populations but are increasingly seen in the United States, males, and older patients. Choledochal cysts are classified by their anatomic location; most involve solitary fusiform dilatation of the extrahepatic biliary tree. Their presentation in Western series is similar to that of symptomatic cholelithiasis. They can be easily seen on ultrasound—provided the ultrasonographer evaluates the biliary tree in addition to the gallbladder.

Choledochal cysts are associated with a 70-fold increased incidence of cholangiocarcinoma, so surgical resection is indicated when discovered. Operative treatment involves resection of the entire extrahepatic biliary tree, cholecystectomy, and reconstruction with a Roux-en-Y hepaticojejunostomy. Surgical resection is considered curative; Edil et al. (2008) reported no subsequent malignancy over 30 years in patients without cancer at the time of cyst excision.

Edil BH, Cameron JL, Reddy S, et al. Choledochal cyst disease in children and adults: a 30-year single institution experience. *J Am Coll Surg.* 2008;206:1000–1005. [PMID: 18471743]

Cholangiocarcinoma

For various reasons, cholangiocarcinomas along with other RUQ malignancies are associated with very poor survival: (1) these lesions often present late and are not amenable to resection; (2) their biological activity is not well understood, and systemic therapy offers little benefit; and (3) operative resection is technically difficult, and patients need to be seen in specialized centers.

The vast majority of cholangiocarcinomas present with jaundice, sometimes in the setting of cholangitis. Ultrasound will often show a dilated proximal biliary tree. ERCP and EUS are useful to delineate the tumor. Preoperative endoscopic brushings are often nondiagnostic and should not be aggressively pursued in patients with resectable disease on cross-sectional imaging. While most proximal cholangiocarcinomas (70%) are not amenable to resection, approximately half of distal tumors may be resected. Resection involves pancreaticoduodenectomy for distal tumors and extrahepatic biliary resection with Roux-en-Y hepaticojejunostomy for proximal disease. The 5-year survival rate remains poor even after complete resection (20–25%). For patients with unresectable disease, survival is again measured in weeks or months.

Fong Y, Blumgart LH, Lin E, et al. Outcome of treatment for distal bile duct cancer. *Br J Surg.* 1996;83:1712–1715. [PMID: 9038548]

Jarnigan WR, Fong Y, DeMatteo RP, et al. Staging, resectability and outcome in 225 patients with hilar cholangiocarcinoma. *Ann Surg.* 2001;234:507–517. [PMID: 11573044]

LeFemina J, Jarnagin WR. Surgical management of proximal bile duct cancers. *Langenbecks Arch Surg.* 2012;397(6):869–879. [PMID: 22391776]

▼ LIVER DISEASE

Samuel C. Matheny, MD, MPH

VIRAL HEPATITIS

ESSENTIALS OF DIAGNOSIS

▶ Variable prodromal signs and symptoms.

▶ Positive specific viral hepatitis tests.

▶ Elevation of serum aspartate aminotransferase (AST) and alanine aminotransferase (ALT).

Acute viral hepatitis is a worldwide problem, and in the United States alone, there are probably between 200,000 and 700,000 cases per year according to the Centers for Disease Control and Prevention (CDC). Over 32% of cases are caused by hepatitis A virus (HAV), 43% by hepatitis B virus (HBV), 21% by hepatitis C virus (HCV), and the remainder are not identified. Although few deaths (~250) due to acute hepatitis are reported annually, considerable morbidity can result from chronic hepatitis caused by HBV and HCV infections, and mortality from complications can be pronounced for years to come.

Hepatitis A

General Considerations

HAV, first identified in 1973, is the prototype for the former diagnosis of *infectious hepatitis*. Over the past several decades, the incidence of HAV infection has varied considerably, and a high number of cases have gone unreported. HAV is a very small viral particle that is its own unique genus (*Hepatovirus*).

Most individuals infected worldwide are children. In general, there are four patterns of HAV distribution (high, moderate, low, and very low), which roughly correspond to differing socioeconomic and hygienic conditions. Countries with poor sanitation have the highest rates of infection. Most children age <9 years in these countries manifest evidence of HAV infection. Countries with moderate rates of infection have the highest incidence in later childhood; food- and waterborne outbreaks are more common. In countries with low endemicity, the peak age of infection is likely to be at early adulthood, and in very low endemic countries, outbreaks are uncommon.

Hepatitis A is usually transmitted by ingestion of contaminated fecal material of an infected person by a susceptible individual. Contaminated food or water can be the source of infection, but occasionally infection can occur by contamination of different types of raw shellfish from areas contaminated by sewage. The virus can survive for 3–10 months in water. Other cases of infection by blood exposures have been reported but are less common. The incubation period for HAV averages 30 days, with a range of 15–50 days.

In countries of low endemicity, persons at greatest risk for infection include travelers to intermediate and high-HAV-endemic countries, men who have sex with men (MSMs), injection or noninjection drug users, persons with occupational risks of infection, household members and other close personal contacts of adopted children newly arriving from the countries mentioned, persons with clotting factor disorders, persons with chronic liver disease, including those who have received transplants, and persons who have direct contact with persons infected with hepatitis A. In areas of high endemicity, all young children are at increased risk.

Prevention

Currently in the United States, the CDC recommends that certain populations at increased risk be considered for pre-exposure vaccination; these include the groups listed earlier. In addition, the CDC now recommends universal immunization for all children age ≥1 year. The immunization schedule consists of three doses for children and adolescents and two for adults. In groups with the potential for high risk of exposure, including any adult age >40 years, prevaccination testing for prior exposure may be cost effective. The appropriate test is the total anti-HAV. Travelers age <40 years who receive the vaccine may assume to be protected after receiving the first dose, although the second dose is desired for long-term protection. For certain travelers (older adults and those with underlying medical conditions), immunoglobulin (Ig) may be given in a different site for additional protection within 2 weeks of travel. A combination vaccine with HBV is available for persons age >18 years who are immunocompetent and is used on the same three-dose schedule as HBV.

Ig or hepatitis A vaccine (if previously unvaccinated) may also be used for postexposure prophylaxis in healthy patients between 12 months and 40 years of age, if given within 14 days, and would most often be used for household or intimate contacts of an infected person, in some institutional settings, or if a common source is identified. For persons with chronic illness or those age <12 months or >40 years, Ig is preferred.

Clinical Findings

A. Symptoms and Signs

The symptoms and signs of acute viral hepatitis are quite similar regardless of type and are difficult to distinguish on the basis of clinical findings. The prodrome for viral hepatitis is variable and may be manifested by anorexia, including changes in olfaction and taste, as well as nausea and vomiting, fatigue, malaise, myalgias, headache, photophobia, pharyngitis, cough, coryza, and fever. Dark urine and clay-colored stools may be noticed 1–5 days before jaundice.

Clinical jaundice varies considerably and may range from an anicteric state to rare hepatic coma. In acute HAV infection, jaundice is usually more pronounced in older age groups (ie, 70–80% in those age 14 years) and rare in children age <6 years (<10%). Weight loss may also be present, as well as an enlarged liver (70%) and splenomegaly (20%). Spider angiomata may be present without acute liver failure. Patients may also report a loss of desire for cigarette smoking or alcohol.

B. Laboratory Findings

Usually, the onset of symptoms coincides with the first evidence of abnormal laboratory values. Acute elevations of ALT and AST are seen, with levels as high as 4000 units or more in some patients. The ALT level is usually higher than the AST. When the bilirubin level is >2.5, jaundice may be obvious. Bilirubin levels may go from 5 to 20, usually with an equal elevation of conjugated and unconjugated forms. The prothrombin time is usually normal. If significantly elevated, it may signal a poor prognosis. The complete blood count may demonstrate a relative neutropenia, lymphopenia, or atypical lymphocytosis. Urobilinogen may be present in urine in the late preicteric stage.

Serum IgM antibody (anti-HAV) is present in the acute phase and usually disappears within 3 months, although occasionally it persists longer. IgG anti-HAV is used to detect previous exposure and persists for the lifetime of the patient. The more commonly available test for IgG anti-HAV is the total anti-HAV.

▶ Treatment

Treatment for the most part is symptomatic, with many clinicians prohibiting only alcohol during the acute illness phase. Most patients can be treated at home.

▶ Prognosis

In the vast majority of patients with HAV, the disease resolves uneventfully within 3–6 months. Rarely, fulminant hepatitis may develop, with acute liver failure and high mortality rates. Rare cases of cholestatic hepatitis, with persistent bilirubin elevations, have also been reported. Some patients develop relapsing hepatitis, in which HAV is reactivated and shed in the stool. Affected patients demonstrate liver function test abnormalities, but virtually all recover completely. HAV does not progress to chronic hepatitis.

Hepatitis B

▶ General Considerations

HBV is a double-shelled DNA virus. The outer shell contains the hepatitis B surface (HBsAg). The inner core contains several other particles, including hepatitis core antigen (HBcAg) and hepatitis B e antigen (HBeAg). These antigens and their subsequent antibodies are described in more detail later.

Worldwide, >400 million people are infected with HBV, but the distribution is quite varied. More than 45% of the global population live in areas of high incidence (infections in >8% of population). There, the lifetime risk of infection is >60%, and early childhood infections are very common. Intermediate-risk areas (infections in 2–7% of the population) represent 43% of the global population. The lifetime risk of infection in these areas is between 20% and 60%, and infections occur in various age groups. In low-risk areas (infections in <2%), which represent ~12% of the global population, the lifetime risk of infection is <20% and is usually limited to specific adult risk groups.

In the United States, HBV is normally a disease of young adults. The largest numbers of cases are reported in adults age 20–39 years, but many cases in younger age groups may be asymptomatic and go unreported. Of the specific risk groups in the United States, >50% in recent studies are those with sexual risk factors (more than one sex partner in the past 6 months, sexual relations with an infected person, or MSM transmission). Over 15% had a history of injection drug use, and 4% had other risk factors such as a household contact with HBV or a healthcare exposure. The mode of transmission can thus be sexual, parenteral, or perinatal, through contact of the infant's mucous membranes with maternal infected blood at delivery.

Body fluids with the highest degree of concentration of HBV are blood, serum, and wound exudates. Moderate concentrations are found in semen, vaginal fluid, and saliva, and low or nondetectable amounts are found in urine, feces, sweat, tears, or breast milk. Saliva can be implicated in transmission through bites, but not by kissing.

The average incubation period for HBV is between 60 and 90 days, with a range of 45–180 days. Although the incidence of jaundice increases with age (<10% of children <5 years old demonstrate icterus compared with 30–50% of those age >35 years), the likelihood of chronic infection with HBV is greater when infection is contracted at a younger age. Between 30% and 90% of all children who contract HBV before the age of 5 years develop chronic disease, compared with 2–10% of those age >35 years.

▶ Prevention

Current immunization recommendations in the United States call for routine immunization of all infants, children, adolescents, and adults in high-risk groups, including all diabetic patients age 19–58 years and all patients with chronic liver disease, including those with chronic hepatitis C and/or significantly elevated liver enzymes. Acknowledgment of a specific risk factor is not a requirement for immunizations. These recommendations include immunizing all children at birth within 24 hours if birth weight is ≥2000 g and at 1 and 6 months. Additionally, all high-risk groups should be screened, as well as all pregnant women. Prevaccination testing of patients in low-risk groups is probably not necessary, but in high-risk groups, this may be cost effective. As illustrated in the first test scenario of Table 33–2, a negative HBsAg titer and a negative anti-HBs titer are evidence of susceptibility to HBV.

The vaccine contains components of HBsAg. Pretesting with anti-HB core antibody (anti-HBc) is probably the single best test, because it would identify those who are infected and those who have been exposed. Posttesting for vaccine is seldom recommended, except for individuals who may have difficulty mounting an immune response (eg, immunocompromised patients). In these patients, the hepatitis B surface antibody (anti-HBs) would be the appropriate test. Some authorities recommend revaccinating high-risk individuals if titer levels have fallen below 10 IU/L after 5–10 years or if they have failed to mount an appropriate immune response with the standard dosing and schedule.

Children born to women of unknown hepatitis B status should receive a first dose of hepatitis B vaccine within 12 hours of birth as well as hepatitis B immune globulin (HBIG) and HBIG within 7 days for infants ≥2000 g if maternal blood is positive. Repeat testing of all infants born to HBV-infected mothers should be performed at 9–18 months with HBsAg

Table 33–2. Interpretation of the hepatitis B panel.

Tests	Results	Interpretation
HBsAg Anti-HBc Anti-HBs	Negative Negative Negative	Susceptible
HBsAg Anti-HBc Anti-HBs	Negative Positive Positive	Immune because of natural factors
HBsAg Anti-HBc Anti-HBs	Negative Negative Positive	Immune because of hepatitis B vaccination
HBsAg Anti-HBc IgM anti-HBc Anti-HBs	Positive Positive Positive Negative	Acutely infected
HBsAg Anti-HBc IgM anti-HBc Anti-HBs	Positive Positive Negative Negative	Chronically infected
HBsAg Anti-HBc Anti-HBs	Negative Positive Negative	Four interpretations possible[a]

[a]May be (1) recovering from acute hepatitis B virus infection, (2) distantly immune and the test is not sensitive enough to detect very low levels of anti-HBs in serum, (3) susceptible with a false-positive anti-HB; or (4) an undetectable level of HBsAg is present in the serum and the person is actually a carrier.

and anti-HBs. Infants born to HBV-infected mothers should receive both the first dose of hepatitis B vaccine at birth as well as 0.5 mL of HBIG in separate sites within 12 hours after birth. Recommendations for postexposure prophylaxis of HBV can be reviewed in the current CDC recommendations.

Clinical Findings

Acute infection may range from an asymptomatic infection to cholestatic hepatitis to fulminant hepatic failure. HBsAg and other markers usually become positive about 6 weeks after infection and remain positive into the clinical signs of illness. Other biochemical abnormalities begin to show abnormalities in the prodromal phase and may persist for several months, even with a resolving disease process. Anti-HB core IgM becomes positive early, with onset of symptoms, and both anti-HB core IgM and anti-HB core IgG may persist for many months or years. Anti-HBs is the last antibody to appear and may indicate resolving infection. The presence of HBeAg indicates active viral replication and increased infectivity (Figure 33–1). Liver function tests should be obtained early in the course of infection, and

evidence of prolonged prothrombin time (international normalized ratio >1.5) should raise concern for hepatic failure. Patients who remain chronically infected may demonstrate HBsAg and HBeAg for at least 6 months, with a usual trend in liver function tests toward normal levels, although results may remain persistently elevated (Figure 33–2). Extrahepatic manifestations of HBV infection may occur and include serum sickness, polyarteritis nodosa, and membranoproliferative glomerulonephritis.

Complications

Complications of chronic infection may include progression to cirrhosis and hepatocellular carcinoma (HCC). Patients with active viral replication are at highest risk of chronic disease, with 15–20% developing progressive disease over a 5-year period. Continued positivity for HBeAg is associated with an increased risk of HCC. Most patients who are chronically infected remain HBsAg positive for their lifetime. There is no general agreement concerning the appropriate screening for patients with chronic infection for HCC. Guidance statements recommend screening all patients with cirrhosis with ultrasonography with or without α-fetoprotein every 6 months.

Treatment

Treatment for chronic disease depends on evidence of viral activity, HBeAg status, human immunodeficiency virus (HIV) and HCV comorbidity, histologic evidence of liver injury, and elevated liver function tests. Currently approved treatment modalities include interferon-alfa, pegylated interferon, and nucleoside(tide) analogs, such as lamivudine, telbivudine, adefovir, tenofovir disproxil, tenofovir alfenamide, and entecavir. Other new antiviral agents are currently being tested. Sensitive tests for determination of response to therapy, such as covalently closed circular DNA, may be more readily available in the future, although most patients will receive treatment indefinitely.

Hepatitis C

General Considerations

HCV has become the most common bloodborne infection as well as the leading cause of chronic liver disease and, subsequently, liver transplantation in the United States. Worldwide, >180 million people are infected, but the infection rates vary considerably. In the United States, it is estimated that approximately 4 million people may be infected with HCV; it is the main cause of death from liver disease. The responsible virus is an RNA virus of the Flaviviridae family. Six major genotypes, numbered 1 through 6, are known, with additional subtypes. There are varying distributions of these genotypes, and they may affect the progression of disease and the response to treatment regimens.

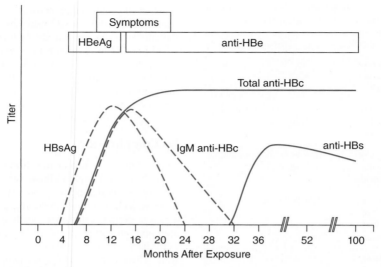

▲ **Figure 33–1.** Acute hepatitis B virus infection with recovery.

Hepatitis C is spread primarily through percutaneous exposure to blood. Since 1992, all donated blood has been screened for HCV. Injection drug use is responsible for >50% of new cases. Within 1–3 months after a first incident of needle sharing, 50–60% of intravenous drug users are infected. Other risk factors include use of intranasal cocaine, hemodialysis, tattooing (debatable), and vertical transmission, which is rare. Breastfeeding carries a low risk of transmission. Sexual transmission is uncertain but is probably 1–3% over the lifetime of a monogamous couple, one of whom is infected. Healthcare workers are at particular risk following a percutaneous exposure (1.8% average incidence).

One-time screening of all individuals born between 1945 and 1965 has been recommended by the CDC, along with screening of patients with known risk factors.

▶ **Prevention**

No immunizations are currently available for HCV infections. Prevention consists mainly of reduction of risk factors,

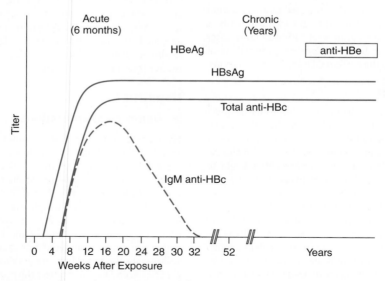

▲ **Figure 33–2.** Progression to chronic hepatitis B virus infection.

including screening of blood and blood products, caution to prevent percutaneous injuries, and reduction in intravenous drug use.

▶ Clinical Findings

A. Symptoms and Signs

1. Acute hepatitis—The incubation period for HCV varies between 2 and 26 weeks, but most commonly is 6–7 weeks. Most patients with HCV are asymptomatic at the time of infection. However, >20% of all recognized cases of acute hepatitis in the United States are caused by HCV, and as many as 30% of adults who are infected may present with jaundice. Acute, fulminant hepatic failure is rare.

2. Chronic hepatitis—In contrast to HAV and HBV, most people infected with HCV (85%) develop a chronic infection. The incidence of significant liver disease is 20–30% for cirrhosis and 4% for liver failure; >1–4% of patients with chronic infection develop HCC annually, or 11–19% over 4–11 years in one study. It appears that certain risk factors increase the likelihood of progression to serious disease. These include increased alcohol intake, age >40 years, HIV coinfection, and possibly male gender and other liver coinfections.

Extrahepatic manifestations of chronic infection are fairly common and are similar to those of HBV, including autoimmune conditions and renal conditions such as membranous glomerulonephritis.

B. Laboratory Findings

Patients in a high-risk category for HCV should be tested with both an approved HCV antibody test such as the Ora-Quick HCV Rapid Antibody test or other approved tests and a confirmatory test by a sensitive HCV RNA test if positive. All patients with HCV infection should have a quantitative HCV-RNA test as well as HCV genotyping prior to therapy in order to select the recommended treatment regimen and predict a therapeutic response, as well as duration of therapy. Evaluation of the stage of fibrosis, for concomitant infection with HIV or hepatitis B or A, and for potential for renal disease and pregnancy is also important.

▶ Treatment

Treatment for both acute and chronic HCV has undergone major strides in recent years. A recent study documents the conversion of a significant number of patients to negative serology when treated in the acute phase of infection; treatment is now recommended for all patients with chronic HCV infection with few exceptions. Virologic cure can be expected in most patients. The development of direct-acting antivirals, such as NS3 protease inhibitors, NS5A inhibitors, and NS5B polymerase inhibitors, has dramatically changed the response rate to therapy in all of the genotypes. It is important to check guidelines for the latest recommendation for specific subtypes of HCV disease. Many of these regimens are interferon and ribavirin free, which greatly simplifies the therapy and decreases the incidence of therapeutic complications. Therapy is usually given for 12 weeks, and sustained viral load can be expected in at least 95% of patients at this time. Other new treatments are currently under investigation.

It is important to immunize patients with chronic HCV infection for HAV, because the incidence of fulminant hepatitis A has been shown to be significantly increased in this population. Patients infected with HCV should also abstain from alcohol. It has also been recommended that HCV-infected individuals be vaccinated for HBV, owing to the poor prognosis of coinfected individuals. Chronic hepatitis C can also progress to cirrhosis and HCC, and appropriate screening measures as discussed in the section on hepatitis B apply to hepatitis C–infected patients as well.

Other Types of Infectious Hepatitis

Over 97% of cases of viral hepatitis in the United States are either A, B, or C. Other types of viral hepatitis occur much less frequently, although worldwide, they may be more important.

Hepatitis D

Hepatitis D virus (HDV) can replicate only in the presence of HBV infection. HDV infection can occur either as a coinfection with HBV or as a superinfection in a chronically infected individual with HBV. Although coinfection can produce more severe acute disease, a superinfection poses the risk of more significant chronic disease, with 70–80% of patients developing cirrhosis. The mode of transmission is most commonly percutaneous. The only tests commercially available in the United States are total (IgG and IgM)–anti-HDV. Prevention of HDV depends on prevention of HBV. There are no products currently available to prevent HDV infection in patients infected with HBV.

Hepatitis E

Hepatitis E virus (HEV) is the most common cause of enterically transmitted non-A, non-B hepatitis. Acute HEV infection is similar to other forms of viral hepatitis; no chronic form is known. Severity of illness increases with age, and for reasons that are unclear, case fatality rates are particularly high in pregnant women. Most cases of HEV reported in the United States have occurred in travelers returning from areas of high endemicity. In certain areas of the world (Mexico, North Africa, the Middle East, and Asia), epidemics of HEV may be common. Prevention includes avoidance of drinking water and other beverages of unknown purity, uncooked shellfish, and uncooked vegetables and fruits. Vaccines for hepatitis E are not universally available.

Acute Hepatitis: A Cost-Effective Approach

Because the vast majority of viral hepatitis cases are caused by HAV, HBV, or HCV, tests to determine the precise etiology are necessary for appropriate primary and secondary prevention for the patient, as well as potential for therapy. If these tests fail to indicate a diagnosis, the etiology may be due to less frequent causes of viral hepatitis such as Epstein-Barr virus, in which jaundice rarely accompanies infectious mononucleosis; cytomegalovirus or herpesvirus in immunocompromised patients; or other nonviral etiologies, such as alcoholic hepatitis, drug toxicity, Wilson disease, or an autoimmune hepatitis.

Centers for Disease Control and Prevention. Testing for HCV Infection: an update of guidance for clinicians and laboratorians. *MMWR Morb Mortal Wkly Rep.* 2013;62(18):362–365. [PMID: 23657112]

Heimbach J, Kulik L, Finn R, et al. AASLD guidelines for the treatment of hepatocellular carcinoma. *Hepatology.* 2018;67: 358–380. [PMID: 28130846]

Kuhar D, Henderson D, Struble K, et al. Updated U.S. public health service guidelines for the management of occupational exposures to HIV and recommendations for postexposure prophylaxis. *MMWR Recomm Rep.* 2005;54(RR-9):1–17. [PMID: 16195697]

Matheny S, Kingery J. Hepatitis A. *Am Fam Physician.* 2012; 86(11):1027–1034. [PMID: 231998670]

Schillie S, Vellozzi C, Reingold A, et al. Prevention of hepatitis B virus infection in the United States: recommendations of the Advisory Committee on Immunization Practices. *MMWR Recomm Rep.* 2018;67(1):1–31.

Soriano V, Barreiro P, Benitez L, et al. New antivirals for the treatment of chronic hepatitis B. *Expert Opin Investig Drugs.* 2017;26(7):843–851. [PMID: 28521532]

Tang L, Covert E, Wilson E, Kottillil S. Chronic hepatitis B infection: a review. *JAMA.* 2018;319(17):1802–1813. [PMID: 29715359]

Terrault N, Lok A, McMahon BJ, et al. Update on prevention, diagnosis, and treatment of chronic hepatitis B: AASLD 2018 Hepatitis B guidance. *Hepatology.* 2018;67(4):1560–1599. [PMID: 29405329]

US Public Health Service. Updated US Public Health Service guidelines for the management of occupational exposures to HBV, HCV, and HIV and recommendations for postexposure prophylaxis. *MMWR Recomm Rep.* 2001;50(RR-11):1–52. [PMID: 11442229]

Workowski K, Bolan GA. Sexually transmitted diseases treatment guidelines 2015. *MMWR Recomm Rep.* 2015;64(RR-03):1–137. [PMID: 26042815]

Websites

American Association for the Study of Liver Disease: HCV Guidance: Recommendations for Testing, Managing, and Treating Hepatitis C. hcvguidelines.org

American Liver Foundation. Liver Update: Function and Disease (excellent survey of issues pertaining to hepatitis). http://www.liverfoundation.org

Centers for Disease Control and Prevention: Hepatitis information (references for immunization and testing, as well as patient information in several languages). http://www.cdc.gov/hepatitis/

ALCOHOLIC LIVER DISEASE

 ESSENTIALS OF DIAGNOSIS

▶ History of alcohol use.
▶ Mildly elevated serum ALT and AST.
▶ Variable clinical signs (may include jaundice, hepatomegaly).

▶ General Considerations

Alcoholic liver disease (ALD) includes several different disease entities, spanning a large clinical spectrum. These diseases range from the syndrome of acute fatty liver to severe liver damage as manifested by cirrhosis. *Fatty liver* is usually asymptomatic except for occasional hepatomegaly and is the histologic result of excessive use of alcohol over a several-day period. In *perivenular fibrosis*, fibrous tissue is deposited in the central areas of the liver, particularly the central veins; this indicates that the individual may then rapidly progress to more severe forms of liver disease. Patients can progress from this stage directly to cirrhosis. *Alcoholic hepatitis* is a condition in which necrosis of hepatic cells occurs as part of an inflammatory response, which includes polymorphonuclear cells, along with evidence of fibrosis. *Cirrhosis* may result from continued progression of disease from alcoholic hepatitis or may occur without evidence of prior alcoholic hepatitis. Cirrhosis is characterized by distortion of the liver structure, with bands of connective tissue forming between portal and central zones. Changes in hepatic blood circulation may also occur, resulting in portal hypertension. Additionally, evidence of abnormal fat metabolism, inflammation, and cholestasis may be seen. Progression to HCC may also occur, although the exact risk of cirrhosis itself in the progression to HCC is not clear.

It is known that women are more likely than men to develop severe end-stage ALD, although the reasons for this phenomenon are only now being clarified. There may be additional genetic factors, most notably in specific enzyme systems, such as the metabolism of tumor necrosis factor (TNF) and alcohol-metabolizing systems, which affect the development of disease. Concomitant diseases, such as HCV infection, obesity, metabolic syndrome, and malnutrition, may also be additional risk factors.

▶ Clinical Findings

A. Symptoms and Signs

A history of drinking alcohol in excess of >3 drinks/day for men and >2 drinks/day for women is related to an increased risk for ALD. Numerous questionnaires have been designed for detection of excessive drinking, but the CAGE questionnaire (**c**ut down, **a**nnoyed by criticism, **g**uilty about drinking, **e**ye-opener drinks) and the Alcohol Use Disorders Inventory Test (AUDIT) are probably the most useful.

Clinical findings may be limited at this stage to occasional hepatomegaly. Patients with alcoholic hepatitis may present with classic signs and symptoms of acute hepatitis, including weight loss, anorexia, fatigue, nausea, and vomiting. Hepatomegaly may be evident, as well as other signs of more advanced disease, such as cirrhosis, because the development of cirrhosis may occur concomitant with a new episode of alcoholic hepatitis. These signs include jaundice, splenomegaly, ascites, spider angiomas, and signs of other organ damage secondary to alcoholism (eg, dementia, cardiomyopathy, or peripheral neuropathy).

B. Laboratory Findings

Various commercially available laboratory tests have been used to detect excessive alcohol intake in the early stages. The sensitivity and specificity of these tests vary. Liver function tests for elevations of AST, ALT, and γ-glutamyl transferase are frequently used. Elevation of mean corpuscular volume (MCV) has also been noted in patients with early-stage disease.

Transaminase levels are usually only mildly elevated in pure alcoholic hepatitis unless other disease processes, such as concomitant viral hepatitis, or acetaminophen ingestion, are present; AST is usually elevated to ≤200 IU/L, and AST to ≤500 IU/L. An AST/ALT ratio >1.5 is usually present. Elevated prothrombin time and bilirubin levels have a significant negative prognostic indication. *The presence of jaundice may have special significance in any actively drinking person and should be carefully evaluated.* Several instruments have been used for evaluation of severity, but the most common is the Maddrey discriminant function (MDF) or the Model for End-State Liver Disease (MELD) score. An MDF score >32 or a MELD score of >2 is indicative of severe disease.

▶ Treatment

Abstinence from alcohol is essential and is probably the most important of all therapies. Recovery from the acute episode is associated with an 80% 7-year survival rate in patients who can abstain from alcohol versus 50% survival in those who continue drinking. The use of naltrexone or acamprosate in conjunction with counseling and support groups to prevent recidivism should be considered.

Initial treatment of the acutely ill patient centers on ensuring adequate volume replacement, with concern for the ability to handle normal saline. Diuretics should be used cautiously. Patients should be assessed for protein-calorie malnutrition and vitamin and mineral deficiencies. Adequate nutrition should be given to patients with severe disease,

parenterally if necessary. There is no indication that avoidance of protein is helpful in patients with encephalopathy. Broad-spectrum antibiotics should be considered early in the treatment course. Many patients develop spontaneous peritonitis, pneumonia, or cellulitis, which should be treated aggressively. Corticosteroids have been suggested as beneficial, but considerable debate still ensues as to whether there is any benefit to survival, although current recommendations are that patients with severe disease (MDF ≥32) with or without encephalopathy and without contraindications for steroid use should be considered for a 4-week course of prednisone followed by a 2-week taper. Corticosteroids may increase the risk for infection in the treatment of alcoholic hepatitis. Pentoxifylline, which modifies TNFα, may also be considered, especially if steroids are contraindicated.

Liver transplantation may be an option. ALD is currently the second most common reason for liver transplantation in the United States. To be considered for transplantation, patients should have remained sober for >6 months and should have had addictive treatment. Recent studies have suggested that patients with severe alcoholic hepatitis should also be considered as eligible. The prognosis is excellent if relapse from drinking can be avoided. Relapse occurs in 15–30% of patients.

Other treatment methodologies in various stages of testing include other TNFα modifiers; antioxidant therapy with agents such as *S*-adenosyl-L-methionine (SAM-e), silymarin, or vitamin E; antifibrotics such as polyenylphosphatidylcholine (PPC); or other medications. Further studies are needed before these therapies can be recommended.

Singal AK, Bataller R, Ahn J, et al. ACG clinical guidelines: alcoholic liver disease. *Am J Gastroenterol.* 2018;113:175–194. [PMID: 29336434]

Singh S, Osna N, Kharbanda K. Treatment options for alcoholic and non-alcoholic fatty liver disease: a review. *World J Gastroenterol.* 2017;23(36):6549–6570. [PMID: 29085205]

Websites

Alcoholic Use Disorders Identification Test (AUDIT) website. https://www.drugabuse.gov/sites/default/files/files/AUDIT.pdf

OTHER LIVER DISEASES

Nonalcoholic Fatty Liver Disease

A relatively new condition described around 1980, nonalcoholic fatty liver disease (NAFLD) encompasses a wide clinical spectrum of patients whose liver histology is similar to those of patients with alcohol-induced hepatitis but without the requisite history. Women are affected more frequently than men. Many of these patients progress to cirrhosis. NAFLD is now the most common liver disease in the United States, occurring in ≤20% of the population in some studies. This condition is common in obese patients, as well as in patients with type 2 diabetes mellitus. It may be a part of syndrome X, which includes obesity, diabetes mellitus, dyslipidemia, and hypertension. Clinical features include hepatomegaly (75%) and splenomegaly (25%), but there are no pathognomonic laboratory markers. Elevations of ALT and AST may be ≤5 times normal, with an AST/ALT ratio of <1. Evidence of steatosis can be seen on hepatic ultrasonography. Treatment includes weight reduction, treatment of diabetes, and treatment of lipid disorders. Specific pharmacologic therapy, such as incretin analogs, pentoxifylline, and other modalities, may be recommended in the future.

Wilson Disease

Wilson disease, which is characterized by hepatolenticular degeneration, is caused by abnormal metabolism of copper. It is inherited in an autosomal recessive pattern and has a prevalence in the general population of approximately 1 in 30,000. Although patients in asymptomatic stages may manifest only transaminasemia or Kayser-Fleischer rings (golden-greenish granular deposits in the limbus), hepatomegaly or splenomegaly may already be present. In most symptomatic patients (96%), the serum ceruloplasmin level is <20 mg/d. Patients >55 years of age who present with persistently elevated AST and ALT levels should probably be screened for Wilson disease with ceruloplasmin levels. In patients with more advanced disease, symptoms of acute hepatitis or cirrhosis may be present. Neurologic signs include dysarthria, tremors, abnormal movements, and psychological disturbances. HCC may occur in patients with advanced disease. Treatment includes penicillamine, trientine, or zinc salts.

Hemochromatosis

An inborn error of iron metabolism leading to increased iron absorption from the diet, hemochromatosis is associated with diabetes, bronze skin pigmentation, hepatomegaly, loss of libido, and arthropathy. Patients may also show signs of cardiac or endocrine disorders. Symptoms usually first manifest between 40 and 60 years of age, and men are 10 times more likely than women to be affected. Hemochromatosis is the most common inherited liver disease in people of European descent. Physical signs include hepatomegaly (95% of symptomatic patients), which precedes abnormal liver function tests. Cardiac involvement includes congestive heart failure and arrhythmias. Many patients have cirrhosis by the time they are symptomatic (50–70%), 20% have fibrosis, and 10–20% have neither. HCC is common in patients with cirrhosis (30%) and is now the most common cause of death. Laboratory findings include elevated serum iron concentration, serum ferritin, and transferrin saturation. Therapy involves treatment of the complications of hemochromatosis, removal of excess iron by phlebotomy, and, in patients with cirrhosis, surveillance for HCC and treatment of hepatic and cardiac failure.

Autoimmune Hepatitis

Autoimmune hepatitis is a hepatocellular inflammatory disease of unknown etiology. Diagnosis is based on histologic examination, hypergammaglobulinemia, and presence of serum autoantibodies. The condition may be difficult to discern from other causes of chronic liver disease, which need to be excluded before diagnosis. This condition may also occur with other autoimmune conditions such as Sjogren syndrome, psoriasis, ulcerative colitis, or hypothyroidism. Immunoserologic tests that are essential for diagnosis are assays for antinuclear antibodies (ANAs), smooth muscle antibodies (SMAs), antibodies to liver and kidney microsome type 1 (anti-LKM1), and anti-liver cytosol type 1 (anti-LC1), as well as perinuclear antineutrophil cytoplasmic antibodies (pANCAs). Treatment, when indicated, is usually immunosuppressive with either prednisone, azathioprine, or both.

Drug-Induced Liver Disease

More than 600 drugs or other medicinals have been implicated in liver disease. Worldwide, drug-induced liver disease represents approximately 3% of all adverse drug reactions; in the United States, >20% of cases of jaundice in the elderly are caused by drugs. Acetaminophen and other drugs account for 25–40% of fulminant hepatic failure. Diagnosis is based on the discovery of abnormalities in hepatic enzymes or the development of a hepatitis-like syndrome or jaundice. Most cases occur within 1 week to 3 months of exposure, and symptoms rapidly subside after cessation of the drug, returning to normal within 4 weeks of acute hepatocellular injury. Hepatic damage may manifest as acute hepatocellular injury (isoniazid, acetaminophen), cholestatic injury (contraceptive steroids, chlorpromazine), granulomatous hepatitis (allopurinol, phenylbutazone), chronic hepatitis (methotrexate), vascular injury (herbal tea preparations with toxic plant alkaloids), or neoplastic lesions (oral contraceptive steroids).

Statins, on the other hand, are widely used and can commonly cause mild liver enzyme elevations, but mild elevations of ALT or AST (<3 times the upper limit of normal) do not appear to contribute to liver toxicity.

A resource of use to determine the potential for hepatotoxicity of a supplement or drug is the following website: livertox.nih.gov.

Primary Biliary Cholangitis (Formerly Termed Primary Biliary Cirrhosis)

This autoimmune disease of uncertain etiology is manifested by inflammation and destruction of interlobular and septal bile ducts, which can cause chronic cholestasis and biliary cirrhosis. It is predominantly a disease of middle-aged women (female-to-male ratio of 9:1) and is particularly prevalent in northern Europe. The condition may be diagnosed on routine testing or be suspected in women with symptoms of fatigue or pruritus, or in susceptible individuals with elevated serum alkaline phosphatase, cholesterol, and IgM levels. Antimitochondrial antibodies are frequently found. Ursodeoxycholic acid is the only therapy currently available, although some patients may benefit from liver transplantation.

Hepatic Tumors & Cysts

HCC is the most common malignant tumor of the liver; it is the fifth most common cancer in men and the eighth most common in women. Incidence increases with age, but the mean age in ethnic Chinese and African populations is lower. Signs of worsening cirrhosis may alert the clinician to consider HCC, but in many cases, the onset is subtle. There are no specific hepatic function tests to detect HCC, but elevated serum tumor markers, most notably α-fetoprotein, are useful. Ultrasonography can detect the majority of HCC but may not distinguish it from other solid lesions. CT and magnetic resonance imaging (MRI) are also helpful in making the diagnosis. Risk factors for HCC include HBV, HCV, all etiologic forms of cirrhosis, ingestion of foods with aflatoxin B_1, and smoking. In suspected HCC, diagnosis with CT scans or MRI is recommended. In moderate-risk patients, ultrasound studies every 6 months and possibly biopsies may be recommended if a definitive diagnosis cannot be made (see previous discussion in the sections on hepatitis).

Benign Tumors

Benign tumors include hepatocellular adenomas, which have become more common with the use of oral contraceptive steroids, and hepatic hemangiomas, which may occur with pregnancy or oral contraceptive steroid use and are the most common benign tumors of the liver.

Liver Abscesses

Liver abscesses can be the result of infections of the biliary tract or can have an extrahepatic source such as diverticulitis or inflammatory bowel disease. In ~40% of cases, no source of infection is found. The most common organisms are *Escherichia coli*, *Klebsiella*, *Proteus*, *Pseudomonas*, and *Streptococcus* species. Amebic liver abscesses are the most common extraintestinal manifestation of amebiasis, which occurs in >10% of the world's population and is most prevalent in the United States in young Hispanic adults. Amebic abscesses may have an acute presentation, with symptoms present for several weeks; few patients report typical intestinal symptoms such as diarrhea. Ultrasonography or CT scans with serologic tests such as enzyme-linked immunosorbent assay (ELISA) or indirect fluorescent antibody tests help confirm the diagnosis.

Bacon B, Adams P, Kowdley K, et al. Diagnosis and management of hemochromatosis: 2011 practice guidelines by the American Association for the Study of Liver Disease. *Hepatology*. 2011;54(1):328-343. [PMID: 21452290]

Manns MP, Czaja AJ, Gorham JD, et al. Diagnosis and management of autoimmune hepatitis. *Hepatology*. 2010;51(6): 2103–2213. [PMID: 20513004]

Onusko E. Statins and elevated liver tests: what's the fuss? *J Fam Pract*. 2009;67(7):449–452. [PMID: 18625167]

▼ PANCREATIC DISEASE

Samuel C. Matheny, MD, MPH

ACUTE PANCREATITIS

 ESSENTIALS OF DIAGNOSIS

► Sudden, severe, abdominal pain in epigastric area, with frequent radiation to the back.

► Elevated serum amylase and lipase.

► Elevated ALT (biliary pancreatitis).

► Evidence of etiology on ultrasound (biliary causes) or CT and MRI (other causes).

▶ General Considerations

Hospital admissions for acute pancreatitis are fairly frequent, and the most common causes vary with the age and sex of the patient. In the United States, gallstones and alcohol abuse are the most frequent etiologies (20–30%), but infectious causes such as mumps virus or parasitic disease should be considered, as well as medications, tumors, trauma, and metabolic conditions. Approximately 20% of cases are idiopathic. It is important to determine the etiology of pancreatitis because early recognition of acute biliary pancreatitis in particular may be important in selecting the appropriate therapeutic approach.

A more detailed discussion of gallstone pancreatitis appears earlier in this chapter.

▶ Clinical Findings

A. Symptoms and Signs

Abdominal pain—usually epigastric, which may radiate to the back—is an common presenting sign. However, the pain may not be significant, and some cases of acute pancreatitis are missed or diagnosed after more significant complications have occurred. Abdominal tenderness ranging from rigidity to mild tenderness may be present. Lack of a specific diagnostic test may affect the accuracy of an early diagnosis.

B. Laboratory Findings

Useful laboratory tests include serum amylase (elevated 3–5 times above normal), serum lipase (more than twice normal), and, for determining the etiology, liver function tests, especially ALT. Serum amylases that are significantly elevated in the presence of epigastric pain are strong indicators of pancreatitis. However, amylase clears rapidly from the blood, and levels may be normal even in patients with severe pancreatitis. A urine dipstick test for trypsinogen-2 may also be useful. The triglyceride levels should be checked, as well as calcium, in an attempt to identify pancreatitis associated with hyperlipemia and hyperparathyroidism.

C. Prognostic Tests and Patient Assessment

Over 20% of patients have a severe case of pancreatitis, and of these, a significant number die. It is therefore important to accurately assess and monitor the severity of the illness and treat accordingly. Attempts to quantify severity of disease have led to certain scoring criteria, but no specific scoring mechanism is reliable enough by itself to predict severity. A careful physician and laboratory assessment to ascertain fluid loss, hypovolemic shock, and organ dysfunction is crucial, and the American College of Gastroenterology states that the following patient-related risk factors for the development of severe disease need to be considered: patient age, comorbid health problems, body mass index, presence of systemic inflammatory response syndrome (SIRS), signs of hypovolemia such as elevated blood urea nitrogen and hematocrit, presence of pleural effusions and/or infiltrates, and altered mental status. Elevated pulse, respiratory rate, temperature, and white blood cell count are concerning for persistent SIRS.

D. Imaging Studies

Ultrasonography of the RUQ is helpful in identifying the etiology of pancreatitis and is usually the initial imaging study of choice. However, it has limited value in staging the severity of disease. (See the discussion earlier in the chapter on gallstone pancreatitis). Contrast-enhanced CT is the most common currently available imaging technique for staging the severity of pancreatitis and can determine the presence of glandular enlargement, intra- and extrapancreatic fluid collections, inflammation, necrosis, and abscesses. This study may not be necessary for patients with mild disease. MRCP may be just as accurate and has some advantages over contrast-enhanced CT in certain patients. MRI is an alternative when CT is not helpful or feasible.

▶ Complications

Complications include organ failure, cardiovascular collapse, and fluid collections around the pancreas. The latter may be asymptomatic or they may enlarge, causing pain, fever, and infection. Extrapancreatic infections, either bacteremia or pneumonia, have recently been shown to complicate the management of acute pancreatitis in a significant number of patients, usually within the first 2 weeks. Pancreatic pseudocysts may occur in patients with very high amylase levels and obstruction of the pancreatic duct. Pancreatic necrosis may also occur and can be fatal. Infection of necrotic tissue should be suspected in patients with unexpected deterioration, fever, and leukocytosis, and confirmed by CT scan and fine-needle aspiration. Sterile necrosis should probably be managed nonoperatively unless progressive deterioration occurs. Septic necrosis usually requires surgical débridement.

▶ Treatment

Patients who have the potential to develop severe pancreatitis, or who already have severe pain, dehydration, or vomiting, should be hospitalized and their hydration needs monitored closely. These patients should receive nothing by mouth and should be given intravenous pain medication. Patients should be monitored carefully to assess adequate renal function, because renal failure is a major cause of morbidity and mortality. Signs of worsening condition include rising hematocrit, tachycardia, and lack of symptom improvement in 48 hours.

Nutritional treatment has evolved in recent years, but areas of controversy remain. Increasing evidence indicates that in cases of mild pancreatitis, there is no benefit to nasogastric suction, and patients who are not vomiting may continue on oral fluids or resume oral fluids after the first week. There is also growing evidence that in severe pancreatitis, early enteral feeding within the first week may lower endotoxin absorption and reduce other complications. If patients cannot absorb adequate quantities via the enteric route, then parenteral feeding may be necessary. Total parenteral nutrition should otherwise be avoided in patients with mild and even severe pancreatitis.

The use of antibiotics is also controversial. Prophylactic antibiotics have been used in severe pancreatitis, but there is some concern that they may predispose patients to fungal infections. The general consensus is to use antibiotics, preferably broad-spectrum agents, for extrapancreatic infection or infected pancreatic necrosis, but not routinely.

Chronic Pancreatitis

Progression of inflammation and fibrotic changes can lead to a condition of chronic pancreatitis, impairing both exocrine and endocrine function. There is some debate regarding whether acute pancreatitis can eventually lead to chronic pancreatitis or whether chronic pancreatitis and recurrent acute pancreatitis are separate entities. Clinical conditions can vary, including abdominal pain, with occasional fat malabsorption and steatorrhea. Glucose intolerance and diabetes mellitus can also result. Alcohol, smoking, anatomic and obstructive abnormalities, and genetic factors may be implicated as risk factors. Diagnosis is based on the clinical history, laboratory tests, and imaging, but sometimes the diagnosis is difficult, since there is an inconsistent picture regarding reliable clinical markers and sensitivity of imaging. However, CT imaging is the best initial imaging test. Treatment consists of pain management, lifestyle changes, enzymatic therapy if necessary, and invasive management if there are anatomic complications or obstructive stones.

Banks PA, Bollen TL, Dervenis C, et al. Classification of acute pancreatitis—2012: revision of Atlanta classification and definitions by international consensus. *Gut.* 2013;62:102–111. [PMID: 23100216]

Forsmark, C, Vege SS, Wilcox CM. Acute pancreatitis. *N Engl J Med.* 2016;375:1972–1981. [PMID: 27959604]

Lew D, Afghani E, Pandol S. Chronic pancreatitis: current status and challenges for prevention and treatment. *Dig Dis Sci.* 2017: 62(7):1702–1712. [PMID: 28501969]

PANCREATIC CANCER

 ESSENTIALS OF DIAGNOSIS

▶ Anorexia, jaundice, weight loss, epigastric pain radiating to back, dark urine, and light stools.

▶ Spiral CT of the abdomen or EUS showing evidence of tumor.

▶ CA 19-9 serum tumor marker.

▶ General Considerations

Although pancreatic cancer is diagnosed in only 30,000 patients each year in the United States, it is the fourth most common cause of death from cancer and the second most common gastrointestinal malignancy. Pancreatic cancer has a very poor prognosis: >80% of patients die within the first year, and the 5-year survival rate is <4%. In the vast majority of patients, the cancer is discovered at too late a stage to benefit from resection, and the response to chemotherapy is very poor. Over 90% of pancreatic cancers are ductal adenocarcinoma.

Cigarette smoking is the major risk factor established to date. Diet may also be a factor, with high intake of fat or meat and obesity associated with an increased risk; fruits, vegetables, and exercise help protect against pancreatic cancer. Likewise, a history of chronic pancreatitis is considered a risk factor, along with surgery for peptic ulcer disease, hereditary pancreatitis, and some genetic mutations (eg, *BRCA2*, associated with hereditary breast cancer). No guidelines currently exist regarding screening of the general population for pancreatic cancer, although some experts feel that patients with a family history of hereditary pancreatitis should be screened.

▶ Clinical Findings

A. Symptoms and Signs

The clinical presentation of pancreatic cancer can vary widely; tumors that occur in the head of the pancreas (two-thirds of all pancreatic cancer) may produce early signs of obstructive jaundice. Tumors in the body and tail of the pancreas may grow quite large and cause fewer signs of obstruction. Symptoms more likely to be associated with pancreatic cancer include abdominal pain, jaundice, dark urine, light-colored stools, and weight loss. Pain may be worse when the patient is lying flat or eating. Other physical signs associated with pancreatic cancer include Courvoisier sign (palpable, nontender gallbladder in a patient with jaundice).

B. Laboratory Findings

Laboratory evaluation should include liver function tests. The serum tumor antigen CA 19-9 may be useful in confirming a diagnosis but is not an appropriate screening tool. Other markers are under consideration.

C. Imaging Studies

There is some debate as to the best imaging study. RUQ transabdominal ultrasound is useful if patients present with abdominal pain and jaundice. If pancreatitis is included in the differential diagnosis, then contrast-enhanced CT scan may be more useful.

▶ Treatment

Because the only hope for a cure is surgical resection, staging of pancreatic tumors is important for management. The difficulty lies in identifying the small fraction of patients (<20%) who will benefit from surgery from those who will not—patients with metastatic disease who would otherwise be subjected to unnecessary invasive procedures and the resultant increased morbidity and mortality.

For patients with metastatic disease, chemotherapy and palliative care should be offered; surgery is avoided. Patients with advanced local disease but no metastases may benefit from radiotherapy and chemotherapy, and those without invasion or metastases may be candidates for resection. Even with resection, the outlook is poor (5-year survival rates of <25%). Radiation therapy may be useful in some patients with localized but nonresectable tumors, and chemotherapy (5-fluorouracil and gemcitabine) has some limited success.

Pain management can be a significant problem, and various modalities may need to be used. Biliary decompression may be required for jaundice.

Cohen S, Kagen AC. Pre-operative evaluation of a pancreatic mass: diagnostic options. *Surg Clin North Am.* 2018;98(1):13–23. [PMID: 29191270]

Kamisawa T, Wood LD, Itoi T, Takaori K. Pancreatic cancer. *Lancet.* 2016;388(10039):73–85. [PMID: 26830752]

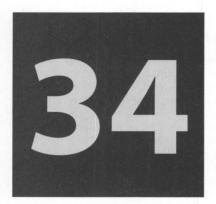

Abnormal Uterine Bleeding

Shannon Voogt, MD

Patricia Evans, MD, MA

ESSENTIALS OF DIAGNOSIS

▶ A clinical history of a menstrual cycle pattern outside the normal parameters.

▶ The normal menstrual cycle is generally 24–38 days in length, with a menstrual flow lasting 4–8 days and a total menstrual blood loss of 5–80 mL.

▶ General Considerations

Abnormal uterine bleeding (AUB), defined as premenopausal menstrual bleeding outside of the normal parameters of volume, duration, regularity, or frequency, affects 10–30% of women at some time during their lives. In 2011, the American College of Obstetricians and Gynecologists (ACOG) adopted a classification system known by the acronym PALM–COEIN, which classifies AUB by its causes: structural (**p**olyp, **a**denomyosis, **l**eiomyoma, **m**alignancy, and hyperplasia) and nonstructural (**c**oagulopathy, **o**vulatory dysfunction, **e**ndometrial, **i**atrogenic, and **n**ot yet classified). The recommendation of ACOG is to pair the term *abnormal uterine bleeding* with the letter denoting the cause in order to achieve uniformity in nomenclature and to eliminate the terminology of dysfunctional uterine bleeding. In addition, descriptive terms should be used instead of traditional Latin terms, such as *heavy menstrual bleeding* instead of *menorrhagia, intermenstrual bleeding* instead of *metrorrhagia,* and *infrequent* or *anovulatory bleeding* instead of *oligomenorrhea.*

American College of Obstetricians and Gynecologists. Diagnosis of abnormal uterine bleeding in reproductive-aged women. ACOG Practice Bulletin No. 128. *Obstet Gynecol.* 2012;120(1):197–206. (Reaffirmed 2016). [PMID: 22914421]

Munro MG, Critchley HO, Border MS, Fraser IS. FIGO classification system (PALM-COEIN) for causes of abnormal uterine bleeding in nongravid women of reproductive age. FIGO Working Group on Menstrual Disorders. *Int J Gynaecol Obstet.* 2011;113:3–13. [PMID: 21345435]
Wouk N, Helton M. Abnormal uterine bleeding in premenopausal women. *Am Fam Physician.* 2019;99(7):435–443. [PMID: 30932448]

▶ Clinical Findings

A. Symptoms and Signs

1. History—The physician should try to establish whether the patient's pattern is cyclic or anovulatory. If the patient menstruates every 24–38 days, the cycle is consistent with an ovulatory pattern of bleeding. Patients often report breast discomfort or premenstrual symptoms with ovulatory bleeding. Although cycles may vary in length by several days, >10 days of variance raises the suspicion of anovulatory cycles. The patient should be asked to describe the current vaginal bleeding in terms of onset, frequency, duration, and severity. Although heavy menstrual bleeding is defined by >80 mL of blood loss, in practice, it is determined by patient report of excessive bleeding. Age, parity, sexual history, previous gynecologic disease, and obstetrical history will further assist the physician in focusing the evaluation of the woman with vaginal bleeding. The physician should ask about medications, including contraceptives, prescription medications, and over-the-counter (OTC) medications and supplements. The patient should be asked about any OTC preparations she might be taking. Patients may not be aware that herbal preparations may contribute to vaginal bleeding. Ginseng, which has estrogenic properties, can cause vaginal bleeding, and St. John's wort can interact with oral contraceptives to cause breakthrough bleeding. A review of symptoms should include questions regarding fever, fatigue, abdominal pain, hirsutism, galactorrhea, changes in bowel movements, and heat/cold intolerance. A careful family history will aid in identifying patients with a predisposition to bleeding disorders, polycystic ovarian syndrome (PCOS), congenital adrenal hyperplasia, thyroid disease, fibroids, and cancer.

2. Physical examination—The physical examination for women complaining of AUB should begin with an evaluation of the patient's vital signs, body mass index, thyroid gland, and features of excess androgen (eg, hirsutism or acne). The pelvic examination will aid in identifying many causes of bleeding, including other sources of bleeding, anatomic abnormalities, infections, pregnancy, and signs of fibroids.

B. Evaluation

The evaluation of patients presenting with AUB includes a combination of laboratory testing, imaging studies, and sampling techniques. The evaluation is directed by both patient presentation and a risk evaluation for endometrial cancer.

C. Laboratory Findings

All patients presenting with AUB should be evaluated with a complete blood count, thyroid-stimulating hormone, urine or serum pregnancy test, and cervical cancer screening if due. If suggested by history or exam, testing for the sexually transmitted diseases gonorrhea, *Chlamydia,* and *Trichomonas* should be performed. Adolescents presenting with menorrhagia at menarche and patients with significant heavy bleeding or anemia should have an evaluation for coagulopathies, including platelet count, prothrombin time, and partial thromboplastin time. If no coagulation abnormality is found, then a test for von Willebrand disease (eg, von Willebrand factor antigen, ristocetin cofactor activity, or factor VIII) should be obtained. In patients with anovulatory bleeding and symptoms suggestive of PCOS or obesity, it is reasonable to check for testosterone and dehydroepiandrosterone sulfate. However, the diagnosis of PCOS may be made without laboratory testing if clinical hyperandrogenism is present with anovulatory cycles. In patients with significant hirsutism, a basal 17-hydroxyprogesterone (17-HP) should also be tested to screen for congenital adrenal hyperplasia.

D. Imaging Studies

1. Transvaginal ultrasound—Transvaginal ultrasonography can be used to evaluate the ovaries, uterus, and endometrial lining for abnormalities. An evaluation of the ovaries can assist in the diagnosis of PCOS because many patients with PCOS will have enlarged ovaries with multiple, small follicles. Transvaginal ultrasound is also useful for evaluating an enlarged uterus for the presence of fibroids. Fibroids will appear as hypoechoic, solid masses seen within the borders of the uterus. Serosal fibroids can be pedunculated and therefore can be seen outside the borders of the uterus.

In postmenopausal patients, an endovaginal ultrasound can be used to evaluate the thickness of the endometrial stripe. Postmenopausal patients with an endometrial stripe thicker than 4–5 mm should have a histologic biopsy. Evaluation of endometrial thickness in premenopausal patients has limited value due to the variations of endometrial thickness during the menstrual cycle. Premenopausal and perimenopausal patients with AUB at risk for endometrial cancer (eg, prolonged anovulation, over age 45) should have histologic sampling performed regardless of endometrial thickness. Hormone replacement therapy can also cause proliferation of a patient's endometrium, rendering an endovaginal evaluation less specific. The endovaginal ultrasound examination is less likely to detect intracavitary lesions, such as submucosal fibroids and polyps.

2. Sonohysterography—Saline infusion sonohysterography involves performing a transvaginal ultrasound following installation of saline into the uterus. This study is most useful in differentiating focal from diffuse endometrial abnormalities and for diagnosing intracavitary lesions. Detection of a focal abnormality indicates need for evaluation by hysteroscopy, and detection of an endometrial abnormality indicates the need to perform an endometrial biopsy or dilation and curettage (D&C). This can be considered as a study of first choice in premenopausal women with AUB given its higher sensitivity and specificity for uterine structural abnormalities than transvaginal ultrasound alone.

3. Magnetic resonance imaging—Magnetic resonance imaging (MRI) can be used to evaluate the uterine structure. The endometrium can be evaluated with an MRI, but the endometrial area seen on MRI does not correspond exactly to the endometrial stripe measured with ultrasound. In most situations, a transvaginal ultrasound is the preferred imaging modality, but if the patient cannot tolerate the procedure, MRI does provide an option for evaluation. MRI is better than ultrasound in distinguishing adenomyosis from fibroids, so if the history and examination suggest adenomyosis, an MRI may be the best first choice. MRI is also sometimes used to evaluate fibroids prior to uterine artery embolization or to map multiple myomas.

E. Special Examinations: Endometrial Sampling

The workup for endometrial cancer should be pursued most aggressively with patients at greatest risk for the disease, such as postmenopausal patients who present with vaginal bleeding and patients over 45 with any AUB. In these patients, the endometrium should be sampled using office-based endometrial biopsy or hysteroscopic dilatation and curettage if office sampling is inadequate or cannot be done. Alternatively, patients with postmenopausal bleeding can be evaluated with vaginal ultrasound initially, with endometrial biopsy if the endometrial stripe is >4 mm. In patients age <45 years, endometrial cancer is usually seen in obese patients and/or patients who are chronically anovulatory. Therefore, patients under age 45 (particularly patients age 35–45) with risk factors for endometrial carcinoma (eg, obesity, PCOS, prolonged anovulatory cycles, or prolonged unopposed estrogen stimulation) or bleeding that does not respond to therapy should be evaluated for hyperplasia and neoplasm with an endometrial sample.

1. Endometrial biopsy—An endometrial biopsy is an adequate method of sampling the endometrial lining to identify histologic abnormalities. The rates of obtaining an adequate endometrial sample depend on the age of the patient. Many postmenopausal women will have an atrophic endometrium, so sampling in this group will more often result in an inadequate endometrial specimen for examination. In this situation, the clinician must use additional diagnostic studies to fully evaluate the cause of the vaginal bleeding.

2. Dilation and curettage—D&C provides a blind sampling of the endometrium. The D&C generally will provide sampling of less than half of the uterine cavity. The D&C is useful in patients with cervical stenosis or other anatomic factors that prevent an adequate endometrial biopsy.

3. Diagnostic hysteroscopy—Direct exploration of the uterus is useful in identifying structural abnormalities such as fibroids and endometrial polyps. In general, diagnostic hysteroscopy is combined with a D&C or endometrial biopsy to maximize identification of abnormalities.

American College of Obstetricians and Gynecologists. Diagnosis of abnormal uterine bleeding in reproductive-aged women. ACOG Practice Bulletin No. 128. *Obstet Gynecol.* 2012;120(1): 197–206. (Reaffirmed 2016). [PMID: 22914421]

American College of Obstetricians and Gynecologists. Management of abnormal uterine bleeding associated with ovulatory dysfunction. ACOG Practice Bulletin No. 136. *Obstet Gynecol.* 2013;122(1):176–185. [PMID: 23787936]

Goldstein S. Sonography in postmenopausal bleeding. *J Ultrasound Med.* 2012;31:333–336. [PMID: 22298878]

McLucas B. Diagnosis, imaging and anatomical classification of uterine fibroids. *Best Practice Res Clin Obstet Gynaecol.* 2008;22:627–642. [PMID: 18328787]

Svirsky R, Smorgick N, Rozowski U, et al. Can we rely on endometrial biopsy for detection of focal intrauterine pathology? *Am J Obstet Gynecol.* 2008;199:115. [PMID 18456238]

Williams T, Mortada R, Portado S. Diagnosis and treatment of polycystic ovary syndrome. *Am Fam Physician.* 2016;94(2): 106–113. [PMID: 27419327]

Wouk N, Helton M. Abnormal uterine bleeding in premenopausal women. *Am Fam Physician.* 2019;99(7):435–443. [PMID: 30932448]

▶ Differential Diagnosis

The differential diagnosis of AUB, excluding pregnancy-related bleeding, encompasses a wide range of possible etiologies (Table 34–1).

Table 34–1. Differential diagnosis of abnormal uterine bleeding in the nonpregnant patient.

Diagnosis	Clinical Presentation
Structural Fibroids Adenomyosis Endometrial polyp Cervical polyp Endometriosis	Heavy, painful menstrual bleeding Intermenstrual spotting (polyps) Abnormal transvaginal ultrasound or sonohysterogram
Endometrial malignancy or hyperplasia	Anovulatory cycles Risk factors for endometrial cancer (age >35, obesity, PCOS, unopposed estrogen) Postmenopausal bleeding
Cervical cancer	Abnormal cervical pap smear Postcoital bleeding, irregular spotting
Bleeding disorder	Asymptomatic mucocutaneous bleeding, easy bruising Heavy menstrual bleeding since menarche
Physiologic anovulation	Adolescence Lactation Perimenopause
PCOS, adult-onset CAH	Hirsutism, acne, central obesity, and anovulatory cycles
Hyperthyroidism	Nervousness, heat intolerance, diarrhea, palpitations, weight loss
Hypothyroidism	Fatigue, cold intolerance, dry skin, hair loss, constipation, weight gain
Iatrogenic Hormonal contraceptives Hormone replacement Copper IUD Antipsychotics Anticoagulants	Bleeding correlating with medication use
Pelvic inflammatory disease Atypical presentation of *Chlamydia* cervicitis	High-risk sexual behavior, fever, pelvic pain, tenderness
Endometrial cause	Regular, heavy menses No structural cause found; may occur with menarche

CAH, congenital adrenal hyperplasia; IUD, intrauterine device; PCOS, polycystic ovarian syndrome.

A. Bleeding Secondary to Medications (Iatrogenic)

1. Hormonal contraception—Vaginal bleeding is a common side effect of all forms of contraception. Many patients starting oral contraceptive pills (OCPs) experience breakthrough bleeding in the initial months. Lower estrogen OCPs have higher rates of spotting and breakthrough bleeding. Breakthrough bleeding is common among users of extended OCP regimens, and having the patient institute a 3-day hormone-free interval at the onset of breakthrough bleeding is an effective treatment for this side effect.

Irregular bleeding is also a common side effect of progestin-only contraceptive methods, such as progestin-only pills, depot medroxyprogesterone acetate (Depo-Provera), subdermal etonogestrel implants (Nexplanon), and levonorgestrel intrauterine devices (IUDs). Although prevalence is difficult to estimate, most patients experience unscheduled bleeding with initiation, and although bleeding generally decreases with time, unscheduled bleeding is the most common reason for discontinuation of progestin-only methods.

2. Other medications—The copper IUD (Paragard) is known to cause heavier menstrual bleeding and dysmenorrhea, although this can improve with time. It does not affect menstrual cycles. Anticoagulants and dopamine antagonists can also affect bleeding.

3. Hormone replacement therapy—Bleeding is common with hormone replacement therapy and can occur with both the continuous and sequential regimens. Approximately 40% of women starting continuous regimens will experience bleeding in the first 4–6 months after starting treatment.

B. Structural Causes

1. Endometrial and cervical polyps—Endometrial polyps can cause intermenstrual spotting, irregular bleeding, and/or heavy bleeding. Cervical polyps usually cause intermenstrual spotting or postcoital bleeding.

2. Adenomyosis—Adenomyosis is defined as the presence of endometrial glands within the myometrium. This is usually asymptomatic, but patients can present with heavy or prolonged menstrual bleeding as well as dysmenorrhea. The dysmenorrhea can be severe and begin ≤1 week prior to menstruation. The appearance of symptoms usually occurs after age 40.

3. Fibroids—Fibroids, also called leiomyomas or myomas, are benign uterine tumors that are often asymptomatic. The most common symptoms associated with fibroid tumors are pelvic discomfort and AUB. Most commonly, patients with symptomatic fibroids experience either heavy or prolonged periods.

4. Malignancy and hyperplasia—Endometrial hyperplasia is an overgrowth of the glandular epithelium of the endometrial lining. This usually occurs when a patient is exposed to unopposed estrogen, either iatrogenically, from obesity, or because of anovulation. The rate of neoplasms found with simple hyperplasia is 1%, and the rate with complex hyperplasia reaches almost 30% when atypia is present. Patients having hyperplasia with atypia should have a hysterectomy because of the high incidence of subsequent endometrial cancer. Most patients without atypia will respond to progesterone treatment. Endometrial ablation may also play a role in the treatment of hyperplasia.

Uterine cancer is the fourth most common cancer in women. Risk factors for endometrial cancer include nulliparity, late menopause (after age 52), obesity, diabetes, PCOS, unopposed estrogen therapy, tamoxifen, and a history of atypical endometrial hyperplasia. Endometrial cancer most often presents as postmenopausal bleeding, although overall, only 10% of patients with postmenopausal bleeding will have endometrial cancer. In the perimenopausal period, endometrial cancer can present as irregular, typically heavy bleeding. The risk of endometrial cancer in premenopausal patients is low, but it can occur in patients who are obese with a long history of anovulatory cycles.

Vaginal bleeding is the most common symptom in patients with cervical cancer. The increased cervical friability associated with cervical cancer usually results in postcoital bleeding, but it also can appear as irregular or postmenopausal bleeding.

C. Nonstructural Causes

1. Coagulopathy—Formation of the platelet plug is the first step in hemostasis during menstruation. Patients with disorders that interfere with the formation of a normal platelet plug can experience heavy bleeding. The two most common disorders are von Willebrand disease and thrombocytopenia. It has been estimated that 13–20% of patients with heavy menstrual bleeding have a coagulopathy, and this number is higher in adolescents.

2. Ovulatory

A. ANOVULATORY BLEEDING—There are multiple causes of anovulation, including physiologic and pathologic etiologies. During the first year following menarche, anovulation is a normal result of an immature hypothalamic-pituitary-gonadal axis. Irregular ovulation is also a normal physiologic result of declining ovarian function during the perimenopausal years and the hormonal changes associated with lactation. Hyperandrogenic causes of anovulation include PCOS, adult-onset congenital adrenal hyperplasia, and androgen-producing tumors. Confirming the diagnosis of PCOS involves the evaluation of clinical features and endocrine abnormalities and the exclusion of other etiologies. Patients with PCOS present with irregular, sometimes heavy bleeding due to prolonged estrogen stimulation and anovulation. In addition, patients can have hirsutism, acne, and central obesity. Endocrinologically, they can have increased testosterone activity, elevated luteinizing hormone concentration with a normal follicle-stimulating hormone level, and hyperinsulinemia due to insulin resistance. PCOS usually begins during puberty, and so patients often report a long history of irregular periods. Elevated body mass index alone without a diagnosis of PCOS may be a contributor to anovulation, and weight loss is generally recommended to help regulate menses.

Adult-onset congenital adrenal hyperplasia results from an enzyme defect in the adrenal gland, most commonly a deficiency of 21-hydroxylase. Phenotypically, patients can present in a variety of ways: with PCOS symptoms, with hirsutism alone, or with hyperandrogenic laboratory work but no hyperandrogenic symptoms.

B. ENDOCRINE ABNORMALITIES—Both hyper- and hypothyroidism can cause changes in the menstrual cycle. A variety of changes can be seen, including irregular menses, amenorrhea, or heavy bleeding. Menstrual abnormalities occur more frequently with severe than with mild hypothyroidism.

3. Endometrial—Regular, cyclic menses with heavy bleeding with no other cause may be attributed to a primary disorder of endometrium, which has not been well described.

4. Infection—Pelvic inflammatory disease in its classic form presents with fever, pelvic discomfort, cervical motion tenderness, and adnexal tenderness. Patients can present atypically with merely a change in their bleeding pattern. Cervical inflammation from *Trichomonas* and gonorrheal and chlamydial cervicitis can cause intermenstrual spotting and postcoital bleeding.

Furness S, Roberts H, Marjoribanks J, Lethaby A. Hormone therapy in postmenopausal women and risk of endometrial hyperplasia. *Cochrane Database Syst Rev.* 2012;8:CD000402. [PMID: 22895916]

Lacey JV, Chia VM. Endometrial hyperplasia and the risk of progression to carcinoma. *Maturitas.* 2009;63:39–44. [PMID: 19285814]

Munro MG, Critchley HO, Border MS, Fraser IS. FIGO classification system (PALM-COEIN) for causes of abnormal uterine bleeding in nongravid women of reproductive age. FIGO Working Group on Menstrual Disorders. *Int J Gynaecol Obstet.* 2011;113:3–13. [PMID: 21345435]

Sasaki RSA, Approbato MS, Maia MCS, Fleury e Ferreira EAB, Zanluchi N. Ovulatory status of overweight women without polycystic ovary syndrome. *JBRA Assist Reprod.* 2019;23(1):2–6. [PMID: 30614235]

Soresky JI. Endometrial cancer. *Obstet Gynecol.* 2008;111:436–447. [PMID: 18238985]

Teede H, Deeks A, Moran L. Polycystic ovary syndrome: a complex condition with psychological, reproductive and metabolic manifestations that impacts on health across the lifespan. *BMC Med.* 2010;8:41. [PMID: 20591140]

Wouk N, Helton M. Abnormal uterine bleeding in premenopausal women. *Am Fam Physician.* 2019;99(7):435–443. [PMID: 30932448]

Zigler RE, McNicholas C. Unscheduled vaginal bleeding with progestin-only contraceptive use. *Am J Obstet Gynecol.* 2017;216(5): 443–450. [PMID: 27988268]

▶ **Treatment**

The treatment for AUB should be directed at the underlying cause once it is identified. Most types of AUB (with the exception of cancer) can be initially treated with hormonal medications, nonsteroidal anti-inflammatory drugs (NSAIDs), or tranexamic acid (Lysteda). Acute bleeding may require emergent evaluation and treatment, including vaginal packing and intravenous (IV) conjugated estrogen (Table 34–2).

A. Bleeding From Contraception

All formulations of OCPs share the characteristic of a higher incidence of intermenstrual bleeding during the first cycle of use. Therefore, one of the most important things physicians can do is to reassure the patient and encourage continued use. Physicians often change formulations of OCPs to higher estrogen versions to decrease the incidence of intermenstrual bleeding. The physician can also try adding exogenous estrogen daily for 7–10 days to control prolonged intermenstrual bleeding.

Similarly, bleeding is common with progestin-only methods, especially early during treatment. Reassurance and patience should be the initial treatment of any bleeding, as well as NSAIDs (eg, naproxen 500 mg twice daily). Levonorgestrel IUDs and depot medroxyprogesterone acetate have the highest rates of amenorrhea, especially after 6 months, and levonorgestrel 52 mg (Mirena) is a first-line treatment for AUB. Etonogestrel subdermal implants have unpredictable bleeding patterns, and if bleeding occurs, it may not improve with time, although a waiting period of 3 months would still be appropriate. With continued bleeding, physicians can consider adding low-dose estrogen for 1–2 weeks or a combined oral contraceptive for 1–3 months. Typically, however, bleeding will recur when the estrogen is stopped.

B. Nonstructural (Ovulatory) Abnormal Uterine Bleeding

Treatment goals include control of the current bleeding episode and reduction of subsequent blood loss. Choice of treatment will depend on whether cycles are ovulatory, the desire for fertility, and underlying medical problems. Treatment options include NSAIDs, estrogen (for acute bleeding episodes), contraceptive methods, cyclic progestins, and tranexamic acid. Those failing medical management have surgical options, including hysterectomy and endometrial ablation.

Blood loss can be reduced by 50% in women treated with NSAIDs, which inhibit prostaglandin synthesis, decreasing menstrual pain and bleeding. Because many of the studies evaluating the role of NSAIDs were completed in women with ovulatory cycles, the results cannot be directly applied to women with anovulatory bleeding. In addition, this treatment

Table 34–2. Nonsurgical treatments for abnormal uterine bleeding.

Treatment	Examples of Dosing	Notes
Acute bleeding		
Conjugated equine estrogen (Premarin)	25 mg IV every 4–6 hours, up to 24 hours 2.5 mg orally every 6 hours, up to 21 days	For acute bleeding only. Reserve oral dosing for hemodynamically stable patients. Follow treatment with progestin to induce withdrawal bleed. Do not use in patients with thrombosis risk.
Oral contraceptive pills	Regular dose (ethinyl estradiol 35 µg), taken 3 times daily for up to 7 days, then taper to once daily	May need to treat nausea. Shorter taper can be used if bleeding is less severe. Do not use in patients with thrombosis risk.
Progestins	Medroxyprogesterone acetate (Provera), 20 mg 3 times daily for 7 days, tapering to 10 mg once daily Norethindrone 5 mg 3 times daily for 7 days	Bleeding will occur when medication is stopped.
Tranexamic acid	10 mg per kg IV every 8 hours 1300 mg orally 3 times daily for 5 days	Avoid in patients with thrombosis risk.
Chronic bleeding		
Levonorgestrel IUD	52 µg device (Mirena)	Effective for most types of bleeding. Light bleeding or spotting may occur for up to 8 weeks after placement.
Depot medroxyprogesterone acetate (Depo-Provera)	Injection every 13 weeks	Irregular bleeding may occur initially.
Oral progestin	Medroxyprogesterone acetate (Provera), 10–20 mg daily, or days 16–26 of cycle Norethindrone 2.5–5 mg daily	Use lowest effective dose. Note that the progesterone-only contraceptive pill (Micronor) is a much lower dosage of norethindrone (0.35 mg) and will not control bleeding.
Combined estrogen-progestin oral contraception	Oral, vaginal ring, or patch Can be used as directed or extended cycle (skipping placebo weeks)	Avoid in patients with thrombosis risk, migraines with aura, or other contraindications to estrogen. Most effective treatment for PCOS.
Tranexamic acid	1300 mg 3 times daily for 5 days	Begin at the onset of menses. Likely safe if trying to become pregnant.
NSAIDs	Multiple formulations. Naproxen 500 mg every 12 hours, or ibuprofen 800 mg every 8 hours, or others	Begin the day before menses if possible, otherwise at onset. Continue for first 3–5 days of menses to reduce pain and bleeding.

IUD, intrauterine device; IV, intravenous; NSAID, nonsteroidal anti-inflammatory drug; PCOS, polycystic ovarian syndrome.

does not address the issue of irregular bleeding and decreasing future health risks due to anovulation.

Estrogen alone is generally used to treat an acute episode of heavy uterine bleeding. IV conjugated estrogen will temporarily stop most uterine bleeding, regardless of the cause. The dose commonly used is 25 mg of conjugated estrogen every 4 hours for up to 24 hours. Nausea limits using high doses of estrogen orally, but lower doses can be used in a patient with acute heavy bleeding who is hemodynamically stable. One suggested regimen is 2.5 mg of conjugated estrogen every 6 hours for 21 days. After acute bleeding is controlled, the physician should add a progestin to the treatment regimen to induce withdrawal bleeding. Alternative hormonal options include combined OCPs, with a regimen of one monophasic pill containing 35 µg of ethinyl estradiol 3 times daily for 7 days, then tapering down to once daily. Progestins, such as medroxyprogesterone acetate (Provera), can be used at 10–20 mg 3 times daily for 7 days, tapering down to once daily. The only nonhormonal option is tranexamic acid, at 1.3 g 3 times daily for 5 days (it can also be given IV).

A long-term regimen should be chosen to regulate future bleeding. The most effective medical therapy is the levonorgestrel 52-mg IUD. In a meta-analysis of 21 randomized controlled trials, the levonorgestrel IUD system was more effective at controlling heavy menstrual bleeding than any other medication. Other effective therapies include OCPs, extended-cycle OCPs (skipping placebo days), daily or cyclic oral progestin, tranexamic acid, and NSAIDs. Progestins can be dosed cyclically, given during the luteal phase only (for 10 days starting on day 16 of the menstrual cycle), or given daily if bleeding is not controlled or if this dosing is difficult for patients. Patients with a history of thromboembolism, cerebrovascular disease, coronary artery disease, breast cancer, or active liver disease should not be started on an estrogen-containing medication. Relative contraindications to estrogen include migraine headache with aura, hypertension, diabetes, age >35 years in a smoking patient, and active gallbladder disease. For those desiring pregnancy, the only options are tranexamic acid and NSAIDs. Tranexamic acid and NSAIDs should be taken during the first 5 days of menses, and both should be avoided in patients with renal disease. Tranexamic acid should also be avoided in patients with risks for thromboembolism.

Patients who fail hormonal management can consider endometrial ablation. Initially used exclusively in patients with menorrhagia, these treatments are now also used in women with anovulatory bleeding. Because endometrial glands often persist after ablative treatment, few women will experience long-term amenorrhea after treatment. The risk of endometrial cancer is not eliminated after treatment, so women at risk for endometrial cancer from long-term unopposed estrogen exposure still need preventive treatment. Because pregnancies have occurred after endometrial ablation, some form of contraception may be needed after the procedure. Hysterectomy is the most effective treatment for heavy menstrual bleeding, although it is generally reserved for patients who do not respond to more conservative therapies due to cost and risks of surgery.

C. Structural Abnormal Uterine Bleeding

Medical management options for fibroids and adenomyosis are similar to those for ovulatory dysfunction. The 52-mg levonorgestrel IUD is more effective than OCPs, but both are options because they both reduce menstrual blood loss. NSAIDs and tranexamic acid can also be used. Evidence on injectable and oral progestins for uterine fibroids is limited. Mifepristone, ulipristal, aromatase inhibitors, and estrogen receptor agonists have been studied and may be available as treatment options after further study. Administration of a gonadotropin-releasing hormone agonist can greatly reduce the volume of a patient's fibroids. Because this effect is temporary, this treatment is largely reserved for preoperative

therapy to facilitate the removal of the uterus or fibroid. Pretreatment can also improve the patient's hematologic parameters by decreasing vaginal bleeding prior to surgery.

If patients fail these medical approaches, surgical options include myomectomy, hysterectomy, or uterine artery embolization. Myomectomy is a good option for the patient who desires future childbearing. The risk exists for the growth of new fibroids and the growth of fibroids too small for removal at the time of surgery. Women undergoing hysterectomies may have the option of an abdominal or vaginal hysterectomy. Vaginal hysterectomies involve fewer complications and shorter hospital stays. The size of the uterus at the time of surgery determines the feasibility of this approach because the surgeon must be able to remove the uterus completely through a vaginal incision.

Women wanting to avoid hysterectomy have the option of uterine fibroid embolization. In this procedure, an interventional radiologist injects tiny polyvinyl alcohol particles into the uterine arteries. Because the hypervascular fibroids have no collateral vascular supply, they undergo ischemic necrosis. Women with pedunculated or subserosal fibroids are not considered ideal candidates for this procedure. In addition, because the effects of uterine artery embolization on childbearing are not well known, the procedure is generally not done on women desiring future fertility.

American College of Obstetricians and Gynecologists. Management of abnormal uterine bleeding associated with ovulatory dysfunction. ACOG Practice Bulletin No. 136. *Obstet Gynecol.* 2013;122(1):176–185. [PMID: 23787936]

American College of Obstetricians and Gynecologists. Management of acute abnormal uterine bleeding in nonpregnant reproductive-aged women. ACOG Practice Bulletin No. 557. *Obstet Gynecol.* 2013;121:891–896. (Reaffirmed 2017). [PMID: 23635706]

Damlo S. ACOG guidelines on endometrial ablation. *Am Fam Physician.* 2008;77:545–549. [No PMID]

De La Cruz MSD, Buchanan EM. Uterine fibroids: diagnosis and treatment. *Am Fam Physician.* 2017;95(2):100–107. [PMID: 28084714]

Guiahi M, McBride M, Sheeder J, Teal S. Short-term treatment of bothersome bleeding for etonogestrel implant users using a 14-day oral contraceptive pill regimen. *Obstet Gynecol.* 2015;126(3):508–513. [PMID: 26181091]

Lethaby A, Hussain M, Rishworth JR, Rees MC. Progesterone or progestogen-releasing intrauterine systems for heavy menstrual bleeding. *Cochrane Database Syst Rev.* 2015;4:CD002126. [PMID: 25924648]

Matteson KA, Rahn DD, Wheeler TL, et al. Non-surgical management of heavy menstrual bleeding: a systematic review and practice guidelines. *Obstet Gynecol.* 2013;121(3):632–643. [PMID: 23635628]

Wouk N, Helton M. Abnormal uterine bleeding in premenopausal women. *Am Fam Physician.* 2019;99(7):435–443. [PMID: 30932448]

Hypertension

Maureen O'Hara Padden, MD, MPH, FAAFP

Kevin M. Bernstein, MD, MMS, CAQSM, FAAFP

Kerry Sadler, MD

Courtney M. Saint, DO

Joseph Sapoval, DO

▶ General Considerations

The definition of "hypertension" remains controversial between multiple organizations with the publications of the 2014 Evidence-Based Guideline for the Management of High Blood Pressure in Adults by the Eighth Joint National Committee (JNC-8) followed by the 2017 American College of Cardiology (ACC)/American Heart Association (AHA) Clinical Practice Guideline for High Blood Pressure in Adults (Table 35–1). The American Academy of Family Physicians continues to support the JNC-8 recommendations after a thorough review and has chosen not to endorse the ACC/AHA guidelines. The ACC/AHA guidelines substantially increase the number of people diagnosed with hypertension, resulting in a small increase in the percentage of US adults recommended to begin antihypertensive medication as well as recommending more intensive therapy and blood pressure lowering for those already taking antihypertensive medications.

According to the National Center for Health Statistics, approximately 33% of people age ≥20 years in the United States have *hypertension*, which they define as an average systolic blood pressure of ≥140 mmHg, a diastolic blood pressure of ≥90 mmHg, or the current use of blood pressure–lowering medication(s). According to the National Health and Nutrition Examination Survey (NHANES) data from 2011 to 2014, 46% of adults age 18 years and older (103 million Americans) met the criteria for hypertension, defined as people currently using blood pressure–lowering medications, systolic blood pressure ≥130 mmHg, and/or diastolic blood pressure ≥90 mmHg. The incidence of hypertension increases with age. If an individual is normotensive at age 55, the lifetime risk for hypertension is 90%. High blood pressure resulted in the death of 61,005 Americans in 2008. From 1998 to 2008, the death rate from hypertension rose by 20.2%, and the actual number of deaths rose by 49.7%. Of persons with high blood pressure, 84.1% are aware of their diagnosis.

Within this group, 76.1% are under treatment, and only 47.2% are well controlled. A higher percentage of men than women have hypertension until the age of 45. Beyond the age of 45, a higher percentage of women than men have hypertension. About 3% of children and adolescents are diagnosed with hypertension. Prevalence is higher in children and adolescents with chronic medical conditions including obesity, sleep-disordered breathing, chronic kidney disease, and those with a history of preterm birth. As childhood obesity continues to increase in prevalence, hypertension and other obesity-related comorbidities are expected to increase in the United States. Hypertension is most prevalent among African Americans, affecting about 43% of the population. Non-Hispanic African Americans and Mexican Americans are also more likely to suffer from high blood pressure than non-Hispanic whites. From 2012 to 2013, the economic cost of hypertensive disease was estimated at $51.2 billion per year, and the total cost of cardiovascular disease was estimated at $316.1 billion per year. Statistics regarding deaths from essential hypertension and hypertensive renal disease are listed in Table 35–2.

The National High Blood Pressure Education Program (NHBPEP), which is coordinated by the National Heart, Lung, and Blood Institute (NHBLI) of the National Institutes of Health, was established in 1972. The program was designed to increase awareness, prevention, treatment, and control of hypertension. Data from NHANES, conducted between 1976 and 2008, revealed that of patients aware of their high blood pressure and under treatment, the number who had achieved control of their high blood pressure had increased. Coincident with these positive changes was a dramatic reduction in morbidity and mortality (40–60%), including stroke and myocardial infarction (MI) secondary to hypertension. However, the most recent series of NHANES surveys conducted between 2007 and 2008 continues to show a leveling off of improvement.

Table 35-1. Classification and management of blood pressure in adults.[a]

JNC-8

BP Classification	SBP[a] (mmHg)	DBP[a] (mmHg)	Lifestyle Modification	Initial Drug Therapy — Without Compelling Indication	Initial Drug Therapy — With Compelling Indication (see Table 35-6)
Normal	<120	and <80	Encourage	No antihypertensive drug indicated	Drug(s) for compelling indications[b]
Prehypertension	120–129	or <80	Yes		
Stage 1 hypertension	130–139	or 80–89	Yes	No specific medication is recommended as first line—most important is to control blood pressure; start with ACE inhibitors for most; also, thiazide-type diuretics, ARB, β-blocker, calcium channel blocker, or combination	Drug(s) for compelling indications[c,d]; other antihypertensive drugs (diuretics, ACE inhibitors, β-blockers, calcium channel blockers) as needed

ACC/AHA

BP Classification	SBP[a] (mmHg)	DBP[a] (mmHg)	Lifestyle Modification	Initial Drug Therapy — Without Compelling Indication	Initial Drug Therapy — With Compelling Indication (see Table 35-6)
Normal	<120	and <80	Encourage	No antihypertensive drug indicated; repeat BP evaluation annually	Drug(s) for compelling indications[b,c]
Elevated	120–129	and <80	Yes		
Stage 1 hypertension	130–139	or 80–89	Yes	Without clinical ASCVD or 10-year CVD risk ≤10%: No antihypertensive drug indicated; repeat BP evaluation in 3–6 months. With clinical ASCVD or 10-year CVD risk ≥10%: BP-lowering medication. Single agent recommended; first-line agents include thiazide-type diuretics, calcium channel blockers, ACE inhibitors, or ARBs; Repeat BP evaluation in 1 month	Drug(s) for compelling indications[c,d]; other antihypertensive drugs (diuretics, ACE inhibitors, β-blockers, calcium channel blockers) as needed

	SBP	DBP	Initiate therapy	Management
Stage 2 hypertension	≥140	or ≥90	Yes	Two-drug combination for most[d] (usually ACE inhibitor and calcium channel blocker; or thiazide-type diuretic or ARB or β-blocker)
Stage 2 hypertension	≥140	or ≥90	Yes	Two first-line agents of different classes, either as separate agents or in a fixed-dose combination, are recommended; repeat BP evaluation in 1 month

[a]Treatment determined by highest BP category.

[b]Treat patients with chronic kidney disease or diabetes to BP goal of <130/80 mmHg.

[c]Treat patients with known CVD or 10-year ASCVD risk ≥10% to goal BP of ≤130/80 mmHg; consider treating patients without known CVD to goal BP ≤130/80 mmHg.

[d]Initial combined therapy should be used cautiously in those at risk for orthostatic hypotension.

ACC, American College of Cardiology; ACE, angiotensin-converting enzyme; AHA, American Heart Association; ARB, angiotensin II receptor blocker; ASCVD, atherosclerotic cardiovascular disease; BP, blood pressure; CVD, cardiovascular disease; DBP, diastolic blood pressure; JNC-8, Eighth Joint National Committee on Prevention, Detection, Evaluation, and Treatment of High Blood Pressure; SBP, systolic blood pressure.

Data from The Seventh Report of the Joint National Committee on Prevention, Detection, Evaluation, and Treatment of High Blood Pressure. National High Blood Pressure Education Program. Bethesda (MD): National Heart, Lung, and Blood Institute (US); 2004 Aug. Report No.: 04-5230; Jamerson K, Weber MA, Bakris GL, et al: Benazepril plus amlodipine or hydrochlorothiazide for hypertension in high-risk patients. N Engl J Med. 2008 Dec 4;359(23):2417–2428; Whelton PK, Carey RM, Aronow WS, et al: ACC/AHA/AAPA/ABC/ACPM/AGS/APhA/ASH/ASPC/NMA/PCNA Guideline for the Prevention, Detection, Evaluation, and Management of High Blood Pressure in Adults: A Report of the American College of Cardiology/American Heart Association Task Force on Clinical Practice Guidelines. J Am Coll Cardiol. 2018 May 15;71(19):e127–e248.

Table 35–2. Essential hypertension and hypertensive renal disease deaths: final data for 2015.

Deaths/100,000 Individuals	Race/Gender
13	African American/male
9.6	White/male
14.4	African American/female
12.8	White/female

Data from Murphy SL, Xu J, Kochanek KD, et al: Deaths: Final Data for 2015, *Natl Vital Stat Rep.* 2017 Nov;66(6):1–75.

High blood pressure is easily detected and usually well controlled with appropriate intervention. Of patients with high blood pressure, 81% are aware of their diagnosis. Among this group, only 72% are under treatment. Approximately 70% of patients being treated were controlled to <140/90 mmHg, and roughly 47% of patients were controlled to <130/80 mmHg. Coincident to these finding, the incidence of end-stage renal disease and the prevalence of heart failure continues to increase. Both conditions have been linked to uncontrolled hypertension. Absolute risk for coronary heart disease and stroke increases in patients with hypertension who have multiple cardiovascular risk factors.

Charles L, Triscott J, Dobbs B. Secondary hypertension: discovering the underlying cause. *Am Fam Physician.* 2017;96(7):453–461. [PMID: 29094913]

Flynn JT, Kaelber DC, Baker-Smith CM, et al. Clinical practice guideline for screening and management of high blood pressure in children and adolescents. *Pediatrics.* 2017;140(3):e20181904. [PMID: 28827377]

James PA, Oparil S, Carter BL, et al. 2014 evidence-based guideline for the management of high blood pressure in adults: report from panel members appointed to the Eighth Joint National Committee (JNC 8). *JAMA.* 2014;311(5):507–520. [PMID: 24352797]

National Center for Health Statistics. *Health, United States, 2016: With Chartbook on Long-term Trends in Health.* Hyattsville, MD: National Center for Health Statistics; 2017. [PMID: 28910066]

Viera AJ, Hinderliter, AL. Evaluation and management of the patient with difficult-to-control or resistant hypertension. *Am Fam Physician.* 2009;79(10):863–869. [PMID: 19496385]

Wang G, Grosse SD, Schooley MW. Conducting research on the economics of hypertension to improve cardiovascular health. *Am J Prev Med.* 2017;53(6 Suppl 2):S115–S117. [PMID: 29153111]

Whelton PK, Carey RM, Aronow WS, et al. 2017 ACC/AHA/AAPA/ABC/ACPM/AGS/APhA/ASH/ASPC/NMA/PCNA Guideline for the Prevention, Detection, Evaluation, and Management of High Blood Pressure in Adults: executive summary: a report of the American College of Cardiology/American Heart Association Task Force on Clinical Practice Guidelines. *Hypertension.* 2018;71(6):1269–1324. [PMID: 29133354]

Pathogenesis

A. Primary or Essential Hypertension

In 90–95% of cases of hypertension, no cause is identified. The pathogenesis of essential hypertension is poorly understood but likely multifactorial, resulting from environmental and genetic influences. A role for genetics has been implicated in the development of high blood pressure (eg, hypertension is more prevalent in some families and in African Americans). Additional risk factors include increased salt intake, excess alcohol intake, obesity, sedentary lifestyle, dyslipidemia, depression, vitamin D deficiency, and certain personality traits, including aggressiveness and poor stress coping skills.

B. Secondary Hypertension

It is reasonable to look for an underlying cause in patients diagnosed with hypertension even though a specific condition can be found in only 2–10% of cases. History or physical examination may suggest an underlying etiology, or the first clue may come later when patients fail to respond appropriately to standard drug therapy. In addition, secondary hypertension should be considered in those with sudden-onset hypertension, severe or resistant hypertension, or suddenly uncontrolled blood pressure that had previously been well controlled, and in patients age <30 years without a family history of hypertension.

Although likely etiologies of secondary hypertension differ by age group, the most common causes across all adult ages include renovascular hypertension, renal disease, aldosteronism, and obstructive sleep apnea (OSA). Etiologies that must be considered in the appropriate patient include use of certain medications such as oral contraceptives, sympathomimetics, decongestants, nonsteroidal anti-inflammatory drugs (NSAIDs), appetite suppressants, antidepressants, atypical antipsychotics, adrenal steroids, cyclosporine, erythropoietin, and certain chemotherapeutic agents. All of these medications can contribute to an elevation in blood pressure. Drug interactions, particularly between monoamine oxidase inhibitors and tricyclic antidepressants, antihistamines, or tyramine-containing food, can also cause an elevation in blood pressure. Additionally, hypertension can be related to excessive use of caffeine, nicotine, decongestants containing ephedrine, alcohol, excessive ingestion of black licorice, or use of illicit drugs such as cocaine or amphetamines. Other over-the-counter (OTC) formulations including weight-loss products, energy drinks, and anabolic steroids and other body-building supplements should also be considered.

Hypertension can also occur secondary to acute and chronic kidney disease, which might be suggested by flank mass, elevated creatinine level, or abnormal findings such as proteinuria, hematuria, or casts on routine urinalysis. Rarely, hypertension may be related to renal artery stenosis, particularly if onset occurs at age <20 or >50 years. In young women, fibromuscular dysplasia can contribute to renovascular hypertension, and in children, renal parenchymal disease is the most common cause of hypertension in preadolescent children. Abdominal bruits with radiation to the renal area may be heard. Other causes to consider in the differential diagnosis include white coat hypertension, postoperative hypertension, hypo- or hyperthyroidism, hyperparathyroidism, primary hyperaldosteronism, Cushing syndrome, coarctation of the aorta, vasculitis, collagen vascular disease, central nervous system (CNS) trauma, spinal cord disorders, pheochromocytoma, pregnancy-induced hypertension, and sleep apnea syndrome in the appropriate clinical presentation. When such causes are entertained, appropriate evaluation should be undertaken.

▶ Prevention

A healthy lifestyle is hailed as both prevention and initial therapy for hypertension (Table 35–3). Clinical trials assessing both prevention (Trials of Hypertension Prevention–Phase II, TONE) and nonpharmacologic treatment of mild hypertension (TOMHS, DAH, Low-Sodium DASH, PREMIER) support the positive impact of maintaining optimal weight; a regular aerobic exercise program; strength training with either dynamic or isometric exercise; and a diet low in sodium, saturated fat, and total fats and rich in fruits and vegetables. Excessive alcohol intake should be reduced and smoking cessation encouraged.

▶ Clinical Findings

Before patients with hypertension can be offered adequate treatment, they must be properly diagnosed. Because patients are often asymptomatic, the risk factors for hypertension must be understood and appropriate patients screened. In addition to the modifiable risk factors noted earlier, there are nonmodifiable factors, including African American race, family history of hypertension, and increasing age.

A. Symptoms and Signs

There are usually no physical findings early in the course of hypertension. In some patients, the presence of hypertension may be signaled by early-morning headaches or, in those with severe hypertension, by signs or symptoms associated with target organ damage. Such symptoms might include nausea, vomiting, visual disturbance, chest pain, or confusion. More typically, the first indication is an elevated blood pressure measurement taken with a sphygmomanometer during a routine visit to a medical provider or after the patient has had a stroke or MI.

For proper measurement of blood pressure, the patient should be seated in a chair with the back supported and the arm bared and supported at heart level. Exercise, caffeine, tobacco, and other stimulants including supplements that are known to increase blood pressure should be avoided in the 30 minutes preceding measurement, and measurement should begin after 5 minutes of rest. The cuff size should be appropriate for the patient's arm, defined by a cuff bladder that encircles 80% of the arm. It is important that the

Table 35–3. Lifestyle modifications to manage hypertension.[a]

Modification	Recommendation[b]	Approximate SBP Reduction (Average)
Weight reduction	Maintain normal body weight (BMI 18.5–24.9 kg/m^2)	1 mmHg/1 kg weight loss
Adopt DASH eating plan	Consume a diet rich in fruits, vegetables, and low-fat dairy products with a reduced content of saturated and total fat	11 mmHg
Increase dietary potassium	4700 mg daily intake optimal in diet, which is met by DASH diet; potassium chloride supplement is what is studied and extrapolated to dietary recommendations	4–5 mmHg
Physical activity	Dynamic exercise or isometric exercise: performed most days of the week	5–8 mmHg
Moderation of alcohol consumption	Dose-dependent response. Limit consumption to ≤2 drinks (1 oz or 30 mL ethanol; eg, 24 oz beer, 10 oz wine, or 3 oz 80-proof whiskey) per day in most men and to ≤1 drink per day in women and lighter weight persons. If >3 drinks/day, cut by half	5.5 mmHg

[a]For overall cardiovascular risk reduction, stop smoking.
[b]The effects of implementing these modifications are dose and time dependent and could be greater for some individuals.
BMI, body mass index; DASH, Dietary Approaches to Stop Hypertension; SBP, systolic blood pressure.
Data from Whelton PK, Carey RM, Aronow WS, et al: 2017 ACC/AHA/AAPA/ABC/ACPM/AGS/APhA/ASH/ASPC/NMA/PCNA Guideline for the Prevention, Detection, Evaluation, and Management of High Blood Pressure in Adults: Executive Summary: A Report of the American College of Cardiology/American Heart Association Task Force on Clinical Practice Guidelines. *Hypertension*. 2018 Jun;71(6):1269–1324.

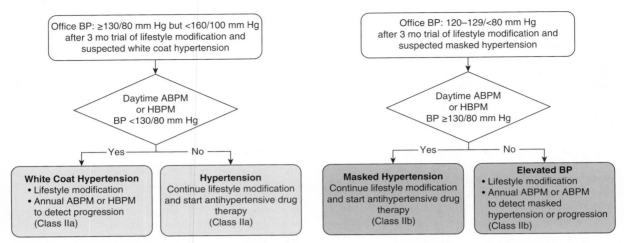

▲ Figure 35–1. White coat hypertension or masked hypertension. ABPM, ambulatory blood pressure monitoring; BP, blood pressure; HBPM, home blood pressure monitoring. (Reproduced with permission from Whelton PK, Carey RM, Aronow WS, et al: 2017 ACC/AHA/AAPA/ABC/ACPM/AGS/APhA/ASH/ASPC/NMA/PCNA Guideline for the Prevention, Detection, Evaluation, and Management of High Blood Pressure in Adults: Executive Summary: A Report of the American College of Cardiology/American Heart Association Task Force on Clinical Practice Guidelines. *Hypertension.* 2018 Jun;71(6):1269–1324.)

diagnosis be made after the elevation of blood pressure is documented with three separate readings, on three different occasions, unless the elevation is severe or is associated with symptoms requiring immediate attention (hypertensive urgency or emergency). Although transient elevation of blood pressure secondary to pain or anxiety, as experienced by some patients when they enter a physician's office ("white coat syndrome"), is a possibility, new evidence reveals that ambulatory blood pressure readings may be a stronger predictor of all-cause mortality than clinic blood pressure measurements and should be considered to further aid in diagnosis (Figure 35–1). This is especially true in patients being treated with antihypertensive medications who are normotensive in clinic to ensure they do not have elevated blood pressure outside of clinic, also known as masked hypertension, which is associated with an all-cause mortality that is twice as high as normotensive patients and similar to that of patients with sustained hypertension.

1. Classification of blood pressure—The 2014 JNC-8 guidelines made no changes to the diagnosis of hypertension. The JNC-8 and 2017 ACC/AHA guidelines each classify the diagnosis of hypertension differently (see Table 35–1). Classifications are based on the average of two or more provider-obtained blood pressure measurements from a seated patient.

2. Self-monitoring—Patients should be encouraged to self-monitor their blood pressure at home. Many easy-to-use blood pressure monitors are commercially available at reasonable cost for use at home. Validated electronic devices are

recommended, and independent reviews of available devices, such as those published by Consumer Reports, are available to assist the consumer. These devices should be periodically checked for accuracy. Self-measurement can be helpful not only in establishing the diagnosis of hypertension, but also in assessing response to medical therapy and in encouraging patient compliance with therapy by providing regular feedback on therapy response.

B. Evaluation

Patients with documented hypertension must undergo a thorough evaluation, including assessment of lifestyle and identification of cardiovascular risk factors, identification of comorbidities that would guide therapy, and surveillance for identifiable causes of high blood pressure. Patients also need to be evaluated to establish whether they already manifest evidence of target end-organ damage.

1. History—A thorough history should be obtained. Any prior history of hypertension should be elicited, as well as response and side effects to any previous hypertension therapy. It is important to inquire about any history or symptoms suggestive of coronary artery disease or other significant comorbidities, including diabetes mellitus, heart failure, dyslipidemia, renal disease, and peripheral vascular disease. The family history should also be reviewed, with special attention to the presence or absence of hypertension, premature coronary artery disease, diabetes, renal disease, dyslipidemia, or stroke. Use of tobacco, alcohol, or illicit drugs should be documented, as well as dietary intake of

Table 35–4. Physical examination: hypertension.

Component of Examination	Assessment Focus
General	Baseline height, weight, and waist circumference Upper and lower extremity blood pressure measurement to assess for coarctation of the aorta Features of Cushing syndrome
Eyes	Funduscopic examination for signs of hypertensive retinopathy (eg, arteriolar narrowing, focal arteriolar constriction, atrioventricular nicking, hemorrhages, exudates)
Neck	Carotid bruits Neck vein distention or thyroid gland enlargement
Heart	Abnormalities in rate, rhythm, murmurs, or extra heart sounds
Lungs	Rales, rhonchi, or wheezes
Abdomen	Abdominal bruits suggestive of renal artery stenosis Enlargement of kidneys (mass) or aortic pulsation suggesting aneurysm
Extremities	Diminished or absent peripheral arterial pulsations Edema Signs of vascular compromise
Neurologic	Neurologic deficits

sodium, saturated fat, and caffeine. Recent changes in weight and exercise level should be queried. Current medications used by the patient should be reviewed, including OTC medications, supplements, and herbal formulations.

2. Physical examination—The initial physical examination should be comprehensive, with careful attention to the areas outlined in Table 35–4.

C. Laboratory and Diagnostic Studies

The 2017 ACC/AHA Guidelines recommend that the following tests be performed: electrocardiogram (ECG), urinalysis, fasting blood glucose level, thyroid-stimulating hormone, potassium level, creatinine level, calcium level, and fasting lipid panel. Urinalysis should be assessed for evidence of hematuria, proteinuria, or casts suggestive of intrinsic renal disease. The complete blood count is helpful to rule out anemia or polycythemia. Potassium levels help assess for hyperaldosteronism, and creatinine levels reflect renal function. The fasting blood glucose level is used to asses for diabetes mellitus, and the lipid profile is an indicator of cardiovascular risk. Further testing is warranted if blood pressure control is not achieved. Additional tests to consider include hemoglobin A1c, urine microalbumin, creatinine

clearance, and 24-hour urine for protein. Echocardiograms and chest x-rays are not routinely recommended for evaluation of hypertensive patients. In certain cases, however, an echocardiogram may prove useful in guiding therapy when baseline abnormalities are found on the ECG (eg, left ventricular hypertrophy or signs of previous silent MI). A chest radiograph may be useful if there are abnormal findings on physical examination. Tests that evaluate for rare causes of hypertension, such as renal artery stenosis (renal ultrasound) or pheochromocytoma (24-hour urine for catecholamines), should be ordered only in patients whose history and physical examination findings raise suspicion.

▶ Treatment

A. Cardiovascular Risk Stratification

In treating hypertension, the public health goal is reduction of cardiovascular and renal morbidity and mortality. Hypertension is clearly important, but it is not the only risk factor. JNC-8 and ACC/AHA define specific components of cardiovascular risk and recommend evaluation of patients for evidence of target organ damage in performing risk stratification and in considering recommendations for therapy.

The JNC-8 guidelines include an algorithm for use when considering initial therapy for patients with hypertension (see algorithm by visiting https://jamanetwork.com/journals/jama/fullarticle/1791497). The 2017 ACC/AHA guidelines (Figure 35–2) recommend the use of 10-year atherosclerotic cardiovascular disease (ASCVD) risk assessment to guide treatment, which can be accessed at http://www.cvriskcalculator.com/. According to both guidelines, lifestyle modification may be used initially if blood pressure is 130–140/80–90 mmHg in patients <60 years of age without diabetes mellitus or chronic kidney disease and with a 10-year estimated ASCVD risk <10%. These patients have a blood pressure goal of <140/90 mmHg. Patients who are not in this population have differing treatment options depending on the guideline being followed.

According to the 2017 ACC/AHA guidelines (see Figure 35–2), "Use of BP [blood pressure]-lowering medications is recommended for secondary prevention of recurrent CVD [cardiovascular disease] events in patients with clinical CVD and an average SBP [systolic blood pressure] of 130 mm Hg or higher or an average DBP [diastolic blood pressure] of 80 mm Hg or higher, and for primary prevention in adults with an estimated 10-year ASCVD risk of 10% or higher and an average SBP 130 mm Hg or higher or an average DBP 80 mm Hg or higher. Use of BP-lowering medication is recommended for primary prevention of CVD in adults with no history of CVD and with an estimated 10-year ASCVD risk <10% and an SBP of 140 mm Hg or higher or a DBP of 90 mm Hg or higher."

When lifestyle modification is used as initial therapy but successful control is not achieved, drug therapy should be

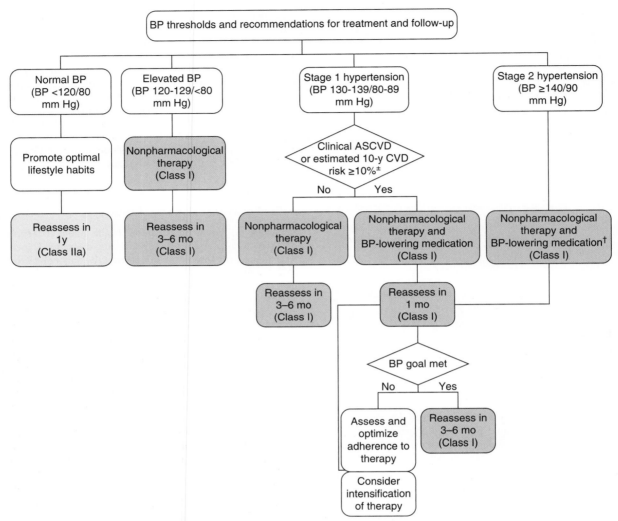

*Using the ACC/AHA Risk Calculator. Note that patients with DM or CKD are automatically placed in the high-risk category. For initiation of RAS inhibitor or diuretic therapy, assess blood tests for electrolytes and renal function 2 to 4 weeks after initiating therapy.

†Consider initiation of pharmacological therapy for stage 2 hypertension with 2 antihypertensive agents of different classes. Patients with stage 2 hypertension and BP ≥160/100 mm Hg should be promptly treated, carefully monitored, and subject to upward medication dose adjustment as necessary to control BP. Reassessment includes BP measurement, detection of orthostatic hypotension in selected patients (eg, older or with postural symptoms), identification of white coat hypertension or a white coat effect, documentation of adherence, monitoring of the response to therapy, reinforcement of the importance of adherence, reinforcement of the importance of treatment, and assistance with treatment to achieve BP target.

▲ **Figure 35–2.** American College of Cardiology/American Heart Association 2017 hypertension guidelines algorithm. ASCVD, atherosclerotic cardiovascular disease; BP, blood pressure; CVD, cardiovascular disease. (Reproduced with permission from Whelton PK, Carey RM, Aronow WS, et al: 2017 ACC/AHA/AAPA/ABC/ACPM/AGS/APhA/ASH/ASPC/NMA/PCNA Guideline for the Prevention, Detection, Evaluation, and Management of High Blood Pressure in Adults: Executive Summary: A Report of the American College of Cardiology/American Heart Association Task Force on Clinical Practice Guidelines. *Hypertension.* 2018 Jun;71(6):1269–1324.)

initiated (see section on pharmacotherapy, later). Further reassessments should consider optimization or titration of the drug regimen in terms of dosage or combinations, as well as reinforcing adherence to lifestyle modification. Follow-up visits should occur at approximately monthly intervals until the blood pressure goal is reached, or more frequently in patients with significant comorbidities. Once patients reach their goal, 3- to 6-month intervals for visits are appropriate. Each guideline defines their goals. The ACC/AHA 2017 guidelines have a blood pressure goal of <130/80 mmHg for all populations. For JNC-8, see algorithm by visiting https://jamanetwork.com/journals/jama/fullarticle/1791497.

If the blood pressure goal is not achieved with triple-drug therapy (ie, agents from different classes, including a diuretic), further investigation must ensue. A lack of motivation on the patient's part can undo the most effective regimen; however, this outcome can be minimized through positive experiences with the clinician to address misunderstandings about the condition and treatment. Poor response to therapy by patients receiving a triple regimen of antihypertensive drugs should also prompt consideration of referral to a hypertension specialist for evaluation and recommendations concerning treatment.

B. Lifestyle Modification

The Joint National Committee and many other organizations cite the adoption of lifestyle modifications as critical, not only for the prevention of hypertension, but also in the treatment thereof. Major recommendations include encouraging the overweight patient to lose weight. Even small amounts of weight loss (10 lb [4.5 kg]) can improve blood pressure control and reduce cardiovascular risk. Weight loss can be facilitated through dietary changes and increased exercise. Patients should be encouraged to set their weekly aerobic exercise goal of ≥150 minutes of moderate-intensity physical activity or 75 minutes of vigorous-intensity exercise as outlined by *Healthy People 2020*. Adoption of the Dietary Approaches to Stop Hypertension (DASH) eating plan is also recommended. This plan promotes potassium and calcium intake, reduced sodium and fat intake, exercise, and moderation of alcohol consumption. The blood pressure reduction gained is roughly equivalent to that of single-drug therapy. However, patients taking angiotensin-converting enzyme inhibitors (ACEIs) or angiotensin II receptor blockers (ARBs) should be cautioned regarding potassium intake, because these medications can result in potassium retention. Any use of tobacco should be discouraged, and patients currently using tobacco should be counseled to quit, as this may help lower blood pressure.

C. Pharmacotherapy

Many medications are available to treat hypertension. Medication should be initiated at a low dose and titrated slowly to achieve desired blood pressure control. When available, formulations available in once-daily dosing are preferred because of increased patient compliance. Also useful are the many combination formulations now available that incorporate two different classes of drugs. Good clinical outcomes and trial data exist demonstrating reduction in complications of hypertension with blood pressure lowering by ACEIs, ARBs, thiazide diuretics, calcium channel blockers, and β-blockers. When selecting a medication, in addition to following guidelines, side effect profile and patient comorbidities should help guide choice as well as the possible out-of-pocket cost that the patient may have to incur as a result of varying economic status and insurance coverage, depending on the patient population being treated (please see to Table 35–5 for price comparisons).

Favorable effects of selective antihypertensive agents may increase interest in their use. Thiazide diuretics slow demineralization in osteoporosis. β-Blockers are useful for atrial arrhythmias and fibrillation, migraine headache prophylaxis, thyrotoxicosis, and essential tremor. Calcium channel blockers are useful in Raynaud syndrome and some arrhythmias, and α-blockers are helpful in prostatism.

Unfavorable effects include cautions for the use of thiazide diuretics in patients with gout or a history of hyponatremia. β-Blockers should be avoided in patients with asthma or with second- or third-degree heart block. ACEIs and ARBs have the potential to cause birth defects and thus should be avoided in women likely to become pregnant and discontinued in those who do become pregnant. Hyperkalemia may be caused by aldosterone antagonists and potassium-sparing diuretics.

The JNC-8 guidelines, which were published in 2014 and are currently the accepted hypertensive guidelines by the American Academy of Family Physicians, have several recommendations for initial therapy. Of note, these recommendations on initial pharmacologic agents are reinforced in the latest 2017 guidelines published by the ACC and AHA. These recommendations are based on studies performed in particular populations, which are broken down into the following groups: (1) general nonblack population, including diabetes; (2) general black population including diabetes; and (3) age >18 with chronic kidney disease and hypertension.

When considering initial pharmacotherapy, the JNC-8 and ACC/AHA 2017 guidelines both support consideration of initiating either single- or dual-drug therapy. Treatment decisions should be individually based and made according to the most recent supported guidelines. In general, the amount of blood pressure reduction is more important than the choice of antihypertensive drug(s) in the appropriate patient population. A number of recent trials (CAPPP, STOP-Hypertension-2, NORDIL, CAMELOT, UKPDS, and INSIGHT) found little to no difference in outcomes between older and newer antihypertensive drugs. Typically, monotherapy for hypertension will consist of an ACEI/ARB, calcium channel blocker, or

Table 35–5. Pricing chart of drugs.

Class	Drug	Price[a]	Class	Drug	Price[a]
Diuretic (thiazide)	Chlorthalidone	$$$	β-Blocker (CONT.)	Metoprolol succinate	$$$
	Hydrochlorothiazide	$$		Metoprolol tartrate	$$
	Indapamide	$$		Timolol	$$$
	Metolazone	$$$			
Diuretic (loop)	Furosemide	$	α$_2$-Agonist (central)	Clonidine	$
	Torsemide	$$		Methyldopa	$
	Bumetanide	$$$			
Diuretic	Triamterene	$$$$	α$_1$-Blocker (peripheral)	Doxazosin	$$$
(potassium-sparing)	Amiloride	$$$		Prazosin	$$
angiotensin-	Ramipril	$$$		Terazosin	$
converting enzyme	Captopril	$$			
inhibitor	Lisinopril	$$	Calcium channel blocker	Nifedipine	$$$
	Enalapril	$$	(dihydropyridine)	Felodipine	$$
	Benazepril	$$$		Amlodipine	$$$
	Fosinopril	$$$		Isradipine	$$$
	Quinapril	$$$		Nisoldipine	$$$$
Angiotensin receptor	Candesartan	$$$$	Calcium channel	Verapamil	$
blocker	Olmesartan	$$$$	blocker (nondihy-	Diltiazem	$
	Irbesartan	$$$$	dropyridine)		
	Losartan	$$$	Aldosterone antagonist	Spironolactone	$$
	Telmisartan	$$$$		Eplerenone	$$$$
	Valsartan	$$$$	Renin inhibitor	Aliskiren	$$$$
β-Blocker	Atenolol	$$	Vasodilator	Hydralazine	$
	Labetalol	$$		Minoxidil	$$
	Propranolol	$	Angiotensin receptor– neprilysin inhibitor	Sacubitril/valsartan	$$$$

[a]Values based on estimates from Epocrates (http://www.epocrates.com/) and are only for a brief comparison of common generic medicines used within separate classes. They are intended to provide a crude idea of price when prescribing various medications and are in no way a reflection of efficacy, side effect profile, or current treatment recommendations. *Key:* $, <$30/90–100 tablets; $$, $30–$70/90–100 tablets; $$$, $70–$200/90–100 tablets; $$$$, >$200/90–100 tablets.

Note: Combination tablets exist between most of the classes listed above, vary in pricing, and offer convenience for patients on multiple medications. They also may enhance compliance and prevent medication errors, especially in the elderly and in patients with polypharmacy.

thiazide diuretic. Unless specifically recommended for another condition, β-blockers should be avoided as initial monotherapy; β-blockers and α-blockers are excluded from initial therapy for numerous reasons. Studies including β-blockers compared to other classes of drugs showed a higher rate of primary outcomes including cardiovascular death, MI, or stroke. α-Blockers also showed a higher rate of cerebrovascular disease, cardiovascular disease, and heart failure as compared to other classes of drugs. If a single drug does not achieve control, a second drug from a different class should be added.

There are three strategies offered in the JNC-8 guidelines that give guidance on how to titrate and add drugs to achieve effective and timely control. The first strategy includes initiation of a single agent followed by titration of the single agent to the maximum dose tolerated and then addition of a second class of drugs if the blood pressure is still not at goal.

The second strategy outlines the initiation of a single agent, but instead of titration to the maximum dose, this strategy recommends the addition of a second agent as next-line and subsequent titration of both agents as needed. The final strategy for obtaining blood pressure control is the initiation of two agents at the outset followed by titration and addition of a third agent for control. This final strategy was given as a recommendation for those whose blood pressure was initially >160/100 mmHg in particular. Drugs with a similar mechanism of action or clinical effects should not be used simultaneously (eg, combining ACEIs, ARBs, and renin inhibitors). Effective and timely control for most patients will be accomplished with at least two antihypertensive medications. The clinician should advise patients—especially those who are diabetic, have autonomic dysfunction, or are elderly—of the risk for orthostatic hypotension.

Ethnic differences have been noted in the blood pressure response to monotherapy. African Americans, who have increased prevalence and severity of hypertension, have demonstrated blunted response to monotherapy, such as β-blockers and ACEIs versus diuretics or calcium channel blockers. As such, most guidelines support thiazide diuretics or calcium channel blockers for initial pharmacotherapy in this population. In particular, the Antihypertensive and Lipid-Lowering Treatment to Prevent Heart Attack Trial (ALLHAT) concluded that the use of thiazide diuretics in this population decreased the risk of cerebrovascular disease, heart failure, and cardiovascular events as compared to ACEIs. In particular, the rate of stroke was 51% higher in the ACEI group as compared to the thiazide group. Calcium channel blockers were shown to also reduce cerebrovascular and cardiovascular events but were not as effective in the prevention of heart failure as compared to a thiazide diuretic. Overall mortality was unchanged between the two groups.

The recommendations that follow are summarized in Table 35–6 and are based on a number of major trials that were reviewed extensively by JNC-8 as well as by the ACC/AHA while developing their guidelines.

1. Drugs affecting the renin-angiotensin-aldosterone system—ACEIs, ARBs, and renin inhibitors are all drugs that target the renin-angiotensin-aldosterone system to lower blood pressure. These will be discussed further in the following sections. Remember, drugs in this class should not be combined, especially in patients with chronic kidney disease or diabetes, as this combination can lead to further renal impairment, hypotension, and hyperkalemia. These medications should also be avoided in pregnancy; therefore, make certain that any woman of childbearing age has an appropriate birth control method prior to prescribing these agents.

A. ACEIs—ACEIs stimulate vasodilation by blocking the renin-angiotensin-aldosterone system and inhibiting degradation of bradykinin. In several randomized controlled clinical trials, these agents have been shown to reduce cardiovascular events in hypertensive patients (CAPPP trial), including particular subgroups (high-risk patients age >55 years [HOPE study], older men [ANBP study], and diabetic patients [FACET and ACAPP trials]). Compelling indications exist for use of ACEIs as first-line treatment in patients with diabetes mellitus, congestive heart failure, a history of ST-segment elevation MI, a history of non–ST-segment elevation anterior MI, and chronic kidney disease. ACEIs have been shown to reduce progression of renal disease in African Americans (AASK trial) and diabetics, but may increase the risk of stroke when used as monotherapy in African Americans (ALLHAT trial). These agents are more effective in promoting regression of left ventricular hypertrophy than diuretics, β-blockers, or calcium channel blockers. Left ventricular hypertrophy is considered one of the best predictors of cardiovascular events in patients with hypertension. They also have been shown to help slow cardiac remodeling in the setting of congestive heart failure, thus preventing further decline.

ACEIs have relatively few side effects and are well tolerated by most patients. A dry cough may be reported in as many as 25% of patients, which is reversible upon cessation of the medication. Hyperkalemia is a side effect known of the renin-angiotensin class of medications; therefore, patients who are also receiving potassium-sparing diuretics should undergo periodic monitoring of electrolytes and serum creatinine.

ACEIs must be used cautiously in patients with known renovascular disease and, when used, may need dose adjustment because of reduced drug clearance. When creatinine elevations exceed 30% above baseline, temporary cessation or reduction of dose is warranted. These agents should be used with extreme caution, if at all, in patients whose serum creatinine level exceeds 3.0 mg/mL. Fosinopril is a good option in patients with renovascular disease because it is the only ACEI that is excreted by both the liver and the kidney. However, ACEIs should not be used in patients with bilateral renal artery stenosis. Angioedema is also a commonly reported side effect, with this complication reported 2–4 times more frequently in African Americans.

B. ARBs—ARBs selectively block angiotensin II activation of AT_1 receptors, which are responsible for mediating vasoconstriction, salt and water retention, and central and sympathetic activation, among others. Angiotensin II is still able to activate AT_2-blockers, facilitating vasodilation and production of bradykinin, which aids in reduction of blood pressure. This class of medication is well tolerated and has a favorable side effect profile. ARBs are a good alternative for patients who cannot tolerate ACEI-associated cough but should be avoided in patients with ACEI-associated edema. Current guidelines state that either ACEIs or ARBs can be used for initial therapy in treatment of hypertension. ARBs have been shown to be more effective than β-blockers in preventing cardiovascular events in hypertensive patients with left ventricular hypertrophy, both with and without diabetes (LIFE trial). Renal protective effects of ARBs have been shown clinically to reduce the progression of nephropathy in diabetic hypertensive patients (RENAAL trial) and to reduce the incidence of new-onset diabetes (VALUE trial). In addition, it has been demonstrated that ARBs reduce subsequent events in patients with acute ischemic stroke (ACCESS study).

C. Renin inhibitors—Aliskiren, a renin inhibitor, works by blinding renin to block the conversion of angiotensinogen to angiotensin I, the rate-limiting step of the renin-angiotensin-aldosterone system. It is the only renin inhibitor available on the market and is typically used in patients who do not tolerate ACEIs or ARBs. They should not be used in

Table 35–6. Clinical trial guideline basis for compelling indications for individual drug classes.

Compelling Indication[a]	Recommended Drugs							Clinical Trial Basis[b]
	D	BB	ACEI	ARB	CCB	Aldo ANT	ARNI	
Heart failure	•	•	•	•		•	*	ACC/AHA Heart Failure Guideline, MERIT-HF, COPERNICUS, CIBIS, SOLVD, AIRE, TRACE, ValHEFT, RALES, ACCOMPLISH, SPRINT, 2017 ACC/AHA/HFSA Guideline, Paradigm-HF, ACCF/AHA Guideline for the Management of Heart Failure
Post-MI		•	•			•		ACC/AHA Post-MI Guideline, BHAT, SAVE, Capricorn, EPHESUS
High coronary disease risk	•	•	•		•			ALLHAT, HOPE, ANBP2, LIFE, CONVINCE, ACCOMPLISH, SPRINT
Diabetes mellitus	•	•	•	•	•			NKF-ADA Guideline, UKPDS, ALLHAT, ACCOMPLISH, ACCORD, 2017 ACC/AHA/HFSA Guideline
Chronic kidney disease			•	•				NKF Guideline, Captopril Trial, RENAAL, IDNT, REIN, AASK, SPRINT
Recurrent stroke prevention	•		•	•				PROGRESS, PATS, SPRINT, 2017 ACC/AHA/HFSA Guideline

[a]Compelling indications for antihypertensive drugs are based on benefits from outcome studies or existing clinical guidelines; the compelling indication is managed in parallel with the blood pressure.

[b]Conditions for which clinical trials demonstrate benefit of specific classes of antihypertensive drugs.

ACC, American College of Cardiology; ACCF, American College of Cardiology Foundation; ACEI, angiotensin-converting enzyme inhibitor; ADA, American Diabetes Association; AHA, American Heart Association; Aldo ANT, aldosterone antagonist; ARB, angiotensin II receptor blocker; ARNI, angiotensin receptor–neprilysin inhibitor; BB, β-blocker; CCB, calcium channel blocker; D, diuretic; HFSA, Heart Failure Society of America; MI, myocardial infarction; NKF, National Kidney Foundation.

Reproduced with permission from The Seventh Report of the Joint National Committee on Prevention, Detection, Evaluation, and Treatment of High Blood Pressure. National High Blood Pressure Education Program. Bethesda (MD): National Heart, Lung, and Blood Institute (US); 2004 Aug. Report No.: 04-5230.

conjunction with these medications because the ACC/AHA guidelines recommend avoiding multiple renin-angiotensin-aldosterone system agents.

2. Calcium channel blockers—There are two classes of calcium channel blockers: (1) the dihydropryidine calcium channel blockers, which vasodilate (nifedipine, amlodipine, felodipine) and (2) the rate-lowering calcium channel blockers (verapamil, diltiazem). They have relatively few side effects but may cause headache, nausea, rash, or flushing in some patients. There are no specific absolute indications for calcium channel blockers, and both JNC-8 and the 2017 AHA/ACC guidelines support the use of dihydropyridine calcium channel blockers as first-line therapy. They should be considered in patients with obstructive airway diseases and as an alternative or adjunct to β-blockers in patients with stable angina in ischemic heart disease. The 2017 AHA/ACC guidelines recommend the use of calcium channel blockers beginning 3 years after MI in patients with coronary artery disease who have both hypertension and angina. In diabetics, nondihydropyridines, with their negative inotropic and chronotropic actions, have a beneficial role in atrial fibrillation and supraventricular tachyarrhythmias. Since nondihydropyridine calcium channel blockers have myocardial depressant activity and several clinical trials have shown no benefit or worse outcomes in patients with heart failure, they are not recommended in patients with hypertension and heart failure with reduced ejection fraction.

Data for the use of calcium channel blockers in the elderly are mixed. The Systolic Hypertension in Europe (SYSEUR) trial, released in 1997, randomized 5000 elderly patients with isolated systolic hypertension to treatment with either placebo or the long-acting dihydropyridine calcium channel blocker nitrendipine. In 2 years of follow-up, there was significant reduction in stroke and cardiovascular events. Similar benefits were reported in elderly patients with hypertension and diabetes using nitrendipine, although the findings were not superior to other antihypertensive agents. In African Americans, response to monotherapy using β-blockers, ACEIs, and ARBs is blunted, which is not seen when using calcium channel blockers or diuretics. Therefore, in African Americans, calcium channel blockers and thiazide diuretics have been shown to be more effective for blood pressure control. Use of combination regimens with a diuretic eliminates these differential responses.

The ACCOMPLISH trial combined benazepril with amlodipine and showed a substantial advantage over combination therapy consisting of benazepril with hydrochlorothiazide, thereby making amlodipine a highly recommended first-line add-on therapy to ACEIs for combination therapy as well as making amlodipine a viable first-line monotherapy option. The ASCOT trial found a decrease in cardiovascular disease and death with amlodipine (calcium channel blocker) versus atenolol (β-blocker). The VALUE trial comparing amlodipine versus valsartan (ARB) found better outcomes with blood pressure control but no difference in rates of cardiovascular events.

Cushman WC, Reda DJ, Perry HM, et al. Regional and racial differences in response to antihypertensive medication use in a randomized controlled trial of men with hypertension in the United States. Department of Veterans Affairs Cooperative Study Group on Antihypertensive Agents. *Arch Intern Med.* 2000;160:825–831. [PMID: 10737282]

Goldstein RE, Boccuzzi SJ, Cruess D, et al. Diltiazem increases late-onset congestive heart failure in postinfarction patients with early reduction in ejection fraction. The Adverse Experience Committee; and the Multicenter Diltiazem Postinfarction Research Group. *Circulation.* 1991;83:52–60. [PMID: 1984898]

Jamerson K, DeQuattro V. The impact of ethnicity on response to antihypertensive therapy. *Am J Med.* 1996;101:22S–32S. [PMID: 8876472]

Saunders E, Weir MR, Kong BW, et al. A comparison of the efficacy and safety of a beta-blocker, a calcium channel blocker, and a converting enzyme inhibitor in hypertensive blacks. *Arch Intern Med.* 1990;150:1707–1713. [PMID: 2200382]

3. Diuretics—Both JNC-8 and the 2017 ACC/AHA guidelines list thiazide diuretics as an option for initial treatment of hypertension. This strong recommendation is based on the many randomized controlled trials that have demonstrated a superior response for diuretics in reduction of morbidity—including stroke, coronary artery disease, and congestive heart failure—and total mortality. ALLHAT was one of the largest such trials. It compared diuretics, calcium channel blockers, and ACEIs as initial therapies in a population with a large number of African American participants. The authors concluded that regardless of age, sex, or race, the use of diuretics in hypertensive, high-cardiovascular-risk patients was associated with similar risk of cardiovascular events equivalent to that of calcium channel blockers and ACEIs, but was superior in performance in patients with underlying heart conditions including heart failure. ACCOMPLISH compared combination therapy in patients at high risk for cardiovascular events with benazepril plus either amlodipine or hydrochlorothiazide and was terminated early because of a substantial disadvantage in combination therapy with hydrochlorothiazide. Because of this large, well-designed study, along with a number of other well-designed studies showing similar efficacy across different antihypertensive classes, initial monotherapy with a specific agent, specifically a diuretic, became controversial and has led to a difference in opinion regarding the use of a specific agent for monotherapy. This ultimately resulted in JNC-8 and ACC/AHA listing thiazide diuretics as one of multiple options for initial monotherapy.

Diuretics should be used cautiously in patients with gout, as worsening hyperuricemia can result. They may also cause muscle cramps or impotence in some individuals. Diuretics may be effective at lower doses in patients with dyslipidemia and diabetes mellitus, but patients placed on higher doses must be observed closely for worsening hyperglycemia or hyperlipidema. The thiazide diuretics are most commonly used in the treatment of hypertension, because loop diuretics are more likely to lead to electrolyte abnormalities such as hypokalemia and to have a shorter duration of action. However, loop diuretics can sometimes be useful in the treatment of hypertension in patients with chronic renal disease and a serum creatinine level of >2.5 mg/dL. The loop diuretics have found most utility in the treatment of congestive heart failure.

ALLHAT Officers Coordinating for the ALLHAT Collaborative Research Group. Major outcomes in high-risk hypertensive patients randomized to angiotensin-converting enzyme inhibitor or calcium channel blocker vs diuretic: the Antihypertensive and Lipid-Lowering treatment to prevent Heart Attack Trial (ALLHAT). *JAMA.* 2002;288:2981. [PMID: 12479763]

Jamerson K, Weber MA, Bakris GL, et al. Benazepril plus amlodipine or hydrochlorothiazide for hypertension in high-risk patients: the Avoiding Cardiovascular Events in Combination Therapy with Systolic Hypertension (ACCOMPLISH) trial. *N Engl J Med.* 2008;359(23):2417. [PMID: 19052124]

4. β-Blockers—According to the newest guidelines, β-blockers should not be used as initial therapy, unless the patient has known history of congestive heart failure or ischemic heart disease. Of course, there are always considerations for treating multiple conditions at one time to decrease a patient's overall pill burden. For example, β-blockers have favorable effects on migraine headache, hyperthyroidism, and anxiety. The most effective β-blockers in controlling hypertension include metoprolol and bisoprolol, which are all cardiac selective, as well as carvedilol, which has both α and β receptor activity. All patients with congestive heart failure should be treated with β-blockers lacking intrinsic sympathomimetic activity, including the three mentioned earlier. Careful use of these agents leads to reduction in overall mortality, improved ejection fraction, and slowed cardiac remodeling associated with congestive heart failure. The side effect profile of these medications is directly related to coexisting conditions of the patient. These agents should be used with caution, if at all, in patients with a history of depression, asthma or reactive airway disease, second- or third-degree heart block, or peripheral vascular disease. In patients with mild to moderate reactive airway disease, β-blockers do not produce adverse effects in the short term. In particular, consider the use of the cardiac selective β-blockers in a patient with known reactive airway disease. The United Kingdom Prospective Diabetes Study (UKPDS) demonstrated that β-blockers can be used safely and effectively for type 2 diabetes mellitus, although there is

concern that hypoglycemic episodes might be masked. Any patient with diabetes mellitus placed on a β-blocker should, therefore, be carefully monitored. Lastly, patients should be informed that β-blockers may cause sexual dysfunction.

5. Other drugs—Other drugs, including α₁-blockers and direct vasodilators, are used to treat hypertension, although less commonly than the other classes of drugs. They are typically used as second- or third-line agents because of increased side effects. The ALLHAT trial suggested that α₁-blockers and direct vasodilators such as doxazosin may increase the risk of stroke and congestive heart failure when used in the treatment of hypertension, resulting in discontinuation of that arm of the trial. These agents are more commonly associated with orthostatic hypotension and should be used with caution in the elderly. However, they may be effective in patients who also have a history of benign prostatic hypertrophy. Clonidine, which is a centrally acting α₁-agonist should be reserved as a last-line agent because of the significant side effect profile. In older patients, this drug is known to cause significant CNS adverse effects. If initiated, clonidine should not be stopped abruptly because of its tendency to lead to rebound hypertension and hypertensive crisis. Clonidine should always be tapered off slowly to avoid these side effects.

6. Combination therapy—Combination therapy allows patients who are on a multidrug regimen to take fewer pills. This has been done with various antihypertensive classes such as combining an ACEI and a calcium channel blocker (ACCOMPLISH). Because the 2017 AHA/ACC guidelines recommend starting two agents in adults with stage 2 hypertension and based on other guidelines, many patients will eventually require a multidrug regimen; thus, prescribing fewer pills can improve compliance. Studies have examined the value of combining medications, especially in the elderly, who often take many pills per day. One study showed favorable outcomes with an ACEI-diuretic combination in the elderly over the course of 1 year. The drug was well tolerated, and compliance was improved.

These medications tend to be more expensive for patients, so it is important to weigh cost and compliance issues to maximize the likelihood of successful treatment. This is where the family physician's role is crucial to the overall care of the patient.

D. Special Considerations

The drug selections noted in Table 35–6 are based on favorable outcome data from clinical trials and should be considered in light of current medications, tolerability, and blood pressure target goal.

1. Ischemic heart disease—According to the ACC/AHA guidelines, a goal blood pressure of <130/80 mmHg is recommended for patient with a history of ischemic heart disease. ACEIs, ARBs, and β-blockers are considered first-line drugs for patients with heart disease because they have been proven to reduce all-cause mortality by >20%. If blood pressure is uncontrolled on those agents alone, the addition of a long-acting calcium channel blocker may be considered. Both β-blockers and calcium channel blockers are considered effective antianginal drugs as well in the setting of stable angina.

2. Heart failure—Strict blood pressure goals of <130/80 mmHg are recommended for this population as well, according to the ACC/AHA guidelines. Heart failure with reduced ejection fraction has the most evidence supporting the use of specific blood pressure agents. ACEIs and β-blockers are recommended first line for asymptomatic patients with ventricular dysfunction. The β-blockers recommended include carvedilol, metoprolol, and bisoprolol. Symptomatic or end-stage heart disease should be treated with ACEIs, β-blockers, ARBs, aldosterone blockers, and loop diuretics. The nondihydropyridine calcium channel blockers, diltiazem and verapamil, should not be used in this population because they have been shown to have myocardial depressant activity. In select patients with stable, mild to moderate, New York Heart Association class II to III heart failure with reduced ejection fraction ≤40% who have demonstrated that they can tolerate an ACEI or an ARB, consideration should be given to replacing their ACEI or ARB with an angiotensin receptor–neprilysin inhibitor (ARNI) containing sacubitril/valsartan. In the Paradigm-HF trial, sacubitril/valsartan was shown to decrease cardiovascular mortality, hospitalization and all-cause mortality. Because there is little experience with this drug to date, recommendations for initiation and use are continuing to evolve. Side effects of this ARNI can include hypotension, hyperkalemia, cough, dizziness, renal failure, and rarely angioedema. In contrast, patients with heart failure with preserved ejection fraction obtain the most beneficial blood pressure control with the use of diuretics such as chlorthalidone.

McMurray JJ, Packer M, Desai AS, et al. Angiotensin-neprilysin inhibition versus enalapril in heart failure. *N Engl J Med.* 2014;371:993–1004. [PMID: 25176015]

Writing Committee Members, Yancy CW, Jessup M, et al. 2016 ACC/AHA/HFSA focused update on new pharmacological therapy for heart failure: an update of the 2013 ACCF/AHA guideline for the management of heart failure: a report of the American College of Cardiology/American Heart Association Task Force on Clinical Practice Guidelines and the Heart Failure Society of America. *Circulation.* 2016;134:e282–e293. [PMID: 27208050]

3. Diabetes mellitus—All first-line classes of antihypertensive medications have proved beneficial in reducing the incidence of cardiovascular disease and stroke in diabetic patients. Often combination therapy is needed because patients with diabetes and hypertension have more difficulty achieving the recommended goal of <130/80 mmHg according to the ACC/AHA. The progression of diabetic nephropathy in the presence of albuminuria is reduced with ACEIs or ARBs.

4. Chronic kidney disease—Goals for these patients include slowing deterioration of renal function and preventing cardiovascular disease. Typically, a combination of three drugs is needed to accomplish aggressive blood pressure management. The current recommendations for any patient with evidence of chronic kidney disease, with or without proteinuria, include the addition of an ACEI or ARB regardless of race or diabetic status. This recommendation is based on evidence that shows an improvement in kidney outcomes and decreased progression to end-stage renal disease. Studies including the African American population with chronic kidney disease and proteinuria benefitted the most from the addition of an ACEI or ARB initially as compared to thiazide or calcium channel blocker therapy; therefore, this is considered a different population under the JNC-8 recommendations. ACEIs and ARBs should be used and may be continued in patients with an increase in serum creatinine clearance of 35% above baselines unless hyperkalemia develops. Increasing doses of loop diuretics are usually needed once the creatinine level reaches 2.5–3.0 mg/dL.

5. Cerebrovascular disease—During the period of an acute ischemic stroke, permissive elevation in blood pressure should be allowed initially with a goal of 15% reduction in the first 24 hours. Intravenous blood pressure medications should be used. For secondary stroke prevention, the goal blood pressure according to the ACC/AHA guidelines is <130/80 mmHg. The combination of an ACEI and thiazide diuretic has been shown to lower recurrent stroke rates.

6. Pregnancy—Hypertensive disorders complicate up to 10% of pregnancies worldwide and constitute a significant cause of maternal and perinatal morbidity and mortality. Preeclampsia remains a risk factor for future cardiovascular disease for women, with the increased risk ranging from doubling in all cases to eightfold increase in women with preeclampsia who gave birth before 34 0/7 weeks of gestation. The American College of Obstetricians and Gynecologists (ACOG) Hypertensive Task Force identifies four distinct categories of hypertensive disorders in pregnancy: (1) preeclampsia-eclampsia, (2) chronic hypertension, (3) chronic hypertension with superimposed preeclampsia, and (4) gestational hypertension.

Preeclampsia is defined as systolic blood pressure ≥140 mmHg or diastolic blood pressure ≥90 mmHg on two occasions at least 4 hours apart after 20 weeks of gestation in a woman with previously normal blood pressure *and* proteinuria (defined as ≥300 mg/24-hour urine collection or protein/creatinine ratio ≥0.3). Or, in the absence of proteinuria, the diagnosis can be made with new-onset hypertension with a platelet count <100,000/μL, serum creatinine >1.1 mg/dL or the doubling of serum creatinine in the absence of other renal disease, elevated liver transaminases to twice normal concentrations, pulmonary edema, or cerebral or visual symptoms. Severe features of preeclampsia include systolic blood pressure ≥160 mmHg or diastolic blood pressure ≥110 mmHg, thrombocytopenia, impaired liver function, renal insufficiency, pulmonary edema and new-onset cerebral or visual disturbances. For women with preeclampsia with severe hypertension, antihypertensive therapy is recommended, and intrapartum-postpartum magnesium sulfate therapy should be administered.

Gestational hypertension is characterized as new-onset blood pressure elevations after 20 weeks of gestation in the absence of proteinuria or other features of preeclampsia, and the failure of blood pressure to normalize in the postpartum period should raise concern for chronic hypertension. *Chronic* hypertension in pregnancy, defined as hypertension present before pregnancy or before 20 weeks of gestation, is present in up to 5% of pregnant women. The use of antihypertensive medication before pregnancy or the persistence of high blood pressure beyond the "usual" postpartum period may also help differentiate chronic hypertension from other hypertensive disorders of pregnancy.

Mild hypertension is considered a systolic blood pressure ≥140 mmHg and/or diastolic blood pressure >90 mmHg. *Severe* is considered a systolic blood pressure ≥160 mmHg and diastolic blood pressure >110 mmHg. Women with mild hypertension who are doing well generally do not need medication. Current evidence has yet to show whether antihypertensive therapy at this level improves perinatal outcomes. Studies have shown that outcomes are improved and thus medications are indicated when necessary to keep blood pressure <160/105 mmHg.

If the patient has not had a previous evaluation, the ACOG Hypertensive Task Force recommends a workup for secondary hypertension and end-organ damage at the time of diagnosis. Although there is limited evidence addressing thresholds at which to institute antihypertensive therapy, the task force recommends initiating pharmacologic therapy when blood pressure is ≥160/105 mmHg. Initial pharmacologic therapy includes labetalol, nifedipine, and methyldopa.

To urgently lower severe range blood pressures, hydralazine demonstrated improvement in outcomes. There is little difference in outcome when comparing these medications. Pharmacologic therapy for chronic therapy includes methyldopa, nifedipine, and labetalol. The use of β-blockers has been associated with a higher rate of babies who are small for

gestational age. According to the NHBPEP Working Group on High Blood Pressure in Pregnancy, diuretics can potentiate the positive effects of other antihypertensives and are not contraindicated unless uteroplacental perfusion is already present as a result of another issue such as preeclampsia or intrauterine growth restriction. ACEIs are considered category D, and this class is contraindicated in the second and third trimesters because of an association with teratogenic effects, including severely underdeveloped calvarial bone, renal failure, oligohydramnios, anuria, renal dysgenesis, and others, including death.

In the postpartum period, ACOG recommends replacing NSAIDs with other analgesics in women with hypertension that persists for >1 day postpartum since they can increase blood pressure. ACOG recommends blood pressure monitoring in the hospital or outpatient setting for at least 72 hours postpartum and again 7–10 days after delivery. For women with persistent postpartum hypertension, blood pressure ≥150/100 mmHg on at least two occasions 4 hours apart warrants antihypertensive therapy. Women with a history of preeclampsia and preterm delivery or with recurrent preeclampsia should have annual blood pressure, lipids, fasting blood glucose, and body mass index assessments.

American College of Obstetricians and Gynecologists; Task Force on Hypertension in Pregnancy. Hypertension in pregnancy. Report of the American College of Obstetricians and Gynecologists' Task Force on Hypertension in Pregnancy. *Obstet Gynecol.* 2013;122(5):1122–1131. [PMID: 24150027]

7. Children and adolescents—The American Academy of Pediatrics (AAP) released updated hypertension guidelines in 2017 and noted a 3.5% prevalence of hypertension in children. With an increase in childhood obesity and its associated medical conditions including hypertension, there is a growing concern for identifying, diagnosing, and treating hypertension in this population given the growing amount of evidence showing an early development of cardiovascular disease within this population. In this population, hypertension diagnosis is based on percentiles for height versus age determined by an NHANES study of >50,000 children in the outpatient setting. The definitions for hypertension for children age 1–13 years and >13 years according to the AAP are listed in Table 35–7.

Blood pressure should be checked on all children >3 years old annually or at every visit if they have obesity, chronic kidney disease, diabetes, or congenital aortic arch abnormalities, *even if surgically corrected.* Diagnosis is made by three confirmed blood pressure values meeting criteria for stage 1 hypertension at separate visits. Among children who are obese, ≤30% will have hypertension. Given that hypertension in this population is uncommon, secondary causes of hypertension should be higher on the differential versus the adult

Table 35–7. Updated definitions of blood pressure (BP) categories and stages for children and adolescents.

For Children Age 1–13 Years	For Children Age >13 Years
Normal BP: <90th percentile	Normal BP: <120/<80 mmHg
Elevated BP: ≥90th percentile to <95th percentile or 120/80 mmHg to <95th percentile (whichever is lower)	Elevated BP: 120/<80 to 129/<80 mmHg
Stage 1 hypertension (HTN): ≥95th percentile to <95th percentile + 12 mmHg, or 130/80 to 139/89 mmHg (whichever is lower)	Stage 1 HTN: 130/80 to 139/89 mmHg
Stage 2 HTN: ≥95th percentile + 12 mmHg, or ≥140/90 mmHg (whichever is lower)	Stage 2 HTN: ≥140/90 mmHg

Reproduced with permission from Flynn JT, Kaelber DC, Baker-Smith CM, et al: Clinical Practice Guideline for Screening and Management of High Blood Pressure in Children and Adolescents. *Pediatrics.* 2017 Sep;140(3). pii: e20171904.

population when performing a diagnostic workup on a child or adolescent with hypertension. These children should be tested for complete blood count, blood urea nitrogen, and creatinine levels; urinalysis; and renal ultrasound within their initial hypertension workup. Additionally, children and adolescents with hypertension should also be screened for hyperlipidemia and diabetes mellitus. Obese children with hypertension should be screened for OSA. Lifestyle modifications in this population are first-line treatment for hypertension. However, in children and adolescents with symptomatic hypertension, secondary hypertension, evidence of end-organ damage, diabetes, or persistent hypertension despite nonpharmacologic measures, antihypertensive medication should be initiated. Goals for treatment vary. In children with primary, uncomplicated hypertension, goal blood pressure is below the 95th percentile. In children with chronic renal disease, diabetes, or evidence of target organ damage, the blood pressure goal is below the 90th percentile. As in adults, lifestyle modifications should strongly be encouraged, including the DASH diet, weight loss, exercise, and proper sleep hygiene. When considering pharmacotherapy, there is currently no consensus for a specific initial drug of choice for monotherapy. Initial therapy should factor in the child's concurrent medical conditions because most drugs are well tolerated and achieve similar goals. Titration and addition of additional agents are similar to those of adults, and agents are typically dosed according to the child's weight. Pregnancy status, testing, and counseling in adolescent females should also be factored in when initiating pharmacotherapy (see section on pharmacotherapy in pregnancy, earlier).

Flynn JT, Kaelber DC, Baker-Smith CM, et al. Clinical practice guideline for screening and management of high blood pressure in children and adolescents. *Pediatrics.* 2017;140(3):e20171904. [PMID: 28827377]

E. Hypertensive Urgency and Emergency

Hypertensive urgencies are situations in which the blood pressure must be lowered within several hours, because of either (1) an asymptomatic, severely elevated blood pressure (>200/130 mmHg) or (2) a moderately elevated blood pressure (>200/120 mmHg) with associated symptoms, including angina, headache, and congestive heart failure. When such symptoms are present, even lower blood pressures may warrant more urgent treatment. Oral therapy can often be used with good response. The current recommendation is to restart previously prescribed medication and/or intensify current treatment with close follow-up.

Hypertensive emergencies require treatment of elevated blood pressures within 1 hour to avoid significant morbidity and mortality. The symptomatology with which the patient presents warrants the immediate attention, not the actual blood pressure value itself. Such patients show evidence of end-organ damage from the elevated blood pressure, including encephalopathy (headache, irritability, confusion, coma), renal failure, pulmonary edema, unstable angina, MI, aortic dissection, and intracranial hemorrhage. Hypertensive emergency is an indication for hospital admission to the intensive care unit, and such patients require intravenous therapy with antihypertensives to slowly control blood pressure.

The initial goal of therapy is reduction of blood pressure by 25% within the first hour. Next, blood pressure should be maintained <160/110 mmHg during hours 2 through 6 and normalized over the following hours and days. Blood pressure should not be lowered too quickly, because doing so can result in hypoperfusion of the brain and myocardium. Once initial treatment goals are achieved, blood pressure can subsequently be reduced gradually to more appropriate levels.

According to the most recent guidelines, there are very few controlled drug trials that compared patient outcomes between classes of medications. Therefore, drug choices should be tailored to the patient's condition and comorbidities. The authors involved with ACC/AHA guidelines seem to favor intravenous nicardipine drip. When myocardial ischemia is present, intravenous nitroglycerin or intravenous β-blockers such as labetalol or esmolol are preferred. Once blood pressure has been brought under control using intravenous therapy, oral agents should be initiated slowly as intravenous therapy is gradually withdrawn. Whether a patient is being treated for hypertensive urgency, hypertensive emergency, or benign hypertension, long-term therapy and lifestyle modification are essential. Patients must receive regular follow-up and meet the treatment goals established by the aforementioned guidelines.

Diabetes Mellitus

36

Belinda Vail, MD, MS, FAAFP

ESSENTIALS OF DIAGNOSIS

► Random plasma glucose ≥200 mg/dL with polydipsia, polyuria, polyphagia, and/or weight loss.

► Fasting plasma glucose ≥126 mg/dL.

► Two-hour oral glucose tolerance test (75-g glucose) ≥200 mg/dL.

► Hemoglobin A1c ≥6.5%.

► A confirmatory, repeat test or alternate test is required.

General Considerations

The age-adjusted prevalence of diabetes has doubled in the United States since the late 1990s. The adoption of a Western diet and the resulting worldwide explosion of obesity have led to an epidemic of diabetes with >422 million people worldwide afflicted. It is a major cause of blindness, renal failure, lower extremity amputations, cardiovascular disease (CVD), and congenital malformations. Rates are disproportionately high in African Americans, Native Americans, Pacific Islanders, Hispanics, and Asians. Only 14% of patients meet targets for glucose, blood pressure, and cholesterol while also not smoking. With one in eight persons developing diabetes and 90% of patients receiving their care from primary care physicians, diabetes management requires a chronic care model with an informed patient and an interactive team. The team should include lay health or community health workers if available.

American Diabetes Association's Standards of Medical Care in Diabetes—2018. *Diabetes Care*. 2018;41(Suppl 1):S1–S159. [No PMID]

Centers for Disease Control and Prevention. Diabetes fact sheet. https://www.cdc.gov/diabetes/library/factsheets.html. Accessed November 18, 2019.

National Institute of Diabetes and Digestive and Kidney Diseases. http://www2.niddk.nih.gov/. Accessed November 18, 2019.

World Health Organization. Diabetes fact sheet. https://www.who.int/news-room/fact-sheets/detail/diabetes. Accessed November 18, 2019.

Pathogenesis

Type 1 diabetes is the result of an autoimmune destruction of the pancreatic β cells with an inability of the body to produce insulin. Type 2 diabetes develops from an increasing cellular resistance to insulin, a process that is accelerated by obesity and inactivity, and is becoming increasingly common in adolescents and children. This insulin resistance increases atherosclerotic CVD, polycystic ovarian syndrome, and nonalcoholic steatohepatitis. A small percentage of patients will develop a more insidious onset of autoimmune diabetes, latent autoimmune diabetes of adulthood (LADA), that may respond for a short period of time to oral medications but progresses to insulin dependence. Some older patients may develop diabetes with mild metabolic changes. Maturity-onset diabetes of the young refers to a group of hereditary diabetes disorders that often do not require insulin. A recently added type 3c results from pancreatitis and resulting destruction of the pancreatic β cells.

Prevention

Patients with metabolic syndrome or a hemoglobin A1c (HbA1c) of 5.7–6.4% (prediabetes) should be targeted for intensive lifestyle intervention. The following interventions have been shown to be more effective than medications and improve blood pressure and lipids, leading to greater reductions in cardiovascular risk:

1. Conversion to a Mediterranean style diet

2. Reduction in screen time to <2 hours per day

3. At least 150 minutes of moderate-intensity exercise weekly (more exercise = greater risk reduction)

4. Weight reduction of at least 5%

5. Smoking cessation

Medications that may also slow progression to diabetes include metformin (cheapest and fewest side effects), acarbose, pioglitazone, liraglutide, and SGLT-2 inhibitors. Tight control of hyperglycemia and blood pressure reduces the complications of diabetes, and a sustained reduction in HbA1c is associated with significant cost savings within 1–2 years.

Burnet DL, Jones R, Freeman C, et al. Can diabetes prevention programs be translated effectively into real-world settings and still deliver improved outcomes? A synthesis of evidence. *Diabet Med.* 2013;30(1):3–15. [PMID: PMC3555428]

Hardt PD, Brendel MD, Kloer HU, et al. Is pancreatic diabetes (type 3c diabetes) underdiagnosed and misdiagnosed? *Diabetes Care.* 2008;31(suppl 2):S165–S169. [PMID: 18227480]

▶ Screening

Fasting glucose is the preferred screening method, although a random glucose or HbA1c is acceptable. The US Preventive Services Task Force (USPSTF) recommends screening for abnormal blood glucose as part of a cardiovascular risk assessment in adults age 40–70 years who are overweight or obese. Earlier screening is recommended in populations and/or individuals at risk. The American Diabetes Association (ADA) recommends universal screening every 3 years beginning at age 45 or any adults with a body mass index (BMI) of ≥25 kg/m² (≥ 23 kg/m² in Asian Americans) and one of the following diabetes risk factors:

- Physical inactivity
- First-degree relative with diabetes
- High-risk race/ethnicity (Native Americans, African Americans, Asians, Hispanics, or Pacific Islanders)
- Previous gestational diabetes or a baby weighing >9 lb
- Hypertension (≥140/90 mmHg)
- High-density lipoprotein (HDL) cholesterol <35 mg/dL and/or triglycerides >250 mg/dL
- Polycystic ovary syndrome
- HbA1c ≥5.7%, impaired fasting glucose, or impaired glucose tolerance
- Signs of insulin resistance (acanthosis nigricans, fatty liver)
- History of CVD

If normal, testing should be repeated every 3 years. Patients with prediabetes should be tested yearly.

A consensus panel has recommended screening of overweight children (weight >120% of ideal or a BMI >85th percentile) every 2 years beginning at age 10 or the onset of puberty who have two of the following risk factors:

- Family history of diabetes in first- or second-degree relative
- High-risk racial or ethnic group (same as listed earlier)
- Signs of, or conditions associated with, insulin resistance (eg, acanthosis nigricans, hypertension, dyslipidemia, and polycystic ovarian syndrome)
- History of high birth weight or maternal gestational diabetes during pregnancy

The USPSTF recommends screening for gestational diabetes in asymptomatic pregnant women after 24 weeks' gestation. Currently, a 2-hour glucose tolerance test (GTT) is recommended, but a 1-hour GTT, followed by a 3-hour confirmatory GTT, is acceptable.

Table 36–1 lists the diagnostic criteria in pregnancy. Women with diabetes prior to pregnancy are at risk for miscarriage and congenital abnormalities. The most common complication of gestational diabetes is macrosomia.

American Diabetes Association. ADA releases 2018 standards of medical care in diabetes, with notable new recommendations for people with cardiovascular disease and diabetes. https://www.prnewswire.com/news-releases/american-diabetes-association-releases-2018-standards-of-medical-care-in-diabetes-with-notable-new-recommendations-for-people-with-cardiovascular-disease-and-diabetes-300569091.html. Accessed November 18, 2019.

Table 36–1. Diabetes in pregnancy.

Risk factors
Age >25 years
High-risk racial or ethnic group
Body mass index ≥25
History of abnormal glucose tolerance test
Previous history of adverse pregnancy outcomes usually associated with gestational diabetes
Diabetes in a first-degree relative

Criteria for diagnosis
2-hour glucose tolerance test (GTT)
  75-g glucose load at 24 weeks' gestation (or sooner if indicated)
  Criteria for diagnosis is one abnormal value:
    fasting >95 mg/d
    1 hour >180 mg/dL
    2 hours >155 mg/dL
Also acceptable:
  The two-step method does not require fasting for the initial test
  Initial screen: 1-hour GTT[a]
    50-g glucose load
    Positive screen ≥135–140 mg/dL
  Diagnosis: 3-hour GTT with a 100-g glucose load
    After an overnight fast with two abnormal values
      Fasting ≥95 mg/dL
      1 hour ≥190 mg/dL
      2 hours ≥165 mg/dL
      3 hours ≥140 mg/dL

A. Signs and Symptoms

The classic symptoms of diabetes are polyuria, polydipsia, and polyphagia, but the first signs may be subtle and nonspecific. Patients with type 1 diabetes exhibit fatigue, malaise, nausea and vomiting, irritability, abdominal pain, and weight loss. They present early in the disease process but usually are quite ill at presentation, with arguably approximately 25% of patients with ketoacidosis. Signs and symptoms of ketoacidosis include tachypnea, labored respirations with the classic "fruity" breath, abdominal pain, confusion, and symptoms associated with dehydration (dry skin and mucous membranes, decreased skin turgor, tachycardia, and hypotension).

Signs of type 2 diabetes are seen well after onset of the disease and may be due to complications. The classic symptoms may be present, but patients may also complain of fatigue, irritability, and drowsiness; blurred vision; numbness or tingling in the extremities; slow wound healing; frequent infections of the skin or gums; or urinary tract infections.

B. History and Physical Examination

A personal or family history of autoimmune disorders may aid in the diagnosis (Table 36–2). Type 1 diabetes usually occurs in children and adolescents, whereas type 2 becomes more common as individuals age. A BMI of <25 kg/m² is more frequently seen in type 1 and LADA, whereas BMI >30 kg/m² is usually indicative of type 2; however, neither age nor BMI should be used as criteria for diagnosis. Hypertension, retinal changes of cotton-wool spots and hemorrhages, decreased sensation in the extremities, and evidence of CVD may also be found at presentation.

C. Laboratory Findings

Serum glucose and HbA1c levels are elevated and are usually higher in type 2 diabetes because the development is more insidious. Serum glucose is often in the 400–600 mg/dL range. Sodium levels are low, resulting from dilution as water follows glucose into the extracellular fluid. A dyslipidemia with low HDL and high triglycerides is common in type 2 diabetes. Increased albumin in the urine represents damage to the glomerular endothelium, and serum creatinine may be elevated. An HbA1c level of ≥6.5% is recognized as the diagnosis of diabetes, but care must be exercised because levels can be influenced by a number of factors. The HbA1c can be falsely elevated in the presence of hypertriglyceridemia,

Table 36–2. Initial history and screening and physical.

Diabetes history including age at onset, previous treatments, and hospitalizations
Family history of diabetes or autoimmune diseases
History of complications and treatment:
  Blood pressure
  Cholesterol
  Eye exams and complications (within 5 years of diagnosis in type 1, immediately in type 2)
  Dental history
  Peripheral and autonomic neuropathy
  Renal complications
  Cardiovascular complications
  Hemoglobinopathies
Lifestyle history
  Diet and exercise patterns
  Sleep and screen for sleep apnea
  Substance use, tobacco, and alcohol
Medications, supplements
Vaccinations (and update)
Glucose monitoring
Screen for:
  Hypoglycemia
  Hypertension
  Hyperlipidemia
  Microalbuminuria
  Depression
  Cognitive impairment
  Contraception
Physical examination
  Height, weight, and body mass index
  Blood pressure and pulse (including orthostatic measurements if indicated)
  Fundoscopic examination with retinal scan or referral for dilated eye exam
  Thyroid exam
  Cardiovascular exam
  Brief skin examination
  Foot examination including monofilament, pulses, vibratory, and temperature perception
Laboratory evaluation
  Hemoglobin A1c
  Lipid profile
  Electrolytes if on diuretics or angiotensin-converting enzyme inhibitors
  Serum creatinine and microalbumin/creatinine ratio
  Liver function tests
  Thyroid-stimulating hormone and celiac disease screen in type 1
  Vitamin B₁₂ if on metformin
Immunizations
  Yearly influenza
  Pneumococcus (Pneumovax) once and repeat at age 65
  Tdap
  Hepatitis B (especially if <age 60)
  Shingles vaccine >age 50

hyperbilirubinemia, splenectomy, renal failure, iron-deficiency anemia, and aplastic anemia and can be falsely lowered by human immunodeficiency virus medications, liver disease, blood loss, hemolytic anemia, and hemoglobin variants like sickle cell.

For diagnosis, C-terminal peptide (C-peptide), the cleaved end of native insulin, is high in type 2 diabetes as the body increases insulin production to overcome resistance. It is extremely low in type 1 diabetes as insulin levels fall and is usually low to low-normal in LADA. Antibody testing is useful in diagnosing type 1 diabetes. Glutamic acid decarboxylase antibody is most commonly tested, along with islet cell antibodies and insulin antibodies. Insulinoma-associated antigen (IA-2) is more predictive but less frequently found. Antibodies against zinc transporter 8 may also be useful in diagnosis of LADA.

In ketoacidosis (usually in type 1), serum glucose is >250 mg/dL (commonly 500–800 mg/dL). Blood pH is <7.30 with an increased anion gap (>10). Bicarbonate is <18 mEq/L. Serum and urine ketones are high, but high β-hydroxybutyrate is a more accurate evaluation of the degree of ketosis.

Patients (usually with type 2) who present with a hyperosmolar hyperglycemic state have very high serum glucose levels (600–1200 mg/dL), but do not have metabolic acidosis (pH >7.30 and serum bicarbonate >15 mEq/L). Serum osmolality is >320 mOsm/kg.

► Complications

Preventing and delaying progression of all complications in patients with diabetes is dependent on lifestyle modification, tight control of blood glucose and blood pressure, and smoking cessation. The ACCORD trial, however, found that intensive glycemic control (HgbA1c ≤6%) did not lower the incidence of adverse microvascular outcomes.

A. Cardiovascular Disease

Heart disease is the leading cause of death in patients with diabetes. Men have double and women 4–5 times the risk for myocardial infarction (MI) as well as a higher incidence of diffuse, multivessel disease, plaque rupture, superimposed thrombosis, and in-hospital mortality. Five-year survival following angioplasty or coronary artery bypass graft (CABG) is lower in patients with diabetes, but survival rates are higher with CABG. Low-dose aspirin therapy is reasonable in adults with diabetes and no history of vascular disease, whose 10-year risk of coronary heart disease (CHD) events is >10%, and who are not at increased risk of bleeding (ie, no history of gastrointestinal bleeding or peptic ulcer disease and no concurrent use of other medications that increase bleeding risk). Adults with diabetes who are at increased risk of CHD events include most men >50 years old and women >60 years old who have at least one additional major risk factor (ie, smoking, hypertension, dyslipidemia, albuminuria, or family history of premature CVD).

Pignone M, Alberts MJ, Colwell JA, et al. Aspirin for primary prevention of cardiovascular events in people with diabetes. https://ahajournals.org/doi/full/10.1161/cir.0b013e3181e3b133. Accessed November 18, 2019.

Smoking cessation is imperative. There are no specific guidelines for cardiac evaluation. An electrocardiogram and stress echocardiogram are recommended for symptoms and may be considered with the onset of microalbuminuria as it often begins concurrently.

Peripheral vascular disease is quite common in patients with diabetes and 80% more common in Hispanic Americans. Treatment focuses on slowing progression and improving symptoms. Besides smoking cessation, regular exercise, and aspirin therapy, cilostazol (Pletal) can improve blood flow. Other choices with limited evidence include pentoxifylline (Trental) and gingko biloba.

1. Hypertension—Angiotensin-converting enzyme (ACE) inhibitors have been the first line of treatment in patients with diabetes, producing a significant decrease in stroke, MI, cardiac death, post-MI mortality, and ischemic events following revascularization procedures. In the HOPE trial, the use of ACE inhibitors correlated with a 34% reduction in the onset of new cases of diabetes and a mild improvement in lipid profiles. They may be used in all diabetic patients with renal disease and a systolic blood pressure >100 mmHg or with hypertension and signs of insulin resistance. Eighth Joint National Committee recommendations are to start antihypertensive medication if the blood pressure is ≥140/90 mmHg. The American College of Cardiology and the American Heart Association recommend starting treatment at blood pressures ≥130/80 mmHg. Thiazides and calcium channel blockers are preferred in blacks unless there is renal damage. There is no specific creatinine level at which ACE inhibitors must be stopped, but the continued use of an ACE inhibitor may be limited by rising potassium levels. The most troublesome side effect is a bradykinin-induced dry cough; they may also cause angioedema and are contraindicated in pregnancy. Angiotensin receptor blockers (ARBs) have similar data for cardiovascular risk reduction, and they are better tolerated than ACE inhibitors.

Thiazide diuretics and β-blockers are effective in lowering blood pressure and have been shown to reduce cardiovascular morbidity and mortality. Although they can have some effect on glucose control, they are acceptable for use in diabetes.

James PA, Oparil S, Carter BL, et al. 2014 evidence-based guideline for the management of high blood pressure in adults. Report from the Panel Members Appointed to the Eighth Joint National Committee (JNC 8). https://jamanetwork.com/journals/jama/fullarticle/1791497. Accessed November 18, 2019.

Stone NJ, Robinson JG, Lichtenstein AH, et al. 2013 ACC/AHA guideline on the treatment of blood cholesterol to reduce atherosclerotic cardiovascular risk in adults: a report of the American College of Cardiology/American Heart Association Task Force on Practice Guidelines. *J Am Coll Cardiol.* 2014; 63(25 Pt B):2889–2934. [PMID: 24239923]

2. Hyperlipidemia—Patients with type 2 diabetes often have a distinct triad of elevated triglyceride and low-density lipoprotein (LDL) levels with decreased HDL levels. Each of these abnormalities has been shown to be an independent factor in atherogenesis. Hydroxymethylglutaryl–coenzyme A reductase inhibitors (statins) reduce cardiovascular events by 25–37%. Current recommendations from the ADA include high-dose statin therapy for all patients with diabetes and a history of atherosclerotic CVD, multiple risk factors, or a 10-year risk > 20%. Moderate dose statins are recommended for anyone > age 40 (best evidence for ages 40–75) and those < age 40 with atherosclerotic CVD risk factors (Table 36–3). If cholesterol is ≥ 70 mg/dL with maximal tolerated statin dose, consider adding ezetimibe or a PCSK9 inhibitor. The JUPITER study suggests an increased incidence in diabetes in patients taking statins, but the outcomes are still improved. Statins are contraindicated in pregnancy and must be used with caution in adolescents. Fish oil is helpful for reducing triglycerides but does not improve outcomes.

B. Microvascular Complications

1. Nephropathy—Diabetic nephropathy is the most common cause of end-stage renal disease (ESRD) in the United States, and the rates are highest in Asian and African Americans. The incidence is much higher in type 1 diabetes, but the prevalence is higher in type 2 diabetes. Glomerular hyperfiltration is an early indication of impending deterioration, and an increase in systolic blood pressure may indicate the onset of microalbuminuria. All patients should be screened yearly with a microalbumin or a microalbumin/creatinine ratio.

Table 36–3. Moderate- and high-intensity statins (daily dosage).

Moderate-Intensity Statins	High-Intensity Statins
Atorvastatin (Lipitor) 10–20 mg	Atorvastatin 40–80 mg
Rosuvastatin (Crestor) 5–10 mg	Rosuvastatin 20–40 mg
Simvastatin (Zocor) 20–40 mg	
Pravastatin (Pravachol 40–80 mg	
Lovastatin (Mevacor) 40 mg	
Fluvastatin XL (Lescol XL) 80 mg	
Fluvastatin 40 mg twice a day	
Pitavastatin (Livalo) 2–4 mg	

Microalbuminuria is defined as 30–300 mg of protein in a 24-hour urine collection, a more accurate but cumbersome test. More than 300 mg per 24 hours constitutes macroalbuminuria or nephropathy.

ACE inhibitors are the drugs of choice for treatment of microalbuminuria. Ramipril has been shown to reduce ESRD and death by 41% and proteinuria by 20% compared with amlodipine. ARBs have comparable efficacy and should be used when the use of ACE inhibitors is limited. They are not recommended in the absence of renal disease or hypertension and should not be used in combination.

2. Retinopathy—Approximately 20% of patients with type 2 diabetes show signs of retinopathy at the time of diagnosis. Progression is orderly from mild abnormalities (small retinal hemorrhages) to proliferative retinopathy with growth of new vessels on the retina and into the vitreous culminating in vision loss. Monocular vision loss is usually from vitreous hemorrhage. The risk of retinopathy increases with increasing HbA1c and duration of disease, but African Americans develop retinopathy at lower HbA1c levels. Patients with proliferative retinopathy should not participate in highly exertional activities like power lifting. In the ACCORD trial, intensive therapy lowered retinopathy but not ultimate vision loss. Patients with type 1 diabetes may begin yearly ophthalmology visits 5 years after diagnosis, but patients with type 2 should begin office visits with diagnosis. Screening may occur every other year if normal, but any abnormality warrants at least yearly follow-up. Panretinal laser photocoagulation therapy has been the standard treatment, but invasive and subconjunctival injection of monoclonal antibodies has been shown to be noninferior. Aflibercept (Eylea) injections last about 2 months. Bevacizumab (Avastin) is the cheapest treatment and is comparable to ranibizumab (Lucentis), both lasting about 4 weeks. All treatment is an attempt to decrease vision loss.

3. Neuropathy—*Peripheral neuropathy* leads to a loss of sensation and pain in the extremities and is the major cause of foot problems in patients with diabetes. Treatment of peripheral neuropathy remains symptomatic. Pregabalin (Lyrica) and duloxetine (Cymbalta) are US Food and Drug Administration approved for treatment, but other treatment options that have efficacy data include antidepressants (amitriptyline, nortriptyline, venlafaxine), anticonvulsants (gabapentin, carbamazepine, lamotrigine, topiramate), topical capsaicin cream, botulinum toxin, lidocaine patches, and tapentadol. Opioids, tramadol, transcutaneous electrical nerve stimulation, and alternative therapies (relaxation therapy, biofeedback, α-lipoic acid, and evening primrose oil) are third-line treatments.

Autonomic neuropathy is common, and patients should be asked about symptoms of nausea, diarrhea or constipation, lightheadedness, incontinence, impotence, and heat intolerance. It is also important to check for any of the following: resting tachycardia, orthostatic hypotension, dependent edema (to assess impaired venoarteriolar reflex), and decreased diameter of dark-adapted pupil. Gastrointestinal motility may be improved with metoclopramide or erythromycin.

C. Ketoacidosis and Hyperglycemic Hyperosmolar Syndrome

Ketoacidosis occurs when there is insufficient insulin to meet the body's needs, leading to increased gluconeogenesis, fatty acid oxidation, and ketogenesis, and resulting in a high ion gap metabolic acidosis, osmotic diuresis, and dehydration. It is a leading cause of death in children, and the incidence is highest for children with poor control, inadequate insurance, or psychiatric disorders.

Treatment involves rehydration with normal saline and an intravenous insulin infusion. Potassium is replaced as it starts to fall near the upper limits of normal. Glucose is added to fluids when serum glucose approaches 250 mg/dL. Patients should be in a monitored bed, and labs should initially be drawn hourly. The insulin infusion is continued until acidosis is resolved and ketones are cleared. Subcutaneous insulin is started prior to stopping the insulin infusion.

Hyperglycemic hyperosmolar syndrome is most commonly seen in type 2 diabetes and results from a relative deficiency of insulin, leading to extremely high blood glucose levels (>600 mg/dL and often >1000 mg/dL). Because insulin is present, the production of ketone bodies is minimal, but there is a profound increase in osmolarity. Idiogenic osmoles in the brain preserve the intravascular volume but, in the presence of rapid glucose correction, can produce cerebral edema. Confusion is common and clears with correction of serum glucose. Treatment is initiated with isotonic fluid, and sugars are controlled slowly with an insulin infusion.

D. Infections

Patients with diabetes are at greater risk for infections, including community-acquired pneumonia (particularly pneumococcal), influenza, periodontal disease, cholecystitis, urinary tract infections, and pyelonephritis. Persistent fever and flank pain for more than 3–4 days despite appropriate antibiotic treatment should elicit an evaluation (preferably by computed tomography) for a perinephric abscess. Fungal infections are frequently seen, especially vaginal candidiasis, but eye and skin infections can also be present. Foot infections include cellulitis, osteomyelitis, plantar abscesses, and necrotizing fasciitis.

E. Diabetic Foot

Diabetes is the leading nontraumatic cause of foot amputation and Charcot foot in the United States, due to the combination of neuropathy, altered foot structure, and vasculopathy. Overall, 15% of patients with diabetes will have a foot ulcer, and 20% of these will lead to amputation. Native Americans have the highest rates of foot infection. Feet should be examined at every office visit and patients instructed in good foot care. Yearly examination with a 10-g monofilament is most predictive of neuropathy. Vibratory sensation and temperature or pinprick sensation should also be assessed. Medicare will pay for special shoes and the fitting of these shoes by a podiatrist or orthotist; however, careful attention to foot care by primary providers was found to be more effective at preventing ulcers than special shoes or inserts.

Treatment of diabetic foot ulcers requires removing pressure on the ulcer and good wound care with deep debridement and appropriate dressings. The best indication of ability to heal is an intact pulse, and decreased pulses or symptoms of claudication should be assessed with an ankle-brachial index. Revascularization may be necessary. Antibiotics should be used only if infection is clearly present as they have been shown to retard healing in the noninfected foot. Wound cultures almost always yield multiple organisms and are not helpful unless taken from the bone in osteomyelitis. The test of choice for diagnosis of osteomyelitis is magnetic resonance imaging, although bone scans are an alternative. Treatment efficacy can be followed by monitoring the sedimentation rate.

Pasquel FJ, Umpierrez GE. Hyperosmolar hyperglycemic state: a historic review of the clinical presentation, diagnosis, and treatment. *Diabetes Care.* 2014;37(11):3124–3131. [PMID: 25342831]

Vinik AI, Caselini CM. Guidelines in the management of diabetic nerve pain: clinical utility of pregabalin. *Diabetes Metab Syndr Obes.* 2013;6:57–78. [PMID: 23467255]

Westerberg DP. Diabetic ketoacidosis: evaluation and treatment. *Am Fam Physician.* 2013;87(5):337–346. [PMID: 23547550]

F. Other

A variety of other conditions are seen more frequently in patients with diabetes. Diabetes is associated with an increased risk of cancer of the liver, pancreas, colon, bladder, breast, and uterus (all cancers also associated with obesity and sedentary lifestyle). Fatty liver disease, hip fractures, obstructive sleep apnea, Dupuytren contracture and trigger finger, and frozen shoulder are all more common in patients with diabetes. Older patients with diabetes have a higher incidence of all-cause dementia, Alzheimer disease, and vascular dementia. Patients ≥65 years old should be screened yearly, as appropriate, for depression and dementia.

▶ Treatment

Management goals should be individualized according to the patient's age, life expectancy, and comorbid conditions. ADA recommendations are to maintain fasting glucose levels of 80–100 mg/dL. HbA1c levels of <7% have been traditionally recommended but are now individualized. Patients with a new diagnosis should attempt to keep HbA1c levels low. The American College of Endocrinology recommends a 2-hour postprandial glucose <140 mg/dL and has set a goal for HbA1c at <6.5%. Patients older than 65 and/or with long-standing diabetes may have a goal HbA1c of <8 mg/dL, and those near end of life will be liberalized to <8.5 mg/dL. An HbA1c goal of <7.5% has been established for all pediatric patients. Blood pressure should be maintained below 140/90 mmHg, but reasonable evidence suggests lower levels for most individuals.

The initial and ongoing evaluation for diabetes includes counseling regarding lifestyle and self-management including smoking cessation, goals and motivation, psychosocial issues, and compliance, family support, and self-image. Education and ownership are imperative for self-management, and include lifestyle changes, smoking cessation, home monitoring, management of blood pressure and lipids, knowledge of medications and side effects, and skin and foot care. Providers are encouraged to employ community resources and assess patients for the social determinants of health. Patients should have structured education at diagnosis, annually, when complications arise, and during transitions in care.

Every visit should include the following:

Weight and BMI

Blood pressure measurement

Funduscopic examination

Basic physical exam concentrating on cardiovascular evaluation

Brief skin examination

Visual examination of feet

Regular screening and laboratory measurements include the following:

HbA1c level every 3 months (every 6 months if usually well controlled)

Verbal or written screen for depression

Yearly dilated retinal exam to screen for retinopathy (every 2 years if normal)

Yearly microalbumin to screen for nephropathy

Yearly foot exam including monofilament, vibratory, and evaluation of pulses

Yearly fasting lipid profile

Yearly electrolytes, blood urea nitrogen, creatinine, and urinalysis

Immunizations should be updated

Use of guidelines, electronic health records, patient management systems, checklists and questionnaires, standing orders (Table 36–4), and a team approach can increase

Table 36–4. Standing orders for diabetic patients.

1. Update the electronic record or place an updated flowsheet in the patient's chart.
2. Monitor and record blood pressure in the same arm at each visit.
3. Measure and record the patient's weight and record with body mass index.
4. If hemoglobin A1c has not been evaluated in the past 6 months, order.
5. If urinalysis and microalbumin testing have not been done in the past year:
   a. Perform a urine dipstick and record the results on the flowsheet.
   b. Order a urine microalbumin test.
6. If a lipid profile has not been obtained in the past year, order.
7. If a dilated eye examination has not been performed in the past year, complete a referral for an ophthalmology examination.
8. Ask the patient to remove his/her shoes and socks.
   a. Palpate dorsalis pedis and posterior tibial pulses.
   b. Inspect the skin for any skin breakdown.
   c. Record the findings on the patient's flowsheet.
9. Check to see if patient has received a pneumococcal vaccine, a dT or Tdap vaccine in the last 10 years, or a flu shot for the current season, and has completed a hepatitis B series. If patient has not received the flu shot, administer following standard clinic protocol.

Physician Signature: _____ Date: _____

efficiency and provide more comprehensive care for patients with diabetes.

Centers for Disease Control and Prevention. CDC recommendations for hepatitis B vaccination among adults with diabetes: grading of scientific evidence in support of key recommendations. Last update August 6, 2012. http://www.cdc.gov/vaccines/acip/recs/GRADE/hepB-vac-adults-diabetes.html. Accessed November 19, 2019.

A. Nutrition

Individualization of nutrition therapy is necessary to achieve glucose and lipid goals, health, and well-being. A Mediterranean-style diet rich in monounsaturated fats is recommended with limited alcohol (7 kcal/g) and decreased fat and overall calorie intake, leading to a modest weight loss of 10–15%. When combined with abstinence from tobacco, it can lower mortality by 50%. Individuals receiving fixed daily doses of insulin should try to maintain a consistent daily caloric intake. Those on intensive insulin therapy should adjust their insulin according to the carbohydrate content of their meals. Increasing protein can counteract hypoglycemia, and the glycemic index can be helpful in choosing appropriate carbohydrates.

B. Exercise

Exercise increases strength and endurance, HDL cholesterol, and insulin sensitivity; reduces stress; improves circulation, digestion, sleep, energy levels, and self-esteem; controls appetite and reduces weight; and lowers heart rate, blood pressure, lipid levels, and blood glucose, thereby delaying the onset of diabetes and reducing the risk of CVD. Prescribe a regular exercise program, adapted to complications, for all patients, including moderate aerobic activity for 20–60 minutes most days (at least 150 min/wk) with resistance training twice a week. Children should be active at least 60 minutes a day. Older patients and those at increased risk of coronary artery disease should have a careful physical examination and an exercise stress test prior to beginning or significantly advancing an exercise program and should avoid sudden strenuous exercise. Recommendations for children include at least 1 hour of daily exercise and no more than 2 hours of non–school-related screen time daily. Athletes with type 1 diabetes may not participate in strenuous exercise when their blood glucose is >300 mg/dL or >250 mg/dL with urine ketones.

C. Weight Loss

Weight loss is best achieved with lifestyle changes including intake of fewer calories and increased exercise. The majority of patients are unable to maintain a sustained weight loss, and weight loss medications are indicated for a BMI ≥27 kg/m^2. Currently available weight loss medications are listed in Table 36–5. Recommendations call for more aggressive treatment of obesity because a 5–10% weight loss (current recommendation is 7%) can significantly delay the onset of diabetes.

Metabolic (bariatric) surgery is a recommended treatment option for patients with a BMI ≥40 kg/m^2 (or ≥37.5 kg/m^2 in Asian Americans). In observational studies, it has been shown to decrease the incidence of diabetes, with ≥75% of patients reverting to a normal HbA1c. Gastric sleeve is largely replacing laparoscopic adjustable gastric banding. Roux-en-Y surgery is most effective because it has both a restrictive and a malabsorptive component. It also requires much closer monitoring and replacement of nutrients. Surgery should be performed at high-volume centers where improved outcomes have been demonstrated.

Dixon JB, Zimmet P, Alberti KG, et al. Bariatric surgery: an IDF statement for obese type 2 diabetes. *Diabetic Med.* 2011;28(6):628–642. [PMID: 21480973]

Gropler RJ. Lost in translation: modulation of the metabolic-functional relation in the diabetic human heart. *Circulation.* 2009;119:2020–2022. [PMID: 19380631]

Kooy A, de Jager J, Lehert P, et al. Long-term effects of metformin on metabolism and microvascular and macrovascular disease in patients with type 2 diabetes mellitus. *Arch Intern Med.* 2009;169:616–625. [PMID: 19307526]

D. Home Monitoring

Although patients should learn to monitor their own glucose levels, the benefit of home monitoring for patients with reasonably controlled blood sugars disappears after 1 year. It does not improve HbA1c levels or quality of life in patients who are not using insulin. If patients are using insulin, sulfonylureas, or corticosteroids; are ill; or are changing therapy, home monitoring may be beneficial. New recommendations include home blood pressure monitoring to identify white coat syndrome and improve blood pressure control.

Table 36–5. Weight loss medications.

Drug	Dosage Range	Mechanism of Action	Advantages	Side Effects and Precautions	Cost
Orlistat (Xenical)	60 mg/d nonprescription 120 mg/d prescription	Blocks fat breakdown and absorption in intestine	Over the counter	May affect absorption of fat-soluble vitamins Flatulence and stool incontinence	Generic $
Lorcaserin (Belviq)	10 mg twice a day	5-HT$_{2c}$ receptor agonist	Promotes satiety	Dizziness, fatigue, headaches Possible serotonin syndrome if used with selective serotonin reuptake inhibitor	$$
Phentermine (Adipex)	15, 30, 37.5 mg/d	Appetite suppressant	Low cost	Short-term use only Not in hypertension	Generic $
Phentermine/ topiramate (Qsymia)	3.75/23–7.5/46 mg/d	Appetite suppressant	Long-term use Very effective	Numbness, dizziness, insomnia, constipation Contraindicated in pregnancy	$$$
Bupropion/naltrexone (Contrave)	8/90 mg twice a day	Decreases appetite and food cravings	Antidepressant effect and craving control	Increases seizure and suicide risk	$$$
Liraglutide (Saxenda)	0.6–3 mg/d subcutaneously	Glucagon-like peptide-1 receptor agonist	Effective Little central nervous system effect	Injectable	$$$

E. Pharmacologic Therapy

In type 2 diabetics with an HbA1c <9%, metformin, if tolerated, is the initial treatment. If HbA1c is >9%, consider adding another medication, and if >10%, consider adding insulin. If the patient has established CVD, consider adding an SGLT-2 (sodium-glucose cotransporter-2) inhibitor or liraglutide. If the HbA1c is not adequately controlled after 3 months, another oral medication or an injectable medication may be added. Generally, no more than three oral medications are used together, and they should have different mechanisms of action. Efficacy is variable between drugs and individuals, but expected lowering of HbA1c is 0.5–2.0%. Choices of medication should be made to maximize efficacy and minimize side effects (Table 36–6).

1. Biguanides—Metformin is the initial choice in type 2 diabetes (especially with obesity); it should be continued if possible when insulin or other oral medications are added because it reduces cardiovascular deaths and all-cause mortality. It is the only oral medication indicated in children (but not in breastfeeding).

2. Sulfonylureas—The oldest oral medications for diabetes, they can be used in patients with hepatic or renal insufficiency but cautiously in the elderly. They should be taken 1 hour before meals to induce insulin secretion or at bedtime where they limit hepatic glucose production. Approximately 20% of patients will not respond, and sulfonylureas lose efficacy over time. Glyburide has the greatest potential for hypoglycemia and cannot be used in renal failure, but it is a category B medication in pregnancy. Glimepiride has a more rapid onset and longer duration of action but induces less hypoglycemia and may be the best choice in patients with known coronary disease.

3. Meglitinides—These rapid-acting medications are taken only with meals and are useful in patients whose fasting glucose levels are well controlled but who have high postprandial values or for patients who eat few or irregular meals. Nateglinide has a more rapid onset and shorter duration of action than repaglinide.

4. Thiazolidinediones—These agents are useful as an adjunct medication or with marked insulin resistance. Pioglitazone decreases triglyceride levels by 33%, increases HDL cholesterol, and may reduce the risk for stroke after a transient ischemic attack but causes volume overload and cannot be used in significant heart failure. It may take 12 weeks for the medication to reach its maximum potential, so dosage should be increased only after several weeks.

5. α-Glucosidase inhibitors—Taken only with meals, they blunt postprandial hyperglycemia. Therapy should be initiated at a low dose and increased slowly to minimize side effects. If they are used with a sulfonylurea or insulin and hypoglycemia occurs, treatment must utilize simple sugars (glucose or lactose), not sucrose. Efficacy is altered with digestive enzymes, antacids, or cholestyramine. Serum transaminase levels must be followed every 3 months for the first year, and they must be stopped when the serum creatinine reaches 2 mg/dL.

6. Dipeptidyl peptidase-4 (DPP4) inhibitors—Glucagon-like peptide 1 (GLP-1) stimulates insulin secretion and biosynthesis and inhibits glucagon secretion and gastric emptying. It is degraded by DPP4. These inhibitors of DPP4 effectively increase GLP-1 and decrease postprandial glucose levels. They are well tolerated with once-daily dosing, but they do carry a risk for pancreatitis and a rare debilitating joint pain.

7. GLP-1 receptor agonists—These synthetic incretins are given by subcutaneous injection and carry the same warning for pancreatitis. They have a black box warning for thyroid tumors. Injections vary from twice a week to weekly. Daily liraglutide is also licensed in a larger dose as a weight loss medication. They all increase insulin in response to glucose at meals, promote satiety, slow gastric emptying, and may lead to significant weight loss.

8. SGLT-2 inhibitors—SGLT-2 inhibitors reduce the reabsorption of filtered glucose in the kidney and lower the reabsorption concentration at the proximal tubule, causing more excretion of glucose in the urine. They also induce weight reduction and lower systolic blood pressure with improved cardiovascular outcomes. But they also can induce postural hypotension and ketoacidosis and have a black box warning for increased amputations.

9. Combination therapy—Combining drugs with different mechanisms of action is most efficacious, but caution must be exercised in combining drugs with similar side effects (thiazolidinediones and α-glucosidase inhibitors are both hepatotoxic). Metformin can be combined with any of the other medications, and there are now multiple commercial combinations of metformin, thiazolidinediones, sulfonylureas, DPP4 inhibitors, and SGLT-2 inhibitors.

George CM, Bruijn LL, Will K, et al. Management of blood glucose with noninsulin therapies in type 2 diabetes. *Am Fam Physician.* 2015;92(1):27–34. [PMID: 26132124]

Gourgari E, Wilhelm EE, Hassanzadeh H, et al. A comprehensive review of the FDA-approved labels of diabetes drugs: indications, safety, and emerging cardiovascular safety data. *J Diabetes Complications.* 2017;31:1719–1727. [PMID: 28939018]

Zheng SL, Roddick AJ, Aghar-Jaffar R, et al. Association between use of sodium-glucose cotransporter 2 inhibitors, glucagon-like peptide 1 agonists, and dipeptidyl peptidase 4 inhibitors with all-cause mortality in patients with type 2 diabetes. *JAMA.* 2018;319(15):1580–1591. [PMID: 29677303]

Table 36–6. Medications for the treatment of diabetes.

Drug	Dosage Range (mg/d)	Mechanism of Action	Advantages	Side Effects and Precautions	Cost
Biguanides Metformin (Glucophage) Metformin XR (Glucophage XR)	Daily or BID 500–2500 500–2000	↓ gluconeogenesis in liver ↑ insulin sensitivity	Decreases mortality No hypoglycemia Lowers insulin levels Possible weight loss Improves lipids and endothelial function Category B in pregnancy Can be used in children	Nausea and diarrhea Hold before and after IV contrast Stop if GFR <30 and do not initiate if <45 Caution with heart failure and hepatic dysfunction Vitamin B_{12} deficiency	Generic $
Sulfonylureas Glipizide (Glucotrol) Glipizide XL (Glucotrol XL) Glyburide (DiaBeta, Micronase) Glyburide, micronized (Glynase) Glimepiride (Amaryl)	Daily or BID 5–40 2.5–20 2.5–20 1–8 1–6	Induce insulin secretion from pancreatic β cells	Can be used in renal (except glyburide) or hepatic failure	Hypoglycemia Weight gain	Generic $
Meglitinides Repaglinide (Prandin) Nateglinide (Starlix)	TID dosing 1.5–16 180–360	Induce secretion of insulin from pancreatic β cells	Rapid onset and short half-life; can use in renal insufficiency	Caution in hepatic insufficiency	$$
Thiazolidinedione Pioglitazone (Actos) Rosiglitazone (Avandia)	Daily dosing 15–45 4–5	Primarily insulin sensitizers in muscle and adipose tissue ↓ gluconeogenesis in the liver	May prevent stroke after TIA	Black box warning: do not use in class III or IV heart failure Monitor LFTs Risk of bladder cancer Distal limb fractures in women Not for use in pregnancy	$
SGLT-2 inhibitor Canagliflozin (Invokana) Dapagliflozin (Farxiga) Empagliflozin (Jardiance)	Daily dosing 100–300 5–10	Block renal reabsorption of glucose, causing urinary excretion	Weight loss Decreased mortality	Orthostatic hypotension, urinary tract and vaginal yeast infections May induce ketoacidosis Contraindicated with GFR <30 Black box warning for risk of amputation (canagliflozin)	$$$
α-Glucosidase inhibitors Acarbose (Precose) Miglitol (Glyset)	TID dosing 75–300 75–300	Inhibit breakdown of disaccharides and delay carbohydrate absorption in brush border of small intestine	No hypoglycemia	Flatulence Cannot use with GI disorders, cirrhosis, Cr >2 mg/dL	$$
DPP4 inhibitor Sitagliptin (Januvia) Saxagliptin (Onglyza) Linagliptin (Tradjenta) Alogliptin (Nesina)	Daily dosing 100 (25–50 renal impairment) 2.5–5 5 (long half-life) 25–400	Block the breakdown of natural incretins	No hypoglycemia Lowers postprandial glucose	Nausea and vomiting Must decrease dose in renal impairment (except linagliptin) No improved outcomes data Rare debilitating joint pain	$$$
GLP-1 receptor agonists Exenatide (Byetta) Liraglutide (Victoza) Albiglutide (Tanzeum) Dulaglutide (Trulicity) Lixisenatide (Adlyxin) **Synthetic amylin** Pramlintide (Symlin)	All subcutaneous 5–10 µg (or 70 µg/wk) 0.6–1.8 µg 30–50 mg/wk 0.75–15 mg/wk 10-20 µg 15–120 µg	Enhance glucose-dependent insulin secretion Suppress inappropriate glucagon secretion and slow gastric emptying	Early satiety and weight loss Improved cardiovascular outcomes (liraglutide)	Nausea, vomiting, diarrhea Hemorrhagic or necrotizing pancreatitis Black box warning for thyroid C-cell tumor Contraindicated with GFR <30 (except liraglutide) Category C in pregnancy Severe hypoglycemia	$$$

BID, twice a day; Cr, creatinine; GFR, glomerular filtration rate; GI, gastrointestinal; GLP-1, glucagon-like peptide-1; IV, intravenous; LFT, liver function test; TIA, transient ischemic attack; TID, 3 times a day.

10. Insulin—The United Kingdom Prospective Diabetes Study (UKPDS) did not show any increase in CVD due to the use of insulin but did demonstrate a significant improvement in all complications of diabetes with tight control. A long-acting insulin provides a basal rate that minimizes hepatic glucose production. A rapid-acting insulin is used with meals to minimize the postprandial insulin peak.

The synthetic insulins, lispro, aspart, and glulisine, have a short onset, rapid peak, and 2- to 4-hour duration of action, more closely mimicking the pharmacokinetics of human insulin in vivo (Table 36–7). They are preferred over regular insulin with its slower onset and longer duration of action, necessitating regular snacking. Inhaled insulin, with pharmacokinetics similar to the rapid-acting insulins, has returned to the market. The long-acting insulin analogs glargine, detemir, and degludec are relatively peakless insulins with a consistent 24-hour duration. They are less soluble in subcutaneous tissue, prolong absorption, and can be used with oral medications or with any of the short-acting insulins (but not mixed in the same syringe). They are usually taken once a day but may be divided into two doses (especially helpful when giving >100 U). Neutral protamine Hagedorn (NPH) insulin has a duration of <24 hours, necessitating twice-daily dosing, with peaks occurring in the afternoon and early morning. Dosage changes are made based on fingersticks taken approximately 8 hours following the dose. Its primary utility lies in its low cost or when used with a rapid-acting insulin in a 70/30 premix for twice-a-day dosing.

In type 2 diabetes, insulin is generally initiated as a daily basal dose, starting at 10 U/d or 0.1–0.2 U/kg/d. If the HbA1c is not controlled, there are three options:

Add a rapid-acting insulin (4 units or 0.1 U/kg) before the largest meal

Add a GLP-1 receptor agonist

Change to premixed insulin twice daily (two-thirds in morning and one-third in evening or half in morning and half in evening)

If goals are still unmet, the rapid-acting insulin can be increased to every meal or the premixed insulin can also be given at noon.

When initiating insulin therapy in type 1 diabetics, the total insulin requirement for 24 hours should be estimated. Half of this amount may be given as a long-acting insulin and the other half as a rapid-acting insulin. Adjustments in the long-acting insulin dosage are based primarily on fasting glucose levels. The rapid-acting portion can be divided, with 40% given before breakfast, 40% before dinner, and the remaining 20% prior to lunch. It should then be adjusted according to caloric intake and resulting postprandial fingerstick glucose levels.

Bioavailability with insulin changes with the site of injection, with the abdomen being the fastest. It is recommended that injections be rotated within the same area.

Insulin pumps allow for continuous use of short-acting insulin with a more consistent absorption rate. Half of the insulin is given continuously as a basal dose, and the other half is divided into mealtime boluses. Many are now used in conjunction with continuous glucose monitoring. They allow for a more normal lifestyle with fewer episodes of severe hypoglycemia, a reduction of total insulin usage, and less weight gain. Particularly good candidates for insulin pump therapy are patients who are difficult to control or have wide glucose swings, have erratic schedules, or have a significant dawn phenomenon; pregnant women and teenagers with poor control and/or frequent episodes of ketoacidosis are also good candidates.

Table 36–7. Available insulins.

Drug	Onset of Action	Peak (hours)	Duration (hours)	Cost
Rapid-acting				
Lispro (Humalog)	15 minutes	0.5–1.5	2–4	$$
Aspart (NovoLog)	15 minutes	1–3	3–5	$$
Glulisine (Apidra)	15 minutes	1–1.5	5	$$$
Inhaled insulin (Afrezza)	12–15 minutes	<1	2–5	$$$
Short-acting				
Regular (Humulin)	30 minutes	2–4	5.8	$
Intermediate				
NPH (Novolin)	1–3 hours	5–7	16–18	$
Long-acting				
Glargine (Lantus)	1 hour	None	24	$$
Detemir (Levemir)	1 hour	6–8 (minimal)	20	$$$
Degludec (Tresiba)	1 hour	None	>24	$$$

NPH, neutral protamine Hagedorn.

▶ Prognosis

The risk of premature death in patients with diabetes is twice that of the general population. Overall, 15% of patients with type 1 diabetes will die before age 40, which is 20 times the rate of the general population. Patients with type 1 diabetes die from ketoacidosis, renal failure, and coronary artery disease. Individuals who develop type 2 diabetes after age 40 have a decreased life expectancy of 5–10 years, and 80% of all patients with type 2 diabetes die from cardiovascular causes. The prognosis improves with significant lifestyle change, control of blood sugar and blood pressure, and smoking cessation.

American Diabetes Association's Standards of Medical Care in Diabetes—2018. *Diabetes Care.* 2018;41(suppl 1):S1–S159. [No PMID]
National Institute of Diabetes and Digestive and Kidney Diseases. http://www2.niddk.nih.gov/. Accessed November 18, 2019.

Websites

American Diabetes Association (ADA). http://www.diabetes.org/
Centers for Disease Control and Prevention (CDC), Division of Diabetes. https://www.cdc.gov/diabetes/index.html
Joslin Diabetes Center. http://www.joslin.org/
National Diabetes Education Program. http://www.ndep.nih.gov/

Endocrine Disorders

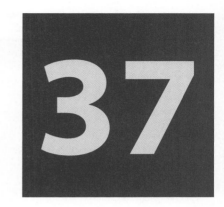

Pamela Allweiss, MD, MSPH

Peter J. Carek, MD, MS

▼ THYROID DISORDERS

Thyroid disorders affect approximately 1 in 200 adults but are more common in women and with advancing age. About 4.6% of people have hypothyroidism, and about 1.2% have hyperthyroidism. Hypothyroidism is much more common than hyperthyroidism, nodular disease, or thyroid cancer. Epidemiologic studies have shown the prevalence of palpable thyroid nodules to be approximately 5% in women and 1% in men living in iodine-sufficient parts of the world. High-resolution ultrasound, however, may detect thyroid nodules in 19–68% of randomly selected people. Nodules are more common in women and the elderly.

Thyroid disease is more common in people who have conditions such as diabetes or other autoimmune diseases (eg, lupus); in those with a family history of thyroid disease or a history of head and neck irradiation; and in patients who use certain medications, including amiodarone and lithium.

National Institute of Diabetes and Digestive and Kidney Diseases. Hyperthyroidism. https://www.niddk.nih.gov/health-information/endocrine-diseases/hyperthyroidism. Accessed November 19, 2019.

National Institute of Diabetes and Digestive and Kidney Diseases. Hypothyroidism. https://www.niddk.nih.gov/health-information/endocrine-diseases/hypothyroidism. Accessed November 19, 2019.

HYPOTHYROIDISM

▶ General Considerations

Causes of hypothyroidism are outlined in Table 37–1. The most common noniatrogenic condition causing hypothyroidism in the United States is Hashimoto thyroiditis. Other common causes are post–Graves disease, thyroid irradiation, and surgical removal of the thyroid. Hypothyroidism may also occur secondary to hypothalamic or pituitary dysfunction, most commonly in patients who have received intracranial irradiation or surgical removal of a pituitary adenoma. In addition, some patients may have mild elevations of thyroid-stimulating hormone (TSH) despite normal thyroxine levels, a condition termed *subclinical hypothyroidism.*

▶ Clinical Findings

A. Symptoms and Signs

Patients with hypothyroidism present with a constellation of symptoms that can involve every organ system. Symptoms include lethargy, weight gain, hair loss, dry skin, slowed mentation or forgetfulness, depressed affect, cold intolerance, constipation, hair loss, muscle weakness, abnormal menstrual periods (or infertility), and fluid retention. Because of the range of symptoms seen in hypothyroidism, clinicians must have a high index of suspicion, especially in high-risk populations. In older patients, hypothyroidism can be confused with Alzheimer disease or other conditions that cause dementia. In women, hypothyroidism is often confused with depression.

Physical findings that can occur with hypothyroidism include low blood pressure, bradycardia, nonpitting edema, generalized hair thinning along with hair loss in the outer third of the eyebrows, skin drying, and a diminished relaxation phase of reflexes. The thyroid gland in a patient with chronic thyroiditis may be enlarged, atrophic, or of normal size. Thyroid nodules are common in patients with Hashimoto thyroiditis.

B. Laboratory Findings

The most valuable test for hypothyroidism is the sensitive TSH assay. Measurement of the free thyroxine (T_4) level may also be helpful. TSH is elevated and free T_4 decreased in overt hypothyroidism (Table 37–2). Other laboratory findings may include hyperlipidemia and hyponatremia. Hashimoto

Table 37–1. Causes of hypothyroidism.

Primary hypothyroidism (95% of cases)
Idiopathic hypothyroidism (probably old Hashimoto thyroiditis)
Hashimoto thyroiditis
Postthyroid irradiation
Postsurgical
Late-stage invasive fibrous thyroiditis
Iodine deficiency
Drugs (lithium, interferon)
Infiltrative diseases (sarcoidosis, amyloid, scleroderma, hemochromatosis)
Secondary hypothyroidism (5% of cases)
Pituitary or hypothalamic neoplasms
Congenital hypopituitarism
Pituitary necrosis (Sheehan syndrome)

thyroiditis, an autoimmune condition, is one of the most common causes of hypothyroidism. Testing for thyroid autoantibodies (antiperoxidase, antithyroglobulin) is positive in 95% of patients with Hashimoto thyroiditis.

Patients with subclinical hypothyroidism have a high TSH level (usually in the 5–10 mIU/mL range) in conjunction with normal free T_4 level. Between 3% and 20% of these patients will eventually develop overt hypothyroidism. Patients who test positive for thyroid antibodies are at increased risk.

▶ **Treatment**

In patients with primary hypothyroidism, therapy should begin with thyroid hormone replacement, usually L-thyroxine. In patients with secondary hypothyroidism, further investigation with provocative testing of the pituitary can be performed to determine whether the cause is a hypothalamic or pituitary problem.

Most healthy adult patients with hypothyroidism require 1.6 µg/kg of thyroid replacement, with requirements falling to 1 µg/kg for the elderly. The initial dosage may range from 12.5 µg to a full replacement dose of 100–150 µg of L-thyroxine. Doses will vary depending on age, weight, cardiac status, duration, and severity of the hypothyroidism. Therapy should be titrated after at least 6 weeks following any change in levothyroxine dose. The serum TSH level is the most important measure to gauge the dose.

Treatment of subclinical hypothyroidism remains controversial. Subclinical hypothyroidism is characterized by a serum TSH above the upper reference limit in combination with a normal free thyroxine (T_4) at a time when thyroid function has been stable for several weeks, the hypothalamic-pituitary-thyroid axis is normal, and there is no recent or ongoing severe illness. The prevalence of subclinical hypothyroidism is 5–10% more common in white older women. The American Association of Clinical Endocrinologists (AACE) guidelines suggest treating patients with TSH levels of >10 mIU/mL as well as those with TSH levels between 5 and 10 mIU/mL in conjunction with goiter or positive antithyroid peroxidase antibodies, or both (level of evidence for American Thyroid Association recommendations: level 3 or 4, clinical consensus based on the literature). Others base any therapeutic intervention on the individual situation (eg, pregnancy status, cardiovascular risk factors).

Once the TSH level reaches the normal range, the frequency of testing can be decreased. Each patient's regimen must be individualized, but the usual follow-up after TSH is stable is at 6 months; the history and physical examination should be repeated on a routine basis thereafter.

Thyroid hormone absorption can be affected by malabsorption, age, and concomitant medications such as cholestyramine, ferrous sulfate, sucralfate, calcium, and some antacids containing aluminum hydroxide. Drugs such as anticonvulsants affect thyroid hormone binding, whereas others such as rifampin and sertraline hydrochloride may accelerate levothyroxine metabolism, necessitating a higher replacement dose. The thyroid dose may also need to be

Table 37–2. Laboratory changes in hypothyroidism.

TSH	Free T₄	Free T₃	Likely Diagnosis
High	Low	Low	Primary hypothyroidism
High (>10 µIU/mL)	Normal	Normal	Not consistent with the American Association of Clinical Endocrinologists guideline mentioned previously; subclinical hypothyroidism with high risk for future development of overt hypothyroidism
High (6–10 µIU/mL)	Normal	Normal	Subclinical hypothyroidism with low risk for future development of overt hypothyroidism
High	High	Low	Congenital absence of T_4/T_3-converting enzyme or amiodarone effect
High	High	High	Peripheral thyroid hormone resistance
Low	Low	Low	Pituitary thyroid deficiency or recent withdrawal of thyroid replacement after excessive replacement

T_3, triiodothyronine; T_4, thyroxine; TSH, thyroid-stimulating hormone.

adjusted during pregnancy. There has been some interest in using a combination of T_4 and triiodothyronine (T_3) or natural thyroid preparations in pregnant women with hypothyroidism, but studies to date have been small and findings inconsistent.

Pregnant women with thyroid dysfunction need close attention. Overt maternal hypothyroidism is known to have serious adverse effects on the fetus. The American Thyroid Association has developed practice guidelines that address the management of thyroid dysfunction during pregnancy and postpartum.

American Association of Clinical Endocrinologists, American Thyroid Association. Clinical practice guidelines for hypothyroidism in adults. *Endocr Pract*. 2012;18:989–1027. [PMID: 23246686]

American Thyroid Association. Guidelines for the diagnosis and management of thyroid disease during pregnancy and the postpartum. *Thyroid*. 2017;27(3):315–389. [PMID: 28056690]

American Thyroid Association Task Force on Thyroid Hormone Replacement. Guidelines for the treatment of hypothyroidism. *Thyroid*. 2014;24(12):1670–1751. [PMID: 25266247]

Franklyn J. The thyroid—too much and too little across the ages. *Clin Endocrinol*. 2013;78(1):1–8. [PMID: 22891671]

Johnson J, Duick D. Diabetes and thyroid disease: a likely combination. *Diabetes Spectrum*. 2002;15:140–142. [No PMID]

Surks MI, Ortiz E, Daniels GH, et al. Subclinical thyroid disease: scientific review and guidelines for diagnosis and management. *JAMA*. 2004;291:228–238. [PMID: 14722150]

HYPERTHYROIDISM

▶ General Considerations

Hyperthyroidism has several causes. The most common is toxic diffuse goiter (Graves disease), an autoimmune disorder caused by thyrotropin receptor antibodies (TRAbs) that stimulate the TSH receptor, increasing thyroid hormone production and release. Other causes include toxic adenoma; toxic multinodular goiter; painful subacute thyroiditis; silent thyroiditis, including lymphocytic and postpartum thyroiditis; iodine-induced hyperthyroidism (eg, related to amiodarone therapy); oversecretion of pituitary TSH; trophoblastic disease (very rare); and excess exogenous thyroid hormone secretion.

▶ Clinical Findings

A. Symptoms and Signs

Patients with hyperthyroidism usually present with progressive nervousness, tremor, palpitations, weight loss, dyspnea on exertion, fatigue, difficulty concentrating, heat intolerance, and frequent bowel movements or diarrhea. Physical findings include a rapid pulse and elevated blood pressure, with the systolic pressure increasing to a greater extent than the diastolic pressure, creating a wide pulse-pressure hypertension. Exophthalmos (in patients with Graves disease), muscle weakness, sudden paralysis, dependent low extremity edema, or pretibial myxedema may also be present. Cardiac arrhythmias such as atrial fibrillation may be evident on physical examination or electrocardiogram, and a resting tremor may be noted on physical examination.

In patients with subacute thyroiditis, symptoms of hyperthyroidism are generally transient and resolve in a matter of weeks. There may be a recent history of a head and neck infection, fever, and severe neck tenderness. Postpartum thyroiditis may occur in the first few months after delivery. Both types of thyroiditis may have a transient hyperthyroid phase, a euthyroid phase, and occasionally a later hypothyroid phase.

B. Laboratory and Imaging Evaluation

Serum TSH measurement should be used as the initial screening test since it has the highest sensitivity and specificity of any single blood test used in the evaluation of suspected thyrotoxicosis. Confirmatory tests at the initial evaluation if there is a high suspicion of hyperthyroidism in addition to a TSH may include free T_4, and total T_3. In overt hyperthyroidism, serum free T_4, T_3, or both are elevated, and serum TSH is subnormal (usually <0.01 mU/L in a third-generation assay). In mild hyperthyroidism, serum T_4 and free T_4 may be normal, and only serum T_3 may be elevated, and serum TSH will be low or undetectable, a condition called T_3 toxicosis, which may indicate the earliest stages of hyperthyroidism caused by Graves disease or an autonomously functioning thyroid nodule. TRAbs may be used to diagnose Graves disease.

Once hyperthyroidism is identified, radionucleotide uptake and scanning of the thyroid, preferably with iodine-123, are useful to determine whether hyperthyroidism is secondary to Graves disease, an autonomous nodule, or thyroiditis (ie, by showing activity and anatomy of the thyroid). In scans of patients with Graves disease, there is increased uptake on radionucleotide imaging with diffuse hyperactivity. In contrast, nodules demonstrate limited areas of uptake with surrounding hypoactivity, and in subacute thyroiditis, uptake is patchy and decreased overall. Recent exposure (past 1–2 months) to iodinated contrast or ingestion of a diet high in iodine such as kelp or iodine supplements may also cause low iodine uptake.

▶ Complications

Thyroid storm represents an acute hypermetabolic state associated with the sudden release of large amounts of thyroid hormone. This occurs most often in Graves disease but can occur in acute thyroiditis. Individuals with thyroid storm present with confusion, fever, restlessness, and sometimes psychosis-like symptoms. Physical examination shows tachycardia, elevated blood pressure, and sometimes fever.

Cardiac dysrhythmias may be present or develop. Patients will have other signs of high-output heart failure (dyspnea on exertion, peripheral vasoconstriction) and may exhibit signs of cardiac or cerebral ischemia. Thyroid storm is a medical crisis requiring prompt attention and reversal of the metabolic demands from the acute hyperthyroidism.

▶ Treatment

β-Adrenergic blockade is recommended in all patients with symptomatic thyrotoxicosis, especially elderly patients and thyrotoxic patients with resting heart rates in excess of 90 bpm or coexistent cardiovascular disease.

A. Treatment of Graves Disease

Patients with Graves disease may be treated with radioactive iodine (RAI) therapy, antithyroid drugs (ATDs), or surgery depending on the patient's comorbidities and age.

RAI therapy would be appropriate in women planning a pregnancy in the future (>6 months after RAI administration, provided thyroid hormone levels are normal), individuals with increased surgical risk, patients with prior neck surgery, and patients with contraindications to ATDs or who have a history of not achieving a remission with prior use of ATDs.

Pretreatment with methimazole prior to RAI therapy for Graves disease should be considered in patients who are at increased risk for complications due to worsening of hyperthyroidism. Methimazole should be discontinued 2–3 days prior to RAI and then resumed 3–7 days after RAI administration.

Iodine-131 (^{131}I) has also been used on an individual basis in patients <20 years old. To date, studies have shown no evidence of adverse effects on fertility, congenital malformations, or increased risk of cancer in women who were treated with RAI during their childbearing years or in their offspring. Patients should be advised to postpone pregnancy for at least 6 months after ablation therapy.

RAI should not be used in breastfeeding mothers. There is also concern that the administration of RAI in patients with active ophthalmopathy may accelerate progression of eye disease. For this reason, some experts initially treat Graves disease with oral suppressive therapy until the ophthalmologic disease has stabilized.

ATDs are well tolerated and successful at blocking the production and release of thyroid hormone in patients with Graves disease. These drugs work by blocking the organification of iodine. ATDs would be preferred in patients who may be more likely to have a remission (people, especially women, with mild disease, small goiters, and negative or low-titer TRAb); pregnant patients; the elderly or others with increased surgical risk or with limited life expectancy; individuals in nursing homes or other care facilities who may have limited longevity and are unable to follow radiation safety regulations; and patients with a history of prior neck surgery. Methimazole is the drug of choice except during the first trimester of pregnancy when propylthiouracil is preferred, in the treatment of thyroid storm, and in patients with minor reactions to methimazole who refuse RAI therapy or surgery. Side effects include rash and rare but serious allergic/toxic events such as agranulocytosis, vasculitis, or hepatic damage. Patients need a baseline complete blood count, including white blood cell count with differential, and a liver profile including bilirubin and transaminases before starting ATD therapy for Graves disease.

Surgery may be preferred in women planning a pregnancy in <6 months provided thyroid hormone levels are normal (possibly before thyroid hormone levels are normal if RAI is chosen as therapy); patients with symptomatic compression or large goiters (≥80 g); patients with relatively low uptake of RAI; if thyroid malignancy is documented or suspected; or patients with large thyroid nodules (>4 cm), coexisting hyperparathyroidism requiring surgery, or moderate to severe active Graves orbitopathy.

B. Therapy for Toxic Multinodular Goiter or Toxic Adenoma

Therapies for toxic multinodular goiter or toxic adenoma include RAI therapy or surgery depending on individual patient factors such as clinical and demographic characteristics.

C. Treatment of Thyroid Storm

For patients with thyroid storm, aggressive initial therapy is essential to prevent complications. Treatment should include the administration of high doses of propylthiouracil (100 mg every 6 hours) to quickly block thyroid release and reduce peripheral conversion of T_4 to T_3. In addition, high doses of β-blockers (propranolol, 1–5 mg intravenously or 20–80 mg orally every 4 hours) can be used to control tachycardia and other peripheral symptoms of thyrotoxicosis. Hydrocortisone (200–300 mg/d) is used to prevent possible adrenal crisis.

D. Post–Radioactive Iodine Therapy Follow-Up

Follow-up is necessary to evaluate possible hypothyroidism after ablation. Follow-up can begin 6 weeks after therapy and continue on a regular basis until there is evidence of early hypothyroidism, as confirmed by an elevated TSH level. Therapy should then be started as described earlier in the discussion of hypothyroidism.

American Thyroid Association. Guidelines for diagnosis and management of hyperthyroidism and other causes of thyrotoxicosis. *Thyroid.* 2016;26(10):1343–1421. [PMID: 21510801]

American Thyroid Association. Guidelines for the diagnosis and management of thyroid disease during pregnancy and the postpartum. *Thyroid.* 2017;27(3):315–389. [PMID: 28056690]

THYROID NODULES

General Considerations

Thyroid nodules are a common clinical finding. Palpable nodules may be discovered on a routine physical examination. Other nonpalpable or "incidental" thyroid nodules may be discovered by ultrasound or other imaging studies for the evaluation of either thyroid or nonthyroid neck conditions. By age 60, about one-half of all people have a thyroid nodule that can be found either through examination or with imaging. Thyroid nodules are more common in the elderly, patients with a history of head and neck irradiation, and those with a history of iodine deficiency. Over 85% of nodules are benign; only 7–15% are malignant.

Pathogenesis

Thyroid nodules may be associated with benign or malignant conditions. Benign causes include multinodular goiter, Hashimoto thyroiditis, simple or hemorrhagic cysts, follicular adenomas, and subacute thyroiditis. Malignant causes include carcinoma (papillary, follicular, Hürthle cell, medullary, or anaplastic), primary thyroid lymphoma, and metastatic malignant lesions.

Clinical Findings

A. Symptoms and Signs

Many patients with thyroid nodules are asymptomatic. Often the nodule is discovered incidentally on physical examination or by imaging studies ordered for unrelated reasons. Evaluation is needed to rule out malignancy. A thorough history should be obtained, including any history of benign or malignant thyroid disease (see sections on hyper- and hypothyroidism, earlier) and head or neck irradiation. Patients should be asked about recent pregnancy, characteristics of the nodule, and any neck symptoms (eg, pain, rate of swelling, hoarseness, swelling of lymph nodes).

Several features of the history are associated with an increased risk of malignancy in a thyroid nodule. These include prior head and neck irradiation, family history of medullary carcinoma or multiple endocrine neoplasia syndrome type 2, age <20 years or >70 years, and rapid growth of a nodule. Physical findings that should raise clinical suspicion of malignancy include firm consistency, cervical lymphadenopathy, and symptoms such as persistent hoarseness, dysphonia, dysphagia, or dyspnea.

B. Laboratory and Diagnostic Findings

The American Thyroid Association has released guidelines on evaluating thyroid nodules. Laboratory and diagnostic evaluation relies on ultrasound, measurement of TSH level, and fine-needle aspiration (FNA).

1. Serum thyrotropin (TSH) should be measured during the initial evaluation of a patient with a thyroid nodule. If the serum TSH is subnormal, which may indicate hyperthyroidism, a radionuclide (preferably iodine-123) thyroid scan should be performed.

2. Diagnostic thyroid/neck ultrasound should be performed in all patients with a suspected thyroid nodule, nodular goiter, or radiographic abnormality suggesting a thyroid nodule incidentally detected on another imaging study such as computed tomography (CT) or magnetic resonance imaging (MRI) or thyroidal uptake on ^{18}F fluorodeoxyglucose–positron emission tomography scan. If the serum TSH is normal or elevated, a radionuclide scan should not be performed as the initial imaging evaluation.

The guidelines focus on the use of the sonographic risk pattern, followed by size to help guide which nodules should undergo FNA biopsy and which nodules do not need biopsy. There are five basic malignancy risk patterns ranging from 1 (high suspicion) to 5 (benign).

High-risk ultrasound features include solid hypoechoic nodule or solid hypoechoic component of a partially cystic nodule *with* one or more of the following features: irregular margins (infiltrative, microlobulated), microcalcifications, taller than wide shape, or rim calcifications with small extrusive soft tissue. An FNA should be done on all high-risk nodules ≥1 cm.

Low-risk features include purely cystic without any solid component. This would be considered benign, and an FNA biopsy is not indicated.

Generally, only nodules >1 cm should be evaluated, since they have a greater potential to be clinically significant cancers. Occasionally, there may be nodules <1 cm that require further evaluation because of clinical symptoms or associated lymphadenopathy. In very rare cases, some nodules <1 cm lack these sonographic and clinical warning signs yet may nonetheless cause future morbidity and mortality

If FNA reveals malignant cells, surgical intervention is indicated, and further treatment will be based on the characteristics noted at surgery (eg, pathologic findings, positive lymph nodes).

Treatment

Patients with malignant thyroid nodules should be referred to surgical and medical oncologists familiar with the management of these tumors.

Patients with very large nodules may require surgery, especially if symptoms secondary to the size (eg, dysphagia) are present. If there is a change in size of the nodule, a repeat FNA should be performed.

Ultrasound-guided percutaneous ethanol injection (PEI) is a therapeutic option for patients with benign nodules that have a large fluid component (thyroid cysts). Aspiration (eg, during FNA) itself may drain a cyst and shrink the size, but recurrences are common. Surgery is sometimes needed if the cyst is very large. Some data show that PEI is more effective in decreasing the size of a nodule than aspiration alone.

American Thyroid Association. Management guidelines for adult patients with thyroid nodules and differentiated thyroid cancer. *Thyroid*. 2016;26(1):1–133. [PMID: 26462967]

Haugen B. 2015 American Thyroid Association management guidelines for adult patients with thyroid nodules and differentiated thyroid cancer: what is new and what has changed. *Cancer*. 2017;123:372–381. [PMID: 27741354]

Knox M. Thyroid nodules. *Am Fam Physician*. 2013;88(3): 193–196. [PMID: 23939698]

Nabhan F, Ringel MD. Thyroid nodules and cancer management guidelines: comparisons and controversies. *Endocr Relat Cancer*. 2017;24(2):R13–R26. [PMID: 27965276]

▼ ADRENAL DISORDERS

ADRENAL INSUFFICIENCY

▶ General Considerations

The most common cause of primary adrenal insufficiency is autoimmune adrenalitis (Addison disease). Other possible causes include infections and diseases that impact adrenal structure and function. Secondary adrenal insufficiency may result from pituitary or hypothalamic disease. Iatrogenic tertiary adrenal insufficiency caused by suppression of hypothalamic-pituitary-adrenal function secondary to glucocorticoid administration is a more common secondary cause of adrenal insufficiency (Table 37–3).

▶ Clinical Findings

A. Symptoms and Signs

Adrenal insufficiency presents with a wide range of symptoms and signs, including weakness, malaise, anorexia, hyperpigmentation (especially of the gingival mucosa, scars, and skin creases), vitiligo, postural hypotension, abdominal pain, nausea and vomiting, diarrhea, constipation, myalgia, and arthralgia. The most specific sign of primary adrenal insufficiency is hyperpigmentation of the skin and mucosal surfaces. Another specific symptom of adrenal insufficiency is a craving for salt. Autoimmune adrenal disease can be accompanied by other autoimmune endocrine deficiencies, such as thyroid disease, diabetes mellitus, pernicious anemia, hypoparathyroidism, and ovarian failure.

In acute adrenal failure, adrenal crisis occurs. Adrenal crisis is characterized by hypotension, bradycardia, fever,

Table 37–3. Causes of adrenal insufficiency.

Primary
Autoimmune adrenalitis
Infectious (tuberculosis, AIDS, fungal, syphilis)
Hemorrhage, necrosis, or thrombosis
Metastatic carcinoma
Infiltration (primary adrenal lymphoma, amyloidosis, hemochromatosis)
Drug induced (anticoagulants, ketoconazole, fluconazole, phenobarbital, phenytoin)
Genetic disorders
Secondary
Pituitary or metastatic tumor
Craniopharyngioma
Pituitary surgery or radiation
Lymphocytic hypophysitis
Sarcoidosis
Histiocytosis
Empty sella syndrome
Hypothalamic tumors
Long-term glucocorticoid therapy
Postpartum pituitary necrosis (Sheehan syndrome)
Necrosis or bleeding into pituitary macroadenoma
Head trauma, lesions of the pituitary stalk
Pituitary or adrenal surgery for Cushing syndrome

AIDS, acquired immunodeficiency syndrome.
(Data from Oelkers W: Adrenal insufficiency. *N Engl J Med*. 1996 Oct 17; 335(16):1206–1212 and Charmandari E, Nicolaides NC, Chrousos GP: Adrenal insufficiency. *Lancet*. 2014 Jun 21;383(9935):2152–2167.)

hypoglycemia, and a progressive deterioration in mental status. Abdominal pain, vomiting, and diarrhea also may be present. In the patient with spontaneous adrenal insufficiency, acute adrenal hemorrhage and adrenal vein thrombosis should be considered.

B. Laboratory Findings

Laboratory abnormalities occur in nearly all patients and include hyponatremia, hyperkalemia, acidosis, slightly elevated plasma creatinine concentrations, hypoglycemia, hypercalcemia, mild normocytic anemia, lymphocytosis, and mild eosinophilia. The diagnosis of adrenal insufficiency relies on a finding of inadequate cortisol production. Plasma cortisol concentration fluctuates throughout the day in a diurnal pattern that is normally high in the early morning and low in the late afternoon. Cortisol levels also increase with stress. A low plasma cortisol level of <3 μ/dL (<83 nmol/L) either in the morning or at a time of stress provides presumptive evidence of adrenal insufficiency. Conversely, a level of ≥20 μg/dL (≥550 nmol/L) rules out adrenal insufficiency. An intermediate plasma cortisol level of 3–19 μg/dL (83–525 nmol/L) is not diagnostic.

For most patients in whom adrenal insufficiency is considered, a corticotropin stimulation test should be performed. In this test, a low dose of corticotropin (250 μg for adults and children ≥2 years of age, 15 μg/kg for infants, and 125 μg for children <2 years of age) is given, and the patient's blood is tested 30–60 minutes later to confirm a corresponding increase in plasma cortisol. Peak cortisol levels below 500 nmol/L (18 μg/dL) at either 30 or 60 minutes indicate adrenal insufficiency. If a corticotropin stimulation test is not feasible or available, a morning cortisol <140 nmol/L (5 μg/dL) in combination with adrenocorticotropic hormone (ACTH) as a preliminary test suggestive of adrenal insufficiency may be used.

C. Imaging Studies

In patients with adrenal insufficiency, radiologic studies may be indicated. In patients having headaches and visual disturbances, an MRI scan should be performed to investigate for a possible pituitary or hypothalamic tumor. In patients with suspected primary adrenal insufficiency, a CT scan of the adrenal glands should be performed to rule out hemorrhage, adrenal vein thrombosis, or metastatic disease as the cause of the adrenal dysfunction.

▶ Treatment

For patients with symptomatic adrenal insufficiency, fluid management, correction of other metabolic abnormalities such as hypoglycemia and hyperkalemia, and the administration of corticosteroids are primary concerns. An approach to managing this condition is shown in Table 37–4.

While providing fluid resuscitation and addressing other metabolic emergencies, the practitioner should administer emergency doses of hydrocortisone. Once the patient is stabilized, corticosteroid maintenance should be provided in

divided doses early in the morning and afternoon to simulate the diurnal release of cortisol by the adrenal gland. The smallest dose that relieves the patient's symptoms should be used to minimize weight gain and risk of osteoporosis. During febrile illnesses, acute injury, or other periods of physiologic stress, the dose of hydrocortisone should be doubled or tripled temporarily. Patients with primary adrenal insufficiency should also receive fludrocortisone as a substitute for aldosterone.

▶ Corticosteroid Dependence and Tapering

A. Causes

Systemic corticosteroid therapy is indicated for many disease states. After several weeks of therapy with corticosteroids, the hypothalamic-pituitary-adrenal axis may become depressed. In this situation, the corticosteroid dose must be reduced gradually to limit the adverse effects of corticosteroid therapy withdrawal.

Several factors should be considered when determining whether a "tapering" regimen should be implemented: the length and amount of steroid and whether a single dose or divided doses were given. Currently, the general consensus is that if high doses are given for >7–10 days, symptomatic adrenal suppression may occur.

B. Management

Initially, the dose of corticosteroid should be gradually reduced until the patient can safely tolerate a dosage equivalent of 20 mg of hydrocortisone (or 5–7.5 mg of prednisone) per day. Although currently no evidence-based guidelines for tapering of corticosteroid exist, suggested tapering regimens are present (Table 37–5).

During this taper, the patient may experience some mild withdrawal symptoms, including fatigue, anorexia, nausea, and orthostatic light-headedness. If the patient experiences acute stress during this period (eg, minor surgery, infection), the steroid dose should be increased to 100–500 mg of hydrocortisone in divided doses, depending on the situation. Once the stress has resolved, the corticosteroid dosage should again be tapered to a dosage equivalent of 20 mg of hydrocortisone per day. This dosage should be continued for at least 4 weeks.

Table 37–4. Initial doses of medications used in treating adrenal insufficiency.

Replacement	
Hydrocortisone	15–25 mg divided into two or three doses per day
Prednisone	3–5 mg once daily
Dexamethasone	0.5 mg once daily
Fludrocortisone	0.05–0.2 mg once daily
Emergency therapy	
Hydrocortisone	100 mg bolus dose followed by infusion of 100–200 mg/24 h

Data from Oelkers W: Adrenal insufficiency. *N Engl J Med.* 1996 Oct 17; 335(16):1206–1212 and Michels A, Michels N: Addison disease: early detection and treatment principles. *Am Fam Physician.* 2014 Apr 1; 89(7):563–568.

Bornstein SR, Allolio B, Arlt W, et al. Diagnosis and treatment of primary adrenal insufficiency: an Endocrine Society clinical practice. *J Clin Endocrinol Metab.* 2016;101(2):364–389. [PMID: 26760044]

Burton C, Cottrell E, Edwards J. Addison's disease: identification and management in primary care. *Br J Gen Pract.* 2015;65: 488–490. [PMID: 26324491]

Charmandari E, Nicolaides NC, Chrousos GP. Adrenal insufficiency. *Lancet.* 2014;383:2152–2167. [PMID: 24503135]

Table 37–5. Corticosteroid taper regimen.

1. Reduce dose by 2.5- to 5.0-mg decrements every 3–7 days until physiologic dose (5–7.5 mg of prednisone per day) is reached.
2. Switch to hydrocortisone 20 mg once daily in the morning.
3. Gradually reduce hydrocortisone dose by 2.5 mg over several weeks to months.
4. Discontinue/continue hydrocortisone based on assessment of morning cortisol:
   - <85 nmol/L: HPA axis has not recovered.
     - Continue hydrocortisone.
     - Reevaluate patient in 4–6 weeks.
   - 85–275 nmol/L: Suspicious for adrenal suppression.
     - Continue hydrocortisone.
     - Further testing of HPA axis or reevaluate in 4–6 weeks.
   - 276–500 nmol/L: HPA axis function is likely adequate for activities of daily living in a nonstressed physiologic state but may be inadequate for preventing adrenal crisis at times of physiologic stress or illness.
     - Discontinue hydrocortisone.
     - Monitor for signs and symptoms of adrenal suppression.
     - Consider further evaluation of HPA axis to determine if function is also adequate for stressed states, or consider empiric therapy with high-dose steroids during times of stress.
   - 500 nmol/L: HPA axis is intact.
     - Discontinue hydrocortisone.

HPA, hypothalamic-pituitary-adrenal.
Adapted with permission from Liu D, Ahmet A, Ward L, et al: A practical guide to the monitoring and management of the complications of systemic corticosteroid therapy. *Allergy Asthma Clin Immunol.* 2013 Aug 15;9(1):30.

Husebye E, Allolio B, Arlt W, et al. Consensus statement on the diagnosis, treatment and follow-up of patients with primary adrenal insufficiency. *J Int Med.* 2014;275(4):104–115. [PMID: 24330030]

Michels A, Michels N. Addison disease: early detection and treatment principles. *Am Fam Physician.* 2014;89(7):563–568. [PMID: 24695602]

Oelkers W. Adrenal insufficiency. *N Engl J Med.* 1996;335;1206–1212. [PMID: 8815944]

Ten S, New M, Maclaren N. Addison's disease 2001. *J Clin Endocrinol Metab.* 2001;86:2909–2922. [PMID: 11443143]

CUSHING SYNDROME

▶ General Considerations

Cushing syndrome refers to overproduction of cortisol due to any cause (eg, adrenal hyperplasia, exogenous steroid use). *Cushing disease* is a more specific term that refers to excessive cortisol resulting from excessive ACTH produced by pituitary corticotropic tumors. ACTH-producing tumors account for 80% of cases of Cushing syndrome. The remaining 20% are caused by adrenal tumors, such as adenomas, carcinomas, and micronodular and macronodular hyperplasia, associated with autonomous production of glucocorticoids.

Cushing syndrome is rare, with a prevalence estimated at 40–80 per 1 million persons. Cushing disease is at least 3 times more prevalent in women than in men, whereas ectopic ACTH secretion is more common in men, largely due to the higher incidence in men of bronchogenic lung cancers that produce ACTH.

▶ Clinical Findings

A. Symptoms and Signs

The most common signs of Cushing syndrome are sudden onset of central weight gain, often accompanied by thickening of the facial fat, which rounds the facial contour ("moon facies"), and a florid complexion due to telangiectasia. Other concomitant signs include an enlarged fat pad ("buffalo hump"), hypertension, glucose intolerance, oligomenorrhea or amenorrhea in premenopausal women, decreased libido in men, and spontaneous ecchymoses (Table 37–6).

B. Laboratory Findings

The evaluation of suspected excessive glucocorticoid production includes screening and confirmatory tests for the

Table 37–6. Clinical symptoms and signs of Cushing syndrome.

General
  Central obesity
  Proximal muscle weakness
  Hypertension
  Headaches
  Psychiatric disorders
Skin
  Wide (>1 cm), purple striae
  Spontaneous ecchymoses
  Facial plethora
  Hyperpigmentation
  Acne
  Hirsutism
  Fungal skin infections
Endocrine and metabolic derangements
  Hypokalemic alkalosis
  Osteopenia
  Delayed bone age in children
  Menstrual disorders, decreased libido, impotence
  Glucose intolerance, diabetes mellitus
  Kidney stones
  Polyuria
Elevated white blood cell count

diagnosis and localization of the source of hormone excess. The Endocrine Society recommends the initial use of one test with high diagnostic accuracy (24-hour urine free cortisol, late-night salivary cortisol, 1-mg overnight [or 2-mg 48-hour] dexamethasone suppression test). Patients with an abnormal result should undergo a second test, either one of the tests just listed or, in some cases, a serum midnight cortisol or dexamethasone–corticotropin-releasing hormone test.

Affective psychiatric disorders (eg, major depression) and alcoholism can be associated with the biochemical features of Cushing syndrome and, therefore, may decrease the reliability of test results.

C. Imaging Studies

Following confirmation of Cushing syndrome, imaging studies should be performed to look for adenomas (MRI scan) or adrenal tumors (CT scan). If both of these studies are negative, chest radiography or CT scanning should be performed to look for ectopic sources of ACTH production.

▶ Treatment

For patients with a pituitary adenoma (Cushing disease) in whom a circumscribed microadenoma can be identified and resected, the treatment of choice is transsphenoidal microadenomectomy. If an adenoma cannot be clearly identified, patients should undergo a subtotal (85–90%) resection of the anterior pituitary gland. Patients who wish to preserve pituitary function (ie, in order to have children) should be treated with pituitary irradiation. If radiation does not decrease exogenous ACTH production, bilateral total adrenalectomy is a final treatment option. For adult patients not cured by transsphenoidal surgery, pituitary irradiation is the most appropriate choice for the next treatment.

Patients who have a nonpituitary tumor that secretes ACTH are cured by resection of the tumor. Unfortunately, nonpituitary tumors that secrete ACTH are seldom amenable to resection. In these cases, cortisol excess can be controlled with adrenal enzyme inhibitors, alone or in combination, with the proper dose determined by measurements of plasma and urinary cortisol.

For patients with adrenal hyperplasia, bilateral total adrenalectomy is required. Patients with an adrenal adenoma or carcinoma can be managed with unilateral adrenalectomy. Patients with hyperplasia or adenomas almost invariably have recurrences that are not amenable to either radiation or chemotherapy.

The Endocrine Society guidelines recommend that all patients receive monitoring and adjunctive treatment for cortisol-dependent comorbidities (psychiatric disorders, diabetes, hypertension, hypokalemia, infections, dyslipidemia, osteoporosis, and poor physical fitness). Patients should

also be evaluated for risk factors of venous thrombosis and receive perioperative prophylaxis for venous thromboembolism if they undergo surgery. Because of the increased risk of infections, clinicians should recommend and offer age-appropriate vaccinations to Cushing syndrome patients.

Patients who are taking corticosteroids for prolonged periods of time may exhibit signs or symptoms of Cushing syndrome. Once the primary problem for which steroids are being prescribed is controlled, patients should be withdrawn from their corticosteroid treatment slowly to avoid symptoms from adrenal suppression. There are few studies evaluating methods of withdrawal from chronic steroid use, however. Clinicians should be guided by the severity of the underlying condition, the duration that steroids have been used, and the dosage of steroids in determining how quickly dosages of steroids should be reduced.

Lacroiz A, Feelders RA, Statakis CA, Neiman LK. Cushing's syndrome. *Lancet.* 2015;386:913–927. [PMID: 26004339]

Loriaux DL. Diagnosis and differential diagnosis of Cushing's syndrome. *N Engl J Med.* 2017;376:1451–1459. [PMID: 28402781]

Newell-Price J, Bertagna X, Grossman AB, Nieman LK. Cushing's syndrome. *Lancet.* 2006;367:1605–1617. [PMID: 16698415]

Nieman LK, Biller BMK, Findling JW, et al. The diagnosis of Cushing's syndrome: an Endocrine Society clinical practice guideline. *J Clin Endocrinol Metab.* 2008;93(5):1526–1540. [PMID: 18334580]

Nieman L, Biller B, Findling J, et al. Treatment of Cushing's syndrome: an Endocrine Society clinical practice guideline. *J Clin Endocrinol Metab,* 2015;100(8):2807–2831. [PMID: 26222757]

Nieman LK, Ilias I. Evaluation and treatment of Cushing's syndrome. *Am J Med.* 2005;118:1340. [PMID: 16378774]

HYPERALDOSTERONISM

▶ General Considerations

Primary hyperaldosteronism accounts for 70–80% of all cases of hyperaldosteronism and is usually caused by a solitary unilateral adrenal adenoma. Other causes of hyperaldosteronism include bilateral adrenal hyperplasia, so-called idiopathic hyperaldosteronism, and glucocorticoid-remediable hyperaldosteronism. Adrenal carcinoma and unilateral adrenal hyperplasia are rare causes.

▶ Clinical Findings

A. Symptoms and Signs

Patients with hyperaldosteronism present with hypertension and hypokalemia. Other complaints include headaches, muscular weakness or flaccid paralysis caused by hypokalemia, or polyuria. Inappropriate hypersecretion of aldosterone is an uncommon cause of hypertension, accounting for <1% of cases. Any patient presenting with hypertension and unprovoked hypokalemia should be considered for the evaluation of hyperaldosteronism. Hypertension may be severe, although malignant hypertension is rare. Specifically, the following patients should be evaluated for hyperaldosteronism: patients with sustained blood pressure above 150/100 mmHg on each of three measurements obtained on different days, with hypertension (blood pressure >140/90 mmHg) resistant to three conventional antihypertensive drugs (including a diuretic), or controlled blood pressure (<140/90 mmHg) on four or more antihypertensive drugs; hypertension and spontaneous or diuretic-induced hypokalemia; hypertension and adrenal incidentaloma; hypertension and sleep apnea; or hypertension and a family history of early-onset hypertension or cerebrovascular accident at a young age (<40 years); and all hypertensive first-degree relatives of patients with primary aldosteronism. The peak incidence occurs between 30 and 50 years of age, and most patients are women.

B. Laboratory Findings

Initially, laboratory evaluation is used to document hyperaldosteronemia and suppressed renin activity. Further diagnostic tests, including imaging procedures, are used to determine whether the etiology is amenable to surgical intervention or requires medical management.

Plasma aldosterone/renin ratio (ARR) is the recommended screening test. Plasma aldosterone is usually measured after 4 hours of upright posture. Plasma renin activity should be measured in the same sample. A ratio of plasma aldosterone concentration to plasma renin activity of >20–40 is very suspicious for hyperaldosteronism.

Patients with a positive ARR should undergo one or more confirmatory tests in most cases. If the patient has spontaneous hypokalemia, plasma renin below detection levels, and plasma aldosterone concentration >20 ng/dL, no confirmatory test is needed. Four confirmatory tests are available: oral sodium loading, saline infusion, fludrocortisone suppression, and captopril challenge. No definitive evidence is present that one test is preferred compared to the others.

C. Imaging Studies

Imaging procedures can assist in differentiating causes of hyperaldosteronism and lateralizing adenomas. The diagnostic accuracy of high-resolution CT scans is only approximately 70% for aldosterone-producing adenomas, largely because of the occurrence of nonfunctioning adenomas. MRI is no better than CT in differentiating aldosterone-secreting tumors from other adrenal tumors. Scintigraphic imaging with ^{131}I-labeled cholesterol derivatives during dexamethasone suppression provides an image based on functional properties of the adrenal gland. Asymmetric uptake after 48 hours indicates an adenoma, whereas symmetric uptake after 72 hours indicates bilateral hyperplasia. Diagnostic accuracy is 72%. However, if the adrenal

CT scan is normal, iodocholesterol scanning is unlikely to be helpful.

▶ Treatment

For adrenal adenoma, total unilateral adrenalectomy is the treatment of choice and provides a cure in most cases. Although some patients with primary bilateral hyperplasia may benefit from subtotal adrenalectomy, these patients cannot be accurately identified preoperatively. Following surgery, the electrolyte imbalances usually correct rapidly, whereas blood pressure control may take several weeks to months.

Medical therapy is indicated for most patients with bilateral adrenal hyperplasia or for patients with adrenal adenomas who are unable to undergo adrenalectomy. Spironolactone controls the hyperkalemia, although it is not a very potent antihypertensive agent. Amiloride and calcium channel blockers are often used to control blood pressure.

Bravo EL. Primary aldosteronism. Issues in diagnosis and management. *Endocrinol Metab Clin North Am.* 1994;23:271. [PMID: 8070422]

Funder J, Carey R, Mantero F, et al. The management of primary aldosteronism: case detection, diagnosis, and treatment: an Endocrine Society clinical practice guideline. *J Clin Endocr Metab.* 2016;101(5):1889–1916. [PMID: 26934393]

▼ PARATHYROID DISORDERS

HYPERPARATHYROIDISM

▶ General Considerations

Hyperparathyroidism refers to excessive production of parathyroid hormone (PTH). *Primary* hyperparathyroidism is the overproduction of PTH in an inappropriate fashion, usually resulting in hypercalcemia. Primary hyperparathyroidism is more common in postmenopausal women. The most common cause is a benign solitary parathyroid adenoma (80% of all cases). Another 15% of patients have diffuse hyperplasia of the parathyroid glands, a condition that tends to be familial. Carcinoma of the parathyroid occurs in <1% of cases.

In secondary hyperparathyroidism, patients have appropriate additional production of PTH because of hypocalcemia related to other metabolic conditions such as renal failure, calcium absorption problems, or vitamin D deficiency.

▶ Clinical Findings

A. Symptoms and Signs

Most patients have nonspecific complaints that may include aches and pains, constipation, muscle fatigue, generalized weakness, psychiatric disturbances, polydipsia, and polyuria. The hypercalcemia can cause nausea and vomiting, thirst, and anorexia. A history of peptic ulcer disease or hypertension may be present, as well as accompanying constipation, anemia, and weight loss. Precipitation of calcium in the corneas may produce a band keratopathy, and patients may also experience recurrent pancreatitis. Finally, skeletal problems can result in pathologic fractures.

B. Laboratory Findings

Hypercalcemia (serum calcium level >10.5 mg/dL when corrected for serum albumin level) is the most important clue to the diagnosis. In patients who have an elevated calcium level with no apparent cause, serum PTH should be determined using a two-site immunometric assay. An elevated PTH level in the presence of hypercalcemia confirms the diagnosis of primary hyperparathyroidism.

Other findings may include a low serum phosphate level (<2.5 mg/dL) with excessive phosphaturia. Urine calcium excretion may be high or normal. Alkaline phosphatase levels are elevated only in the presence of bone disease, and elevated plasma chloride and uric acid levels may be seen.

C. Imaging Studies

With chronic hyperparathyroidism, diffuse bone demineralization, loss of the dental lamina dura, and subperiosteal resorption of bone (particularly in the radial aspects of the fingers) may be apparent on x-rays. Cysts may be noted throughout the skeleton, and "salt-and-pepper" appearance of the skull may be seen. Pathologic fractures can occur, and renal calculi and soft tissue calcification may be visualized.

Imaging studies are usually reserved for patients with resistant or recurrent disease. In these cases, ultrasonography, CT scanning, MRI, and thallium-201–technetium-99m scanning may help locate ectopic parathyroid tissue.

▶ Treatment

Treatment of severe hypercalcemia and parathyroidectomy are the mainstays for therapy. When hypercalcemia is severe, treatment includes aggressive hydration. Correction of any underlying hyponatremia and hypokalemia should be initiated, along with administration of a loop diuretic to accelerate calcium clearance. Other medications that can be effective in reducing hypercalcemia include etidronate, plicamycin, and calcitonin. Any medications or other products that increase calcium levels, such as estrogens, thiazides, vitamins A and D, and milk, should be avoided.

In addition to management of acute hypercalcemia, surgical removal of parathyroid tissue should be undertaken. Surgical resection provides the most rapid and effective method of reducing serum calcium in these patients.

Hyperplasia of all glands requires removal of three glands along with subtotal resection of the fourth. Surgical success is directly related to the experience and expertise of the operating surgeon.

For mild cases and poor surgical candidates, conservative therapy with adequate hydration and long-term pharmacologic therapy is recommended. Patients should avoid drugs and products that elevate calcium and should have their serum calcium monitored closely.

American Association of Clinical Endocrinologists, American Association of Endocrine Surgeons. Position statement on the diagnosis and management of hyperparathyroidism. *Endocr Pract.* 2005;11:49–54. [PMID: 16033736]

HYPOPARATHYROIDISM

▶ General Considerations

Hypoparathyroidism results from underproduction of PTH. The most common cause is the removal of the parathyroid glands during a thyroidectomy or following surgery for primary hyperparathyroidism. Less commonly, hypoparathyroidism is idiopathic, familial, or the result of a congenital absence of the parathyroid glands (DiGeorge syndrome). Patients with idiopathic hypoparathyroidism often have antibodies against parathyroid and other tissues, and an autoimmune component may play a role. Other unusual causes of hypoparathyroidism include previous neck irradiation, magnesium deficiency, metastatic cancer, and infiltrative diseases.

▶ Clinical Findings

A. Symptoms and Signs

The lack of PTH results in hypocalcemia, which produces most of the symptoms associated with hypoparathyroidism. Symptoms associated with hypocalcemia include tetany, carpopedal spasms, paresthesias of the lips and hands, and a positive Chvostek sign or Trousseau sign. Patients may also exhibit less specific symptoms such as anxiety, depression, or fatigue. Additionally, hyperventilation, respiratory alkalosis with or without respiratory compromise, laryngospasm, hypotension, and seizures may occur with severe hypocalcemia.

B. Laboratory Findings

On laboratory evaluation, patients with hypoparathyroidism have low serum calcium and elevated serum phosphate levels, with a normal alkaline phosphatase level. Urinary levels of calcium and phosphate are decreased. The key finding is a low to absent PTH value.

▶ Treatment

Acute hypocalcemia with tetany requires aggressive therapy with multiple drugs. Therapy should be started with calcium gluconate administered intravenously in a 10% solution. The infusion is given slowly until tetany resolves. Oral calcium along with vitamin D supplementation should be given after the acute crisis has resolved. Hypomagnesemia should be corrected with intravenous magnesium sulfate administered at a dose of 1–2 g every 6 hours. Chronic replacement of magnesium can be accomplished using 600-mg magnesium oxide tablets once or twice daily.

For the maintenance of normal calcium, vitamin D supplementation along with oral calcium should be given. Calcium in the form of calcium carbonate (40% elemental calcium) is the drug of choice, administered in a dose of 1–2 g of calcium per day. Serial calcium levels should be obtained regularly (every 3–6 months), and "spot" urine calcium levels should be maintained below 30 mg/dL.

Acute Musculoskeletal Complaints

Jeanne Doperak, DO
Kelley Anderson, DO

▼ UPPER EXTREMITY

ROTATOR CUFF IMPINGEMENT

ESSENTIALS OF DIAGNOSIS

- ▶ Anterior shoulder pain that is often atraumatic.
- ▶ Discomfort frequently worse with repetitive or overhead activities.
- ▶ Strength often maintained on exam.

▶ General Considerations

The term subacromial *impingement syndrome* defines any entity that compromises the subacromial space and irritates the enclosed rotator cuff tendons. It is not clearly or consistently defined and may represent a variety of disorders from subacromial bursitis to calcific tendinosis. Often these entities arise in a similar fashion and may be difficult to differentiate. Diagnosis is based on a meticulous history and physical exam and appropriate imaging.

▶ Clinical Findings

A. Symptoms and Signs

Diagnosis of subacromial impingement is primarily clinical. The patient complains of dull shoulder pain of insidious onset over weeks to months. Less often, these symptoms arise following trauma. Pain is typically localized to the anterolateral acromion and radiates to the lateral deltoid. Pain is often aggravated by repetitive overhead activities, such as a carpenter swinging a hammer or a baseball player throwing a ball. Individuals often complain of pain when they roll onto

the shoulder at night and will awaken with symptoms if the arm is positioned over the head.

Physical exam usually reveals normal RoM, although the patient may experience pain on reaching the maximum forward flexion and abduction. Muscular weakness can be seen but is often secondary to pain and not secondary to loss of function. In other words, a patient who is coached to try to resist on manual muscle testing despite pain will often exhibit near-full strength. The maintenance of strength can help differentiate between inflammation and a high-grade cuff tear.

B. Imaging Studies

Radiographs that may aid in diagnosis include anteroposterior (AP), outlet, and axillary views of the affected shoulder. The outlet view provides visualization of acromial morphology exhibiting curvature or spurs that may contribute to the underlying pathology. Plain films may also provide evidence of tendon calcification, underlying degenerative disease, and cystic changes in the humeral head. Magnetic resonance imaging (MRI) can confirm the diagnosis but seldom changes the treatment plan. Musculoskeletal ultrasound can be a useful and less expensive point-of-care imaging tool. In the hands of a trained provider, musculoskeletal ultrasound can dynamically illustrate tendon bunching and excessive bursal fluid, suggesting inflammation.

C. Special Tests

Provocative testing includes the Neer test and the Hawkins test. The Neer test involves passive elevation of an internally rotated, forward-flexed arm. In the Hawkins test, the arm is positioned in 90° of forward flexion and is internally rotated with a bent elbow. These motions cause "impingement" of the supraspinatus tendon against the acromion. Pain with either maneuver is considered a positive test; however, these tests may also be positive in patients with other pathology.

▶ Differential Diagnosis

Differential diagnosis includes acromioclavicular joint arthritis, rotator cuff tear, glenohumeral instability, arthritis, supraspinatus nerve entrapment, and cervical disk disease.

▶ Treatment

Nonsurgical management of shoulder impingement continues to be successful in most patients. Evidence supports early initiation of physical therapy aimed at eccentric strengthening of the shoulder complex, including the scapular stabilizers for restoration of function and improvement of symptoms. A subacromial steroid injection can be used to help control pain initially if discomfort is a barrier to starting manual exercise therapy. Addition of nonsteroidal anti-inflammatory drugs (NSAIDs) can aid in pain control when necessary. Modification of offending activities may be needed for a period of time; for instance, swimmers may need a kickboard in the pool, or a pitcher may need to modify pitch counts. Surgical intervention is considered only after failure of conservative treatment.

Rhon DI, Boyles RB, Cleland JA. One-year outcome of subacromial corticosteroid injection compared with manual physical therapy for the management of the unilateral shoulder impingement syndrome: a pragmatic randomized trial. *Ann Intern Med.* 2014;161(3):161–169. [PMID: 25089860]

Simons S, Kruse D, Dixon JB. Shoulder impingement syndrome. https://www.uptodate.com/contents/shoulder-impingement-syndrome. Accessed November 15, 2019.

ROTATOR CUFF TEARS

ESSENTIALS OF DIAGNOSIS

- ▶ Frequently traumatic shoulder pain in a middle-aged individual.
- ▶ Significant loss of function in affected arm especially overhead.
- ▶ Pain often radiates to lateral deltoid.
- ▶ Rare in young athletes.

▶ General Considerations

Rotator cuff tears are often patients' perceived source of shoulder pain. In reality, this pathology is exceedingly rare in young athletes and often asymptomatic in older adults, with several studies illustrating cuff tears in >50% of individuals age >60 years. This epidemiology leads to challenges in treatment plans that are often individualized.

The rotator cuff complex contains four muscles (the SITS muscles): the subscapularis, infraspinatus, teres minor, and supraspinatus. Biomechanically the cuff assists in abduction and internal and external rotation of the humerus, and together, the muscles facilitate stabilization of the humeral head in the glenoid. Disruption of any part of this complex can result in shoulder dysfunction and pain.

▶ Clinical Findings

A. Signs and Symptoms

Many rotator cuff tears are asymptomatic, especially in older individuals. If symptoms are present, a careful history will often reveal a single event such as a fall onto an outstretched arm or picking up a large bag, resulting in an audible pop and sudden pain. This pain is often located in the front of the shoulder or over the lateral deltoid. Weakness and stiffness are frequently described, especially with overhead motion or internal rotation of the shoulder. Patients will complain of difficulty brushing their hair or fastening a bra strap and/or seatbelt.

Careful examination may demonstrate subtle atrophy of the shoulder musculature, which suggests a chronic problem. Patients will have limitations in active RoM and pain as the arm is raised over 90° in flexion, in abduction, and sometimes in internal rotation when the subscapularis tendon is involved. The affected arm can be passively taken through a full RoM suggesting an extraarticular process. Manual muscle testing will typically display pronounced weakness in the plane of the torn tendon.

B. Imaging Studies

Plain films can be useful to rule out other causes of shoulder pain such as osteoarthritis or fracture. Changes seen on plain films that may be consistent with rotator cuff tears can include loss of space between the humeral head and acromion and cystic changes in the greater tuberosity. Ultrasound can diagnose a rotator cuff tear if performed and read by an experienced individual, but the MRI arthrogram is considered the gold standard in the diagnostic imaging of rotator cuff disease. The injection of dye at the time of MRI increases the sensitivity and specificity of the test significantly.

C. Special Tests

Testing for the most commonly torn rotator cuff tendon, the supraspinatus, includes the empty-can test. The examiner positions the patient's arm in 70° abduction and 30° forward flexion, and internally rotates it so that the thumb points down (as if emptying a held can). The examiner then pushes down against resistance. Pain and weakness are considered a positive test.

The lift-off test evaluates the subscapularis. The patient rotates the arm behind the back at approximately the mid-lumbar level and attempts to push the examiner's hand away from the back. As with the empty-can test, weakness and pain indicate a positive test.

Treatment

Treatment focuses on eliminating pain and restoring function. In light of the age-related epidemiologic data presented earlier, treatment is not a one-size-fits-all algorithm. If a rotator cuff tear has been confirmed in an individual <60 years old, in most cases, a timely referral to an orthopedic surgeon should be made.

Previously, the majority of individuals over 60 with rotator cuff tears were treated with conservative therapy and surgery was reserved only for those who were unable to restore daily function. This paradigm has changed in recent years. With a more active aging population, surgical decisions are being made based on expectation of performance rather than on year of birth. For instance, a 70-year-old CrossFit competitor would most likely require surgery to continue to participate at the level the patient demands and anticipates. This example may seem extreme, but one of our goals as providers should be keeping our patient population as active as possible, even as they age. With an ever increasing body of evidence that exercise is medicine, restoration of function is one the best disease preventions we can offer.

Sambandam SN, Vishesh K, Gul A, Mounasamy V. Rotator cuff tears: an evidence based approach. *World J Orthop.* 2015;6(11): 902–918. [PMID: 26716086]

ACROMIOCLAVICULAR JOINT SPRAIN

ESSENTIALS OF DIAGNOSIS

▶ Pain and deformity over top of shoulder.
▶ Pain usually occurs after a fall onto the lateral shoulder with patient's arm at the side.

General Considerations

The acromioclavicular (AC) joint is the articulation between the distal clavicle and scapula. This is a common injury in young active individuals after a fall onto the lateral aspect of their shoulder with the arm at the side. Classification of the injury is based on the extent of soft tissue injury. In a type 1 sprain, the joint remains intact, and there is no clavicle displacement on shoulder inspection or radiographically. Type 2 injury involves the AC ligaments that are torn. In a type 2 injury, the distal clavicle is slightly widened on radiograph, but there is no vertical displacement on inspection as the coracoclavicular (CC) ligaments are maintained. Type 3 injury involves both the AC and CC ligaments and results in elevation of the distal clavicle that can be enough to tent the skin. Type 4–6 injuries are extremely rare and always surgical.

Clinical Findings

A. Symptoms and Signs

Patients with AC joint injuries will present with pain that localizes to the top of the shoulder. Based on the extent of injury, there may be notable asymmetry when compared to the unaffected side. Pain is often worse with overhead or cross-body shoulder motions. This discomfort will often lead to limited range of motion (RoM) and weakness on exam.

B. Imaging Studies

Plain radiographs are sufficient to view and evaluate the AC joint. The Zanca view is the most accurate. It is helpful to get bilateral Zanca views on the same cassette to compare one side to the other.

C. Special Tests

The cross-arm adduction test evaluates the AC joint. The involved arm is brought across the body in the horizontal plane so that the elbow points forward. Pain at the AC joint in this position is a positive test.

Treatment

Type 1–3 injuries are typically treated nonsurgically. A brief period of sling immobilization for comfort should be followed by early initiation of RoM exercises. NSAIDs may be used for early pain control. Return to play for athletes is based on restoration of strength, motion, and function. Treatment of type 3 injuries remains controversial and should be evaluated on a case-by-case basis. Type 4–6 injuries should be referred urgently to an orthopedic surgeon.

Sirin E, Aydin N, Topkar OM. Acromioclavicular joint injuries: diagnosis, classification and ligamentoplasty procedures. July 17, 2018. https://online.boneandjoint.org.uk/doi/full/10.1302/2058-5241.3.170027. Accessed November 15, 2019.

RUPTURE OF BICEPS TENDON

ESSENTIALS OF DIAGNOSIS

▶ Associated with eccentric load and reported "pop."
▶ Proximal lesion with residual "Popeye" muscle deformity.
▶ Distal lesion with elbow swelling and ecchymosis.

General Considerations

The biceps muscle of the arm functions to flex and supinate at the elbow. Injury to the biceps tendons can occur at either the distal attachment at the radial tuberosity or at the proximal attachment where the long head of the biceps tendon inserts at the supraglenoid tubercle. These injuries are both associated with a sudden eccentric load and occur most commonly in middle-aged men. Smoking and corticosteroid use are risk factors.

▶ Clinical Findings

A. Symptoms and Signs

Patients with distal ruptures will present with variable pain patterns. Some individuals complain of anterior shoulder pain, whereas others will be pain free. Nearly all distal ruptures will exhibit bunching of the biceps muscle in the distal arm—a "Popeye" muscle.

Patients with proximal ruptures will present with pain, swelling, and ecchymosis at the elbow. Often there is weakness with manual muscle testing, and a positive hook test will be present (see special tests, eg, hook test, discussed later).

B. Imaging Studies

Plain radiographs of the shoulder and elbow would be necessary only to rule out concurrent injury. MRI will confirm the diagnosis either proximally or distally. Ultrasound can be a quick tool in the office to directly observe and evaluate the bicep tendon and muscle along its entire length.

C. Special Tests

The hook test is performed to evaluate for a distal biceps tendon rupture. The patient actively supinates the flexed elbow. An intact hook test permits the examiner to hook her or his finger under the intact biceps tendon from the lateral side. With an avulsion, there is no cordlike structure to palpate or hook. Absence of the tendon is a positive test.

▶ Treatment

A proximal biceps tendon rupture is usually treated nonsurgically with a period of activity modification and physical therapy. Anti-inflammatories can be used for pain control if needed. Patients do not have persistent strength deficits as the short head of the muscle remains attached. Keep in mind that, relative to the location of the tear and mechanism of injury, there may be overlapping pathology (cuff/labral tear) that may need to be considered if the patient does not improve as expected over time.

A distal biceps tendon rupture is nearly always operative because the patient will lose >50% strength with flexion and supination over time. This injury should be referred to an orthopedic surgeon in a timely manner for best results.

Alentorn-Geli E, Assenmacher AT, Sanchez-Sotelo J. Distal biceps tendon injuries a clinically relevant current concepts review. *EFFORT Open Rev.* 2016;1(9):316–324. [PMID: 28461963]

Thomas JR, Lawton JN. Biceps and triceps ruptures in athletes. *Hand Clin.* 2017;33:35–46. [PMID: 27886838]

SHOULDER INSTABILITY

 ESSENTIALS OF DIAGNOSIS

▶ Encompasses a large continuum of disorders with traumatic, congenital, and biomechanical causes.

▶ Patient reports feeling of looseness or slipping of shoulder.

▶ Excessive motion can be subtle to gross with complete disarticulation of the humeral head at the glenoid.

▶ General Considerations

Shoulder instability can be viewed as any condition in which the balance of various stabilizing structures in the shoulder is disrupted, resulting in increased humeral head translation. This excessive motion at the humeral head can be partial, as in a subluxation, or grossly unstable with complete disarticulation of the humeral head at the glenoid. By far, most complete dislocations are anterior, but they can be posterior and, on rare occasions, inferior. In younger patients, instability can be due to trauma, congenital laxity, weakness, poor biomechanics, or a combination of each of these entities. In older patients, instability is most often caused by trauma, specifically falls.

▶ Clinical Findings

A. Symptoms and Signs

Patients with acute anterior dislocations that have not self-reduced will present with shoulder pain, an unwillingness to move the affected arm, and a tendency to cradle the arm. Inspection will reveal a bulge (due to the displaced humeral head) as well as dimpling inferior to the acromion where the humeral head should be.

If a patient is not dislocated at the time of the exam but reports a recent dislocation, the exam usually reveals limited RoM, weakness, and global pain complaints. If the patient has more subtle instability with no true dislocation, the exam will often reveal hypermobility with an increased arc of motion and retained strength. Special tests, described later, will help with the diagnosis.

B. Imaging Studies

Radiographs will confirm a shoulder dislocation but will often be normal with more subtle chronic subluxations. AP and outlet views are standard, but an axillary view shows the relationship of the humeral head to the glenoid fossa and is more accurate when assessing for joint congruency. Occasionally a bony defect is seen in the posterolateral portion of the humeral head, called a *Hill-Sachs lesion*. The axillary view will also allow the examiner to assess for any glenoid fractures after a dislocation; these fractures are called *Bankart lesions*.

MRI is often warranted to assess for cuff pathology in older individuals and labral pathology in younger patients. An MRI arthrogram is the gold standard.

C. Special Tests

The apprehension test helps determine anterior shoulder instability. The patient is placed supine with the arm in 90° of abduction. The examiner then applies an external rotation stress. Patient apprehension due to subluxation of the humeral head is considered a positive test. Posterior pressure on the proximal humeral head can provide relief of symptoms if shoulder instability is the cause of the pain (relocation test).

▶ Treatment

In episodes of acute dislocation, the initial treatment is to reduce the shoulder pain and swelling. Once reduced, the patient may be placed in a sling for comfort, but there is no evidence that immobilization in internal rotation prevents recurrent instability. Anti-inflammatories can be given for pain control, and early rehab should focus on RoM, cuff strength, and scapular stabilization. Return to play for athletes is when full function (strength and RoM) is regained.

In episodes of more subtle chronic instability without frank dislocation, a trial of physical therapy should be the initial treatment. If the patient has recurrent episodes of dislocation or ongoing pain/dysfunction after physical therapy, more aggressive surgical options should be pursued. Younger patients (<25 years old) are known to have a greater incidence of recurrence; therefore, the practitioner's threshold for surgical opinions should be much lower.

Sofu H, Gursu S, Koçkara N, et al. Recurrent anterior shoulder instability: review of the literature and current concepts. *World J Clin Cases.* 2014;2(11):676–682. [PMID: 25405191]

LATERAL & MEDIAL EPICONDYLITIS

ESSENTIALS OF DIAGNOSIS

▶ Gradual onset of elbow pain often related to repetitive stress.

▶ Pain localizes to the epicondyles of the humerus and is worse with flexion/extension of the wrist, based on medial or lateral pathology.

▶ General Considerations

For many years, epicondylitis was attributed to inflammation at the tendon origin; however, recent evidence shows that it is actually due to a breakdown of collagen from aging, microtrauma, or vascular compromise. Although properly termed *tendinosis*, the condition is referred to by its longstanding, more common name *epicondylitis* throughout this discussion to avoid confusion. Lateral and medial epicondylitis occur at the elbow and are primarily overuse or repetitive stress disorders.

▶ Clinical Findings

A. Signs and Symptoms

Lateral epicondylitis is a tendinosis at the origin of the extensor tendons on the lateral epicondyle of the humerus. It is commonly known as "tennis elbow" because it is seen in activities that involve repetitive wrist extension (such as a backhand stroke in tennis). Patients complain of pain over the lateral elbow that may radiate down the forearm. There is tenderness to palpation over the origin of the extensor carpi radialis brevis tendon, which is anterior and distal to the lateral epicondyle. Pain is aggravated with wrist extension or forearm supination.

Medial epicondylitis, also known as "golfer's elbow," is seen after repetitive use of the flexor and pronator muscles of the wrist and hand (as occurs when playing golf, using a screwdriver, or hitting an overhand tennis stroke). Pain is insidious at the medial elbow and worsens with resisted forearm pronation and wrist flexion. Patients may complain of a weak grasp. Tenderness to palpation occurs just distal and anterior to the medial epicondyle.

B. Imaging Studies

Radiographs will confirm that there is no other overlapping pathology such as degenerative joint disease. Ultrasound can be used in the office to help evaluate the tendon integrity at the insertions. However, imaging is not necessary to make this diagnosis.

▶ Treatment

Although epicondylitis is not challenging to diagnose, it can be very difficult to treat. Conservative treatment is the mainstay of treatment, and the natural history of this problem shows that 70–80% of patients will improve in 1 year even in the absence of treatment. Few patients like to wait that long, and there are interventions that may help speed recovery. Activity modification with reduction of the offending activity is key in improvement. NSAIDs can help with early pain management, and a rehabilitation program focusing on eccentric exercises will promote healing. Corticosteroid injections are often requested by patients because they provide short-term relief, but studies have shown that after 6 weeks, those receiving injections had higher recurrence of symptoms. Forearm bands can be worn in order to relieve tension at the tendon insertion. Although patients will report relief with the orthoses, there is no evidence to support their efficacy. Nitroglycerine patches are used topically and applied over the painful area to act as a local and systemic vasodilator. Limited studies have shown improved outcomes in the first 6 months but not longer-term improvements. The prescriber should be aware that patches must be used "off label" and cut into smaller doses and can cause significant side effects, especially in older individuals. Patch treatment should be reserved for a very specific patient population. Autologous platelet-rich plasma (PRP) injections are the newest treatment option and remain controversial. PRP injections involve drawing blood from the patient, centrifuging the sample, and then injecting the PRP layer at the site of injury. There is mixed evidence regarding this newer treatment, which can be quite expensive, making it typically not a first-line therapy. Surgery should be considered only in those who have failed a sustained period of conservative treatment.

Ahmad Z, Siddiqui N, Malik S, et al. Lateral epicondylitis a review of pathology and management. *Bone Joint J.* 2013;95-B(9): 1158–1164. [PMID: 23997125]

DE QUERVAIN TENOSYNOVITIS

ESSENTIALS OF DIAGNOSIS

▶ Atraumatic pain at first dorsal compartment of wrist radiating into thumb and forearm.

▶ Often caused by repetitive activity.

▶ General Considerations

De Quervain tenosynovitis involves the abductor pollicis longus and the extensor pollicis brevis of the thumb. Although this was once assumed to be an inflammatory condition, recent evidence has shown that degeneration of the tendon is present. The condition can arise with repetitive activity that requires grasping or repetitive thumb use.

▶ Clinical Findings

A. Symptoms and Signs

Diagnosis is largely clinical. Patients may complain of difficulty gripping items and often rub the area over the radial styloid. Pain is located on the radial side of the wrist and thumb and occasionally radiates proximally or distally.

There is tenderness to palpation just distal to the radial styloid. Pain can also be reproduced with resisted thumb abduction and extension, or with thumb adduction into a closed fist and passive ulnar deviation (Finkelstein test). Pain over the tendons represents a positive test; however, other conditions can cause a positive test such as arthritis of the first carpometacarpal joint.

B. Imaging Studies

Radiographs are not necessary for diagnosis but can be useful to rule other pathology such as osteoarthritis or a fracture.

▶ Treatment

The goals of treatment are to decrease inflammation, prevent adhesion formation, and prevent recurrent tendonitis. Brief periods of icing and use of NSAIDs are helpful initially, and the patient should be placed in a thumb-restricting splint (thumb spica splint). If pain continues, a corticosteroid injection may be considered. In most patients, symptoms resolve after a single steroid injection. Steroid injection may be repeated after 8–12 weeks if symptoms are not 50% improved. If no improvement occurs after two injections within the year, a referral for surgical consultation should be obtained.

Shehab R, Mirabilli MH. Evaluation and diagnosis of wrist pain: a case-based approach. *Am Fam Physician.* 2013;87(8):568–573. [PMID: 23668446]

ULNAR COLLATERAL LIGAMENT INJURY OF THE THUMB

ESSENTIALS OF DIAGNOSIS

▶ Pain at medial aspect of metacarpophalangeal (MCP) joint of thumb.

▶ History of valgus force to thumb.

▶ General Considerations

The collateral ligaments of the MCP joint of the thumb stabilize the joint to both valgus- and volar-directed forces. Injury to the medial collateral ligament is extremely common and reported to be 86% of all injuries to the base of the thumb. The term *gamekeeper's thumb* was initially applied to this pathology as a result of Scottish gamekeepers with ligament rupture due to chronic valgus stresses. These days, the injury is more accurately described as *skier's thumb* as it typically occurs secondary to a fall onto an outstretched hand with an abducted thumb receiving a valgus force (as would occur when falling holding a ski pole). However, it is important to recognize that this injury occurs in many other sports and settings. Identification of the injury and timely treatment will result in more favorable outcomes.

▶ Clinical Findings

A. Symptoms and Signs

The patient with an acute ulnar collateral ligament (UCL) tear typically describes a specific event of a valgus-directed force onto an abducted thumb. This results in pain, swelling, and occasionally ecchymosis over the ulnar aspect of the MCP joint of the thumb. A mass or lump can occasionally be palpated at the site of tenderness, which might suggest a Stener lesion. A Stener lesion occurs when the ruptured ligament displaces in such a manner that the adductor aponeurosis becomes interposed between the ligament and bone. This prevents healing and typically requires surgical repair.

The gold standard for testing the UCL has been to compare laxity at the joint to that at the contralateral side. The thumb should be held proximal and distal to the MCP joint and a gentle valgus force applied at both 30° joint flexion and full extension. If laxity is seen only at 30° of MCP joint flexion, partial tear is suggested. When there is laxity at both 30° flexion and full extension, a complete rupture is likely.

B. Imaging Studies

Although diagnosis of UCL injury of the thumb is based largely on history and physical exam, radiographs should be obtained to rule out other coexisting pathology. Plain films of the thumb in the AP and lateral planes can be evaluated for fracture. An MRI of the thumb may be ordered to confirm the diagnosis.

▶ Treatment

If the MCP joint is stable on exam and only a partial tear is suspected, nonsurgical management is often successful. The injured thumb should be immobilized in a hand-based thumb spica splint for 4 weeks. After this period of immobilization, physical therapy can help the patient regain thumb function. If the MCP joint is not stable on exam and a complete rupture is diagnosed, the patient should be referred to an orthopedic surgeon for surgical repair. If this injury is left untreated, chronic instability will lead to arthritic changes of the MCP joint, which in most cases are irreversible.

Ritting AW, Baldwin PC, Rodner CM. Ulnar collateral ligament injury of the thumb metacarpophalangeal joint. *Clin J Sport Med*. 2010;20(2):106–112. [PMID: 20215892]

▼ LOWER EXTREMITY

PATELLAR TENDINOPATHY

ESSENTIALS OF DIAGNOSIS

▶ Pain at inferior pole of patella.

▶ Results from overuse/overloading the patella tendon.

▶ Initially occurs after activity, but can progress over time.

▶ General Considerations

The patellar tendon is an extension of the quadriceps femoris tendon and traverses from the inferior pole of the patella to its anchor point at the tibial tuberosity. *Patellar tendinopathy*, sometimes referred to as *jumper's knee*, causes pain at the inferior pole of the patella and usually results from recurrent overload of the knee during running, jumping, or lunging. Historically, this process was thought to be a result of inflammation. However, as with most tendinopathies, we now know that the pain results from strain and micro-tearing. Diagnosis is made clinically through history and physical exam.

▶ Clinical Findings

A. Symptoms and Signs

Clinically, patellar tendinopathy presents with the insidious onset of well-localized anterior knee pain focused at the inferior pole of the patella. Pain is often exacerbated by activities such as jumping, lunging, ascending/descending stairs, and kneeling. Onset of pain typically begins after exertion but can progress over time to encompass the entire activity.

On physical exam, the most consistent finding is tenderness to palpation over the tendon at the inferior pole of the patella and pain with resisted knee extension. As an extraarticular process, this diagnosis should not cause a knee effusion or mechanical symptoms. RoM is typically preserved but can be painful at end points.

In adolescents, overloading the patellar tendon can lead to Osgood-Schlatter disease (epiphysitis resulting in fragmentation of the tibial tubercle) or Sinding-Larsen-Johansson syndrome (epiphysitis involving fragmentation of the inferior pole of the patella), both of which will have open growth plates on plain radiographs.

B. Imaging Studies

Standard knee radiographs including AP, posteroanterior weight bearing with 45° flexion, lateral, and merchant views. These are helpful to assess for tendon calcification, underlying degenerative changes, or other bony pathology. MRI is confirmatory but will unlikely change the treatment plan. Musculoskeletal ultrasound can also be used in the office to evaluate and diagnose tendon injury/pathology and can be more cost-effective.

▶ Differential Diagnosis

Differential diagnosis includes patellofemoral pain syndrome, fat pad impingement, Osgood-Schlatter disease, Sinding-Larsen-Johansson syndrome, chondromalacia, patellar subluxation/dislocation, and patellar tendon rupture.

▶ Treatment

Previously, tendon pain was treated with rest and anti-inflammatories. More recent evidence has changed our approach to address the underlying degenerative, micro-tearing pathology. Initial treatment should include a rehab program focused on hip and quadriceps strengthening (specifically eccentric exercises). Activities should be modified to offload the anterior knee, and biomechanical abnormalities should be addressed. Although limited evidence exists, patients may experience pain relief wearing a patellar tendon strap. Corticosteroid injections should be avoided in weight-bearing tendons secondary to risk of rupture. Some clinicians are using PRP and nitroglycerine patch therapy to treat this difficult diagnosis. However, both are off-label uses of the product, and scientific evidence is still limited. Modalities such as shockwave therapy and Tenex are also being used for treatment of pain related to chronic tendon damage. Recovery can be prolonged, but after 6 months of failed conservative treatment, surgical options can be considered. It is important to educate patients that the literature shows similar outcomes in surgical and conservative treatment groups.

Aaron S, Watson JN, Hutchinson MR. Patellar tendinopathy. *Sports Health*. 2015;7(5):415–420. [PMID: 26502416]

PATELLOFEMORAL PAIN SYNDROME

ESSENTIALS OF DIAGNOSIS

▶ Overuse injury presents with anterior knee pain.
▶ Often occurs after a recent change in activity type, intensity, and frequency.

▶ General Considerations

Patellofemoral pain syndrome (PFPS) is the most common condition that prompts active people to seek treatment for anterior knee pain. The pain is typically described behind the patella and/or at the anterior medial aspect of the knee.

The patella articulates with the femur in the trochlear groove. It is stabilized by its attachments with the quadriceps femoris, vastus lateralis, vastus medialis, and medial and lateral retinacula. Weakness of these supporting structures can lead to biomechanical changes in patellar alignment, resulting in lateral tracking and causing irritation to the chondral surfaces.

Three major contributing factors have been evaluated in relation to PFPS: malalignment of the lower extremity, muscular imbalances within the quadriceps, and overactivity. Lower extremity alignment factors associated with PFPS include torsion of the femur or tibia, genu valgum, genu recurvatum, increased Q angle, femoral anteversion, and foot

pronation. Each of these factors has the potential to draw the patella laterally and contribute to abnormal patellar tracking.

▶ Clinical Findings

A. Symptoms and Signs

Historically, patients with PFPS present with an insidious onset of diffuse, aching, anterior knee pain often described as around and/or behind the patella. Pain can be bilateral and is aggravated by climbing stairs, ascending hills, squatting, or sitting for a prolonged period of time ("theater" sign). The patient sometimes reports a sensation of popping or grinding with activity.

Although the extent of their contributions is unclear, alignment, gait, and stance should be assessed and gross abnormalities addressed. On exam, there is often tenderness with palpation of the posteromedial or posterolateral patellar facets, as well as a positive "patellar grind" or Clarke sign (pain with slight compression of the patella that is exacerbated by quadriceps contraction). Although not typically in end-stage disease, a knee effusion can be present with mechanical symptoms.

B. Imaging Studies

Radiographs are seldom indicated unless pain is prolonged or associated with trauma or if bony pathology is suspected. A typical knee series includes a bilateral standing AP view, a lateral view, a bilateral posteroanterior flexion weight-bearing or tunnel view (45° of flexion), and a patellar profile (Merchant or skyline) view. The images are used to evaluate patella height, joint space narrowing, lateral patella deviation, or other bony abnormality such as a tumor.

▶ Differential Diagnosis

Differential diagnosis includes patellar tendinopathy, patellofemoral osteoarthritis, osteochondral defect of the trochlear or patellar surface, iliotibial band syndrome, anterior fat pad inflammation, synovial plica, retinacular strain, and epiphysitis. (*Note:* It is important to rule out referred pain from hip pathology in children.)

▶ Treatment

Treatment is directed at correcting patellar maltracking and abnormal biomechanical factors and modifying activities that cause symptoms. Exercises designed to strengthen the medial quadriceps and hip muscles and stretch the hamstrings and iliotibial bands have shown success in restoring normal function. The use of foot orthotics can be considered for those with pes planus, pes cavus, and significant hind foot eversion. Patients often perceive relief with bracing or taping, which helps guide the patella medially, especially during activities. Limited evidence exists for the effectiveness of NSAIDs, and their utility is questioned in patients with this disorder. Viscosupplementation has been found to provide pain relief in patients with more advanced disease and significant chondral damage from chronic maltracking. Surgery is reserved for patients with significant damage to the chondral surface and for those who have failed prolonged conservative therapy.

Petersen W, Ellermann A, Gösele-Koppenburg A, et al. Patellofemoral pain syndrome. *Knee Surg Sports Traumatol Arthrosc.* 2014;22(10):2264–2274. [PMID: 24221245]

LIGAMENTOUS INJURIES OF THE KNEE

The knee is a modified hinge joint that is stabilized by the anterior cruciate ligament (ACL), posterior cruciate ligament (PCL), medial collateral ligament (MCL), lateral collateral ligament (LCL), menisci, capsule, and surrounding musculature. Injury to one or more of these ligaments can lead to knee joint instability.

Anterior Cruciate Ligament Injury

 ESSENTIALS OF DIAGNOSIS

▶ Acute trauma resulting in immediate joint effusion and pain.
▶ Positive Lachman test.

▶ **General Considerations**

An intact ACL prevents anterior translation of the tibia on the femur and creates rotational stability. Injury to the ACL commonly results when there is an abrupt deceleration combined with a twisting mechanism, typically during cutting or pivoting after the foot is planted. Less commonly, it can occur after forced hyperextension.

▶ **Clinical Findings**

A. Symptoms and Signs

This injury typically occurs with a sudden change in direction and 70% of the time without contact. The patient often hears or feels a "pop." Swelling is usually rapid (minutes to hours) as a large hemarthrosis develops within the joint along with pain and decreased RoM. Without the restraint of an intact ACL, the tibia displaces anteriorly as the patient ambulates and causes a sensation of instability or giving way, particularly with pivoting motions.

An acute ACL injury can often be diagnosed immediately; however, the majority of patients present a day or more after the injury. By that time, muscle spasm and pain may limit the examination and make clinical diagnosis difficult. In the setting of an acute knee injury with effusion, the Lachman test is the most sensitive test to rule in or out an ACL tear.

B. Imaging Studies

Although radiographs are of limited value in diagnosing ACL tears, a *standard knee series* is recommended to rule out other bony pathology. A fracture of the lateral tibial plateau (Segond fracture) is pathognomonic of an ACL tear. MRI is the imaging modality of choice to confirm a clinically suspected ACL tear. The typical bone bruise pattern occurs in the medial femoral condyle and lateral tibial plateau. There may be associated articular cartilage damage, meniscus pathology, and multiple ligament injuries.

C. Special Tests

With either of the following tests, significant anterior translation of the tibia or lack of a discrete end point indicates a positive test; the injured knee must always be compared to the uninjured side as the patient may have some inherent laxity:

Lachman test: With the patient supine and the knee relaxed in 30° of flexion with just slight external rotation of the hip, the examiner stabilizes the distal femur with one hand, grasps the proximal tibia with the other, and attempts to sublux the tibia anteriorly.

Anterior drawer test: Less sensitive than the Lachman test, the anterior drawer test is performed with the patient supine and the knee flexed to 90°. The examiner stabilizes the relaxed leg by sitting on the patient's foot, grasps the tibial plateau with both thumbs on the tibial tubercle, and applies an anteriorly directed force.

▶ **Treatment**

Initial treatment includes a hinged knee brace, protected weight bearing for comfort, cryotherapy, early RoM exercises, quadriceps sets, and straight leg raises. The majority of active individuals should be referred for surgical consultation. In a very specific subset of patients, nonsurgical treatment is a viable option. These patients are typically older and not active in "cutting" sports. They have to accept some degree of chronic instability and the potential for further meniscal and articular surface injuries.

Posterior Cruciate Ligament Injury

 ESSENTIALS OF DIAGNOSIS

▶ Posterior force on flexed knee.
▶ Positive posterior drawer and "sag" sign.

General Considerations

The PCL limits posterior displacement of the tibia on the femur. PCL tears are less common than ACL tears and often go undetected. The usual mechanism of injury is a posteriorly directed force on the proximal tibia typically in hyperflexion as when a flexed knee strikes a dashboard in a vehicle accident. When seen in the emergency department, 95% of PCL injuries are found in combination with other pathology.

Clinical Findings

A. Symptoms and Signs

Unlike the scenario with ACL tears, patients rarely report a "pop." The initial trauma may be subtle, and subsequent symptoms can be vague. Patients present with knee pain, effusion, and difficulty with the final 10°–20° of flexion. Unsteadiness may be a complaint, but significant instability is more likely to be reported with combined ligamentous injuries. The posterior drawer test is the most accurate test for assessing PCL integrity.

B. Imaging Studies

Imaging preferences are the same as with suspected ACL injuries, and MRI is up to 100% sensitive and 84–100% specific in determining complete PCL tear. A typical bone bruise pattern is found in the anterior tibia. It is imperative that a careful vascular exam be completed, given possible injury to the popliteal artery with PCL tears.

C. Special Tests

The posterior drawer test is performed with the patient supine with the knee flexed to 90°. The examiner stabilizes the relaxed leg by sitting on the patient's foot, grasps the tibial plateau with both thumbs on the tibial tubercle, and applies a posterior-directed force. If significant posterior translation of the tibia or lack of a discrete end point is greater than that of the unaffected limb, the test is positive.

Treatment

Nonsurgical management is acceptable for chronic and/or isolated, low-grade, acute PCL tears. The PCL has greater healing potential than the ACL and can heal over time. Initial treatment for a low-grade PCL injury involves early RoM and emphasizes quadriceps strengthening and partial weight bearing with protection against posterior sag (a brace can be useful and can be locked in extension for 1–2 weeks). A complete tear is treated initially with 2–4 weeks of immobilization in full extension. Indications for expeditious surgical referral include combined ligamentous injury (eg, posterolateral corner), significant laxity, and avulsion fractures. Guidelines for conservative versus surgical management of PCL injuries are still being debated.

Injuries of the Medial Collateral & Lateral Collateral Ligaments

ESSENTIALS OF DIAGNOSIS

► MCL tear results from valgus force causing medial knee pain and laxity.
► LCL tear results from varus force causing lateral knee pain and laxity.
► If effusion is present, consider combined pathology.

General Considerations

The MCL is the most commonly injured stabilizing ligament of the knee. A medially directed or valgus force is the most common cause of MCL disruption. Isolated LCL disruption is relatively rare and occurs with a blow to the anteromedial knee with a varus force.

Clinical Findings

A. Symptoms and Signs

Patients with an isolated collateral ligament tear generally present with a classic mechanism of injury and may report the sensation of a "pop." Patients complain of localized pain and tenderness over the damaged ligament but rarely report significant instability or locking. Localized swelling may be seen with isolated tears, but a significant effusion is uncommon.

B. Imaging Studies

Radiographs are helpful in ruling out other bony pathology but are seldom necessary for diagnosis of isolated tears of the MCL or LCL. X-ray findings may reveal calcification, more commonly in the proximal origin, with chronic injury (Pellegrini-Stieda lesion). MRI is the gold standard for diagnosis and is useful when examination findings are equivocal and can also show associated posterior oblique ligament involvement, bone bruising, or trabecular microfractures that can be found in the lateral femoral condyle or lateral tibial plateau, which typically resolve spontaneously by 4 months.

C. Special Tests

Valgus and varus stress testing, to evaluate the MCL and LCL respectively, is performed at full extension (0°) and 30°. Laxity that is apparent only at 30° of flexion suggests an isolated MCL or LCL injury (first or second degree). Additional laxity in full extension (third degree) suggests concomitant soft tissue injury (ACL or PCL).

▶ Treatment

Treatment of isolated collateral ligament tears is primarily conservative. Ice and use of a compression wrap help to control local swelling. Achieving stability using a hinged knee brace locked in extension is appropriate for 1–2 weeks in a second-degree injury and 3–6 weeks for third-degree injury. However, regardless of severity, the patient must be encouraged to gradually increase weight bearing as soon as possible. Prior to full return to sports, athletes should have achieved full nonpainful RoM and strength and completed a functional rehabilitation program. PRP injections for this injury are still being investigated but have promising early results. Recovery may vary from days to weeks, but nonsurgical management is routinely favored. Surgical fixation is reserved for failed conservative therapy in isolated injuries, which are typically tibial-sided injuries.

Kocher MS, Shore B, Nasreddine A, Heyworth BE. Treatment of posterior cruciate ligament injuries in pediatric and adolescent patients. *J Pediatr Orthop.* 2012;32(6):553–560. [PMID: 22892615]

Levine JW, Kiapour AM, Quatman CE, et al. Clinically relevant injury patterns after an anterior cruciate ligament injury provide insight into injury mechanisms. *Am J Sports Med.* 2013;41:385–394. [PMID: 23144366]

Muyamoto RG, Bosco JA, Sherman OH. Treatment of medial collateral ligament injuries. *J Am Acad Orthop Surg.* 2009;17:152–161. [PMID: 19264708]

MENISCAL TEARS

ESSENTIALS OF DIAGNOSIS

▶ Mechanism of injury is typically a pivoting motion with the foot planted.

▶ Swelling is likely to occur, and pain can be palpated along the joint line.

▶ Patient may describe a clicking or locking sensation in the knee.

▶ General Considerations

The lateral and medial menisci are C-shaped wedges of cartilage that act as shock absorbers between the femur and the tibia. They attach at the anterior and posterior aspects of the tibial plateau and help with load bearing and distribution. In addition, they contribute to overall joint stability and proprioception. The medial meniscus sustains more force during weight bearing and is fused with the MCL, which renders it much less mobile than the lateral meniscus and therefore more susceptible to tearing. Active patients are more prone to acute tears and often have associated ligamentous injuries

that occur with sudden twists or turns during activity. As one ages, the meniscus thins and weakens, which can lead to degenerative tears that require less force.

▶ Clinical Findings

A. Symptoms and Signs

Acute, isolated meniscal tears result primarily from shearing forces during a twisting or hyperflexion injury with the foot planted. Patients describe a "pop" and pain initially. An effusion will likely develop over 24–48 hours. Patients often complain of pain with squatting, mechanical symptoms such as locking or catching, and instability.

Occasionally, a fragment will break off or a large bucket-handle tear will displace into the joint and become lodged within it, preventing full extension and creating a "locked knee." This presentation requires early surgical referral.

Patients with degenerative tears tend to present with an insidious onset of pain, mechanical symptoms, and only mild intermittent swelling. These patients have a more arthritic presentation.

Exam should focus on RoM to ensure that there is no loss of extension or flexion. Joint line tenderness over the affected meniscus is the best clinical indicator of a meniscal tear. Several provocative maneuvers have been developed to re-create impingement of the torn fragment. Examples are the McMurray, Apley, and Thessaly tests, which are helpful but only marginally sensitive or specific.

B. Imaging Studies

Although radiographs cannot confirm the diagnosis of a meniscal tear, a standard knee series (see section on ACL injury, earlier) is obtained to rule out additional bony pathology and to examine for joint space narrowing. It is important to be aware that the amount of joint space narrowing and degenerative change will help direct treatment in older individuals. MRI is the confirmatory imaging modality of choice and may show increased uptake within the meniscus and possible extrusion.

▶ Treatment

Initial treatment for isolated meniscal pathology includes cryotherapy, RoM exercises, NSAIDs, and weight bearing as tolerated. In a young, active individual, early surgical referral should be considered. Depending on activity level and goals, in those middle-aged and older, a course of conservative treatment including physical therapy, corticosteroid injection, and bracing can be initially prescribed. Indications for surgical referral include failure to respond to nonsurgical treatment or recurrent episodes of catching, locking, or giving way. When radiographs show substantial degenerative change, meniscal tears should be treated similarly to arthritis.

Raj MA, Bubnis MA. Knee meniscal tears. StatPearls. Last Updated: October 27, 2018. https://www.statpearls.com/kb/viewarticle/23936/. Accessed November 15, 2019.

Osteoarthritis of the Knee

 ESSENTIALS OF DIAGNOSIS

▸ Insidious onset of joint pain and decreased RoM.

▸ Pain and stiffness are worst after prolonged immobilization and activity.

▸ Joint line pain, grinding, effusion, and muscle weakness are common on physical exam.

▸ General Considerations

Osteoarthritis (OA) is a degenerative condition that affects >20 million people in the United States. It is often progressive, and risk factors include increasing age, female gender, genetics, ethnicity, nutrition, obesity, previous joint injury/trauma, malalignment, and excessive exercise. OA involves the articular surfaces of bones. Typically, over time with normal wear and tear, the cartilage degrades and results in focal loss and joint space narrowing. This causes pain and stiffness, especially after prolonged periods of immobilization and activity. It is often seen in the weight-bearing or larger joints such as the knees and hips; however, it can occur along any articular surface.

▸ Clinical Findings

A. Symptoms and Signs

Onset of pain usually occurs over months to years. Patients typically complain of pain and stiffness in the morning or after prolonged immobilization and activity. They may also describe a "grinding" sensation and complain of intermittent joint swelling. Pain is often diffuse and described in many ways, such as aching, burning, sharp, or dull. It is not unusual for the pain to radiate proximally or distally.

Physical examination of the knee may reveal a decreased RoM and effusion. Pain may be palpated along the length of the joint line, usually medially more than laterally. There is likely associated muscle weakness in the supporting musculature. Crepitus can usually be palpated with joint motion.

B. Imaging Studies

Standard radiographs of the knee are obtained with close attention to views of the weight-bearing joints. Joint space narrowing, osteophytes, subchondral sclerosis, and cyst formation are the most common findings.

C. Lab Studies

If other rheumatologic disorders are suspected, a laboratory analysis should be obtained. A complete blood count, complete metabolic panel, urinalysis, erythrocyte sedimentation rate (ESR), C-reactive protein (CRP), rheumatoid factor, anti–cyclic citrullinated peptide, and antinuclear antibody should be considered for initial screening. The inflammatory markers ESR and CRP may be slightly elevated during the symptomatic phase; all others should be normal.

▸ Differential Diagnosis

Differential diagnosis includes rheumatoid arthritis, meniscal tears, gout, pseudogout, bursitis, psoriatic arthritis, avascular necrosis, and insufficiency fracture.

▸ Treatment

Treatment of OA is aimed at conservative therapy. Topical NSAIDs or other topical analgesics should be first line and may be beneficial in the early stages. Acetaminophen, aspirin, and NSAIDs are commonly used medications for pain relief in OA. A nonimpact exercise program is important to maintain RoM and strength. In cases of increased body mass index (BMI), weight reduction alone can aid in pain relief and decrease further risk of advancing arthritis. Hydrotherapy is a great way to get active without significant joint stress. With aerobic exercise on land, bracing can be used for overall support. Certain braces are able to offload the medial or lateral joint, and other braces facilitate patellar tracking. Glucosamine and chondroitin sulfate are beneficial for some people in reducing OA pain, but their true benefit/efficacy is still being determined.

If a significant effusion is present, an aspiration and an intraarticular corticosteroid injection can aid in temporary pain relief. Risk-benefit profile of corticosteroids in uncontrolled diabetics must be considered given the temporary increase in glucose that occurs. Viscosupplementation with intraarticular hyaluronic acid provides prolonged benefit in some patients and can be repeated every 6 months if effective. Clinicians are still investigating the use and benefits of PRP intraarticular injections for OA of the knee. When conservative therapy is exhausted and daily activities are limited secondary to pain and decreased mobility, then partial or full joint replacement should be considered and referral to an orthopedic surgeon should be initiated.

Bhatia D, Bejarano T, Novo M. Current interventions in the management of knee osteoarthritis. *J Pharm Bioallied Sci.* 2013;5(1):30–38. [PMID: 23559821]

ANKLE SPRAINS

ESSENTIALS OF DIAGNOSIS

▸ Mechanism of injury is forced inversion and plantar flexion (lateral sprain) or forced eversion and dorsiflexion (medial and/or high ankle sprain).

▸ Pain with palpation over the affected ligaments.

▸ Pain worse with ambulation, swelling, and ecchymosis over the lateral or medial ankle with instability of the ankle joint are common physical findings.

▸ General Considerations

Ankle ligament sprains are the most common ankle injuries, and the majority (80%) involve the lateral ankle ligaments: the anterior talofibular ligament (ATFL), calcaneofibular ligament (CFL), and posterior talofibular ligament. They occur after the ankle is placed under extreme inversion and plantar flexion. Syndesmotic or "high" ankle sprains occur when the ankle is dorsiflexed and everted. The recovery from a syndesmotic sprain can be prolonged and is important to identify. Medial ankle sprains are less common and involve the deltoid ligament complex.

▸ Clinical Findings

A. Symptoms and Signs

Patients present with pain over the injured ligaments after "rolling" their ankle and sometimes hearing a "pop." Swelling, ecchymosis, and difficulty with weight bearing are the typical presentation findings but can be variable.

On physical examination, it is important to observe the patient's gait. Often pain can be palpated over the injured ligaments. RoM is often decreased. A complete exam should include palpating the proximal fibula and foot for concurrent injury.

B. Imaging Studies

The Ottawa ankle rules provide high-yield criteria for ordering radiographs (sensitivity 94–100%). Indications for radiographs include bony tenderness at the distal (6 cm), posterior portions of the lateral or medial malleoli, inability to bear weight immediately and take four steps in the emergency department or office, and pain with palpation of the navicular or base of the fifth metatarsal. Routine radiographs include anterior, lateral, and weight-bearing mortise views to assess for fracture, widening of the mortise (indicates instability of the joint), or osteochondritis dissecans injury. MRI is considered to evaluate the ligaments in patients with chronic instability, and computed tomography (CT) scan is used if occult fracture is suspected.

C. Special Tests

Anterior drawer: Stabilize the distal tibia with one hand, and then grasp the calcaneus in the palm of the other hand and apply an anterior force. Excessive anterior motion or a "clunk" suggests disruption of the ATFL.

Talar tilt: Stabilize the tibia with one hand, and then grasp the calcaneus in the palm of the opposite hand and invert the hind foot. Significant laxity with inversion suggests disruption of the ATFL and CFL. A reverse talar tilt assesses for laxity of the deltoid ligament.

▸ Differential Diagnosis

Differential diagnosis includes tibia or fibula fracture, talus or calcaneus fracture, osteochondral defect in the talus, or anterior or posterior ankle impingement.

▸ Treatment

Initial treatment of isolated, acute lateral ankle sprains consists of RICE: rest, ice, compression or support, and elevation. Occasionally, crutches, a posterior splint, cast, or walking boot is required if there is concern for fracture or significant instability. Once fracture has been ruled out, early motion and weight bearing have been shown to facilitate return to activity. This includes a timely physical therapy referral for rehabilitation focusing on restoring motion, strength, and flexibility. Return to play is allowed after full, pain-free strength and RoM are achieved and there are no limitations with sport-specific activities. Often athletes will benefit from taping or a lace-up ankle support once functional.

Syndesmotic sprains require early diagnosis and a more conservative treatment course. If the weight-bearing mortise view shows clear space widening, immediate surgical referral is indicated. If the joint is stable, there is some variability in treatment protocols. This injury can be treated with a brief period of immobilization in a tall walking boot for 1–2 weeks prior to initiating an aggressive rehab program. It is important to inform your patient that this injury will take longer to recover than a typical ankle sprain.

McGovern RP, Martin RL. Managing ankle ligament sprains and tears: current opinions. *Open Access J Sports Med*. 2016;7:33–42. [PMID: 27042147]

MEDIAL TIBIAL STRESS SYNDROME

ESSENTIALS OF DIAGNOSIS

▸ Distal, posteromedial tibia pain worse at the beginning of and after activity, and resolves with rest.

▸ If untreated, pain can advance and occur during activity.

▸ Pain is diffuse as opposed to localized.

General Considerations

Medial tibial stress syndrome (MTSS) is a common overuse injury that causes activity-related pain over the posteromedial aspect of the distal two-thirds of the tibia. Runners are most commonly affected, but MTSS is also quite prevalent in athletes who participate in jumping sports such as basketball, tennis, volleyball, and gymnastics. Risk factors may be pes planus, leg length discrepancy, tight Achilles tendons, higher BMI, female sex, excess hind foot valgus, and recent change in footwear, running surface, or activity intensity.

Clinical Findings

A. Symptoms and Signs

Initially, patients may present with pain at the beginning of a workout or physical activity that may be relieved with continued activity or rest. However, as the injury progresses, pain may last throughout the duration of activity and continue during rest. The pain is referred to as a dull ache over the distal one-third of the posteromedial tibia.

Physical examination reveals diffuse tenderness along the posteromedial border of the distal tibia. In some cases, swelling may be present. Pain is reproduced with passive dorsiflexion and plantar flexion, standing toe raises, and one- or two-legged hop.

B. Imaging Studies

Radiographs of the tibia (AP and lateral) are typically negative but should be obtained to evaluate for stress fracture or tumor. If conservative therapy fails, an MRI or three-phase bone scan should be obtained for further assessment. An MRI is considered the gold standard because it shows greater anatomic detail.

Differential Diagnosis

Differential diagnosis of exertional leg pain includes MTSS, deep venous thrombosis, fascial herniations, muscle strains, posterior tibial tendinitis, nerve or artery entrapment, chronic exertional compartment syndrome, stress fracture, and neoplasm.

Treatment

Initial treatment of MTSS consists of activity modification and avoidance of aggravating factors using pain as a guide. Cross-training activities such as swimming, biking, and jumping are encouraged to maintain cardiovascular fitness during the recovery phase. Impact activities can be increased gradually thereafter, advancing only if asymptomatic at each stage. Ice massage, NSAIDs, shock-absorbent inserts, heel cord stretching, and correction of malalignment can aid in treatment and pain relief. Physical therapy with massage, electrical stimulation, ultrasound, and iontophoresis

should be considered. Surgical referral for posteromedial fasciotomy is reserved for patients with extraordinarily resistant and painful symptoms and after compartment pressure testing has been completed. A clinician must have a high index of suspicion for stress fracture in the setting of MTSS and consider early imaging if any doubt exists.

Reinking MF, Austin TM, Richter RR, Kreiger MM. Medial tibial stress syndrome in active individuals: a systematic review and meta-analysis of risk factors. *Sports Health*. 2017;9(3):252–261. [PMID: 27729482]

PLANTAR FASCIITIS

 ESSENTIALS OF DIAGNOSIS

▸ Heel pain at the medial, plantar aspect of the calcaneus.

▸ Heel pain and tightness with first steps of morning.

General Considerations

The plantar fascia is the fibrous aponeurosis that provides static support and dynamic shock absorption for the longitudinal arch of the foot. After a recent change in distance, intensity, or duration of activity, the plantar fascia can develop microtears and eventually chronic degenerative changes as a result of overuse. This is referred to as *plantar fasciitis*, a common cause of heel pain. Risk factors include pes cavus or pes planus, prolonged standing, excessive training, decreased flexibility of the Achilles tendon and intrinsic foot muscles, obesity, and sedentary lifestyle. Diagnosis is based primarily on history and physical examination. Typically patients have heel pain in their first steps in the morning and with palpation of the medial aspect of the anterior calcaneus.

Clinical Findings

A. Symptoms and Signs

Classically, patients present with insidious onset of pain on the plantar surface of the heel that is worse with the first steps in the morning or when standing after a prolonged period of rest. Pain usually diminishes with rest but may recur at the end of the day. Athletes report that running, hill climbing, and sprinting exacerbate the pain.

Physical examination generally demonstrates tenderness along the anteromedial aspect of the calcaneus that intensifies with stretching of the plantar fascia by passive dorsiflexion of the toes. Limited ankle dorsiflexion associated with a tight heel cord may also be noted.

B. Imaging Studies

Radiographs are rarely indicated for the initial diagnosis and treatment of plantar fasciitis. Heel spurs on the anterior calcaneus can be misleading; these are present in 15–25% of the general population without symptoms, and many symptomatic patients do not have spurs. For chronic, recalcitrant cases, radiographs of the foot (AP, lateral, and oblique views) can guide further treatment plans. Musculoskeletal ultrasound can be used for in-office evaluation and diagnosis.

Differential Diagnosis

The differential diagnosis of heel pain includes calcaneal stress fracture, plantar fascia rupture, fat pad atrophy, retrocalcaneal bursitis, nerve entrapment syndromes, arthropathies, Achilles or flexor hallucis tendinopathy, posterior tibial tendinitis, heel contusion, calcaneal apophysitis, or even tumor.

Treatment

Plantar fasciitis is a self-limiting condition, and regardless of therapy, most cases will resolve within a year and 90% of patients will improve with conservative treatment. This includes activity modification, NSAIDs, heel cushions or arch supports, and an aggressive Achilles and plantar fascia stretching program. Deep myofascial massage and iontophoresis have been used by physical therapists with positive benefit in many cases, and shockwave therapy can be considered. Corticosteroid injections may provide short-term benefit but can cause fat pad atrophy or plantar fascia rupture. PRP is also being considered for pain control, and the literature is beginning to show support for this. Custom orthotics in combination with night splints may be beneficial in patients with recalcitrant symptoms. After 6 months of conservative therapy, extracorporeal shockwave therapy is a promising option but seldom covered by medical insurance. After a prolonged period of conservative treatment with continued pain, surgical release or fasciotomy can also be considered.

Aiyer A. Plantar fasciitis. Orthobullets. Updated: October 26, 2016. https://www.orthobullets.com/foot-and-ankle/7025/plantar-fasciitis. Accessed November 15, 2019.

Greater Trochanteric Bursitis

ESSENTIALS OF DIAGNOSIS

► Pain over lateral aspect of hip.
► Symptoms worsened with pressure on lateral hip such as rolling onto side at night.

General Considerations

The greater trochanteric bursa is located on the lateral aspect of the hip and can be a source of pain for individuals of all ages. Inflammation can be either the result of direct trauma or insidious. Historically this pathology has been described as a single source of pain, the bursa. However, more recent evidence suggests broader inflammation and involvement of the iliotibial band and gluteus medius muscle.

Clinical Findings

A. Signs and Symptoms

Patients will complain primarily of lateral hip pain with tenderness to palpation at the greater trochanteric bursa. The patient typically has full hip RoM and full strength; however, both extremes of motion and manual muscle testing may bring on symptoms.

B. Imaging Studies

Plain radiographs of the hip and pelvis help rule out other pathology such as OA or bony hip deformities. Musculoskeletal ultrasound can be used to visualize the bursa for both diagnosis and treatment (injection).

Treatment

Initial treatment includes physical therapy with a focus on iliotibial band stretching and hip strengthening. Often, adding the modality of a foam roller can be helpful in treating this entity. Pain should be controlled with ice and NSAIDs. For most patients, a single corticosteroid injection provides improvement of symptoms. A cure rate with conservative interventions can be expected to exceed 90%. However, recurrence is common, and for those with ongoing pain after an extended course of conservative care, surgery may be considered.

Reid D. The management of greater trochanteric pain syndrome: a systematic literature review. *J Orthop.* 2016;12(1):15–28. [PMID: 26955229]

Hip Impingement/Labral Tear

ESSENTIALS OF DIAGNOSIS

► Deep anterior groin pain.
► Reproduced with flexion and internal rotation of the hip.

General Considerations

Femoroacetabular hip impingement (FAI) and labral tears are modern orthopedic concepts with a constantly expanding body of literature. The two pathologies are intimately related in that a large majority of patients with impingement are found to have labral tears.

Hip impingement is described as an osseous abnormality of femoral head-neck offset (cam) or excessive coverage of the acetabular rim (pincer) resulting in early chondrolabral damage, OA, and hip pain. The cause of the bony abnormalities remains unclear at this time.

A labral tear has been found to frequently coexist with hip impingement. The labrum of the hip is a triangular fibrocartilaginous structure located circumferentially around the bony acetabulum that plays a crucial role in hip mechanics. The etiology of tears falls into four categories: traumatic, degenerative, idiopathic, and congenital.

▶ Clinical Findings

A. Symptoms and Signs

The majority of patients with both impingement and labral tears will present with anterior groin pain. The majority will be insidious (50–65%), but some will follow a traumatic event. Patients will occasionally complain of mechanical symptoms such as clicking, catching, locking, or giving way. Most will have decreased hip motion and weakness on exam. Symptoms typically worsen with activity. Nearly all patients will have a positive anterior impingement (flexion, adduction, and internal rotation [FADIR]) test, which is described later.

B. Imaging Studies

Plain radiographs will demonstrate the abnormal morphology of impingement. AP weight-bearing pelvis and cross-table lateral views should be ordered. The cross-table lateral view will show a classic "pistol-grip deformity" in cam impingement. The "crossover sign" suggests acetabular overcoverage as is seen in pincer impingement.

An MRI arthrogram of the hip is necessary to visualize labral pathology and is considered the gold standard diagnostic study.

C. Special Tests

The anterior impingement test is a provocative test that is commonly used and is nearly always positive in patients with FAI and labral tears. However, it must be interpreted with caution as it is also positive in many other situations such as hip OA. The patient is positioned supine, and the hip is passively flexed to 90° followed by forced adduction and internal rotation (FADIR). The presence of anterior groin pain during this maneuver is considered a positive test.

▶ Treatment

Initial treatment should be conservative, combining physical therapy focusing on hip strengthening, NSAIDs, and activity modification. An intraarticular injection of a long-acting anesthetic combined with a corticosteroid can be both therapeutic and diagnostic for this pathology. If the injection relieves symptoms, even for a brief period, the pain generator is presumed to be intraarticular. A patient who continues to have symptoms after 6–8 weeks of conservative treatment should be referred to an orthopedic surgeon who is experienced in hip arthroscopy for further evaluation.

Pun S, Kumar D, Lane NE. Femoroacetabular impingement. *Arthritis Rheumatol.* 2015;67(1):17–27. [PMID: 25308887]

▼ PEDIATRIC AND ADOLESCENT MUSCULOSKELETAL DISORDERS SPONDYLOLYSIS

 ESSENTIALS OF DIAGNOSIS

▶ Lumbar pain that worsens with extension.

▶ General Considerations

Spondylolysis is one of the most common causes of back pain in active young children and adolescents. It is defined as a defect, or *stress fracture*, in the pars interarticularis of the posterior neural arch of the vertebrae. It occurs at the L5 level in ≤95% of cases and is bilateral in approximately 80% of cases. The etiology is typically repetitive hyperextension of the lumbar spine as is seen in sports such as gymnastics, football, diving, and pole vaulting.

▶ Clinical Findings

A. Symptoms and Signs

Spondylolysis is usually characterized by the insidious onset of low back pain that increases with activity and lumbar extension. Pain may be severe at times, but neurologic symptoms and radiculopathy are rare. Physical examination may be relatively normal, or the patient may have localized lumbosacral tenderness or reproducible pain with gentle extension.

B. Imaging Studies

The initial imaging for suspected spondylolysis includes AP, lateral, and right and left oblique radiographs of the lumbar spine. The most common radiographic finding is a fracture through the collar of the "Scotty dog" on oblique radiographs. If clinical suspicion remains high despite normal radiographs, more advanced imaging is warranted. Several other modalities have proved useful in detecting pars defects, including bone scan, single-photon emission CT, conventional CT, and MRI.

C. Special Tests

The "stork test" is performed by standing on one leg while hyperextending the spine. Reproduction of pain indicates a positive test.

Differential Diagnosis

The differential diagnosis of acute low back pain in the pediatric population includes spondylolisthesis, scoliosis, lumbosacral strain, and discogenic pain. Inflammatory arthropathies should be considered in the context of chronic pain. Night pain, fever, or other systemic symptoms should prompt an evaluation for infection or neoplasm.

Treatment

Treatment of symptomatic spondylolysis generally involves a combination of activity modification, bracing, and rehabilitation. Antilordotic bracing will often reduce pain. Rehab protocols should focus on core strengthening and hamstring stretching. Finally, a gradual return to play will result in 95% of patients returning to their preinjury activity level. Surgical management is indicated if pain persists despite conservative treatment.

Donnally CJ III, Varacallo M. Lumbar spondylolysis and spondylolisthesis. StatPearls. Last Updated: October 27, 2018. https://www.statpearls.com/kb/viewarticle/24467/. Accessed November 15, 2019.

LEGG-CALVE-PERTHES DISEASE & SLIPPED CAPITAL FEMORAL EPIPHYSIS

ESSENTIALS OF DIAGNOSIS

▶ Adolescent, often overweight male, presents with limp and diffuse hip pain.

General Considerations

Legg-Calves-Perthes disease (LCPD) is defined as idiopathic osteonecrosis and collapse of the femoral head. Most cases occur between 4 and 8 years of age. Boys are more commonly affected. Slipped capital femoral epiphysis (SCFE) is defined as the posterior and inferior slippage of the proximal femoral epiphysis on the metaphysis (femoral neck), which occurs through the epiphyseal plate (growth plate). The peak incidence occurs in early adolescence at 12–13 years of age. There is predominance in overweight males. The etiology of SCFE is assumed to be multifactorial and may include obesity, growth surges, and less commonly, endocrine disorders. Both conditions may be found bilaterally in the same individual.

Clinical Findings

A. Signs and Symptoms

The presentations of both LCPD and SCFE are characterized by diffuse aching pain in the groin, medial thigh, or knee.

Pain is often accompanied by an altered gait or limp, and it is usually worsened by activity. SCFE may present as knee pain in ≤23% of cases, and it cannot be overstated that the investigation of knee pain in children should include a history and physical examination that addresses the hips as well.

Physical examination may produce pain at the extremes of motion, particularly in hip abduction and internal rotation. Both disorders will present with loss of normal motion, particularly in internal rotation.

B. Imaging Studies

AP and frog-leg lateral and/or cross-table lateral radiographs of both hips should be obtained. Plain radiographs nearly always confirm the diagnosis of SCFE by demonstrating displacement of the femoral head. The LCPD radiographic findings present a continuum of changes as the disease progresses. In the early stages of LCPD, plain radiographs may be normal. However, over time, there can be widening of the joint space, sclerosis of the femoral head, cystic changes, and coxa magna, which is defined as flattening and widening of the femoral head.

Differential Diagnosis

The differential diagnosis includes developmental dysplasia of the hip, septic arthritis, transient synovitis, labral pathology, and benign or malignant neoplasms. Inflammatory causes (juvenile rheumatoid arthritis, spondyloarthropathies, Lyme disease arthritis) are possible as well.

Treatment

LCPD is a self-limiting condition, but symptoms may persist for ≤4 years. The primary goal of treatment for LCPD is pain reduction, and this sometimes requires bracing/casting and protected weight bearing. Operative intervention may be indicated in older patients or those with advanced disease. Surgery is the preferred treatment for SCFE and typically involves emergent stabilization of the femoral head with metallic fixation devices. Delays in treatment may lead to further displacement and osteonecrosis, ultimately compromising postoperative outcomes.

Peck DM, Voss LM, Voss TT. Slipped capital femoral epiphysis: diagnosis and management. *Am Fam Physician.* 2017;95(12): 779–784. [PMID: 28671425]

OSTEOCHONDRITIS DISSECANS

ESSENTIALS OF DIAGNOSIS

▶ Active adolescent with poorly localized joint pain.

General Considerations

Osteochondritis dissecans (OCD) is described as an idiopathic lesion of the cartilage and subchondral bone in the skeletally immature patient. The "classic" location for this lesion is the lateral aspect of the medial femoral condyle; however, it can also be seen in the other knee compartments, ankle, and elbow. The pathology is not entirely understood, but the etiology is believed to be repetitive trauma. There is a male predominance.

Clinical Findings

A. Symptoms and Signs

The clinical presentation is poorly localized knee pain that is worsened by activity. There may be a mild limp. In more advanced disease, the patient may report mechanical symptoms, such as locking or catching. An effusion is present in only <20% of patients and thus should not be used to rule in or out this pathology. Wilson's test has been described for this lesion; however, evidence shows it to be positive in only 16% of knees with proven OCD lesions and thus should not be considered a dependable test. During Wilson's test, the patient's knee rests at 90 degrees of flexion, the examiner internally rotates the tibia, and the patient slowly extends the knee. A positive test occurs when pain is worse on knee extension to 30° from flexion and pain is relieved with external rotation of tibia.

B. Imaging Studies

Most OCD lesions can be diagnosed on plain radiographs. Lesions can be difficult to visualize on standard views, so four views of the knee should be ordered: AP, lateral, tunnel, and Merchant views. There should be a low threshold for imaging the contralateral knee for comparison and the possibility of bilateral lesions. MRI is recommended to assess the size, location, and character of the OCD lesion.

Treatment

To classify treatment, two points need to be determined: (1) whether the patient is skeletally mature and (2) whether the lesion is stable. If the lesion is stable and the patient is skeletally immature, then nonsurgical treatment should be first-line. There is no exact timetable, but most clinicians agree on a period of restricting sports participation (perhaps with casting) for 6 weeks. As the lesion heals radiographically, gradual return to activity is allowed. This is a very subjective process that is open for broad interpretation. Those lesions that are unstable or do not respond to conservative care should be treated surgically.

Jones MH, Williams AM. Osteochondritis dissecans of the knee: a practical guide for surgeons. *Bone Joint J.* 2016;98-B(6): 723–729. [PMID: 27235511]

APOPHYSEAL INJURIES

ESSENTIALS OF DIAGNOSIS

▶ Insidious pain over growth plate in skeletally immature individual.

▶ Overuse injury.

General Considerations

An *apophysis* is a growing bony prominence at which secondary ossification occurs in the skeletally immature individual. Apophysitis is a painful, inflammatory condition at the tendinous insertion of these bony prominences. This condition is unique to active youth and, by definition, not existent in skeletally mature individuals. Repetitive stress and traction on the apophysis ("overuse") are the offending causes. There seems to be a period of risk surrounding growth spurts. The most common sites of apophysitis are the tibial tuberosity (Osgood-Schlatter disease), inferior patella (Sinding-Larsen-Johansson syndrome), posterior calcaneus (Sever disease), medial epicondyle of elbow ("Little League elbow"), and humeral head ("Little League shoulder"). It is important to note that tendinopathies are unusual in children since the apophysis is intrinsically weaker and more susceptible to injury than the tendon.

Clinical Findings

A. Symptoms and Signs

These conditions are diagnosed clinically by history and physical examination. Patients generally describe an insidious onset of well-localized pain at the site of injury or inflammation. Pain is uniformly present during or shortly after activity. Tenderness is easily elicited by palpation. The presence of mechanical symptoms (locking, catching, or loss of motion), particularly in the elbow, should prompt consideration of an alternate diagnosis.

B. Imaging Studies

Although plain radiographs may serve to exclude other causes of pain, they are not routinely necessary in establishing the diagnosis.

▶ Treatment

Apophysitis is generally self-limited and resolves once skeletal maturity is reached and the apophysis fuses. In the meantime, treatment is accomplished by activity modification, ice, NSAIDs, and rehab focused on stretching and strengthening. In most cases, a candid discussion with the athlete and her or his family will reveal training patterns that can be altered to prevent further injury. In the case of baseball pitchers, proper throwing mechanics and adhering to pitch count recommendations will be helpful.

Longo UG, Ciuffreda M, Locher J, Maffulli N, Denaro V. Apophyseal injuries in children's and youth sports. *Br Med Bull.* 2016;120(1):139–159. [PMID: 27941042]

39

Common Upper & Lower Extremity Fractures

Wade M. Rankin, DO, CAQSM

Richard A. Okragly, MD, FAMSSM

Michael A. Fitzgerald, DO

Kelly Evans-Rankin, MD, CAQSM

Amanda C. Goodale, DO

Steven Sanker, DO

Tyler K. Drewry, MD, CAQSM

▼ UPPER EXTREMITY FRACTURES

CLAVICLE FRACTURES

▶ Clinical Findings

A. Symptoms and Signs

Clavicle fractures (Figure 39–1) are relatively common as a result of sports injury or direct trauma, accounting for 2–5% of all fractures in adults. The typical mechanism of injury is a fall directly on the shoulder with the arm at the side. Rarely, fractures may also occur from a direct blow or fall onto an outstretched hand. The patient will complain of pain involving the affected shoulder and will typically hold the arm in adduction and internal rotation, avoiding any motion. There may be swelling, discoloration, deformity, and crepitus on palpation at the fracture site. Displaced fractures may cause visible tenting of the skin.

B. Imaging Studies

Clavicle fractures are best seen on an anteroposterior (AP) view. An AP view with the beam directed 30°–45° cephalad is sometimes necessary to lessen rib interference. A serendipity view may also be obtained to assess for sternoclavicular dislocations. A computed tomography (CT) scan can better visualize poorly seen medial or lateral one-third fractures. Additional x-rays of the ipsilateral shoulder may be necessary to evaluate for associated injuries. All x-rays need to be carefully examined for the presence of a concomitant scapular fracture resulting in a floating shoulder.

▶ Complications

Complications may include injuries to the subclavian blood vessels or brachial plexus. Associated pneumothorax is also a rare complication. Fractures displaced ≥100% appear to be at increased risk for nonunion. Excessive callus formation can lead to cosmetic deformity or, more rarely, compromise of neurovascular structures. It may require years for a large callus to remodel. Intraarticular fractures on either the medial or lateral end can lead to degenerative arthritis. Other long-term sequelae include pain both at rest and with activity, weakness, and paresthesias.

▶ Treatment

Nonsurgical management is the treatment of choice for most clavicle fractures and usually involves a sling for 2–6 weeks, analgesics, and avoidance of overhead activity. A sling is primarily used instead of a figure-of-eight bandage due to comfort. Clavicle fractures can be categorized using the Allman classification.

Middle one-third clavicle fractures (group I) account for approximately 80% of fractures. Treatment for displacement or overlapping of >2 cm is controversial, but minimally displaced midshaft fractures can be treated conservatively. Distal one-third clavicle fractures (group II) include multiple different subtypes that depend on fracture location in relation to the coracoclavicular ligaments. The vast majority may be treated conservatively, but certain subtypes may need orthopedic referral. Medial one-third fractures (group III) are the least common clavicular fractures and are almost always treated nonoperatively using a sling. They are most commonly associated with multisystem trauma. If posterior sternoclavicular dislocation is suspected, the patient should be transferred to the emergency department and should receive CT to rule out damage to the great vessels and pulmonary system.

Indications for operative management include open fractures, fractures that compromise the airway or neurovascular structures, the presence of significant displacement and/or tenting of the skin, or a floating shoulder. Radiographs should be obtained at 2-week follow-up to assess for

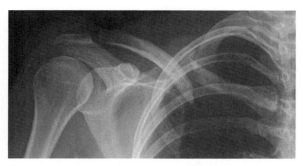

▲ **Figure 39–1.** Clavicle midshaft fracture. (Used with permission from Justin Montgomery, MD; University of Kentucky Radiology.)

displacement and angulation. Visible callus typically forms between 4 and 6 weeks, coinciding with significant clinical improvement. Once the fracture is clinically and radiographically healed, radiographs can be discontinued. The patient may return to normal activity when the clavicle is painless, the fracture is healed on radiograph, and the shoulder has a full range of motion and near-normal strength. Noncontact sports may often be resumed at 6 weeks, but return to contact sports may require 2–4 months.

Monica J, Vredenburgh Z, Korsh J, Gatt C. Acute shoulder injuries in adults. *Am Fam Physician.* 2016;94(2):119–127. [PMID: 27419328]
Pecci M, Kreher JB. Clavicle fractures. *Am Fam Physician.* 2008;77(1):65–70. [PMID: 18236824]
Van der Meijden OA, Gaskill TR, Millet PJ. Treatment of clavicle fractures: current concepts review. *J Shoulder Elbow Surg.* 2012; 21:423–429. [PMID: 22063756]

PROXIMAL HUMERUS FRACTURE

▶ Clinical Findings

A. Symptoms and Signs

Falls from standing height are the main cause of proximal humerus fractures in adults. The incidence increases with age, particularly over age 65. Women are affected 2–3 times as often as men. Less common injury patterns include direct trauma or sudden muscle contraction. Patients typically present with pain and swelling in the shoulder that is worse with shoulder movement. On examination, patients may hold the affected extremity adducted against their body. Neurovascular status must be evaluated in patients with this injury.

B. Imaging Studies

Plain radiographs of the affected shoulder are the initial imaging study in a patient with a suspected proximal humerus fracture. The typical views include a true AP view, a scapular-Y view, and an axillary view. Modified axillary views may be necessary if the patient cannot abduct their arm >60°. CT scan with three-dimensional reconstructions may be indicated if x-rays are nondiagnostic in a patient with a high index of suspicion for a fracture. The Neer classification scheme is used most commonly to describe proximal humerus fractures based on the four anatomic segments of the proximal humerus. They include the articular part, the greater tuberosity, the lesser tuberosity, and the humeral shaft. Neer described one-, two-, three-, and four-part fractures if the segments were displaced by 1 cm or angulated 45 degrees from each other.

▶ Complications

Varying degrees of decreased shoulder range of motion may result from proximal humerus fractures. This can include adhesive capsulitis. Other complications can include injuries to the brachial plexus and axillary and suprascapular nerve compression. More severe injuries can include joint dislocation or acute compartment syndrome. Injury to the anterior and posterior circumflex arteries can lead to avascular necrosis of the humeral head. With any fracture, malunion and nonunion are of concern.

▶ Treatment

A vast majority of proximal humerus fractures are nondisplaced or minimally displaced and therefore can be treated conservatively. Nonsurgical treatment of Neer one-part fractures involves a period of immobilization with an arm sling and referral to physical therapy at approximately the 2-week mark to improve range of motion and strength deficits. There is moderately high-quality evidence that surgery for patients with one-part fractures does not result in a better outcome at 1 and 2 years after injury compared with nonsurgical treatment. Complex proximal humerus fractures (defined as Neer two-part and higher) and fractures of the anatomic neck (higher risk of avascular necrosis) should be immobilized in a sling and referred to an orthopedic surgeon. In addition, orthopedic referral should be sought if there is concern for neurovascular compromise, if there is presence of a shoulder dislocation, or if the treating physician lacks experience in fracture management. In addition, there is insufficient evidence regarding the different nonsurgical, surgical, or rehabilitation interventions for these fractures.

Handoll HH, Brorson S. Interventions for treatment proximal humerus fractures. *Cochrane Database Syst Rev.* 2015; 11:CD000434. [PMID: 26560014]
Handoll HH, Keding A, Corbacho B, et al. Five-year follow-up results of the PROFHER trial comparing operative and nonoperative treatment of adults with displaced fracture of the proximal humerus. *Bone Joint J.* 2017;99-B:383–392. [PMID: 28249980]

MIDSHAFT HUMERUS FRACTURES

▶ Clinical Findings

A. Symptoms and Signs

Midshaft humerus fractures occur from a direct blow or a bending force to the humerus. In addition, a fall-on-outstretched-hand (FOOSH) injury or fall on the elbow with the arm in abduction can lead to a midshaft humerus fracture, particularly in females over the age of 60 years. Less commonly, high-velocity throwing or other activities that cause forceful muscle contractions can lead to fracture. Patients typically present with severe pain in the upper arm. There may be referred pain to the shoulder or elbow. Deformity of the midarm may be appreciated on examination. A detailed neurovascular examination of the affected arm is imperative in the evaluation of a suspected midshaft humerus fracture. Both motor and sensory function of the radial, median, and ulnar nerves should be tested. Radial and ulnar pulses should be assessed as well.

B. Imaging Studies

Imaging requires at least AP and lateral radiographs. Additional oblique views may be required to fully assess the extent of the fracture. Fracture patterns include spiral, oblique, and transverse. The AO classification scheme is generally used to classify the various types of fractures: type A fractures are simple fractures with the humeral shaft is broken in two; type B are wedge fractures; and type C are complex fractures that have multiple fragments (comminuted). Displacement occurs because of the pull of the deltoid, biceps, triceps, and pectoralis muscles.

▶ Complications

Fractures of the humerus shaft are often complicated by radial nerve injury. The incidence of radial nerve injury is roughly 11%, making it the most common peripheral nerve injury associated with bone fractures. The radial nerve is most susceptible at the posterior midshaft, where it lies in contact with the humerus, and at the distal lateral humerus, where it pierces the lateral intermuscular septum. Intact radial nerve motor function includes active extension of the wrist, fingers, and thumb at the metacarpal-phalangeal joints. Radial nerve sensation is tested at the dorsal radial aspect of the hand at the thumb/index finger webspace. Median and ulnar nerve injuries are uncommon following midshaft humerus fractures. Nonunion can also occur, particularly with transverse fractures and severely comminuted fractures.

▶ Treatment

The initial treatment of humeral shaft fractures involves immobilization in an upper arm sugar-tong splint (coaptation splint). Alternately, a long-arm posterior splint can be used. There may be an indication for the use of traction with some spiral, oblique, and comminuted fractures, prior to splinting, to obtain satisfactory alignment. This can be achieved with a hanging cast, collar and cuff sling, or an upper arm sugar-tong splint. Orthopedic referral should be sought if midshaft humerus fractures cannot be maintained in adequate alignment, defined as <20° of anterior/posterior angulation, <30° of varus angulation, and <3 cm of shortening. Surgical referral is indicated with open fractures, fractures with vascular compromise, fracture-dislocations, and pathologic fractures. Orthopedic referral should be considered in unstable transverse fractures, in patients who are noncompliant with splinting or bracing, and when the treating physician lacks experience in fracture management. Functional bracing is the currently accepted gold standard for definitive treatment. Timing for functional bracing depends on the degree of swelling in the arm but is typically 1–2 weeks after injury, and braces are worn for 4–6 weeks. There is no high-quality evidence showing any differences in patient outcomes between nonsurgical and surgical interventions. There is no evidence to support one nonsurgical method over another. In addition, if surgical intervention is undertaken, there is no evidence to favor plate fixation over intramedullary nailing.

Clement ND. Management of humeral stress fractures; non-operative versus operative. *Arch Trauma Res.* 2015;4(2):e28013. [No PMID]

Gosler MW, Testroote M, Morrnhof JW, Janzing HM. Surgical versus non-surgical interventions for treating humeral shaft fractures in fractures. *Cochrane Database Syst Rev.* 2012;1:CD008832. [PMID: 22258990]

Rocchi M, Tarallo L, Mugnai, Adani R. Humerus shaft fracture complicated by radial nerve palsy: is surgical exploration necessary? *Musculoskelet Surg.* 2016;100(Suppl 1):S53–S60. [PMID: 27900704]

RADIAL HEAD FRACTURES

▶ Clinical Findings

A. Symptoms and Signs

Radial head fractures account for up to one-third of all elbow fractures. The typical mechanism of injury is a FOOSH with a pronated forearm or with the elbow in slight flexion. Alternatively, a direct blow to the lateral elbow can also produce these fractures. Patients present with elbow pain, swelling, and pain on movement of the forearm. The elbow will be tender to palpation over the radial head, just distal to the lateral epicondyle.

B. Imaging Studies

AP and lateral x-rays of the elbow are generally adequate to detect a fracture, although an oblique or radiocapitellar view may be necessary for visualization of subtle fractures or

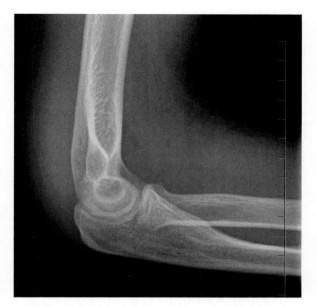

▲ **Figure 39–2.** Fat pad sign with a proximal radial head fracture. (Used with permission from Justin Montgomery, MD; University of Kentucky Radiology.)

to better evaluate displacement. Sometimes, an elbow joint effusion (sail sign and/or visualization of the posterior fat pad) is the only x-ray evidence of a fracture (Figure 39–2). CT scan may better show degree of displacement and angulation for surgical considerations.

The Mason classification system is as follows:

Type I: nondisplaced fracture; no mechanical obstruction to movement

Type II: displacement >2 mm or angulation >30°

Type III: comminuted fractures

Type IV: fracture with associated elbow dislocation

▶ Complications

Loss of elbow motion, specifically decreased elbow extension, is the most common complication. For this reason, elbow movement is encouraged as early as possible according to the type of fracture (see Mason classification below) and the patient's symptoms. Additional complications can include posttraumatic arthritis, heterotopic ossification, complex regional pain syndrome, and wrist pain from an associated distal radioulnar joint injury.

▶ Treatment

Mason type I fractures can be managed conservatively without orthopedic referral. The elbow can be placed in a posterior splint or sling for ≤7 days as needed to control pain. Early movement should be encouraged. If symptoms allow, these fractures can also be treated without immobilization with patients allowed movement of the elbow as tolerated. Repeat x-rays in 1–2 weeks to ensure alignment has been maintained. Resolution of pain and return of normal elbow function are usually obtained by 2–3 months. Any mechanical restriction to rotation is an indication for surgery.

Orthopedic referral is generally indicated for Mason type II–IV fractures. Mason type II fractures with slight displacement may be managed without surgery. More significant displacement or angulation generally requires open reduction with internal fixation or excision. Mason type III fractures require surgical correction with fixation, excision, or replacement of the comminuted radial head depending on the degree of comminution.

Black WS, Becker JA. Common forearm fractures in adults. *Am Fam Physician.* 2009;80(10):1096–1102. [PMID: 19904894]

Kodde IF, Kaas L, Flipsen M, van den Bekerom MP, Eygendaal D. Current concepts in the management of radial head fractures. *World J Orthop.* 2015;6(11):954–960. [PMID: 26716091]

COLLES FRACTURES (DISTAL RADIUS FRACTURES)

▶ Clinical Findings

A. Symptoms and Signs

Fracture of the distal radius, commonly referred to as a Colles fracture, is typically the result of a FOOSH injury (Figure 39–3). Patients present with swelling, ecchymosis, tenderness, and painful range of motion of the distal forearm. On examination, the classic "dinner fork" deformity (dorsal displacement of the distal fragment and volar angulation of the distal intact radius with radial shortening) may be identified; however, the extremity may appear normal.

B. Imaging Studies

Imaging confirms fracture severity, determines stability, and guides the treatment approach. Plain radiographs should include posteroanterior (PA) and lateral views of the wrist, as well as oblique views for further fracture definition. Accurate assessment of radiographic measurements is crucial for appropriate management and includes radial inclination (average of 23°), radial height (average of 11 mm), and volar tilt (average of 11°). CT scans are helpful for evaluating the extent of intraarticular involvement, as well as for surgical planning.

▶ Complications

Early complications may include median nerve neuropathy, extensor pollicis longus tendon rupture, and compartment

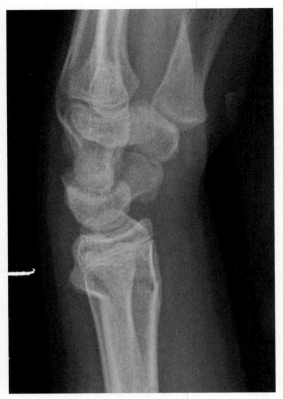

▲ **Figure 39–3.** Colles fracture with dinner fork deformity. (Used with permission from Justin Montgomery, MD; University of Kentucky Radiology.)

syndrome. Late complications may include radiocarpal arthrosis, complex regional pain syndrome, cosmetic changes of the wrist, and fracture malunion or nonunion.

▶ Treatment

Distal radius fractures may be treated nonoperatively or operatively, depending on various factors. Indications for emergent orthopedic consultation include open fractures, fractures with associated acute neuropathy or compartment syndrome, or suspected vascular compromise.

Nondisplaced extraarticular fractures are relatively stable and are treated nonoperatively with a long-arm splint acutely to allow for swelling, then transitioned to a short-arm cast. The usual duration of immobilization is 6 weeks, with serial x-rays performed weekly for the first several weeks to monitor for displacement.

Displaced fractures should undergo an attempt at closed reduction followed by immobilization in a long-arm sugartong splint acutely. Postreduction radiographs must be obtained to assess the quality of the reduction. If the fracture reduction is acceptable, the patient may remain in the splint and be followed up with serial radiographs to ensure reduction is maintained. Given the reduction is well maintained, the splint may be transitioned to a cast for a total of 6 weeks of immobilization.

Surgical fixation is indicated for distal radius fractures that fail to meet acceptable alignment criteria (see the following list). Various methods include closed reduction percutaneous pinning, external fixation, and open reduction internal fixation (ORIF). Postoperatively, most patients will be cleared for activities as tolerated by 10–12 weeks.

Acceptable criteria for distal radius fractures include the following:

- Radial height: <5 mm of shortening
- Radial inclination: <5° change
- Articular step off: <2-mm step-off
- Volar tilt: Dorsal angulation <5° or within 20° of contralateral distal radius

Hsu H, Nallamothu SV. Fracture, wrist. [Updated 2018 May 13]. In: StatPearls [Internet]. Treasure Island, FL: StatPearls Publishing; 2018. https://www.ncbi.nlm.nih.gov/books/NBK499972/. Accessed November 19, 2019.

SCAPHOID FRACTURES

▶ Clinical Findings

A. Symptoms and Signs

Scaphoid fractures should be suspected in any patient who presents after sustaining a FOOSH injury and reports radial-sided wrist pain. The most common mechanism of injury is an axial load across a dorsiflexed and radially deviated wrist. Potential fracture sites include the scaphoid waist (65%), proximal pole (15%), distal pole (10%), and tubercle (8%). Bone healing occurs at different rates depending on the location of the fracture. Regardless of fracture location, patients will present with a painful wrist and may report swelling, ecchymosis, or paresthesias of the affected hand. On examination, there is maximal tenderness in the anatomic snuffbox, pain with radial deviation of the wrist, and pain with axial compression of the thumb.

B. Imaging Studies

Evaluation of suspected scaphoid fractures begins with standard radiography including PA, lateral, and oblique wrist films. A dedicated scaphoid view (PA view with wrist in ulnar deviation) is often obtained for better visualization as well. Initial radiographs are normal in approximately 25% of patients. Typically, these patients are placed into a short-arm thumb spica cast and followed up in 1–14 days for repeat imaging. If repeat radiographs are negative and fracture suspicion remains, magnetic resonance imaging (MRI) can be obtained to rule out occult fracture. CT scans are quite useful in guiding treatment and assessing for fracture union, which can be misleading on radiographs.

▶ Complications

Approximately 80% of the scaphoid is covered by cartilage, thus providing few entrances for vascularity. This unique and tenuous blood supply places the scaphoid at higher risk for complications. The dorsal carpal branch of the radial artery supplies a majority of the scaphoid through the distal pole and then proceeds to the proximal pole in a retrograde fashion. Consequently, blood supply to the proximal pole is fragile and can be easily disrupted by a fracture, which significantly increases the risk of nonunion.

A delay in the diagnosis of a scaphoid fracture can lead to several complications including delayed union (no healing at 3 months), avascular necrosis, compartment syndrome, compressive neuropathy, and nonunion (no healing at 4–6 months). Malunion or nonunion resulting in a humpback deformity (radiographically defined as an intrascaphoid angle of >35°) can lead to carpal instability, loss of wrist extension, weak grip, carpal collapse, and degenerative changes in the wrist. Scaphoid injuries can be associated with additional wrist ligamentous injury, resulting in perilunar instability and need for urgent surgical referral.

▶ Treatment

Treatment of acute scaphoid fractures is dependent on numerous factors including patient activity/occupation, fracture displacement, comminution, and anatomic location. Nondisplaced scaphoid fractures can be effectively treated nonoperatively with high union rates similar to those of a surgical procedure (Grade A recommendation). Indications for nonoperative management include nondisplaced or minimally displaced distal pole or waist fractures (Figure 39–4). There is no universally preferred method of cast immobilization; a long-arm or short-arm cast, including or not including the thumb, leads to equivalent outcomes in the treatment of scaphoid fractures with immobilization (Grade A recommendation). Length of immobilization is often determined by follow-up radiographs and clinical examination but typically is 8–12 weeks. Immobilization may be required for up to 12–14 weeks in those with high risk of nonunion.

Indications for operative management include fracture instability, angulation, displacement, malrotation, and fracture of the proximal pole. The most commonly used surgical method is screw fixation, which has been shown to lead to faster time to union, reduced risk of nonunion, improved functional outcomes, and earlier return to work.

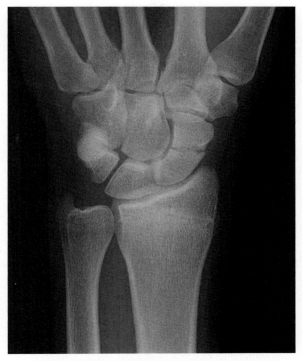

▲ **Figure 39–4.** Scaphoid waist fracture. (Used with permission from Justin Montgomery, MD; University of Kentucky Radiology.)

Boles CA. Scaphoid fracture imaging. *eMedicine.* https://emedicine.medscape.com/article/397230-overview. Accessed May 24, 2018.

Seitz WH Jr, Papandrea RF. Fractures and dislocations of the wrist. In Bucholz RW, Heckman JD, eds. *Rockwood and Green's Fractures in Adults.* 5th ed. Philadelphia, PA: Lippincott Williams & Wilkins; 2002.

Tait MA, Bracey JW, Gaston RG. Acute scaphoid fractures: a critical analysis review. *JBJS Rev.* 2016;4(9):01874474-201609000-00004. [PMID: 27760075]

Winston MJ, Weiland AJ. Scaphoid fractures in the athlete. *Curr Rev Musculoskeletal Med.* 2017;10(1):38–44. [PMID: 28251560]

METACARPAL FRACTURES

▶ Clinical Findings

A. Symptoms and Signs

Metacarpal fractures encompass 30–40% of all hand fractures and are usually the result of a direct blow to the hand or a fall. These fractures are classified by their anatomic location (head, neck, shaft, or base), with the neck and shaft being the most common sites for fracture of metacarpals

2 through 5, whereas the first metacarpal is typically fractured at the base. A Bennett fracture is the most common fracture involving the thumb and refers to an intraarticular fracture that separates the palmar ulnar aspect of the first metacarpal base from the remaining first metacarpal. A boxer's fracture refers to a fifth metacarpal neck fracture.

Patients present with localized tenderness and swelling, decreased grip strength, and decreased range of motion. The examiner should pay particular attention when evaluating for bony deformity, malrotation (evidenced by scissoring on exam), skin integrity, and neurovascular integrity of the hand.

B. Imaging Studies

Standard hand radiographs including AP, lateral, and oblique views are recommended. If first metacarpal injury is suspected, dedicated views of the thumb can be obtained to provide additional information such as the Roberts view (true AP view of the first carpal-metacarpal joint). A CT scan may be helpful for fractures of the metacarpal head and base and intraarticular fractures.

▶ Complications

Common complications associated with metacarpal fractures include decreased grip strength, joint stiffness, painful grip, prolonged dorsal swelling, arthrosis, malunion, and nonunion. The risk of these complications can be minimized with initiating early range-of-motion exercises, confirming absence of malrotation (most common cause of malunion), and appropriately treating associated soft tissue injuries and infections (most common cause of nonunion and arthrosis).

▶ Treatment

Specific considerations for metacarpal fracture treatment depend on the metacarpal involved, location, ability of the fracture to be reduced, and ultimate stability once reduction is obtained. Most extraarticular metacarpal fractures can be treated nonoperatively with the expectation of good hand function. Indications for nonoperative management include stable fracture pattern, absence of rotation deformity, and acceptable angulation and shortening. Metacarpal shaft fractures of the index and long fingers can tolerate up to 20° of angulation, whereas the ring and small fingers can tolerate up to 30 and 40° of angulation, respectively (Figure 39–5). For thumb metacarpal fractures, up to 30° of angulation is acceptable because of the mobility of the trapeziometacarpal joint. If closed reduction alone is unable to maintain these cited angulations, surgical management must be considered. Nonoperative management involves approximately 3 weeks

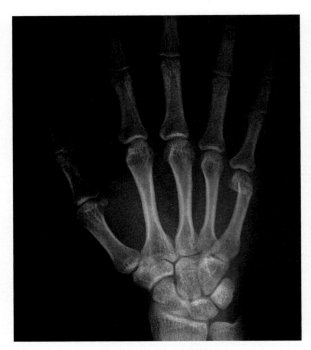

▲ **Figure 39–5.** Boxer's fracture of the fifth metacarpal. (Used with permission from Justin Montgomery, MD; University of Kentucky Radiology.)

of immobilization, with range-of-motion activities beginning thereafter. A 2-week follow-up radiograph should be checked to ensure fracture stability. Bridging callus should be seen at 4–6 weeks.

Indications for operative management of metacarpal fractures include any degree of rotational malalignment, metacarpal shortening >5 mm, articular surface step-off >1 mm, >25% articular involvement, presence of multiple metacarpal fractures, open fractures, and intraarticular base fractures. The Bennett fracture is inherently unstable, and surgical fixation is recommended when there is an articular step-off ≥1 mm. Surgical treatment of Bennett fractures is varied but generally consists of either closed reduction with percutaneous pinning or open reduction with either pins or interfragmentary screws. Treatment for a boxer's fracture varies depending on whether the fracture is open versus closed, the degree of angulation, rotation, and other associated injuries. Immobilization with an ulnar gutter splint may be the definitive treatment for closed, nondisplaced fractures without angulation or rotation, whereas referral to a hand surgeon would be indicated for management of open fractures, significantly angulated or malrotated fractures, or those involving injury to neurovascular structures.

Ben-Amotz O, Sammer DM. Practical management of metacarpal fractures. *Plast Reconstr Surg.* 2015;136(3):370e–379e. [PMID: 26313842]

Carter KR, Nallamothu SV. Fracture, Bennett. Updated May 13, 2018. In: StatPearls [Internet]. Treasure Island, FL: StatPearls Publishing; 2018 January. https://www.ncbi.nlm.nih.gov/books/NBK500035/?report=classic. Accessed November 19, 2019.

Cotterell IH, Richard MJ. Metacarpal and phalangeal fractures in athletes. *Clin Sports Med.* 2015;34(1):69–98. [PMID: 25455397]

Wong VW, Higgins JP. Evidence-based medicine: management of metacarpal fractures. *Plast Reconstr Surg.* 2017;140(1):140e–151e. [PMID: 28654615]

PHALANGEAL FRACTURES

▶ Clinical Findings

A. Symptoms and Signs

Phalangeal fractures are common fractures that most primary care physicians will encounter in their clinical practice. Fractures of the proximal, middle, and distal phalangeal shafts are common. Pain, swelling, and deformity of the affected digit are typical findings of phalangeal fractures. Distal tuft fractures typically result from crush injuries and are associated with subungual hematoma or laceration of the nail matrix and/or pulp. Mallet fractures result from avulsion of the dorsal base of the distal phalanx by the extensor tendon. The classic physical exam finding of a mallet fracture is the inability to actively extend the distal interphalangeal (DIP) joint.

B. Imaging Studies

Standard plain radiographic imaging of phalangeal fractures includes an AP, lateral, and oblique view of the affected digit. Occasionally, advanced imaging with CT is required in more extensive fractures.

▶ Complications

A vast majority of finger fractures heal without complication. Complications that may occur include joint stiffness, numbness, hypersensitivity, deformity of the nail and nail bed, nonunion, and malunion. Permanent loss of function can occur with improper treatment of fractures.

▶ Treatment

Most phalangeal fractures can be treated nonoperatively using a variety of techniques including casting, functional bracing, dorsal block splinting, or buddy strapping depending on the location of the fracture. The typical "safe" position of immobilization places the metacarpophalangeal joints in 70° of flexion and the proximal interphalangeal joints in full extension. This position is used to prevent collateral ligament and volar plate contractures. Orthopedic referral is indicated for open fractures and unstable fractures, which are defined as short oblique, spiral, or comminuted fractures; fractures with displacement or malrotation; articular surface incongruity; and fractures of the subcondylar proximal phalanx. Special consideration is warranted for distal tuft fractures. Restoration of the soft tissue envelope usually is enough to stabilize the fracture. Immobilization of the DIP joint with unrestricted movement of the proximal interphalangeal joint for 10–14 days will support fracture healing. Mallet fractures should be treated nonoperatively for 6–8 weeks, with the DIP joint in a hyperextension splint. Care must be taken to not allow the DIP joint to flex past neutral during the period of immobilization to ensure healing without an extension lag.

Carpenter S, Rohde RS. Treatment of phalangeal fractures. *Hand Clin.* 2013;29:519–534. [PMID: 24209951]

Cotterell IH, Richard MJ. Metacarpal and phalangeal fractures in athletes. *Clin Sports Med.* 2015;34(1):69–98. [PMID: 25455397]

▼ LOWER EXTREMITY FRACTURES

STRESS FRACTURES

▶ General Considerations

Management of traumatic fractures of the lower extremity long bones is relatively straightforward if a few simple rules are recognized. Orthopedic referral is required for any traumatic fracture that is displaced or involves a joint line. The goal of this section is to guide the primary care physician through a basic understanding of concepts surrounding bone stress pathogenesis, including epidemiology, clinical signs and symptoms, physical examination, radiographic diagnostic aids, and treatment of four difficult-to-treat areas of stress reaction in the lower extremities. The population most at risk for stress reaction is athletes. This population presents therapeutic challenges secondary to their increased activity, predilection to overuse injury, and desire to return to competition as quickly as possible, which may lead them to compete before the stress injury fully resolves.

Stress fractures are estimated to make up 10% of all athletic injuries. Ninety-five percent of stress injuries occur in the lower extremities secondary to the extreme repetitive weight-bearing loads placed on these bones. In one military study that included >31,000 cases, lower extremity stress fractures were most commonly observed in the tibia/fibula, followed by the metatarsals. The peak incidence occurs in people age 18–25 years. Two well-established risk factors for lower extremity stress fracture are female sex and previous history of stress fracture. There is a decreased incidence of stress fracture in men secondary to greater lean body mass and overall bone structure. It has been estimated that female military recruits have a relative risk of stress fracture that is 1.2–10 times greater than men while engaging in the same level of training. In athletic populations, a gender difference is not as evident, possibly because athletic women are more fit and better conditioned. Incidence is estimated to be comparable for all races.

Stress fracture is most common after changes in an athlete's training regimen. A review of 671 stress fractures in collegiate student-athletes found rates were highest in endurance sports including cross-country, track, and soccer. Injury is especially prevalent in unconditioned runners who increase their training regimen. Training error, which can include increased quantity or intensity of training, introduction of a new activity, poor equipment, and change in environment (ie, surface), is the most important risk factor for stress injury. Low bone density, dietary deficiency, low body mass index, menstrual irregularities, hormonal imbalance, sleep deprivation, and biomechanical abnormalities also place athletes at risk. Keeping this in mind and recognizing the increasing incidence of the female athletic triad (amenorrhea/oligomenorrhea, disordered eating [or low energy availability], and low bone mineral density [osteoporosis/osteopenia]), it is easy to understand why women can have an increased risk for stress injury.

▶ Clinical Findings

A. Symptoms and Signs

Stress fractures are related to a maladaptive process between bone injury and bone remodeling. Bone reacts to stress by early osteoclastic activity (old-bone resorption) followed by strengthening osteoblastic activity (new-bone formation). With continued stress, bone resorption outpaces new-bone formation, and a self-perpetuating cycle occurs, with continued activity allowing weakened bone to be more susceptible to continued microfracture and ultimately progressing to frank fracture. The initiation of stress reaction is unclear. It has been postulated that excessive forces are transmitted to bone when surrounding muscles fatigue. The highly concentrated muscle forces act across localized area of bone, causing mechanical insults above the stress-bearing capacity of bone.

Athletic stress fracture follows a crescendo process. Symptoms start insidiously with dull, gnawing pain at the end of physical activity. Pain increases over days to the point where the activity cannot be continued. At first, pain decreases with rest; then shorter and shorter duration of activity causes pain. More time is then needed for pain to dissipate until it is present with minimal activity and at night. After a few days of rest, pain resolves, only to return once again with resumption of activity. More specific historical and physical examination findings are discussed later in the chapter in conjunction with specific anatomic regions.

B. Imaging Studies

The diagnosis of stress fracture is primarily clinical and is based on history and physical examination. It is prudent to start with plain radiographs, which have poor sensitivity but high specificity, as the initial study. The presence of stress reaction is confirmed by the presence of periosteal reaction, intramedullary sclerosis, callus, or obvious fracture line. Plain films typically fail to reveal a bony abnormality unless symptoms have been present for at least 2–3 weeks.

The technetium triple-phase bone scan is often used to improve diagnostic power. Stress reactions can often be visualized within 48–72 hours from symptom onset. Triple-phase bone scan can differentiate soft tissue and bone injuries. All three phases can be positive in an acute fracture. In soft tissue injuries with no bony involvement, the first two phases are often positive, whereas the delayed image shows minimal or no increased uptake. In conditions such as medial tibial stress syndrome (MTSS), in which there is early bony stress reaction, the first two phases are negative and the delayed image is positive. Nuclear medicine bone scans should not be used to monitor fracture healing because the fracture line is not clearly visualized and delayed images continue to demonstrate increased uptake for ≥12 months after initial studies.

CT scans can identify conditions that mimic stress fracture on bone scan, confirm fracture suspected on bone scan, or help to make treatment decisions as with navicular stress fractures.

MRI offers the advantage of visualizing soft tissue changes in anatomic regions in which the soft tissue structures often cloud the differential diagnosis. Clinically, the high sensitivity of bone scan and MRI is necessary only when the diagnosis of stress fracture is in question or the exact location or extent of injury must be known in order to determine treatment. MRI is currently the gold standard for stress fracture imaging.

Kaeding CC, Najarian RG. Stress fractures: classification and management. *Phys Sportsmed* 2010;38(3):45–54. [PMID: 20959695]

Knapp TP, Garrett WE. Stress fractures: general concepts. *Clin Sports Med*. 1997;16:339. [PMID: 9238314]

Rizzone KH, Ackerman KE, Roos KG, Dompier TP, Kerr ZY. The epidemiology of stress fractures in collegiate student-athletes, 2004-2005 through 2013-2014 academic years. *J Athl Train*. 2017;52(10):966–975. [PMID: 28937802]

Waterman BR, Gun B, Bader JO, et al. Epidemiology of lower extremity stress fractures in the United States Military. *Mil Med*. 2016;181:1308–1313. [PMID: 27753569]

Wright AA, Taylor JB, Ford KR, et al. Risk factors associated with lower extremity stress fractures in runners: a systematic review with meta-analysis. *Br J Sports Med*. 2015;49(23):1517–1523. [PMID: 26582192]

Femoral Stress Fractures

▶ General Considerations

Stress fractures involving the femur can occur in a variety of locations, most commonly the femoral shaft and neck. One study that looked at 320 athletes with bone scan–positive stress fractures revealed the femur to be the fourth most frequent site of injury.

▶ Differential Diagnosis

The symptom most commonly encountered with stress fractures of the femur is pain at the anterior aspect of the hip. Differentiating the diagnosis can be difficult secondary to the multiple number of structures in the hip that have the potential to produce similar pain syndromes and the deep non-palpable structures of the anatomic region. Diagnosis can be made complex by the multitude of structures in this region from which pain may emanate; thus, the physician must be attuned to the history to narrow the differential down to a list in which stress fracture is prominent. This is important in order to avoid severe complications associated with fractures of the femoral neck.

▶ Femoral Shaft Fractures

Femoral shaft stress fractures, although less common than femoral neck stress fractures, are overall more common than expected, with an incidence of 3.7% among athletes. Onset of pain can be gradual over a period of days to weeks. Average time from symptom onset to diagnosis is approximately 2 weeks. The fulcrum test is well suited to act as a guide for ordering radiologic tests and thereby decreasing time to diagnosis. It is also a useful clinical test to assess healing. For this test, the athlete is seated on the examination table with legs dangling as the examiner's arm is used as a fulcrum under the thigh. The examiner's arm is moved from the distal to proximal thigh as gentle pressure is applied to the dorsum of the knee with the opposite hand. A positive test is elicited by sharp pain or apprehension at the site of the fracture. Plain films are rarely sensitive in detecting stress fractures within the first 2–3 weeks of symptoms. Bone scan or MRI may be useful in this time period to aid in diagnosis. The most common site of injury in athletes is the midmedial or posteromedial cortex of the proximal femur.

Once diagnosis is confirmed, treatment depends on the underlying causes responsible for the injury. If the fracture is consistent with a compression-sided fracture (Figure 39–6), treatment consists of rest with gradual resumption of activity. This usually is adequate for healing of nondisplaced fractures. Treatment protocols are based on empiric data gathered from clinical observation. An example of a treatment protocol may consist of rest for a period of 1–4 weeks, with toe-touch weight bearing progressing to full weight bearing. This would be followed by a phase of low-impact activity (ie, biking, swimming). Once patients are able to perform low-impact activity for a prolonged time without pain, they may gradually advance to high impact. Resumption of full activity averages between 8 and 16 weeks. Surgical treatment should be considered if there is displacement

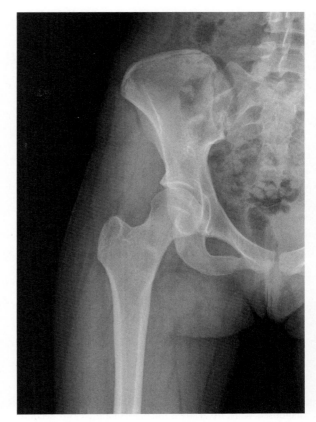

▲ **Figure 39–6.** Compression-sided stress fracture of the right femoral neck. Note sclerotic line perpendicular to medial cortex. (Used with permission from Justin Montgomery, MD; University of Kentucky Radiology.)

of the fracture, delayed union, or nonunion following conservative therapy.

▶ Femoral Neck Fractures

Stress fractures of the femoral neck make up an estimated 9% of all stress injuries. Although uncommon, they carry a high complication rate if the diagnosis is missed or the fracture is improperly treated. The primary presenting symptom is pain at the site of the groin, anterior thigh, or knee. Pain is exacerbated by weight bearing or physical activity. The athlete may have an antalgic gait or painful, limited hip range of motion in internal rotation or external rotation. MRI is the diagnostic modality of choice for evaluating femoral neck stress fractures.

Stress fractures of the femoral neck are divided into two categories: compression (occurring along the inferior or medial border of the neck) and tension (along the superior or lateral neck) type. Compression fractures are more common in younger patients. The fracture line, if seen on the radiograph, can propagate across the femoral neck. A nondisplaced, incomplete compression fracture is treated with rest until the patient is pain free with full motion. Non-weight-bearing ambulation with the patient on crutches follows until radiographic healing as shown on plain films is complete. Frequent radiographs may need to be obtained to monitor propagation of the fracture. If the compression fracture becomes complete or fails to heal with rest, then internal fixation may be necessary. Patients treated nonsurgically may not achieve full activity for several months. Tension (distraction)-sided femoral neck fractures are an emergency because of the potential for complications (ie, nonunion or avascular necrosis). The patient is immediately rendered non–weight bearing and will acutely need internal fixation. If the fracture is displaced, the patient will need open reduction and internal fixation urgently.

McCormick F, Nwachukwu BU, Provencher MT. Stress fractures in runners. *Clin Sports Med.* 2012;31:291–306. [PMID: 22341018]
Waterman BR, Gun B, Bader JO, et al. Epidemiology of lower extremity stress fractures in the United States Military. *Mil Med.* 2016;181:1308–1313. [PMID: 27753569]

Tibial Stress Fracture

▶ General Considerations

Tibial stress fractures account for half of all stress fractures diagnosed. Most tibial stress fractures in athletes are secondary to running. It is estimated that they make up 4% of all running-related injuries and are the most common type of stress fracture in runners. Increased risk of tibial stress injury is associated with lower muscle mass, higher body fat, thinner and small bones, and foot anomalies (either pes planus or pes cavus). Two sites located within the tibia are most commonly associated with stress fractures. The first of these is located between the middle and distal third of the tibia along the posteromedial border. This type of injury is most often associated with running. The second site is along the middle third of the anterior cortex. This injury is most commonly associated with activities involving a great deal of jumping (eg, dancing, basketball, gymnastics).

▶ Clinical Findings

A. Symptoms and Signs

On history, the patient commonly describes pain occurring in the region of the fracture with activity (eg, running or jumping) and resolving with rest. The pain eventually progresses and lasts longer after the activity until the patient is symptomatic at rest. Physical examination often reveals localized pain to palpation. Sometimes persistent thickening, secondary to periosteal reaction, can be appreciated by palpation along the tibia.

B. Imaging Studies

Diagnosis by radiographic plain film may be possible if symptoms have been present for at least 4–6 weeks. Triple-phase bone scan is very sensitive and may allow diagnosis within 48–72 hours of symptom onset. Tibial stress fractures can be seen clearly on MRI with sensitivity comparable to that of triple-phase bone scan. Both bone scan and MRI allow differentiation of MTSS and stress fracture.

▶ Differential Diagnosis

MTSS is the most commonly confused diagnosis in the classification of tibial stress injuries with stress fracture. MTSS usually occurs diffusely along the middle and distal third of the posteromedial tibia and is commonly seen in runners. This condition, however, can also be seen with activities involving persistent jumping. The symptom spectrum commonly progresses, as does that of stress fractures, with continued activity. MTSS represents a stress reaction within bone whereby the usual remodeling process becomes maladaptive. This injury responds well to rest in a shorter time period as compared with stress fracture and is easily differentiated from stress fracture on triple-phase bone scan.

▶ Treatment

Once the diagnosis of tibial stress fracture has been made, a distinction between a compression versus tension-sided injury must be made. Fractures along the posteromedial border are considered compression stress injuries and respond well to conservative therapy (Figure 39–7). The average recovery time for this injury is approximately 12 weeks when the patient is treated with rest alone. Most guidelines for treatment of this injury involve relative or absolute rest. These stress fractures can be effectively treated in a pneumatic leg brace. Athletes treated in the pneumatic brace (long-leg air cast) showed decreased time to pain-free symptoms (14 ± 6 days) and time to competitive participation (21 ± 2 days) versus traditional mode non–weight-bearing treatment (77 ± 7 days). Athletes in the brace may continue exercising, but modifications of the training routine must be made to maintain pain-free activities. Patients are treated on the basis of a functional activity progression as outlined by Swenson and colleagues.

Tibial stress fractures of the midanterior cortex, also known as "the dreaded black line" radiographically (Figure 39–8), are very difficult to manage conservatively. This fracture occurs at the tension side of the tibial cortex, most commonly in athletes who jump. Delayed union and complete fracture are two significant complications associated with this area. A systemic review by Robertson and

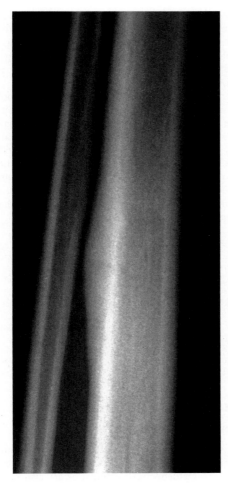

▲ **Figure 39–7.** Periosteal stress reaction at the posterior medial aspect of the tibia.

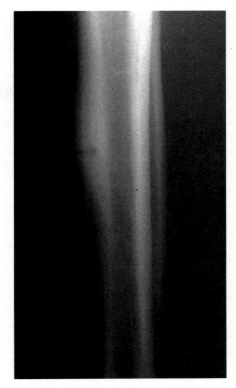

▲ **Figure 39–8.** Dreaded black line at the anterior medial aspect of the tibia.

Wood noted that anterior tibial stress fractures require longer healing time and are more likely to result in surgical management. The average time to symptom-free return to activity from symptom onset is 3–10 months with conservative care. Conservative treatment revolves around rest, immobilization, or both. Patients who do not respond to conservative treatment or are involved in activities (career or competitive athletics) would benefit from surgical treatment with tibial intramedullary nailing. Patients with these fractures should be referred to a sports medicine specialist.

Arnold MJ, Moody AL. Common running injuries: evaluation and management. *Am Fam Physician.* 2018;97(8):510–516. [PMID: 29671490]

Beck BR, Rudolph K, Matheson GO, et al. Risk factors for tibial stress injuries: a case-control study. *Clin J Sport Med.* 2015;25: 230–236. [PMID: 24977954]

McCormick F, Nwachukwu BU, Provencher MT. Stress fractures in runners. *Clin Sports Med.* 2012;31:291–306. [PMID: 22341018]

Robertson GA, Wood AM. Return to sports after stress fractures of the tibial diaphysis: a systematic review. *Br Med Bull.* 2015; 114:95–111. [PMID: 25712999]

Shindle MK, Endo Y, Warren RF, et al. Stress fractures about the tibia, foot, and ankle. *J Am Acad Orthop Surg.* 2012;20(3): 167–176. [PMID: 22382289]

Tarsal Navicular Stress Fracture

▶ General Considerations

Tarsal navicular stress fractures are an underdiagnosed source of prolonged, disabling foot pain predominantly seen in active athletes involved in sprinting and jumping. One study involving 111 competitive track and field athletes found that navicular stress fractures are the second most common lower extremity stress fracture. Certain anatomic variants, including metatarsus adductus, as well as a combination of short first metatarsal and long second metatarsal, are associated with increased incidence of navicular stress fracture.

Clinical Findings

A. Symptoms and Signs

These fractures are prone to misdiagnosis secondary to the vague nature of the pain. A review by Saxena et al estimates that the average time between symptom onset and definitive treatment is nearly 9 months. The pain may radiate along the medial arch and not directly over the talonavicular joint. Sometimes pain radiates distally, causing the physician to suspect a Morton neuroma or metatarsalgia. The pain often disappears with a few days of rest, often tricking the athlete into not believing the potential seriousness of the diffuse foot pain. The diagnosis is also clouded because the fractures are rarely seen on plain film.

Symptoms suggesting a clinical diagnosis consist of (1) insidious onset of vague pain over the dorsum of the medial midfoot or over the medial aspect of the longitudinal arch; (2) ill-defined pain, soreness, or cramping aggravated by activity and relieved by rest; (3) well-localized tenderness to palpation over the navicular bone or medial arch; and (4) little swelling or discoloration. Certain foot abnormalities, including short first metatarsal and metatarsus adductor and limited dorsiflexion of the ankle, may concentrate stress on the tarsal navicular region, predisposing to stress.

B. Imaging Studies

Initial imaging for tarsal navicular stress fractures includes plain radiographs. Plain radiographs should be obtained in AP, lateral, and oblique standing positions. Unfortunately, sensitivity is low because a majority of these fractures are incomplete and therefore difficult to see on plain radiographs. Also, bony resorption requires 10 days to 3 weeks to allow visualization. Most fractures are located in the central third of bone along the proximal articular surface, which is a relatively avascular region.

The next recommended diagnostic procedure is a triple-phase bone scan. These are positive at an early stage and almost 100% sensitive. CT scanning is the gold standard for optimal evaluation once bone scan has demonstrated increased uptake in the navicular bone. The best images are obtained with ≤1.5-mm slices. As imaging devices and technique have improved, MRI has been used with increased frequency and is almost as sensitive as bone scan in the detection of these fractures. MRI carries the additional advantage of no radiation exposure and evaluation of surrounding structures.

Treatment

Data indicate that 6–8 weeks of non–weight-bearing cast immobilization compares favorably with surgical treatment for failed weight-bearing treatment. Surgery is recommended

for a displaced complete fracture with a small transverse fragment (ossicle), a fracture line extending from the dorsal to plantar cortex, or failure of conservative management. Surgical treatment often consists of either bone graft or screw fixation followed by non–weight-bearing cast immobilization for 6 weeks.

After 6 weeks of non–weight-bearing cast immobilization, fracture healing is followed clinically by palpation of the fracture site along the dorsal proximal region of the navicular bone. Persistent tenderness over this "N" spot requires an additional 2 weeks of non–weight-bearing immobilization before reassessment. If the fracture site is not tender after casting, the patient may begin weight bearing. Imaging may remain positive up to 6 months following the injury. For this reason, the recommendation is not to repeat imaging but, instead, to rely on clinical examination (palpation of the N spot).

Fowler JR, Gaughan JP, Boden BP, Pavolov H, Torg JS. The non-surgical and surgical treatment of tarsal navicular stress fractures. *Sports Med*. 2011;41(8):613–619. [PMID: 21780848]

Gross CE, Nunley JA 2nd. Navicular stress fractures. *Foot Ankle Int*. 2015;36:1117–1122. [PMID: 26276132]

Khan KM, Fuller PJ, Brukner PD, et al. Outcome of conservative and surgical management of navicular stress fracture in athletes: eighty-six cases proven with computerized tomography. *Am J Sports Med*. 1992;20:657–666. [PMID: 1456359]

Saxena A, Behan SA, Valerio DL, Frosch DL. Navicular stress fracture outcomes in athletes: analysis of 62 injuries. *J Foot Ankle Surg*. 2017;56:943–948. [PMID: 28842101]

Metatarsal Stress Fractures

General Considerations

Metatarsal stress fractures in athletes are very common. Depending on the study referenced, they are either third or fourth in incidence. These fractures are also known as "march fractures" because of the large numbers of military recruits who obtained these fractures after sudden increases in their level of activity. The second metatarsal is the most common location, followed by the third and fourth metatarsals. The second metatarsal is subjected to 3–4 times body weight during loading and push-off phases of gait.

Clinical Findings

A. Symptoms and Signs

Clinical suspicion for this injury is raised when the athlete complains of forefoot or midfoot pain of insidious onset. On examination, these injuries present as areas of point tenderness overlying the metatarsal shaft.

B. Imaging Studies

Radiographs are usually sufficient to document stress fracture, which is visualized as a frank fracture or periosteal reaction at the affected site. As with most stress fractures, the patient may be symptomatic 2–4 weeks prior to visualizing the fracture on radiograph. If the diagnosis is in question, bone scan and MRI have significantly higher sensitivity and specificity for detecting these injuries at an earlier timeframe.

▶ Treatment

Treatment is easily managed by the primary care physician. The injury is treated symptomatically, allowing the athlete to participate in activities that are not painful. Immobilization in the form of a steel shank insole or stiff, wooden-soled shoe may be necessary for a limited time, until the pain disappears. At times, the patient may benefit from a short-leg walking cast or removable walking boot for severe pain. Four weeks of rest are usually sufficient for healing. During these 4 weeks, the athlete may continue modified conditioning with non–weight-bearing exercises (eg, swimming and pool running), followed by cycling and stair climbing.

Although most of these fractures heal well with conservative management, fractures of the proximal fifth metatarsal have a high incidence of delayed union and nonunion. A thorough understanding of the classification and anatomy of fractures in this location is required for proper identification to determine conservative versus surgical treatment.

FRACTURES OF THE PROXIMAL FIFTH METATARSAL

The fifth metatarsal consists of a base tuberosity, shaft (diaphysis), neck, and head (Figure 39–9). Fractures of the proximal fifth metatarsal include tuberosity avulsion fractures, acute Jones fractures, and diaphyseal stress fractures.

Tuberosity Avulsion Fractures

Tuberosity fractures are typically known as "dancer fractures" because they are usually associated with an ankle inversion plantar flexion injury. This injury is likely secondary to the plantar aponeurosis pulling from the base of the fifth metatarsal. Nondisplaced fracture carries an excellent prognosis, almost always healing in 4–6 weeks with conservative therapy. The athlete's treatment consists of limited weight bearing to pain with modified activity such as that used with second, third, and fourth metatarsal injuries. If needed, the athlete can be immobilized in a walking cast, wooden (or steel shank)-soled shoe, or walking boot. The immobilization can usually be removed by 3 weeks (average 3–6 weeks) in favor of modified footwear if pain has diminished. The patient then may gradually return to vigorous activity; most athletes return to full sports activity in 6–8 weeks. Bony union usually takes place by 8 weeks. Orthopedic referral is needed for displaced fractures or comminuted fractures >3 mm or involving >60% of the cubometatarsal articular surface or with step-off of >2 mm. Sometimes small displaced fractures at this site may require surgical removal if bony union does not occur secondary to chronic irritation.

Jones Fractures

Jones fractures consist of a transverse fracture at the junction of the diaphysis and metaphysis (Figure 39–10). The Jones fracture is believed to occur when the ankle is in plantar flexion and a large adduction force is applied to the forefoot. It is important to realize that this is a midfoot injury with no prodromal symptoms. Therefore, the injury is classified as acute.

Torg and colleagues showed that this fracture, in nonathletes, could heal in 6–8 weeks with strict non–weight-bearing immobilization. However, secondary to low vascularization and high stresses at the site of the Jones fracture, the injury is associated with a poor outcome. A meta-analysis by Yates et al concluded that nonsurgical treatment resulted in significantly higher rate of fracture nonunion and prolonged healing time and return to activity. That being said, those who do undergo conservative treatment are placed on a

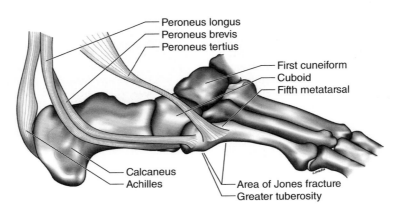

Peroneus longus
Peroneus brevis
Peroneus tertius

First cuneiform
Cuboid
Fifth metatarsal

Calcaneus
Achilles

Area of Jones fracture
Greater tuberosity

▲ **Figure 39–9.** Anatomy of the proximal fifth metatarsal. (Used with permission from Ellsworth C. Seeley, MD.)

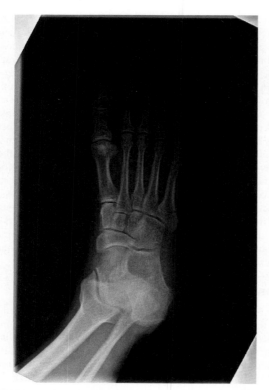

▲ **Figure 39–10.** The Jones fracture. (Used with permission from Justin Montgomery, MD; University of Kentucky Radiology.)

non–weight-bearing immobilization protocol and in a plaster cast for 6–8 weeks. If there is lack of clinical healing by 6–8 weeks, therapy is individualized. If clinical healing is present by 6–8 weeks, immobilization is continued in a fracture brace with range of motion and gradual weight bearing. Orthopedic referral should be considered for displacement >2 mm, for radiographic nonunion after 12 weeks of conservative treatment, or in persons with a high activity level. In these instances, treatment must be individualized either with continued cast immobilization or surgical intervention. Surgical intervention for Jones fracture consists of either intramedullary screw fixation or bone grafting.

Diaphyseal Fractures

Stress fractures distal to the site of Jones fractures and acute-on-chronic fractures occurring in the same position as Jones fractures are commonly seen in athletes who run. Pain is usually over the lateral aspect of the foot, over the fifth metatarsal base. Usually no significant trauma has been associated with these fractures. Prodromal symptoms occurring weeks to months in advance of an acute injury can often be elicited in the history.

Treatment of choice for acute nondisplaced diaphyseal stress fracture is non–weight-bearing immobilization. More extensive fractures require individualized treatment. Conservative treatment may take ≤20 weeks and result in nonunion. Complications of prolonged immobilization include recurrence of fracture and significant dysfunction from muscle atrophy and loss of range of motion. For athletes, surgical options are recommended. Casting and prolonged immobilization of acute or chronic fractures frequently fail, giving rise to delayed or nonunion fractures. Orthopedic referral is indicated for open fractures, fracture-dislocations, intraarticular fractures, or multiple metatarsal fractures. In these instances, surgery is often needed and is the recommended procedure of choice.

The difference between screw fixation and bone grafting is recovery time. It takes up to 12 weeks to return to prefracture activity with grafting versus 6–8 weeks with screw fixation. Grafting carries a higher failure rate. Screw fixation is now recommended first, with bone grafting if fixation fails.

Bica D, Sprouse RA, Armen J. Diagnosis and management of common foot fractures. *Am Fam Physician*. 2016;93(3):183–191. [PMID: 26926612]

Kerkhoffs GM, Versteegh VE, Sierevelt IN, Kloen P, van Dijk CN. Treatment of proximal metatarsal V fractures in athletes and non-athletes. *Br J Sports Med*. 2012;46:644–648. [PMID: 22247296]

Polzer H, Polzer S, Mutschler W, Prall W. Acute fractures to the proximal fifth metatarsal bone: development of classification and treatment recommendations based on the current evidence. *Injury*. 2012;43:1626–1632. [PMID: 22465516]

Shindle MK, Endo Y, Warren RF, et al. Stress fractures about the tibia, foot, and ankle. *J Am Acad Orthop Surg*. 2012;20(3):167–176. [PMID: 22382289]

Yates J, Feeley I, Sasikumar S, et al. Jones fracture of the fifth metatarsal: is operative intervention justified? A systematic review of the literature and meta-analysis of results. *Foot (Edinb)*. 2015;25:251–257. [PMID: 26481787]

Healthy Aging & Geriatric Assessment

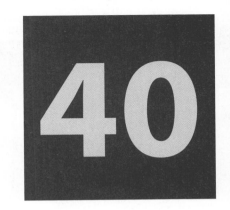

Lora Cox-Vance, MD, CMD

CHARACTERISTICS OF AGING

The population of the United States, like that of other industrialized nations, is aging. The US population of adults age ≥65 years increased at a faster rate (15.1%) between 2000 and 2010 than did the total US population (9.7%). Between the years 2010 and 2050, the number of Americans ≥65 years old is projected to have doubled. In the rapidly changing arena of healthcare financing and delivery, services that promote or improve functional abilities, prevent or delay disease progression, and improve the overall health status of this aging population are essential. This chapter defines successful and healthy aging, highlights recommendations for health promotion and disease prevention, and describes key elements in geriatric assessment.

Aging is a physiologic process. The term *healthy aging* does not imply an absence of limitations, but rather an adaptation to the changes associated with the aging process that is acceptable to the individual. Successful or healthy aging is characterized by (1) low burden of disease and disability, (2) higher cognitive and physical functioning, and (3) an active engagement with life (Table 40–1). Healthcare providers can promote healthy aging by assisting older adults in developing competence in directing and managing their health and promoting their autonomy and quality of life.

Although there are common physiologic changes associated with aging, the geriatric population is a highly heterogeneous group with varying degrees of chronic disease and physical and cognitive disability within individuals. Many chronic conditions commonly affect this population (Table 40–2). The overall health status and well-being of older adults are highly complex and result from many interacting processes, including risk factor exposure (tobacco, alcohol, illicit drugs, diet, sedentary lifestyle, environmental toxins), biological age-related changes, and the development and consequences of functional impairments. Many of the conditions previously considered "normal aging" are now

known to be modifiable or even preventable with appropriate disease prevention and health promotion strategies.

Bryant LL, Corbett KK, Kutner JS. In their own words: a model of healthy aging. *Soc Sci Med.* 2001;53:927–941. [PMID: 11522138]
Fried LP. Epidemiology of aging. *Epidemiol Rev.* 2000;22:95. [PMID: 10939013]
Kyle L. A concept analysis of healthy aging. *Nurs Forum.* 2005;40: 45–57. [PMID: 16053504]
Peel N, McClure RJ, Bartlett HP. Behavioral determinants of healthy aging. *Am J Prevent Med.* 2005;28:298–304. [PMID: 15766620]
US Census Bureau. *2010 Census Briefs; The Older Population: 2010.* November 2011. https://www.census.gov/prod/cen2010/briefs/c2010br-09.pdf. Accessed November 19, 2019.
US Census Bureau. *The Next Four Decades. The Older Population in the United States: 2010 to 2050.* May 2010. https://www.census.gov/prod/2010pubs/p25-1138.pdf. Accessed September 3, 2018.

PREVENTION & HEALTH PROMOTION

Prevention in geriatrics attempts to delay morbidity and disability and should be a primary goal of any medical practice caring for older individuals. The primary strategy for prevention lies in the alteration of lifestyle and environmental factors that contribute to the development or progression of chronic disease. A prospective cohort study of older adults with an average baseline age of 68 years found that participants with fewer lifestyle risk factors experienced lower disability and mortality, with the benefits persisting through the ninth decade of life.

Frailty is a complex geriatric syndrome associated with several chronic conditions, many of which may be preventable (Table 40–3). Important evidence of frailty includes slow walking speed, low physical activity, weight loss, and cognitive impairment. Preventive services for older adults should be implemented with a goal of preventing frailty, preserving function, and optimizing quality of life.

Table 40–1. Factors associated with healthy aging.

"Going and doing" is worthwhile and desirable to the individual
  Social activities
  Reading
  Travel
  Housework
  Fishing
  Creative outlets: eg, music, arts, dance, needlework
Sufficient abilities to accomplish valued activities
  Mobility
  Vision
  Cognitive functioning
  Coping
  Independence
Having appropriate resources to support the activity
  Valued relationships: friends and family
  Healthcare and health information
Optimistic attitude
  Self-esteem, self-efficacy, self-confidence

Data from Bryant LL, Corbett KK, Kutner JS: In their own words: a model of healthy aging. *Soc Sci Med.* 2001 Oct;53(7):927–941.

Table 40–2. Most common conditions associated with aging.

Arthritis
Hypertension
Heart disease
Hearing loss
Influenza
Injuries
Orthopedic impairments
Cataracts
Chronic sinusitis
Depression
Cancer
Diabetes mellitus
Visual impairments
Urinary incontinence
Varicose veins

Table 40–3. Conditions associated with frailty.

Advanced age, usually ≥85 years
Functional decline
Falls and associated injuries (hip fracture)
Polypharmacy
Chronic disease
Dementia and depression
Social dependence
Institutionalization or hospitalization
Nutritional impairment

Data from Hamerman D: Toward an understanding of frailty. *Ann Intern Med.* 1999 Jun 1;130(11):945–950.

Health promotion is a broad term that encompasses the objective of improving or enhancing the individual's current health status. The purpose of health promotion, especially as applied to the elderly, is the prevention of avoidable decline, frailty, and dependence, thereby promoting healthy aging.

For health promotion to be effective with older adults, it must be individualized, factoring in age, functional status, comorbid conditions, life expectancy, patient goals and preferences, and culture. Culture is important in understanding the older adult's health belief system. Without this understanding, a healthcare provider may be unable to negotiate a health promotion and prevention strategy that is acceptable to the patient and the provider.

Ahmed N, Mandel R, Fain MJ. Frailty: an emerging geriatric syndrome. *Am J Med.* 2007;120:748–753. [PMID: 17765039]
Chakravarty EF, Hubert HB, Krishnan E, et al. Lifestyle risk factors predict disability and death in healthy aging adults. *Am J Med.* 2012;125(2):190–197. [PMID: 22269623]
Rothman MD, Leo-Summers L, Gill TM. Prognostic significance of potential frailty criteria. *J Am Geriatr Soc.* 2008;56:2211–2216. [PMID: 19093920]

HEALTH PROMOTION & SCREENING

Many of the leading causes of death in the geriatric population (Table 40–4) are amenable to both primary and secondary preventive strategies, especially if targeted early in life. The major targets of prevention should therefore be focused at the major causes of death—including coronary heart

Table 40–4. Leading causes of death in those age ≥65 years, United States, 2010.

Cause of Death	Number
Cardiovascular disease	477,338
Cancer	396,670
Lung disease	160,877
Stroke	109,990
Alzheimer disease	82,616
Diabetes mellitus	49,191
Nephritis	41,994
Unintentional injury	41,300

Data from National Center for Health Statistics. Leading Causes of Death Reports.

disease, cancer, lung disease, and stroke—with the goals of reducing premature mortality caused by acute and chronic illness, maintaining function, enhancing quality of life, and extending active life expectancy. A priority in screening should be given to preventive services that are both easy to deliver and associated with beneficial outcomes.

Primary, secondary, and tertiary preventive efforts should be considered in older adults as enthusiastically as they are employed in younger adults. In developing screening and preventive strategies for individual patients, several factors must be considered, including major causes of death and related risk factors, the burden of comorbidity, functional ability, cognitive status, life expectancy, and patients' goal and preferences. These considerations should guide the patient-provider discussion and decision making.

A review of the literature reveals controversy and variation in some specific recommendations across sponsoring medical specialties. This is largely related to a lack of randomized clinical trials in patients age >75 years. As the number of quality clinical trials including older adults increases, these recommendations will further evolve.

The US Preventive Services Task Force (USPSTF) has set the standard for providing recommendations for clinical practice on preventive interventions, including screening tests, counseling interventions, immunizations, and chemoprophylactic regimens. These standards are established by a review of the scientific evidence for the clinical effectiveness of each preventive service. A detailed discussion of health promotion and preventive screening strategies relevant to the geriatric population, including recommendations from the USPSTF, can be found in Chapter 15, on health maintenance for adults. The Agency for Healthcare Research and Quality provides an electronic resource, the Electronic Preventive Services Selector, to assist providers in identifying age-appropriate preventive and screening measures. This tool is available online at http://epss.ahrq.gov.

Albert RH, Clark MM. Cancer screening in the older patient. *Am Fam Physician.* 2008;78:1369–1374. [PMID: 19119555]
US Department of Health and Human Services. AHRQ Electronic Preventive Services Selector. http://epss.ahrq.gov. Accessed August 3, 2018.

PHYSICAL ACTIVITY & EXERCISE IN OLDER ADULTS

Exercise and physical activity as forms of primary prevention have many benefits, even for sedentary older adults. Even leisure activities can serve as a form of primary prevention and have many benefits in older adults. The Leisure World Cohort Study of activities and mortality in the elderly suggests that as little as 15 minutes of leisure physical activity per day decreases mortality risk, with the greatest reduction

noted at 45 minutes of physical activity per day. A specific aim of the US Government Healthy People 2020 Initiative is to increase the proportion of older adults with reduced physical or cognitive function who engage in leisure-time physical activities by 10%.

A meta-analysis of physical activity and well-being in advanced age concluded that the maximum benefit of physical activity was in self-efficacy and that improvements in cardiovascular status, strength, and functional capacity also improved well-being. Engaging in leisurely physical activities has been shown to increase levels of exercise in sedentary populations.

The American Heart Association (AHA) and American College of Sports Medicine (ACSM) recommend the following exercise goals for older adults: (1) moderate aerobic activity for 30 minutes on 5 days per week, (2) 10 repetitions of 8–10 strength training exercises at least 2 days per week, and (3) stretching or other activities to maintain flexibility for at least 10 minutes twice per week. When engaging in moderate aerobic exercise, the older adult should be advised to work hard enough to sweat but below the point at which increased breathing efforts make conversation difficult.

The AHA recommends a preparticipation history and physical exam (Table 40–5) for sedentary older adults planning to begin an exercise program. The ACSM recommends exercise stress testing for older adults before engaging in a vigorous exercise program such as strenuous cycling or running (Table 40–6). Conditions that are absolute and relative contraindications to exercise stress testing or embarking on an exercise program should be evaluated (Table 40–7).

Table 40–5. Contents of a physical activity preparticipation evaluation for older adults.

History, to include
Patient's lifelong pattern of activities and interests
Activity level in past 2–3 months to determine a current baseline
Concerns and perceived barriers regarding exercise and physical activity:
Lack of time
Unsafe environment
Cardiovascular risks
Limitations of existing chronic diseases
Level of interest and motivation for exercise
Social preferences regarding exercise
Physical examination, with emphasis on
Cardiopulmonary systems
Musculoskeletal and sensory impairments

Data from Fletcher GF, Balady GJ, Amsterdam EA, et al: Exercise standards for testing and training: a statement for healthcare professionals from the American Heart Association. *Circulation.* 2001 Oct 2;104(14):1694–1740.

Table 40–6. Graded exercise test (GXT) recommendations according to coronary heart disease (CHD) risk factors[a] and exercise stratification.

Risk	Moderate-Intensity Exercise	Vigorous-Intensity Exercise
	Walking at 3–4 mph Cycling for pleasure <10 mph Moderate effort swimming Racket sports; pulling or carrying golf clubs	Walking briskly uphill or with a load Cycling fast or racing >10 mph Swimming, fast tread or crawl Singles tennis or racquetball
Low Men age <45 years and women age <55 years with ≤1 CHD risk factor and asymptomatic	GXT not necessary GXT not necessary	GXT not necessary GXT recommended
Moderate Men age ≥54 years and women age ≥55 years or those with ≥2 CHD risk factors	GXT not necessary	GXT recommended
High Individuals with symptoms of disease or known metabolic, cardiovascular, or pulmonary disease	GXT recommended	GXT recommended

[a]CHD risk factors: family history, cigarette smoking, hypertension, dyslipidemia, impaired fasting glucose tolerance, obesity, sedentary lifestyle. Data from American College of Sports Medicine. *ACSM's Guidelines for Exercise Testing and Prescription.* 6th ed. Philadelphia, PA: Lippincott Williams & Wilkins; 2000.

Recommendations for exercise should be provided to older patients in writing and include the frequency, intensity, type, and duration of exercise. It is important for older adults to gradually increase their physical activity levels over time and for providers to set realistic and obtainable goals as part of each exercise prescription. Older adults should be advised to increases their exercises every 1–2 weeks and have follow-up arranged every 4–6 weeks when initiating an exercise program.

Promotion of an active lifestyle is important at all ages, and the benefits to older adults are numerous. Providers should help older adults understand that exercise need not be strenuous or prolonged to be beneficial. Just encouraging patients to get up out of their chairs and start moving will improve not only the quality but also the quantity of disability-free years.

Table 40–7. Absolute and relative contraindications to exercise stress testing or starting an exercise program.

Absolute Contraindications	Relative Contraindications
Acute myocardial infarction within 2 days Critical or severe aortic stenosis Active endocarditis Decompensated heart failure High-risk unstable angina Active myocarditis or pericarditis Acute pulmonary embolism or infarction Serious cardiac arrhythmias causing hemodynamic compromise; acute noncardiac condition that may affect exercise performance or may exacerbate the condition (infection, renal failure, thyrotoxicosis) Physical disability that precludes safe and adequate test performance Inability to obtain consent	Left main coronary stenosis Moderate stenotic valvular heart disease Tachyarrhythmias or bradyarrhythmias Atrial fibrillation with uncontrolled ventricular rate Hypertrophic cardiomyopathy Electrolyte abnormalities Mental impairment leading to an inability to cooperate High-degree atrioventricular block

Adapted with permission from Fletcher GF, Balady GJ, Amsterdam EA, et al: Exercise standards for testing and training: a statement for healthcare professionals from the American Heart Association. *Circulation.* 2001 Oct 2;104(14):1694–1740.

American College of Sports Medicine. Exercise and physical activity for older adults. *Med Sci Sports Exerc.* 2009;41:1510–1530. [PMID: 19516148]

Metkus TS Jr. Exercise prescription and primary prevention of cardiovascular disease *Circulation.* 2010;121(23):2601–2604. [PMID: 20547940]

Nelson M, Rejeski WJ, Blair SN, et al. Physical activity and public health in older adults: recommendation from the American College of Sports Medicine and the American Heart Association. *Med Sci Sports Exerc.* 2007;39(8):1435–1445. [PMID: 17762378]

Netz Y, Wu MJ, Becker BJ, et al. Physical activity and psychological well-being in advanced age: a meta-analysis of intervention studies. *Psychol Aging.* 2005;20:272–284. [PMID: 16029091]

Paganini-Hill A, Kawas CH, Corrada MM. Activities and mortality in the elderly: the World Leisure Cohort Study. *J Gerontol A Biol Med Sci.* 2011;66A(5):559–567. [PMID: 21350247]

Pescatello LS. Exercising for health: the merits of lifestyle physical activity. *West J Med.* 2001;174:114. [PMID: 11156922]

US Department of Health and Human Services. *Healthy People 2020.* https://www.healthypeople.gov. Accessed September 3, 2018.

NUTRITION IN OLDER ADULTS

Achieving healthy nutrition and weight status in older adults is a priority, according to *Healthy People 2020*. As individuals age, chronic diseases, functional impairments, polypharmacy, and age-related physiologic and socioeconomic changes may all act in concert to place an older adult at risk for malnutrition and undernutrition. *Malnutrition* is defined as a state in which a deficiency, excess, or imbalance of energy or other nutrients causes adverse physiologic effects. Malnutrition is a major factor associated with mortality in older persons. Several interrelated factors can place an older adult at nutritional risk (Tables 40–8 and 40–9). Poor nutritional status may be the result of insufficient dietary intake, leading to undernutrition; excess dietary content for actual expenditure, leading to obesity; and inappropriate dietary intake, exacerbating such conditions as diabetes, hypertension, and renal insufficiency.

Weight tends to increase with aging until the seventh decade, when it stabilizes or begins to decline. Obesity tends to be a problem for patients age <75 years, whereas undernutrition is commonly encountered in those age <85 years. Energy requirements decrease in the elderly. The recommended daily allowance of 2300 kcal for a 77-kg man and 1900 kcal for a 65-kg woman should be reduced by 10%, based on basal energy expenditure between ages 51 and 75 years, with an additional 10–15% reduction after age 75. Although animal studies have indicated increased longevity with lower body weight and caloric restriction without malnutrition, studies on the relative risk of obesity to mortality in older adults are inconsistent, ranging from a protective effect for hip fractures to increased functional disability.

Weight loss should be considered clinically significant when the change in baseline weight is >5% in 3 months or >10% in 6 months. An older adult with a body mass index (BMI) of <17 kg/m^2 also warrants further evaluation. Because anorexia, weight loss, and undernutrition in older persons have such deleterious effects, identification of causative factors that can be treated or reversed is of major importance. Often, a review of the status of underlying medical conditions, medications, functional limitations, and socioeconomic circumstances will reveal reversible factors contributing to weight loss. Use of oral supplements has been shown to produce small but consistent increases in weight in older adults. Use of appetite-stimulating agents such as megestrol, dronabinol, and oral steroids to promote weight gain is controversial, given the known side effects of these drugs and the absence of quality studies to support their use in most elderly patients. These medications are not recommended as part of a routine strategy to address weight loss in older adults.

The significance of mild to moderate obesity in the elderly is unclear. Height/weight charts for ideal body weight based on life insurance tables are probably less accurate in older adults, and BMI calculations may underestimate body fat, especially in those with reduced muscle mass. Older adults with rapid weight gain should be assessed for underlying congestive heart failure, renal disease, and other such illness. For those with chronic obesity, recommending weight loss should be done with caution and consideration of patient-specific factors. For patients age <70 years who are 20% above ideal body weight, a weight loss strategy including dietary modification and increased physical activity should be recommended. For patients age >70 years, weight loss should be recommended if a medical condition such as hypertension, diabetes, or degenerative joint disease exists and is likely to be significantly improved. A nutritionist can further assist the primary care physician in formulating a weight loss program for older patients, with a goal of 0.5–1 lb of weight loss per week.

Promotion of a balanced, healthy diet for all older adults, including recognition and remediation of macronutrient deficiencies, should be incorporated into the health promotion strategies of all primary care physicians caring for older adults. To be most beneficial, nutritional assessments and body weight measurements of older adults should be performed on a periodic basis. Levels of sodium, protein, fiber, fluid, and micronutrient intake are all important factors in providing nutritional counseling to older adults with recommendations tailored to individuals. The US Department of Agriculture (USDA) *2015–2020 Dietary Guidelines for America* and the USDA MyPlate (www.ChooseMyPlate.gov) methods offer specific food guidelines useful for both patients and providers.

Table 40–8. Nutrient requirements in older adults, with signs of excess and deficiency.

Nutrient	Requirement	Signs of Deficiency	Signs of Excess
Vitamin A	Requirements decrease with advancing age; 3333 IU for men, 2667 IU for women	Loss of bright, moist appearance; dry conjunctiva; gingivitis	Toxic effects include headache, lassitude, anorexia, reduced white blood cell count, impaired hepatic function, and bone pain with hypercalcemia; hip fracture
Vitamin B₁ (thiamine)	1.1–1.2 mg/d	Common in alcoholic elderly and institutionalized elderly; disordered cognition (delirium), neuropathies, and cardiomegaly	Liver damage and exacerbation of peptic ulcer disease, especially with those using megadoses
Vitamin B₂ (riboflavin)	1.1–1.3 mg/d	Cheilosis, angular stomatitis, gingivitis; changes to tongue papillae	
Vitamin B₆ (pyroxidine)	1.5–1.7 mg/d	Glossitis, peripheral neuropathy, and dementia especially related to alcohol abuse	Liver damage and nervous system dysfunction, especially with those using megadoses
Vitamin B₁₂	2.4 µg/d	Pallor, optic neuritis, hyporeflexia, ataxia, anorexia; loss of proprioception, vibratory sense, and memory loss; megaloblastic anemia	
Vitamin C		Gingival hypertrophy, bleeding gums, petechiae, and ecchymoses	Megadose use can cause diarrhea, oxalate kidney, and bladder stones; result in impaired absorption of vitamin B₁₂; interfere with serum and urine glucose testing; produce false-negative hemoccult testing
Vitamin D	10–15 µg/d (400–600 IU/d)	Osteomalacia; severe bone pain and osteoporosis; muscular hypotonia; pulmonary macrophage dysfunction	Nausea, headache, anorexia, weakness, and fatigue; interferes with vitamin K absorption
Vitamin K	Widely distributed in food and provided by synthesis of intestinal bacteria; supplements advised for fat malabsorption syndromes and long-term antibiotic therapy	Hemorrhages in skin or gastrointestinal tract; unexplained prolongation of prothrombin time	Unknown
Folic acid	400 µg/d	Pallor, stomatitis, glossitis, memory impairment, depression	
Vitamin E	400 IU/d	Deficiency is rare; abundant in diet	Interferes with vitamin K metabolism; thrombophlebitis; gastrointestinal (GI) distress; possible reduction in wound healing
Niacin	14–16 mg/d	Fissured tongue; dry, thickened, scaling, hyperpigmented skin; diarrhea; dementia	Histamine flush; liver toxicity
Calcium	1200–1500 mg/d	Osteoporosis	
Iron		Rare secondary to increased iron stores; usually secondary to pathologic blood loss	Constipation; excess iron usually given when anemia of chronic disease is misdiagnosed as iron-deficiency anemia; some association between neoplasia and coronary artery disease
Zinc		Impaired wound healing; diarrhea; decreased vision, olfaction, insulin, and immune function; anorexia; impotence	GI disturbance; sideroblastic anemia from impaired copper absorption; adverse effect on cellular immunity; interferes with other vitamin absorption

Data from Morley JE: The Science of Geriatrics. New York, NY: Springer Publishing; 2000 and Dwyer JT, Gallo JJ, Reichel W: Assessing nutritional status in elderly patients. *Am Fam Physician*. 1993 Feb 15;47(3):613–20.

Table 40–9. Factors associated with undernutrition in the elderly.

Depression
Dementia
Anorexia
Poor dental health
Medications
Pain
Fatigue
Sensory alterations
Impaired function
Dietary restrictions (more common in women)
Social isolation
Impecuniousness, alcoholism
Swallowing dysfunction
Dieting (low fat, low cholesterol)

Data from Stechmiller JK. Early nutritional screening of older adults: review of nutritional support. *J Infus Nurs.* 2003 May-Jun;26(3):170–177 and Morley JE. Anorexia and weight loss in older persons. *J Gerontol A Biol Sci Med Sci.* 2003 Feb;58(2):131–137.

Alibhai SM, Greenwood C, Payette H. An approach to the management of unintentional weight loss in elderly people. *Can Med Assoc J.* 2005;172:773–780. [PMID: 15767612]

American Dietetic Association. Position of the American Dietetic Association: nutrition, aging and the continuum of care. *J Am Diet Assoc.* 2000;100:580. [PMID: 10812387]

De Castro JM. Age-related changes in the social, psychological, and temporal influences on food intake in free-living, healthy, adult humans. *J Gerontol A Biol Sci Med Sci.* 2002;57:M368. [PMID: 12023266]

Kennedy RL, Chokkalingham K, Srinivasan R. Obesity in the elderly: who should we be treating, and why, and how? *Curr Opin Clin Nutr Metab Care.* 2004;7:3–9. [PMID: 1509896]

Loreck E, Chimakurthi R, Steinle N. Nutritional assessment of the geriatric patient: a comprehensive approach toward evaluating and managing nutrition. *Clin Geriatr.* 2012;20(4):20–26. [No PMID]

Lui L, Bopp MM, Roberson PK, et al. Undernutrition and risk of mortality in elderly patients within 1 year of hospital discharge. *J Gerontol A Biol Sci Med Sci.* 2002; 57:M741. [PMID: 12403803]

US Department of Health and Human Services. *Healthy People 2020.* https://www.healthypeople.gov. Accessed September 3, 2018.

Vollmer W, Sacks FM, Ard J, et al. Effects of diet and sodium intake on blood pressure: subgroup analysis of the DASH-sodium trial. *Ann Intern Med.* 2001;135(12):1019–1028. [PMID: 11747380]

GERIATRIC ASSESSMENT

The geriatric assessment is a multidimensional assessment designed to evaluate an older adult's physical and mental health, functional abilities, cognitive status, and social circumstances (Table 40–10). Older adults may be affected by several chronic conditions and syndromes (Table 40–11) that place them at higher risk for impairment. Healthcare providers can identify severe functional impairments by clinical

Table 40–10. Goals of geriatric assessment.

To define the functional capabilities and disabilities of older patients
To appropriately manage acute and chronic diseases of frail elders
To promote prevention and health
To establish preferences for care in various situations (advanced care planning)
To understand financial resources available for care
To understand social networks and family support systems for care
To evaluate an older patient's mental and emotional strengths and weaknesses

observation alone but often have difficulty identifying mild to moderate impairments. Geriatric assessment helps to identify older adults at risk for increasing frailty and provides an opportunity to intervene in a manner that may enhance general health, function, and quality of life. Social assessment is important in the development of an effective care plan.

Not all older adults will require a comprehensive geriatric assessment. Rather, this tool should be employed in older adults with chronic conditions and syndromes that place them at risk to screen for impairments. A useful validated self-administered screening tool, the Vulnerable Elders Survey-13 (VES-13), can be used to assess the functional and health status of community-dwelling older adults. (The VES-13 can be accessed online at http://www.rand.org/health/projects/acove/survey.html.) An additional screening tool that can be used by office staff to screen ambulatory older patients can be found in Table 40–12.

Table 40–11. Common chronic syndromes among the vulnerable elderly.

Dementia
Depression
Diabetes mellitus
Falls and mobility disorders
Hearing impairment
Heart failure
Hypertension
Ischemic heart disease
Malnutrition
Osteoarthritis
Osteoporosis
Pneumonia and influenza
Pressure ulcers
Stroke and atrial fibrillation
Urinary incontinence
Vision impairment

Data from Wenger NS, Shekelle, PG, MacLean CH, et al. Quality indicators for assessing care of vulnerable elders. *Ann Intern Med.* 2001;135[Suppl (8; Pt 2)]:653.

Table 40–12. A geriatric screening for impaired ambulatory elderly.

1. Medications
   Did the patient bring in all bottles or a list of medications?
   List all medications.
   Remember to ask about over-the-counter medications.
   Remember to ask about supplements and herbs.
2. Nutrition
   Weigh patient and record.
   Have you lost >10 lb in the past 6 months?
   Positive screen: 10 lb weight loss or <100 lb.
   Intervention: Further evaluation with the Mini-Nutritional Assessment.
3. Hearing
   Use handheld audioscope at 40 dB and screen both ears at 1000 and 2000 Hz.
   Positive screen: Patient unable to hear 1000 or 2000 Hz frequency in both ears or unable to hear the 1000 and 2000 Hz frequency in *one* ear.
   Intervention: Evaluate for cerumen impaction; refer to audiology.
4. Vision
   Ask: "Do you have any problems driving, watching TV, reading, or doing any of your activities because of your eyesight?"
   If *yes*:
   Do Snellen eye chart
   Positive screen: 20/40 or greater
   Intervention: Refer to optometry or ophthalmology
5. Mental status
   Ask to remember three objects: "ball, car, and flag" (have them repeat objects after you)
   Positive screen: Unable to remember all three items after 1 min
   Intervention: Administer more formal mental status testing such as the 7-Minute Neurocognitive Screening Battery or Mini-Mental State Examination; assess for causes of cognitive impairment including delirium, depression, and medications
6. Depression
   Ask: "Are you depressed?" or "Do you often feel sad or depressed?"
   Positive screen: Yes.
   Intervention: Perform a more thorough depression screen (Geriatric Depression Scale); evaluate medications; consider pharmacologic treatment; and/or refer to psychiatry.
7. Urinary incontinence
   Ask: In the past year, have you ever lost urine or gotten wet? If *yes*:
   Ask: Have you lost urine on at least 6 separate days?
   Positive screen: Yes to both
   Intervention: Initiate workup for incontinence; consider urology referral.
8. Physical disability
   Ask: Are you able to do strenuous activities like fast walking or biking? Heavy work around the house like washing windows, floors, and walls? Go shopping for groceries or clothes? Get to places out of walking distance? Bathe, either sponge bath, tub bath, or shower? Dress, like putting on a shirt, buttoning and zipping, and putting on your shoes?
   Positive screen: Unable to do any of the above independently or able to do only with assistance from another.
   Intervention: Corroborate responses if accuracy uncertain with caregivers; determine reason for inability to perform task; institute appropriate medical, social, and environmental interventions; patient may benefit from physical and/or occupational therapy and a home visit.
9. Mobility
   Ask: Do you fall or feel unbalanced when walking or standing?
   Positive screen: Yes.
   Intervention: "Get up and go" test: Get up from the chair, walk 20 feet, turn, walk back to the chair, and sit down (walk at normal, comfortable pace).
   Positive screen: Unable to complete the task in 15 s
   Intervention: Refer to physical therapy for gait evaluation and assistance with use of appropriate adaptive devices; home safety evaluation; patient may need to be instructed in strengthening of both upper and lower extremities.
10. Home environment
   Ask: Do you have trouble with stairs either inside or outside of your house? Do you feel safe at home?
   Positive Screen: Yes.
   Intervention: Supply the older patient or caregiver with a home safety self-assessment checklist; consider making a home visit or use a visiting nurse or other community resource to evaluate the home; make appropriate referrals to help remediate safety issues.
11. Social support
   Ask: Who would be able to help you in case of an illness or emergency?
   Record identified person(s) in medical record with contact information.
   Intervention: Become familiar with available resources for the elderly within your community or know who can provide you with that assistance.

Data from Lachs MS, Feinstein AR, Cooney LM, et al: A simple procedure for general screening for functional disability in elderly patients. *Ann Intern Med.* 1990 May 1;112(9):699–706 and Moore AA, Siu AL: Screening for common problems in ambulatory elderly: clinical confirmation of a screening instrument. *Am J Med.* 1996 Apr;100(4):438–443.

Table 40–13. Components of geriatric assessment.

A. Functional assessment
  1. Basic activities of daily living (BADLs): fundamental to self-care:
     Bathing
     Dressing
     Toileting
     Transfers
     Continence
     Feeding
  2. Instrumental activities of daily living (IADLs): complex daily activities fundamental to independent community living and interactions)[a]:
     Housework: Can you do your own housework?
     Traveling: Can you get places outside of walking distance?
     Shopping: Can you go shopping for food and clothing?
     Money: Can you handle your own money?
     Meal preparation: Can you prepare your own meals?
  3. Advanced activities of daily living (AADLs): "functional signature"
     Gait-mobility and balance
     Upper extremity evaluation
B. Cognitive and affective assessment
     Dementia
     Depression
     Suicide
     Alcohol misuse
     Sensory impairments
     Nutrition
     Incontinence
C. Social assessment (caregivers, environment, finances)
     Driving
     Sexuality
     Advance care planning

[a]In order of most difficult to least difficult—knowing a person can perform one item indicates they can perform item below it.
Data from Gallo JJ, Fulmer T, Paveza G, et al. Handbook of Geriatric Assessment. 4th ed. New York, NY: Jones & Bartlett; 2005; Katz S, Ford AB, Moskowitz RW, et al. Studies of illness in the aged: the index of ADL: a standardized measure of biological and psychosocial function. *JAMA*. 1963 Sep 21;185:914–919; Fillenbaum G. Screening the elderly: a brief instrumental activities of daily living measure. *J Am Geriatr Soc.* 1985 Oct;33(10):698–706.

Family physicians who care for older adults should strive to incorporate the geriatric assessment tool into their clinical practice. If impairments are identified as part of the geriatric assessment, a comprehensive, interdisciplinary approach should be employed to address those impairments, optimize function, and improve quality of life. Table 40–13 outlines several components of the geriatric assessment, and a more detailed discussion of several of these components follows in the remainder of this chapter.

Elsawy B, Higgins KE. The geriatric assessment. *Am Fam Physician.* 2011;83(1):48–56. [PMID: 21888128]
Ensberg M, Gerstenlauer C. Incremental geriatric assessment. *Prim Care Clin Office Practice.* 2005;32:619. [PMID: 16140119]

Saliba D, Elliott M, Rubenstein LZ, et al. The Vulnerable Elders Survey: a tool for identifying vulnerable older people in the community. *J Am Geriatr Soc.* 2001;49:1691–1699. [PMID: 11844005]

Functional Assessment

A. Predictors of Functional Decline

The ability to function independently in the community is an important public health and quality-of-life issue for all older adults. A recent trend toward declining disability has been noted among older persons, especially those with higher levels of education. For example, older adults who walk a mile at least once a week show decreasing decline in functional limitations and disability than their sedentary counterparts. However, these trends are not indicative of the total population. Older adults of African American and Hispanic background generally report more functional limitations and disability and represent vulnerable subpopulations within the United States.

Several predictors of functional decline and mortality have been reported. Health status belief and decreased abilities in activities of daily living (ADLs) appear to be important predictors of mortality. Older adults with depression have increased risk of ADL disability because it appears that depressive symptoms undermine efforts to maintain physical functioning.

Kivela SL, Pahkala K. Depressive disorder as a predictor of physical disability in old age. *J Am Geriatr Soc.* 2001;49:290–296. [PMID: 11300240]
Ostchega Y, Harris TB, Hirsch R, et al. The prevalence of functional limitations and disability in older persons in the US: data from the National Health and Nutrition Examination Survey III. *J Am Geriatr Soc.* 2000;48:1132–1135. [PMID: 10983915]

B. Evaluation of Functional Status

The capacity to perform functional tasks necessary for daily living can be used as a surrogate measure of independence or a predictor of decline and institutionalization. Functional status needs to be assessed objectively and independently of medical, laboratory, and cognitive evaluation because specific functional loss is not disease specific and cognitive impairment does not necessarily imply inability to function independently in a familiar environment. Limitations noted on functional assessment should prompt the search for contributing and modifiable conditions, including musculoskeletal dysfunction, cognitive impairment, depression, substance abuse, adverse medication reactions, or sensory impairment.

Knowledge of how older adults spend their time can give physicians a reference point for potential functional decline at subsequent visits. Functional assessment can be considered as a hierarchy ranging from advanced, independent, and basic ADLs. An older adult may be fully independent, require assistance, or be fully dependent in any or all of these activities. Individuals may move across levels of assistance or dependence, especially during and after an acute illness. Assessment of these activities allows providers to match services to needs.

The advanced activities of daily living (AADLs) include very-high-level tasks that may be considered the functional signature of a well community-dwelling older individual. These tasks include voluntary social, occupational, or recreational activities. An older person who does not successfully participate in such activities may not be impaired, but the presence of significant involuntary loss of AADLs may be an important risk factor for further functional losses.

The instrumental activities of daily living (IADLs) are intermediate-level activities (Table 40–13) and are required for independent living. Older adults living in the community who cannot perform IADLs may have difficulty functioning at home and may be appropriate for assisted living or personal care home settings.

The basic activities of daily living (BADLs) include self-care activities (Table 40–13) that are at the most basic level of functioning. Loss of BADLs tends to progress from those involving lower extremity strength to those activities that rely on upper extremity strength, such that mobility and toileting are lost before dressing and feeding. Dependence for toileting has been shown to be an indicator of overall poor performance that should alert the provider to the need for increased care. Older adults requiring assistance for BADLs may be appropriate for a nursing home setting.

De Vriendt P, Gorus E, Cornelis E, et al. The process of decline in advanced activities of daily living: a qualitative explorative study in mild cognitive impairment. *Int Psychogeriatr.* 2012;24(6):974–986. [PMID: 22301014]

Katz S, Ford AB, Moskowitz RW, et al. Studies of illness in the aged: the index of ADL. *JAMA.* 1963;185:914–919. [PMID: 14044222]

Lawton MP, Brody EM. Assessment of older people: self-maintaining and instrumental activities of daily living. *Gerontologist.* 1969;9(3):179–186. [PMID: 5349366]

Sherman FT. Functional assessment: easy-to-use screening tools to speed initial office work-up. *Geriatrics.* 2001;56:36. [PMID: 11505859]

C. Other Geriatric Assessment Elements

Issues relating to mobility and balance (Chapter 41), incontinence (Chapter 42), depression (Chapter 56), and sensory impairments (Chapter 45) are covered in this book, and the reader is referred to those chapters for more detailed information. The remainder of this chapter focuses on issues that need to be addressed in the evaluation of older adults.

Table 40–14. Social support screening.

How many relatives do you see or hear from in the course of a month?
Tell me about the relative with whom you have the most contact.
How many relatives do you feel close to—such as to discuss private matters?
How many friends do you see or hear from in the course of a month?
Tell me about the friend with whom you have the most contact.
When you have an important decision to make, do you have someone you can talk to about it?
Do you rely on anybody to assist you with shopping, cooking, doing repairs, cleaning house, etc?
Do you help others with shopping, cooking, transportation, childcare, etc?
Do you live alone?
With whom do you live?

Data from Gallo JJ, Fulmer T, Paveza G, et al. *Handbook of Geriatric Assessment.* 4th ed. New York, NY: Jones & Bartlett; 2005.

1. Social support—Social networks consist of informal supports such as family and close longtime friends, formal supports including social services and healthcare delivery agencies, and semiformal supports such as church groups and neighborhood organizations. Relationships with family and friends may be complex and can have important implications for the vulnerable elder. The availability of assistance from family or friends frequently influences whether a functionally dependent older adult remains at home or is institutionalized. Table 40–14 contains questions that may be incorporated into social support screening.

2. Caregiver burden—Adults providing care for a frail or cognitively impaired person can face overwhelming demands. Older adults may be either the provider or recipient of such caregiving. Caregiver burden describes the strain or load borne by these providers. A caregiver's perceived burden is closely linked to the caregiver's ability to cope and handle stress. Caregivers are at higher risk for mortality if there is increased mental or emotional strain. Physicians should be vigilant for signs of possible caregiver burnout in any caregiver. These signs include multiple somatic complaints, anxiety or depression, social isolation, and weight loss. Formal assessment tools include the Caregiver Strain Index and the Zarit Burden Interview.

Bedard M, Molloy DW, Squire L, et al. The Zarit Burden Interview: a short version and screening version. *Gerontologist.* 2001;41: 652–657. [PMID: 11574710]

Kasuya RT, Polgar-Bailey P, Takeuchi R. Caregiver burden and burnout: a guide for primary care physicians. *Postgrad Med.* 2000;108:119–123. [PMID: 1126138]

Schulz R, Beach SR. Caregiving as a risk factor for mortality: the Caregiver Health Effects Study. *JAMA.* 1999;282:2215–2219. [PMID: 10605972]

3. Economic factors—Economic factors have important consequences with respect to an older adult's health, nutrition, and living environment. Economic factors may influence an older adult's access to food, medications, assistive technology, and various healthcare services. The physician can inquire as to whether older individuals have sufficient financial resources to meet their needs and whether proposed treatments or interventions will cause the patient an economic burden. The primary care provider should have a working knowledge of Medicare and be familiar with state and local resources.

4. Physical environment—An older adult's physical environment, including their home, neighborhood, and transportation system, is critical to maintaining independence. Environmental hazards within the home are common and can place an older adult at increased risk for falls and injury. Common, modifiable home hazards include loose throw rugs, obstructed pathways, poor lighting, absence of stair handrails, absence of bathroom grab bars, and low or loose toilet seats. The physician should inquire about the safety of the neighborhood and if older adults have access to transportation or transportation services. This is especially important for older adults who are dependent on caregivers for IADLs and are still living within the community.

Environmental hazards are not easily detected during an office visit. A home visit either by the physician or a community agency provider can reveal problems in the living situation, such as wandering, household hazards, social isolation and loneliness, family stress, nutrition problems, financial concerns, and even alcohol abuse. An environmental home safety checklist can be provided to the older adult or a caregiver to complete a self-assessment within the home.

Kao H, Conant R, Soriano T, et al. The past, present, and future of house calls. *Clin Geriatr Med.* 2009;25:19–34. [PMID: 19217490]

5. Driving competence—The number of older adults who drive will continue to increase as the general population of the United States increases. The ability to drive allows the older adult to maintain important links within the community and is closely linked to independence and self-esteem. Older adults who are unable to drive or who stop driving risk social isolation, depression, and functional decline. Many older drivers voluntarily modify their driving habits by driving shorter distances; driving only during daylight; and avoiding rush hour, major highways, and inclement weather.

Older drivers should be counseled on the importance of safety restraints, obeying speed limits, use of a helmet if riding a motorcycle or bicycle, taking a driving refresher course, and avoidance of alcohol and use of mobile phones while driving. Adults age ≥65 years account for 16% of all traffic fatalities. Driving accidents with older adults are less likely to involve high speeds or alcohol, but are more likely to involve visual-spatial difficulties and cognitive and motor

skills. Heart disease and hearing impairment are also commonly associated with adverse driving events.

Evaluating the driving competence of an older adult is challenging. Driving involves a set of complex tasks that require not only physical but also mental integrity. Chronic illness, functional status, or even cognitive status cannot consistently predict adverse driving events. Assessment of the older driver should include a review of the driving record, medications, alcohol use, and functional measures including vision, hearing, attention, visual-spatial skills, muscle strength, and joint flexibility. Providers can consider use of the 4Cs screening tool (crash history, family concerns, clinical condition, and cognitive functions) to identify at at-risk drivers. Primary care providers must be familiar with state laws regarding required reporting of driving safety concerns and reportable medical conditions.

American Geriatrics Society, Pomidor A, eds. *Clinician's Guide to Assessing and Counseling Older Drivers.* 3rd ed. Report No. DOT HS 812 228. Washington, DC: National Highway Traffic Safety Administration; 2016.
Carr DB, Duchek JM, Meuser TM, et al. Older drivers with cognitive impairment. *Am Fam Physician.* 2006;73:1029–1034. [PMID: 16570737]
Hogan DB. Which older patients are competent to drive? Approaches to office-based assessment. *Can Fam Physician.* 2005;51:362–368. [PMID: 15794021]
O'Connor M, Kapust LR, Lin B, et al. The 4Cs (crash history, family concerns, clinical condition, and cognitive functions): a screening tool for the evaluation of the at-Risk driver. *J Am Geriatr Soc.* 2010;58:1104–1108. [PMID: 20487078]

6. Alcohol misuse—Approximately 40% of adults over age 65 consume alcohol. In the primary care setting, alcohol misuse is identified in approximately 10.5% of older men and 3.9% of older women. Alcohol misuse places an older adult at increased risk for falls, accidental injury, hypertension, and cognitive impairment. The National Institute on Alcohol Abuse and Alcoholism recommends that people age >65 years have no more than seven drinks a week and no more than three drinks on any one day. Preventive care should include screening all elders at least once to detect problems or hazardous drinking by taking a history of alcohol use and using a standard screening questionnaire, such as the 4-item CAGE or the 10-item AUDIT. (Information for older adults about alcohol misuse can be found at http://www.nia .nih.gov/health/publication/alcohol-use-older-people.)

Blow F, Barry KL. Alcohol and substance misuse in older adults. *Curr Psychiatr Rep.* 2012;14:310–319. [PMID: 22660897]
National Institute on Alcohol Abuse and Alcoholism. *Older Adults.* http://www.niaaa.nih.gov/alcohol-health/special-populations-co-occurring-disorders/older-adults. Accessed September 12, 2018.
Ringler SK. Alcoholism in the elderly. *Am Fam Physician.* 2000;61:1710–1716. [PMID: 10750878]

7. Sexual health—Sexual health remains an important consideration in older adults. Older adults may not initiate discussions about sexual health on their own; thus, the provider should routinely include discussion of sexual health in their assessment. Using open-ended questions allows the individual to give as much or as little information as is comfortable. The clinician needs to understand the older adult's previous and present normal sexual patterns and interests and whether any changes that have occurred affect sexual functioning and intimacy. These may include medical conditions, medications, physical disabilities, mood disturbance, or cognitive impairment. Sexual assessment may include questions about quality of erection and orgasm for men and lubrication and orgasm for women. If a problem is uncovered, a more thorough assessment and evaluation should be undertaken. All sexually active older adults should be counseled on safer sex practices.

Evidence shows that lesbian, gay, bisexual, and transgender (LGBT) older adults may be less likely to share their sexual orientation or seek care for sexual health issues.

Clinicians must be astute and maintain awareness of the unique challenges faced by these adults to provide the most appropriate screening and prevention interventions.

Gingold H. The graying of sex. *NYS Psychologist*. 2007;9(4):8–23. [No PMID]

Gott M, Hinchliff S. Barriers to seeking treatment for sexual problems in primary care: a qualitative study with older people. *Fam Practice*. 2003;20:690–695. [PMID: 14701894]

National LGBT Education Center. *Improving the Lives of Gay, Lesbian, Bisexual and Transgender Older Adults, 2010*. Boston, MA: National LGBT Education Center; 2010.

Taylor A, Gosney MA. Sexuality in older age: essential considerations for healthcare professionals. *Age Ageing*. 2011;40:538–543. [PMID: 21778176]

8. Spirituality—Information about an older adult's spirituality can provide insight into factors affecting their care decisions and help providers understand the patient's resources to cope with illness and other stressors. The spiritual assessment may include questions about their concept of God or

Table 40–15. Five steps to successful advanced care planning.

Steps	Process
1. Introduce the topic	During a wellness visit or some other time when the individual is in a good state of health, explain the purpose and nature of the discussion Inquire into how familiar the individual is with advanced care planning and define terms as necessary Be aware of the comfort level of the patient—give information and be supportive Suggest that family members, friends, or even members of the community explore how to manage potential burdens Discuss the identification of a proxy decision maker Encourage the patient to bring the proxy decision maker to the next visit
2. Engage in structured discussions	Convey commitment to patients to follow their wishes and protect patients from unwanted treatment or undertreatment Involve the potential proxy decision maker in discussions and planning Allow the patient to specify the role he/she would like the proxy to assume if the patient is incapacitated—follow patient's explicit wishes, or allow the proxy to decide according to the patient's best interests Elicit the patient's values and goals
3. Document patient preferences	Review advanced directives with patient and proxy for inconsistencies and misunderstandings Enter the advanced directives into the medical record Recommend statutory documents be completed by the patient that comply with state statutes Distribute directives to hospital, patient, proxy decision maker, family members, and all healthcare providers Include advanced directives in the care plan
4. Review and update the directive regularly	
5. Apply directives to actual circumstances	Most advanced directives go into effect when the patient can no longer direct her/his own medical care Assess the patient's decision-making capacity Never assume advanced directive content without reading it thoroughly Advanced directives should be interpreted in view of the clinical facts of the case Physician and proxy decision maker will need to work together to resolve ambiguous or uncertain situations If disagreements between physician and proxy cannot be resolved, seek the assistance of an ethics consultant or committee

Data from Emanuel LL, von Gunten CF, Ferris FD: Advance care planning. *Arch Fam Med*. 2000 Nov-Dec;9(10):1181–1187.

deity, afterlife, value and meaning in life, and any specific religious practices. Older adults can suffer from spiritual distress that may be expressed as depression; crying; fear of abandonment; or hopelessness, anxiety, and despair. This distress may occur in the setting of illness, after the loss of a significant other, following a family or personal disaster, or when there is a disruption in the usual religious activities. Inquiring into the spirituality of patients requires empathy on the part of the physician, strong interpersonal skills, and a closely established physician-patient relationship.

Sulmasy DP. Spirituality, religion and clinical care. *Chest*. 2009; 135:1634–1642. [PMID: 19497898]

9. Advanced care planning—Advanced care planning is the process of planning for the medical future in which the patient's preferences will guide the nature and intensity of future medical care, particularly if the patient is unable to make independent decisions. It is important for the physician to learn about the patient's personal values, goals, and preferences for care (Table 40–15).

Older adults should indicate the type or level of care that they would and would not want to receive in various situations. Advanced care planning is designed to ensure that the patient's wishes are known and respected. Older adults should be encouraged to share their wishes with family members, and the provider can assist in facilitating this discussion.

Fried TR, Bullock K, Iannone L, et al. Understanding advance care planning as a process of health behavior change. *J Am Geriatr Soc.* 2009;9:1547–1555. [PMID: 19682120]
Kahana B, Dan A, Kahana E, Kercher K. The personal and social context of planning end-of-life care. *J Am Geriatr Soc.* 2004;52:1163–1167. [PMID: 15209656]

Websites

Administration on Aging. https://acl.gov/about-acl/administration-aging
American Geriatrics Society Foundation for Health in Aging. https://www.healthinaging.org/health-aging-foundation
American Association of Retired Persons. http://www.aarp.org
American Geriatrics Society. http://www.americangeriatrics.org
American Society of Consultant Pharmacists. http://www.ascp.com
Centers for Disease Control and Prevention National Prevention Information Network. http://www.cdcnpin.org
Children of Aging Parents. http://www.caps4caregivers.org
Family Caregiver Alliance. http://www.caregiver.org
Medicare Hotline. http://www.medicare.gov
National Adult Day Services Association. http://www.nadsa.org
National Center on Elder Abuse. https://ncea.acl.gov/
National Council on the Aging. http://www.ncoa.org
National Institute on Aging. http://www.nia.nih.gov

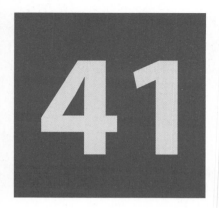

Common Geriatric Problems

Robert B. Allison II, DO

Providing care for individuals across all age demographics is not the same. Just as providing care for infants and adolescents differs from that of an adult, so too is caring for the elderly. Geriatric medicine is not simply general medicine for those >65 years old. Aging individuals develop a constellation of medial comorbidities that involve a myriad of treatment options. Individuals pursue a wide range of treatments attempting to preserve their current level of independence, maintain a certain quality of life, and limit the potential for functional and cognitive decline. Multimorbidity, frailty, and polypharmacy seem to interlace themselves across the continuum of care when treating older adults. As the current population continues to live longer, providers need to develop a balanced approach to treating multiple comorbidities with appropriate therapeutic interventions all while preserving their patients' current level of independence and quality of life.

MULTIMORBIDITY

ESSENTIALS OF DIAGNOSIS

▶ Identify and incorporate patient preferences into medical decision making.

▶ Discuss medical decision making as a balance between expected benefit, potential risk, and treatment burden.

▶ Develop a collaborative plan with an acceptable level of complexity.

▶ Optimize treatment benefit while reducing harm and enhancing quality of life.

More than half of older adults have three or more chronic diseases that can have a cumulative impact on their health.

Individuals who are diagnosed with multiple chronic conditions, or multimorbidity, have higher rates of morbidity, mortality, polypharmacy, adverse drug effects, and institutionalization; higher healthcare costs; and a lower quality of life. Unfortunately, older individuals with multimorbidity are commonly excluded, or poorly represented, in clinical trials and observational studies. This makes data analysis and clinical recommendations difficult to interpret for these patients. Moreover, most practice guidelines only focus on the management of an isolated disease. Older adults with multimorbidity are heterogeneous in terms of illness severity, functional status, prognosis, personal priorities, and risk of adverse events even when diagnosed with the same pattern of conditions. One of the unique challenges in providing quality care to older adults is the interpretation of clinical trials and guideline recommendations and translating those results into a treatment plan that is acceptable for each patient. Developing a treatment plan for multimorbidity patients involves five key elements: establishing patient preferences; reviewing pertinent literature; determining the disease prognosis; constructing a management plan; and optimizing quality of life.

▶ Establishing Patient Preferences

Older individuals with multimorbidity face many more treatment decisions than their peers without such medical complexity. There is an ever-growing number of clinical guidelines, all directed to improve the outcome of one specific disease state. Unfortunately, limited data are available to guide the management of several disease states coinciding with one another, and providers who simply adhere to the guidelines may not adequately account for individual patient preferences. Those with multimorbidity should evaluate and prioritize treatment options within the constructs of personal and cultural desires. Some decisions may be straightforward and may not require much input from the provider. Other decisions may be more complex, and patients may turn to the provider for guidance. Figure 41–1 outlines a stepwise approach to best assure providers are eliciting patient preferences during complex decision making. Older adults with multimorbidity are more likely to confront preference-sensitive decisions because the decision to treat one disease has the potential to affect the homeostatic balance of their

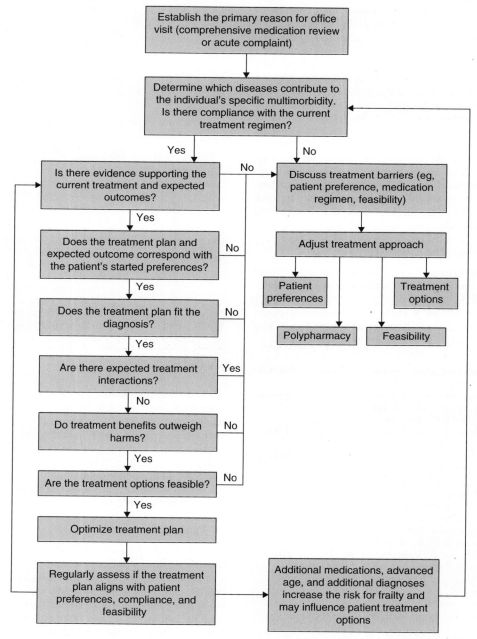

▲ **Figure 41–1.** A stepwise approach to best assure providers are eliciting patient preferences during complex decision making.

other ailments. This risk-reward paradigm is never greater when weighing the potential for clinical improvement against the burden of treatment.

An important step in eliciting preference is to assure the patient adequately understands the information presented. Only then can patients begin to develop their preferences based on personal values and priorities. For individuals with cognitive impairment, a surrogate decision maker should be appointed to make decisions on behalf of the patient. When it comes to making treatment decisions, some patients will defer to the provider, some wish to make decisions on their own, and others want to make shared decisions with family, friends, and caregivers; however, virtually all patients want their opinion to guide the process. This does not imply that patients can demand any treatment if there is no expectation of some meaningful benefit. The continually evolving health of older adults with multimorbidity will generate periodic changes in patient preferences. Previous decisions should be reexamined by both the patient and the provider, and new preferences should be established moving forward. Table 41–1 summarizes the key concepts to establishing patient preferences.

▶ Interpreting the Evidence

The interaction between varying disease states is a constant theme when caring for older adults with multimorbidity. The continual interaction is unpredictable, thus making multimorbidity difficult to study. Consequently, determining whether the individual will benefit from a particular

Table 41–2. Interpreting the evidence.

Applicability of evidence	Are older adults included in sufficient numbers? Does the study account for multimorbidity? Does the study design encompass the population to which it is being applied?
Outcomes	Are the outcomes reported meaningful and applicable to the population for which it is being applied?
Harms and burdens	Were adverse events reported? Did investigators look for potential effects, positive or negative, on other comorbid conditions? How were variable treatment interactions documented? Were funding, financial burden, and treatment complexity disclosed?
Absolute risk reduction	Baseline risk assessment in older adults with multimorbidity may vary, and when that risk falls outside the established risk for the trial, it is difficult to apply the study effectively.
Time horizon to benefit	Studies look for a defined time to accrue observable, clinically meaningful risk reduction for a specific outcome. Providers should account for the time needed to expect a clinical outcome when making management decisions. Patients and providers should decide if anticipated benefits warrant potential treatment harms.

Table 41–1. Eliciting patient preferences.

1. Recognize when an older adult is facing a preference-sensitive decision.
   A. Electing to treat one condition may exacerbate another.
   B. Interventions that provide long-term benefit may cause short-term harm.
   C. Initiating medications may provide targeted improvement but lead to broad complications.
2. Adequately inform older adults about the expected risk and benefit of a specific treatment option.
   A. Don't minimize adverse effects.
   B. Avoid words such as "rarely" or "frequently."
   C. Provide the numerical likelihood of an event to occur.
   D. Absolute risk reduction is preferred to relative risk reduction.
   E. Discuss an event as either "occurring" or "not occurring" to avoid positive or negative bias.
3. Elicit patient preferences after patient has been sufficiently informed.
   A. Future treatment options are guided by clearly stated goals of care (eg, longevity, quality, comfort, function).
   B. Visual aids help in decision making (eg, decision tree, visual analog scale).
   C. Decision-making tools are framed by personal preference (eg, standard gamble, time trade-off).

treatment is complicated. A key fundamental of evidence-based medicine is whether the study represents the patient demographic for which it is being applied. Unfortunately, there is a paucity of research involving older adults, and the research that is available tends to exclude individuals with multiple comorbidities. When evaluating data and applying it to older adults with multimorbidity, the provider should ask several important questions and identify the key concepts outlined in Table 41–2.

▶ Prognosis

An individual's prognosis should guide, but not dictate, clinical decisions within the context of patient preference. The provider should evaluate the prognosis by considering the individual's potential life expectancy and what impact the prognosis would have on the patient's quality of life if the patient elected treatment or conservative therapy. Treatment decisions must weigh potential risks, benefits, and overall burden against that individual's treatment preferences, as previously discussed. The time horizon to benefit, as outlined earlier, may be longer than the individual's projected life span. In this case, treatment may consist of multiple medications (polypharmacy), adverse drugs reactions, potential loss of independence, and decreased quality of life without improving the original disease state. The same concept is true for disease-specific screening tests that may be invalid based on the older adult's multimorbidity and current prognosis. These are a few of the issues a provider must consider when incorporating prognosis into clinical decision making.

Most older adults wish to discuss prognosis. However, when entering into a conversation about prognosis, the provider must be culturally sensitive and ethical in approach. The ethical principles of autonomy, beneficence, nonmaleficence, and justice should be at the forefront of a patient-provider discussion about prognosis. Providers can also prioritize their decision recommendations by categorizing life expectancy as short term (within 1 year), mid term (within 5 years), and long term (>5 years). Using such categories allows the provider to offer treatment options to older adults with multimorbidity that will confer the most benefit while reducing potential treatment harms.

Understanding the prognosis can help patients make decisions across a variety of settings. Determining disease prevention through screening exams (eg, colon cancer screening) may be more appropriate for someone discussing a mid-term or long-term prognosis, whereas someone given a short-term prognosis may forgo treating a disease whose time horizon to benefit is greater than the patient's current life expectancy (eg, statin therapy for primary prevention; tight glycemic control for macrovascular risk reduction). However, discussing prognosis can also be difficult for patients, often leading to discussions about end-of-life care and mortality. The provider can use this time to facilitate a discussion about advanced care planning, understand an individual's treatment rationale, and review the patient's therapy preferences.

▶ Clinical Feasibility

The more complex a treatment regimen is for an adult with multimorbidity, the higher is the likelihood of nonadherence, adverse drug reactions, decreased quality of life, increased financial burden, and added stress for identified caregivers. Providers should use a stepwise approach to break down the treatment complexity: obtain informed consent to treat; decide on the number of treatment choices provided; identify how many steps are needed to complete each treatment; and determine how easy it will be to integrate the new treatment plan into the current treatment regimen. Providers must also be aware that an individual's medication compliance is influenced by external psychosocial factors and internal perception of need, cost, and current symptom management. Once a treatment plan has been selected, providers should

conduct regular assessments and continual education for their patients. When done in a variety of different ways, such teaching can reaffirm the treatment regimen, because older adults with multimorbidity generally do not recall discussions with the provider.

One way to assess compliance is to assemble an interdisciplinary care team. This team can use tools such as the Medication Management Instrument for Deficiencies in the Elderly (MedMaIDE), Drug Regimen Unassisted Grading Scale (DRUGS), Hopkins Medication Schedule (HMS), and Medication Management Ability Assessment (MMAA). Conducting a comprehensive medication review and assisting with medication management on a regular basis has been shown to decrease hospitalizations. Discussing the care plan with an individual's support system, including family and caregivers, will also add to compliance, particularly in cases where cognitive impairment affects adherence. Healthcare transitions (eg, home–hospital, hospital–skilled nursing facility, skilled nursing facility–home) are important opportunities to reevaluate treatment feasibility and compliance.

Patient preference and clinical feasibility have a large influence on treatment choice. Providing educational programs to encourage self-management skills and improve self-efficacy improve compliance. Mutual engagement between patients and provider also generates increased adherence, persistence, and motivation to continue their current treatment plan.

▶ Optimizing Therapies and Care Plans

Older adults with multimorbidity have a higher likelihood of adverse outcomes when treatments and interventions are not optimized to assure feasibility or are not aligned with patient preference. Providers can improve treatment benefit by prioritizing the most essential pharmacologic and nonpharmacologic interventions. Polypharmacy and suboptimal medication use lead to decreased medication compliance and less benefit from otherwise appropriate medications, respectively. The age-related changes in pharmacokinetics and pharmacodynamics lead to a greater likelihood of adverse drug reactions in this population. Reducing the number of medications, or deprescribing, can decrease the likelihood of adverse drug reactions and improve adherence.

In an attempt to optimize therapy, providers should first identify treatments, procedures, and other nonpharmacologic interventions that may not be appropriate based on prognosis and patient preference. Conducting a thorough medication reconciliation at each healthcare transition can help identify potentially harmful medications and lead to deprescribing. There are several different tools to aid in such medication management, which are outlined later in this chapter. Polypharmacy in older adults with multimorbidity is intrinsically related to reduced therapeutic benefit, increased adverse drug events, larger financial and caregiver burden, and reduced patient compliance. Similar steps should be taken when it comes to determining the need for further nonpharmacologic interventions (eg, lab work, procedures, implantable cardiovascular devices). For older adults with multimorbidity and variable life expectancy, achievable treatment benefit may be offset by the potential for adverse events and the burden such treatment would impose on their quality of life.

Establishing patient preferences in the context of available, evidence-based research and developing a feasible treatment plan congruent with the patient's prognosis are the cornerstone of providing quality care for older adults with multimorbidity. Feasibility and treatment optimization should be based on the individual's preferences while recognizing treatment risks, benefits, and burden. Providers should reassess treatment plans on a regular basis given the inevitable progression of disease. A change in disease state or the addition of a new diagnosis may alter the prognosis and ultimately influence patient preference. Providing care for older adults with multimorbidity is ever changing, but by establishing patient preferences and clear treatment expectations, providers can formulate feasible treatment plans that are goal oriented and patient centered.

American Geriatrics Society Expert Panel on the Care of Older Adults With Multimorbidity. Patient-centered care for older adults with multiple chronic conditions: a stepwise approach from the American Geriatrics Society: American Geriatrics Society Expert Panel on the Care of Older Adults with Multimorbidity. *J Am Geriatr Soc*. 2012;60(10):1957–1968. [PMID: 22994844]

FRAILTY

ESSENTIALS OF DIAGNOSIS

▶ Frailty is a cumulative decline in multiple physiologic systems over a lifetime, which can potentiate a state of vulnerability to sudden changes in health. These changes are triggered by a stressful event and result in poor a resolution of homeostasis, thus increasing the risk for adverse outcomes.

▶ The frailty phenotype and Frailty Index are the two most commonly accepted frailty models.

▶ Frail older adults are at increased risk for disability, falls, hospitalizations, and mortality.

▶ A comprehensive geriatric assessment and treatment plan, in conjunction with exercise, can preserve independence and improve functional ability.

The world population is aging at an exponential rate, from roughly 460 million people over the age of 65 years old in 2004 to an estimated 2 billion people by 2050, according to reports by the Population Reference Bureau in Washington, DC, in 2005 and the United Nations Department of Economic and Social Affairs in 1999. Healthcare providers will be faced with a multitude of evolving disease states and comorbidities, but the most inclusive expression of population aging and disease complexity is the clinical condition of frailty. Described as a cumulative decline in multiple physiologic systems over a lifetime that can potentiate a state of vulnerability to sudden changes in health that are triggered by a stressful event and result in poor resolution of homeostasis, frailty assessment tools are multiple, but universally accepted clinical criteria still remain undefined. It is a long-established clinical expression that implies concern over an older adult's vulnerability and prognosis.

There are two universally accepted frailty models from which all further research has been extrapolated. The frailty phenotype, suggested by Fried and colleagues, was developed from a secondary analysis of the American Cardiovascular Health Study. The researchers identified five independent variables: unintentional weight loss, self-reported exhaustion, slow gait speed, poor grip strength, and low energy expenditure. Older adults with three of these five factors were considered frail, those with one to two factors were considered as prefrail, and those with no factors were considered as robust. Individuals identified as frail had more adverse outcomes (increased falls, decreased mobility/function, increased hospitalizations, increased mortality) than those categorized as robust, whereas those diagnosed as prefrail had outcomes between the two. The frailty phenotype objectifies specific signs and symptoms to generate a dichotomous result: frail or not frail. The frailty phenotype can be seen as an inherent syndrome that stresses external forces and results in measurable decline in function.

The Frailty Index was derived by Rockwood and colleagues by analyzing the Canadian Study of Health and Aging. They established 92 baseline parameters of signs, symptoms, lab values, disease states, and disabilities to define frailty. The Frailty Index is calculated by adding the total number of variables present and dividing the sum by the total number of variables available. Thus, frailty represents a cumulative effect of individual deficits where no one trait is singularly responsible for adverse outcomes but the accumulation of multiple insults generates a graded scale of frailty. This model accounts for the vulnerability seen in older adults and the inability to restore homeostasis after accumulated stressors. Frailty is not defined by a cluster of specific traits, but by a summation of equally weighted deficits.

▶ Epidemiology

Frailty has repeatedly been observed more commonly in women than in men. However, frail men have a higher mortality rate than frail women. Frailty increases steadily with age. Transitioning to a level of greater frailty is more common than clinical improvement; thus, frail older adults are at increased risk for worsening disability, falls, hospitalizations, and mortality.

Pathophysiology

The loss of physiologic reserve is a normal expectation of the aging continuum. Aging is thought to be the result of molecular and cellular damage that has accumulated over time. It is unclear what level of cellular damage will lead to organ damage, particularly because many organ systems exhibit considerable redundancy. This physiologic reserve is what provides an individual the ability to compensate for disease-related changes and the natural aging process.

In frailty, the physiologic reserve is exhausted much more quickly and the ability to preserve homeostatic balance fails. The disruption of multiple interrelated physiologic systems causes a cumulative decline in function, which gradually wears down the ability to maintain homeostasis. Frailty is most likely not the decline of one particular organ system, but the aggregate loss of multiple systems, leading to decline in physiologic reserve. This accelerated loss of reserve creates vulnerability. Subsequently, older adults are more susceptible to minor stressful events that lead to a disproportionate change in their health. The intrinsic connections between the brain, endocrine system, immune system, and skeletal muscle system are the areas most commonly researched in the study of frailty.

There are characteristic structural and functional changes in the brain as individuals age, and typically, the loss of individual neurons in the cortex is minimal. However, when there is loss in metabolically active regions of the brain like the hippocampal pyramidal region, there are altered levels of cognitive function and a decreased ability to manage the stress response. Physiologic aging also leads to changes to microglial cells, particularly their structure and function as immune cells of the central nervous system. These cells typically respond to major brain injuries, localized irritation, or systemic inflammation. Throughout the aging process, these cells need less stimuli to activate, resulting in cellular damage and neuronal death. Primed microglial cells are thought to play an important role in the pathophysiology of delirium. Delirium, mild cognitive impairment, and dementia are all associated with frailty. Older adults identified as frail have an increased risk of delirium and subsequent increase in mortality. Increased rates of frailty have also been associated with faster rates of cognitive decline.

The endocrine system is intrinsically linked to the brain through the hypothalamic-pituitary axis to provide homeostasis through a series of regulatory hormones. The aging process is responsible for the decline in three major regulatory hormones. Insulin-like growth factor 1 (IGF-1) is a small peptide that increases anabolic activity in many cells and is particularly important in neuronal plasticity and increased skeletal muscle strength. The decline in growth hormone synthesis by the pituitary causes a reduction in IGF-1 by the liver and other organs. In addition, the decline in estradiol and testosterone causes increased release of luteinizing hormone and follicle-stimulating hormone. Finally, dehydroepiandrosterone (DHEA) and DHEA sulfate (DHEAS) levels decrease while cortisol levels increase because of reduced adrenocortical cell activity. Changes in the levels of all of these hormones are considered important in frailty; however, stronger evidence is needed to fully establish their exact relationship. Of note, persistently high levels of cortisol have been associated with increased catabolism that leads to decreased muscle mass, weight loss, anorexia, and reduced energy expenditure, which are hallmark features of the frailty phenotype.

Reduced phagocytic activity of neutrophils, macrophages, and natural killer cells is just one trait of an aging immune system. Blunted B-cell antibody response, alterations in T-cell lymphocyte production, and a decline in stem cells are also observed. The aging immune system may function adequately in the quiescent state but may not properly respond to times of heightened stress and inflammation. The pathophysiology of frailty is described as an abnormal response to low-grade inflammation. This response is both exaggerated and prolonged even after the initial stimulus has resolved. The senescent immune system is slow to restore hemostasis and has limited resources to provide protection from the next minor stressor.

Glycosylation of proteins, lipids, and nucleic acids generates advanced glycation end products (AGEs) that have been associated with aging, chronic disease, and mortality. AGEs are thought to play an important role in frailty because they cause widespread cellular damage by upregulation of inflammation. This cycle of repeated inflammation is associated with anorexia and breakdown of both skeletal muscle and adipose tissue. The end result of this inflammatory pathway leads to nutritional deficits, muscle weakness, and weight loss, which characterize frailty.

Sarcopenia, defined as loss of skeletal muscle mass, strength, and power, is considered a key component of frailty. Normal muscle homeostasis is maintained through a balance of new muscle cell formation, hypertrophy, and protein loss. The musculoskeletal system is influenced by nutritional factors and physical activity, whereas low levels of inflammatory cytokines such as interleukin-6 and tumor necrosis factor-α activate muscle breakdown to generate amino acids for energy and cleave antigenic peptides. The delicate balance of cell formation, muscle hypertrophy, and apoptosis is regulated by the brain, endocrine system, and immune system. The disruption of these regulatory systems, often seen as contributors to frailty, alters the homeostatic balance in the

Table 41–3. Frailty phenotype gait speed cutoff time (walk 15 ft).

Men (height in cm)	Time (in seconds)
≤173 cm	≤7
>173 cm	≤6
Women (height in cm)	Time (in seconds)
≤159 cm	≤7
>159 cm	≤6

musculoskeletal system, increases inflammatory cytokines, and accelerates the development of sarcopenia.

Physical Exam

Frailty, as defined by either the frailty phenotype or Frailty Index, is a constellation of signs and symptoms rather than the presence or absence of specific physical exam findings. The frailty phenotype consists of five independent variables. Weight loss can either be a self-reported loss of 10 lb in the past year or a documented weight loss of ≥5% annually. Gait speed is calculated by measuring how many seconds it takes to walk 15 ft. Values are compared to established standards outlined in Table 41–3. Grip strength is measured in kilograms on a handheld dynamometer. The average of three attempts is compared to established standards, outlined in Table 41–4. Exhaustion is documented by an individual's response to two statements on the Center for Epidemiological Studies

Table 41–4. Frailty phenotype grip strength cutoff.

Men (BMI)	Strength (in kg)
≤24	≤29
24.1-26	≤30
26.1-28	≤30
>28	≤32
Women (BMI)	Strength (in kg)
≤23	≤17
23.1-26	≤17.3
26.1-29	≤18
>29	≤21

BMI, body mass index.

Depression (CES-D) scale. Responses to the statements "I felt that everything I did was an effort" and "I could not get going" are scored as 0 (rarely or none of the time), 1 (some or little of the time), 2 (a moderate amount of the time), or 3 (most of the time). Patients answering 2 or 3 are categorized as frail. Physical activity is measured by calorie expenditure per week. Calories are calculated using a standardized algorithm based on a patient's responses to the 18 activities outlined in the short version of the Minnesota Leisure Time Activity Questionnaire. Men who expend <383 kcal/wk are frail. Women who expend <270 kcal/wk are frail.

The Frailty Index variables are listed in Table 41–5.

There are several other assessment tools used to identify frailty. The Timed-Up-and-Go Test (TUGT), hand grip strength, and pulmonary function testing have been suggested but lack diagnostic accuracy. The Edmonton Frail Scale is a multidimensional assessment tool that includes the TUGT and a cognitive assessment test. It lacks diagnostic accuracy but is quick, valid, and reliable for routine use by nongeriatricians. A comprehensive geriatric assessment (CGA) has become the gold standard to assess older adults in clinical practice. This multidisciplinary approach evaluates an individual's medical, psychological, and functional capacity to develop a treatment plan and guide follow-up visits. This is a very time-intensive assessment that requires some level of advanced experience in the care of older adults and is beyond the scope of this chapter.

Frailty Outcomes

Frailty, comorbidity, and disability share several similarities, but frailty is an independent diagnosis. Comorbidity is simply defined as two or more disease states, whereas disability is defined as the restriction in at least one activity of daily living. Frailty is a much more inclusive diagnosis that involves disease, functional ability, and physical exam findings. Although there are notable areas of overlap between comorbidity, disability, and frailty, an older adult does not need to be diagnosed with multiple diseases or be disabled to meet the definition of frail. However, a lager disease burden and a greater need of assistance may suggest a higher likelihood of frailty.

Reducing the severity of frailty or decreasing the prevalence can have large benefits for patients, their family members, and the global healthcare system. Frail older adults have increased rates of falling, loss of mobility, hospitalizations, institutionalization, and mortality. Frail adults who are admitted to a hospital and receive an inpatient CGA are more likely to return home, are less likely to experience cognitive or functional decline, and have lower in-hospital mortality. Research also suggests that community-dwelling adults who follow the established CGA plan can preserve their independence by continuing to live at home, can reduce the need for institutionalization, and can reduce falls.

Table 41–5. Variables of the Frailty Index.

Disruption of Independence	**Systemic Diseases (Cont.)**
Difficulty with instrumental activities of daily living (ADLs)	Gastrointestinal complaints
Difficulty with ADLs	Urinary complaints
Difficulty with toileting	Kidney trouble
Difficulty with bath	Stroke or effect of stroke
Difficulty with grooming	Seizure disorder
Difficulty with getting dressed	Chronic headaches
Difficulty with cooking	**Physical Exam (normal or abnormal)**
Difficulty with going out	Head and neck
Urinary incontinence	Thyroid
Stool incontinence	Breast
Impaired mobility	Lungs
Changes in Mood	Cardiovascular
Mood problems	Peripheral pulses
History of depression	Abdomen
Feels sad, blue, or depressed	Rectum
Changes in sleep	Skin
Paranoia	Frontal release signs
Cognitive clouding/delirium	**Neurologic Exam (presence or absence)**
Changes in Memory	Sucking reflex
Memory changes	Snout reflex
Impaired judgement/cognition	Palmomental reflex
Impaired or abstract thinking	Muscle bulk difficulties
Aphasia	Poor neck tone
Apraxia	Poor limb tone
Agnosia	**Consequences of Cerebral Vascular Accident**
Movement Disorders	History of stroke
Resting tremor	Recent headaches
Intention tremor	Chronic visual loss
Dyskinesia/chorea	Decreased hearing
Akinesia	**Laboratory Testing (normal or abnormal)**
History of Parkinson disease	Glucose
Bradykinesia of the face	Sodium
Bradykinesia of the limbs	Potassium
Change in limb coordination	Blood urea nitrogen
Change in trunk coordination	Creatinine
Change in posture/standing	Calcium
Changes in vibratory sensation	Phosphate
Systemic Diseases	Inorganic phosphate
History of malignancy	Thyroid-stimulating hormone
History of thyroid disease	Vitamin B_{12}
History of diabetes mellitus	Folate
History of syncope	Red blood cell folate
Heart and circulation problems	Total protein
Arterial hypertension	Albumin
Cardiac symptoms (congestive heart failure/arrythmia)	Venereal Disease Research Laboratory (VDRL)
Respiratory complaints	

Exercise has positive effects on the brain, endocrine system, immune system, and musculoskeletal system. Studies evaluating both home-based and group-based exercise routines have concluded that exercise improves outcomes in mobility and functional ability for frail older adults. The effect size is small to moderate, and the most effective intensity of such programs is uncertain. There is a paucity of evidence to suggest nutritional interventions impact the nutritional deficits and weight loss recognized in frailty.

There are limited pharmacologic studies targeted at improving frailty. Angiotensin-converting enzymes inhibitors may slow down, or even stop, the decline in skeletal muscle strength by improving the musculoskeletal structure and biochemical function. Although testosterone improves muscle strength, its adverse effect on cardiovascular and pulmonary outcomes cannot be understated. The general use of vitamin D supplementation in older adults remains controversial.

Clegg A, Young J, Iliffe S, Rikkert MO, Rockwood K. Frailty in elderly people. *Lancet.* 2013;381(9868):752–762. [PMID: 23395245]

Fried LP, Tangen CM, Walston J, et al. Frailty in older adults: evidence for a phenotype. *J Gerontol A Biol Sci Med Sci.* 2001; 56:M146–156. [PMID: 11253156]

Mitnitski AB, Mogilner AJ, Rockwood K. Accumulation of deficits as a proxy measure of aging. *Sci World J.* 2001;1:323–336. [PMID: 12806071]

POLYPHARMACY

ESSENTIALS OF DIAGNOSIS

▶ Polypharmacy is a neutral descriptor of an individual's current medication regimen.

▶ In clinical practice, providers must compare appropriate multidrug regimens against potentially inappropriate medications.

▶ Polypharmacy is associated with a decline in functional status, increased falls, and cognitive impairment.

▶ The American Geriatrics Society Beers Criteria and the Screening Tool of Older People's Prescriptions criteria are two commonly used tools targeted at reducing potentially inappropriate medications.

Treating a disease state has become synonymous with taking medication. The accumulation of disease generates an extended medication list, although taking more medication can lead to poor health outcomes. Many older adults have multimorbidity and, subsequently, take multiple medications. *Polypharmacy* is the standard term used to describe taking multiple medications. The term *polypharmacy* is a neutral descriptor of an individual's current medication regimen; however, it is commonly used to describe negative outcomes for those taking multiple medications. There is no universally agreed upon number of medications someone takes to define polypharmacy, although several studies have operationalized five or more medications as an arbitrary cut point.

Although the quantitative approach has been used in several research studies that look at adverse outcomes, there are likely situations that necessitate a multidrug regimen to properly treat the disease. If such a regimen has appropriate indications that are evidence based, adverse drug events are carefully monitored, and the patient achieves the desired health outcome, then such polypharmacy may be considered appropriate. An alternative definition that moves away from quantity and recognizes the quality of prescribing is a timelier representation of polypharmacy given the increasing number of adults with multimorbidity. Polypharmacy can also be described as the administration of multiple unnecessary medications, the use of more medication than is clinically warranted, or the use of unnecessary infective or habit-forming medications. In current practice, there are clinical scenarios that require providers to compare such problematic polypharmacy against appropriate multidrug regimens, and there are also scenarios when simply reducing the current pill burden is the appropriate therapeutic decision.

▶ Adverse Outcomes

Older adults with multimorbidity are at increased risk for adverse outcomes. These individuals typically take multiple medications that are often prescribed by more than one provider. Increasing the number of medications leads to a greater likelihood of drug combinations, which inherently leads to higher likelihood of adverse drug reactions and drug-disease interactions. Adverse drug events are observed across the healthcare landscape. From the emergency room to long-term care facilities and even in the ambulatory setting, older adults taking multiple medications are at increased risk for poor outcomes. The risk of drug-disease interactions increases with an increased number of medications.

Polypharmacy has been associated with a decline in functional status. The inability to perform instrumental activities of daily living, a decrease in functional ability, and an increase in the number of falls have all been associated with adults taking multiple medications. Falls are associated with increased morbidity and mortality in older adults with polypharmacy.

Other comorbidities such as urinary incontinence and poor nutrition have also been associated with polypharmacy. Many medications are known to increase urinary frequency because of their pharmacodynamics. Individuals with urinary incontinence may also experience urinary frequency, and often these symptoms can be associated with potentially inappropriate medications (PIMs). Regarding nutritional status, older adults taking 10 or more medications are at risk for malnutrition, hypercholesterolemia, hyperglycemia, increased sodium intake, and a decrease in fat-soluble vitamins, minerals, and fiber.

Finally, older adults taking multiple medications are at increased risk for cognitive impairment and medication nonadherence. Polypharmacy, whether taking multiple medications or PIMs, is a well-known risk factor for delirium.

There is a higher likelihood of cognitive impairment according to the number of medications prescribed. Prescription complexity, dosage frequency, and PIMs all contribute to medication nonadherence. Individuals who are nonadherent to their medication regimen have an associated risk of disease progression, treatment failure, and hospitalizations, which increase the risk of adverse outcomes.

Potentially Inappropriate Medications

As older adults live longer, they develop a variety of comorbid disease combinations. The aggregate of different disease combinations is intrinsically linked to the prescribing of multiple medications. Medication use is associated with increasing age and the number of chronic medical conditions. Each drug combination may vary slightly from the next, but there are subtle commonalities that exist among several mediation classes. Providers who care for older adults should recognize PIMs because these medications are associated with a series adverse health outcomes, drug-drug interactions, drug-disease interactions, economic burden, and time to horizon benefit. Some PIM classes are outlined in Table 41–6.

Prescribing Strategies

There have been several different attempts to stratify PIMs into clinically applicable categories. Medications are considered potentially inappropriate when the risk of adverse effects outweighs the potential clinical benefit. Providers caring for older adults should recognize PIMs because these

Table 41–6. Possible adverse drugs effects.

Anticholinergic medications: xerostomia, constipation, urinary retention, falls, and cognitive impairment

Central α-blockers: orthostatic hypotension, bradycardia, and adverse central nervous system effects

Benzodiazepines: falls, fractures, cognitive impairment, delirium, and motor vehicle accidents

Sedative/hypnotics: falls, fractures, cognitive impairment, delirium, increased emergency department visits and hospitalizations, motor vehicle crashes

Antipsychotics: cause considerable harm without improving care outcomes for delirium and dementia; avoid antipsychotic medications for behavioral treatment in adults with delirium or dementia unless nonpharmacologic interventions (behavioral modifications) have failed and the individual is a physical harm to him- or herself or others

Hormone replacement (eg, methyltestosterone, testosterone, estrogen): potential for cardiac problems; contraindicated in men with prostate cancer; potential carcinogenic (breast and uterine)

Nonsteroidal anti-inflammatory drugs: peptic ulcer disease, gastrointestinal bleed (when used in adults >75 years old, coadministration with oral or parenteral corticosteroids, antiplatelet agents, or anticoagulants)

Skeletal muscle relaxers: constipation, urinary retention, sedation, fractures

medications are associated with serious adverse health outcomes; drug-drug interactions, drug-disease interactions, economic burden, and time to horizon benefit are just some of the potential outcomes that providers need to consider when starting each prescription.

The Screening Tool of Older People's Prescriptions (STOPP) criteria was developed in 2008 and updated in 2015. These guidelines were developed and have been regularly used in Europe but have been applied worldwide and include an exhaustive list of PIMs. The same organization that developed the STOPP criteria also developed the Screening Tool to Alert to Right Treatment (START) criteria. Although the STOPP criteria recognize potentially inappropriate prescribing, START criteria make suggestions regarding potential prescribing omissions. STOPP/START criteria have been developed to minimize inappropriate prescribing for older adults. These criteria are based on a European panel of experts who reviewed of the most updated literature to develop these consensus statement.

The STOPP criteria have modest overlap with the American Geriatrics Society Beers Criteria for Potentially Inappropriate Medication Use in Older Adults. The Beers Criteria were initially developed for long-term nursing home residents in 1991, but the criteria have been revised several times and expanded to include hospitalized patients and those who are community dwelling. The 2019 Beers Criteria is the most current edition and categorizes potentially inappropriate medications into several different tables). These tables arrange medications based on: their intended therapeutic use (along with the potential adverse drug reaction); by organ system or disease (identifying which drugs are contraindicated or exacerbate that disease state); medications to be used with caution (because their risk may outweigh their benefit); drug-drug interactions that should be avoided (because of specific adverse events); medications that should be avoided or have their dosage reduced based on renal function; drugs with strong anticholinergic properties. There are also tables that identify medications that have been removed, added, or modified since 2015 American Geriatric Society Beers Criteria. The Beers Criteria is used to improve medication selection, reduce adverse drug reactions, educate providers, and ultimately reduce patient exposure to potentially inappropriate mediations. However, there are several other tools used to address polypharmacy.

Several polypharmacy reduction strategies have been developed to help providers effectively manage polypharmacy. These approaches are described as either implicit based or explicit based. The implicit-based approach is based on a provider's clinical judgement and relies on clinical information for interpretation for assessment. This approach is highly individualized and relies on the provider's proper assessment and clinical experience, thus making it difficult to apply this approach across a large patient population. The Assess, Review, Minimize, Optimize, Reassess (ARMOR) protocol, used in long-term care settings, and the Prescribing Optimization Method (POM), developed for general practitioners to use in the outpatient setting, are both implicit-based tools for prescribing. Explicit-based tools require a minimal amount of clinical expertise to improve medication appropriateness. Both STOPP/START and the American Geriatrics Society Beers Criteria are explicit-based approaches used to reduce PIMs. Explicit-based tools are more objective and easier to apply consistently across a larger patient population. Choosing between an implicit-based or explicit based approach is provider dependent, but the shared focus is reducing PIMs and improving overall patient outcomes. Common treatment approaches using implicit-based and explicit-based tools are outlined in Table 41–7.

Addressing polypharmacy should be part of the routine assessment for providers taking care of older adults. The use of implicit- or explicit-based tools should serve as a construct to begin the conversation about medication management, but these tools should not be viewed as punitive measures or strict guidelines. They are merely one component in a

Table 41–7. Implicit- and explicit-based approach to reducing polypharmacy.

Implicit-Based Tool Techniques	Explicit-Based Tool Techniques
Define the clinical indication for all medications.	Define the clinical indication for all medications (*implicit criteria—applies only to STOPP criteria).
Assess relative risks and benefits of each medication.	Assess relative risks and benefits of each medication.
Identify adverse drug events or reactions.	Evaluate drug-drug interactions.
Evaluate drug-drug and drug-disease interactions.	Evaluate drug-disease or syndrome interactions.
Adjust dosage for renal function.	Adjust dosage for renal function.
	Consider duration of use.
	Check for drug duplication (*implicit criteria—applies only to STOPP criteria).
	Promote nonpharmacologic approaches when applicable.

STOPP, Screening Tool of Older People's Prescriptions.

comprehensive approach to reducing PIMs and adverse drug events, all while attempting to improve functional capacity and preserve independence for older adults.

Levy HB. Polypharmacy reduction strategies: tips on incorporating American Geriatrics Society Beers and Screening Tool of Older People's Prescriptions criteria. *Clin Geriatr Med.* 2017;33(2):177–187. [PMID: 28364990]

Maher RL Jr, Hanlon JT, Hajjar ER. Clinical consequences of polypharmacy in elderly. *Expert Opin Drug Saf.* 2014;13(1):57–65. [PMID: 24073682]

O'Mahony D, O'Sullivan D, Byrne S, et al. STOPP/START criteria for potentially inappropriate prescribing in older people: version 2. *Age Ageing.* 2015;44:213–218. [PMID: 25324330]

The 2019 American Geriatrics Society Beers Criteria Update Expert Panel. American Geriatrics Society 2019 updated Beers criteria for potentially inappropriate medication use in older adults. *J Am Geriatr Soc.* 2019;67:674–694.

Health care has been operationalized to deliver care in disease-specific silos. Multimorbidity, frailty, and polypharmacy are all obstacles that practitioners providing care for older adults must address outside of their silos by integrating a comprehensive disease management strategy centered around patient preference. Older adults with multimorbidity should be offered to partake in their care planning, and the provider should develop a collaborative plan with an acceptable level of complexity based on their disease burden and degree of frailty. However, frailty is not synonymous with multimorbidity, and older adults do not need multiple comorbidities to be frail. Frailty is a cumulative decline over time, which then leads to a certain vulnerability to sudden changes in health that can lead to an increased risk of adverse outcomes. Healthcare providers attempt to avoid adverse outcomes by prescribing medications, and older adults electively take over-the-counter preparations for a multitude of reasons. Although polypharmacy may be appropriate in certain situations, PIMs can also lead to adverse outcomes. Addressing multimorbidity, recognizing frailty, and orchestrating a proper medication regimen are the key elements to providing quality care for adults as they age across the healthcare continuum and should not be viewed as independent variables, but rather essential elements that make up complete geriatric care.

Urinary Incontinence

Robert J. Carr, MD

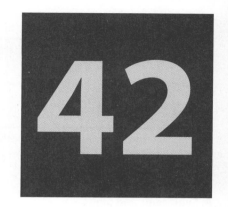

PHYSIOLOGY OF NORMAL URINATION

Urinary incontinence is the involuntary loss of urine that is so severe as to have social or hygienic consequences. A basic understanding of the normal physiology of urination is important to understand the potential causes of incontinence and the various strategies for effective treatment.

The lower urinary tract consists primarily of the bladder (detrusor muscle) and the urethra. The urethra contains two sphincters: the internal urethral sphincter (IUS), composed predominantly of smooth muscle, and the external urethral sphincter (EUS), which is primarily voluntary muscle. The detrusor muscle of the bladder is innervated predominantly by cholinergic (muscarinic) neurons from the parasympathetic nervous system, the stimulation of which leads to bladder contraction. The sympathetic nervous system innervates both the bladder and the IUS. Sympathetic innervation in the bladder is primarily β-adrenergic and leads to bladder relaxation, whereas α-adrenergic receptors predominate in the IUS, leading to sphincter contraction. Thus, in general, sympathetic stimulation promotes bladder filling (relaxation of the detrusor with contraction of the sphincter), whereas parasympathetic stimulation leads to bladder emptying (detrusor contraction and sphincter relaxation).

The EUS, on the other hand, is striated muscle and under primarily voluntary (somatic) control. This allows for some ability to voluntarily postpone urination by tightening the sphincter and inhibiting the flow of urine. Additional voluntary control is provided by the central nervous system (CNS) through the pontine micturition center. This allows for central inhibition of the autonomic processes described earlier and for further voluntary postponement of the need to urinate until the circumstances are more socially appropriate or until necessary facilities are available.

The physiologic factors influencing normal urination, summarized in Table 42–1, are important considerations when discussing urinary disorders and treatment.

AGE-RELATED CHANGES

Contrary to common perception, urinary incontinence is not inevitable with aging. Most elderly patients remain continent throughout their lifetimes, and a complaint of incontinence at any age should receive a thorough evaluation and not be dismissed as "normal for age." Nonetheless, many common age-related changes predispose elderly patients to incontinence and increase the likelihood of its development with advancing age.

The frequency of involuntary bladder contractions (detrusor hyperactivity) increases in both men and women with aging. In addition, total bladder capacity decreases, causing the voiding urge to occur at lower volumes. Bladder contractility decreases, leading to increased postvoid residuals and increased sensation of urgency or fullness. Elderly patients excrete a larger percentage of their fluid volume later in the day than younger persons. This, in addition to the other changes listed, often leads to an increase in the incidence of nocturia with aging and more frequent nighttime awakenings.

In women, menopausal estrogen decline leads to urogenital atrophy and a decrease in the sensitivity of α-receptors in the IUS. In men, prostatic hypertrophy can lead to increased urethral resistance and varying degrees of urethral obstruction.

It is important to remember that these age-related changes are found in many healthy, continent persons as well as those who develop incontinence. It is not completely understood why the predisposition to urinary problems is stronger in some patients than in others, which emphasizes the multifactorial basis of incontinence.

Table 42–1. Physiologic factors influencing normal urination.

Bladder filling	Sympathetic nervous system	β-Adrenergic α-Adrenergic	Detrusor relaxation IUS contraction
Bladder emptying	Parasympathetic nervous system	Cholinergic	Detrusor contraction
Voluntary control	Somatic nervous system Central nervous system	Striated muscle Pontine micturition center	EUS contraction Central inhibition of urinary reflex

EUS, external urethral sphincter; IUS, internal urethral sphincter.

> ## Clinical Findings

A. Symptoms and Signs

1. Incontinence outside the urinary tract—Incontinence is often classified according to whether it is related to specific urogenital pathology or to factors outside the urinary tract. Terms such as *transient versus established, acute versus persistent,* and *primary versus secondary* have been used to highlight this distinction. The mnemonic DIAPPERS is helpful in remembering the many causes of incontinence that occur outside the urinary tract (Table 42–2). These "extraurinary" causes are very common in the elderly, and it is important to identify them or rule them out before proceeding to a more invasive search for primary urogenital etiologies.

Delirium, depression, and disorders of excessive urinary output generally require medical or behavioral management of the primary cause rather than strategies relating to the bladder. Once the primary causes are corrected, the incontinence often resolves. Urinary tract infections, although easily treated if discovered, are a relatively infrequent cause of urinary incontinence in the absence of other classic symptoms (eg, dysuria, urgency, frequency). Asymptomatic bacteriuria, which is common even in well elderly, does not cause incontinence.

Pharmaceuticals are a particularly important and very common cause of incontinence. Because of the many neural receptors involved in urination (see Table 42–1), it is easy to understand why so many medications used to treat other common problems can readily affect continence. Medications frequently associated with incontinence are listed in Table 42–3.

Table 42–2. Causes of urinary incontinence without specific urogenital pathology.[a]

D	Delirium/confusional state
I	Infection (symptomatic)
A	Atrophic urethritis/vaginitis
P	Pharmaceuticals
P	Psychiatric causes (especially depression)
E	Excessive urinary output (hyperglycemia, hypercalcemia, congestive heart failure)
R	Restricted mobility
S	Stool impaction

[a]Also known as *transient, acute,* or *secondary incontinence.*

Table 42–3. Pharmaceuticals contributing to incontinence.

Pharmaceutical	Mechanism	Effect
α-Adrenergic agonists	IUS contraction	Urinary retention
α-Adrenergic blockers	IUS relaxation	Urinary leakage
Anticholinergic agents	Inhibit bladder contraction, sedation, immobility	Urinary retention and/or functional incontinence
Antidepressants		
Antihistamines		
Antipsychotics		
Sedatives		
β-Adrenergic agonists	Inhibits bladder contraction	Urinary retention
β-Adrenergic blockers	Inhibits bladder relaxation	Urinary leakage, urgency
Calcium channel blockers	Relaxes bladder	Urinary retention
Diuretics	Increases urinary frequency, urgency	Polyuria
Narcotic analgesics	Relaxes bladder, fecal impaction, sedation	Urinary retention and/or functional incontinence

IUS, internal urethral sphincter.

Table 42–4. Nonprescription agents contributing to incontinence.

Agent	Mechanism	Effect	Common Examples
Alcohol	Diuretic effect, sedation, immobility	Polyuria and/or functional incontinence	Beer, wine, liquor, some liquid cold medicines
α-Agonists	IUS contraction	Urinary retention	Decongestants, diet pills
Antihistamines	Inhibit bladder contraction, sedation	Urinary retention and/or functional incontinence	Allergy tablets, sleeping pills, antinausea medications
α-Agonist/antihistamine combinations	IUS contraction and inhibition of bladder contraction	Marked urinary retention	Multisymptom cold tablets
Caffeine	Diuretic effects	Polyuria	Coffee, soft drinks, analgesics

IUS, internal urethral sphincter.

Many of these medications are available over the counter and in combination (Table 42–4). In addition, commonly used substances such as caffeine and alcohol can contribute to incontinence by virtue of their diuretic effects or their effects on mental status. For this reason, the association between medications and substances associated with incontinence may not be obvious to the patient or readily volunteered during a medication history unless the physician specifically asks about them.

Restricted mobility or the inability to physically get to the bathroom in time to avoid incontinence is also referred to as "functional" incontinence. The incontinence may be temporary or chronic, depending on the nature of the physical or cognitive disability involved. Physical therapy or strength and flexibility training may be helpful, as well as simple measures such as a bedside commode or urinal.

Stool impaction is very common in the elderly and may cause incontinence either through its local mass effect or by stimulation of opioid receptors in the bowel. It has been reported to be a causative factor in ≤10% of patients referred to incontinence clinics for evaluation. Continence can often be restored by a simple disimpaction.

2. Urologic causes of incontinence—Once secondary or transient causes have been investigated and ruled out, further evaluation should focus on specific urologic pathology that may be causing incontinence.

The urinary tract has two basic functions: the emptying of urine during voiding and the storage of urine between voiding. A defect in either of these basic functions can cause incontinence, and it is useful to initially classify incontinence according to whether it is primarily a defect of storage or of emptying. An *inability to store* urine occurs when the bladder contracts too often (or at inappropriate times) or when the sphincter(s) cannot contract sufficiently to allow the bladder to store urine and keep it from leaking. In these situations, the bladder rarely, if ever, fills to capacity and the patient's symptoms are generally characterized by frequent incontinent episodes of relatively small volume. An *inability to empty* urine occurs when the bladder is unable to contract appropriately or when the outlet or sphincter(s) is (are) partially obstructed (either physically or physiologically). Thus, the bladder continues to fill beyond its normal capacity and eventually overflows, causing the patient to experience abdominal distention and continual or frequent leakage.

Whether the primary problem is the inability to store or the inability to empty can often be determined easily during the history and physical examination according to the patient's incontinence pattern (intermittent or continuous) and whether abdominal (bladder) distention is present. Determination of postvoid residual is also helpful in making this distinction (see section on history and physical findings, later). This initial classification is important in narrowing down the specific etiology of the incontinence and in ultimately deciding on the appropriate management strategy.

3. Symptomatic classification—Once it is determined whether the primary problem is with storage or with emptying, incontinence can be further classified according to the type of symptoms that it causes in the patient. The most common categories are discussed in the following sections. The first two types, urge incontinence and stress incontinence, result from an inability to store urine. The third type, incontinence associated with chronic urinary retention, results from an inability to empty urine. This was traditionally referred to as *overflow incontinence*, a term that is no longer commonly used. A patient may have a single type of incontinence or a combination of more than one type (mixed incontinence). Table 42–5 summarizes the major categories of incontinence, the underlying urodynamic findings, and the most common etiologies for each.

A. URGE INCONTINENCE—Urge incontinence is the most common type of incontinence in the elderly.

Table 42–5. Types and classification of urinary incontinence.

Underlying Defect	Symptomatic Classification	Most Common Urodynamics	Possible Etiologies
Inability to store urine	Urge (U)	Detrusor hyperactivity	Uninhibited contractions; local irritation (cystitis, stone, tumor); central nervous system causes
	Stress (S)	Sphincter incompetence	Urethral hypermobility; sphincter damage (trauma, radiation, surgery)
Inability to empty urine	Chronic urinary retention (overflow)	Outlet obstruction	Physical (benign prostatic hyperplasia, tumor, stricture); neurologic lesions, medications
		Detrusor hypoactivity	Neurogenic bladder (diabetes, alcoholism, disk disease)
	Functional (F)	Normal	Immobility problems; cognitive deficits
	Mixed	U + S, U + F	

Patients complain of a strong, and often immediate, urge to void followed by an involuntary loss of urine. It is rarely possible to reach the bathroom in time to avoid incontinence once the urge occurs, and patients often lose urine while rushing toward a bathroom or trying to locate one. Urge incontinence is most frequently caused by involuntary contractions of the bladder, often referred to as *detrusor instability*. These involuntary contractions increase in frequency with age, as does the ability to voluntarily inhibit them. Although the symptoms of urgency are a hallmark feature of this type of incontinence, detrusor instability can sometimes result in incontinence without these symptoms. Although most patients with detrusor instability are neurologically normal, uninhibited contractions can also occur as the result of neurologic disorders such as stroke, dementia, or spinal cord injury. In these cases, it is often referred to as *detrusor hyperreflexia*. Detrusor instability and urgency can also be caused by local irritation of the bladder as with infection, bladder stones, or tumors. The term *overactive bladder syndrome* (OABS) is now commonly used to describe the symptoms of urgency caused by detrusor instability and to emphasize that they can occur either with or *without* incontinence. OABS is described by the International Continence Society as voiding ≥8 times during a 24-hour period and awakening ≥2 times during the night. Treatment of OABS is similar regardless of whether incontinence is present.

B. STRESS INCONTINENCE—Stress incontinence is much more common among women than men and is defined as a loss of urine associated with increases in intraabdominal pressure (Valsalva maneuver). Patients complain of leakage of urine (usually small amounts) during coughing, laughing, sneezing, or exercising. In women, stress incontinence is most often caused by urethral hypermobility resulting from weakness of the pelvic floor musculature, but it can also be caused by intrinsic weakness of the urethral sphincter(s), most commonly following trauma, radiation,

or surgery. Stress incontinence is rare in men, unless they have suffered damage to the sphincter through surgery or trauma. In diagnosing stress incontinence, it is important to ascertain that the leakage occurs exactly *coincident* with the stress maneuver. If the leakage occurs several seconds after the maneuver, it is more likely caused by an uninhibited bladder contraction that has been triggered by the stress maneuver and is urodynamically more similar to urge incontinence. This is sometimes known as *stress-induced detrusor instability*.

C. INCOMPLETE BLADDER EMPTYING (OVERFLOW INCONTINENCE)—This is a loss of urine associated with overdistention of the bladder. Patients complain of frequent or constant leakage or dribbling, or they may lose large amounts of urine without warning. Incomplete emptying may result either from a defect in the bladder's ability to contract (*detrusor hypoactivity*) or from obstruction of the bladder outlet or urethra. Detrusor hypoactivity is most commonly the result of a *neurogenic bladder* secondary to diabetes mellitus, chronic alcoholism, or disk disease. It can also be caused by medications, primarily muscle relaxants and β-adrenergic blockers. Outlet obstruction can be physical (prostatic enlargement, tumor, stricture), neurologic (spinal cord lesions, pelvic surgery), or pharmacologic (α-adrenergic agonists). Because neurogenic bladder is relatively rare in the geriatric population, it is important to rule out possible causes of obstruction whenever the diagnosis of overflow incontinence is made.

D. FUNCTIONAL INCONTINENCE—The term *functional incontinence* is used to describe physical or cognitive impairments that interfere with continence even in patients with normal urinary tracts (see section on incontinence outside the urinary tract, Table 42–2, and the DIAPPERS mnemonic, earlier).

E. MIXED INCONTINENCE—*Mixed incontinence* describes various combinations of the preceding four types.

When present, it can make the diagnosis and management of incontinence more difficult. The term is most frequently used to describe patients who present with a combination of stress and urge incontinence, although other combinations are also possible. Functional incontinence, for example, can coexist with stress, urge, or overflow incontinence, further complicating the treatment of these patients. Side effects of medications being used to treat other comorbidities can also cause a mixed picture when combined with underlying incontinence of any type. Mixed stress and urge incontinence is particularly common among elderly women. When present, it is helpful to focus on the symptom that is most bothersome to the patient and to direct the initial therapeutic interventions in that direction.

B. Screening

Because of its high prevalence, low degree of self-reporting, and adverse effects on health and well-being, annual screening of women for urinary incontinence is recommended. Screening should assess whether women experience incontinence and whether it affects their activities and quality of life. Several screening tools have been developed for this purpose, among the most well validated of which is the Michigan Incontinence Symptom Index (M-ISI).

C. History and Physical Findings

The history and physical examination of a patient presenting with incontinence should have the following goals:

1. To evaluate for and rule out causes of incontinence outside the urinary tract (DIAPPERS)
2. To determine whether the primary defect is an inability to store urine or an inability to empty urine
3. To determine the type of incontinence according to the patient's symptoms and likely etiologies
4. To determine the pattern of incontinence episodes and its effect on the patient's functional ability and quality of life

1. History—A thorough medical history should include a special focus on the neurologic and genitourinary history of the patient as well as any other medical problems that may be contributing factors (see Table 42–2). Information on any previous evaluation(s) for incontinence, as well as their degree of success or failure, can be helpful in guiding the current evaluation and in determining patient expectations. A careful medication history is very important, focusing on the categories of medications listed in Table 42–3 and remembering to include nonprescription substances (see Table 42–4). Finally, the pattern of incontinence is important in helping to classify its type and in planning appropriate therapy. While many urinary symptoms (eg, dribbling,

frequency, hesitancy, nocturia) may lack diagnostic specificity, symptoms of urgency (the sudden urge to void with leakage before reaching the toilet) are very sensitive and specific for the diagnosis of urge incontinence. Urine leakage with coughing or other stress maneuvers is a sensitive indicator of stress incontinence but is less specific than urge because of overlap with other conditions. A voiding diary or bladder record can be a very useful tool in obtaining additional diagnostic information. The patient or caregiver is given a set of forms and is asked to keep a written record of each incontinent episode for several days. A sample form is shown in Table 42–6, and a smartphone app (*iP Voiding Diary*) is also available. Incontinent episodes are recorded in terms of time, estimated volume (small or large), and precipitating factors. Fluid intake, as well as any episode of urination in the toilet, is also recorded. When completed accurately, the bladder record can often elucidate the most likely type of incontinence and provide a clue to possible precipitating factors. Continuous leakage, for example, may be more consistent with overflow incontinence, whereas multiple, large-volume episodes may be more consistent with urge. Smaller-volume episodes associated with coughing or exercise may be more consistent with stress incontinence, whereas incontinence occurring only at specific times each day may suggest an association with a medication or other non–urinary tract cause. Although other information from the physical and laboratory evaluations will obviously be needed, the physician can often make significant progress toward determining the type of incontinence and possible precipitating factors from the history and voiding record alone.

2. Physical examination—In addition to a thorough search for nonurologic causes of incontinence, the physical examination should focus on the cardiovascular, abdominal, genitourinary, and rectal areas. Cardiovascular examination should focus on signs of fluid overload. Evidence of bladder distention on abdominal examination should raise suspicion for overflow incontinence. Genital examination should include a pelvic examination in women to assess for evidence of atrophy or mass, as well as any signs of uterine prolapse, cystocele, or rectocele. A rectal examination is helpful in ruling out stool impaction or mass, as well as in evaluating sphincter tone and perineal sensation for evidence of a neurologic deficit. A prostate examination is usually included, but several studies have demonstrated a poor correlation between prostate size and urinary obstruction. A neurologic examination focusing on the lumbosacral area is helpful in ruling out a spinal cord lesion or other neurologic deficits.

3. Special tests—Two additional tests, specific to the diagnosis of incontinence, should be added to the general physical examination.

Table 42–6. Sample voiding record.

Bladder Record

Name: _____

Date: _____

Instructions: Place a check in the appropriate column next to the time you urinated in the toilet or when an incontinence episode occurred. Note the reason for the incontinence and describe your liquid intake (for example, coffee, water) and estimate the amount (for example, one cup).

Time Interval	Urinated in Toilet	Had a Small Incontinent Episode	Had a Large Incontinent Episode	Reason for Incontinent Episode	Type/Amount of Liquid Intake
6-8 a.m.					
8-10 a.m.					
10-noon					
Noon-2 p.m.					
2-4 p.m.					
4-6 p.m.					
6-8 p.m.					
8-10 p.m.					
10-midnight					
Overnight					

Number of pads used today: _____

Number of episodes: _____

Comments: _____

A. Cough stress test—This test attempts to reproduce the symptoms of incontinence under the direct visualization of the physician and is useful in differentiating stress from urge incontinence. The patient should have a full bladder and preferably be in a standing position (although a lithotomy position is also acceptable for patients unable to stand). The patient should be told to relax and then to cough vigorously while the physician observes for urine loss. If leakage occurs simultaneously with the cough, a diagnosis of stress incontinence is likely. A delay between the cough and the leakage is more likely caused by a reflex bladder contraction and is more consistent with urge incontinence.

B. Postvoid residual (PVR)—Measurement of PVR is not recommended routinely, but can be useful for patients suspected of (or at increased risk for) urinary retention or outlet obstruction. This includes men with severe urinary symptoms, women with prior gynecologic or pelvic surgery, persons with neurologic disorders or diabetes, and those who have failed initial empiric therapy. PVR measurement is traditionally done by urinary catheterization; however, portable ultrasound scanners for this purpose are now available that also provide very accurate readings. These ultrasound devices minimize the risks of instrumentation and infection that are inherent in catheterization, especially in male patients. Prior to measurement, the patient should be asked to empty the bladder as completely as possible. Residual urine in the bladder should be measured within a few minutes after emptying using either in-and-out catheterization or ultrasound. A PVR of <50 mL is normal; >200 mL indicates inadequate bladder emptying and is consistent with overflow incontinence. PVRs between 50 and 199 mL can sometimes be normal but may also exist with chronic urinary retention, and results should be interpreted in light of the clinical picture. Patients with elevated PVRs should generally be referred for further evaluation and to rule out obstruction prior to treatment of the incontinence symptoms.

C. Other diagnostic maneuvers—Other maneuvers, or "bedside urodynamics," have often been recommended to help in the diagnosis of incontinence. The best known of these are the Q-tip test to diagnose pelvic laxity and the Bonney (Marshall) test to determine whether surgical intervention will be helpful. Although these tests may be useful in some settings, recent studies have cast doubt on their predictive value, and in the family medicine setting, they are unlikely to add clinically useful information that would help in sorting out the small percentage of patients whose diagnosis remains unclear after a thorough history and physical examination.

Multichannel urodynamic testing is not routinely recommended in the diagnosis of incontinence and has not been shown to be any more predictive of surgical or nonsurgical outcomes than diagnosis by patients' symptom reports.

C. Laboratory and Imaging Evaluation

Like the history and physical examination, the laboratory evaluation should be focused on ruling out the nonurologic causes of incontinence. A urinalysis is very helpful in screening for infection as well as in evaluating for hematuria, proteinuria, or glucosuria. It must be remembered, however, that asymptomatic bacteriuria is very common in the elderly and is not a cause of incontinence. Antibiotic treatment of asymptomatic bacteriuria has not been shown to reduce morbidity or to improve incontinence in either the institutionalized elderly or ambulatory women. Thus, antibiotic treatment in the face of incontinence and bacteriuria should be reserved for patients whose incontinence is of recent onset, has recently worsened, or is accompanied by other signs of infection. Hematuria, in the absence of infection, should be referred for further evaluation to rule out carcinoma.

Additional laboratory studies that are recommended and may be helpful in selected patients include measurement of renal function (blood urea nitrogen and creatinine) and evaluation for metabolic causes of polyuria (hypercalcemia, hyperglycemia). Radiologic studies are not routinely recommended in the initial evaluation of most patients with incontinence; however, a renal ultrasound study is useful in patients with obstruction to evaluate for hydronephrosis.

Abrams P, Cardozo L, Khoury S, et al, eds. *Incontinence*. 3rd ed. Plymouth, MA: Health Publications; 2005.
Abrutyn E, Mossey J, Berlin JA, et al. Does asymptomatic bacteriuria predict mortality and does antimicrobial treatment reduce mortality in elderly ambulatory women? *Ann Intern Med*. 1994;121:827–833. [PMID: 7818631]
American College of Obstetricians and Gynecologists. Evaluation of uncomplicated stress urinary incontinence in women before surgical treatment. Committee Opinion No. 603. *Obstet Gynecol*. 2014;123:1403–1407 (reaffirmed 2017). [PMID: 24848922]

Fantl JA, Newman DK. *Urinary Incontinence in Adults: Acute and Chronic Management*. Clinical Practice Guideline 2, 1996 update. AHCPR Publication 96-0682. Rockville, MD: US Department of Health and Human Services, Public Health Service, Agency for Health Care Policy and Research; 1996.
Holroyd-Leduc JM, Tannenbaum C, Thorpe KE, et al. What type of urinary incontinence does this woman have? *JAMA*. 2008;299:1446–1456. [PMID: 18364487]
O'Reilly N, Nelson HD, Conry JM, et al. Screening for urinary incontinence in women: a recommendation from the Women's Preventive Services Initiative. *Ann Intern Med*. 2018;169:320–328. [PMID: 30105360]
Ouslander JG. Management of overactive bladder. *N Engl J Med*. 2004;350:786. [PMID: 14973214]
Resnick NM. Urinary incontinence. *Lancet*. 1995;346:94–99. [PMID: 7603221]
Suskind AM, Dunn RL, Morgan DM, et al. A screening tool for clinically relevant urinary incontinence. *Neurourol Urodyn*. 2015;34(4):332–335. [PMID: 24464849]

▶ Treatment

If nonurologic or functional causes are found as major contributors to the patient's incontinence, treatment should be targeted at the underlying illnesses and improving any functional disability. In addition to medical management of the underlying disorder(s), physical therapy and the use of assistive devices may be helpful in improving the patient's level of function and ability to reach the bathroom prior to having an incontinent episode. For the ambulatory patient, a home visit is often useful in assessing for any environmental hazards that may be contributing to functional incontinence.

Simple lifestyle modifications may be helpful in mild cases of urinary incontinence. Fluid restriction and avoidance of caffeine and alcohol, especially in the evening, can be recommended as an initial step. Weight loss can be recommended if the patient is obese, and the use of a bedside commode or urinal can also be helpful. For patients with more severe incontinence, however, including most patients with urologic causes, further treatment measures are usually necessary.

Treatment for urinary incontinence is divided into three categories: behavioral and nonpharmacologic therapies, pharmacotherapy, and surgical intervention.

A. Behavioral and Nonpharmacologic Therapies

Lifestyle measures and behavioral therapies should be the first-line treatments in most patients with urge or stress incontinence, as they have the advantages of being effective in a large percentage of patients with few, if any, side effects. Lifestyle measures include limiting excessive fluid intake, avoiding caffeinated and alcoholic beverages, and attaining a healthy weight. Weight loss in overweight and obese women has been shown to be effective in reducing episodes of stress incontinence, but urge incontinence was not decreased. Behavioral therapies range from those designed to treat the underlying problem and restore continence (eg, bladder training, pelvic muscle exercises) to those designed simply to promote dryness through increased attention from a caregiver (eg, timed voiding, prompted voiding). The former category requires a motivated patient who is cognitively intact, whereas the latter category can be used even in patients with significant cognitive impairment.

1. Bladder training—This technique is designed to help patients control their voiding reflex by teaching them to void at scheduled times. The patient is asked to keep a voiding record for approximately 1 week to determine the pattern of incontinence and the interval between incontinent episodes. A voiding schedule is then developed with a scheduled voiding interval significantly shorter than the patient's usual incontinence interval. (For example, if the usual time between incontinent episodes is 1–2 hours, the patient should be scheduled to void every 30–60 minutes.) The patient is asked to empty the bladder as completely as possible at each scheduled void regardless of whether an urge is felt. Patients who have the urge to void at unscheduled times should try to stop the urge through relaxation or distraction techniques until the urge passes and then void at the next scheduled time. If the urge between scheduled voids becomes too uncomfortable, the patient should go ahead and void, but should still void again as completely as possible at the next scheduled time. As the number of incontinent episodes decreases, the scheduled voiding intervals should be gradually extended each week, until a comfortable voiding interval is reached.

Fantl and colleagues (1991), in a well-publicized albeit relatively small trial of bladder retraining, demonstrated significant improvement in both the number of incontinent episodes and the amount of fluid lost in incontinent elderly women by this method. Although the benefit was greatest in women with urge incontinence, women with stress incontinence also demonstrated improvement. In a later study, their group also demonstrated a significant improvement in quality of life following institution of bladder training. Studies in a family practice setting, in a home nursing program, and in a health maintenance organization also demonstrated significant benefit from a program of bladder training. The latter, a randomized controlled trial published in 2002, included patients with stress, urge, and mixed incontinence. Overall, patients had a 40% decrease in their incontinent episodes, with 31% being 100% improved, 41% at least 75% improved, and 52% at least 50% improved.

2. Pelvic floor muscle training (PFMT)—These exercises, also known as *Kegel exercises*, are designed to strengthen the periurethral and perivaginal muscles. They are most useful in the treatment of stress incontinence but may also be effective in urge and mixed incontinence. Patients are initially taught to recognize the muscles to contract by being asked to squeeze the muscles in the genital area as if they were trying to stop the flow of urine from the urethra. While doing this, they should ensure that only the muscles in the front of the pelvis are being contracted, with minimal or no contraction of the abdominal, pelvic, or thigh muscles. Once the correct muscles are identified, patients should be taught to hold the contraction for 5–10 seconds and then relax for the same period. At least three sets of 8–10 contractions per day are often recommended, although the optimal duration and frequency have not been conclusively determined. Patients are then taught to contract their pelvic muscles before and during situations in which urinary leakage may occur to prevent their incontinent episodes from occurring.

A systematic review of 43 published clinical trials concluded that pelvic muscle exercises are effective for both stress and mixed incontinence but that their effectiveness for urge incontinence remains unclear. Biofeedback has been used effectively to improve patients' recognition and contraction of pelvic floor muscles, but the required equipment and expertise can make this impractical in a primary care setting. Weighted vaginal cones and electrical stimulation have also been used to enhance pelvic muscle exercises. These modalities are provided by many physical therapy or geriatric departments and can be considered as additional options for women who are unsuccessful with pelvic muscle exercises or who have obtained only partial improvement. The Cochrane group concluded that weighted vaginal cones, electrostimulation, and pelvic muscle exercises are probably similar in effectiveness. There was some evidence that women who received biofeedback in addition to PFMT reported higher rates of cure or improvement compared to PFMT alone. The effectiveness of pelvic muscle exercises has not been well studied in men, but pelvic muscle exercises have been shown to improve incontinence following prostatectomy.

3. Timed voiding—Timed voiding is a passive toileting assistance program that is caregiver dependent and can be used for patients who are either unable or unmotivated to participate in more active therapies. Its goal is to prevent incontinent episodes rather than to restore bladder function. The caregiver provides scheduled toileting for the patient on a fixed schedule (usually every 2–4 hours), including at night. There is no attempt to motivate the patient to delay voiding or resist the urge to void as there is in bladder training. The technique can be used for patients who can toilet independently as well as those who require assistance. It has been used with success in both male and female patients and has achieved improvements of ≤85%. Timed voiding has also been used effectively in postprostatectomy patients as well as in patients with neurogenic bladder.

A variation of timed voiding, known as *habit training*, uses a voiding schedule that is modified according to the patient's usual voiding pattern rather than an arbitrarily fixed interval. The goal of habit training is to preempt incontinent episodes by scheduling the patient's toileting interval to be shorter than the usual voiding interval. Both timed voiding and habit training are most commonly used in nursing homes but may also be used in the home if a motivated caregiver is available.

4. Prompted voiding—Prompted voiding is a technique that can be used for patients with or without cognitive impairment; it has been studied most frequently in the nursing home setting. Its goal is to teach patients to initiate their own toileting through requests for help and positive reinforcement from caregivers. Approximately every 2 hours, caregivers prompt the patients by asking whether they are wet or dry and suggesting that they attempt to void. Patients are then assisted to the toilet if necessary and praised for trying to use the toilet and for staying dry. A recent systemic analysis of controlled trials of prompted voiding concluded that the evidence was suggestive, although inconclusive, that prompted voiding provided at least short-term benefit to incontinent patients. The addition of oxybutynin to a prompted voiding program may provide additional benefit for some patients. Prompted voiding has been shown to be most effective for reducing daytime incontinence, and routine nighttime toileting has not been shown to be effective in reducing incontinent episodes during the night.

B. Pharmacotherapy

Medications may be used alone or in conjunction with behavioral therapy when degree of improvement has been insufficient. There are very few studies comparing drug therapy with behavioral therapy, but both have been found to be more effective than placebo. An accurate diagnosis of the type of incontinence is necessary in order to choose appropriate pharmacotherapy for each patient.

1. Urge incontinence—There are currently two approved drug classes for treating urge incontinence and overactive bladder: anticholinergic agents and β-agonists. Anticholinergic medications are usually the drugs of first choice because of lower cost and generic availability. Six anticholinergic medications are now available for this indication (Table 42–7). Evidence is insufficient to compare most these medications against one another for safety and efficacy. All of the anticholinergic medications have significant side effects including dry mouth, blurred vision, dizziness, palpitations, constipation, and headache, resulting in a substantial discontinuation rate. They also have significant drug interactions, especially when combined with other medications with cholinergic properties (eg, antihistamines, antipsychotics, muscle relaxants). There is some evidence that prolonged exposure to anticholinergic medications may increase the risk for dementia.

Table 42–7. Medications for urge incontinence.

	Generic Name	Trade Name	Formulations	Starting Dose	Dosing Interval
Anticholinergics					
	Oxybutynin	Ditropan Ditropan XL Oxytrol	Immediate Extended Transdermal	5 mg 5 mg 3.9 mg patch	2-4 times a day Once a day 2 times a week
	Tolterodine	Detrol Detrol LA	Immediate Extended	1 mg 2 mg	2 times a day Once a day
	Trospium	Santura	Immediate Extended	20 mg 60 mg	2 times a day Once a day
	Solifenacin	Vesicare	Extended	5 mg	Once a day
	Darifenacin	Enablex	Extended	7.5 mg	Once a day
	Fesoterodine	Toviaz	Extended	4 mg	Once a day
β₃-Agonist					
	Mirabegron	Myrbetriq	Extended		Once a day

In comparative trials, solifenacin, darifenacin, and tolterodine had the lowest rates of discontinuation due to adverse effects, and oxybutynin had the highest rate. Oxybutynin is also available in an over-the-counter transdermal patch with a lower incidence of adverse effects than the oral formulation.

Trospium (Sanctura) offers the advantage of fewer drug-drug interactions because it is not metabolized by the cytochrome P450 system and is cleared by the kidney. Solifenacin (Vesicare) and darifenacin (Enablex) are more selective for the M3 muscarinic receptors in the bladder than the more traditional agents. M3 receptors are found preferentially in smooth muscle, the salivary glands, and the eyes. This selectivity may lead to a lower incidence of drowsiness and dizziness in some patients; the most common side effects are dry mouth and constipation. Fesoterodine (Toviaz), released in 2009, is similar to long-acting tolterodine and has the same active metabolite. It is supplied in a higher-dose formulation (8 mg), which may increase its efficacy but also its side effects.

Mirabegron (Myrbetriq), released in 2012, is the first β_3-agonist for use in OABS and urge incontinence. Stimulation of β_3-receptors helps to relax the bladder and increase storage capacity, and this drug can be used as an alternative to anticholinergics for patients who do not tolerate or respond adequately to them. Mirabegron has been shown to slightly increase heart rate and blood pressure, so these parameters should be monitored in patients on this drug. In addition, mirabegron can lead to increased drug levels of digoxin, metoprolol, desipramine, and other medications metabolized by the cytochrome P450-2D6 system. Mirabegron is approved as monotherapy or as combination therapy with solifenacin (new in 2018).

The tricyclic antidepressant imipramine has traditionally been widely used to treat urge incontinence, but its use has now largely been supplanted by these newer agents with more favorable side effect profiles and better documented efficacy.

2. Stress incontinence—There are currently no US Food and Drug Administration (FDA)–approved pharmacologic treatments for stress incontinence, and treatment of stress incontinence with systemic pharmacologic therapy is generally not recommended.

Traditionally, estrogen therapy was used in conjunction with α-agonists to increase α-adrenergic responsiveness and improve urethral mucosa and smooth muscle tone. However, the Heart and Estrogen/Progestin Replacement Study (HERS) demonstrated estrogen therapy to be less effective than placebo for symptoms of urinary incontinence, with only 20.9% of the treatment group reporting improvement and 38.8% reporting worsening of their incontinence (compared with 26% improvement and 27% worsening in the placebo group). In addition, data from the Women's Health Initiative study indicated that patients on an estrogen-progestin combination demonstrated increased risk for heart disease, stroke, breast cancer, and pulmonary embolism. Although systemic estrogen therapy is not recommended for the treatment of urinary incontinence, there is some evidence that intravaginal formulations (but not transdermal patches or implants) may improve continence in women with stress incontinence.

α-Adrenergic agents such as pseudoephedrine are no longer recommended as they are only minimally more effective than placebo and have substantial adverse effects.

Duloxetine is approved for stress incontinence in Europe, but efficacy data in the United States have not been compelling. It may be a reasonable choice for treating depression in patients who also have stress incontinence.

3. Overflow incontinence—Overflow incontinence associated with outlet obstruction is seldom treated with medications because the primary therapy is removal of the obstruction. In men, outlet obstruction is most commonly caused by prostatic enlargement secondary to infection (prostatitis), benign prostatic hyperplasia, or prostate cancer. Prostatitis can be treated with a 2- to 4-week course of a fluoroquinolone or trimethoprim-sulfamethoxazole. Once prostate cancer has been ruled out, benign prostatic hyperplasia may be treated with α-blockers, finasteride, surgery, or transurethral microwave thermotherapy. α-Blockers have been shown to be ineffective in "prostatism-like" symptoms in elderly women.

Medical treatment of overflow incontinence caused by bladder contractility problems is rarely efficacious. The cholinergic agonist bethanechol may be useful subcutaneously for temporary contractility problems following an overdistention injury but is generally ineffective when given orally or when used on a long-term basis.

C. Surgical Intervention

Surgical therapy may be indicated for patients with incontinence resulting from anatomic abnormalities (eg, cystocele, prolapse), patients with outlet obstruction resulting in urinary retention, or patients in whom more conservative methods of treatment have not provided sufficient relief. Beyond the correction of anatomic abnormalities or obstruction, surgical therapy is most effective for stress incontinence or for mixed incontinence in which stress incontinence is a primary component. Numerous surgical options are available for the management of stress incontinence, including injection of periurethral bulking agents, transvaginal suspensions, retropubic suspensions, slings, and sphincter prostheses. Choice of procedure is based on the relative contributions of urethral hypermobility versus intrinsic sphincter deficiency, urodynamic findings, the need for other concomitant surgery, the patient's medical condition and lifestyle, and the experience of the surgeon.

D. Electrical Stimulation

These devices are sometimes used to treat incontinence that has been refractory to other methods. The goals are to stimulate contractions of the pelvic floor muscles and/or inhibit overactive bladder contractions. Noninvasive stimulation electrodes can be placed in either the vagina or the anus. Current evidence does not support the efficacy of these methods as being better than behavioral training alone. Electrodes can also be implanted in the sacral nerve roots, the bladder, or the peripheral tibial nerve. These appear to be more effective than noninvasive stimulation but are reserved for carefully selected patients who have been refractory to less invasive measures.

E. Pads, Garments, Catheterization, and Pessaries

The use of absorbent pads and undergarments is extremely common among the elderly. Although they are not recommended as primary therapy before other measures have been tried, they may be useful in patients whose incontinence is infrequent and predictable, who cannot tolerate the side effects of medications, or who are not good candidates for surgical therapy. The main purpose of these pads and garments is to contain urine loss and prevent skin breakdown. However, very few studies have compared the numerous absorbent products available and their degree of success or failure in meeting these objectives. A Cochrane review concluded that disposable products may be more effective than nondisposable products in decreasing the incidence of skin problems and that superabsorbent products may perform better than fluff pulp products. More comparative studies are needed in this area to assist patients and caregivers in making better-informed decisions.

Although urethral catheterization should be avoided as a general rule, it is sometimes indicated in cases of overflow incontinence or in patients for whom no other measures have been effective. External collection devices (eg, Texas catheters) are preferable to indwelling catheters, but acceptable external devices are not widely available for women, and adverse reactions such as skin abrasion, necrosis, and urinary tract infection may occur. When internal catheterization is needed, intermittent or suprapubic catheterization has been shown to be preferable to indwelling catheterization in reducing the incidence of bacteriuria and its consequent complications. Indwelling urethral catheterization should be limited to very few circumstances, including as a comfort measure for the terminally ill, for prevention of contamination of pressure ulcers, and for patients with inoperable outflow obstruction.

Pessaries are intravaginal devices used to maintain or restore the position of the pelvic organs in patients with genitourethral prolapse. Although there are few comparative data on their use in incontinence, they can sometimes be useful in patients with intractable stress incontinence who are poor candidates for, or who do not desire, surgery.

F. Incontinence in Men

Although discussion of urinary incontinence is usually focused on women, men can also experience urinary incontinence. Urge is the most common type of male incontinence, and male stress incontinence is usually limited to men with a history of prostate surgery, spinal cord disorders, or pelvic trauma. Evaluation in men is similar to that in women with the additions of penile and prostate examinations. As with women, treatment progresses from lifestyle changes and behavioral therapies to medications and more invasive strategies as needed. As with women, anticholinergic agents are considered the first-line medications for urge incontinence in men. There are no FDA-approved medications for male stress incontinence, although duloxetine is sometimes tried.

G. Primary Care Treatment Versus Referral

Once the information from the history, physical examination, and initial diagnostic testing is available, a presumptive diagnosis can be made in the large majority of patients. If the patient has uncomplicated urge or stress incontinence, or a mixture of urge and stress, primary treatment can be initiated by the family physician. If the patient has overflow incontinence, manifested by urinary retention, referral is indicated to rule out obstruction prior to attempting medical or behavioral management. In the minority of patients in whom the type or cause of incontinence remains unclear, referral for urodynamic testing may be indicated if a specific diagnosis will be helpful in guiding therapy. Urodynamic testing in the routine evaluation of incontinence is not indicated because studies have not shown an improvement in clinical outcome between patients diagnosed by urodynamics and patients whose treatment was based on history and physical examination.

Other indications for referral include incontinence associated with recurrent symptomatic urinary tract infections, hematuria without infection, history of prior pelvic surgery or irradiation, marked pelvic prolapse, suspicion of prostate cancer, lack of correlation between symptoms and physical findings, and failure to respond to therapeutic interventions as would be expected from the presumptive diagnosis.

H. Evidence-Based Guideline Summary

In 2014, the American College of Physicians published evidence-based clinical guidelines for management of urinary incontinence in women. These guidelines are as follows:

1. PFMT is first-line treatment for stress incontinence.

2. Bladder training is recommended for urge incontinence.

3. PFMT with bladder training is recommended for mixed incontinence.

4. Systemic pharmacologic treatment for stress incontinence is not recommended.

5. Pharmacologic treatment is recommended for urge incontinence if bladder training is unsuccessful.

6. Weight loss and exercise are recommended for obese women with urinary incontinence.

Appell RA, Sand P, Dmochowski R, et al. Prospective randomized controlled trial of extended-release oxybutynin chloride and tolterodine tartrate in the treatment of overactive bladder: results of the OBJECT study. *Mayo Clin Proc.* 2001;76:358–363. [PMID: 11322350]

Benson JT. New therapeutic options for urge incontinence. *Curr Womens Health Rep.* 2001;1:61. [PMID: 12112953]

Culbertson S, Davis AM. Nonsurgical management of urinary incontinence in women. *JAMA.* 2017;317:79–80. [PMID: 28030686]

Drake MJ, Chapple C, Esen AA, et al. Efficacy and safety of mirabegron add-on therapy to solifenacin in incontinent overactive bladder patients with an inadequate response to initial 4-week solifenacin monotherapy: a randomised double-blind multicentre phase 3B study (BESIDE). *Eur Urol* 2016;70(1):136–145. [PMID: 26965560]

Eustice S, Roe B, Paterson J. Prompted voiding for the management of urinary incontinence in adults. *Cochrane Database Syst Rev.* 2000;2:CD002113. [PMID: 10795861]

Fantl JA, Wyman JF, McClish DK, et al. Efficacy of bladder training in older women with urinary incontinence. *JAMA.* 1991;265:609–613. [PMID: 1987410]

Fink HA, Taylor BC, Tacklind JW, et al. Treatment interventions in nursing home residents with urinary incontinence: a systemic review of randomized trials. *Mayo Clin Proc.* 2008;83:1332–1343. [PMID: 19046552]

Glazener CM, Lapitan MC. Urodynamic investigations for management of urinary incontinence in adults. *Cochrane Database Syst Rev.* 2002;3:CD003195. [PMID: 12137680]

Godec CJ. "Timed voiding"—a useful tool in the treatment of urinary incontinence. *Urology.* 1994;23:97. [PMID: 6691214]

Grady D, Brown JS, Vittinghoff E, et al. Postmenopausal hormones and incontinence: the Heart and Estrogen/Progestin Replacement Study. *Obstet Gynecol.* 2001;97:116–120. [PMID: 11152919]

Harvey MA, Baker K, Wells GA. Tolterodine versus oxybutynin in the treatment of urge urinary incontinence: a meta-analysis. *Am J Obstet Gynecol.* 2001;185:56–61. [PMID: 11483904]

Hay-Smith EJ, Herderschee R, Dumoulin C, et al. Comparisons of approaches to pelvic floor muscle training for urinary incontinence in women. *Cochrane Database Syst Rev* 2011;12:CD009508. [PMID: 22161451]

Herderschee R, Hay-Smith EJ, Herbison GP, et al. Feedback or biofeedback to augment pelvic floor muscle training for urinary incontinence in women. *Cochrane Database Syst Rev.* 2011;7:CD009252. [PMID: 21735442]

MacDonald R, Fink HA, Huckabay C, et al. Pelvic floor muscle training to improve urinary incontinence after radical prostatectomy; a systematic review of effectiveness. *BJU Int.* 2007;100(1):76–81. [PMID: 17433028].

Madersbacher H, Richter R. Conservative management in the neuropathic patient. In Abrams P, Khoury S, Wein A, et al, eds. *Incontinence: First International Consultation on Incontinence. Recommendations of the International Scientific Committee: The Evaluation and Treatment of Urinary Incontinence.* Plymouth, United Kingdom: Health Publication Ltd; 1999.

Malallah MA, Al-Shaiji TF. Pharmacological treatment of pure stress urinary incontinence: a narrative review. *Int Urogynecol J.* 2015;26:477–485. [PMID: 25630399]

Pharmacist's Letter Detail-Document. *Medications for Overactive Bladder.* Pharmacist's Letter/Prescriber's Letter; October 2012. https://pharmacist.therapeuticresearch.com/Content/Segments/PRL/2012/Oct/Medications-for-Overactive-Bladder-4819. Accessed November 19, 2019.

Qaseem A, Dallas P, Forciea MA, et al. Nonsurgical management of urinary incontinence in women: a clinical practice guideline from the American College of Physicians. *Ann Intern Med.* 2014;161:429–440. [PMID: 25222388]

Rossouw JE, Anderson GL, Prentice RL, et al. Risks and benefits of estrogen plus progestin in healthy postmenopausal women: principal results from the Women's Health Initiative randomized controlled trial. *JAMA.* 2002;288:321–333. [PMID: 12117397]

Shamliyan T, Wyman JF, Ramakrishnan R, Sainfort F, Kane RL. Benefits and harms of pharmacologic treatment for urinary incontinence in women: a systematic review. *Ann Intern Med.* 2012;156:861–874. [PMID: 22711079]

Shirran E, Brazzelli M. Absorbent products for the containment of urinary and/or faecal incontinence in adults. *Cochrane Database Syst Rev.* 2000;2:CD001406. [PMID: 10796783]

Subak LL, Quesenberry CP, Posner SF, et al. The effect of behavioral therapy on urinary incontinence: a randomized controlled trial. *Obstet Gynecol.* 2002;100:72–78. [PMID: 12100806]

Subak LL, Wing R, West DS, et al. Weight loss to treat urinary incontinence in overweight and obese women. *N Engl J Med.* 2009;360:481–490. [PMID: 19179316]

Elder Abuse

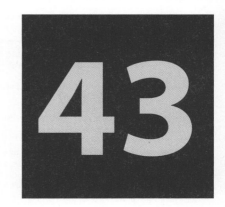

David Yuan, MD, MS
Katherine Wilhelmy, MD
Matthew Koperwas, MD

▶ General Considerations

As hidden as the other forms of family violence may be, domestic elder abuse is even more concealed within our society. As the baby boomers age, the number of elders in the United States will continue to increase. The societal cost for the identification and treatment of elder abuse is also projected to rise as the baby boomers enter the elder years. Elder abuse is now recognized as a pervasive and growing problem. Vastly underreported, for every case of elder abuse and neglect that is reported to authorities, as many as five cases are not reported.

Many physicians feel ill-equipped to address this important social and medical problem. The most common reporters of abuse are family members (17%) and social services agency staff (11%). Physicians reported only 1.4% of the cases. Healthcare professionals consistently underestimate the prevalence of elder abuse. Concerns for patient safety and retaliation by the caregiver; violation of the physician-patient relationship; and patient autonomy, confidentiality, and trust issues are quoted as reasons for low reporting. Studies have shown that healthcare professionals attest to viewing cases of suspected elder abuse but yet fail to report them. One study revealed that physicians report only 2% of all suspected cases.

Older victims who suffer from neglect or physical abuse are likely to seek care from their primary care physician or gain entry into the medical care system through an emergency department. Except for the older person's caregivers, physicians may be the only ones to see an abused elderly patient.

Cooper C, Selwood A, Livingston G. Knowledge detection and reporting of abuse by health and social care professionals: a systematic review. *Am J Geriatr Psychiatry.* 2009;17(10):826–838. [PMID: 19916205]

Dong XQ. Elder abuse: systemic review and implications for practice. *J Am Geriatr Soc.* 2015;63(6):1214–1238. [PMID: 26096395]

Lachs MS, Pillemer K. Elder abuse. *Lancet.* 2004;364:1263. [PMID: 15464188]

Schmeidel AN, Daly JM, Rosenbaum ME, et al. Health care professionals' perspectives on barriers to elder abuse detection and reporting in primary care settings. *J Elder Abuse Negl.* 2012;24(1):17–36. [PMID: 22206510]

A. Definition and Types of Abuse

Elder abuse encompasses all types of mistreatment and abusive behaviors toward older adults. The mistreatment can be either acts of commission (abuse) or acts of omission (neglect). The National Center on Elder Abuse (NCEA) describes seven different types of elder abuse: physical abuse, sexual abuse, emotional abuse, self-neglect, financial exploitation, neglect, and abandonment (Table 43–1). Self-neglect is defined as the behavior of an elderly person that threatens her/his own health and safety. Labeling a behavior as abusive, neglectful, or exploitative is difficult and can depend on the frequency, duration, intensity, severity, consequences, and cultural context. Currently, state laws define elder abuse, and definitions vary considerably from one jurisdiction to another.

Hoover RM, Polson M. Detecting elder abuse and neglect: assessment and intervention. *Am Fam Physician.* 2014;89(6): 453–460. [PMID: 24695564]

Wood EF. *The Availability and Utility of Interdisciplinary Data on Elder Abuse: A White Paper for the National Center on Elder Abuse.* Chicago, IL: American Bar Association Commission on Law and Aging for the National Center on Elder Abuse. National Center on Elder Abuse at American Public Human Services Association; 2006.

B. Prevalence

It is estimated that 4% of adults >65 years old are subjected to mistreatment in the United States. In almost 90% of cases,

Table 43–1. Elder abuse: definitions.

Physical abuse	Use of physical force that may result in bodily injury, physical pain, or impairment
Sexual abuse	Nonconsensual sexual contact of any kind with an elderly person
Emotional abuse	Infliction of anguish, pain, or distress through verbal or nonverbal acts
Financial/material exploitation	Illegal or improper use of an elder's funds, property, or assets
Neglect	Refusal, or failure, to fulfill any part of a person's obligations or duties to an elderly person
Abandonment	Desertion of an elderly person by an individual who has physical custody of the elder or who has assumed responsibility for providing care to the elder
Self-neglect	Behaviors of an elderly person that threaten the elder's health or safety

Data from National Center on Elder Abuse. *Major Types of Elder Abuse.*

the perpetrator of the abuse is known, and in two-thirds of cases, the perpetrators are spouses or adult children. Because of underreporting, poor detection, and differing definitions, the true estimate of elder abuse may be far greater. In a 2017 study, the prevalence of emotional abuse was 27.1%, physical abuse 6.9%, sexual abuse 3.4%, neglect 33.5%, and financial exploitation 34.5%. Psychological abuse is more prevalent than physical abuse. Neglect—the failure of a designated caregiver to meet the needs of a dependent elderly person—is the more common form of elder maltreatment. The prevalence of elder financial abuse is difficult to gauge. One researcher estimates that for every known case of financial exploitation, 24 go unreported. Elder self-neglect is an important public health concern that is the most common form of elder abuse and neglect reported to social services.

Acierno R, Hernandez MA, Amstadter AB, et al. Prevalence and correlates of emotional, physical, sexual, and financial abuse and potential neglect in the United States: the National Elder Mistreatment Study. *Am J Public Health.* 2010;100(2):292–297. [PMID: 20019303]

Gibson SC, Greene E. Assessing knowledge of elder financial abuse: a first step in enhancing prosecutions. *J Elder Abuse Negl.* 2013;25(2):162–182. [PMID: 23473298]

Mosqueda L, Dong X. Elder abuse and self-neglect. *JAMA.* 2011;306(5):532–540. [PMID: 21813431]

Williams J, Racette EH, Hernandez-Tejada MA, et al. Prevalence of elder polyvictimization in the United States: data from the National Elder Mistreatment Study. *J Interpers Violence.* 2017;1:886260517715604. [PMID: 29294807]

C. Risk Factors

Several explanations have been proposed to explain the origins of elder mistreatment. These explanations have focused on overburdened or mentally disturbed caregivers, dependent elders, a history of childhood abuse and neglect, and the marginalization of elders in society. Abuse among older adults with cognitive impairment is markedly higher than for unimpaired adults. In a recent systematic review, caregiver burden/stress was a significant risk factor. Care setting also seems to influence risk of elder abuse. Most elder abuse and neglect occur in the home. Paid home care has a relatively high rate of verbal abuse, and assisted-living settings have an unexpectedly high rate of neglect. Moving from paid home care to nursing homes has been shown to more than triple the odds of the elder experiencing neglect. In one study, >70% of nursing home staff reported that they had behaved at least once in an abusive or neglectful way toward residents over a 1-year period. Risk factors commonly cited for elder mistreatment are listed in Table 43–2.

A typology of abusers has also been suggested to better delineate who may perpetrate abuse. Five types of offenders have been postulated:

1. *Overwhelmed offenders* are well intentioned and enter caregiving expecting to provide adequate care; however, when the amount of care expected exceeds their comfort level, they lash out verbally or physically.

2. *Impaired offenders* are well intentioned but have problems that render them unqualified to provide adequate care. The caregiver may be of advanced age, have physical or mental illness, or have developmental disabilities.

3. *Narcissistic offenders* are motivated by anticipated personal gain and not the desire to help others. These individuals tend to be socially sophisticated and gain a position of trust over the vulnerable elder.

Table 43–2. Risk factors for elder abuse.

Cognitive impairment
Aggressive behaviors
Psychological distress
Lower levels of social network and social support
Lower household income
Need for activities of daily living assistance
Shared living environment
Younger age

Data from Mosqueda L, Dong X: Elder abuse and self-neglect: "I don't care anything about going to the doctor, to be honest..." *JAMA.* 2011 Aug 3;306(5):532–540 and Rosay A, Mulford CF: Prevalence estimates and correlates of elder abuse in the United States: The National Intimate Partner and Sexual Violence Survey. *J Elder Abuse Negl.* 2017 Jan–Feb;29(1):1–14.

Maltreatment is usually in the form of neglect and financial exploitation.

4. *Domineering or bullying offenders* are motivated by power and control and are prone to outbursts of rage. This abuse may be chronic and multifaceted, including physical, psychological, and even forced sexual coercion.

5. *Sadistic offenders* derive feelings of power and importance by humiliating, terrifying, and harming others. Signs of this type of abuse include bite, burn, and restraint marks and other signs of physical and sexual assault.

Each of these categories is not exclusively independent of the others.

Johannesen M, LoGiudice D. Elder abuse: a systematic review of risk factors in community-dwelling elders. *Age Ageing.* 2013;42(3):292–298. [PMID: 23343837]

McDonald L, Beaulieu M, Harbison J, et al. Institutional abuse of older adults: what we know, what we need to know. *J Elder Abuse Negl.* 2012;24(2):138–160. [PMID: 22471513]

Page C, Conner T, Prokhorov A, et al. The effect of care setting on elder abuse: results from a Michigan survey. *J Elder Abuse Negl.* 2009;21(3):239–252. [PMID: 19827327].

Ramsey-Klawsnik H. Elder-abuse offenders: a typology. *Generations.* 2000;24:17. [No PMID]

▶ Clinical Findings

Several medical and social factors make the detection of elder abuse more difficult than other forms of family violence. The elderly dependent patient may fear retaliation from the abuser and may be reluctant to come forward with information. Given the higher prevalence of chronic diseases in older adults, signs and symptoms of mistreatment may be misattributed to chronic disease, leading to "false negatives," such as fractures that are ascribed to osteoporosis instead of physical assault. Alternatively, sequelae of many chronic diseases may be misattributed to elder mistreatment, creating "false positives," such as weight loss because of cancer erroneously ascribed to intentional withholding of food.

A. Screening

The US Preventive Services Task Force (USPSTF) found insufficient evidence to recommend for or against routine screening of older adults or their caregivers for elder abuse. The American Medical Association recommends that older patients be asked about family violence even when evidence of such abuse does not appear to exist. A careful history is crucial to determining whether suspected abuse or neglect exists. The physician should interview the patient and caregiver separately, and if the caregiver does not allow this, abuse potential should be considered. A physician's suspicions should be heightened if the caregiver dominates the medical interview. General questions about feeling safe at home and who prepares meals and handles finances can open the door to more specific questions. Ask if the caregiver is yelling or hitting, making the elder wait for meals and medications, confining the elder to a room, or threatening institutionalization. It is also important to inquire about the possibility of sexual abuse (unwanted touching) or financial abuse (stolen money, being coerced to sign legal documents without understanding the consequences). Self-neglect may be present if the patient begins to miss appointments, gets lost on the way to appointments, or is unable to take medications correctly. Table 43–3 lists important questions to ask when screening for suspected abuse.

Table 43–3. Elder Abuse Suspicion Index.

Within the past 12 months			
1. Have you relied on people for any of the following: bathing, dressing, shopping, banking, or meals?	Yes	No	Did not answer
2. Has anyone prevented you from getting food, clothes, medication, glasses, hearing aids, or medical care, or from being with people you wanted to be with?	Yes	No	Did not answer
3. Have you been upset because someone talked to you in a way that made you feel shamed or threatened?	Yes	No	Did not answer
4. Has anyone tried to force you to sign papers or to use your money against your will?	Yes	No	Did not answer
5. Has anyone made you afraid, touched you in ways you did not want, or hurt you physically?	Yes	No	Did not answer
6. Physician: Elder abuse may be associated with findings such as poor eye contact, withdrawn nature, malnourishment, hygiene issues, cuts, bruises, inappropriate clothing, or medication compliance issues. Did you notice any of these today or in the past 12 months?	Yes	No	Did not answer

Data from Yaffe MJ, Wolfson C, Lithwick M, et al: Development and validation of a tool to improve physician identification of elder abuse: the Elder Abuse Suspicion Index (EASI). *J Elder Abuse Negl.* 2008;20(3):276–300.

Avoid confrontation and blame when interviewing the caregiver. Ask about caregiver burden. Be alert if a caregiver has poor knowledge of a patient's medical problems. If a caregiver has excessive concerns about costs or is financially dependent on the elder, be alert for financial abuse. A study of 2800 older adults found that elder mistreatment was associated with an increased risk for nursing home placement and all-cause mortality. Self-neglect is associated with increased rates of hospitalization and mortality as well.

Dong X, Simon M, Mendes de Leon C, et al. Elder self neglect and abuse and mortality risk in a community-dwelling population. *JAMA*. 2009;302(5):517–526. [PMID: 19654386]

US Preventive Services Task Force. *Screening for Intimate Partner Violence and Abuse of Elderly and Vulnerable Adults.* http://www.uspreventiveservicestaskforce.org. Accessed 2013.

B. Physical Examination

There are no pathognomonic signs of elder abuse, and physical abuse is not the most common type of elder abuse. Yet a thorough physical examination is critical because the elder victim may not be forthcoming about the abuse. Particular attention to the functional and cognitive status of the elder is important to understanding the degree of dependence that the elder may have. Neglect or self-neglect should be suspected when a patient appears disheveled or has evidence of poor hygiene. Table 43–4 lists findings suggestive of physical abuse.

Detailed documentation of the physical examination is important as it may be used as evidence in a criminal trial. Documentation must be complete and legible, with accurate descriptions and annotations on sketches or, when possible, with the use of photographic documentation.

Lachs MS, Pillemer KA. Elder abuse. *N Engl J Med*. 2015;373: 1947–1956. [PMID: 26559573]

Palmer M, Brodell RT, Mostow EN. Elder abuse: dermatologic clues and critical solutions. *J Am Acad Dermatol*. 2013;62(2):e37–e42. [PMID: 23058875]

US Administration on Aging. *National Center on Elder Abuse Administration on Aging.* https://ncea.acl.gov/. Accessed November 18, 2019.

▶ Intervention & Reporting

Barriers to reporting elder abuse are listed in Table 43–5. Forty-four US states have mandatory reporting laws that require healthcare professionals to report a reasonable suspicion of abuse or self-neglect. Most states have anonymous reporting and Good Samaritan laws that can offer an alternative to a direct physician report if there are significant concerns for maintaining the physician-patient relationship. By emphasizing the treatment of the health consequences of the abuse, the elderly patient and caregiver may feel less threatened. Reporting should be done in a caring and compassionate manner in order to protect the autonomy and self-worth of the elder while ensuring his or her continued safety.

The victim should be told that a referral will be made to Adult Protective Services (APS). Involving the caregiver in the discussion must be carefully considered with regard to potential retaliation on the victim. The law enforcement implications of APS should be downplayed, and the social support and services offered by APS should be offered as part of the medical management of the victim. Victims may deny the possibility of abuse or fail to recognize its threat to their personal safety. In financial abuse, the victim, the offender, or both may not acknowledge the abuse. If the victim refuses the APS referral, the clinician may explain that she or he is

Table 43–4. Findings suggestive of physical abuse.

Finding	Bruising	Burns
Size	>5 cm	
Shape	Resembling implement used, eg, hand, shoe, belt, or cane	Resembling implement used, eg, cigarette, clothing iron
Location	Face, side of right arm, or back of torso	Immersion burns may appear in stocking/glove distribution
Miscellaneous	Color not indicative of age of bruise	Characteristic similar to burns seen in children

Modified with permission from Palmer M, Brodell RT, Mostow EN: Elder abuse: dermatologic clues and critical solutions. *J Am Acad Dermatol*. 2013 Feb;68(2):e37–e42.

Table 43–5. Factors affecting the reporting and recognition of elder abuse and neglect.

Medical care providers might not report abuse for the following reasons:
Might not recognize the abuse/neglect and therefore attribute the patient's medical condition to another cause
Might feel constrained by time
Might be concerned about offending the patient and family or in denial that a family member is abusing, especially if the potential abuser is also a patient of the physician
Is unfamiliar with mandatory reporting laws
Is unfamiliar with available resources
Is concerned about personal safety and is afraid of involvement
Is unfamiliar with screening tools
Misinterprets the patient's signs as indicative of another disease process

Data from Abbey L: Elder abuse and neglect: when home is not safe. *Clin Geriatr Med*. 2009 Feb;25(1):47–60 and Dong XQ. Elder Abuse: Systematic Review and Implications for Practice. *J Am Geriatr Soc*. 2015 Jun;63(6):1214–1238.

bound to adhere to state regulations and that the regulations were developed to help older persons who were not receiving the care they needed.

The safety of the patient is the most important consideration in any case of suspected abuse. If the abuse is felt to be escalating, as may occur with physical abuse, law enforcement and APS should be contacted. Hospitalization of the elder may be a temporary solution to removing the victim from the abuser.

If elders have decision-making capacity, their wishes to either accept interventions for suspected abuse or refuse those interventions must be respected. If an abused elder refuses to leave an abusive environment, the primary care physician can still help. This may include helping the older victim to develop a safety plan, such as when to call 911, or installing a lifeline emergency alert system. Close follow-up should be offered.

If older victims no longer retain decision-making capacity, the courts may need to appoint a guardian or conservator to make decisions about living arrangements, finances, and care. This is typically coordinated through APS. The physician's role is to provide documentation of impaired decision-making capacity and of the findings of abuse.

Intervention can be complicated when self-neglect is suspected. Patients may be capable of understanding their actions even if their choices disagree with recommendations of family or professionals. Assessment of cognition and decision-making capacity is critical and may be challenging if individuals refuse assessment. Behavioral health professionals, ethics committees, the guardianship process, and court system are invaluable in assisting families and physicians. Because of confidentiality guidelines, it may be difficult to enlist clergy and other community organizations for help.

As the size of the elderly population continues to grow, physicians need to be vigilant in identifying patients at risk for elder abuse. The physician's role is to recognize elder abuse and self-neglect, treat any associated medical problems, and provide a safe disposition for the patient.

Bond MC, Butler KH. Elder abuse and neglect: definitions, epidemiology, and approaches to emergency department screening. *Clin Geriatr Med.* 2013;29(1):257–273. [PMID: 23177610]

Cooper C, Selwood A, Livingston G. Knowledge, detection, and reporting of abuse by health and social care professionals: a systemic review. *Am J Geriatr Psychiatry.* 2009;17:826–838. [PMID: 19916205]

Movement Disorders

Yaqin Xia, MD, MHPE

Movement disorders (MDs) are a broad spectrum of motor and nonmotor disturbances arising from the dysfunction of subcortical motor control circuitry, including basal ganglia and thalamus, as well as other parts of the nervous system, involving the cortex, cerebellum, and central and peripheral autonomic nervous systems. Patients suffering from MDs have normal muscle strength and sensation, but their normal voluntary motor activities are influenced or impaired by involuntary movement, alteration in muscle tone or posture, and loss of coordination or regulation—either facilitation or inhibition—of pyramidal motor activities as a result of malfunction. MDs can be classified into the following categories on the basis of their clinical manifestations: tremor, chorea and choreoathetosis, dystonia, myoclonus, tics, and ataxia. MDs involve less movement (hypokinesia or akinesia), excessive movement (hyperkinesias), or both (Table 44–1).

PARKINSON DISEASE

ESSENTIALS OF DIAGNOSIS

▶ Cardinal motor parkinsonism syndrome features (Appendix 1).
  ▶ Bradykinesia
  ▶ Rest tremor, rigidity, or both.
▶ Absence of secondary causes or atypical symptoms.
▶ At lease two supportive criteria: response to dopaminergic therapy, presence of levodopa treatment complications, rest tremor of a limb, positive olfactory loss, or metaiodobenzylguanidine scintigraphy cardiac test.

General Considerations

Parkinson disease (PD) is the second most common progressive neurodegenerative disorder after Alzheimer disease but remains the only neurodegenerative disease for which symptoms can be effectively controlled medically. It affects 1% of the global population age 65 years or older and may double in 2030 with aging of the population. Numerous hypotheses have been explored to explain the process of the neurodegeneration. With the significant improvement in understanding PD and its pathologic process, researches are still in the process of exploring its etiologies, the disease process including the premotor stage before its diagnosis, its treatment, and its prevention. Aging is the greatest risk factor associated with PD. Approximately 95% of PD cases are idiopathic/sporadic and occur in people age >50 years. The incidence of PD is 1.5 times higher in males. In the United States, its prevalence is 128 per 100,000 persons age 50–64 years, 550 per 100,000 persons age 65–74 years, and 958 per 100,000 persons age 75 years and older, with 340,000 total patients with PD in 2005. It is projected that this number will double to 610,000 in 2030. Around 5–10% of PD cases are genetically inherited. An individual may have a doubled risk if there is a family history in a first-degree relative. Genetic therapies targeting α-synuclein (SNCA), glucocerebrosidase (GBA), and leucine-rich repeat kinase 2 (LRRK2) are under investigation.

Pathogenesis

The pathogenesis of PD is considered the result of progressive and degenerative loss of dopaminergic projection neurons and axons in the substantia nigra (SN) and striatum from α-synuclein toxicity as a result of multifactorial etiologies, which may include environmental, genetic, toxic, oxidation stress, activation of immune system, and inflammatory response. Another, yet to be proven pathologic process is the potential cell-to-cell transmission through exosome excretion and endocytosis uptake. The spread of α-synuclein in the nervous system may be in a prion-like fashion, starting from the olfactory and vagal nerves and progressing toward the central nervous system (CNS). Patients will become

Table 44–1. Classification of movement disorders.

Hypokinetic Disorders	Hyperkinetic Disorders
Neurodegenerative parkinsonian syndrome	Tremor
Parkinson disease (idiopathic)	Tics (Tourette syndrome)
DLB	Chorea (Huntington disease)
PSP	Myoclonus
MSA (Shy-Drager, OPCA, SND)	Dystonia/athetosis
CBGD	Ataxia
Spinal muscular atrophy	Akathisia (almost always
Wilson's disease	affects the legs)
Secondary nondegenerative parkinsonism	Hemiballismus
syndrome	Stereotype
Drug-induced parkinsonism	Restless legs syndrome
Vascular parkinsonism	Dyskinesia
Normal pressure hydrocephalus	Gait disorders
Other: infections, toxins,	
Metabolic disorders	
Psychogenic	

CBGD, corticobasal ganglionic degeneration; DLB, dementia with Lewy bodies; MSA, multisystem atrophy; OPCA, olivopontocerebellar atrophy; PSP, progressive supranuclear palsy; SND, striatonigral degeneration.

symptomatic when a significant amount (~50%) of dopaminergic SN neurons or their axon terminals are impaired or lost. One side of the SN is usually more severely affected than the other, which results in more prominent symptoms on one side of the body.

Lewy bodies, typical α-synuclein (αSyn) immunoreactive intracytoplasmic eosinophilic inclusions in neurons, are a neuropathologic hallmark of PD. PD may also involve the CNS and peripheral and enteric nervous systems, with Lewy bodies located in the olfactory nucleus, amygdala, brainstem, neocortex, vagal nerve nucleus, and sympathetic nervous system. αSyn is also found in the intramural enteric nervous system, skin, retina, submandibular gland, cardiac nervous system, and other visceral organ nervous systems. Lewy bodies are also associated with Alzheimer disease, Down syndrome, and other neurologic diseases. Mutations in the *SNCA* (dominant inherited PD), *GBA*, transmembrane protein lymphocyte-activation gene 3 (*LAG3*), *LRRK2* (age-dependent penetration), and *PARK/PINK1/DJ1* genes (recessively inherited PD) are related to increased risk of PD.

▶ **Clinical Findings**

A. Symptoms and Signs

Based on the significant advances in PD research and clinical expertise over the past two decades, the Movement Disorder Society (MDS) Task Force published the MDS Clinical Diagnostic Criteria for Parkinson's Disease in 2015 (Appendix 1). The diagnosis of PD is clinical, based on parkinsonism cardinal symptoms examined according to the motor examination recommended in the 2008 version of the MDS Unified Parkinson Disease Rating Scale (UPDRS). It is crucial to differentiate PD from other neurodegenerative and nondegenerative/secondary parkinsonism syndromes (PS) and other diseases with tremor (see Table 44–1). PS cardinal motor symptoms are prerequisite criteria, including bradykinesia and rest tremor, rigidity, or both. They are not the result of infections or primary visual, vestibular, cerebellar, proprioceptive, or other neurodegenerative disorders (absence of absolute exclusion criteria and red flags Appendix 1). At least two of the supportive criteria should be met. The patients' excellent and sustained response to dopaminergic treatment and end-of-dose wearing off support the diagnosis. The most common initial finding is an asymmetric resting tremor in an upper extremity. The cardinal signs may eventually become bilateral after several years but will remain more prominent on one side of the body. Early referral to PD specialists is necessary when a patient has atypical or secondary parkinsonism. A diagnosis of possible PD is considered if there are two or fewer red flags, each counterbalanced by at least one supportive criterion. (Please consult the MDS-UPDRS form for detailed evaluation items for PD.)

1. Cardinal motor signs—Bradykinesia is decrease in speed (bradykinesia) and amplitude (akinesia/hypokinesia) of voluntary movement. Limb bradykinesia must be documented to diagnose PD, and it can be evaluated by finger/toe/foot tapping or hand pronation/supination movements. Patients cannot perform rapid repetitive movements, such as tapping the fingers or heels repeatedly. Bradykinesia may also involve the eyes (masklike stare, infrequent blink) or face (hypomimia) or manifest as micrographia, soft voice, or slow walking. Patients may make short, shuffling steps with a decreased arm swing, freezing gait, or difficulty turning in bed.

Rigidity is the "lead-pipe," velocity-independent resistance to passive movement of limbs and neck. It is checked when the patient is in a relaxed condition. Cogwheel phenomenon may or may not be present, but isolated cogwheel phenomenon without lead-pipe rigidity cannot be defined as PD rigidity.

Rest tremor in PD is a characteristic oscillating or pill-rolling movement of one hand at a regular rhythm (4–6 Hz). It is the presenting symptoms in 50–70% of patients, with hands, fingers, forearms, and feet most frequently affected. Other parts of the body such as the jaw or face may also be affected. The tremor diminishes during sleep and voluntary movement and reemerges at rest.

Patients with PD may experience impaired balance and postural reflexes when standing, known as *postural instability*, which will increase the risk of falls. It is not PD diagnostic criteria, and early presentation suggests other diagnoses instead of PD.

2. Nonmotor/premotor symptoms—PD affects both dopaminergic (motor) and nondopaminergic (nonmotor) neurons. Nondopaminergic central and peripheral nervous system involvement is present in most PD patients and may begin subtly, several years before the motor signs start. These symptoms affect patients' emotional, cognitive, behavioral, and general health. Nondopaminergic features, such as falling and dementia, are the major source of PD disability. Recognizing these premotor or nonmotor symptoms may aid in the early diagnosis of PD and its morbidities, so preventive measures and treatment can be started early to achieve more favorable results. The major nonmotor/premotor features are listed in Table 44–2. The significance of these nonmotor features in early diagnosis of PD requires further investigation.

Olfactory impairment precedes motor features of PD by many years in most patients with PD. Olfactory testing is not specific but may be used to identify people either at risk for developing PD or in a presymptomatic stage of PD. Rapid eye movement (REM) behavior disorder is another early nonmotor feature and specific for neurodegenerative processes including PD. Excessive daytime sleepiness affects 20–60% of patients and is increased with dopamine agonist use. Insomnia affects 37–60% of PD patients.

Dementia, which is 2–6 times more likely in PD patients than in the healthy population, may occur early in PD and is not an exclusive criterion, except the frontotemporal type. About 50% of PD patients develop PD dementia 10 years after disease onset. Mild cognitive impairment and PD dementia diagnosis criteria have been set by the International Parkinson and Movement Disorder Society. Lewy body deposition is associated with dementia in PD. Risk factors of dementia include hallucinations, older age, severity of motor symptoms, speech and gait impairment, lower education, depression, and male gender. It can also be a result of medications with anticholinergic properties or other medical conditions that can affect patients' mental status, such as infection, dehydration, or intracranial bleeding. Major depression is seen in approximately 17% of PD patients, with milder depression seen in another approximately 35% of PD patients. The somatic and cognitive symptoms in PD, such as psychomotor retardation or anhedonia resulting from inability to perform usual activities, overlap with those of depression, which makes it difficult to diagnose. Risk factors include use of antidepressants, cognitive impairment, longer disease duration, motor fluctuations, female sex, and younger age. The Hamilton Depression Rating Scale or the Montgomery-Asberg Depression Rating Scale should be used in conjunction with a structured patient interview in all circumstances to eliminate *Diagnostic and Statistical Manual of Mental Disorders* exclusion criteria.

Hallucinations can occur early or before motor symptoms start. Visual hallucinations are the most common clinical manifestation. They have a significant impact on the quality of life of patients and their caregivers, with higher mortality and nursing home placement. Auditory, tactile, olfactory, and somatic hallucinations are less frequent and may occur concomitantly with visual hallucinations. Vivid dreaming, illusions, or delusions may also occur. Psychosis occurs late (10 years after the diagnosis) in the disease process. These symptoms are often the side effects of antiparkinsonian medications. Both dopaminergic and dopamine receptor agonists pose a higher risk for psychosis, which is independent of dosage and treatment duration. Other underlying disease processes, for example, dementia, advanced age, depression, insomnia, and preexisting psychiatric conditions (which usually occur early in PD), are also risk factors for psychosis. Autonomic dysfunction is common in PD, such as constipation, daytime urinary urgency (not simply nocturia), and symptomatic orthostasis. Severe autonomic dysfunction in the first 5 years of the PD diagnosis suggests another etiology other than PD.

Table 44–2. Common nonmotor/premotor symptoms of Parkinson disease (PD).

Clinical Areas Involved	Clinical Features and Potential Complications
Hyposmia	Impairment of odor detection, identification, and discrimination (90% of cases)
Autonomic dysfunction	Orthostatic hypotension (late presentation), hyperhidrosis Genitourinary: daytime bladder urgency, frequency and nocturia, erectile dysfunction and anorgasmia Gastrointestinal: gastroparesis, constipation (60–80%), diarrhea
Cognitive symptoms	Frontal executive dysfunction PD dementia
Sleep	Sleep-maintenance insomnia Rapid eye movement sleep behavior disorder Excessive daytime somnolence RLS/PLMS (30–80%)
Neurologic symptoms	Impaired color discrimination, pain (50%), paresthesias (40%) Fatigue Speech and voice disorders (89%) Nocturnal akinesia
Psychiatric disorders	Stress from the illness Anxiety Depression (50%) Psychosis (20–40%) Hallucinations (sensory) Apathy

PLMS, periodic limb movement disorder; RLS, restless leg syndrome.

The Non-Motor Symptoms Questionnaire can help with evaluating PD nonmotor symptoms and signs.

B. Laboratory Findings

Genetic tests should be considered in patients with a family history or early onset of PD before age 40 years.

C. Ancillary Testing

Neuroimaging tests are not necessary for PD diagnosis but may be considered to help with uncertain cases, such as to differentiate PS from other causes of tremor and dementia. Olfactory loss and/or metaiodobenzylguanidine (MIBG) scintigraphy positive for cardiac sympathetic denervation have been added to supportive criteria. They may differentiate PD from other PS with a specificity of >80%. Olfactory testing should be considered in order to differentiate PD from progressive supranuclear palsy and corticobasal degeneration. ^{123}I-FP-CIT single-photon emission computed tomography (CT) may help to differentiate patient with essential tremor. Both CT and magnetic resonance imaging (MRI) can be ordered for atypical clinical presentations to rule out other intracranial pathologic processes; examples are midbrain atrophy in possible progressive supranuclear palsy, cerebellar/brainstem atrophy/gliosis in possible multiple system atrophy (MSA), normal-pressure hydrocephalus, and vascular or other causes of parkinsonism. MRI measurement of iron deposition and transcranial sonography can differentiate PD from progressive supranuclear palsy and MSA by detecting hyperechogenicity of the SN.

Researchers have been trying to identify changes in brain structural and functional imaging studies to assist PD diagnosis, especially in the premotor stage. Early diagnosis is critical in redefining the importance of neuroprotective treatment. Routine use of imaging studies is currently not recommended for PD diagnosis.

▶ Differential Diagnosis

It is important to differentiate PD from other PS neurodegenerative diseases such as progressive supranuclear palsy, dementia with Lewy bodies, MSA, corticobasal degeneration, and other medical conditions with tremor (see Table 44–1). Some medical conditions may have similar but distinctive clinical presentations (see Table 44–1), as listed in the absolute exclusion criteria and red flags in Appendix 1, which are designed to minimize both of these diagnostic errors. Up to 25% of the geriatric population may present with mild PSs without PD. An imaging study of the brain is usually required to rule out other PSs if a patient has an atypical presentation, such as being unresponsive to levodopa, early falls in the disease course, symmetric signs without tremor, rapid disease process, and early dysautonomia. Patients with secondary parkinsonism may have a positive medication or medical

history. Parkinson-plus syndromes related to underlying neurodegenerative conditions are relatively uncommon and have characteristic clinical presentations and different neurologic imaging findings. Progressive supranuclear palsy is the most common Parkinson-plus syndrome. It is characterized by a downward-gaze palsy, minimal tremor, and severe postural instability with frequent falls starting during the first year of the disease process. Corticobasal ganglionic degeneration demonstrates asymmetric symptoms but also severe limb apraxia and dystonia.

▶ Complications

Both motor and nonmotor clinical features of PD cause progressive disability that interferes with daily activities in all age groups and at all stages of the illness. The frequent reasons for hospitalization include motor disturbances, reduced mobility, lack of adherence to treatment, inappropriate use, falls, fractures, and pneumonia. Other potential complications of PD include weight loss, malnutrition and risk of aspiration, cognitive deterioration and depression, problem with speech, worsening of vision, and loss of smell. The risk of osteoporosis may double in PD. Table 44–2 lists common nonmotor symptoms and complications.

Motor complications, dyskinesias, and motor fluctuations usually start 4–6 years after initiation of treatment. They are assumed to be induced by pulsatile plasma levodopa levels. Dyskinesias are involuntary movements that can present as choreiform movements, dystonia, and myoclonus. Patients with motor fluctuations may experience a sudden loss of levodopa effects and switch from an "on" symptom-controlled period to an "off" symptomatic period, an end-dose "wearing-off" effect, and "freezing" during "on" periods. Neuroleptic malignant syndrome may result from a sudden stop of PD treatment and should be avoided.

▶ Treatment

Treatment of PD is aimed at cardinal symptom control, disease process modification, nonmotor manifestation treatment, and management of motor and nonmotor complications in late stages of PD. Motor symptom control is mainly through supplementation of levodopa (L-dopa), or decreased metabolism/degradation of dopamine. Although no treatment has been shown conclusively to slow down progression of the disease, several pharmacologic and surgical therapies are available to control patients' symptoms.

The goals of treatment vary depending on the disease stage. In early PD, treatment goals are to modify the disease process, delay and control motor symptoms, and maintain patients' independent functions; in more advanced PD, the goals are to maximize medication effectiveness, manage motor complications from L-dopa, and control complications due to PD progression. Nonmotor symptom treatment should be started early and monitored throughout the disease process.

Neuroprotection of the dopaminergic neurons in the SN is still under investigation.

A. Pharmacotherapy

When to start PD therapy is a collaborative decision relying on effective communication between the physician, patient, and family. A variety of factors will be considered, such as the degree of impairment and its effect on the patient's daily life and employment, the patient's understanding of PD, and the patient's attitude toward medications. The traditional wait and watch approach (ie, starting treatment when the patient begins to experience functional impairment) has been challenged.

1. Motor symptom therapy—L-dopa with carbidopa, a dopa decarboxylase inhibitor, is the most effective medication for PD symptom control and has a more favorable safety profile compared with other regimens, especially in older patients. However, the motor complications, such as dyskinesia with disabling involuntary movements, motor fluctuation with *on* periods (responding to treatment) and *off* periods, or hypertonia, may appear a few months to several years after initiation of L-dopa. They compromise L-dopa treatment effects and limit its long-term use. High L-dopa exposure based on weight, female sex, low weight, and young age are risk factors for motor complications.

Off time is the return of disabling Parkinson features during L-dopa treatment. It is more common in the morning when patients wake up and in the late afternoon and is partially related to fluctuation of L-dopa blood levels as a result of its short half-life and various gastrointestinal transition times to the jejunum where the medication is absorbed. Strategies to extend L-dopa treatment and minimize motor complications have been explored. Subcutaneous injection of apomorphine, a short-acting D_1/D_2 dopamine agonist, is the only approved rescue therapy for off time. Inhaled L-dopa and sublingual apomorphine rescue formula are under development. Amantadine is an adjunct medication that may decrease dyskinesia risk without increasing off periods. Other medications to treat dyskinesia are under investigation, such as partial dopamine agonists, D_1 agonists, and opioid receptor antagonists. Continuous intrajejunal delivery of L-dopa/carbidopa intestinal suspension or gel has shown significant reduction of off time and dyskinesia. Inhalation L-dopa has been shown to rapidly correct off periods in advanced PD. Continuous subcutaneous infusion is being evaluated for its lower delivery capacity. L-dopa intravenous infusion and patches are not commercially available for technical difficulty and potential side effects.

Sustained-release levodopa has not been shown to decrease motor complications. Adding a dopamine agonist, catechol-O-methyltransferase (COMT) inhibitors, or monoamine oxidase B (MAO-B) inhibitors to L-dopa reduces off periods by limiting dopamine metabolism and prolonging its half-life, but it does not work well in many cases, and in the same manner as increasing dosage or frequency of L-dopa, it may increase the risk of dyskinesia. Domperidone can be used for nausea and vomiting, which are common side effects of L-dopa. The fear of the side effects and motor complications may delay the use of L-dopa and result in undertreatment of PD, but alternative medications may be used as first-line treatment to reduce dyskinesias.

COMT inhibitors increase brain L-dopa availability by inhibiting its peripheral metabolism. Its clinical use has been limited by potential fetal liver toxicity.

Dopamine agonists (DAs) are used by many physicians as the first monotherapy to control PD motor symptoms, especially in younger patients. DAs have shown significant improvement in the UPDRS in early PD with fewer motor side effects, but their other side effects (Table 44–3) have limited their use, especially in those age >65 years or those with alcohol abuse, obsessive compulsive disorder (OCD), or mood disorders. Used together with L-dopa, they decrease dosage of L-dopa, but do not prevent motor complications and the need for surgical intervention. Ergoline DAs, including bromocriptine, pergolide, lisuride, and cabergoline, are almost never used now because they are associated with moderate to severe cardiac valvulopathy and pleural, pericardial, and retroperitoneal serosal fibrosis.

MAO-B inhibitors extend dopamine half-life through irreversibly inhibiting the metabolism of synaptic dopamine. They may reduce oxidative stress of dopamine neurons and provide neuroprotective benefits and slow neurodegeneration. Early use of the irreversible MAO-B inhibitors has shown effectiveness in some clinical trials in controlling motor symptoms and providing disease-modifying, L-dopa–sparing relief when used simultaneously with a DA and causing less functional decline. MAO-B inhibitors, alone or together with a DA, are preferred by some physicians to initiate PD treatment, but they have demonstrated conflicting effectiveness on motor fluctuation. Safinamide is a newly released MAO-B reversible inhibitor to be used as an adjunct to L-dopa to increase on time without increase in dyskinesia.

Amantadine is an *N*-methyl-D-aspartate receptor antagonist. It is the only medication with dyskinesia improvement benefit. Table 44–3 lists the common antiparkinsonian medications.

2. Neuroprotective/disease-modifying therapy—Neuroprotective and disease modification treatments should be the final goal of PD treatment. Ideally, it should be started as soon as the diagnosis of PD has been made or even before the nonmotor or premotor symptoms are identified, targeting α-synuclein aggregation, lysosomal and mitochondrial dysfunction, and possibly the spreading process. The insidious onset and wide variety of possible etiologies render PD difficult to identify and prevent. There is insufficient evidence to support the neuroprotective or modifying effects of the

Table 44–3. Pharmacotherapy for Parkinson disease.

Class/Drug	Clinical Use and Side Effects
Dopaminergic drugs	Nausea and vomiting, dyskinesia, motor fluctuations, somnolence, ICDs and DDS, psychosis, hypotension, peripheral edema, melanoma, weight loss
Precursor amino acid: Levodopa	
Carbidopa/levodopa (Sinemet)	Increase by one tablet every day or every other day to a maximum of eight tablets per day
Controlled release (Sinemet CR)	Increase by one tablet every 3 days to a maximum of eight tablets per day
Continuous PEG-J tube:	Pancreatitis, peritonitis, tube and infusion system malfunction, suicide and polyneuropathy, inconvenience of pump
Duodopa gel: Duodopa suspension: Duopa	Bolus plus continuous infusion
Carbidopa/levodopa/entacapone (Stalevo)	Used when other medications become less effective; increase slowly to a maximum of eight tablets per day
Dopamine agonists	Excessive somnolence (caution with driving), ICDs, hallucinations, orthostatic hypotension, edema, vomiting, dizziness, confusion; higher risk in older patients
Pramipexole	Extended-release form available.
Ropinirole	Adjust every week as needed
Apomorphine	For rescue therapy for "off" episodes; nausea (requires trimethobenzamide initially), hypotension, subcutaneous form (rapidly sulfonated if swallowed)
Rotigotine	Transdermal

MAO-B inhibitor
  Selegiline
  Rasagiline
	Sleep disturbance, lightheadedness, nausea, abdominal pain, confusion, hallucinations; avoid tyramine-containing food, such as aged cheese, sausages, salamis, or soy sauce (cause uncontrolled hypertension); be aware of drug interactions; no dose titration required; possibly neuroprotective

Safinamide	MAO-B inhibitor plus channel blockers

N-Methyl-D-aspartate (NMDA)
  receptor inhibitor
  Amantadine
	Antidyskinetic
	Hallucinations, dry mouth, livedo reticularis, ankle swelling, myoclonic encephalopathy in setting of renal failure; avoid in cognitive impairment; benefits not long lasting
	Insufficient evidence in treatment of early PD

COMT inhibitors	Effective only with levodopa; worsening of levodopa-induced dyskinesias, diarrhea, nausea, vivid dreams, visual hallucinations, sleep disturbances, daytime drowsiness, headache
Tolcapone	Second-line option for fetal hepatotoxicity
Entacapone	Strict licensing criteria; blood level monitoring needed

Anticholinergics
  Trihexyphenidyl
  Biperidine
	Limited use for significant neuropsychiatric and cognitive adverse effects
	Confusion, sleepiness, blurred vision, constipation
	May worsen motor symptoms on discontinuation; tapering needed

COMT, catechol-O-methyltransferase; DDS, dopamine dysregulation syndrome; ICD, impulse control disorder; MAO-B, monoamine oxidase B; PD, Parkinson disease; PEG-J, percutaneous endoscopic transgastric jejunostomy.

MAO-B inhibitors selegiline and rasagiline. Individuals taking nonsteroidal anti-inflammatory drugs have reduced PD incidence, but there is little or no evidence to substantiate the disease-modifying effects of vitamins, anti-inflammatory medications, nutritional supplements, or coenzyme Q10. How to identify at-risk patients and diagnose PD early to start preventive or protective treatment, which is under investigation, also needs to be addressed. Treatments targeting α-synuclein activity are in process, such as active or passive immunizations, inhibition of α-synuclein folding, and glucosylceramide modifications. Other medications such as isradipine, inosine, deferiprone, and exenatide are under

investigation for their potential disease-modifying mechanism. Genetic approaches to control and modify PD process are also under investigation.

3. Nonmotor symptom therapy—Medications and other management methods are chosen based on each specific symptom or problem, such as selective serotonin reuptake inhibitor (SSRI) antidepressants for depression and baclofen for pain and spasm control. Once dementia is detected, it should be treated with rivastigmine or donepezil because of their small but significant effect on the improvement in cognitive scales and activities of daily living. Polypharmacy should be assessed and avoided. Antiparkinsonian medications such as anticholinergics, DAs, amantadine, and MAO-B inhibitors may need to be decreased or discontinued. Control of cardiovascular risk factors, such as using a statin, is important to decrease the risk of dementia in PD patients at risk. Cholinesterase inhibitors may be considered for dementia, but should not be used in PD with dyskinesia or motor fluctuations. Midodrine or fludrocortisone may be used for orthostatic hypotension if avoiding provoking agents, such as antihypertensives, dopaminergics, anticholinergics, and antidepressants, is not working. Sleep disturbance may improve with adjusting L-dopa dosage, discontinuing nighttime use of antiparkinsonian drugs, discontinuing DAs, or starting clonazepam or melatonin. Methylphenidate may help improve gait and decrease the risk of falls. The first step in controlling psychotic symptoms is to decrease the dosage of antiparkinsonian medication or gradually remove some medications, in the following order: anticholinergics, selegiline, amantadine, dopamine receptor agonists, COMT, and finally, L-dopa (switch to short acting). Antipsychotic agents are considered if the patient still has symptoms that are bothersome. The atypical antipsychotic agents clozapine and quetiapine have fewer extrapyramidal and prolactin-elevating adverse effects. Other second-generation antipsychotic medications, such as ziprasidone, risperidone, and olanzapine, and the third-generation antipsychotic aripiprazole are not recommended because they may be not as effective or may have worse extrapyramidal adverse effects. Cholinesterase inhibitors (except rivastigmine), such as donepezil, galantamine, and tacrine, have shown inconsistent results and may worsen PD or have other side effects. Electroconvulsive therapy should be used as a last resort for psychiatric disorders or depression when medications are not effective. By stimulating the D_3 dopamine receptors in the mesolimbic pathways, ropinirole has been shown to control motor symptoms and mood fluctuation, including depression and anxiety in patients with motor fluctuations.

B. Surgical Intervention

Surgery is an effective treatment option in more advanced PD. Subthalamic nucleus and globus pallidus internus deep-brain stimulation (DBS) are effective in improving motor function and alleviating motor complications including off periods and dyskinesia. DBS is reserved for advanced PD and motor complications from L-dopa treatment. DBS can also improve psychological, behavioral, and cognitive changes. Patients with better preoperative response to L-dopa challenge are more likely to improve from DBS. Potential neuro-restoration with dopaminergic or stem cell replacement may also bring hope in controlling dopamine deficiency–related disabilities. Other options such as unilateral thalamotomy and pallidotomy are effective in controlling motor complications but can cause destructive lesions.

C. Ancillary Treatment and Supportive Measures

Once the diagnosis of PD is made, patients and their caregivers should be involved and empowered in the decision making of the treatment and care. Both oral and written communication should be implemented because of possible cognitive impairment. The clinical care team, including physician, nurse, physiotherapist (early referral), occupational therapist, speech therapist, nutritionist, case managers, and social workers with expertise in Parkinson management, should work with patients and caregivers to provide comprehensive clinical treatment as well as supportive care. Suspected patients should be referred to PD specialists untreated to confirm the diagnosis. Patients are encouraged to have discussions with the Department of Transportation regarding their driving license. Psychological counseling and therapy, such as cognitive behavioral therapy, supportive therapy, and coping skill development, may help patients with psychiatric manifestations.

Supportive treatment is important in terms of maintaining function and general health. It includes allied health interventions; occupational therapy; physical therapy; and speech, swallowing, and voice therapy. Physical exercise is an important component in PD treatment. It can improve PD patients' motor performance as well as their learning, memory, and mental health. It may repair or reverse the neurochemical damage through facilitating synaptogenesis and neurotrophy. Providing support to the family and caregivers is also crucial. Information regarding PD and other resources should be provided to caregivers. Patients and their families can be referred to various support groups, including the American Parkinson Disease Association (https://www.apdaparkinson.org), the Parkinson's Foundation (http://www.parkinson.org), and the Michael J. Fox Foundation for Parkinson Research (http://www.michaeljfox.org). Another website providing PD information is the International Parkinson and Movement Disorder Society website (http://www.movementdisorders.org/).

▶ Prevention

So far, monogenetic etiologies are rare causes of PD, and other factors have contributed to the PD process. Environmental toxins may also play a minor role in increasing the risk of PD, such as exposure to pesticides from farming, living in rural areas, and drinking well water; manganese from welding; or ephedrone recreational use. Physical activity is associated with decreased risk of PD. Some potential protective factors with negative associations with PD have been identified in some studies, such as caffeine, alcohol, and smoking (not recommended as preventive use); calcium channel blockers; and statins. Continuous explorations of PD preventive factors, such as ibuprofen, diet, and inosine, for example, are in process.

Prognosis & Disease Process Monitoring

PD is a chronic and progressive disease with a mean survival of >10 years. Older age at onset and the presence of rigidity or hypokinesia as initial symptoms predict a more rapid rate of motor progression, as do other associated morbidities such as stroke, auditory deficits, visual impairments, gait disturbances, and male sex.

Caring for PD patients involves a long-term assessment of disease progress and monitoring for the effectiveness and adverse effects of treatment in order to modify the management plan as needed. Clinical rating scales can be used to evaluate patients' function, satisfaction, and severity of motor and non-motor symptoms. The UPDRS is widely used and contains six sections to assess mood and cognition; activities of daily living in both on and off states; motor abilities; complications of therapy; disease severity; and global function, including level of disability, mood, and both disease- and treatment-related manifestations of PD. Other monitoring/evaluating instruments include the Parkinson Psychosis Rating Scale (PPRS), Mini-Mental State Examination (MMSE), and the Parkinson Disease Quality of Life Questionnaire (PDQL), to name only a few.

Antonini A, Moro E, Godeiro C, Reichmann H. Medical and surgical management of advanced Parkinson's disease. *Mov Disord.* 2018;33(6):900–908. [PMID: 29570862]

Ascherio A, Schwarzschild MA. The epidemiology of Parkinson's disease: risk factors and prevention. *Neurology.* 2016;15:1257–1272. [PMID: 27751556]

Berg D, Postuma RB, Adler CH, et al. MDS research criteria for prodromal Parkinson's disease. *Mov Disord.* 2015;30(12):1600–1611. [PMID: 26474317]

Dorsey ER, Constantinescu R, Thompson JP, et al. Projected number of people with Parkinson disease in the most populous nations, 2005 through 2030. *Neurology.* 2007;68:384–386. [PMID: 17082464]

International Parkinson and Movement Disorder Society. https://www.movementdisorders.org/MDS.htm. Accessed November 25, 2019.

Jankovic J, Poewe W. Therapies in Parkinson's disease. *Curr Opin Neurol.* 2012;25:433–447. [PMID: 22691758]

Lang AE, Espay AJ. Disease modification in Parkinson's disease: current approaches, challenges, and future considerations. *Mov Disord.* 2018;33:660–677. [PMID: 29644751]

Marinus J, Zhu K, Marras C, et al. Risk factors for non-motor symptoms in Parkinson's disease. *Lancet Neurol.* 2018;17(6):559–568. [PMID: 29699914]

National Institute for Health and Care Excellence. Parkinson's disease in adults. https://www.nice.org.uk/guidance/ng71. Accessed November 25, 2019.

Noyce AJ, Lees AJ, Schrag AE. The prediagnostic phase of Parkinson's disease. *J Neurol Neurosurg Psychiatry.* 2016;87:871–878. [PMID: 26848171]

Olanow CW, Stocchi F. Levodopa: a new look at an old friend. *Mov Disord.* 2018;33(6):859–866. [PMID: 29178365]

Postuma RB, Berg D, Stern M, et al. MDS clinical diagnostic criteria for Parkinson's disease. *Mov Disord.* 2015;30(12):1591–1601. [PMID: 26474316]

Scottish Intercollegiate Guidelines Network. Diagnosis and pharmacological management of Parkinson's disease. https://www.sign.ac.uk/assets/sign113.pdf. Accessed November 25, 2019.

Subramaniam RM, Frey KA, Hunt CH, et al. ACR-ACNM practice parameter for the performance of dopamine transporter (DaT) single photon emission computed tomography (SPECT) imaging for movement disorders. *Clin Nucl Med.* 2017;42:847–852. [PMID: 28922189]

TREMOR

Tremor is an involuntary, rhythmic oscillation of one part of the body from regular contractions of reciprocally innervated antagonistic muscles. It is the most common MD. Tremor can occur at rest (rest tremor), while voluntarily maintaining a position against gravity (postural tremor), or during voluntary movement (kinetic tremors). Table 44–4 lists different types of tremor due to different physiologic or pathologic etiologies based on activation conditions. In 2017, the International Parkinson and Movement Disorder Society published the Consensus Statement on the Classification of Tremors and recommended revisions in classification based on clinical characteristics (axis 1) and etiology (axis 2: acquired, genetic, or idiopathic). Axis 1 includes historical features (age at onset, family history, and temporal evolution), tremor characteristics (body distribution, activation condition), associated signs (systemic, neurologic), and laboratory tests (electrophysiology, imaging). This new classification involves more extensive aspects of tremors with opportunities for defining tremor syndromes, including action/rest tremors, focal tremors, task- and position-specific tremors, orthostatic tremors, tremors with prominent additional signs, and others. Detailed information is expected after more applications in the clinic setting.

ESSENTIAL TREMOR

ESSENTIALS OF DIAGNOSIS

► Core criteria:
  ► Isolated postural or kinetic action tremor of bilateral upper limbs.
  ► At least 3 years' duration.
  ► Absence of other neurologic signs, such as dystonia, ataxia, or parkinsonism.
► Exclusion criteria of essential tremor.
  ► Isolated focal tremors (voice, head).
  ► Orthostatic tremor with a frequency >12 Hz.
  ► Task- and position-specific tremors.
  ► Sudden onset and stepwise deterioration.

Table 44–4. Classification of tremors (based on activation conditions).

Category	Tremor Characteristics	Medical Conditions
Action tremor		
Postural tremor	Occurs when a body part (limb) is maintaining a posture against the force of gravity (4–12 Hz[a]) Position independent Position dependent	(Enhanced) physiologic tremor: most common tremor Essential tremor (second most common) Orthostatic tremor Writing tremor Musician's tremor Psychogenic tremor Cerebellar tremor Rubral tremor Neuropathic tremor Dystonic tremor
Kinetic: Simple kinetic tremor	Occurs with voluntary but non–target-directed movement of extremities (3–10 Hz)	For example, tremor throughout pronation-supination or flexion-extension wrist movement, waiving hand at a slow speed
Intention tremor	Occurs with target-directed movement (finger-to-nose) (<5 Hz),	Cerebellar and cerebellar outflow tract disease: eg, MS, trauma, stroke tumor, vascular, Wilson, drugs, toxins, rubral tremor
Task-specific kinetic tremor	Involves task-specific, skilled, highly learned motor acts (eg, writing, sewing, playing musical instruments) (5–7 Hz)	Primary writing tremor, musician's tremor
Isometric tremor	Occurs with muscle contraction against a stationary object (eg, squeezing examiner's fingers) (4–6 Hz)	
Rest tremor	Frequency: low to medium (3–6 Hz)	Parkinsonism (third most common) Rubral (midbrain) tremor Wilson disease: 5–40 years of age, wing-beating tremor Severe essential tremor
Miscellaneous		Myoclonus Convulsions Asterixis Fasciculation Clonus Psychogenic: abrupt onset, different tremor features, absence of neurologic findings, psychiatric history Tremors exaggerated by medication: atorvastatin, albuterol, caffeine, stimulant, metoclopramide, corticosteroids, fluoxetine, haloperidol, hypoglycemic agents, thyroid hormones, etc

[a]Hz, hertz; the number of tremor cycles per second.

General Considerations

Essential tremor (ET) is the most common pathologic MD. It starts at a mean age of 45 years and affects approximately 4% of those age >40 years, and the prevalence increases with age. It affects both males and females. ET is a chronic and slowly progressive disorder with both upper extremities most commonly affected. It is postural and kinetic in nature and can be disabling and affect quality of life. ET is considered to be associated with GABAergic dysfunction in a cortico-thalamo-olivo-cerebellar circuit as a result of genetic and/or environmental toxins. Family aggregation is noted in more than half of patients and seems to follow an autosomal dominant pattern of inheritance. Linkage of genes on chromosomal regions 13q13 (ETM1 [ET monogenetic locus]), 2p24.1 (ETM2), and 6p23 to ET and their and other genetic clinical significance need to be further investigated. Environmental factors such as β-carboline alkaloids, which include harmine and harmane, may also play a role in the development of ET.

Clinical Findings

A. Symptoms and Signs

ET is diagnosed based on its clinical features compiled through a detailed medical history regarding tremor, family history, social history (alcohol, caffeine, and drug use), and medications, as well as a thorough physical examination. The tremor typically starts from both hands or forearms (~95%) or less commonly from one hand (usually dominant) in 10–15% of cases, with upper extremity involvement as the initial presentation. The tremor can be postural, occurring with outstretched arms, or kinetic, occurring during action such as finger-to-nose movement, pouring and drinking water from a cup, writing, or drawing Archimedean spirals. With more advanced age, the tremor will be slower but have greater amplitude, which can be more disabling. Other parts of the body can be affected concomitantly with hand tremor, such as head (34%), legs (30%), voice (12%), chin, tongue, or trunk. Isolated head and isolated voice tremors can exclude ET diagnosis. The patient may present with head shaking (no-no) or nodding (yes-yes), a shaky or trembling voice, or an unsteady gait (eg, tandem gait disturbance). Ethanol reduces tremor in two-thirds of cases with prompt improvement within 15 minutes. Many tremor scales are available for assessing severity, for example, the tremor rating scale from the Washington Heights–Inwood Genetic Study of Essential Tremor (score 0–5) and the Fahn-Tolosa-Marin tremor rating scale (score 0–40). In Table 44–5, the classic phenomena of ET are described and contrasted with features of tremor resulting from other physiologic and pathologic causes. *ET plus* diagnosis is considered in ET with additional neurologic signs such as impaired tandem gait, memory impairment, questionable dystonic posturing, or other nonspecific signs. Typical ET of <3 years in duration can be followed as indeterminate tremor.

B. Laboratory and Other Tests

Routine laboratory tests such as thyroid function; liver function; electrolytes, including calcium, magnesium, and phosphorous; and blood glucose level may be ordered. Other lab tests or imaging studies should be ordered according to each clinical scenario. In patients whose tremor started before age 40 years, serum ceruloplasmin and 24-hour urine copper levels should be checked to rule out Wilson disease. Physiologic studies such as electromyography and accelerometry are available in specialized labs. They are not part of the routine evaluation but can assist with atypical tremor diagnosis and measure tremor severity and its influence on patients by assessing frequency, rhythmicity, and amplitude of the tremor.

Nonmotor Complications

ET is not as benign as once believed. It can cause substantial physical, cognitive, and psychosocial disability. Patients may lose or have to quit their jobs owing to the uncontrollable tremor and memory and other cognitive impairments. Activities of daily living, as simple as drinking and eating, are significantly affected. The impact of ET on the patient's physical, psychological, and social health status needs to be assessed from the patient's point of view. The health-related quality-of-life evaluation for activities of daily living abilities is also essential to management.

Nonmotor, cognitive-neuropsychological presentations of ET also contribute to the patient's health status and may influence functional disability. Depression, anxiety, low vigor, mild executive dysfunction, possible mild cognitive impairment, and personality changes are some of the nonmotor manifestations of ET. Patients with late onset are more likely to have dementia. A disease-specific questionnaire, for example, the Quality of Life in Essential Tremor Questionnaire, will assist in a comprehensive evaluation of ET to improve management and quality of life.

Treatment

The goal of ET treatment is to decrease functional disability and improve the patient's health status and quality of life. Treatment may be initiated when symptoms are present. Both pharmacologic and surgical approaches are available. The response to medical treatment varies; some patients may not benefit from any medications or have only a partial response. Propranolol and primidone are recommended as initial therapy in ET, either alone or in combination (Table 44–6). In medically refractory patients, patients with disabling ET, or patients unable to tolerate medical treatment, DBS of the thalamus and unilateral thalamotomy have shown marked improvement of tremor. DBS of the ventral intermediate thalamic nucleus has fewer adverse events than thalamotomy and is reversible.

Physical or occupational therapy with lightweight training of wrists may help improve hand stability and function. Behavioral management is important to help ET patients deal with decreased function and social embarrassment.

Prognosis

ET is a slowly progressive disorder with a potential 7% increase in tremor amplitude each year. More than two-thirds of patients reported significant changes in their daily living and socializing, and approximately 15% were seriously disabled, more notably men, in a longitudinal, prospective study. Complications secondary to difficulty in ambulating, falls, pneumonia, and other functional disabilities may contribute to increased mortality.

Bhatia KP, Bain P, Bajaj N, et al. Consensus statement on the classification of tremors. From the Task Force on Tremor of the International Parkinson and Movement Disorder Society. *Mov Disord.* 2018;33(1):75–87. [PMID: 29193359]

Crawford P, Zimmerman EE. Tremor: sorting through the differential diagnosis. *Am Fam Physician.* 2018;97(3):180–186. [PMID: 29431985]

Table 44–5. Clinical and differential diagnosis of tremors.

Tremor	Clinical Features	Diagnostic Tests and Management
Essential tremor	An 8- to 12-Hz tremor is seen in young adults and a 6- to 8-Hz tremor in elderly people; there are negative neurologic signs with normal muscle tone and coordination, worsening with stress, fatigue, and voluntary movement; improves with alcohol ingestion	Only for differential diagnosis or atypical presentations
Enhanced physiologic tremor	High frequency, 8–12 Hz, lower amplitude; involves hands; occurs under various conditions, eg, stress, caffeine intake, fatigue, hypoglycemia, thyroid and adrenal gland disorders, alcohol withdrawal, and medication use; no other neurologic signs; responsive to offending medication or toxin reduction or removal, treatment of endocrine disorders, and stress management	Chemistry profile (glucose, liver function tests); thyroid function tests; review of medications; propranolol prior to stressful events may help
Neurodegenerative disease: Parkinson disease Others	Late age onset; asymmetric; slow (4–7 Hz), high amplitude, rest tremor; pill-rolling; subsides with voluntary movement; additional parkinsonian symptoms Clinical characteristics of multiple system atrophy, progressive supranuclear palsy, spinocerebellar ataxias, corticobasal degeneration, Wilson disease, genes causing Fahr disease, fragile X–associated tremor/ataxia syndrome	See text Illness specific, such as liver function tests; serum ceruloplasmin; urine copper; slit-lamp examination for Kayser-Fleischer rings for Wilson disease
Cerebellar tremor	Intentional tremor on the ipsilateral side of the body; <5 Hz; positive ataxia; dysmetria; nystagmus; other cerebellar signs	Appropriate imaging and other tests
Orthostatic tremor, primary	Occurs exclusively while standing (13–18 Hz); late onset; rare family history; tremor limited to legs and paraspinal muscles; differentiate from the tremor associated with dementia, Parkinson disease, and spinocerebellar ataxia	Electromyographic confirmation of tremor frequency Response to gabapentin, pramipexole, and clonazepam
Neuropathic tremor	Associated with peripheral nerve pathology, eg, hereditary neuropathies, Guillain-Barré syndrome, chronic inflammatory demyelinating polyneuropathy; not responsive to propranolol or other therapy	
Psychogenic/functional tremor	Inconsistent, sudden onset, and widely fluctuating tremor; distractibility; somatization in past history; tremor changes with voluntary movement of contralateral limb	Electrophysiologic testing
Infectious/inflammatory diseases	Multiple sclerosis, encephalitis lethargica, subacute sclerosing panencephalitis, human immunodeficiency virus, tuberculosis, syphilis, measles, typhus, encephalitis	Illness-specific tests and studies.
Task-specific intention tremors	Involves skilled, highly learned motor acts, eg, writing, sewing, playing musical instrument (5–7 Hz)	Treatment: botulinum toxin injection; surgery effective; oral medicine less effective
Toxins and drugs	Mercury, lead, manganese, arsenic, cyanide, toluene, etc Anticonvulsants: valproate, carbamazepine, phenytoin Tetrabenazine, antidepressants, sympathomimetics, bronchodilator, β_2-agonists, lithium, neuroleptics, metoclopramide, amiodarone, thyroid hormone, anticancer drugs, substance withdrawal	

Hopfner F, Helmich RC. The etiology of essential tremor: genes versus environment. *Parkinsonism Relat Disord.* 2018;46(Suppl 1): S92–S96. [PMID: 28735798]

Louis ED. Diagnosis and management of tremor. *Am Acad Neurol.* 2016;22(4):1143–1158. [PMID: 27495202]

Louis ED. Essential tremor. *Clin Geriatr Med.* 2006;22:843–857. [PMID: 17000339]

Louis ED, Benito-León J, Ottman R, et al. A population-based study of mortality in essential tremor. *Neurology.* 2007;69: 1982–1989. [PMID: 18025392]

Louis ED, Ford B, Lee H, et al. Diagnostic criteria for essential tremor: a population perspective. *Arch Neurol.* 1998;55: 823–828. [PMID: 9626774]

Shah B. Essential tremor: a comprehensive overview. *J Neurol Disord.* 2017;5:343. [No PMID]

Zesiewicz TA, Elble RJ, Louis ED, et al. AAN evidence-based guideline update: treatment of essential tremor: report of the Quality Standards Subcommittee of the American Academy of Neurology. *Neurology.* 2011;77(19):1752–1755. [PMID: 22013182]

Table 44–6. Pharmacotherapy for essential tremor.

Class/Drug	Usual Daily Dosage	Clinical Use and Side Effects
α-Adrenergic blockers Propranolol (A[a])	Starting dose 20 mg twice a day Optimal: 160–320 mg/d Long acting with better effect	50% improvement Well tolerated; titrate every 3–7 d Fatigue, mild to moderate bradycardia and reduced blood pressure, exertional dyspnea, depression
Anticonvulsants (GABA receptor) Primidone (A[a])	25–750 mg/d (divided 3 times a day); should be tapered off after 6 months use for suicide thought side effects	50a75% response rate Tolerance may develop Sedation, fatigue, unsteadiness, vomiting, acute toxic reaction, ataxia, vertigo 33–77% improvement in patients who failed first line treatment
Gabapentin (B[a])	100–1800 mg/d	For moderate to severe essential tremor (B[a]) Drowsiness, nausea, dizziness, unsteadiness 22–37% improvement
Topiramate (B[a])	25–300 mg/d	Dizziness, ataxia, somnolence, depression, nausea, weight loss, paresthesia
Benzodiazepines (GABA receptor) Alprazolam (B[a])	0.125–3 mg/d	Sedation and cognitive slowing; potential for abuse May be effective in those who failed first-line treatment. 25–35% improvement
Clonazepam (C[a])	0.5–4 mg/d	Efficacy varies; 26–71% improvement Withdrawal following abrupt discontinuation
Botulinum toxin injection (C[a]) For hand/head/voice tremor		Produces focal weakness; reduces tremor effectively but may not improve function; postinjection pain Significant clinical improvement but no statistical significance

[a]*Level of evidence:* A—at least one high-quality meta-analysis, systematic review of randomized controlled trials (RCTs), or RCT with a very low risk of bias and directly applicable to the target population; B—high-quality systematic reviews of case-control or cohort studies, and high-quality case-control or cohort studies with a very low risk of confounding or bias and a high probability that the relation is causal and that the studies are directly applicable to the target population and with overall consistency of results; C—well-conducted case-control or cohort studies with a low risk of confounding or bias and a moderate probability that the relation is causal and that the studies are directly applicable to the target population and with overall consistency of results; D—nonanalytic studies: case reports, case series, or expert analysis.

TIC DISORDERS: TOURETTE SYNDROME

ESSENTIALS OF DIAGNOSIS

► Two or more motor tics and one or more vocal tics are present (not necessarily concurrent).

► The tics occur many times a day nearly every day over >1 year without a tic-free period of >3 consecutive months.

► Disease onset before age 18 years.

► Other causes of tics ruled out (eg, substance use, stimulants, Huntington disease, CNS infection, stroke).

► General Considerations

Tourette syndrome (TS) is a complex chronic neuropsychiatric disorder. It affects 0.4–3.8% of children 5–18 years of age. Tics typically start early, at 2–5 years of age, and peak around 9–12 years; the severity improves at the end of adolescence. Simple and transient tics are common in children, with 6–20% affected. The mean age of onset is approximately 7 years, with males affected 3–4 times more often than females. Both genetic (research to identify genes is in process) and environmental factors (eg, psychological stress, postinfection autoimmune disease, intrauterine exposure, fetal or neonatal hypoxia, and androgen influences) play a role in the development of TS. Abnormal dopaminergic signaling and the noradrenergic and serotoninergic systems may be involved in the TS pathophysiologic process.

Clinical Findings

A. Symptoms and Signs

Tics are sudden, brief (0.5–1 second), uncontrollable, repetitive, nonrhythmic, stereotyped, and purposeless movements (motor tics) or vocalizations (vocal tics). Tics can be either simple, such as blinking, grimacing, head jerking, shoulder shrugging, and throat clearing or other meaningless utterances/noises, or more coordinated and purposeful complex features, such as jumping, kicking, abdomen thrusting, stuttering, echolalia (involuntary repetition of other people's words), echopraxia (imitating others' gestures), and coprolalia (involuntary speaking obscenities). Ninety percent of patients with TS have premonitory sensations or unpleasant somatosensory urges (burning, tingling, itching, or pain) preceding tics. They are relieved by the execution of tics.

Tics are the only positive findings on neurologic examination in TS. They usually start in the upper body, especially the eyes or other parts of the face, in the form of simple motor or vocal tics. As TS gradually progresses, the tics can involve other parts of the body such as the extremities and torso, where they will become complex in nature and vary in type and combination, severity, and location. The phenotype of TS involves not only tics but also behavioral components and commonly associated comorbidities (Table 44–7). Frustrated or embarrassed by the involuntary and sometimes disabling tics and comorbidities, together with the misconception of family and others that tics can be controlled, patients may develop anxiety, depression, or even social withdrawal, which impairs academic and social performance. Comorbid conditions include obsessions such as repeatedly counting, hand washing, or touching, and the need to scratch out a word. The socially inappropriate behaviors and self-injurious behaviors are common and difficult to treat. A comprehensive physiopsychosocial evaluation (eg, Yale Global Tic Severity Scale, Global Assessment of Functioning, Health-Related Quality of Life Scale, Child Behavior Checklist, or Youth Self-Report) is necessary for children with tics. In TS, the obsessions are usually thoughts of violence, sex, and aggression, with compulsive actions of touching self/others, symmetry, and ordering. Comorbid attention deficit/hyperactivity disorder (ADHD) may impact cognitive performance. A neuropsychological assessment may be considered. Coping strategies for the patient, family, and teachers need to be explored.

B. Laboratory and Other Test Findings

TS is a clinical diagnosis based on a thorough personal and family history, physical examination, and close observation of the disease process. Laboratory tests, electroencephalogram (EEG), and brain imaging studies (CT, MRI, or positron emission tomography [PET]) may be considered to rule out infections or other neurologic conditions that can either cause tics or mimic tics.

Differential Diagnosis

Other medical conditions that may cause tics or be misdiagnosed as tics need to be ruled out before starting treatment. Tics may be mistaken for other hyperkinetic MDs such as chorea, myoclonus, dystonia, tardive dyskinesia, seizure, periodic limb movements of sleep, and restless leg syndrome. Tics can also be caused by other medical conditions such as stroke, infections, dystonia, ET, and dementia.

Treatment

The goal of TS treatment is to control disabling symptoms and comorbidities; improve academic, occupational, or social performance and quality of life; and support patient and family. It is important to prioritize treatment to the most bothersome symptoms and to achieve symptom control to the level at which the patient can function. Patients and families need to realize that complete resolution of symptoms is difficult to achieve. TS with mild symptoms that do not interfere with the patient's daily functioning can be followed clinically without medical treatment.

A. Medical Treatment

Medication treatment should be started only when tics and comorbidities are causing social, emotional, academic,

Table 44–7. Tourette syndrome phenotype and comorbidities.

Tic Component	Simple or Complex Features
Socially inappropriate behaviors	Coprophenomena (coprolalia, mental coprolalia, copropraxia) Echophenomena (echolalia, echopraxia) Paliphenomena (palilalia, palipraxia) spitting, hitting and kicking, self-injury
Compulsive behaviors	Forced touching, repetitive looking at objects, other ritualized behaviors
Comorbidities (90%[a])	ADHD (60%[a]) Obsessive-compulsive behaviors and OCD (50%[a]) Autism spectrum disorder (ASD) Depression Anxiety Hostility Learning disability (20%[a]) Problems with executive planning, organization, and social problem solving

[a]Percentage of the comorbidity in patients diagnosed with Tourette syndrome.
ADHD, attention deficit/hyperactivity disorder; OCD, obsessive-compulsive disorder.

Table 44–8. Pharmacotherapy for Tourette syndrome (TS).

Class	Drug	Clinical Use and Adverse Effects
Nondopaminergic		
α_2-Adrenergic receptor agonists	Clonidine (oral, transdermal)	Initial treatment of TS, helps with ADHD symptoms Sedation, bradycardia, orthostatic hypotension, and constipation Withdrawal: taper over 7–10 days
	Guanfacine	Lightheadedness, fatigue, insomnia, stomachache, irritability. Better tolerated.
GABAergic receptor agonist	Baclofen	Treatment of spasticity
Others	Topiramate Botulinum toxin A Lorazepam	Headache and diarrhea
Dopaminergic blockade		Up to 70% tic reduction Neuroleptic malignant syndrome (NMS), dyskinesia, excessive sedation Metabolic abnormalities, type 2 diabetes, weight gain, hyperprolactinemia, cardio-vascular disease; monitor BMI, BP, liver function, cholesterol, and blood sugar
Typical antipsychotics	Pimozide (calcium channel blocker)	Less dyskinesia and sedation Arrhythmia and prolonged QTc
	Haloperidol Fluphenazine	Effective but higher side effect profile; orthostatic hypotension Increased BP, no QTc change
Atypical antipsychotics	Olanzapine, etc	Better side effect profile than typical antipsychotics
Benzamides	D_2-blocking agents: tiapride, sulpiride, amisulpride	5-HT$_3$ and 5-HT$_4$ blocking Not available in the United States
Benzodiazepine	Clonazepam	Use is limited by increasing tolerance and side effects.

ADHD, attention deficit/hyperactivity disorder; BMI, body mass index; BP, blood pressure.

physical stresses. α_2-Agonists are the current first-line treatment (Table 44–8). They may help reduce tics by approximately 30% and can improve comorbid ADHD symptoms. Antipsychotics are the most effective medication in treating TS, but because of their potential side effects of dopamine blockade, they are usually reserved for moderate to severe TS and after trial of other medications (α_2-agonists, topiramate, baclofen, botulinum toxin A, and tetrabenazine). They can reduce the severity of tics by 25–50%. Acute dystonic reactions may occur with initiation of these agents. Anticholinergics can be added to decrease their risk. Tardive dyskinesia may develop during antipsychotic treatment and is not always reversible after treatment is discontinued. Pergolide, tetrabenazine, and topiramate are also effective in decreasing tics. Stimulants or SSRIs may be started for ADHD, OCD, and other comorbidities.

B. Behavioral Therapy and Counseling

Habit reversal therapy through awareness training and competing response practice is as effective as antipsychotics and supportive therapy. Assertiveness training, cognitive therapy, relaxation therapy, and habit reversal therapy are widely used to improve patients' social functioning and the undesirable behaviors associated with tics. Education should be provided to the family and at school to create a supportive and understanding environment and decrease misconceptions and intolerance.

C. Other Therapies

Botulinum toxin injection and DBS are available for medically refractory tics. Omega-3, *N*-acetylcysteine, ningdong granule, and 5-ling granule may be effective as complementary treatment.

► Prognosis

Tics typically wax and wane, with the most severe tics occurring in children between 8 and 12 years of age. Many patients will experience significant improvement by the age of 18 in motor tics. However, if tics persist into adulthood (20%), TS can cause severe behavioral and social dysfunction. The psychopathologic symptoms worsen with age.

Cath DC, Hedderly T, Ludolph AG, et al. European clinical guidelines for Tourette syndrome and other tic disorders. Part I: assessment. *Eur Child Adolesc Psychiatr.* 2011;20:155–171. [PMID: 21445723]

Quezada J, Coffman KA. Current approaches and new developments in the pharmacological management of Tourette syndrome. *CNS Drugs.* 2018;32(1):33–45. [PMID: 29335879]

Robertson MM. Tourette syndrome in children and adolescents: aetiology, presentation and treatment. *Br J Psych Adv.* 2016;22:165–175. [No PMID]

Robertson MM, Althoff RR, Hafez A, et al. Principal components analysis of a large cohort with Tourette syndrome. *Br J Psychiatr.* 2008;193:31–36. [PMID: 18700215]

Website

Tourette Association of America. https://tourette.org/. Accessed November 25, 2019.

RESTLESS LEGS SYNDROME

ESSENTIALS OF DIAGNOSIS

► Core criteria:
  ► An urge to move the legs, usually accompanied by uncomfortable and unpleasant sensations in the legs.
  ► The urge to move the legs and unpleasant sensations beginning or worsening during periods of rest or inactivity such as lying down or sitting.
  ► The urge to move the legs and unpleasant sensations that are partially or totally relieved by movement, such as walking or stretching, as least as long as the activity continues.
  ► The urge to move the legs and unpleasant sensations during rest or inactivity only occur or are worse in the evening or at night than during the day.
  ► The occurrence of the above features is not solely accounted for as symptoms primary to another medical or a behavioral condition (eg, myalgia, venous stasis, leg edema, arthritis, leg cramps, positional discomfort, habitual foot tapping).
► Supportive features:
  ► Family history of restless legs syndrome (RLS).
  ► Positive response to dopaminergic therapy.
  ► Occurrence of periodic leg movements (PLMs) in sleep (PLMS) or during wakefulness (PLMW).

► Additional diagnostic criteria for children aged 2–12 years:
  ► Children must express leg discomfort in their own words, for example, tickle, bugs, or feeling shaky.
  ► Have two of the following: sleep disturbance, parent with definite RLS, and elevated periodic limb movement index on polysomnography.

General Considerations

RLS is a chronic neurologic sensorimotor disorder with a prevalence of 5–10% in the adult population; it affects approximately 2% of children age 8–17 years. It affects 12 million people in the United States, with a 2:1 female predominance, and it is also more severe in females. Primary RLS is idiopathic and occurs sporadically, but it demonstrates a strong genetic component with familial inheritance (60%). Pathogenesis of RLS is unclear and is considered to be related to low brain iron and the subcortical dopaminergic system. Several genes for RLS have been identified. Secondary RLS can be associated with other medical conditions such as anemia (iron, vitamin B_{12}/folate deficiency), thyroid problems, diabetes, kidney failure, peripheral neuropathy, ADHD, fibromyalgia, rheumatoid arthritis, Sjögren syndrome, pregnancy, ataxia, and PD. Medications and substances that can aggravate RLS symptoms include antinausea drugs (prochlorperazine, metoclopramide), anticonvulsants (phenytoin, droperidol), antipsychotic drugs (haloperidol), tricyclic and SSRI antidepressants, and over-the-counter cold and allergy medications, as well as caffeine, alcohol, and tobacco.

Clinical Findings

A. Symptoms and Signs

Diagnosis of RLS is based on a detailed history, including symptoms, medications, family history, and a thorough neurologic evaluation. The International RLS Study Group (IRLSSG) published and refined essential diagnostic criteria as listed at the beginning of the section. Its typical presentation includes unpleasant sensations due to paresthesias and dysesthesias (burning, itching, tingling, cramping, or aching, but no pain) deep in the legs (calves), which subside only with voluntary movement of the legs. The sensation may present on only one side of the body and may move to another part of the body. The motor restlessness occurs with the urge to relieve the sensation, and the patient may move voluntarily with repetitive stereotypical movements such as pacing, rocking, and stretching. Patients with RLS usually have sleep disturbances, such as difficulty falling asleep or maintaining sleep, leg movement during sleep, and daytime fatigue. PLMS and PLMW are stereotyped, repetitive movements with dorsiflexion of the ankles or big toes. Abnormal physical findings and positive test results may be due to associated conditions in secondary RLS. Smoking, alcohol consumption, poor sleep hygiene, and fatigue may aggravate symptoms of RLS. The IRLSSG Rating Scale can be used for evaluation of RLS severity and response to treatment.

B. Laboratory and Other Test Findings

A complete blood count, ferritin iron level, electrolytes, glucose level, thyroid hormone, and kidney function should be ordered. PLMS can be assessed and monitored by the International Restless Leg Syndrome Scale. Polysomnography is not routinely ordered. It may be considered when the presentation is not diagnostic for RLS, there is suboptimal response to treatment, or other nocturnal conditions such as sleep apnea are suspected.

▶ Differential Diagnosis

Among the many medical conditions that need to be differentiated from RLS, polyneuropathy is the most commonly encountered. The sensory symptoms of polyneuropathy do not improve with movement, and there will be positive findings from the neurologic examination, nerve biopsy, and neurophysiologic examination. The differential diagnosis includes nocturnal leg cramps (with intense foot or calf pain lasting seconds to 10 minutes and resolving spontaneously), obstructive sleep apnea syndrome, intermittent claudication, pathophysiologic insomnia, TS, REM sleep behavior disorder, and orthostatic tremor. Renal comorbidities and diuretics may complicate leg cramps and need to be monitored. Augmentation, or worsening symptoms of RLS, is a common complication of RLS treatment with dopaminergic agents. When augmentation happens, the time of symptoms onset starts 2 or more hours earlier than usual starting time before or in early treatment. The RLS sensory and motor symptoms spread to other body parts or with paradoxical response (symptoms worsen with increased dosage of treatment and lessen with decreased dosage). The treatment effect may become shorter. Augmentation from treatment needs to be differentiated from disease progression of RLS; presence of other aggregating factors, such as sleep deprivation, alcohol use, iron deficiency, or medications; and tolerance to treatment or end-of-dose response (symptoms present in early morning).

▶ Treatment

The goal of RLS treatment is to minimize the unpleasant sensations and motor restlessness, reduce sleep disturbance, and improve quality of life.

A. Nonpharmacotherapy

Identify any conditions that may cause or aggravate RLS, such as offensive medications, caffeine, smoking, and excessive alcohol consumption. Give iron supplementation when ferritin is low and vitamin supplementation. Monitor kidney function. A healthy lifestyle will help alleviate RLS with moderate daily exercise, leg movement and massage, and hot baths. Cognitive behavioral and exercise therapy are under investigation.

B. Pharmacotherapy

Medications should be started when patients are experiencing daily symptoms that are affecting their quality of life. The nonergot DAs ropinirole and pramipexole are the medications of choice for primary RLS (high evidence). DAs are 70–90% effective in relieving symptoms. They can be administered 1–3 hours before the onset of symptoms, and their effect is immediate. Adverse effects include nausea, peripheral edema, daytime somnolence, and impulsivity. L-dopa (high evidence) is fast acting and can be taken 1–2 hours before symptoms start. However, augmentation may develop with long-term use or high doses (>200 mg) of dopaminergic medications, especially carbidopa/L-dopa. It is recommended for treatment of intermittent RLS. L-dopa is less favored as an initial medication than DAs because of its motor side effects as well as augmentation. Gabapentin enacarbil (the prodrug of gabapentin), gabapentin, and pregabalin are effective in RLS treatment. Other medications such as clonidine, bupropion, tramadol, carbamazepine, valproic acid, topiramate, methadone, clonazepam, and zolpidem are under investigation. Table 44–9 lists the effective medications for RLS treatment. Oral iron treatment may reduce RLS symptoms in patients with iron deficiency or refractory RLS (minimal evidence).

Monitoring of RLS augmentation is necessary for all dopaminergic agents. There are limited data on its management. To prevent augmentation, avoiding prolonged use of dopaminergic agents with dosage as low as possible may help, but augmentation has been reported to develop after a couple of months of starting the treatment at any dosage. A nondopaminergic agent can be added. Daily treatment should be deferred as long as possible and start with intermittent treatment. Long-acting DA may cause less augmentation (may gradually wean off current L-dopa). A2δ ligands may be considered as first-line treatment. RLS exacerbating factors need to be eliminated. If ferritin level is <50–75 μg/mL or transferrin saturation is <20%, oral or intravenous iron supplement should be provided. A good history should include enquiring about recent lifestyle changes such as sleep deprivation, alcohol/caffeine use, or new medications (dopamine antagonists, antihistamines, antidepressants). A 10-day washout after gradually weaning off dopamine medication, with a drug-free period of 10 days as tolerated by patients, may allow evaluation of the severity of RLS and transition to another medication.

Table 44–9. Pharmacotherapy for restless legs syndrome (RLS).

Class	Drug	Clinical Use and Adverse Effects
Dopaminergic agents	Levodopa[a]	Also can use in RLS with hemodialysis
Non–ergot-derived dopamine agonists		Long-acting form available
	Rotigotine[a]	3-mg transdermal patch for moderate to severe symptoms
	Ropinirole[a]	4 mg, less hypersomnolence
	Pramipexole[a]	0.5–0.75 mg
		May be less effective in moderate to severe symptoms
a2d Ligands		Dizziness, somnolence, headache; lower dose in geriatrics
	Pregabalin	
	Gabapentin enacarbil	Efficacious at a dose of 1200 mg
	Gabapentin	May use with other medications
Opioids		For short-term treatment only
		Dizziness, nausea, urinary retention, constipation, addictive potential
	Oxycodone-naloxone	For severe treatment-resistant RLS
	Oxycodone	For significant daily symptoms and pain syndromes (use with other nonopioid medications)
		Monitor sleep-related respiratory problems
Antidepressants		
	Bupropion	

[a]Monitoring for augmentation required.

Allen RP, Picchietti D, Hening WA, et al. Restless legs syndrome: diagnostic criteria, special considerations, and epidemiology: a report from the restless legs syndrome diagnosis and epidemiology workshop at the National Institutes of Health. *Sleep Med.* 2003;4(2):101–119. [PMID: 14592341]

Ball E, Caivano CK. Internal medicine: guidance to the diagnosis and management of restless legs syndrome. *South Med J.* 2008;101:631–634. [PMID: 18475241]

Garcia-Borreguero D, Silber MH, Winkelman JW, et al. Guidelines for the first-line treatment of restless legs syndrome/Willis–Ekbom disease, prevention and treatment of dopaminergic augmentation: a combined task force of the IRLSSG, EURLSSG, and the RLS-foundation. *Sleep Med.* 2016;21:1–11. [PMID: 27448465]

Hallegraeff J, de Greef M, Krijnen W, et al. Criteria in diagnosing nocturnal leg cramps: a systematic review. *BMC Fam Pract.* 2017;18(1):29. [PMID: 28241802]

Hening WA, Allen RP. Restless legs syndrome (RLS): the continuing development of diagnostic standards and severity measures. *Sleep Med.* 2003;4(2):95–97. [PMID: 14592339]

Winkelmann J. Treatment of restless legs syndrome: evidence-based review and implications for clinical practice. *Mov Disord.* 2018;33(7):1077–1091. [PMID: 29756335]

Website

International RLS Study Group. Diagnostic criteria. http://irlssg.org/diagnostic-criteria/. Accessed November 25, 2019.

CHOREA

Chorea is an irregular, rapid, involuntary jerky movement that flows randomly to any part of the body. Multiple etiologies, such as Huntington disease (see next section), vascular disorders, electrolyte imbalance, medications (antiparkinsonian, anticonvulsants, cocaine, neuroleptics), infection (HIV, encephalitis), and autoimmune disorders (systemic lupus erythematosus, Sydenham chorea), have been identified as causing chorea by affecting the basal ganglia. Chorea usually affects the hands, feet, face (eg, nose wrinkling), and trunk. Laboratory tests may be ordered to differentiate the causes, such as throat culture and streptococcal blood antigen for Sydenham chorea, liver function tests, complement levels, antinuclear antibody, antiphospholipid antibody titers, thyroid-stimulating hormone, and electrolytes. Brain CT, MRI, and PET scan may also aid in diagnosis.

HUNTINGTON DISEASE

Huntington disease (HD) is an adult-onset (age 35–50 years), fully penetrant autosomal dominant progressive neurodegenerative disorder caused by a mutation with CAG trinucleotide repeats in the huntingtin gene (*HTT*) on chromosome 4. A mutant huntingtin protein, produced as the result of the *HTT*, causes neuron dysfunction in the basal ganglion, thalamus, cerebellum, and other areas of the brain. It affects approximately 1 in 10,000 people. Dopamine and glutamate neurotransmitters are thought to be affected. It is characterized by motor disturbance, cognitive decline, and psychiatric impairment. Its clinical features include early-stage hyperkinetic chorea, hypokinetic phage with dystonia, gait disturbance, dysarthria and dysphagia, eye movement disorders, and associated cognitive and behavioral disorders (dementia, depression, OCD, suicidal ideation). HD diagnosis is made based on positive family history, genetic testing, and motor symptoms defined by the Unified Huntington Disease Rating scale (UHDRS). The UHDRS measures the motor, cognitive, behavioral, and functional impairment in HD. MRI demonstrates intracranial changes in premanifest and clinical stages of HD.

Genetic confirmatory testing may be offered to patients with clear symptoms of HD and a family history of HD. Testing for fatal HD in individuals without symptoms but with a documented family history can cause enormous stress and emotional concerns. Genetic counseling before and after the test regarding implications of possible results and potential family, social, and ethical issues is important for informed decision making and patient and family support. Individuals who have a positive test result will experience a gradually increasing sense of hopelessness as the onset of the disease approaches. Some will suffer severe depression with suicidal ideation. They will demonstrate increased avoidance behaviors, and close monitoring is warranted.

Treatment is mainly symptomatic to control chorea, behavioral comorbidities (by means of antidepressants), and potential complications (rhabdomyolysis, local trauma from falls, and aspiration pneumonia). Tetrabenazine, a monoamine-depleting agent, is the only US Food and Drug Administration–approved drug for HD. It is likely effective in chorea control. Its serious side effects include depression, parkinsonism, prolonged QT interval, and neuroleptic malignant syndrome. Deutetrabenazine has a longer half-life and may have fewer side effects. Sulpiride is a neuroleptic and has been demonstrated to be effective in chorea management. Other neuroleptic medications commonly used include olanzapine, risperidone, and quetiapine. Antidepressants with serotonergic and noradrenergic effects can be used for depression. The effect of methylphenidate, amantadine, and bupropion for apathy needs to be further evaluated in randomized controlled trials. Preclinical preventive treatments are under investigation.

Supportive management and a multidisciplinary approach, including speech, physical, and occupational therapy, are important in maintaining patients' quality of life. Possible new HD treatments include HD genetic treatment and prevention of mutant huntingtin protein production.

Patients can be referred to several national support groups and organizations, including the Huntington Disease Society of America (http://www.hdsa.org) and the Hereditary Disease Foundation (http://www.hdfoundation.org/).

Armstrong MJ. Evidence-based guideline: pharmacologic treatment of chorea in Huntington disease. Report of the Guideline Development Subcommittee of the American Academy of Neurology. *Neurology*. 2012;79:597–603. [PMID: 22815556]

Kalman L, Johnson MA, Beck J, et al. Development of genomic reference materials for Huntington disease genetic testing. *Genet Med*. 2007;9:719–723. [PMID: 18073586]

McColgan P, Tabrizi SJ. Huntington's disease: a clinical review. *Eur J Neurol*. 2018;25:24–34. [PMID: 28817209]

Satija P, Ondo WG. Restless legs syndrome: pathophysiology, diagnosis and treatment. *CNS Drugs*. 2008;22:497–518. [PMID: 18484792]

Timman R, Roos R, Maat-Kievit A, Tibben A. Adverse effects of predictive testing for Huntington disease underestimated: long-term effects 7-10 years after the test. *Health Psychol*. 2004;23:189–197. [PMID: 15008664]

Websites

Huntington's Disease Society of America. http://www.hdsa.org. Accessed November 25, 2019.

Hereditary Disease Foundation. http://www.hdfoundation.org/. Accessed November 25, 2019.

OTHER MOVEMENT DISORDERS

▶ Dystonia

Dystonia is characterized by involuntary, sustained or intermittent, uncoordinated simultaneous agonist and antagonist muscle contractions, which result in repetitive twisting movements, or abnormal postures. It may affect all age groups from infancy to adult and affect one body region (*focal*) to trunk or two or more body regions (*generalized*). Dystonic movements are initiated or worsened with intentional movements and subside at the *null point*, when the affected muscle groups are placed at maximum of pull. Dystonic movements can be triggered by specific actions such as hand cramps with writing, called *task-specific dystonia*; or they can extend beyond the commonly affected body parts, called *overflow dystonia*. Mirror movements may be seen in unaffected extremities when repetitive tasks, such as writing or foot tapping, are performed in the most affected body side; in a more severe form than action dystonia, they can occur at rest, called *rest dystonia*. Finally, the movements become fixed postures or positions, referred to as *permanent contractures*. A sensory trick (*geste antagonistique*) may suppress dystonic movements by touching affected or adjunctive body parts, such as a scarf around the neck for cervical dystonia. Commercial genetic testing of the most common dystonic genes, *DYT-TOR1A* and *DYT-THAP1*, are available.

Combined dystonia is associated with other neurologic phenomena, such as myoclonus, PD, and ataxia; medication offenders (prochlorperazine, metoclopramide, antipsychotics, SSRIs, and serotonin-norepinephrine reuptake inhibitors); or medical conditions such as Wilson disease and GLUT1 deficiency.

The diagnosis of dystonia is based on history, typical clinical presentation, and neurologic examination. Imaging studies may have findings related to associated etiologies. Genetic counseling should be provided to patients and family before and after the testing.

Treatment of dystonia is aimed at underlying causes and symptom control. Medications that may cause dystonia should be evaluated. Carbidopa/L-dopa is used for dopa-responsive dystonia. It may be partially effective in idiopathic, genetic, or acquired dystonia. Anticholinergics (trihexyphenidyl), benzodiazepines, dopamine-depleting agents (tetrabenazine), and baclofen are also used in the treatment. Botulinum toxin injection is the first choice for most focal and segmental dystonias. DBS is the first-line surgical treatment for dystonia. A comprehensive approach to dystonia management includes physical therapy, such as stretching exercises and sensory tricks, to help maintain range of motion or interrupt muscle twisting and psychological supportive treatment.

Shanker V, Bressman SB. Diagnosis and management of dystonia. *Continuum (Minneap Minn)*. 2016;22(4):1227–1245. [PMID: 27495206]

▶ Myoclonus

Myoclonus refers to sudden, brief, jerklike, involuntary spasmodic movements of a muscle or a group of muscles. Positive myoclonus is due to involuntary muscular contractions; negative myoclonus (asterixis) is due to sudden brief loss of muscle tone. It is not preceded by an urge to move and not suppressible. It is not interrupted by a geste antagoniste such as in dystonia. The movements can be focal, segmental, axial, or generalized and arrhythmic, rhythmic, or oscillatory. Based on etiology, myoclonus can be classified into four categories. *Physiologic myoclonus* is a normal and benign movement that occurs commonly, such as hiccups, hypnic jerks, anxiety-induced or exercise-induced jerks, and benign infantile myoclonus with feeding. The movements are usually self-limited and not disabling. *Essential myoclonus* is a multifocal MD, which can be sporadic or hereditary in an autosomal dominant pattern (associated with dystonia). Even though myoclonic movements are the one abnormal clinical finding on neurologic examination, they occur more frequently at any time, affecting patients' daily lives. *Epileptic myoclonus* occurs with seizure activities and demonstrates EEG and electromyographic changes. *Secondary (symptomatic) myoclonus* is the most common type of myoclonus (~70%) and occurs as the result of central or peripheral nervous system insult or damage from a wide variety of medical conditions, which can be metabolic (inborn errors of metabolism, Hashimoto encephalopathy, hepatic failure, hyponatremia, renal failure), neurodegenerative (PD, HD), or due to trauma or infection (Lyme, arbovirus, Whipple), medications (eg, anesthetic agents, opiates, and anticonvulsants), autoimmune (celiac), or toxin exposure (pesticides, gases). Electrophysiologic studies (EEG/electromyography), MRI and transcranial magnetic stimulation can be employed for the diagnosis and to evaluate origin of myoclonus at cortical, subcortical, spinal, and peripheral levels. Laboratory investigations and genetic testing can be ordered based on suspected underlying conditions. Treatment of myoclonus is aimed at the secondary causes such as removal medications or correction of metabolic imbalances. Evidence for symptomatic treatment is disappointing. Different medications are used according to the level of the nervous system involved, such as levetiracetam and piracetam for cortical myoclonus; clonazepam is used in cortical, subcortical, and spinal myoclonus; botulinum toxin injection is used for spinal and peripheral myoclonus. Other medications have been used to control myoclonus, such as lamotrigine, rituximab, adrenocorticotropic hormone, valproic acid, gabapentin, and primidone. DBS may be effective in certain cases of myoclonus.

Borg M. Symptomatic myoclonus. *Neurophysiol Clin.* 2006;36: 309–318. [PMID: 17336775]

Chang VC. Myoclonus. *Curr Treat Options Neurol.* 2008;10: 222–229. [PMID: 18579026]

Dijk JM. Management of patients with myoclonus: available therapies and the need for an evidence-based approach. *Lancet Neurol.* 2010;9:1028–1036. [PMID: 20864054]

Mills K, Mari Z. An update and review of the treatment of myoclonus. *Curr Neurol Neurosci Rep.* 2015;15(1):512. [PMID: 25398378]

Appendix 1. MDS clinical diagnostic criteria for PD—executive summary/completion form.

The first essential criterion is parkinsonism, which is defined as bradykinesia, in combination with at least 1 of rest tremor or rigidity. Examination of all cardinal manifestations should be carried out as described in the MDS–Unified Parkinson Disease Rating Scale.[30] Once parkinsonism has been diagnosed:

Diagnosis of Clinically Established PD requires:

1. Absence of absolute exclusion criteria
2. At least two supportive criteria, and
3. No red flags

Diagnosis of Clinically Probable PD requires:

1. Absence of absolute exclusion criteria
2. Presence of red flags counterbalanced by supportive criteria

   If 1 red flag is present, there must also be at least 1 supportive criterion

   If 2 red flags, at least 2 supportive criteria are needed

   No more than 2 red flags are allowed for this category

Supportive criteria

(Check box if criteria met)

☐ 1. Clear and dramatic beneficial response to dopaminergic therapy. During initial treatment, patient returned to normal or near-normal level of function. In the absence of clear documentation of initial response a dramatic response can be classified as:

   a) Marked improvement with dose increases or marked worsening with dose decreases. Mild changes do not qualify. Document this either objectively (>30% in UPDRS III with change in treatment), or subjectively (clearly-documented history of marked changes from a reliable patient or caregiver).

   b) Unequivocal and marked on/off fluctuations, which must have at some point included predictable end-of-dose wearing off.

☐ 2. Presence of levodopa-induced dyskinesia

☐ 3. Rest tremor of a limb, documented on clinical examination (in past, or on current examination)

☐ 4. The presence of either olfactory loss or cardiac sympathetic denervation on MIBG scintigraphy

Absolute exclusion criteria: The presence of any of these features rules out PD:

☐ 1. Unequivocal cerebellar abnormalities, such as cerebellar gait, limb ataxia, or cerebellar oculomotor abnormalities (eg, sustained gaze evoked nystagmus, macro square wave jerks, hypermetric saccades)

☐ 2. Downward vertical supranuclear gaze palsy, or selective slowing of downward vertical saccades

☐ 3. Diagnosis of probable behavioral variant frontotemporal dementia or primary progressive aphasia, defined according to consensus criteria[31] within the first 5 y of disease

☐ 4. Parkinsonian features restricted to the lower limbs for more than 3 y

☐ 5. Treatment with a dopamine receptor blocker or a dopamine-depleting agent in a dose and time-course consistent with drug-induced parkinsonism

☐ 6. Absence of observable response to high-dose levodopa despite at least moderate severity of disease

☐ 7. Unequivocal cortical sensory loss (ie, graphesthesia, stereognosis with intact primary sensory modalities), clear limb ideomotor apraxia, or progressive aphasia

☐ 8. Normal functional neuroimaging of the presynaptic dopaminergic system

☐ 9. Documentation of an alternative condition known to produce parkinsonism and plausibly connected to the patient's symptoms, or, the expert evaluating physician, based on the full diagnostic assessment feels that an alternative syndrome is *more likely* than PD

Red flags

☐ 1. Rapid progression of gait impairment requiring regular use of wheelchair within 5 y of onset

☐ 2. A complete absence of progression of motor symptoms or signs over 5 or more y unless stability is related to treatment

☐ 3. Early bulbar dysfunction: severe dysphonia or dysarthria (speech unintelligible most of the time) or severe dysphagia (requiring soft food, NG tube, or gastrostomy feeding) within first 5 y

☐ 4. Inspiratory respiratory dysfunction: either diurnal or nocturnal inspiratory stridor or frequent inspiratory sighs

☐ 5. Severe autonomic failure in the first 5 y of disease. This can include:

   a) Orthostatic hypotension[32]—orthostatic decrease of blood pressure within 3 min of standing by at least 30 mm Hg systolic or 15 mm Hg diastolic, in the absence of dehydration, medication, or other diseases that could plausibly explain autonomic dysfunction, or

   b) Severe urinary retention or urinary incontinence in the first 5 y of disease (excluding long-standing or small amount stress incontinence in women), that is not simply functional incontinence. In men, urinary retention must not be attributable to prostate disease, and must be associated with erectile dysfunction

(Continued)

Appendix 1. MDS clinical diagnostic criteria for PD—executive summary/completion form. (*Continued*)

☐ 6. Recurrent (>1/y) falls because of impaired balance within 3 y of onset

☐ 7. Disproportionate anterocollis (dystonic) or contractures of hand or feet within the first 10 y

☐ 8. Absence of any of the common nonmotor features of disease despite 5 y disease duration. These include sleep dysfunction (sleep-maintenance insomnia, excessive daytime somnolence, symptoms of REM sleep behavior disorder), autonomic dysfunction (constipation, daytime urinary urgency, symptomatic orthostasis), hyposmia, or psychiatric dysfunction (depression, anxiety, or hallucinations)

☐ 9. Otherwise-unexplained pyramidal tract signs, defined as pyramidal weakness or clear pathologic hyperreflexia (excluding mild reflex asymmetry and isolated extensor plantar response)

☐ 10. Bilateral symmetric parkinsonism. The patient or caregiver reports bilateral symptom onset with no side predominance, and no side predominance is observed on objective examination

Criteria Application:

1. Does the patient have parkinsonism, as defined by the MDS criteria?   Yes ☐   No ☐

    If no, *neither* probable PD nor clinically established PD can be diagnosed. *If yes:*

2. Are any absolute exclusion criteria present?   Yes ☐   No ☐

    If "yes," *neither* probable PD nor clinically established PD can be diagnosed. *If no:*

3. Number of red flags present _____

4. Number of supportive criteria present _____

5. Are there at least 2 supportive criteria *and* no red flags?   Yes ☐   No ☐

    If yes, patient meets criteira for clinically established PD. *If no:*

6. Are there more than 2 red flags?   Yes ☐   No ☐

    If "yes," probable PD cannot be diagnosed. *If no:*

7. Is the number of red flags equal to, or less than, the number of supportive criteria?   Yes ☐   No ☐

    If yes, patient meets criteria for probable PD

Hearing & Vision Impairment in the Elderly

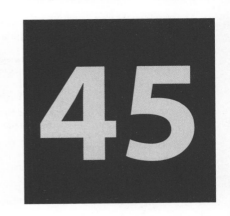

45

Archana M. Kudrimoti, MD

Saranne E. Perman, MD

Nathaniel D. Stewart, MD

Sensory impairment affects up to two-thirds of the geriatric population. Identification, evaluation, and treatment of these conditions (Table 45–1) may improve patients' quality and quantity of life. The impact of sensory impairments is significant. The same objective level of sensory function can result in different levels of disability depending on the needs and expectations of patients. Poor hearing is associated with depression as well as decreased quality of life; poor mental health; and decreased physical, social, and cognitive functioning. Vision impairment increases the risk of death and is associated with an elevated risk of falling and hip fracture, depression, medication errors, dependency, and problems with driving.

Research has yet to demonstrate that community-based screening of asymptomatic older people results in improvements in vision or hearing. The US Preventive Services Task Force (USPSTF) (2012) concluded that there is insufficient evidence to assess the balance of benefits and harms of screening for hearing loss in asymptomatic adults aged 50 years or older (I recommendation). The American Academy of Family Physicians (AAFP) recommends screening persons older than 60 years for hearing loss during periodic health examinations (Strength of Recommendation Taxonomy [SORT] C). AAFP and USPSTF concluded that there is inadequate direct evidence that screening for impairment of visual acuity by primary care physicians improves functional outcomes in the elderly, yet there is adequate evidence that early treatment of refractive error, cataracts, and age-related macular degeneration (AMD) improves or prevents loss of visual acuity.

COMMON CAUSES OF HEARING IMPAIRMENT IN THE ELDERLY

PRESBYCUSIS

 ESSENTIALS OF DIAGNOSIS

▶ Age-related high-frequency sensorineural hearing loss.
▶ Difficulty with speech discrimination.

▶ General Considerations

Presbycusis is the most common form of hearing loss in the elderly, although it often goes unrecognized. It occurs more frequently with advancing age and in patients with a positive family history. This multifactorial disorder is due to a combination of structural and neural degeneration and genetic predisposition. Risk factors for presbycusis include noise exposure, smoking, and medications such as aminoglycoside antibiotics, loop diuretics, and cardiovascular risk factors such as hypertension. Presbycusis is a diagnosis of exclusion.

▶ Prevention

Until the exact pathophysiology of presbycusis is understood, attempts at prevention will be limited. Limitation of noise exposure may reduce the hearing loss. Although several

Table 45–1. Differential diagnosis of geriatric hearing and vision impairment.[a]

Hearing Impairment	Vision Impairment
Presbycusis	**Presbyopia**
Cerumen impaction	**Age-related macular degeneration**
Noise-induced hearing loss	**Glaucoma**
Central auditory processing disorder	**Senile cataract**
Otosclerosis	**Diabetic retinopathy**
Chronic otitis media	Central retinal artery or vein occlusion
Glomus tumor or vascular anomaly	Posterior vitreous or retinal detachment
Cholesteatoma	Vitreous hemorrhage
Autoimmune hearing loss	Temporal arteritis
Perilymph fistula	Optic neuritis
Ménière disease	Corneal pathology
Acoustic neuroma	Iritis

[a]The most common causes are indicated in bold type.

studies have evaluated the role of vitamins, antioxidants, smoking cessation, and diet in preventing presbycusis, there have been no conclusive findings in humans.

▶ Clinical Findings

Patients with this disorder may present with a chief complaint of hearing loss and difficulty understanding speech. However, presbycusis is often diagnosed only after complaints are raised by close patient contacts or hearing loss is noted on routine screening in a patient without hearing-related complaints. The Hearing Handicap Inventory of the Elderly Screening Version (HHIE-S) is a widely accepted subjective screening tool for hearing disability. Abnormalities of the whisper test are found as the level of hearing loss increases. Older patients who report hearing loss can be referred directly for audiometry (SORT C).

An audiogram of a patient with presbycusis typically shows bilaterally symmetric high-frequency hearing loss. Magnetic resonance imaging with contrast is recommended for patients with idiopathic sudden-onset sensorineural hearing loss to evaluate for serious underlying pathology (SORT C).

▶ Treatment

The treatment of presbycusis consists of hearing rehabilitation, which often involves fitting for digital and analog types of hearing aids. Counseling should be provided because patient perceptions and expectations are the most important factors in obtaining and using hearing aids, and referral for assessment for assistive listening devices should be considered for patients who are unable to use hearing aids (SORT C).

Cochlear implantation is reserved for patients with profound hearing loss that is unresponsive to hearing aids. Additional tools include lip-reading classes; television closed captioning; sound-enhancing devices for concerts, church, or other public gatherings; and telephone amplifiers. A combined approach involving the patient, hearing loss specialist, family physician, and close contacts of the patient is likely to produce the best overall treatment plan.

▶ Prognosis

The expectation of slow progression of this hearing loss should be communicated to the patient. Complete deafness, however, is not typical of presbycusis.

NOISE-INDUCED HEARING LOSS

 ESSENTIALS OF DIAGNOSIS

▶ History of occupational or recreational noise exposure.

▶ Bilateral notch of sensorineural hearing loss between 3000 and 6000 Hz on audiogram.

▶ Problems with tinnitus, speech discrimination, and hearing in the presence of background noise.

▶ General Considerations

Noise-induced hearing loss is the second most common sensorineural hearing loss (Table 45–2) after presbycusis. Up to one-third of patients with hearing losses have some component of their deficit that is noise-induced. The degree of hearing loss is related to the level of noise and the duration of exposure. Excessive shear force from loud sounds or long exposure results in cell damage, cell death, and subsequent hearing loss.

▶ Prevention

Hearing protection programs are prevalent in industrial settings and typically include the use of earplugs, intermittent audiograms, and limiting exposure. Patient commitment to

Table 45–2. Causes of hearing loss.

Conductive Hearing Loss	Sensorineural Hearing Loss
Outer ear	**Inner ear**
Otitis externa	Presbycusis
Trauma	Noise exposure
Cerumen	Ménière disease
Osteoma	Ototoxic drugs
Exostosis	Meningitis
Squamous cell carcinoma	Viral cochleitis
	Barotraumas
Middle ear	Acoustic neuroma
Otitis media	Meningioma
Tympanic membrane perforation	Multiple sclerosis
Cholesteatoma	Vascular disease
Otosclerosis	
Glomus tumors	
Temporal bone trauma	
Paget disease	

the use of hearing protection is critical for the success of prevention programs.

Clinical Findings

Patients may present with tinnitus, decreased speech discrimination, and difficulty hearing when background noise is present. Patients identified through hearing protection programs may be asymptomatic. Results of the whisper test or office-based pure-tone audiometry may be normal or abnormal, depending on the degree of hearing loss.

Audiometric evaluation of noise-induced hearing loss reveals a bilateral notch of sensorineural hearing loss between 3000 and 6000 Hz.

Treatment

When prevention fails, treatment involves hearing rehabilitation, as previously outlined in the treatment of presbycusis. Education about the risks of loud noise exposure should begin when patients are young, because hearing loss can occur from significant recreational noise. The importance of adhering to hearing protection programs should also be emphasized.

Prognosis

Nothing can be done to reverse cell death from noise-induced hearing loss; however, some patients exposed to brief episodes of loud noise exhibit only hair cell injury and may recover hearing over time. These patients are more susceptible to noise-induced hearing loss on reexposure.

CERUMEN IMPACTION

ESSENTIALS OF DIAGNOSIS

▶ Mild, reversible conductive hearing loss.

▶ Cerumen buildup in ear canal, limiting sound transmission.

▶ Direct visualization of wax plug confirms diagnosis.

General Considerations

Impaction of wax in the external auditory canal is a common, frequently overlooked problem in the elderly. Removal of cerumen has been shown to significantly improve hearing ability. The incidence of cerumen impactions increases in the elderly population. Chronic skin changes lead to loss of normal migration of skin epithelium leading to exfoliated cell debris accumulation. Cerumen gland atrophy results in drier wax that is more likely to become trapped by the large tragi hairs in the external ear canal. The likelihood of impaction is increased by hearing aid or earplug use.

Prevention

Cerumen impactions may be prevented by the regular use of agents that soften wax. Readily available household agents such as water, mineral oil, cooking oils, hydrogen peroxide, or glycerin may be used. Commercially available ceruminolytic compounds, such as carbamide peroxide, triethanolamine polypeptide, and docusate sodium liquid, are also efficacious, but not more so than less expensive options. Patients should avoid using cotton swabs and ear candling to remove cerumen.

Clinical Findings

Patients presenting with cerumen impaction may complain of sudden or gradual hearing loss, tinnitus affecting one or both the ears, and interference with hearing aids. Examination of the external canal reveals partial or complete occlusion of the ear canal with cerumen.

Complications

Various removal methods are associated with ear discomfort and potential for ear canal trauma. Canal trauma can result in bleeding, canal swelling, or infection. Warm water should be used for ear irrigation, because cold water can induce vertigo.

Treatment

Routine treatment of asymptomatic patients is unnecessary. When the wax is soft, gentle irrigation of the canal with warm water may be sufficient to remove the offending material. In the case of firmer wax, ceruminolytic agents may be applied, followed by irrigation. Any cerumen remaining after these maneuvers may be removed using a curette in combination with an otoscope for direct visualization. The patient may experience an improvement of symptoms even with partial removal of the impaction. Patients should be instructed about ear cleaning techniques and home use of ceruminolytics.

Prognosis

Cerumen impaction has an excellent prognosis, and hearing can be dramatically improved with relatively simple interventions. However, recurrence of impaction is common.

CENTRAL AUDITORY PROCESSING DISORDER

ESSENTIALS OF DIAGNOSIS

▶ Hearing impairment due to insult to central nervous system.

▶ Reduction in speech discrimination exceeds hearing loss.

GENERAL CONSIDERATIONS

Central auditory processing disorder (CAPD) is the general term for hearing impairment that results from central nervous system (CNS) dysfunction. Any insult to the nervous system such as stroke or dementia can cause CAPD. The disorder is characterized by a loss of speech discrimination that is more profound than the associated loss in hearing.

Prevention

It has been postulated that the protection of the CNS provided by aspirin therapy and hypertension control could reduce the incidence of CAPD.

Clinical Findings

Patients with CAPD have difficulty understanding spoken language but may be able to hear sounds well. A patient may have difficulty following verbal instructions but understand written ones. There are no specific physical findings of CAPD, but patients may have other evidence of neurologic abnormalities.

Treatment

Treatment of CAPD is limited. If CNS dysfunction is caused by a reversible entity, then treatment for the underlying cause should be initiated. Identifying and treating other causes of sensory impairment may improve the patient's level of disability; however, CAPD may decrease the effectiveness of auditory rehabilitation. Patient education efforts should focus on educating friends and family about the disorder and options for hearing rehabilitation. The prognosis for patients with CAPD is determined by the underlying disorder.

National Institute on Deafness and Other Communication Disorders. Health information. http://www.nidcd.nih.gov/health/pages/default.aspx. Accessed November 22, 2019.

National Institute on Aging. Hearing loss: a common problem for older adults. www.nia.nih.gov/health/publication/hearing-loss. Accessed November 22, 2019.

Pacala JT. Hearing deficits in the older patient: "I didn't notice anything." *JAMA.* 2012;307(11):1185–1194. [PMID: 22436959]

Schwartz SR. Clinical practice guidelines: ear wax (cerumen impaction) otolar. *Head Neck Surg.* 2017;156:S1–S29. [PMID: 28045591]

Sprinzl GM, Riechelmann H. Current trends in treating hearing loss in elderly people: a review of the technology and treatment options- a mini-review. *Gerontology.* 2010;56(3):351–358. [PMID: 20090297]

Walling AD, Dickson GM. Hearing loss in older adults. *Am Fam Physician.* 2012;85(12):1150–1156. [PMID: 22962895]

COMMON CAUSES OF VISION IMPAIRMENT IN THE ELDERLY

Visual impairment is defined as binocular acuity of 20/40 or worse. Legal blindness is when central visual acuity is worse than 20/200. Older adults with good visual acuity show problems with visual function in real-life situations as testing is usually done in an optimum condition with maximum contrast and illumination with minimal glare. Testing for visual problems with decreased contrast sensitivity, decreased illumination, and increased glare is not practical for primary care providers, and hence it is important that they ask questions routinely to screen for performance under these circumstances. Educating the patient about simple measures to improve the environment may help with their quality of life.

PRESBYOPIA

ESSENTIALS OF DIAGNOSIS

▶ Age-related decrease in near vision.

▶ Distance vision remains unaffected.

General Considerations

Presbyopia is an age-associated progressive loss of the focusing power of the lens. Its incidence increases with age. The cause of this disorder is the ongoing increase in the diameter of the lens as a result of continued growth of the lens fibers with aging. This thickened lens accommodates less responsively to the contraction of muscles in the ciliary body, limiting its ability to focus on near objects.

Clinical Findings

Patients presenting with this disorder frequently complain of eye strain or of blurring of their vision when they quickly change from looking at a nearby object to one that is far away. On examination, the only abnormality noted is a decrease in near vision.

Treatment

Because presbyopia is due to normal age-related changes of the eye, there is no proven prevention. In patients with normal distance vision, treatment for this disorder is as simple as purchasing reading glasses. For patients requiring correction of their distance vision, options include spectacle correction with bifocal or trifocal lenses, monovision contact lenses in which one eye is corrected for distance vision and the other eye for near vision, or contact lens correction of distance vision and simple reading glasses for near vision. Surgical treatment of presbyopia is an evolving science, including procedures on the cornea, lens, and sclera.

Prognosis

All patients should be educated to anticipate a decline in near vision with aging. When left uncorrected, problems may occur with reading, driving, or other activities of daily living.

AGE-RELATED MACULAR DEGENERATION

ESSENTIALS OF DIAGNOSIS

- ▶ Slowly progressive central vision loss with intact peripheral vision.
- ▶ Vision problems in low light intensity and Amsler grid distortion.
- ▶ Drusen located in the macula of the retina.

General Considerations

AMD is the leading cause of severe vision loss in older Americans. It is characterized by atrophy of cells in the central macular region of the retinal pigment epithelium, resulting in the loss of central vision. Peripheral vision generally remains intact. AMD is typically classified as early and intermediate (usually dry type) or advanced/late AMD, which is divided into atrophic or nonneovascular (dry) or exudative or neovascular (wet) forms. The exudative form occurs in only 10% of patients with AMD, but it is responsible for the majority of severe vision loss related to the disease.

Prevention

Of the several risk factors that have been studied, only increasing age and tobacco abuse have been consistently associated with AMD. Because smoking has been strongly implicated as a risk factor (SORT C) and continued tobacco use is associated with a worse response to laser photocoagulation, smoking cessation should be highly recommended to all patients. Hypertension has also been linked to a worse response to laser therapy; thus, effective blood pressure control is desirable. Finally, daily AREDS (Age-Related Eye Disease Study) and AREDS2 vitamin supplementations play a role in delaying vision loss (SORT A). Patients with intermediate AMD or unilateral advanced AMD had an approximate 28% reduction of their risk for developing advanced AMD if treated with a high-dose combination of vitamin C, vitamin E, β-carotene, and zinc. Patients who smoke should only take AREDS2 formulations, which exclude β-carotene, due to increased risk of lung cancer. Patients with early or no AMD did not have the same benefit.

Clinical Findings

A. Symptoms and Signs

Patients may report onset of blurred central vision that is either gradual or acute with difficulty reading in dim light and night driving. Wavy or distorted central vision, known as *metamorphopsia*; intermittent shimmering lights; and central blind spots, termed *scotoma*, may all occur. Clinical findings include decreased visual acuity, Amsler grid distortion, and characteristic abnormalities on dilated funduscopic examination. In early disease, the most common findings are drusen: yellowish-colored deposits deep in the retina. In late disease of the atrophic type, areas of depigmentation are seen in the macula. In the exudative form, abnormal vessels (subretinal neovascularization) leak fluid and blood beneath the macula.

B. Special Examinations

Fluorescein angiography may be used by a specialist to confirm the diagnosis and to help determine whether a patient has atrophic or exudative AMD.

▶ Treatment

A. Referral

An ophthalmologist will play a critical role in care of the patient with known or suspected AMD. Urgent referral to an eye specialist should occur if a patient with suspected or known AMD presents with *acute* visual changes. Treatment of exudative AMD is a rapidly advancing field with many ongoing clinical trials of surgical and pharmaceutical interventions. Current treatment options include laser photocoagulation, photodynamic therapy (Verteporfin), and intravitreal antiangiogenic therapy (anti–vascular endothelial growth factor [VEGF]). In particular, intravitreal injections of VEGF have been shown to stabilize disease (SORT A). No effective treatments exist for patients with dry AMD.

Vision rehabilitation is the cornerstone of helping patients maximize their remaining vision and maintain their level of function for as long as possible. Low-vision professionals along with social workers can be of great assistance in recommending optical aids and devices and accessing local, state, and federal resources for the visually impaired. Direct-illumination devices, magnifiers, high-power reading glasses, telescopes, closed-circuit television, large-print publications, and bold-lined paper are some of the many devices that can be employed.

B. Patient Education

Patient education is important. More information on patient education is provided at http://www.amd.org.

▶ Prognosis

Many patients with mild dry AMD will not experience significant worsening of their vision. It is difficult to predict which patients will develop advancing disease and further loss of central vision. This condition is generally progressive but is not completely blinding. Peripheral vision should not be affected by AMD.

Lim LS, Mitchell P, Seddon JM, et al. Age-related macular degeneration. *Lancet.* 2012;379(9827):1728–1738. [PMID: 22559899]

Yonekawa Y. Age-related macular degeneration: advances in management and diagnosis. *J Clin Med.* 2015;4(2):343–359. [PMID: 26239130]

GLAUCOMA

ESSENTIALS OF DIAGNOSIS

▶ Optic neuropathy with variably progressive vision loss.

▶ Intraocular pressure (IOP) is often elevated but may be normal.

▶ General Considerations

Glaucoma is the second leading cause of blindness in the United States. Although glaucoma is most often associated with elevated IOP, it is the optic neuropathy that defines the disease. Normal IOP is generally accepted to be between 10 and 21 mmHg. The majority of patients with an IOP of >21 mmHg will not develop glaucoma, and 30–50% of patients with glaucoma will have an IOP of <21 mmHg. Despite these facts, it has been clearly shown that as IOP increases, so does the risk of developing glaucoma. The two most common forms of glaucoma are primary open-angle glaucoma (POAG) and primary angle-closure glaucoma (PACG), with the former approximately seven times more common than the latter in the United States and Europe. Other identified risk factors for glaucoma include family history, advancing age, and African American or Hispanic race. Additional possible risk factors include diabetes mellitus, hypertension, and myopia. Patients with PACG may experience acute or subacute events that occur after a sudden rise in intraocular pressure or from chronic PACG that is insidious in onset and largely asymptomatic. Chinese ethnicity, hyperopia, and female sex increase the risk of PACG.

▶ Prevention

The AAFP and the USPSTF do not recommend screening for glaucoma, citing insufficient evidence to recommend for or against routine screening by primary care clinicians for elevated IOP or early glaucoma (I recommendation). The American Academy of Ophthalmology recommends screening for glaucoma by an ophthalmologist every 1–2 years after age 65.

▶ Clinical Findings

A. Symptoms and Signs

Patients with acute angle-closure glaucoma typically present with unilateral intense pain and blurred vision. Patients may report seeing halos around light sources and complain of photophobia, headache, nausea, and vomiting. Physical examination shows a mid-dilated pupil, conjunctival injection, and lid edema. Patients generally have markedly elevated IOP, usually between 60 and 80 mmHg.

POAG is a more insidious disease with a long asymptomatic phase. Patients may notice a gradual loss of peripheral vision.

B. Special Tests

The following five tests are used to diagnose glaucoma: tonometry measures the pressure within the eye; ophthalmoscopy assesses the optic nerve damage (symmetrically enlarged cup-to-disk ratio, cup-to-disk ratio asymmetry between the two eyes, or a highly asymmetric cup in one eye); perimetry assesses the field of vision; gonioscopy measures the angle at which the cornea meets the iris; and pachymetry measures the thickness of the cornea. Highly sophisticated image analysis systems are now available to evaluate the optic nerve and retinal nerve fiber layer, and they include scanning laser tomography, laser polarimetry, and ocular coherence tomography.

▶ Treatment

Patients with significant risk factors or physical findings that raise concern for glaucoma should be referred to an ophthalmologist for further evaluation and confirmation of diagnosis.

A. Acute Angle-Closure Glaucoma

Acute angle-closure glaucoma is a medical emergency that requires immediate referral and treatment to prevent vision loss.

B. Primary Open-Angle Glaucoma

The treatment of POAG consists of pharmacologic and surgical interventions aimed at decreasing the IOP. Although elevated IOP is not required for the diagnosis of glaucoma, it has been shown that reduction of IOP in patients with glaucoma slows the progression of disease. Even patients with normal pressures can benefit from reduction in IOP.

1. Pharmacotherapy—Topical eye drops or oral medications aimed at decreasing aqueous humor production or increasing outflow are used. Topical agents such as β-blockers and prostaglandin analogs are first-line therapy, and α-adrenergic agents and carbonic anhydrase inhibitors are second-line therapy. Topical miotics and epinephrine compounds are now infrequently used. Oral medications include carbonic anhydrase inhibitors such as acetazolamide. Topical glaucoma agents have varying degrees of systemic absorption and are capable of producing systemic side effects and drug-drug interactions. Patients should be educated on the importance of medication side effects, compliance, and routine eye care.

2. Surgical intervention—Laser trabeculoplasty and laser or conventional trabeculectomy are the most commonly performed procedures after failed medical management.

▶ Prognosis

Untreated glaucoma can result in blindness. Treatment of POAG can prevent further loss of vision but typically does not restore lost vision.

Gupta D, Chen PP. Glaucoma. *Am Fam Physician.* 2016;93(8):
668–674. [PMID: 27175839]
Jost BJ, Aung T, Bourne RR, et al. Glaucoma. *Lancet.*
2017;390(10108):2183–2193. [PMID: 28577860]

CATARACTS

ESSENTIALS OF DIAGNOSIS

▶ Opacity or cloudiness of the crystalline lens.

▶ General Considerations

Any opacification of the lens is termed a *cataract*. Cataract disease is the most common cause of blindness worldwide and the most common eye abnormality in the elderly. Risk factors for cataracts include advancing age, exposure to ultraviolet (UV) B light, glaucoma, smoking, alcohol abuse, diabetes, and chronic steroid use. Diet and vitamins do not play a role in development or progression of the disease. Because cataracts tend to develop slowly, the patient may not be fully aware of the degree of vision impairment.

▶ Prevention

Physicians should use steroids at as low a dose when needed for treatment of other conditions and discontinue them when possible. Patients should be advised on how to minimize UV light exposure as well as the benefits of smoking cessation and control of chronic diseases.

▶ Clinical Findings

Patients may report blurring of vision, difficulty seeing in oncoming lights (glare) and difficulty with night driving, and monocular diplopia. The patient may also complain of a decrease in color perception and even note "second sight," which is an improvement in near vision with a nuclear cataract. Examination of the eye reveals opacification of the lens. Cataracts may be easier to see with dilation of the eye and a direct ophthalmoscope.

▶ Treatment

The treatment of cataracts is predominantly surgical. Factors influencing the timing of surgery include life expectancy, current level of disability, status of other medical illnesses, family and social situations, and patient expectations.

Preoperative medical management has been shown to have no benefit and is no longer recommended (SORT A). Cataract surgery is a low-risk procedure and is often accomplished under local anesthesia with minimally invasive techniques. There is no need to discontinue anticoagulation for the procedure. Surgeons should be made aware if patients are taking α-blockers because these drugs are associated with a complication called *intraoperative floppy iris syndrome.*

Prognosis

Cataracts do not resolve and may progress without treatment. The prognosis with surgical treatment is excellent, and ≥95% of patients obtain improved vision after surgery.

Eichenbaum JW. Geriatric vision loss due to cataracts, macular degeneration, and glaucoma. *Mt Sinai J Med.* 2012;79(2):276–294. [PMID: 22499498]
Liu YC, Wilkins M, Kim T, et al. Cataracts. *Lancet.* 2017; 390(10094):600–612. [PMID: 28242111]

DIABETIC RETINOPATHY

 ESSENTIALS OF DIAGNOSIS

▶ Asymptomatic, gradual vision loss or sudden vision loss in a diabetic patient.

▶ Characteristic fundoscopic findings of microaneurysms, flame hemorrhages, exudates, macular edema, and neovascularization.

General Considerations

Diabetic retinopathy (DR) is the leading cause of blindness in adults in the United States. It is important to consider DR as a disease of the aging eye because prevalence increases with duration of diabetes mellitus. The risk of blindness attributable to this disorder is greatest after 30 years of illness. DR is divided into two major forms: nonproliferative DR (NPDR) and proliferative DR, named for the absence or presence of abnormal new blood vessels emanating from the retina, respectively. NPDR can be further classified into mild, moderate, severe, and very severe categories depending on the extent of nerve fiber layer infarcts (cotton-wool spots), intraretinal hemorrhages, hard exudates, and microvascular abnormalities. The severity of proliferative retinopathy can be classified as early, high risk, and severe depending on the severity and extent of neovascularization.

Prevention

Patients with type 2 diabetes mellitus should have a comprehensive eye examination by an ophthalmologist shortly after diagnosis to screen for signs of retinopathy. Meticulous glycemic control decreases the risk of development and progression of retinopathy in all patients with diabetes. In addition, tight control of blood pressure also significantly reduces a patient's risk of developing retinopathy.

Clinical Findings

Many patients presenting with DR are free of symptoms; even those with the severe proliferative form may have 20/20 visual acuity. Others may report decreased vision that has occurred slowly or suddenly, unilaterally or bilaterally. Scotomata or floaters may also be reported. Funduscopic examination reveals any or all of the following: microaneurysms, dot and blot intraretinal hemorrhages, hard exudates, cotton-wool spots, boat-shaped preretinal hemorrhages, neovascularization, venous beading, and macular edema.

Fluorescein angiography may be performed by an ophthalmologist to further assess the degree of disease.

Treatment

Untreated proliferative retinopathy is relentlessly progressive, leading to significant vision impairment and blindness. In addition to maximizing glucose and blood pressure control, focal and panretinal laser photocoagulation surgery or vitrectomy is the mainstay of acute and chronic treatment and may preserve vision in certain patients. Fenofibrate has recently been shown to slow progression of disease and delay time to first surgical treatment (SORT A). There is low-quality evidence that intravitreal anti-VEGF treatment can be used in the management of proliferative DR if standard therapy is ineffective. However, there is strong evidence this treatment does effectively stabilize disease progression of patients with macular edema (SORT A). When vision loss has occurred, vision rehabilitation should be initiated, as described earlier in the discussion of AMD. Topics to review with patients include the importance of an annual, comprehensive eye examination, glycemic control, and hypertension management.

Prognosis

Early diagnosis and treatment and tight glycemic and blood pressure control improve prognosis and prevents blindness.

Antonetti D, Klein R, Gardner TW. Diabetic retinopathy. *N Engl J Med.* 2012;366(13):1227–1239. [PMID: 22455417]
Pelletier AL, Rojas-Roldan L, Coffin J. Vision loss in older adults. *Am Fam Physician.* 2016;94(3):219–226. [PMID: 27479624]
Solomon SD. Diabetic retinopathy: a position statement by the ADA. *Diabetes Care.* 2017;40:412–418. [PMID: 28432087]

Websites

Lighthouse International (health information on vision disorders, treatment, and rehabilitation services). http://www.lighthouse.org
National Institute on Aging (patient education handout on the aging eye and hearing loss). https://www.nia.nih.gov/health/aging-and-your-eyes

Oral Health

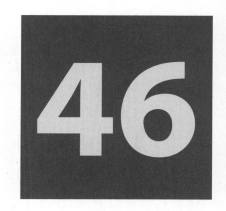

46

Wanda C. Gonsalves, MD

Although the nation's oral health is believed to be the best it has ever been, oral diseases remain common in the United States. In May 2000, the first report on oral health from the US Surgeon General, *Oral Health in America: A Report of the Surgeon General*, called attention to a largely overlooked epidemic of oral diseases that is disproportionately shared by Americans. This epidemic strikes, in particular, the poor, young, and elderly. The report stated that although there are safe and effective measures for preventing oral diseases, these measures are underused. The report called for improved education about oral health, for a renewed understanding of the relationship between oral health and overall health, and for an interdisciplinary approach to oral health that would involve primary care providers.

DENTAL ANATOMY & TOOTH ERUPTION PATTERN

In utero, the 20 primary teeth evolve from the expansion and development of ectodermal and mesodermal tissue at approximately 6 weeks of gestation. The ectoderm forms the dental enamel, and the mesoderm forms the pulp and dentin. As the tooth bud evolves, each unit develops a dental lamina that is responsible for the development of the future permanent tooth. The adult dentition is composed of 32 permanent teeth. Figure 46–1 shows the anatomy of the tooth and supporting structures. Table 46–1 outlines the eruption pattern of the teeth.

DENTAL CARIES

ESSENTIALS OF DIAGNOSIS

▶ Nonlocalized pain when exposed to heat, cold, or sweats.

▶ Painless white spot (demineralized areas of enamel) near gingival margins (white or brown spots).

▶ As infection proceeds to pulp, pain becomes localized.

▶ Visible pits or holes in the teeth.

▶ Poor oral hygiene and frequent snacking between meals are risk factors.

▶ General Considerations

Dental caries (tooth decay) is the single most common chronic childhood disease, 5 times more common than asthma and 7 times more common than hay fever among children age 5–7 years. Minority and low-income children are disproportionately affected. According to the Centers for Disease Control and Prevention (CDC), among children age 2–4 years and 6–8 years, tooth decay is more prevalent in Mexican American and African American than in non-Hispanic white communities. Among adults age 35–44 years in those same communities, untreated tooth decay is 2 times more prevalent than among non-Hispanic whites. In addition, one-third of persons of all ages have untreated tooth decay, 8% of adults age >20 years have lost at least one permanent tooth to dental caries, and many older adults suffer from root caries.

▶ Pathogenesis

Dental caries is a multifactorial, infectious, communicable disease caused by the demineralization of tooth enamel in the presence of a sugar substrate and of acid-forming cariogenic bacteria that are found in the soft gelatinous biofilm plaque (Figure 46–2). Thus, the development of caries requires a susceptible host, an appropriate substrate (sucrose), and the cariogenic bacteria found in plaque. *Streptococcus mutans* (also known as mutans streptococci [MS]) is considered to be the primary strain causing decay. Additionally, when

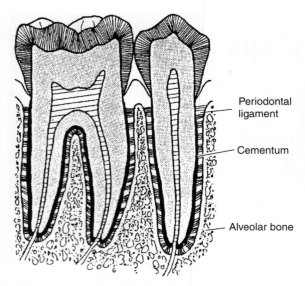

▲ **Figure 46–1.** Anatomy of the tooth and supporting structures.

Periodontal ligament

Cementum

Alveolar bone

Table 46–1. Eruption pattern of teeth.

Teeth	Eruption Date
Primary dentition	
Mandibular central incisor	6 months
Maxillary central incisor	7 months
Mandibular lateral incisor	7 months
Maxillary lateral incisor	9 months
Mandibular first molar	12 months
Maxillary first molar	14 months
Mandibular canine	16 months
Maxillary canine	18 months
Mandibular second molar	20 months
Maxillary second molar	24 months
Permanent dentition	
Mandibular central incisors	6 years
Maxillary first molars	6 years
Mandibular first molars	6 years
Maxillary central incisors	7 years
Mandibular lateral incisors	7 years
Maxillary lateral incisors	8 years
Mandibular canines	9 years
Maxillary first premolars	10 years
Mandibular first premolars	11 years
Maxillary second premolars	11 years
Mandibular second premolars	11 years
Maxillary canines	11 years
Mandibular second molars	12 years
Maxillary second molars	12 years
Mandibular third molars	17–21 years
Maxillary third molars	17–21 years

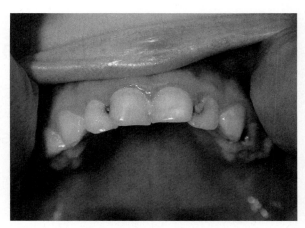

▲ **Figure 46–2.** Dental caries due to plaque.

plaque is not regularly removed, it may calcify to form calculus (tartar) and cause destructive gum disease.

Finally, the development of caries is a dynamic process that involves an imbalance between demineralization and remineralization of enamel. When such an imbalance is caused by environmental factors such as low pH or inadequate formation of saliva, dissolution of enamel occurs and caries result.

▶ **Clinical Findings**

A. Symptoms and Signs

When enamel is repeatedly exposed to the acid formed by the fermentation of sugars in plaque, demineralized areas develop on the tooth surfaces, between teeth, and on pits and fissures. These areas are painless and appear clinically as opaque or brown spots (Figures 46–3 to 46–5). If infection

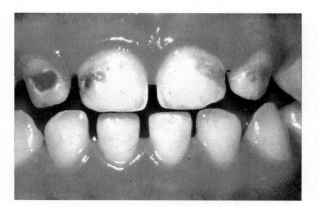

▲ **Figure 46–3.** Brown spots indicating demineralized areas in enamel.

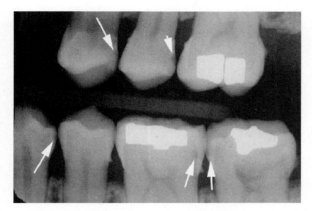

▲ **Figure 46–4.** Opaque areas indicating demineralized areas in enamel.

is allowed to progress, a cavity forms that can spread to and through the dentin (the component of the tooth located below the enamel) and to the pulp (composed of nerves and blood vessels; an infection of the pulp is called *pulpitis*), causing pain, necrosis, and, perhaps, an abscess.

B. Diagnosis

Carious lesions progress at various rates and occur at many different locations on the tooth, including the sites of previous restorations. Demineralized lesions (white or brown spots) generally occur at the margins of the gingiva and can be detected visually; they may not be seen on radiographs. Advanced carious lesions, such as those spread through dentin, can be detected clinically or, if they occur between the teeth, by radiographs. Root caries, commonly seen in older adults, occur in areas from which the gingiva has receded.

Dental professionals use a dental explorer to detect early caries in the grooves and fissures of posterior teeth. To diagnose secondary caries (caries formed at the site of

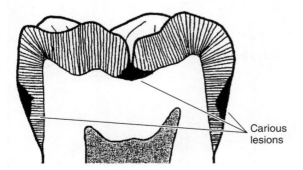

Carious
lesions

▲ **Figure 46–5.** Dental caries.

restorations), dental professionals use digitally acquired and postprocessed images.

▶ Risk Assessment

Caries can develop at any time after tooth eruption. Early teeth are principally susceptible to caries caused by the transmission of MS from the mouth of the caregiver to the mouth of the infant or toddler. This type of caries is called *early childhood caries* (ECC) or *baby bottle tooth decay*. According to the American Academy of Pediatric Dentistry, ECC "is defined as 'the presence of one or more decayed (noncavitated or cavitated lesions), missing (due to caries), or filled tooth surfaces' in any primary tooth in a child 71 months of age or younger." In children age <3 years, any sign of smooth-surface caries is called *severe early childhood caries* (S-ECC). Children with a history of ECC or S-ECC are at a much higher risk of subsequent caries in primary and permanent teeth. (Guidelines on caries risk assessment and management may be found on the American Academy of Pediatric Dentistry website: http://www.aapd.org/media/Policies_Guidelines/G_CariesRiskAssessment.pdf.)

ECC contributes to other health problems, including chronic pain, poor nutritional practices, and low self-esteem, which may lead to lack of self-esteem among older children and a great reduction in their ability to succeed in life.

The risk factors for adult caries are similar to those for childhood caries.

▶ Differential Diagnosis

Developmental defects or pits in the tooth surface or visible groove is the differential diagnosis.

▶ Prevention & Treatment

Fluoride, the ionic form of the element fluorine, is widely accepted as a safe and effective practice for the primary prevention of dental caries. Fluoride slows or reverses the progression of existing tooth decay by (1) being incorporated into the enamel before tooth eruption, (2) inhibiting demineralization, (3) enhancing remineralization, and (4) inhibiting bacterial activity in plaque. Unfortunately, only 75% of the US population has access to community water fluoridation, according to the CDC census in 2012. Systemic fluoride supplements (tablets, drops, lozenges) are recommended for children age 6 months to 16 years who are at high risk of the development of caries; for infants with ECC; for those who live in nonfluoridated water areas; and for adults whose water is not fluoridated or who have diseases that produce a decrease in salivary flow, receding gums, or mental or physical disabilities. A supplemental fluoride dosage schedule is shown in Table 46–2. Topical fluoride supplements such as gels and varnishes are highly concentrated fluoride products that are professionally applied by a dental health provider or

Table 46–2. Supplemental fluoride dosage schedule.

Age	Fluoride Ion Level in Drinking Water (ppm)[a]		
	<0.3 ppm	0.3-0.6 ppm	>0.6 ppm
Birth–6 months	None	None	None
6 months–3 years	0.25 mg/d[b]	None	None
3–6 years	0.50 mg/d	0.25 mg/d	None
6–16 years	1.0 mg/d	0.50 mg/d	None

[a]1 ppm = 1 mg/L.
[b]2.2 mg sodium fluoride contains 1 mg fluoride ion.
Adapted with permission from Fluoride supplementation for children: interim policy recommendations. American Academy of Pediatrics Committee on Nutrition. *Pediatrics*. 1995 May;95(5):777.

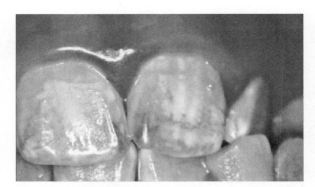

▲ **Figure 46–6.** Fluorosis.

a parent (for gels). Varnishes, which are less toxic than gels and more effective than mouth rinses, are applied 3 times a week, once a year by disposable brushes, cotton-tipped applicators, or cotton pellets. (For more information, see www.smilesforlifeoralhealth.org.)

Before prescribing supplemental fluoride, the primary care provider must determine the fluoride concentration in the child's primary source of drinking water. Other sources of fluoride include well water exposed to fluorite minerals, certain fruits and vegetables grown in soil irrigated with fluoridated water, beverages, and foods such as meats or poultry that may contain 6–7% of total dietary fluoride. Although fluoride supplementation is not recommended for persons who live in communities whose water is optimally fluoridated (0.7–1.2 ppm or >0.6 mg/L), the bottled water used by many families may contain low levels of fluoride. The Department of Health and Human Services proposed to not have a fluoride range, but to limit the fluoride recommendation to the lower limit of 0.7 ppm. Parents and caregivers should be educated about the benefits of fluoride and the possible side effects of too much fluoride, a condition called *fluorosis*. Fluorosis results when too much fluoride is obtained from any source when the permanent tooth is forming (Figure 46–6). Overall, 22% of children and adolescents aged 6–19 years have very mild or greater fluorosis. The benefits and side effects of fluoride use should be weighed against the risk of tooth decay among children at high risk of caries.

A second method of preventing dental caries is proper oral hygiene. Before the teeth erupt, a parent may use a washcloth or cotton gauze to clean an infant's mouth and to transition the child to toothbrushing. Parents should supervise brushing and should discourage children age <6 years from using fluoridated dentifrices because of the risk that toothpaste may be swallowed during brushing. Generally speaking, children age <3 should use no more than a smear

or rice-size amount of fluoridated toothpaste, and no more than a pea-size amount should be used for those between 3 and 6 years. Teeth should be brushed twice a day, and rinsing after brushing should be kept to a minimum or eliminated altogether.

Dental sealants, first introduced in the 1960s, are plastic films that coat the chewing surfaces of primary or permanent teeth. Sealants prevent decay from developing in the pits and fissures of teeth. Dental professionals often use sealants in combination with topical fluorides (Figure 46–7).

Older children and adults should avoid frequent consumption of drinks and snack foods containing sugars. Chewing sugar-free gum or cheese after meals has a saliva buffer effect that may counter plaque acids. Xylitol has been proposed as preventing caries; however, its recommendation lacks consistent evidence.

American Academy of Pediatric Dentistry. Guideline on fluoride therapy. *Pediatr Dent*. 2013;35(5):E165–E168. [PMID: 24290545]

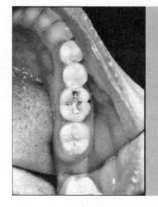
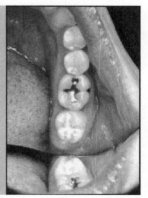

▲ **Figure 46–7.** Dental sealants.

American Academy of Pediatric Dentistry. Policy on use of xylitol in caries prevention. *Pediatr Dent.* 2010;32(special issue):36–38. [PMID: 19216379]

Fontana M, Gonzalez-Cabezasc C. Are we ready for definitive clinical guidelines on xylitol/polyol use? *Adv Dent Res.* 2012;24(2):123–128. [PMID: 22899694]

National Institutes of Health. Diagnosis and management of dental caries throughout life. NIH Consensus Statement Online, March 26–28, 2001;18:1. https://consensus.nih.gov/2001/2001DentalCaries115PDF.pdf. Accessed March 19, 2020.

PERIODONTAL DISEASE

ESSENTIALS OF DIAGNOSIS

► Swelling of the intradental papillae followed by swelling of the gingiva.

► Mild gingivitis is painless, and gums may bleed when brushing or eating hard foods.

► Shifting or loose teeth with associated alveolar bone loss.

► **General Considerations**

Periodontal disease is the most common oral disease in adults, affecting one of every two adults age >30 years, according to the CDC. Three forms exist: gingivitis, chronic periodontitis, and aggressive periodontitis. It is uncommon among young children, affecting <1%; however, in some studies, ≤25% of Hispanic children aged 12–17 years were affected. Like dental caries, periodontal diseases are caused by bacteria in dental plaque that create an inflammatory response in gingival tissues (gingivitis) or in the soft tissue and bone supporting the teeth (periodontitis). Risk factors that contribute to the development of periodontal disease include poor oral hygiene, environmental factors such as crowded teeth and mouth breathing, steroid hormones, smoking, comorbid conditions such as weakened immune status or diabetes, and low income.

Severe gum disease is defined as a 6-mm loss of attachment of the tooth to the adjacent gum tissue. Severe gum disease affects approximately 14% of adults age 45–54 years and 23% of those age 65–74 years. Approximately 25% of adults age ≥65 years no longer have any natural teeth. The severity of periodontal disease does not increase with age. Rather, the disease is believed to occur in random bursts after periods of quiescence.

► **Pathogenesis**

A. Gingivitis

Gingivitis is caused by a reversible inflammatory process that occurs as the result of prolonged exposure of the gingival

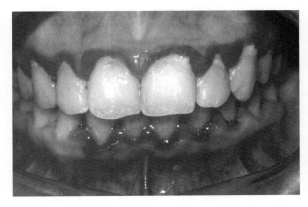

▲ **Figure 46–8.** Gingivitis.

tissues to plaque. Gingivitis may develop as a result of steroid hormones, which encourage the growth of certain bacteria in plaque during puberty and pregnancy and in women taking oral contraceptive pills.

No special tests are needed to diagnose gingivitis; rather, the disease is diagnosed by clinical assessment. Simple or marginal gingivitis may be painless and is treated by good oral hygiene practices such as toothbrushing and flossing. This type of gingivitis occurs in 50% of the population age ≥4 years. The inflammation worsens as mineralized plaque forms calculus (tartar) at and below the gum surface (sulcus). Gingivitis may persist for months or years without progressing to periodontitis; this fact suggests that host susceptibility plays an important role in the development of periodontitis. Additionally, gingivitis (Figure 46–8) can be either acute or chronic. A severe form, acute necrotizing ulcerative gingivitis (ANUG), also known as *Vincent disease* or "trench mouth," is associated with anaerobic fusiform bacteria and spirochetes. ANUG (Figure 46–9) is painful, ulcerative, and

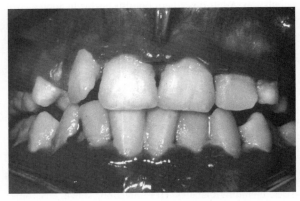

▲ **Figure 46–9.** Acute necrotizing ulcerative gingivitis.

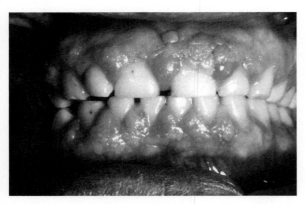

▲ **Figure 46–10.** Gingival enlargement due to drugs.

edematous and produces halitosis and bleeding gingival tissue. Predisposing factors include conditions that contribute to a weakened immune status, such as human immunodeficiency virus (HIV) infection, smoking, malnutrition, viral infections, and, possibly, stress. Chronic gingivitis affects >90% of the population and results in gingival enlargement or hyperplasia that resolves when adequate plaque control is instituted. Generalized gingival enlargement or swelling (gingiva hyperplasia) may be caused by drugs such as calcium channel blockers, phenytoin, and cyclosporine (Figure 46–10); by pregnancy; or by systemic diseases such as leukemia, sarcoidosis, and Crohn disease.

B. Periodontitis

Chronic periodontitis (CP) is caused by chronic inflammation of gingival soft tissue and supporting structures by plaque microorganisms, specifically gram-negative bacteria that affect gingival soft tissues and supporting structures, with resultant loss of periodontal attachment and bony destruction. CP is common in adults, affecting >50% of the population. Adult-onset periodontitis begins in adolescence and is reversible if treated in its early stages, when minimal pockets (gaps) have formed between the tooth and the periodontal attachment. Severe periodontitis is characterized by a 6-mm loss of tooth attachment as detected by the dental health professional by means of dental probes.

If periodontitis is found in children or young adults or if it progresses rapidly, the primary care provider should be alert to the possibility of a systemic cause such as diabetes mellitus, Down syndrome, hypophosphatasia, neutropenia, leukemia, leukocyte adhesion deficiency, or histiocytosis. A less common, rapidly progressing form of adult periodontitis begins in the third or fourth decade of life and is associated with severe gingivitis and rapid bone loss. Several systemic diseases, including diabetes, HIV infection, Down syndrome, and Papillon-Lefèvre syndrome, have been associated with

this rare form of periodontitis. Localized juvenile periodontitis (LJP) and localized prepubertal periodontitis (LPP) are forms of early-onset periodontitis seen in young children and teenagers, respectively, without the evidence of systemic disease. LJP is more common among African American children. It affects the first molars and incisors, with rapid destruction of bone. Although there is some evidence for autosomal transmission, it is likely heterogenous. Both LJP and LPP are believed to be the result of a bacterial infection (specifically implicated is *Actinobacillus actinomycetemcomitans*) and, possibly, host immunologic deficits.

▶ Clinical Findings

A. Symptoms and Signs

Clinical signs of gingivitis and periodontitis include interdental papillae edema, erythema, and bleeding on contact during tooth brushing or dental probing (Figure 46–11). The amount of gingival inflammation and bleeding and the probing depth of gingival pockets determine the severity of periodontal disease. Tartar, gum recession, and loose teeth are characteristics of severe periodontal disease. For children age <4 years, loss of primary teeth may be the first clinical sign of periodontal disease and the systemic manifestation of hypophosphatasia. Dental probing by the dental health professional will detect sulcus depth.

B. Imaging Studies

Bone loss can be detected by radiographs and bone density scans.

▶ Periodontal Health & Systemic Disease

Emerging evidence, particularly from the dental literature, suggests that periodontal disease may be a risk factor for systemic conditions such as cardiovascular disease, diabetes mellitus, and adverse pregnancy outcomes of preterm labor

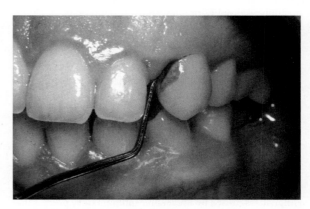

▲ **Figure 46–11.** Gingival inflammation and bleeding.

and low birth weight. Current evidence supports a bidirectional relationship between diabetes and periodontal disease. Periodontal disease is a risk factor for poor glycemic control among diabetic patients, and diabetes is associated with increased severity of periodontal disease. Studies showing the relationship between periodontal disease and cardiovascular disease have proposed that patients with chronic bacterial infection or periodontitis may have (1) a bacteria-induced platelet aggregation defect that contributes to acute thrombolic events, (2) injury to vascular tissue by bacterial toxins, or (3) vascular injury resulting from a host inflammatory response that predisposes the patient to a systemic disorder such as atherosclerosis. Additionally, the link between periodontal disease and preterm labor has several proposed biological mechanisms, one of which is the infection that is mediated by prostaglandins and cytokines among patients with severe periodontitis. This infection causes decreased fetal growth and premature labor.

▶ Differential Diagnosis

Other causes of gingivitis include hormonal changes associated with pregnancy; systemic disease such as diabetes, Addison disease, and HIV; and mechanical injury such as popcorn kernels that might become wedged under the gums.

Gingiva hyperplasia caused by medications such as calcium channel blockers, phenytoin, and cyclosporine causes overgrowth of the gingiva that may occur with or without gingivitis.

▶ Prevention & Treatment

Controlling the bacterial burden is key for the prevention and control of periodontal diseases and can be accomplished by brushing twice daily with American Dental Association/Food and Drug Administration–approved antigingivitis toothpaste and flossing daily or using interdental devices. Gingivitis, the mildest form of periodontal disease, is reversible with regular toothbrushing and flossing. Nonsurgical and surgical treatments are available for periodontitis. Nonsurgical therapies include over-the-counter and prescription antimicrobial mouth rinses, such as a 0.1–0.2% chlorhexidine gluconate aqueous mouthwash used twice a day. Caution is advised when chlorhexidine is used because it causes superficial staining of the teeth and black tongue. Additionally, low-dose doxycycline 20 mg twice a day has been proposed for severe periodontitis.

The gold standard is professional care to remove tartar (scaling and root planing). Some patients may require periodontal surgery.

Because tobacco use is an important risk factor for the development and progression of periodontal disease, patients should be counseled about tobacco cessation. Systemic diseases such as diabetes that may contribute to periodontal disease should be well controlled.

Al-Ghazi, MN, Ciancio SG, Aljada A, et al. Evaluation of efficacy of administration of sub-antimicrobial-dose doxycycline in the treatment of generalized adult periodontitis in diabetics. *J Dent Res.* 2006;82(Spec ISS A):Abstract.
American Academy of Periodontology. https://www.perio.org/. Accessed November 25, 2019.
Engebretson SP, Hey-Hadavi J, Celenti R, Lamster IB. Low-dose doxycycline treatment reduces glycosylated hemoglobin in patients with type 2 diabetes: a randomized controlled trial. *J Dent Res.* 2003;82(Spec ISS A):Abstract no. 1445.
Gonsalves W, Chi A, Neville BW. Common oral lesions: part 1. Superficial mucosal lesions. *Am Fam Physician.* 2007;75:501–507. [PMID: 17323710]
Salvi GE, Lawrence HP, Offenbacher S, et al. Influences of risk factors on the pathogenesis of periodontitis. *Periodontal 2000.* 1997;14:173–201. [PMID: 9567971]
Teng YT, Taylor GW, Scannapieco F, et al. Periodontal health and systemic disorders. *J Can Dent Assoc.* 2002;68:188. [PMID: 11911816]
Zeeman GG, Veth EO, Dennison DK. Focus on primary care: periodontal disease: implications for women's health. *Obstet Gynecol Surv.* 2001;56:43. [PMID: 11140863]

ORAL & OROPHARYNGEAL CANCERS

 ESSENTIALS OF DIAGNOSIS

► White or red patch that may progress to ulcer of mucosal surface, endophytic or exophytic growth.
► Lesions persisting for >2 weeks require biopsy.
► Common distribution of lesions in order of frequency is the tongue, floor of mouth, and lower lip vermilion.
► Risk factors include smoking and alcohol use, human papillomavirus (HPV), lichen planus, and Plummer-Vinson syndrome.

▶ General Considerations

In the United States, cancers of the oral cavity and oropharynx constitute approximately 3% of all cancers among men (the ninth most common cancer among men) and 2% of all cancers among women. The prevalence of these cancers increases with age. Since the 1970s, the incidence of these cancers and the death rates associated with them have been slowly decreasing, except among African American men, for whom the incidence and 5-year mortality estimates are nearly twice as high as for non-Hispanic white men.

The overall survival rate for patients with oral and oropharyngeal cancers is only approximately 51% and has not changed substantially since the early 1990s. However, the 5-year survival estimate for patients with lip carcinoma is >90%; this high survival rate is due in part to early detection.

Most oral and oropharyngeal cancers are squamous cell carcinomas that arise from the lining of the oral mucosa. HPV, the most common sexually transmitted infection in the United States today, is a cause of cervical cancer and approximately 26% of all head and neck and oropharyngeal squamous cell carcinomas. Most HPV infections (low-risk HPV types) will resolve spontaneously and not lead to cervical or oral cancers. High-risk oncogenic HPV subtypes 16 and 18 have been found to be the cause of almost all cases of cervical cancer and 60–70% of newly diagnosed oropharyngeal cancers. HPV-positive oropharyngeal cancers are more frequent in non-Hispanic white men, younger populations (52–56 years), and people who do not use tobacco or alcohol. The tonsil is most commonly affected. These cancers occur most commonly (in order of frequency) on the tongue, the lips, and the floor of the mouth. Approximately 60% of oral cancers are advanced by the time they are detected, and approximately 15% of patients will have another cancer in a nearby area such as the larynx, esophagus, or lungs. Early diagnosis, which has been shown to increase survival rates, depends on the discerning clinician who recognizes risk factors and suspicious symptoms and can identify a lesion at an early stage.

Table 46–3 shows the risk factors associated with oral and oropharyngeal cancers (need to add HPV). Tobacco use and heavy alcohol consumption are the two principal risk factors responsible for 75% of oral cancers. The incidence of oral cancer is higher among persons who smoke or drink heavily than among those who do not.

▶ Prevention

All forms of tobacco, including cigarette, pipe, chewing, and smokeless tobacco products, have been shown to be carcinogenic in the susceptible host. Alcohol has been identified as another important risk factor for oral cancer, both independently and synergistically when heavy consumers of alcohol also smoke. Therefore, primary prevention in the form of

reducing or eliminating the use of tobacco and alcohol has been strongly recommended. The US Preventive Services Task Force has not endorsed annual screening (secondary prevention) for asymptomatic patients, stating that "there is insufficient evidence to recommend for or against routine screening" and "clinicians may wish to include an examination for cancerous and precancerous lesions of the oral cavity in the periodic health examination of persons who chew or smoke tobacco (or did so previously), older persons who drink regularly, and anyone with suspicious symptoms or lesions detected through self-examination." However, the American Cancer Society and the National Cancer Institute's Dental and Craniofacial Research Group support efforts that promote early detection of oral cancers. The American Cancer Society recommends annual oral cancer examinations for persons age ≥40 years

Because primary care providers are more likely than dentists to see patients at high risk of oral and oropharyngeal cancers, providers need to be able to counsel patients about their behaviors and be knowledgeable about performing oral cancer examinations. The primary screening test for oral cancer is the oral cancer examination, which includes inspection and palpation of extraoral and intraoral tissues (Table 46–4). There are currently no recommended

---

Table 46–3. Risk factors associated with oral and oropharyngeal cancer.

Tobacco use (smoking or using smokeless tobacco or snuff)
Excessive consumption of alcohol
Viral infections (HSV, HIV, EBV, HPV)
Chronic actinic exposure
Betel quid use
Lichen planus
Plummer-Vinson or Paterson-Kelly syndrome
Immunosuppression
Dietary factors (low intake of fruits and vegetables)

EBV, Epstein-Barr virus; HIV, human immunodeficiency virus; HPV, human papillomavirus; HSV, herpes simplex virus.

Table 46–4. Components of an oral cancer examination.[a]

Extraoral examination
Inspect head and neck
Bimanually palpate lymph nodes and salivary glands
Lips
Inspect and palpate outer surfaces of lip and vermilion border
Inspect and palpate inner labial mucosa
Buccal mucosa
Inspect and palpate inner cheek lining
Gingiva/alveolar ridge
Inspect maxillary/mandibular gingiva and alveolar ridges on both the buccal and lingual aspects
Tongue
Have patient protrude tongue and inspect dorsal surface
Have patient lift tongue and inspect ventral surface
Grasping tongue with a piece of gauze and pulling it out to each side, inspect lateral borders of tongue from its tip back to lingual tonsil region
Palpate tongue
Floor of mouth
Inspect and palpate floor of mouth
Hard palate
Inspect hard palate
Soft palate and oropharynx
Gently depressing the patient's tongue with a mouth mirror or tongue blade, inspect soft palate and oropharynx

[a]A good oral examination requires an adequate light source, protective gloves, 2 × 2 gauze squares, and a mouth mirror or tongue blade.

screening methods for anal, vulvar, vaginal, penile, or oropharyngeal HPV infections.

▶ Clinical Findings

A. Symptoms and Signs

Early oral cancer and the more common precancerous lesions (leukoplakia) are subtle and asymptomatic. They begin as a white or red patch, progress to a superficial ulceration of the mucosal surface, and later become an endophytic or exophytic growth. Some lesions are solitary lumps. Larger, advanced cancers may be painful and may erode underlying tissue.

According to the definition of the World Health Organization, leukoplakia is "a white patch or plaque that cannot be characterized clinically or pathologically as any other disease." The lesions may be white, red, or a combination of red and white (called *speckled leukoplakia* or *erythroleukoplakia*). Multiple studies have shown that these lesions undergo malignant transformation. Biopsies have shown that erythroplakia and speckled leukoplakia are more likely than other types of leukoplakia to undergo malignant transformation with more severe epithelial dysplasia. Figures 46–12 and 46–13 show leukoplakia.

Oropharyngeal carcinomas can be found in the intraoral cavity, the oral cavity proper, and the oropharyngeal sites. The most common intraoral site is the tongue; lesions frequently develop on its posterior lateral border. Lesions also occur on the floor of the mouth and, less commonly, on the gingiva, buccal mucosa, labial mucosa, or hard palate.

A common cancer of the oral cavity proper is lower lip vermilion carcinoma. These lesions arise from a precancerous lesion called *actinic cheilosis*, which is similar to an actinic keratosis of the skin. Dry, scaly changes appear first and later progress to form a healing ulcer, which is sometimes

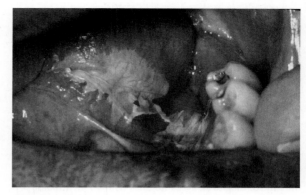

▲ **Figure 46–13.** Leukoplakia.

mistaken for a cold sore or fever blister. Figure 46–14 shows actinic cheilosis.

Oropharyngeal carcinomas commonly arise on the lateral soft palate and the base of the tongue. Presenting symptoms may include dysphagia, painful swallowing (odynophagia), and referred pain to the ear (otalgia). These tumors are often advanced at the time of diagnosis. Oral cancer metastasizes regionally to the contralateral or bilateral cervical and submental lymph nodes. Distant metastases are commonly found in the lungs, but oral cancer may metastasize to any other organ.

B. Diagnosis

All patients whose behaviors put them at risk of oral cancer should undergo a thorough oral examination that involves visual and tactile examination of the mouth; full protrusion

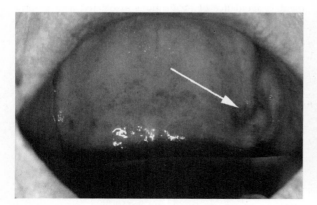

▲ **Figure 46–12.** Leukoplakia.

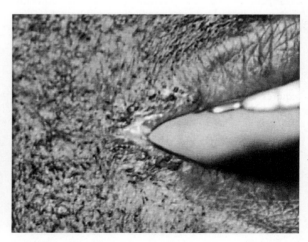

▲ **Figure 46–14.** Actinic cheilosis.

of the tongue with the aid of a gauze wipe; and palpation of the tongue, the floor of the mouth, and the lymph nodes in the neck. Because oral cancer and precancerous lesions are asymptomatic, primary care providers need to carefully examine patients who are at risk of oral or oropharyngeal carcinomas. Using a scalpel or small biopsy forceps, the primary care physician should perform a biopsy of any nonhealing white or red lesion that persists for >2 weeks. Alternatively, the patient may be referred to a dentist, an oral surgeon, or a head and neck specialist, who can perform the biopsy. Patients with large lesions or advanced disease should undergo a complete head and neck examination, because 15% of these patients will have a second primary cancer at the time of diagnosis. Neck nodules with no identifiable primary tumor may be evaluated by fine-needle aspiration.

C. Imaging Studies

Imaging studies such as computed tomography with contrast and magnetic resonance imaging of the head and neck are used to determine the extent of disease and involvement of the cervical lymph nodes for the purposes of staging.

▶ Differential Diagnosis

Precancerous white lesions may be confused with frictional keratosis, lesions that result from chronic chewing of the cheek, and nicotine stomatitis, a condition with hyperkeratotic epithelial changes on the hard palate as a result of cigarette smoking.

Other white lesions include hairy leukoplakia, geographic tongue, and candidiasis, which should be included in the differential of precancerous lesions.

▶ Treatment

Treatment for oral and lip cancers includes chemotherapy, surgery, radiation, or some combination of these therapies, depending on the extent of the disease. These treatments can cause severe stomatitis (inflammation of the mouth), xerostomia (dry mouth), disfigurement, altered speech and mastication, loss of appetite, and increased susceptibility to oral infection. The management of these complications requires a multidisciplinary team approach by the clinician, oral surgeon, oncologist, and speech therapist. Early diagnosis allows better treatment, cosmetic appearance, and functional outcome and increases the probability of survival. Patients should be encouraged to visit their dental health provider before beginning cancer therapy so that existing health problems can be treated and some complications can be prevented.

Burd EM. Human papillomavirus laboratory testing: the changing paradigm. *Clin Microbiol Rev.* 2016;29(2):291–319. [PMID: 26912568]

Cleveland JL, Junger ML, Saraiya M, et al. The connection between human papillomavirus and oropharyngeal squamous cell carcinomas in the United States: implications for dentistry. *J Am Dent Assoc.* 2011;142(8):915–924. [PMID: 21804058]

Kreimer AR, Clifford GM, Boyle P. Human papillomavirus types in head and neck squamous cell carcinomas worldwide: a systematic review. *Cancer Epidemiol Biomarkers Prev.* 2005;14:467–475. [PMID: 15734974]

Mashberg A, Samit A. Early diagnosis of asymptomatic oral and oropharyngeal squamous cancers. *CA Cancer J Clin.* 1995;45:328. [PMID: 7583906]

Neville BW, Day TA. Oral cancer and precancerous lesions. *CA Cancer J Clin.* 2002;52:195–215. [PMID: 12139232]

Silverman S Jr. Demographics and occurrence of oral and pharyngeal cancers. The outcomes, the trends, the challenge. *J Am Dent Assoc.* 2001;132:7S. [PMID: 11803655]

Weinberg MA, Estefan DJ. Assessing oral malignancies. *Am Fam Physician.* 2002;65:1379. [PMID: 11996421]

▶ Oral Effects of Medications

Medications used to treat certain systemic conditions may have oral manifestations. Most commonly these include xerostomia (dry mouth), gingival hyperplasia, dental caries and erosions, and osteonecrosis of the jaw.

Xerostomia, commonly seen in the elderly, is caused by hypofunction of the salivary gland, but has also been caused by antihypertensives, antidepressants, protease inhibitors, antihistamines, and diuretics. Xerostomia increases the risk of denture sores and caries, since saliva is a lubricant with antimicrobial properties. Symptoms include a sensation of dry mouth. Treatment is avoidance of medications known to cause xerostomia and cariogenic foods, good oral hygiene, and salivary substitutes or stimulants.

Gingiva hyperplasia has been associated with calcium channel blockers, methotrexate, cyclosporine, and phenytoin. Dental caries may be caused by syrups such as cough medicines, and dental erosions may follow use of β-blockers, calcium channel blockers, nitrates, and progesterone. Treatment is avoidance of medications associated with gingiva hyperplasia.

Avascular osteonecrosis of the mandible and maxilla have been associated with bisphosphonates. Symptoms include swelling and pain, difficulty eating, bleeding, lower lip paresthesia, and loose and mobile teeth. Since radiographs are nonspecific, lesions should be biopsied for definitive diagnosis. Risk factors include intravenous bisphosphonates, cancer, invasive dental procedures, smoking, steroid use, radiation therapy, and poor dental hygiene. Patients should be advised to avoid dental procedures while taking these medications.

Ghezzi E, Ship J. Systemic diseases and their treatments in the elderly: impact on oral health. *J Public Health Dent.* 2000;60(4):289–296. [PMID: 11243049]

Gonsalves W, Wrightson AS, Henry R. Common oral problems in older patients. *Am Fam Physician.* 2008;78(7):845–852. [PMID: 18841733]

Pazianas M, Miller P, Blumentals WA, et al. A review of the literature on osteonecrosis of the jaw in patients with osteoporosis treated with oral bisphosphonates: prevalence, risk factors, and clinical characteristics. *Clin Ther.* 2007;29(8):1548–1558. [PMID: 17919538]

Peker I, Alkurt MT, Usalan G. Clinical evaluation of medication on oral and dental health. *Int Dent J.* 2008;58:218–222. [PMID: 18783115]

Turner M, Ship J. Dry mouth and its effects on the oral health of elderly people. *J Am Dent Assoc.* 2007;138 (Suppl):15S–20S. [PMID: 17761841]

Global References for Oral Health

Beltram-Aguilar ED, Barker LK, Canto MT, et al. Centers for Disease Control and Prevention: surveillance for dental caries, dental sealants, tooth retention, edentulism and enamel fluorosis—United States, 1988–1994 and 1999–2002. *MMWR Surveill Summ.* 2005;54:1–43. [PMID: 16121123]

Office of Disease Prevention and Health Promotion, US Department of Health and Human Services. Healthy People 2010. http://www.healthypeople.gov/document/html/objectives/21-08.htm. Accessed August 23, 2010.

US Department of Health and Human Services (DHHS). Oral Health in America: A Report of the Surgeon General—Executive Summary. DHHS, National Institute of Dental and Craniofacial Research, National Institutes of Health; 2000. https://www.nidcr.nih.gov/research/data-statistics/surgeon-general. Accessed November 25, 2019.

Websites

Academy of General Dentistry. http://www.agd.org

American Association of Public Health Dentistry. http://www.aaphd.org

American Dental Association. http://www.ada.org

Centers for Disease Control and Prevention. Oral health. http://www.cdc.gov/oralhealth

Children's Dental Health Project. https://www.cdhp.org

Health Resources and Services Administration (HRSA) Oral Health Initiative. http://www.hrsa.gov/oralhealth

National Maternal and Child Oral Health Resource Center. http://www.mchoralhealth.org

Smiles for Life. http://www.smilesfororalhealth.org

US Surgeon General's Report on Children's Oral Health. http://www.nidcr.nih.gov/sgr/sgr.htm

Pharmacotherapy Principles for the Family Physician

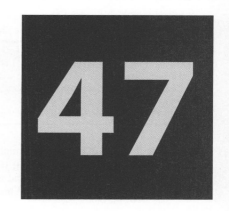

Jennie B. Jarrett, PharmD, BCPS, MMedEd, FCCP

Paul Stranges, PharmD, BCACP

Katie B. Kaczmarski, PharmD, BCACP, AE-C

Medication therapy is an integral element of healthcare interventions. In 2016, >4 billion prescriptions were dispensed in the United States. Pharmacotherapy is often supported by "hard science" of research evidence; clinical practice often shifts to the "soft science" of medicine, combining patients' culture and beliefs, their histories, and medication adherence to provide the best possible care.

Of the billions of prescriptions filled, it is estimated that half are taken improperly. Achieving a balance between "hard" and "soft" sciences—providing evidence-based medication therapy that patients will adhere to—becomes paramount. This chapter explores patient adherence; provider considerations, such as evidence, pharmacokinetics/pharmacodynamics, and safety; and healthcare system factors, such as formulary systems/resources.

Editorial: the soft science of medicine. *Lancet.* 2004;363:1247. [PMID: 15094264]

IMS Institute for Healthcare Informatics. Medicines use and spending in the U.S. http://www.imshealth.com. Accessed June 12, 2018.

TAKING A MEDICATION HISTORY

Discrepancies among documented medication therapy records and actual patient use of medications are common and occur with all classes of medications. Therefore, the first step for the provider in determining optimal medication therapy is to understand what medications patients are actually taking and how they are taking them. In addition to gathering information regarding prescribed medications, it is important for providers to also ensure they review all over-the-counter products, herbal products, and dietary supplements patients may be using regularly. Over 28% of the population regularly takes herbal supplements on a yearly basis, but only 16% of these patients report this to their physician. A thorough medication history is an important

resource to assess for appropriate medication use and to screen for possible medication-related problems. Table 47–1 lists five concise steps to a medication history. To obtain an accurate medication history, the physician should start by asking open-ended questions; for example, "What medications are you taking?" This approach avoids the common mistake of assuming the patient is taking all their medications as prescribed. Conducting an open-ended medication history may take more time up front, but the benefits gained in rapport building and medication optimization are well worth the time and effort, especially when it comes to the risks associated with over- and underprescribing medications. One example of medication optimization is the minimization of polypharmacy; *polypharmacy* is defined as the concurrent use of multiple medications or the prescribing of more medications than are clinically indicated.

Dickinson A, Blatman J, El-Dash N, et al. Consumer usage and reasons for using dietary supplements: report of a series of surveys. *J Am Coll Nutr.* 2014;33(2):176–182. [PMID: 24724775]

Rambhade S, Chakarborty A, Shrivastava A, Patil UK, Rambhade A. A survey on polypharmacy and use of inappropriate medications. *Toxicol Int.* 2012;19(1):68–73. [PMID: 22736907]

Steinke DT, MacDonald TM, Davey PG. The doctor patient relationship and prescribing patterns: a view from primary care. *Pharmacoeconomics.* 1999;16:599–603. [PMID: 10724789]

Tam VC, Knowles SR, Cornish PL, et al. Frequency, type and clinical importance of medication history errors at admission to hospital: a systematic review. *Can Med Assoc J.* 2005; 173(5):510–515. [PMID: 16129874]

▶ Evaluation & Change

A thorough medication history and safety assessment begins to clarify many aspects of a patient's medication regimen and, paired with evidence, can help the clinician make an informed patient-specific decision about a regimen. *Evidence-based medicine* (EBM) is "a model for

Table 47–1. Reviewing a medication regimen.

1. Match the medication with the diagnosis.
2. Review the regimen for duplication of therapy.
3. Elicit from the patient if she or he is taking the medicine.
4. Review laboratory results and patient history for efficacy/toxicity of the regimen.
5. Strive to remove any unnecessary agents from the regimen.

incorporating the tools of clinical epidemiology into clinical practice." This model entails obtaining the best external evidence to support clinical decisions and is, therefore, not restricted solely to randomized trials and meta-analysis.

Kennedy HL. The importance of randomized clinical trials and evidence-based medicine: a clinician's perspective. *Clin Cardiol.* 1999;22:6–12. [PMID: 9929747]

Tilburt JC. Evidence-based medicine beyond the bedside: keeping an eye on context. *J Eval Clin Practice.* 2008;14(5):721–725. [PMID: 19018902]

It is critical to appreciate that EBM does not depend solely on the skills and aptitude of literature evaluation and application of data, but must also incorporate clinical experience. The most commonly reported barrier to practicing EBM is a lack of time. However, the goal of EBM is to provide appropriate allocation of effective and efficient care to all patients. It is estimated that >6 million references have been published in >4000 journals in the National Library of Medicines database, MEDLINE. Slawson and Shaughnessy (2005) propose that the practitioner should approach this "information jungle" with a basic equation:

$$\text{Usefulness} = \frac{\text{Relevance} + \text{Validity}}{\text{Work}}$$

Relevance is directly proportional to its applicability to the physician's practice. Validity relates to the intrinsic methodology, study design, and conclusions. Thus, by maximizing the principles of the usefulness equation, one may locate the best source of information. The mnemonic **p**atient-**o**riented **e**vidence that **m**atters (POEMs) is an easy way for practitioners to focus in on information that can directly affect practice. Table 47–2 lists EBM-related websites.

Duncan B, Ables AZ. Do drug treatment POEMs report data in clinically useful ways? *J Fam Practice.* 2013;62(2):E1–E5. [PMID: 23405382]

Shaughnessy AF, Slawson DC, Becker L. Clinical jazz: harmonizing clinical experience and evidence-based medicine. *J Fam Pract.* 1998;47:425–428. [PMID: 9866666]

Slawson DC, Shaughnessy AF. Becoming an information master. Using "medical poetry" to remove the inequities in health care delivery. *J Fam Pract.* 2001;50:51–56. [PMID: 11195481]

Table 47–2. Evidence-based medicine (EBM) sources.

Clinical Information Internet Sources
Agency for HealthCare Research and Quality:
    http://www.ahrq.gov
Centre for EBM:
    http://www.cebm.net/
The Cochrane Library:
    http://www.cochrane.org
Essential Evidence Plus:
    http://www.essentialevidenceplus.com
Journal of Family Practice POEMS:
    https://www.mdedge.com/familymedicine

Evidence-Based Guideline Websites
Agency for HealthCare Research and Quality:
    http://www.ahrq.gov/clinic
Clinical Evidence, BMJ Publishing Group:
    http://www.clinicalevidence.org
Health Web:
    http://www.health.gov
Institute for Clinical Systems Improvement:
    http://www.ICSI.org
National Guideline Clearinghouse:
    https://www.ahrq.gov/gam/index.html

Slawson DC, Shaughnessy AF. Teaching evidence-based medicine: should we be teaching information management instead? *Acad Med.* 2005;80(7):685–689. [PMID: 15980087]

Zwolsman S, te Pas E, Hooft L, et al. Barriers to GPs' use of evidence-based medicine: a systematic review. *Br J Gen Pract.* 2012;62(600):e511–e521. [PMID: 22781999]

EXPLORING THE EVIDENCE: USE OF GUIDELINES & FORMULARIES

Clinical practice guidelines are defined by the Institute of Medicine as "statements that include recommendations intended to optimize patient care which is informed by a systematic review of evidence and an assessment of the benefits and harms of alternative care options." Clinical practice guidelines are intended to support clinicians' decision making by providing a comprehensive summary and critique of the available evidence. Several types of evidence-based guidelines exist, and the strength of evidence of each is variable. *Evidence-based clinical practice guidelines* incorporate recent literature regarding the effectiveness of therapy and clinical experience. *Expert consensus guidelines* may be the simplest type of guideline; however, limitations to this approach are inherent author bias and limited evidence-based sources. *Outcomes-based guidelines* incorporate measures of effectiveness to validate a positive impact on patient care.

The Cochrane Collaboration produces systematic reviews, maintains a registry of trials, and is a leading provider of evidence-based guidelines. Cochrane reviews may be located in the Cochrane Library, Cochrane Collaboration, or *Cochrane Reviews' Handbook* at the following site: http://www.cochrane.org. In addition to the Cochrane Collaboration, many medical/professional societies, health maintenance organizations, and the Agency for Health Care Policy and Research provide practice guidelines and Internet links to the guidelines.

Coleman CI, Talati R, White CM. A clinician's perspective on rating the strength of evidence of a systematic review. *Pharmacotherapy.* 2009;29:1017–1029. [PMID: 19698007]

Murad MH, Montori VM, Ioannidis JP. How to read a systematic review and meta-analysis and apply the results to patient care: users' guides to the medical literature. *JAMA.* 2014;312(2):171–179. [PMID: 25005654]

Institute of Medicine. Clinical Practice Guidelines We Can Trust. http://www.iom.edu/Reports/2011/Clinical-Practice-Guidelines-We-Can-Trust.aspx. Accessed March 21, 2013.

BALANCING THE EVIDENCE WITH THE PATIENT

▶ Medication Adherence

"Drugs don't work in patients who don't take them."
— C. Everett Koop, MD, former US Surgeon General

Medication adherence, or the degree to which a patient's medication-taking behaviors comply with a prescribed regimen, represents a serious and insidious barrier to optimal patient care. Many factors may affect adherence to a regimen, including perceived acuity of the disease being treated, regimen complexity, sequelae of the patient's underlying illness, and provider-patient relationships. Regardless of the reasons for nonadherence, it is clear that patients may not receive the full benefit of a medication regimen as a consequence of not taking the medication. In the United States, an estimated 33–69% of medication-related hospitalizations result from poor medication adherence.

While many studies report percentages of "adherence" and "nonadherence" as dichotomous and mutually exclusive variables, the true nature of medication adherence more likely resembles a continuum. Recognizing medication nonadherence and acting to improve patient self-efficacy present opportunities to improve both patient care and provider-patient relationships.

Blaschke TF, Osterberg L, Vrijens B, et al. Adherence to medications: insights arising from studies on the unreliable link between prescribed and actual drug dosing histories. *Annu Rev Pharmacol Toxicol.* 2012;52:275–301. [PMID: 21942628]

Osterberg L, Blaschke T. Drug therapy: adherence to medication. *N Engl J Med.* 2005;53:487–497. [PMID: 16079372]

Steiner JF. Rethinking adherence. *Ann Intern Med.* 2012;157:580–585. [PMID: 23070491]

Because it is difficult to predict patient adherence behavior, it is critical to identify barriers to adherence that may be controlled or modified. Many techniques may be used to assess compliance, including directly observed therapy, pill counts, review of prescription refill records, and patient interviews. Directly questioning the patient, while efficient and easy to do in an office visit, may create a bias toward perceived compliance that is not actually true. Douchette and colleagues developed the Drug Adherence Work-Up (DRAW) tool to assess patient adherence to medication and barriers associated with medication administration. Patients are asked the following questions:

1. Please tell me how you take your medication every day.
2. Do you feel like you have too many medications or too many doses per day?
3. Do you sometimes forget to take your medication on routine days?
4. Do you forget on nonroutine days such as weekends or when traveling?
5. Do you have a concern that your medication is not helping you?
6. Do you feel that you do not need this medication?
7. Have you had any side effects?
8. Are you concerned about side effects?
9. Is the cost of this medication too much?

Techniques from motivational interviewing may be additionally useful in eliciting patient responses. In particular, empathizing with patients about their medication regimen may build the provider-patient relationship and be helpful. For example, a physician might ask about medication adherence while providing support, as in the following example: "I know it is difficult to take all of your medications regularly. How many days of the week are you able to take them?" By approaching adherence from the positive perspective of what the patient is able to accomplish, this allows the patient to feel comfortable, and allows the physician to gain useful and truthful information. It is important to meet patients where they are, especially when working together to overcome barriers to adherence.

If nonadherence to a medication regimen is identified, consider assisting patients by helping them to create a medication list or calendar, provide refill reminders, use a pill organizer, develop a medication reminder chart, or consider electronic devices and compliance services. Consider referring patients to their pharmacist for support. Clinical and community pharmacists will be able to provide practical assistance for improving patient adherence as well as support to find the most cost-effective regimen to additionally improve adherence.

Doucette WR, Farris KB, Youland KM, et al. Development of the Drug Adherence Work-up (DRAW) tool. *J Am Pharm Assoc.* 2012;52(6):e199–204. [PMID: 23945734]

Palacio A, Garay D, Langer B, et al. Motivational interviewing improves medication adherence: a systematic review and meta-analysis. *J Gen Intern Med*. 2016;31(8):929–940. [PMID: 27160414]

Clear communication with patients when prescribing new medications is imperative. Improved medication adherence has been associated with patients who receive better general communication, more medication information, and better explanations about how to take medications. Despite the importance of conveying this information, prescribers often fall short. Tarn and colleagues (2006) studied physician communication for new medications and found that physicians failed to describe the medication's name 26% of the time, potential side effects 65% of the time, and cost 88% of the time. Community pharmacists are valuable resources to assist with patient counseling and conveying important information about new medications. However, community pharmacist counseling may be limited due to state regulations and busyness of their practice. Thus, it is important to not simply rely on the community pharmacist to convey this important information to patients.

The measurement tool used by Tarn and colleagues, known as the *medication communication index*, was developed from national guidelines for communication about new medications. This simple five-category index can be used as a guide for the five points to discuss with patients each time a new medication is started: (1) name of the medication, (2) purpose or justification for use, (3) duration of intake, (4) directions for use, and (5) potential adverse effects.

Kripalani S, Osborn CY, Vaccarino V, et al. Development and evaluation of a medication counseling workshop for physicians: can we improve on "take two pills and call me in the morning"? *Med Educ Online*. 2011;16:7133. [PMID: 21915162]

Tarn DM, Heritage J, Paterniti DA, et al. Physician communication when prescribing new medications. *Arch Intern Med*. 2006;166:1855–1862. [PMID: 17000942]

Tarn DM, Paterniti DA, Heritage J, et al. Physician communication about the cost and acquisition of newly prescribed medications. *Am J Managed Care*. 2006;12:657–664. [PMID: 17090222]

Svarstad B, Bultman DC, Mount JK. Patient counseling provided in community pharmacies: effects of state regulation, pharmacist age, and busyness. *J Am Pharm Assoc*. 2004;44:22–29. [PMID: 14965149]

▶ Managing Medication Cost

In 2016, spending on prescription drugs in the United States amounted to $328 billion, or 9.9% of national health expenditures. These costs continue to rise from year to year; between 2010 and 2016, prescription drug spending increased by $75.5 billion (almost 30%). For patients who have trouble affording their prescriptions, there are several ways to combat the high costs of drug therapy.

It is important to know if patients have insurance for prescription medications. Prescription coverage is typically included with most private, employer-based, and Medicaid insurance plans. Medicare patients need either Part D or a Medicare Advantage Plan (also called Medicare Part C) to cover cost of prescription medications. Insurance plans may use different cost-sharing strategies to reduce insurance premiums but increase the price patients pay for medications. Cost-sharing measures include copayments (payment made by the patient in addition to the payment by the insurance) and deductibles (specified amount of money an insured patient must pay before an insurance company will start paying for claims). Prescribing within the payer's formulary may aid in reducing out-of-pocket costs. Many third-party payers now post their formularies online where patients and providers can easily reference them. Prescribing of generic or lowest-tier drugs is encouraged whenever possible. Some retail pharmacy chains provide generic drug pricing plans that can decrease patients' medication costs even further. Coupon or discount programs (eg, goodrx.com) may offer significant savings for patients without insurance or those with high copays or deductibles. Pharmaceutical company coupons are typically for their newer, expensive agents, which is useful in the short term, but typically not a sustainable mechanism for medication procurement. Overall medication burden may also cause financial strain for patients. In this case, a thorough medication regimen review may identify drugs that can be discontinued or changed for lower cost alternatives, if medically appropriate.

Centers for Medicare and Medicaid Services. National Health Fact Sheet. https://www.cms.gov/Research-Statistics-Data-and-Systems/Statistics-Trends-and-Reports/NationalHealth ExpendData/NHE-Fact-Sheet.html. Accessed June 12, 2018.

National Council on Patient Information and Education. Enhancing Prescription Medicine Adherence: A National Action Plan. http://www.talkaboutrx.org/documents/enhancing_prescription_medicine_adherence.pdf. Accessed March 21, 2013.

Formulary systems are fundamental tools of hospitals, health systems, and managed care organizations to designate preferred products and provide rational, cost-effective prescribing decisions. A drug formulary may be defined as "a continuously revised list of medications that are readily available for use within an institution and reflect the current clinical judgment of the medical staff."

Drug formulary policies are based on comparative efficacy, safety, drug interactions, dosing, pharmacology, pharmacokinetics, and cost. Decisions are made by consensus of a pharmacy and therapeutics (P&T) committee made up of healthcare professionals of all major disciplines of practice who serve to represent the medical staff. A P&T committee has been described as "an advisory committee that is responsible for developing, managing, updating, and administering a formulary system." The goal of this body is to guide the appropriate, safe, and cost-effective use of medications.

Boucher BA. Formulary decisions: then and now. *Pharmacotherapy.* 2010;30:35–41. [PMID: 20500042]

Schiff GD, Galanter WL, Duhig J, et al. A prescription for improving drug formulary decision making. *PLoS Med.* 2012;9:1–7. [PMID: 22629233]

Taylor LS, Cole SW, May JR, et al. ASHP statement on the pharmacy and therapeutics committee and the formulary system. *Am J Health Syst Pharm.* 2008;65:2384–2386. [PMID: 18589893]

For patients who do not have insurance, a few options can be pursued to help them obtain medications at a reduced cost:

1. *A patient age ≥65 years can apply for drug coverage through Medicare Part D.* To determine which plans the patient is eligible for, and associated costs, visit www .medicare.gov.

2. *Determine whether your patient qualifies for any federal, state, or military-operated program.* Income restrictions apply.

3. *Have contact information available for state Medicaid programs.*

4. *Consider applying for medication assistance programs sponsored by pharmaceutical manufacturers.* Pharmaceutical manufacturers supplied free or low-cost medications to >5 million people in the United States. Several Internet sites are available to aid in obtaining information on how to use these programs, including www.needymeds.com, www.rxhope.com, and www .injuredcalltoday.com/the-medicine-program.

Felder TM, Palmer NR, Lal LS, et al. What is the evidence for pharmaceutical patient assistance programs? A systematic review. *J Health Care Poor Underserved.* 2011;22:24–49. [PMID: 21317504]

Partnership for Prescription Assistance. Prescription assistance programs. http://www.pparx.org/en/prescription_assistance_ programs. Accessed March 21, 2013.

ENSURING MEDICATION SAFETY

Patient harm as a consequence of a medical error or drug effect is a common, costly, and largely preventable problem. Fatalities related to adverse drug reactions (ADRs) have been estimated to rank between the fourth and sixth leading cause of death in the United States.

During premarketing trials, if ≥1500 patients are exposed to a drug, the most common ADRs will be detected. However, >30,000 patients must be exposed to the drug in the postmarketing period to detect an ADR in one patient with a power of 0.95 to discover an incidence of 1 in 10,000. For both new and older medications alike, primary care providers play an important role in detecting and reporting

unexpected or previously unreported reactions to medications. Physicians can anonymously report ADRs simply by (1) logging onto www.fda.gov/MEDWATCH or calling 800-FDA-1088, or (2) if in a hospital or nursing home setting, contacting the pharmacy or local drug information center. Adverse reactions to vaccines should be reported to the Vaccine Adverse Event Reporting (VAERS) program, which is cosponsored by the Centers for Disease Control and Prevention and US Food and Drug Administration (FDA). Risk Evaluation and Mitigation Strategies (REMS) are activities required by the FDA to ensure the benefit of a drug continues to outweigh the risks. REMS requirements may include providing a medication guide at the time of dispensing or administration, a communication plan, and required activities or interventions. A medication guide is detailed information to help patients use a medication and avoid serious adverse events. Communication plans involve information provided directly from the manufacturer to healthcare providers about serious risks associated with a medication and how to avoid these risks. Required activities and interventions include certifications, documentation, or monitoring that prescribers, pharmacists, or patients must adhere to in order to receive or continue treatment.

Bates DW, Cullen DJ, Laird N, et al. Incidence of adverse drug events and potential adverse drug events: implications for prevention. *JAMA.* 1995;274:29–34. [PMID: 7791255]

Pirmohamed M, Breckenridge AM, Kitteringham NR, et al. Fortnightly review: adverse drug reactions. *Br Med J.* 1998;316:1295–1298. [PMID: 9554902]

US Food and Drug Administration. Safety Information and Adverse Drug Reporting Program. http://www.fda.gov/Safety/ MedWatch/default.htm. Accessed June 30, 2018.

US Food and Drug Administration. What's in a REMS. https:// www.fda.gov/Drugs/DrugSafety/REMS/ucm592636.htm. Accessed June 12, 2018.

Vaccine Adverse Event Reporting System. http://vaers.hhs.gov/ esub/index. Accessed March 22, 2013.

von Lau NC, Schwappach DL, Koeck CM. The epidemiology of preventable adverse drug events: review of the literature. *Wien Klin Wochenschr.* 2003;115(12):407–415. [PMID: 12918183]

MATCH THE PATIENT & THE DRUG: PHARMACOKINETIC & PHARMACODYNAMIC PRINCIPLES

Although a subset of ADRs is unpredictable, those that are preventable include drug-drug interactions. A grasp of basic pharmacokinetic/pharmacodynamic principles is needed to prevent interactions. Pharmacokinetics characterizes the rate and extent of absorption, distribution, metabolism, and elimination of a drug. Pharmacodynamics is the study of the relationship between the drug concentration at the site of action and the patient response. The patient's age, gender, weight, genetics, and comorbid conditions (especially renal and hepatic function) can affect drug pharmacokinetics and pharmacodynamics and should be considered when recommending medications. Pharmacogenomics is the study of the relationship of genetics in drug metabolism and response. In a systematic review by Phillips and colleagues of 27 drugs known to frequently cause ADRs, 59% were known to be influenced by individual patient genetic characteristics.

El Desoky ES. Pharmacokinetic-pharmacodynamic crisis in the elderly. *Am J Ther*. 2007;14(5):488–498. [PMID: 17890940]

Kirchheiner J, Seeringer A. Clinical implications of pharmacogenetics of cytochrome p450 drug metabolizing enzymes. *Biochim Biophys Acta*. 2007;1770(3):489–494. [PMID: 17113714]

Pai MP. Drug dosing based on body surface area: mathematical assumptions and limitations in obese patients. *Pharmacotherapy*. 2012;32:856–868. [PMID: 22711238]

Phillips KA, Veenstra DL, Oren E, Lee JK, Sadee W. Potential Role of Pharmacogenomics in Reducing Adverse Drug Reactions: A Systematic Review. *JAMA*. 2001;286(18):2270–2279. doi:10.1001/jama.286.18.2270.

Schwartz JB. The current state of knowledge on age, sex, and their interactions on clinical pharmacology. *Clin Pharmacol Ther*. 2007;82(1):87–96. [PMID: 17495875]

DRUG-DRUG INTERACTIONS: USING PHARMACOKINETIC & PHARMACODYNAMIC PRINCIPLES

Drug-drug interactions and ADRs can also be avoided by considering how a medication is metabolized and transported in the body. The main enzymatic system responsible for drug metabolism is the cytochrome P450 (CYP) system. Metabolism through the CYP system occurs mainly in the liver, but can also occur in the intestines and other organs. Many medications also rely on transporter proteins for absorption, distribution, metabolism, or elimination. Some examples of transport proteins include P-glycoproteins (P-gp), organic anion transporter proteins (OAT), and ATP-binding cassette transporter proteins (ABC). Understanding these systems allows prediction of drug-drug interactions among many patients. To do this, it is necessary to identify which drugs are being metabolized or transported (substrate), the type of interaction, and the affect and severity of the interaction. Interactions can be placed into two categories:

- **Induction**: The interacting drug increases metabolism or transport of the substrate.

- **Inhibition**: The interacting drug decreases metabolism or transport of the substrate.

The interaction may result in increased or decreased exposure to a drug depending on where the interaction occurs along the pharmacokinetic pathway. A change in drug selection may prevent a drug interaction. Physicians may check for drug-drug interactions using drug information resources.

Gex-Fabry M, Balant-Gorgia AE, Balant LP. Therapeutic drug monitoring databases for postmarketing surveillance of drug-drug interactions. *Drug Safety*. 2001;24:947–959. [PMID: 11735651]

Lynch T, Price A. The effect of cytochrome P450 metabolism on drug response, interactions, and adverse effects. *Am Fam Physician*. 2007;76(3):391–396. [PMID: 17708140]

KEEPING UP WITH THE LITERATURE

Subscribing to survey services is one way to stay current with the pertinent literature, while decreasing the amount of work and time required. Survey services provide an efficient means of reviewing a host of medical journals and articles. However, one should do this cautiously because of the potential for bias toward positive conclusions or embellishment of study results. The conclusions and recommendations presented by such services should be critically evaluated before applying the information in practice.

Castillo DL, Abraham NS. Knowledge management: how to keep up with the literature. *Clin Gastroenterol Hepatol*. 2008;6:1294–1300. [PMID: 18986844]

Three basic categories of survey services exist: (1) abstracting services, (2) review services, and (3) traditional newsletters. Abstracting services for family physicians include, but are not limited to, the *ACP Journal Club*, the *Journal of Family Practice*, and *Journal Watch Online*. All have a goal of providing relevant information in a timely manner. *ACP Journal Club* (http://acpjc.acponline.org/) is published by the American College of Physicians–American Society of Internal Medicine. This service provides brief, high-level summaries of current original articles and systematic reviews in a structured abstract format. The *ACP Journal Club* reviews over 100 journals and uses prestated criteria to select and evaluate data. Pertinent information summaries are provided to subscribers on a bimonthly basis. The *Journal of Family Practice* (https://www.mdedge.com/familymedicine) provides family physicians with timely, reliable information supplemented with expert commentary on clinically applicable topics. *Journal Watch Online* (http://www.jwatch.org) is supported by the publishers of the *New England Journal of Medicine*. This service, similar to the others, provides current summaries of the most important primary literature. An editorial board, composed of physicians from many specialty areas, reviews, analyzes, and summarizes 55–60 critically important articles. The summaries are published on a bimonthly basis. In addition, this service features *Clinical Practice Guidelines Watch* and editorials of the year's top medical stories.

ACP Journal Club. http://acpjc.acponline.org. Accessed June 30, 2018.

Journal Watch Online. http://www.jwatch.org. Accessed June 30, 2018.

The Journal of Family Practice. https://www.mdedge.com/familymedicine. Accessed November 23, 2019.

Review Services provide a succinct summary of a specific topic, rather than a survey of the literature. One example of a review service is *The Medical Letter* (http://www.medletter .com). *The Medical Letter* is published by an independent nonprofit organization and provides critical appraisals of new medications or uses for medications in a clinical context, comparing and contrasting the new medications to similar established agents. This concise publication is printed bimonthly. Another example of a review service is *Primary Care Reports* (https://www.reliasmedia.com/products/346-primary-care-reports-online-1-year-subscription-w-auto-renew). This service is printed bimonthly and is intended to provide review articles on critical issues in primary care; treatment recommendations are provided with each review.

Primary Care Reports. https://www.reliasmedia.com/. Accessed June 30, 2018.
The Medical Letter. http://www.medletter.com. Accessed June 30, 2018.

Traditional newsletters provide brief reviews of current literature with topics from news media and other sources. Examples of this type of newsletter include The *Drug and Therapeutics Bulletin* and *Therapeutics Letter*. The *Drug and Therapeutics Bulletin* (http://www.dtb.bmj.com) is a concise monthly bulletin that provides evaluations of medications and summarizes randomized, controlled, clinical trials and consensus statements. This service provides informed and unbiased assessments of medications and their overall place in therapy. The *Therapeutics Letter* (https://www.ti.ubc.ca/ therapeutics-letter/) is a bimonthly newsletter that targets problematic therapeutic issues and provides evidence-based reviews written and edited by a team of specialists and working groups of the International Society of Drug Bulletins.

Drug and Therapeutics Bulletin. http://dtb.bmj.com. Accessed June 30, 2018.
Therapeutics Initiative. Evidence-based drug therapy. https://www .ti.ubc.ca/therapeutics-letter/. Accessed November 23, 2019.

It is recommended that physicians use these services as filtering tools to determine which primary literature articles are critical to read in-depth. Survey services provide condensed forms of information, but it is the clinician's responsibility to analyze, interpret, and apply this information effectively in patient care decisions.

DRUG INFORMATION/PHARMACOTHERAPY IN THE DIGITAL ERA

Traditionally, textbooks have been the cornerstone reference for physicians for drug information such as the *Physician's Desk Reference* (PDR), *American Hospital Formulary Services*

(AHFS), *Drug Facts and Comparisons* (*Facts & Comparisons*), and the *Drug Information Handbook*. However, as we move into this digital era where instantaneous, accurate information is expected, physicians and residents alike are turning toward their computers and handheld devices for drug information resources.

Cohen JS. Dose discrepancies between the Physician's Desk Reference and the medical literature, and their possible role in the high incidence of dose-related adverse drug events. *Arch Intern Med.* 2001;16:957–964. [PMID: 11295958]

There are numerous drug information resources available to address general or specific pharmaceutical categories (eg, ADRs, drug interactions, therapeutic use, dosing) that are well referenced with the prescribing information from drug manufacturers, counseling tips, and FDA warnings. *MICROMEDEX* is a computerized drug information resource that contains facts from the DRUGDEX Information System. This is a well-referenced, easily searchable, expansive drug information reference, housing information on prescription, nonprescription, and herbal products. *Facts & Comparisons* contains information on prescription and nonprescription medications. This reference provides tables and comparative drug class data along with patient counseling information. *Clinical Pharmacology* is another digital resource available to address drug questions including interaction information and a wide array of printouts available for patient-friendly information. Finally, *Lexicomp* is a thorough drug information resource to search for drug information questions. With a user-friendly mobile application, *Lexicomp* is a widely used resource.

With increases of natural products, *The Natural Medicines Comprehensive Database* and the National Library of Medicine are two electronic references that consistently provide valid natural production information. *ePocrates Rx* has been advocated by insurance companies and government agencies to enhance clinical management and decrease medication errors.

Clinical Pharmacology. http://www.clinicalpharmacology.com/. Accessed June 30, 2018.
ePocrates Rx. http://www.epocrates.com. Accessed June 30, 2018.
Facts and Comparisons. http://www.factsandcomparisons.com/. Accessed June 30, 2018.
Lexicomp. http://www.lexi.com/. Accessed June 30, 2018.
MICROMEDEX 2.0. http://www.micromedex.com/. Accessed June 30, 2018.
Natural Medicines Comprehensive Database. http://www.natural database.com. Accessed June 30, 2018.
Sweet BV, Gay WE, Leady MA, et al. Usefulness of herbal and dietary supplement references. *Ann Pharmacother.* 2003;37:494–499. [PMID: 12659602]

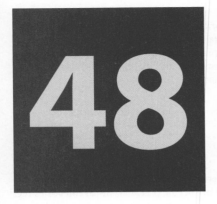

Genetics for Family Physicians

Mylynda B. Massart, MD, PhD

Natasha Robin Berman, MA, MS, MPH, LCGC

INTRODUCTION

In the current era of precision and molecular medicine, it is becoming increasingly important that family medicine providers become familiar with genetics and genomics. There is no longer a field of medicine that has not been impacted by the understanding and advancements in genetics following the sequencing of the human genome. In addition, advances in computational modeling and data analysis have inspired national and international initiatives to better understand the role of genomics coupled with environmental influences to better understand and predict health on the individual level as well as enhance treatment of disease. Precision medicine will allow for the integration of unprecedented amounts of data regarding genetics, family history, environmental exposures, nutrition, and many more "omes" (eg, exposome, genome, microbiome) to complement patient care.

Historically, the field of medical genetics was predominantly practiced as a subspecialty. Medical geneticists diagnosed and cared for individuals with genetic disorders resulting from classic single-gene disorders, chromosome abnormalities, and metabolic diseases. Over the past decade, medical geneticists and genetic counselors have expanded into prenatal care for the identification of at-risk parents and counseling regarding reproductive decision making, as well as oncology, as the identification of genetic cancer-susceptibility testing has become readily available. Recent approval by the US Food and Drug Administration (FDA) of many commercially available direct-to-consumer (DTC) genetic test has created access to this technology online without a physician-driven test order. Initially, these DTC tests were primarily reporting genetic ancestry data or health traits such as whether one can smell asparagus in their urine. However, several companies are now offering increasingly relevant medical data including hereditary cancer risk as well as whole-genome sequencing. Consumers are highly engaged in this level of genetic testing, and in this era of patient-driven

medicine, patients are demanding that their healthcare providers support and be receptive of the integration of these results into their personal healthcare management. The advancements in the identification of genetic-related risk as well as the increasing availability of testing and reimbursement for testing make genetics highly relevant to the average family medicine patient. Genetics is now impacting preventative health decisions, routine prenatal care, medication selection, and identification of risk for many complex chronic diseases. The potential patient population that may benefit from genetics is outgrowing the genetic specialist workforce. There are not enough medical geneticists or genetic counselors to keep up with the increased need for knowledge and resources. In addition, the geographic distribution of genetic specialists primarily near large academic health centers markedly limits access for most patients. Finally, increasing insurance copays and deductibles create an additional barrier to patient access to specialty care genetics. Integration of genetics, genomics, and precision medicine is a logical extension of the services provided by family medicine given the broad relevance of precision medicine to patient care.

To successfully integrate genetics and genomics into the practice of family medicine, physicians need to be familiar with common genetic terminology and concepts as well as current uses of the technology as it applies to pharmacogenomics, prenatal genetics, management of complex chronic disease, and genetic cancer risk assessment. Additionally, providers will need to become comfortable with managing routine genetic cases and recognize which patients will need to be referred to genetic specialist colleagues. Providers will need to become familiar with the types of testing available, identifying appropriate candidates for genetic testing, accessing testing, and integrating the results back into the clinical management of the patient. As this new standard of care is adopted, health system support needs to both expand in the capacity for electronic health records to store genetic data and also trigger real-time clinical decision support and education for providers. This chapter will provide a review of core genetics concepts and considerations, practical integration recommendations, and challenges to the successful integration of genetics into the practice of family medicine.

GENETIC REVIEW

Human genetic information is contained in DNA and is present in nearly every cell in the human body. DNA consists of paired strands of chemical bases called nucleotides, which are compacted into complex structures composed of DNA and proteins to form chromosomes; somatic cells have 46 chromosomes that are arranged in 23 pairs, making up the human genome. The first 22 pairs, called autosomes, contain the genetic information for both men and women. The chromosomes that determine sex (X and Y) are paired as XX for females and XY for males. One chromosome from each pair is inherited from the mother and the other from the father. The germ cells or gametes (sperm and egg cells) contain only 23 chromosomes.

Chromosomes contain the thousands of genes that are the basis of inheritance. It is estimated that the human genome consists of about 20,000 protein-coding genes. Genes consist of short segments of DNA along each chromosome that encode the blueprint for a protein or RNA molecule. These coding regions are known as exons. Additional noncoding regions known as introns are sequences of DNA that are often involved in the control of gene expression. Each gene comes in a pair; one copy of each gene is inherited from an individual's father and the other from his or her mother. The coding region of each gene specifies the instructions for a particular protein or RNA molecule according to the order in which the nucleotides are arranged. Proteins are responsible for the development and function of our bodies. During cell replication and division, errors can occur in the DNA sequence (mutations), resulting in a protein that does not function properly or is present in insufficient amounts. Occasionally errors such as large deletions or rearrangements of chromosome structure occur that affect the function of multiple genes.

The chromosomes themselves can have chemical modifications (acylation, methylation) that contribute to how compactly the chromosomes are packaged into chromatin. This packaging can also impact gene expression and can be modified by environmental factors. The level of packaging can also be inherited in a process we now call epigenetics. There is a vast amount of current research studying epigenetics, inheritance, and health.

In addition to the genetic material contained in the cell nucleus, there is also genetic material stored in the mitochondria, an energy-producing organelle found in our cells. Mitochondrial DNA is stored in a single, circular chromosome and is inherited through the cytoplasm of the maternal gamete. Thus, mitochondrial DNA is maternally inherited only.

GENETIC EVALUATION

▶ Family History

A. The Pedigree: Importance

The pedigree is a quick and easy way to visualize multiple generations worth of health information. It is a tool used by genetics professionals to better visualize inheritance patterns, determine how a disease may be affecting a family, and identify at-risk individuals in the family. Although family medicine providers routinely collect family history information, the details of the family history can be overlooked during a complex and time-limited primary care visit. One of the benefits of an appointment with a genetics professional is increased time to discuss family health history in detail. Because it is not feasible to refer all patients to a genetic specialist, the pedigree can be a quick and easy tool to help determine who needs a higher level genetics consultation. Family medicine providers are the first point of contact for most patients with a genetic concern or risk, and a quick "snap shot" pedigree will allow a provider to rapidly identify potential red flags and initiate appropriate referrals. In an ideal clinical setting, the electronic health record would be capable of integrating annual patient-entered family and personal health history information to generate the pedigree and alert providers to red flags. Until then, pedigree info could be gleaned from the history, assembled into pedigree format, and scanned into the chart with an appropriate annotation in the "problem list" as to where the pedigree is stored. In the setting where drawing a full pedigree is not practical, a standard risk assessment form could be employed at annual and new patient visits.

Nelson HD, Fu R, Goddard K, et al. Risk assessment, genetic counseling, and genetic testing for BRCA-related cancer: systematic review to update the U.S. Preventive Services Task Force Recommendation. Report No.: 12-05164-EF-1. Rockville, MD: Agency for Healthcare Research and Quality; 2013.

Rich EC, Burke W, Heaton CJ, et al. Reconsidering the family history in primary care. *J Gen Intern Med.* 2004;19:273–280. [PMID: 15009784]

Trotter TL, Martin HM. Family history in pediatric primary care. *Pediatrics.* 2007;120:S60–S65. [PMID: 17767006]

B. The Pedigree: Critical Components

This section will review the critical information to obtain from patients and the standard pedigree nomenclature necessary to assemble a pedigree.

Any pedigree should contain at least three generations if possible. This will include the patient's first-degree relatives (children, siblings, and parents) as well as their second-degree relatives (half-siblings, aunts/uncles, nieces/nephews, grandparents, and grandchildren). When possible, third-degree relatives (cousins) are often helpful. Included in this chapter is a sample of current standard nomenclature (Figure 48–1).

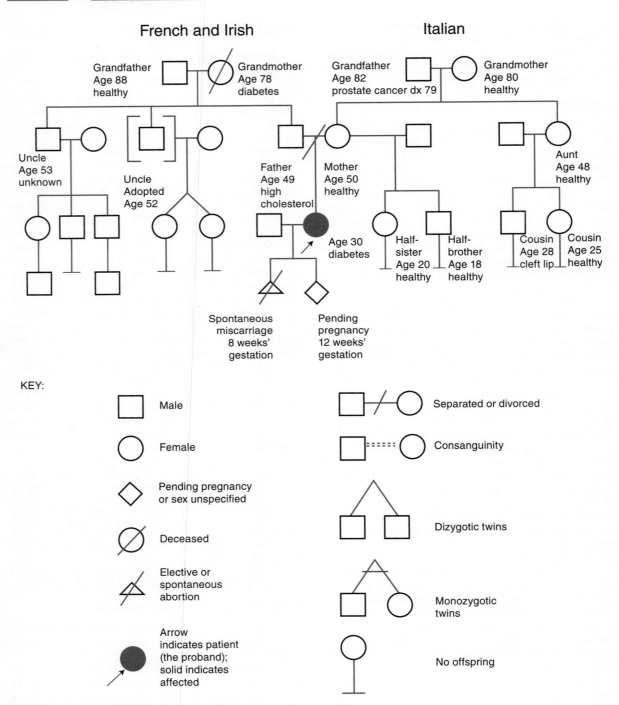

▲ Figure 48–1. Standard pedigree symbols and sample pedigree. dx, diagnosed.

When drawing a pedigree, the most important aspect is that others can read and understand it. The pedigree should note the age of diagnosis, medical issues, and current age of all individuals. It is particularly important to indicate the age of diagnosis, if known. The more information the better, but during a busy clinic, this may not always be possible. Therefore, the following list is provided to assist in obtaining the minimal information necessary for adequate interpretation of the pedigree. Standard information that needs to be gathered includes the following:

- Three-generation pedigree
- Age/year of birth of all family members
- Health status of each individual as well as age of onset/diagnosis of health concerns
- If there are no health concerns for an individual, that should also be indicated
- If possible, identification of ethnic background (can be inquired about by asking if patients know where their family was from prior to coming to the United States)

Bennett RL, French KS, Resta RG, et al. Standardized human pedigree nomenclature: update and assessment of the recommendations of the National Society of Genetic Counselors. *J Genet Couns.* 2008;17:424–433. [PMID: 18792771]

Although producing a pedigree can be time consuming, only updates will be needed in subsequent visits rather than the whole history. Additionally, rather than inquiring if an individual has any health concerns, it may be helpful to ask about major health concerns, following up with questions that may elicit specific indicators for a genetics referral. Ultimately the choice of how to obtain a family health history is the decision of the provider; the most important thing is to identify patients who would benefit most from further evaluation regarding a possible genetic concern or from a referral for conditions such as familial hypercholesterolemia or possible *BRCA* carrier status.

It is also possible to request that patients organize their family health history prior to coming to the clinic and to bring it in for evaluation by a provider. There are several tools available to help patients obtain and organize this information, including the Surgeon General tool My Family Health Portrait website. It is still important to review the information with the patient in person to ensure accuracy. Because family health history is something that changes and evolves over time, it is important that the health record be updated periodically with new diagnoses, births, deaths, or other relevant information. Finally, most current electronic health record programs do not have a designated location for pedigrees or genetic results. Therefore, it is critical to develop institution-wide guidelines about where this information is stored and annotated in the health record.

Centers for Disease Control and Prevention. Public health genomics knowledge base: My Family Health Portrait. https://phgkb.cdc.gov/FHH/html/index.html#. Accessed November 25, 2019.

▶ Inheritance Patterns

There are several core inheritance patterns that are important to recall when interpreting a pedigree (Table 48–1). The classic Mendelian patterns refer to a disease caused by one single gene. There are five common patterns of inheritance for single-gene disorders: autosomal dominant, autosomal recessive, x-linked dominant, x-linked recessive, and mitochondrial. The expression of the allele carrying the mutation can be dominant, recessive, or codominant. Non-Mendelian inheritance refers to any disease that does not follow the laws of simple independent assortment of a single gene.

Table 48–1. Clues to determine patterns of inheritance.

Pattern[a]	Diagnostic Clues
Autosomal dominant	Males and females equally affected Transmission passes from one generation to another (vertical inheritance) 50% risk for each offspring to be affected Variable expressivity: affected individuals in the same family may demonstrate varying degrees of phenotypic expression (severity) Reduced penetrance: some individuals who have inherited a genetic mutation may not express the phenotype ("skipped generations" may be seen)
Autosomal recessive	Males and females equally affected Multiple affected offspring and unaffected parents (horizontal inheritance) 25% risk for each offspring to parents with an affected child
X-linked recessive	Affects more males than females Heterozygous females are usually normal or have mild manifestations Inheritance is through maternal side of the family (diagonal inheritance) Female carriers have a 50% risk for each daughter to be a carrier and a 50% risk for each son to be affected All daughters of an affected male are carriers, and none of his sons are affected
Multifactorial or complex	Risk highest for closest relatives to affected individuals Multiple genes and environmental factors may contribute to risk No well-defined pattern of inheritance in pedigree; "runs in the family"

[a]For more complex patterns of inheritance, see Korf BR: Basic genetics. *Prim Care.* 2004 Sep;31(3):461–478. [PMID: 15331242]

▶ Genetic Variation

In addition to the classic inheritance patterns of genetic changes that lead to disease, there are several additional levels of genetic variation that contribute to health and disease status. The most common is the single nucleotide polymorphism (SNP). An SNP is a single nucleotide variation that occurs at a specific site in the genome. To be considered an SNP, the variation needs to be present in >1% of the population. There are >10 million SNPs in each person's genome. These variations can be linked directly to specific disease states, or they can have no appreciable effect. The process of mapping genetic lineage looks at how SNPs are transmitted from generation to generation to delineate lineage and geographic regions of ancestry. SNPs are also the small variations in the cytochrome P450 genes that lead to variations in drug metabolism and are the basis of pharmacogenomics. Copy number variation is another way that small regions of the genome can vary among individuals; small sequences of DNA can vary in copy number as both short and long sequence repeats, and these copy number variants can lead directly to the manifestation of disease or a modification of normal cellular function.

CLINICAL GENETICS

▶ Genetic Counseling

A. What Is a Genetic Counselor?

Genetic counselors are typically master's-level graduates who have received specialized education related to human genetics and counseling. These genetic counseling programs are accredited by the Accreditation Counsel for Genetic Counseling (ACGC), which outlines specific standards and competencies. These competencies include expertise in genetics, the ability to provide psychosocial support and use counseling skills when interacting with patients, and the ability to educate others about complex genetic information. Their primary service is the interpretation of family and medical histories to assess the chance of disease occurrence or recurrence; provide education about inheritance, testing, management, prevention, resources, and research opportunities; and provide counseling to promote informed choices and adaptation to the risk or condition.

Historically, genetic counselors were primarily employed in pediatric genetics clinics. Over the past several decades, genetic counseling has become a critical part of prenatal and oncology care. In this modern era of genomic medicine, there is a new need for the primary care genetic counselor who can provide support and assistance as part of a primary care multidisciplinary team.

Resta R, Biesecker BB, Bennett RL, et al. A new definition of genetic counseling: National Society of Genetic Counselors' Task Force report. *J Genet Couns.* 2006;15:77–83. [PMID: 16761103]

Genetic counseling at its core is intended to assist individuals with understanding and making decisions about their health as it is impacted by genetics. Family medicine providers may engage in genetic counseling at different levels, based on the clinical circumstance of the patients as well as their own comfort with the material. Ideally, all genetic counseling should include collection of accurate information and interpretation that is accessible to the patient. Genetic counseling should use a nondirective approach with patients due to the sensitive nature of genetics. Any counseling session should strive to empower the patient to make his or her own healthcare decisions. Critical components to integrate into a counseling session are the informed consent process, pre- and posttest counseling, conveying risk, and a discussion of the merits and drawbacks of testing so that the patient can decide which avenue to pursue.

Doyle DL, Awwad RI, Austin JC, et al. 2013 review and update of the genetic counseling practice based competencies by a Task Force of the Accreditation Council for Genetic Counseling. *J Genet Couns.* 2016;25:868–879. [PMID: 27333894]

B. Recognizing Who to Refer to Genetics

As the relevance of genetics to family medicine rapidly increases, the number of patients who may benefit from a genetic specialist consultation will similarly increase. As with all other areas of medicine, it is crucial to know one's expertise and when it is necessary to refer a patient for a specialty consultation. When analyzing a pedigree or family history, it is important to be able to identify patterns and specific red flags that would help determine which individuals would benefit most from a genetics referral. The following list includes several examples that would be appropriate for referral:

- Abnormal results of prenatal screening/testing
- Pattern suspicious for an inherited form of a disease in family history
- Multiple people in the family have similar disease/symptoms
- Known inherited condition that runs in the family
- Patient would like additional information about a prior positive genetic test result and the primary care doctor is not comfortable or familiar with the condition
- Previous children with birth defects or genetic disorders
- Families with history of developmental delays or intellectual disability
- Patient interested in screening/testing options that the primary care doctor is not comfortable or familiar with
- Patient interested in prenatal screening or diagnostic options that the primary care doctor is not comfortable or familiar with

- Individuals with multiple miscarriages (three or more), any stillbirth, or infertility
- Strong history of cancer, either personal or familial
- Multiple family members with the same or similar types of cancers
- Cancers at a young age (<50 years)
- Unusual cancers (like male breast cancer)
- Individuals with multiple primary cancers
- Having a child who may have an undiagnosed genetic condition
- Individuals in the 95th or greater percentile of low-density lipoprotein (LDL) levels

Genetic counselor services across the country can be found online through the National Society of Genetic Counselors. In addition, there is now an increasing amount of genetic counseling services available over the phone and online to provide counseling in geographic areas without direct access to genetic services.

National Society of Genetic Counselors. Find a genetic counselor. https://www.findageneticcounselor.com/. Accessed November 25, 2019.

▶ Methods of Genetic Testing

A. What Are You Testing?

Genetic testing can be used to identify changes in a patient's chromosomes, genes, or proteins. Before ordering testing for heritable disorders, clinicians should carefully consider the relevance and the implications of the testing for their patient.

B. Testing Categories

Genetic testing is typically considered to fall into several major categories, which help to determine how the test can be used for clinical decision making for a patient or her or his family members. **Diagnostic testing** is used to confirm or identify a known or suspected genetic disorder in a symptomatic individual. This type of testing may also include assays that help to inform prognosis and treatment decisions in someone with an established disease diagnosis. **Predictive testing** is offered to an asymptomatic individual with or without a family history of a genetic disorder to better define the patient's risk of developing a given condition. Patients are further defined as presymptomatic if eventual development of symptoms is certain (eg, Huntington disease) or predispositional if eventual development of symptoms is likely but not certain (ie, colon cancer). **Carrier testing** was historically offered to individuals who have a family member with an autosomal recessive or X-linked condition or individuals in an ethnic group known to have a high carrier rate for a particular disorder (eg, sickle cell anemia in the African

American population). Conversely, recent guidelines for expanded carrier testing released by the American College of Obstetricians and Gynecologists (ACOG) in 2017 advocate for carrier screening regardless of ethnicity or family history. **Pharmacogenetic testing** is used to help guide selection and dosing of medications for drug therapy. **Prenatal screening/testing** is performed during a pregnancy and is offered when there is an increased risk of having a child with a genetic condition (eg, quad screen, noninvasive prenatal screen, chorionic villus sampling, amniocentesis). **Preimplantation testing** is performed on early embryos during in vitro fertilization and offered to couples who are at increased risk of having a child with a genetic condition. **Newborn screening** is performed during the newborn period to identify children who may be at increased risk of a specific genetic disorder so that further evaluation and treatment can be initiated as soon as possible.

C. Different Lab Methods

There are three main categories of genetic testing methods. These include cytogenetics, biochemical assays, and molecular testing to detect abnormalities in chromosome structure, protein function, and DNA sequence.

1. Cytogenetics—Cytogenetics is used to identify structural abnormalities within chromosomes. The chromosomes are collected from cells, fixed onto microscope slides, and stained to show specific banding patterns in each chromosome. This technique detects variations in chromosome structure and can be used for white blood cells, bone marrow, and cells in amniotic fluid. Fluorescence in situ hybridization (FISH) is a process that paints chromosomes or portions of chromosomes with fluorescent molecules to identify chromosomal abnormalities such as insertions, deletions, translocations, and amplifications.

2. Biochemical testing—Biochemical testing examines proteins instead of genes. Specific biochemical tests have been developed to look at protein levels and activity as a measure of disease. The most common test is the gas chromatography/mass spectrometry (GC/MS) and tandem mass spectrometry (MS/MS) used in newborn screening to identify inborn errors of metabolism or biochemical genetic diseases.

3. Molecular testing—Molecular tests examine DNA for a disease for which the genetic sequence is already known. These techniques include sequencing, polymerase chain reaction (PCR)–based assays, and hybridization. PCR is used in many genetic tests to amplify targeted segments of DNA for subsequent analysis. Comparative genomic hybridization (CGH), also called chromosomal microarray analysis, is a molecular cytogenetic method to evaluate for gains or losses of parts of a chromosome that are not detectable using karyotyping or FISH. This method is based on comparing fluorescently labeled patient DNA to reference DNA.

CGH can detect small deletions and duplications, but it cannot detect structural chromosomal changes such as balanced reciprocal translocations/inversions or changes in chromosomal copy number.

DNA microarray analysis, also referred to as chip analysis, evaluates actual gene expression. Fluorescently labeled molecules of mRNA hybridize to numerous small segments of DNA that have been fixed to a small microchip. Computer technology can then analyze the bound, labeled markers, allowing for simultaneous testing of thousands of genes from an individual patient. This type of technology also allows for SNP analysis, with the ability to identify single nucleotide differences in binding of patient DNA to reference DNA.

Sequencing the first human genome in 2003 cost an estimated $500 million dollars. Technology continues to increase in speed and decrease in cost. With the use of next-generation sequencing technology, current cost estimates for whole-genome sequencing or whole-exome sequencing, which is just the protein-encoded regions of the genome, are around $500 to $1000. This now brings the cost of the technology to a range where it may be financially beneficial to consider testing and to start discussions of preemptive genetic testing on all patients versus question-specific testing each time a new genetic clinical question arises during the lifetime of a patient.

Genetic Alliance. Understanding Genetics: A New York, Mid-Atlantic Guide for Patients and Health Professionals. https://www.ncbi.nlm.nih.gov/books/NBK115548/. Accessed November 25, 2019.

Schwarze K, Buchanan J, Taylor JC, et al. Are whole-exome and whole-genome sequencing approaches cost-effective? A systematic review of the literature. *Genet Med.* 2018;20(10):1122–1130. [PMID: 29446766]

D. What a Genetic Test Can Reveal

It is critically important for patients to understand the risks of what a genetic test can reveal prior to making a decision to test. Both clinical and DTC genetic testing can lead to unintentional disclosure of one's private data. There can be breach of secure data systems by hacking or inadvertent sharing of information with insurance companies. Although there are some laws currently in place (see next section), there remains risk to individuals if genetic information is disclosed. In addition, patients need to understand their right to decide if they want to know the information or not. Some patients feel very empowered with knowledge, yet others find knowledge to be anxiety provoking.

Genetic data, even when perceived as completely benign (eg, ancestry data), can impact how an individual self-identifies. If the genetic data conflict with the patient's self-image, this can result in significant anxiety and distress. Examples of this include incidental determination of nonpaternity or revelation of previously unknown ethnicity. Genetic testing can also reveal incidental findings or results that the patient was not directly seeking. Patients need to understand the reporting of incidental medical findings for which prevention, treatment, or therapies are not available. Finally, a patient's genetic results may impact other family members who did not get tested and may not want to have this type of genetic information. Genetic findings that can lead to improved health outcomes should be shared with other at-risk family members. This can create significant stress on family dynamics. Insightful decision making about the desire to have the genetic information is important prior to testing.

E. Ethical, Legal, and Social Issues

Many issues can arise when individuals are faced with the diagnosis of or susceptibility to a genetic disorder. Critical issues to consider include the following:

- Privacy (the rights of individuals to control access to information about themselves)

- Informed consent (giving permission to do genetic testing with the knowledge of the risks, benefits, effectiveness, and alternatives to testing)

- Confidentiality (acknowledgment that genetic information is sensitive and that access should be limited to those authorized to receive it)

- Insurance and employment discrimination (In 2008, the Genetic Information Nondiscrimination Act [GINA] became law, providing baseline national protections in the United States that prohibit the use of genetic test results [including family history] to discriminate for employment or health insurance purposes in asymptomatic individuals. It does not prevent the use of such information in life, long-term care, or disability insurance underwriting. Several states have enacted laws to protect individuals from genetic discrimination by insurance companies or in the workplace. The Health Insurance Portability and Accountability Act [HIPAA] also provides some protection from discrimination.)

- Nonpaternity or unknown adoption status

- Duty to warn (the obligation to disclose information to at-risk relatives if they are in clear and imminent danger). On rare occasions, this duty may require a healthcare professional to consider breaching patient confidentiality.

- Patient autonomy (the obligation to respect the decision-making capacities of patients who have been fully informed with accurate and unbiased information)

- Professional limitations (the duty of clinicians to realize the extent of their knowledge, skills, attitudes, or behavior as they pertain to their practice and the laws, rules, regulations, and standards of care)

- Law enforcement (access to genetic data for the purpose of solving criminal cases or immigration status). Several recent public cases have highlighted the need for protection of genetic databases (both commercial and research) from being used by the legal system.

Clayton EW. Ethical, legal, and social implications of genomic medicine. *N Engl J Med.* 2003;349:562–569. [PMID: 12904522]

Hudson, KL, Holohan MK, Collins FS. Keeping pace with the times: the Genetic Information Nondiscrimination Act of 2008. *N Engl J Med.* 2008;358:2661. [PMID: 18565857]

National Human Genome Research Institute. Policy issues in genetics. https://www.genome.gov/about-genomics/policy-issues. Accessed November 25, 2019.

F. DTC Testing

DTC genetic testing has become increasingly available commercially over the past decade. In 2017, the DTC test market was a $99 million industry. In the same year, the FDA approved marketing of several initial health risk reports from 23andMe. It is now estimated that 1 in 25 adults in the United States have access to some form of their genetic data. The likelihood is high that patients will bring this data to the attention of their primary care provider.

There are currently several companies offering DTC testing, involving ancestry/genealogy data, carrier status data, and disease risk information. In addition, there is a blossoming secondary industry developing to provide lifestyle interpretation of these results as well as the raw genetic data (uninterpreted). These companies offer interpretation and recommendations regarding diet and nutrition, exercise, and even wine preferences based on one's genetic results. While this information can be inspiring or fun, it is critical to know and counsel patients regarding the lack of clinical validation for these third-party interpretation applications. Additionally, it is necessary to understand the limits of the use of raw data as this data has not been validated by the DTC companies. When patients do present DTC testing in the office, it is important to ask several questions to determine the following: (1) whether the results are reported directly from the original DTC company; (2) whether the DTC company has Clinical Laboratory Improvement Amendments (CLIA) certification or the results are from a third-party interpretation site of analysis of raw data; and (3) the primary concern or question that prompted the patient to seek genetic testing. To integrate the result into the clinical care of the patient, the result must come from a CLIA-certified lab. There have been numerous examples of errors in third-party interpretation and raw data analysis. If the test result is not CLIA certified, then the test should be repeated in a CLIA-certified lab if relevant to the care of the patient. If the result would not affect patient care, it is important to discuss the underlying motivation of the patient seeking this information and provide the appropriate guidance and/or clinical testing to address this concern. In addition to the DTC model, there is a newer hybrid model that is physician mediated. This model allows for patients to initiate testing independently but requires an additional physician order to complete the testing process. This physician can be provided by the testing company or be the patient's primary care physician.

PRENATAL GENETICS

▶ Carrier Screening

In 2017, ACOG revised their recommendations on carrier screening. Carrier screening, as mentioned earlier in this chapter, is genetic testing performed on an asymptomatic individual who might carry a variant allele of a gene known to cause disease in offspring. Carrier screening should be offered before pregnancy, such that couples are aware of their genetic risk and may make informed reproductive choices. If a patient chooses to test and is found to be positive for a specific mutation, their partner should also be offered testing in order to receive informed genetic counseling about their reproductive options. Genetic carrier screening is an individual choice, and patients have the right to decline screening. Genetic carrier screening in theory need only be done once in a person's lifetime and the results properly stored in the medical record. However, with the advancement in the carrier testing panels that are available, it is recommended to review prior tests and evaluate for new tests with each new pregnancy. Additionally, the cost of panels is often less expensive than the cost of individual disease carrier status testing. Providers should familiarize themselves with the standard of care in this regard in their region and their health system.

Historically, carrier screening has been offered based on ethnic-based screening, such as screening for Tay-Sachs disease in patients of Ashkenazi Jewish descent. However, it is increasingly difficult to define a patient's ancestry, and the patient's genetic ancestry may not be consistent with his or her self-identified ethnic origin. Disorders are also less likely to be limited to certain ethnicities with the degree of ethnic admixture now seen among the population. The current recommendation is to offer pan-ethnic screening as well as expanded carrier screening to everyone, although ethnic-specific panels are still acceptable. Expanded carrier screening can range from a small panel of standard genetic conditions to several hundred conditions (eg, Counsyl or Horizon). All screening should include the following core conditions: spinal muscular atrophy; cystic fibrosis; hemoglobinopathies; fragile X in women with a family history of fragile X, intellectual disability, or unexplained ovarian insufficiency/failure before age 40; and Tay-Sachs if either member of a couple is of Ashkenazi Jewish, French-Canadian, or Cajun descent. Each family medicine provider who provides obstetric care needs to adopt a standardized approach and consistently offer testing to each patient. The determination of whether to test at all should be based on the patient's personal values. If a family has a specific family history for a genetic disorder, it is recommended that they be referred to genetic counseling for further evaluation and consideration.

Committee on Genetics. Committee opinion no. 691: carrier screening for genetic conditions. *Obstet Gynecol*. 2017;129:41–55. [PMID: 28225426]

Noninvasive Prenatal Screening

Noninvasive prenatal screening (NIPS) is now becoming increasingly more available for first-trimester aneuploidy screening or an adjunct to a positive quad screen. As early as 9 weeks of pregnancy, fetal DNA called cell-free DNA (cfDNA) can be isolated from maternal serum, amplified, and analyzed for abnormal chromosome copy number such as trisomy 21 or 18. In the near future, this technology will also likely screen for single gene mutations, although the testing is not yet validated or approved to do so. With NIPS, it is important to understand that this is only a screening test and that the gold standard of testing remains an amniocentesis/chorionic villus sampling for karyotype/FISH analysis.

Genetics Home Reference. What is noninvasive prenatal testing (NIPT) and what disorders can it screen for? https://ghr.nlm.nih.gov/primer/testing/nipt. Accessed November 25, 2019.

HEREDITARY CANCER SYNDROMES

General Considerations

As many as 10% of all cancers are caused by a hereditary cancer syndrome. The family medicine provider plays a critical role in recognizing the family history red flags that may identify patients who are at higher risk for an inherited form of cancer. The identification of these patients allows for enhanced screening to identify and treat cancer at early stages and implement important risk reduction opportunities in the form of prophylactic surgery or medical therapy to reduce their individual risk for developing cancer. Patients with a family history or a personal history of early-onset cancers, bilateral cancers in paired organs, male breast cancer, or cancer affecting multiple generations should be considered for genetic counseling and testing (Table 48–2). Current guidelines suggest that even in the absence of any family history of breast or ovarian cancer that patients personally affected with ovarian, primary peritoneal, and fallopian tube cancers should be referred for genetic counseling and possible *BRCA1/2* mutation testing. In patients of Ashkenazi Jewish descent, a personal history of breast cancer at any age may be considered an indication for genetic testing. Assessing both the maternal and paternal family history is important because the gene mutation, although inherited in an autosomal dominant fashion, may not manifest in a male. Genetic counseling provides the patient a detailed

Table 48–2. Indicators of hereditary cancer susceptibility in a family.

Cancer in two or more first-degree relatives
Multiple cancers in multiple generations
Early age of onset (ie, <50 years for adult-onset cancers)
Multiple cancers in a single individual
Bilateral cancer in a paired organ such as breasts, kidneys, or ovaries
Presence of rare cancers in family (eg, male breast cancer)
Recognition of a known association between etiologically related cancers in the family, such as breast and ovarian cancer (hereditary breast ovarian cancer) or adrenocortical carcinoma and breast cancer (Li-Fraumeni syndrome)
Presence of congenital anomalies associated with an increased cancer risk
Presence of precursor lesions known to be associated with cancers (atypical nevi and risk of malignant melanoma)
Recognizable pattern of inheritance

risk assessment, options for genetic testing, and appropriate interpretation of any completed testing. Patients found to be at risk for a hereditary cancer syndrome should be managed by a multidisciplinary team with expertise in cancer genetics.

Hereditary Breast and Ovarian Cancer

This is a dominantly inherited syndrome most commonly caused by germline mutations in the genes *BRCA1* and *BRCA2*. In the general population, the mutated gene is found in approximately 1 in every 500 persons, but in those of Ashkenazi Jewish ancestry, the cancer frequency is 1 in every 40 individuals. However, the majority of breast and ovarian cancers are sporadic, and only 5–10% of them are caused by a *BRCA1* or *BRCA2* mutation.

Key features strongly suggestive of a *BRCA1/2* mutation would be early onset of breast or ovarian cancer in a patient, a family history with multiple affected members, or the presence in the family history of both breast and ovarian cancer. It is important to recognize that males who carry one of these mutations may be asymptomatic but also are at risk for breast, prostate, and pancreatic cancer. However, even women with the mutation may not develop cancers because the gene is not completely penetrant. For a female with the mutation, there is 40–66% lifetime risk of breast cancer and up to a 46% risk of ovarian cancer. These risks are significantly higher than the US general population risk of 12% for breast cancer and 1.5% for ovarian cancer. In addition, many of these cancers will occur before age 50. Equally of concern is the risk of breast cancer in the contralateral breast, which is between 40% and 65% over a lifetime and up to 30% 10 years after diagnosis.

Patients with early-onset breast or ovarian cancer or those with family histories of these conditions should undergo cancer genetic counseling for evaluation and genetic testing. If the patient is found to carry a pathogenic mutation, an appropriate management plan needs to be developed to include both screening options and prophylactic surgical options based on national guidelines.

The absence of a known pathogenic mutation does not exclude the possibility that the family has a hereditary form of breast and/or ovarian cancer. In addition to the other known syndromes outlined in the following sections, there are likely many other cancer-causing gene mutations that have yet to be discovered. In the presence of a strong family history but negative gene testing, it is essential that the patient understand that his or her risk for developing cancer is not equal to the average population risk; a comprehensive screening plan should be developed for the at-risk patient.

Hereditary Nonpolyposis Colon Cancer (Lynch Syndrome)

A family history of early-onset colon, ovarian, or endometrial cancers should raise suspicion of Lynch syndrome and prompt genetic counseling and gene testing for the DNA mismatch genes that are commonly mutated in this disorder. In addition to the associated gynecologic cancers, a wide variety of other cancers may be found in these families, including gastric, small intestine, biliary, brain, skin, and pancreatic. In the patient identified with Lynch syndrome, a comprehensive screening plan including care by both a gastroenterologist and a gynecologist is essential, as the risk for ovarian cancer and endometrial cancer may be as high as 12% and 60%, respectively.

Li-Fraumeni Syndrome

This condition is highly penetrant, with a 90% risk of cancer by age 60. Most cases are due to germline mutations in the tumor suppression genes *p53* and *CHEK2*. Soft tissue sarcomas, often expressed in children or young adults, are the most common cancers. Breast cancer is commonly associated, as are bone, brain, and adrenal cancers. Unlike most of the other cancer-predisposing genes, the frequency of de novo mutations is quite high (7–20%), and therefore, gene testing may be offered in the absence of a positive family history.

Aarnio M, Sankila R, Pukkala E, et al. Cancer risk in mutation carriers of DNA-mismatch-repair genes. *Int J Cancer.* 1999;81:214–218. [PMID: 10188721]

Chen S, Parmigiani G. Meta-analysis of BRCA1 and BRCA2 penetrance. *J Clin Oncol.* 2007;25:1329–1333. [PMID: 17416853]

Daly MB, Axilbund JE, Buys S, et al. Genetic/familial high-risk assessment: breast and ovarian. *J Natl Compr Canc Netw.* 2010;8:562–594. [PMID: 20495085]

Gonzalez KD, Buzin CH, Noltner KA, et al. High frequency of de novo mutations in Li-Fraumeni syndrome. *J Med Genet.* 2009;46:689–693. [PMID: 19556618]

Kurian AW. BRCA1 and BRCA2 mutations across race and ethnicity: distribution and clinical implications. *Curr Opin Obstet Gynecol.* 2010;22:72–78. [PMID: 19841585]

Peshkin BN, Isaacs C. Evaluation and management of women with BRCA1/2 mutations. *Oncology.* 2005;19:1451–1459. [PMID: 16370446]

GENETIC TESTING FOR HEREDITARY CANCER

When a decision is made to proceed with genetic testing, the testing should first be offered to the person affected by the cancer in question. If that person is positive for one of the known gene mutations, precise testing should be available for other, potentially at-risk, but unaffected relatives. Such testing is equally important for the affected person, as any positive test in a relative increases the individual's risk for a second primary cancer. As a result, an appropriate surveillance plan must be put in place.

If a mutation is identified in the family, a negative test in other relatives removes them from the high-risk category. Of course, they remain at risk for sporadic cancers at the rate of the general population and should have age-appropriate screening. A positive test for a *BRCA1/2* mutation requires a multidisciplinary approach to management. Table 48–3 outlines a sample management plan. These guidelines can change rapidly with new information, and consultation with a cancer genetics professional should always precede implementation of any management plan.

In addition to the development of a management plan, cancer geneticists can address psychological effects of a positive diagnosis and provide information to the patient on implications for other family members who may be at risk.

Table 48–3. Management of a patient with *BRCA1/2* mutation.

Screening for breast cancer
- Monthly breast self-exam beginning at age 18
- Physician breast exams every 6–12 months beginning at age 25
- Mammography beginning at age 25; frequency should be at least annually; more often, and to include breast magnetic resonance imaging, if clinically indicated

Screening for ovarian cancer
- Bimanual pelvic exam every 6–12 months from age 25
- Serum CA-125 at least annually beginning at age 30
- Transvaginal ultrasound with Doppler assessment, beginning at age 35

Risk reduction options
- Consider tamoxifen after age 35
- Consider oral contraceptives for both contraception and ovarian cancer risk reduction
- Consider prophylactic mastectomy
- Oophorectomy is strongly recommended by age 40, or when childbearing is complete

Data from Peshkin BN, Isaacs C. Evaluation and management of women with BRCA1/2 mutations. *Oncology.* 2005 Oct;19(11): 1451–1459.

There are two problematic areas in genetic testing. The first is that of the indeterminate negative. In these families, the family history strongly suggests autosomal dominant inheritance, but no causative mutation is found. These patients should be cautioned against interpreting the failure to find a mutation as a negative result. These patients should be treated as high-risk patients with increased surveillance despite the absence of a common genetic mutation.

The second area of confusion for patients is the indeterminate positive result. Full sequencing of *BRCA1/2* as well as other cancer-susceptibility genes may detect variants of uncertain clinical significance (VUS). These variants, often a single nucleotide change, have an unknown impact on protein function. Population studies will, in some cases, identify the variant as either benign or deleterious, but most will not have been categorized. In general, the finding of a VUS should not be used to modify the care of a patient.

EXAMPLES

▶ Hereditary Cancer

A 30-year-old female patient comes into the clinic and, in describing her family health history, mentions that she has a "lot of cancer" on her father's side. However, because it is breast cancer and "since it is on [her] dad's side," she isn't worried. She mentions that both of her paternal aunts had multiple breast cancers, and both aunts passed away between age 40 and 45 years. The aunt who died at age 45 was diagnosed with breast cancer at age 30 and again with a new cancer at 35. Her other aunt was diagnosed at age 29 with breast cancer and again with breast cancer at 38. She also shares that her paternal grandmother died at age 45 after being diagnosed with breast cancer at 43 and that she has a cousin who was recently diagnosed with ovarian cancer at 30. Figure 48–2 shows the pedigree of her family history.

It is important to explain to this patient that hereditary breast and ovarian cancer syndromes can be passed through both her father or her mother and that it is important for her to consider genetic counseling. Additionally, she should be prepared to find out if anyone in her family has already had genetic testing or might be interested in genetic testing for a hereditary breast and ovarian cancer syndrome. This scenario represents a common misconception among patients that breast cancer cannot be passed down through the paternal genes.

▶ Familial Hypercholesterolemia

A young man who is otherwise healthy and reports a balanced diet and regular exercise is measured to have an LDL level of 200 mg/dL. On exam, he is noted to have xanthomas on his bilateral hands. He indicates that many of his family members have been on statins for much of their lives. His brother has been on statins since his 20s, and his father started statins in his 30s. He reports that his paternal grandfather also had high cholesterol.

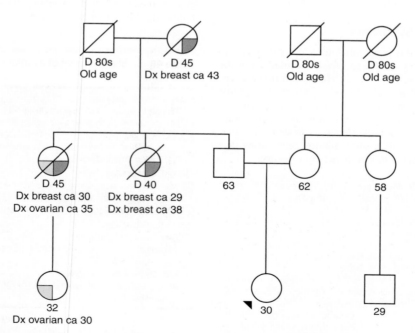

▲ **Figure 48–2.** Hereditary cancer example pedigree. ca, cancer; D, died; Dx, diagnosed.

In this case, it is important to evaluate the patient for genetic hypercholesteremia. Given the clear pattern of high cholesterol in the family. If the patient were to be diagnosed with familial hypercholesteremia, it would be important to provide the patient with information so that all of his first-degree relatives could be tested (cascade testing). This would include testing any children because children with hypercholesteremia are at risk for being symptomatic of coronary artery disease.

CURRENT CHALLENGES AND FUTURE DIRECTIONS

Several implementation challenges still need to be overcome as the field of family medicine moves forward with the integration of genetics and precision medicine. First and foremost, ongoing education both as continuing medical education and point-of-care clinical decision support (the right amount of education at the right time) needs to be developed and expanded across health systems. The availability of genetic testing, the cost, and the reimbursement for tests need to be firmly established. Clinical algorithms for the inclusion of genomic data need to be developed and distributed, and additional randomized controlled trials need to be done to establish the outcomes of precision medicine data and the value to cost reduction and improved outcomes. Finally, significant advances need to occur in the electronic health record to aggregate and interpret the immense amount of data obtained from genomics and precision medicine. Many regional and national precision medicine research efforts such as the National Institutes of Health's All of Us Precision Medicine Research program and the eMERGE network through the National Human Genome Research Institute are striving to advance solutions for each of these challenges and ease this transition. Through genomics and precision medicine, the next decade will bring changes to the practice of medicine and health care that will stretch the imagination.

Websites

Find a Genetic Counselor. http://findageneticcounselor.com/
Genetics Home Reference. https://ghr.nlm.nih.gov/
My Gene Counsel. https://www.mygenecounsel.com
Surgeon General Family Health History. https://www.genome
    .gov/For-Patients-and-Families/Family-Health-History

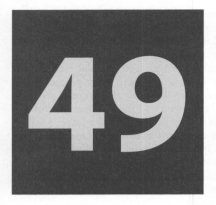

49

Pharmacogenomics

Matthew D. Krasowski, MD, PhD

OVERVIEW OF PHARMACOGENOMICS

Pharmacogenomics (also known as *pharmacogenetics*) is a component of individualized ("personalized") medicine that addresses how genetic factors impact drug therapy, with the goal of optimizing drug therapy and ensuring maximal efficacy with minimal side effects. The effect of drugs is traditionally divided into pharmacokinetics (how drugs are absorbed, distributed, metabolized, and eliminated) and pharmacodynamics (the molecular target or targets underlying the therapeutic effect). In principle, genetic variation can influence pharmacokinetics, pharmacodynamics, or both. Currently, most clinical applications of pharmacogenomics involve drug metabolism, but with a steady rise in applications involving pharmacodynamics. Many of the current pharmacogenomic clinical applications focus on the cytochrome P450 (CYP) enzymes. The sequencing of the human genome and intensive research into how genetic variation affects drug response hold the promise of altering the paradigms for medication therapy. However, current clinical applications using pharmacogenomics are still rather limited primarily due to limited evidence that such testing is cost effective and provides clinical benefit. The coming years should see steady growth in this field that will allow primary care providers and other health professionals to better manage drug therapy.

Genetic Variability

The most common type of genetic variation is single nucleotide polymorphism (SNP), a situation in which some individuals have one nucleotide at a given position while other individuals have another nucleotide (eg, cytosine vs adenosine, C/A). If this occurs in the coding region of a gene (ie, within coding exons), it may result in a change in the amino acid sequence that results when DNA is transcribed into RNA and the RNA is then translated into protein. Other less common types of genetic variation include insertions or deletions (sometimes referred to collectively as *indels*), partial or total gene deletion, alteration of mRNA splicing (ie, the process of removing introns from genomic DNA sequences that contain exons and introns), variation in gene promoters, and gene duplication or multiplication.

Genetic variants are named in a historical but often confusing system to those new to the field. By definition, the normal allele (individual copy of a gene on a chromosome) is defined as *1 (eg, CYP2D6*1). In order of historical discovery, variant alleles were designated *2, *3, *4, and so on added later on. Unfortunately, this nomenclature does not give any clue to the nature of the genetic variation. For instance, *4 and *6 could represent fairly benign genetic variants, whereas *5 could signify a variant that results in complete absence of enzyme activity. However, this nomenclature is what is commonly used.

Pharmacogenomics Involving Drug Metabolism

Although numerous nongenetic factors influence the effects of medications—including disease, organ function, concomitant medications, herbal therapy, age, and gender—there are now many examples in which interindividual differences in medication response are due to variants in genes encoding drug targets, drug-metabolizing enzymes, and drug transporters. Currently, most well-established applications of pharmacogenomics involve drug metabolism. Several organs can metabolize (biotransform) drug molecules, with the liver being the dominant organ for this purpose in humans. The proteins that have been studied in greatest depth are the CYP enzymes, a complicated group of enzymes expressed in liver, intestines, kidneys, lungs, and some other organs. Several CYP enzymes account for the majority of drug metabolism in humans: CYP3A4/5, CYP2D6, CYP2C9, and CYP2C19. CYP3A4, in particular, has been shown to play a role in the metabolism of >50% of the prescribed drugs in the United States.

Genetic variation of CYP2D6 was one of the first classic examples of pharmacogenomics. In the 1970s, the now obsolete antihypertensive drug debrisoquine was being tested in clinical trials. For the majority of individuals, this drug provided safe control of hypertension. However, some individuals developed prolonged hypotension after receiving the drug, with the hypotension lasting for days in some people. Debrisoquine was later found to be metabolized mainly by CYP2D6, an enzyme found in the liver that is now known to metabolize approximately 25% of all drugs currently prescribed in the United States. Of the CYP enzymes, CYP2D6 shows the greatest range of genetic variation, with common genetic variants that include total gene deletion (CYP2D6*5) and gene duplication, with rare individuals documented that have over four functional copies of the CYP2D6 gene (instead of the usual two alleles). Genetic variation of CYP2D6, as will be discussed later, has clinical importance for psychiatric, cardiac, and opiate medications. Individuals with low CYP2D6 activity may experience severe adverse effects to standard doses of certain drugs, whereas those with higher-than-average activity may degrade a drug so quickly that therapeutic concentrations are not achieved with standard doses.

The CYP enzymes also underlie a number of clinically important drug-drug interactions, including herbal drugs. For example, the antibiotic erythromycin is a powerful inhibitor of multiple CYP enzymes, including CYP3A4. Erythromycin thus has potentially dangerous interactions with drugs metabolized by CYP3A4, such as the immunosuppressive drugs cyclosporine and tacrolimus, if appropriate dose reductions are not made. On the contrary, several compounds markedly increase (induce) the expression of CYP enzymes, including rifampin, phenytoin, carbamazepine, phenobarbital, and the herbal antidepressant St. John's wort. By increasing the expression of CYP enzymes and other proteins involved in drug metabolism and elimination, inducers such as rifampin can cause increased metabolism not only of other drugs but also of endogenous compounds such as steroid hormones and vitamin D. This is the mechanism underlying unintended pregnancy that can result in women using estrogen-containing oral contraceptives who also receive a CYP inducer such as rifampin or St. John's wort. CYP inducers greatly increase the metabolism of the estrogen component of combined oral contraceptives, resulting in therapeutic failure. CYP inducers are also known to cause osteomalacia by accelerating the metabolism and clearance of the active form of vitamin D ($1\alpha,25$-dihydroxyvitamin D_3).

There is some nomenclature related to pharmacogenomics of drug-metabolizing enzymes that can be confusing to those new to the field. *Poor metabolizers* represent individuals with little or no enzymatic activity, due either to lack of expression of the enzyme or mutations that reduce enzymatic activity (eg, a mutation that alters the active catalytic site) in both alleles. *Extensive metabolizers* are considered the "normal" situation and generally represent individuals with two normal copies of the enzyme gene on each chromosome. *Intermediate metabolizers* have enzymatic activity roughly half that of extensive metabolizers. The most common genetic reason underlying intermediate activity is one copy of the normal gene and one variant copy associated with low activity (ie, heterozygous for the mutation). *Ultrarapid metabolizers* have enzymatic activity significantly greater than that of the average population. This often results when an individual has more than the normal two copies of a gene. Gene duplication or multiplication is not seen with many genes but can occur with CYP2D6. For example, an individual may have three or more functional copies of the CYP2D6 gene instead of the normal two copies and thus have higher than average enzyme activity.

Two common drugs, clopidogrel and codeine, are *prodrugs* that are inactive until converted to active metabolites by CYP enzymes. Clopidogrel is activated by CYP2C19, and codeine is converted to morphine by CYP2D6. For these prodrugs, poor metabolizers of the respective CYP enzyme will be more likely to show lack of efficacy.

For many other drugs, CYP enzymes inactivate the drug and thus play an important role in clearance. Poor metabolizers may thus experience drug toxicity with standard doses due to slower drug clearance. Ultrarapid metabolizers may see little clinical effect with standard drug doses due to rapid clearance of the drug.

▶ Pharmacogenomics Involving Pharmacodynamics

Understanding the genetic variation involving pharmacodynamics has developed more slowly than that of pharmacokinetics. In part, this is because the molecular targets of certain drugs are incompletely understood. An example of pharmacodynamic genetic variation is for the β_2-adrenergic receptor, the target of β-agonists used in asthma therapy such as albuterol and salmeterol. Genetic variation of the receptor influences how well β-agonist therapy works. However, genetic testing of the β_2-adrenergic receptor has not yet had much impact clinically. The other example of pharmacogenomics involving pharmacodynamics is the molecular target of warfarin, the vitamin K epoxide reductase complex subunit 1 (VKORC1) protein, which will be discussed later. The importance of understanding pharmacodynamic variation is that it holds the potential of predicting therapeutic efficacy (or lack thereof). This could be especially valuable for disorders such as major depression where weeks or even months may be required to determine effectiveness of a drug.

Haga SB, Mills R, Moaddeb J, et al. Patient experiences with pharmacogenetic testing in a primary care setting. *Pharmacogenomics*. 2016;17:1629–1636. [PMID: 27648637]

Table 49–1. Possible indications for pharmacogenomic testing.

Provide guidance for drug and dose selection
Predict drug toxicity
Evaluate cause of adverse drug reaction
Investigate reason for therapeutic failure
Familial testing if other family member known to have pharmacogenomic variant

O'Donnell PH, Ratain MJ. Germline pharmacogenomics in oncology: decoding the patient for targeting therapy. *Mol Oncol.* 2012;6:251–259. [PMID: 22321460]

St Sauver JL, Bielinski SJ, Olson JE, et al. Integrating pharmacogenomics into clinical practice: promise vs reality. *Am J Med.* 2016;129:1093–1099. [PMID: 27155109]

▶ Clinical Applications

Pharmacogenomics may be useful for a number of clinical indications (Table 49–1). Although pharmacogenomics is far from fulfilling its promise of developing a patient-specific pharmacologic profile, there are areas in which genetic testing is being applied clinically. Table 49–2 lists pharmacogenomic associations mentioned in package inserts for approved medications.

▶ Clopidogrel & CYP2C19

Clopidogrel (Plavix) is a commonly used antiplatelet drug administered to reduce risk of myocardial infarction, stroke, and peripheral vascular events. Clopidogrel is converted to an active thiol metabolite mainly by CYP2C19. Patients who are CYP2C19 poor metabolizers (most commonly the *2 and *3 alleles) may show "Plavix resistance" and pose higher risk for therapeutic failure and cardiovascular events while on clopidogrel. The TRITON-TIMI 38 trial demonstrated that patients with CYP2C19 loss-of-function mutations had a relative 53% increased risk of death from cardiovascular causes (myocardial infarction, stroke) and a threefold increased rate of stent thrombosis compared to patients with normal CYP2C19 genotype. The US Food and Drug Administration (FDA) issued a label warning update in March 2010 for CYP2C19 poor metabolizers. The 2013 Clinical Pharmacogenetics Implementation Consortium guidelines recommended that patients who are poor or

Table 49–2. Selected pharmacogenomic biomarkers and drugs with package insert data on pharmacogenomics.

Biomarker	Drug Categories Affected	Specific Drugs
CYP2C9	Analgesics	Celecoxib
CYP2C9, VKORC1	Anticoagulant	Warfarin
CYP2C19	Cardiovascular Neurologic and psychiatric Gastrointestinal	Clopidogrel Carisoprodol, citalopram, clobazam, diazepam Proton pump inhibitors: dexlansoprazole, esomeprazole, lansoprazole, omeprazole, pantoprazole, -rabeprazole
CYP2D6	Analgesics Cardiovascular Neurologic and psychiatric	Codeine Carvedilol, metoprolol, propranolol *Antidepressants* (SSRIs/SNRIs): citalopram, fluoxetine, fluvoxamine, nefazodone, paroxetine, venlafaxine *Antidepressants* (tricyclics): amitriptyline, clomipramine, desipramine, doxepin, imipramine, nortriptyline, protriptyline *Antipsychotics*: aripiprazole, clozapine, iloperidone, perphenazine, risperidone *Other*: atomoxetine, chlordiazepoxide, modafinil
HLA-B*1502	Neurologic	Carbamazepine, phenytoin
HLA-B*5701	Antivirals	Abacavir
TPMT	Oncologic/rheumatologic	Azathioprine, 6-mercaptopurine
UGT1A1	Oncologic	Irinotecan

SNRI, serotonin-norepinephrine reuptake inhibitor; SSRI, selective serotonin reuptake inhibitor.
Data from US Food and Drug Administration.

intermediate metabolizers based on CYP2C19 genotype be prescribed alternate antiplatelet therapy.

However, CYP2C19 genotyping for patients who are candidates for clopidogrel therapy has not been widely adopted. One important point is that the CYP2C19 function is only one factor of many that can influence clopidogrel response, with drug-drug interactions also of importance. In addition, a functional test (platelet aggregometry) can produce similar clinical information. As a result, multiple task forces, including the Veterans Health Administration Clinical Pharmacogenetics Subcommittee, do not recommend routine genetic screening for clopidogrel. CYPC19 genotyping may be clinically useful for patients with high risk for poor outcomes or recurrent coronary events despite ongoing clopidogrel therapy. The related drug prasugrel is an alternative antiplatelet agent for patients with poor clinical response to clopidogrel.

▶ Other Drugs Metabolized by CYP2C19

Several other categories of drugs are inactivated by CYP2C19 metabolism. These include carisoprodol (muscle relaxant), citalopram, clobazam, diazepam, and most of the proton pump inhibitors used to treat gastroesophageal reflux (eg, lansoprazole, omeprazole). CYP2C19 poor metabolizers may experience drug toxicity at standard doses. The frequencies of CYP2C19-inactivating genetic variants are highest in Asians (~15–25%) and Polynesians (up to ~75%) and lower in African American (4%) and white (2–5%) populations. Genotyping of CYP2C19 has been much more widely applied in Japan than in the United States because of the prevalence of CYP2C19 poor metabolism in the Japanese population. CYP2C19 genotyping may be helpful in patients with poor clinical response or unusual toxicity to drugs metabolized by CYP2C19.

Caudle KE, Klein TE, Hoffman JM, et al. Incorporation of pharmacogenomics into routine clinical practice: the Clinical Pharmacogenetics Implementation Consortium (CPIC) guideline development process. *Curr Drug Metab*. 2014;15:209–217. [PMID: 24479687]

Mega JL, Hochholzer W, Frelinger AL 3rd, et al. Dosing clopidogrel based on CYP2C19 genotype and the effect on platelet reactivity in patients with stable cardiovascular disease. *JAMA*. 2011;306:2221–2228. [PMID: 22088980]

Vassy JL, Stone A, Callaghan JT, et al. Pharmacogenetic testing in the Veterans Health Administration (VHA): policy recommendations from the VHA Clinical Pharmacogenetics Subcommittee. *Genet Med*. 2019;21(2):382–390. [PMID: 29858578]

▶ Warfarin

Warfarin remains the most commonly prescribed oral anticoagulant, although the recent introduction of other oral anticoagulants (eg, direct thrombin and factor X inhibitors) has reduced warfarin usage. Warfarin-related bleeding complications occur in approximately 3% of patients in the first 3 months of therapy, with the highest risk also in the first 3 months of therapy. During maintenance therapy, there is a risk of bleeding complications of 7.6–16.5 per 100 patient-years. Thus, there is a need to accurately predict both the initial and maintenance doses of warfarin.

Two major genes are involved in warfarin pharmacogenomics: CYP2C9 and VKORC1. CYP2C9 metabolizes warfarin to an inactive metabolite. VKORC1 is the molecular target inhibited by warfarin, thus reducing the production of vitamin K–dependent clotting factors. CYP2C9 poor metabolizers are at risk for warfarin toxicity at standard doses because of reduced clearance of the drug. The two most common mutations are CYP2C9*2 and *3. VKORC1 has several genetic variants that influence warfarin sensitivity or resistance. Collectively, genetic variation in CYP2C9 and VKORC1 account for approximately one-third of the observed variation in warfarin dosage that leads to stable anticoagulation. Additional proteins involved in warfarin effect include CYP4F2 and gamma-glutamyl carboxylase (GGCX). Genetic variation in the genes for CYP4F2 and GGCX also have an effect on warfarin.

Various algorithms are available to predict optimal warfarin dosage. The most widely used (www.warfarindosage. org) is open access and allows the clinician to input various factors that influence warfarin response (eg, age, gender, concomitant medications such as statins and trimethoprim/sulfamethoxazole, cigarette smoking, weight, CYP2C9 genotype, VKORC1 genotype, CYP4F2 genotype, GGCX genotype). The algorithm does not require genetic information if unavailable. The output of the algorithm is an estimated maintenance dose of warfarin. Large-scale clinical trials evaluating genotype-guided warfarin dosing have produced mixed results, in some cases showing no benefit or even inferiority to standard dosing algorithms. As a consequence, in the United States, warfarin pharmacogenetic testing is generally not covered by health insurance and remains mostly a research tool.

Gage BF, Bass AR, Lin H, et al. Effect of genotype-guided warfarin dosing on clinical events and anticoagulation control among patients undergoing hip or knee arthroplasty: the GIFT randomized clinical trial. *JAMA*. 2017;318:1115–1124. [PMID: 28973620]

Kimmel SE, French B, Kasner SE, et al. A pharmacogenetic versus a clinical algorithm for warfarin dosing. *N Engl J Med*. 2013;369:2283–2293. [PMID: 24251361]

Pirmohamed M, Burnside G, Eriksson N, et al. A randomized trial of genotype-guided dosing of warfarin. *N Engl J Med*. 2013; 369:2294–2303. [PMID: 24251363]

Verhoef TI, Redekop WK, Langenskiold S, et al. Cost-effectiveness of pharmacogenetic-guided dosing of warfarin in the United Kingdom and Sweden. *Pharmacogenomics J*. 2016;16:478–484. [PMID: 27272045]

Codeine & CYP2D6

Codeine is a prodrug that needs to be converted by CYP2D6 to morphine for therapeutic effect. CYP2D6 poor metabolizers are likely to get poor therapeutic effect from codeine due to lack of morphine conversion. Such patients more often benefit from other opiates such as hydrocodone, oxycodone, or morphine itself. However, as mentioned earlier, there are also individuals who are CYP2D6 ultrarapid metabolizers. Such patients convert codeine to morphine rapidly and may even experience morphine toxicity. Life-threatening codeine toxicity due to rapid CYP2D6 metabolism has been especially seen in the pediatric population, with some fatalities. Codeine toxicity may occur in CYP2D6 ultrarapid metabolizing children administered codeine (eg, for pain relief for dental surgery) or in breastfeeding infants whose mothers are CYP2D6 ultrarapid metabolizers prescribed codeine. In either case, the excess of morphine can cause respiratory depression and other symptoms of opiate overdose. The FDA issued separate warnings on use of codeine in breastfeeding mothers and for postsurgical pain management for children in 2007 and 2012, respectively. CYP2D6 pharmacogenetic testing has not become standard of care given alternate analgesic drugs available for poor and ultrarapid metabolizers.

Other Drugs Metabolized by CYP2D6

Numerous other drugs are metabolized by CYP2D6. In contrast to the activation of codeine by CYP2D6, many drugs are inactivated by CYP2D6-mediated metabolism, often representing the major route of elimination for these drugs. The major categories of CYP2D6 substrates include β-adrenergic receptor antagonists (carvedilol, metoprolol, propranolol), antidepressants (including some selective serotonin reuptake inhibitors, serotonin-norepinephrine reuptake inhibitors, and tricyclic antidepressants), and antipsychotics (both typical and atypical agents) (see Table 49–2). For drugs inactivated by CYP2D6, poor metabolizers are at risk for drug toxicity at standard doses, due to slow clearance of the drug. Poor metabolizers may require reduced dosage or use of an alternative drug. Ultrarapid metabolizers may show lack of efficacy at standard dosages and need higher doses to compensate for more rapid metabolism.

Caudle KE, Klein TE, Hoffman JM, et al. Incorporation of pharmacogenomics into routine clinical practice: the Clinical Pharmacogenetics Implementation Consortium (CPIC) guideline development process. *Curr Drug Metab.* 2014;15:209–217. [PMID: 24479687]

St Sauver JL, Bielinski SJ, Olson JE, et al. Integrating pharmacogenomics into clinical practice: promise vs reality. *Am J Med.* 2016;129:1093–1099. [PMID: 27155109]

Vassy JL, Stone A, Callaghan JT, et al. Pharmacogenetic testing in the Veterans Health Administration (VHA): policy recommendations from the VHA Clinical Pharmacogenetics Subcommittee. *Genet Med.* 2019;21(2):382–390. [PMID: 29858578]

Cancer Pharmacogenomics

There are increasing pharmacogenomic applications involving cancer therapy. Some examples are related to drug metabolism, while others involve the mechanism of action.

Azathioprine and 6-mercaptopurine (6MP) are agents used in the treatment of cancers (eg, acute lymphoblastic leukemia) and autoimmune disorders such as rheumatoid arthritis and inflammatory bowel disease. Azathioprine is the prodrug of 6MP. One route for inactivation and clearance of 6MP is by the enzyme thiopurine methyltransferase (TPMT). Although azathioprine and 6MP both have the potential for bone marrow suppression if used in high doses, approximately 1 in 300 whites (less in most other populations) experiences very profound bone marrow toxicity following standard doses of azathioprine and 6MP.

Many of the patients experiencing severe toxicity in response to azathioprine or 6MP therapy have very low TPMT enzymatic activity (they are TPMT poor metabolizers). Several clinical laboratory tests can predict up front whether individuals will have difficulty metabolizing 6MP and azathioprine. In 2004–2005, the package inserts for azathioprine and 6MP were revised to include warnings on toxicity related to genetic variation of TPMT. TPMT poor metabolizers can still receive 6MP or azathioprine but need markedly reduced doses. Functional testing for TPMT enzyme activity in the blood is currently commonly performed prior to initiating therapy with 6MP or azathioprine.

A second oncology application involves the drug irinotecan, a chemotherapeutic agent used in the treatment of colorectal cancer. Irinotecan has complicated metabolism but is inactivated by glucuronidation mediated by UDP-glucuronosyltransferase 1A1 (UGT1A1), an enzyme that also carries out conjugation of bilirubin. A variety of rare, severe mutations in UGT1A1 can result in the Crigler-Najjar syndrome, a devastating disease that can be fatal in childhood unless liver transplantation is performed. A milder mutation, designated UGT1A1*28, is the most common cause of a mostly benign condition called Gilbert syndrome, a condition often diagnosed incidentally in the primary care setting following detection of (usually mild) unconjugated hyperbilirubinemia on routine chemistry laboratory studies or in the workup of jaundice. These individuals are, however, at high risk for severe toxicity following irinotecan therapy. With standard doses, such individuals may develop life-threatening neutropenia or diarrhea poorly responsive to therapy. Genetic testing for UGT1A1*28 is FDA approved, and similar to 6MP and azathioprine, the package insert for irinotecan now includes specific information on UGT1A1 genetic variation. However, genetic screening for UGT1A1 has not been adopted universally.

Pharmacogenomics also finds application in oncology in targeted therapies for certain cancers. One of the best examples is the use of trastuzumab (Herceptin) for breast cancers overexpressing the HER2 protein. In the pathology workup of breast cancer, determination of HER2 expression status determines whether trastuzumab is a therapeutic option.

A recent trend in oncology is the emergence of *paired diagnostics*, where a drug and its companion diagnostic test are approved simultaneously. An example is vemurafenib (Zelboraf), a drug that targets metastatic melanoma with a specific mutation in *BRAF*. Vemurafenib and the companion test to determine *BRAF* mutation status were approved simultaneously by the FDA. Health insurance coverage for vemurafenib generally will occur only if used for cancers with the specific *BRAF* mutation. This is an area that continues to develop rapidly.

Lu CY, Loomer S, Ceccarelli R, et al. Insurance coverage policies for pharmacogenomic and multi-gene testing for cancer. *J Pers Med.* 2018;8:E19. [PMID: 29772692]
Wu AC, Mazor KM, Ceccarelli R, Loomer S, Lu CY. Access to guideline-recommended pharmacogenomic tests for cancer treatments: experience of providers and patients. *J Pers Med.* 2017;7:E17. [PMID: 29140263]

▶ Abacavir & Carbamazepine Hypersensitivity

Drug hypersensitivity is a relatively common problem and may manifest on a spectrum from mild symptoms to more severe presentations such as Stevens-Johnson syndrome and toxic epidermal necrolysis. Genetic variation in the human leukocyte antigen (HLA)-B gene has now been strongly linked to severe hypersensitivity to abacavir (antiviral used to treat human immunodeficiency virus, HIV) and carbamazepine (anticonvulsant).

Approximately 5–8% of HIV patients develop hypersensitivity to abacavir. Presence of the HLA-B*5701 allele carries a high risk of hypersensitivity. If the HLA-B*5701 is absent, the risk of hypersensitivity is very low. Label warning to abacavir was issued in July 2008.

For carbamazepine, the HLA-B*1502 allele is positively correlated to hypersensitivity. This allele occurs mainly in individuals of southeast Asian descent and is uncommon in other populations. Label warning for carbamazepine was issued in December 2007. The HLA-B*1502 is also linked to hypersensitivity to phenytoin and its prodrug fosphenytoin. Pharmacogenetic testing for abacavir and carbamazepine hypersensitivity carry strong recommendations from multiple societies and policy-recommending groups.

Caudle KE, Klein TE, Hoffman JM, et al. Incorporation of pharmacogenomics into routine clinical practice: the Clinical Pharmacogenetics Implementation Consortium (CPIC) guideline development process. *Curr Drug Metab.* 2014;15:209–217. [PMID: 24479687]
Vassy JL, Stone A, Callaghan JT, et al. Pharmacogenetic testing in the Veterans Health Administration (VHA): policy recommendations from the VHA Clinical Pharmacogenetics Subcommittee. *Genet Med.* 2019;21(2):382–390. [PMID: 29858578]

DISCUSSION & FUTURE DIRECTIONS

The clinical application of pharmacogenomics has developed slowly, with so far only small impact on primary care. At present, few studies have clearly demonstrated clinical efficacy and cost-effectiveness of genetic testing to guide pharmacotherapy. Consequently, pharmacogenomic therapy is often used retrospectively to try to determine why a particular patient has experienced toxicity or unexplained lack of efficacy to a drug. Clinicians also need to realize that genetics may account for only a minor portion of variability in response to a drug. Other factors such as concomitant medications or organ failure may be more important in some circumstances. Clinical experience and ongoing research trials should better define useful applications of pharmacogenomics so that testing will become more common in the primary care setting. Evidence demonstrating benefit of pharmacogenomics testing will also be important in whether health insurance will cover the testing.

50

Complementary & Integrative Health

Wayne B. Jonas, MD

Mary P. Guerrera, MD, FAAFP, FAAMA, DABIHM

▶ Background

According to the World Health Organization, between 65% and 80% of the world's health care services are classified as traditional medicine. These practices become relabeled as complementary, alternative, or unconventional medicine when they are used in Western countries. Recently, there has been more of a move to focus on integrating these practices into conventional care and so the terms *integrative medicine* and *integrative health* (when lifestyle and self-care are included) have arisen, and these are now more commonly used. In 1995, a panel of experts, convened at the National Institutes of Health (NIH), defined *complementary and alternative medicine* (CAM) as "a broad domain of healing resources that encompasses all health systems, modalities, practices and their accompanying theories and beliefs, other than those intrinsic to the politically dominant health system of a particular society or culture in a given historical period." Similar definitions have been used since then by other organizations. Surveys of CAM use by the public and health professionals have defined it as those practices used for the prevention and treatment of disease that are not an integral part of conventional care and are neither taught widely in medical schools nor generally available in hospitals. NIH currently "uses the term 'complementary health approaches' when we discuss practices and products of non-mainstream origin. We use 'integrative health' when we talk about incorporating complementary approaches into mainstream health care." Table 50–1 lists the major types and domains of CAM, while recognizing that there can be some overlap, adapted from the National Center for Complementary and Integrative Health (NCCIH) at NIH.

A. Use of CAM

Practices that lie outside the mainstream of "official" or current conventional medicine have always been an important part of the public's management of their personal health. Complementary, alternative, and unconventional medicine

Table 50–1. Complementary and alternative medicine (CAM) systems of health care, therapies, or products.

Major Domains of CAM	Examples Under Each Domain
Whole medical systems	Ayurvedic medicine Homeopathic medicine Native American medicine (eg, sweat lodge, medicine wheel) Naturopathic medicine Traditional Chinese medicine (eg, acupuncture, Chinese herbal medicine) Tibetan medicine
Mind-body medicine	Meditation/mindfulness Hypnosis Yoga and tai chi Guided imagery Dance therapy Music therapy Art therapy Prayer and mental healing Biofeedback
Biology-based therapies	Herbal therapies Dietary supplements Biologics
Manipulative and body-based practices	Massage Chiropractic Osteopathy
Energy therapies	Qigong Reiki Therapeutic touch
Bioelectromagnetic therapies	Magnet therapy Electromagnetic devices

Adapted from the major domains of CAM and examples of each developed by the National Center for Complementary and Alternative Medicine, National Institutes of Health.

has become increasingly popular in the United States. Two identical surveys of unconventional medicine use in the United States, done in 1990 and 1996, showed a 45% increase in use of CAM by the public. Visits to CAM practitioners increased from 400 million to >600 million per year. The amount spent on these practices rose from $14 billion to $27 billion—most of it not reimbursed. More recent data from the 2012 National Health Interview Survey (NHIS) show this estimate has increased to $30.2 billion. Professional organizations are now beginning the "integration" of these practices into mainstream medicine. Overall the use of CAM among US adults (18 years or older) has continued to be estimated at about one-third of the overall population base on national survey data: 32.3% (2002), 35.5% (2007), and 33.2% (2012) (Figure 50–1, A&B). Of note, children's (age 4–17 years) use of CAM was also evaluated via these NHIS studies and was found to be stable at about 12% over the 5-year time span between surveys: 12.0% (2007) and 11.6% (2012) (Figure 50–1, C&D).

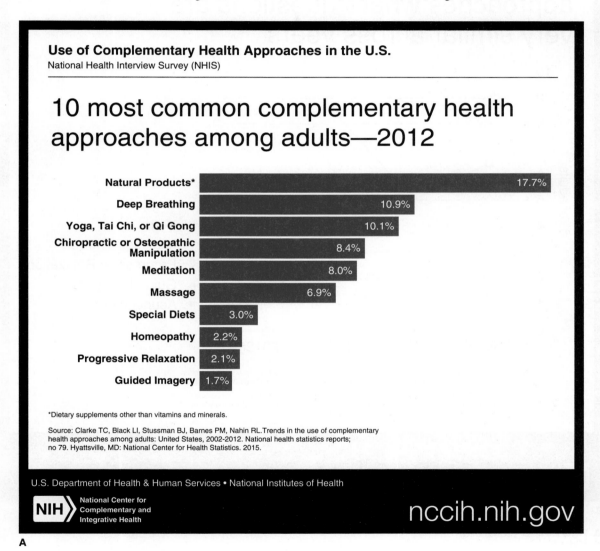

Use of Complementary Health Approaches in the U.S.
National Health Interview Survey (NHIS)

10 most common complementary health approaches among adults—2012

Approach	Percentage
Natural Products*	17.7%
Deep Breathing	10.9%
Yoga, Tai Chi, or Qi Gong	10.1%
Chiropractic or Osteopathic Manipulation	8.4%
Meditation	8.0%
Massage	6.9%
Special Diets	3.0%
Homeopathy	2.2%
Progressive Relaxation	2.1%
Guided Imagery	1.7%

*Dietary supplements other than vitamins and minerals.

Source: Clarke TC, Black LI, Stussman BJ, Barnes PM, Nahin RL.Trends in the use of complementary health approaches among adults: United States, 2002-2012. National health statistics reports; no 79. Hyattsville, MD: National Center for Health Statistics. 2015.

U.S. Department of Health & Human Services • National Institutes of Health

NIH National Center for Complementary and Integrative Health

nccih.nih.gov

A

▲ **Figure 50–1.** Most frequently used complementary and alternative medicine (CAM) modalities and conditions. ADHD, attention deficit/hyperactivity disorder. (Data from Black LI, Clarke TC, Barnes PM, et al: Use of complementary health approaches among children aged 4–17 years in the United States: National Health Interview Survey, 2007–2012, *Natl Health Stat Report.* 2015 Feb 10;(78):1–19.)

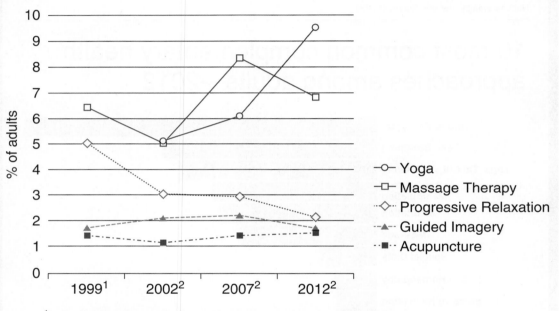

Use of Complementary Health Approaches in the U.S.
National Health Interview Survey (NHIS)

13-year trends for complementary approaches where questions are very similar across years

Legend:
- —○— Yoga
- —□— Massage Therapy
- ···◇··· Progressive Relaxation
- —▲— Guided Imagery
- ···■··· Acupuncture

[1]Citation: Ni H, Simile C, Hardy AM. Utilization of complementary and alternative medicine by United States adults: Results from the 1999 National Health Interview Survey. Med Care 2002; 40(4):353–8.

[2]Citation: Clarke TC, Black LI, Stussman BJ, Barnes PM, Nahin RL. Trends in the use of complementary health approaches among adults: United States, 2002-2012. National health statistics reports; no 79. Hyattsville, MD: National Center for Health Statistics. 2015.

U.S. Department of Health & Human Services • National Institutes of Health

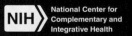
National Center for Complementary and Integrative Health

nccih.nih.gov

B

▲ **Figure 50–1.** (*Continued*)

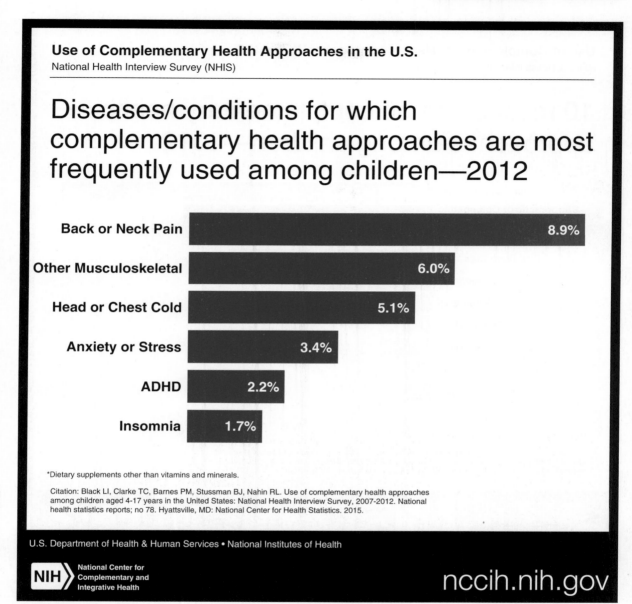

Figure 50–1. (*Continued*)

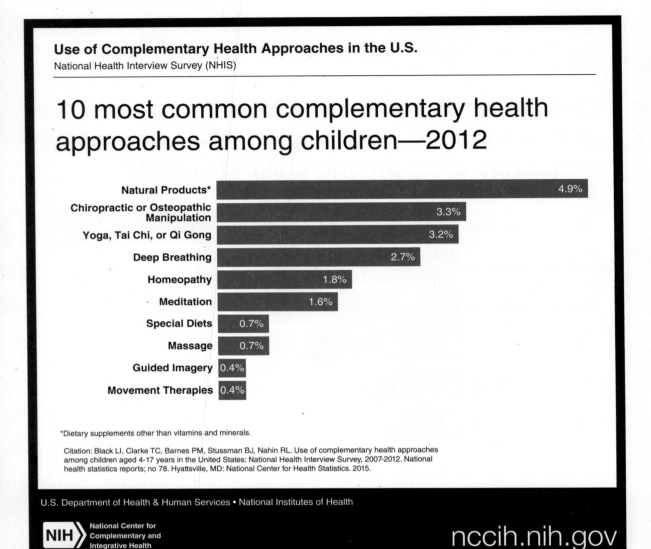

Use of Complementary Health Approaches in the U.S.
National Health Interview Survey (NHIS)

10 most common complementary health approaches among children—2012

Approach	Percentage
Natural Products*	4.9%
Chiropractic or Osteopathic Manipulation	3.3%
Yoga, Tai Chi, or Qi Gong	3.2%
Deep Breathing	2.7%
Homeopathy	1.8%
Meditation	1.6%
Special Diets	0.7%
Massage	0.7%
Guided Imagery	0.4%
Movement Therapies	0.4%

*Dietary supplements other than vitamins and minerals.

Citation: Black LI, Clarke TC, Barnes PM, Stussman BJ, Nahin RL. Use of complementary health approaches among children aged 4-17 years in the United States: National Health Interview Survey, 2007-2012. National health statistics reports; no 78. Hyattsville, MD: National Center for Health Statistics. 2015.

U.S. Department of Health & Human Services • National Institutes of Health

NIH National Center for Complementary and Integrative Health

nccih.nih.gov

D

▲ **Figure 50–1.** (*Continued*)

The public uses these practices for both minor and major problems. Multiple surveys have now been conducted on populations with cancer and human immunodeficiency virus (HIV), minorities, and women on CAM use. Rates of use are significant in all these groups. For example, women, especially those with multiple chronic conditions, were found to be higher users of CAM compared with men. In addition, women's use of CAM during childbearing is common, with one-fifth of currently or recently pregnant women reporting

CAM use for reasons related to pregnancy. Of note surveys have shown that women explore and use CAM both for themselves *and* as healthcare decision makers for their family; thus, the family physician holds a unique and important role when asking and advising women about their, as well as their family's, use of CAM. Cancer survivors, another common group of patients seen by family physicians, reported a 79% use of one or more vitamins/mineral products and/or CAM modality in the prior year. Immigrant populations often use traditional medicines that they experienced in their country of origin and not commonly used in the West.

As the public's use of CAM has grown, so, too, has the call to action of our research institutions and training centers. Will CAM treatments offer hope as we grapple with the growing burden of the opioid crisis, chronic illness, and rising costs that continue to stress our health systems? Are new educational and research training paradigms needed? Such efforts have emerged and are evolving. For example, the NIH has launched new Clinical Trial Demonstration Projects via their Health Care Systems Research Collaboratory to implement cost-effective, large-scale studies. Our current medical and health professions students are the future. How are they learning about the potential healing power and possible pitfalls of CAM? Currently, based on Association of American Medical Colleges data, 129 of the nation's 145 medical schools require their medical students to enroll in required CAM coursework, with 89 offering the topic as an elective. A significant development in residency training, led by family medicine educators, is the Integrative Medicine in Residency (IMR) national curriculum project. Launched in 2008 via eight pilot sites, the IMR was the first time that integrative medicine education became a required component of graduate medical education. Over the past decade, IMR has exponentially grown and has been successfully disseminated to 80 residencies, including family medicine, pediatrics, internal medicine, preventive medicine, and psychiatry. (http://integrativemedicine.arizona.edu/education/imr.html). An increasing percentage of hospitals have developed complementary and integrative medicine programs offering both in- and outpatient services. Some health management organizations have "expanded" benefits packages that include specific alternative practitioners and services with a reimbursement option. A 2011 survey of CAM use in US hospitals showed that 37% of hospitals offered CAM services. Most of these services were offered on an outpatient basis, with massage therapy (54%), acupuncture (35%), and relaxation training (27%) among the most popular. On an inpatient basis, the top modalities offered are pet therapy (46%), massage therapy (40%), and music/art therapy (30%). A more recent survey of CAM use in 43 children's hospitals showed that of the 26 (60%) responders, 92.3% of the hospitals offered one or more CAM service and 38% had a hospital-based CAM center. The top three services offered were pet therapy (81%), music therapy (81%), and massage therapy (69%).

As the interface of CAM and conventional medicine has grown, there has emerged the concept of *integrative medicine (IM)* as a way to bridge the best of both worlds. The Academic Consortium for Integrative Medicine and Health has defined IM and integrative health as the practice of medicine that reaffirms the importance of the relationship between practitioner and patient; focuses on the whole person; is informed by evidence; and makes use of all appropriate therapeutic and lifestyle approaches, healthcare professionals,

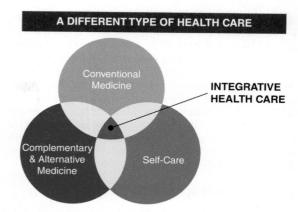

A DIFFERENT TYPE OF HEALTH CARE

Conventional Medicine

INTEGRATIVE HEALTH CARE

Complementary & Alternative Medicine

Self-Care

▲ **Figure 50–2.** Defining integrative medicine and health.

and disciplines to achieve optimal health and healing. The application of IM and integrative health can be defined as the purposeful, coordinative application of appropriate preventive and treatment modalities that support and stimulate the patient's inherent healing and self-recovery capacities. As such, these treatments are derived from various practices and healthcare systems from around the world. Thus, the term *integrative medicine* encompasses concepts from various healing philosophies, such as person-centered care, humanistic medicine, holistic health care, and the medical home. Figure 50–2 illustrates the overlap and distinction of these terms. IM involves the merger of conventional medicine and CAM; lifestyle medicine is the merger of conventional medicine and self-care. We proposed that the term *integrative health* (IH) be used for the merger of all three: conventional medicine, CAM, and self-care.

CAM, and more specifically IM and integrative health, is finding an important and growing place in American medical practice. Indeed, its significance is evidenced by the newly formed American Board of Integrative Medicine (ABOIM) created in 2014 under the auspices of the American Board of Physician Specialties (ABPS) (http://www.abpsus.org/integrative-medicine). In addition, the Veterans Health Administration (VHA), the largest healthcare system in the United States, launched the new Office of Patient-Centered Care and Cultural Transformation to begin to shift from a mostly disease-oriented approach in health care to one focused on prevention and well-being. Since 2012, the program and its signature "Circle of Health" have grown and are being disseminated throughout the VHA's system. The model includes both conventional and complementary approaches in addressing a veteran's whole health. Essentially delivering integrative health care, the model is currently being researched, and initial outcomes appear favorable (eg, decreased use of opioids for pain, cost savings, and increased satisfaction). Undoubtedly, these philosophies and practices will continue to be debated informally among medical staff and physicians and formally in peer-reviewed publications, as well as medical societies, academies, and organizations. More importantly, the individual Western-trained medical physician will continue to be the primary arbitrator and counselor for his or her patient through the time-honored fundamentals of the therapeutic alliance; that is, compassion coupled with trust, integrity, and empathy; concern coupled with caring and active listening; competence coupled with skill, intellect, and common sense; and communication coupled with availability, continuity, and follow-through.

B. Conventional Physician Use of CAM in Practice

Family physicians are frequently faced with questions about CAM. Some also refer patients for CAM treatment and IM consults and, to a lesser extent, provide CAM or IM services. A review of 25 surveys of conventional physician referral and use of CAM found that 43% of physicians had referred patients for acupuncture, 40% for chiropractic services, and 21% for massage. The majority believed in the efficacy of these three practices. Rates of use of CAM practices ranged from 9% (homeopathy) to 19% (chiropractic and massage). National surveys have confirmed that many physicians refer for and fewer incorporate CAM practices into their professional practice. However, as CAM and IM physician training and fellowships programs (eg, the Andrew Weil Center for Integrative Medicine's IM fellowship: http://integrative-medicine.arizona.edu/education/fellowship/index.html; and the ABOIM's listing of current IM fellowships: http://www.abpsus.org/integrative-medicine-fellowships) continue to grow, so will the direct incorporation of CAM and IM into clinical care and training programs.

C. Risks of CAM

The amount of research on CAM systems and practices is relatively small compared with that on conventional medicine. There are >1000 times more citations on conventional cancer treatments in the National Library of Medicine's bibliographic database, MEDLINE, than on alternative cancer treatments. With increasing public use of CAM, inadequate communication between patients and physicians about it, and few studies on the safety and efficacy of most CAM treatments, risks are increased for misuse and harm. Analysis of the 2012 NHIS survey data revealed that 42% of patients using CAM did not disclose such use to their primary care physician, with the primary reason reported to be due to physicians not asking. In response to inadequate communication about CAM use, NIH launched the "Time to Talk" campaign to increase awareness (http://nccam.nih.gov/timetotalk/forpatients.htm?nav=gsa). Many practices, such as acupuncture, homeopathy, and meditation, are low risk but require practitioner competence to avoid inappropriate use.

Botanical preparations can be toxic and produce herb-drug interactions. Contamination and poor quality control also exist with these products, especially those harvested, produced, and shipped from Asia and India.

D. Potential Benefits of CAM

Both CAM and IM practices have value for the way we manage health and disease. In botanical medicine, for example, there is research showing the benefit of herbal products such as *ginkgo biloba* for improving problems due to *circulation* (although not Alzheimer disease), *curcumin* for inflammation and pain in arthritis, and the prevention of heart disease with garlic. A number of placebo-controlled trials have been performed showing that *Hypericum* (St. John's wort) is effective in the treatment of mild to moderate depression. Additional studies report that *Hypericum* is as effective as some conventional antidepressants but produces fewer side effects and costs less. However, the quality of too many of these trials does not reach the standards set for drug research in this country. Thus, physicians need to have and apply basic skills in the evaluation of clinical literature.

Alwhaibi M, Sambamoorthi U. Sex differences in the use of complementary and alternative medicine among adults with multiple chronic conditions. *Evid Based Complement Altern Med.* 2016;2016:2067095. [PMID: 27239207]

Ananth S. More hospitals offering CAM. https://www.hhnmag.com/articles/5496-more-hospitals-offering-cam. Accessed November 25, 2019.

Black LI, Clarke TC, Barnes PM, Stussman BJ, Nahin RL. Use of complementary health approaches among children aged 4–17 years in the United States: National Health Interview Survey, 2007–2012. National Health Statistics Reports No 78. Hyattsville, MD: National Center for Health Statistics; 2015.

Clarke TC, Black LI, Stussman BJ, Barnes PM, Nahin RL. Trends in the use of complementary health approaches among adults: United States, 2002–2012. National Health Statistics Reports No 79. Hyattsville, MD: National Center for Health Statistics; 2015.

Daily JW, Yang M, Park S. Efficacy of turmeric extracts and curcumin for alleviating the symptoms of joint arthritis: a systematic review and meta-analysis of randomized clinical trials. *J Med Food.* 2016;19(8):717–729. [PMID: 27533649]

Falci L, Shi Z, Greenlee H. Multiple chronic conditions and use of complementary and alternative medicine among U.S. adults: results from the 2012 National Health Interview Survey. *Prev Chronic Dis.* 2016;13:E61. [PMID: 27149072]

John GM, Hershman DL, Falci L, et al. Complementary and alternative medicine use among U.S. cancer survivors. *J Cancer Surviv.* 2016;10(5):850–864. [PMID: 26920872]

Johnson PJ, Kozhimannil KB, Jou J, et al. Complementary and alternative medicine use among women of reproductive age in the United States. *Womens Health Issues.* 2016;26(1):40–47. [PMID: 26508093]

Jou J, Johnson PJ. Nondisclosure of complementary and alternative medicine use to primary care physicians: findings from the 2012 National Health Interview Survey. *JAMA Intern Med.* 2016;176(4):545–546. [PMID: 26999670]

Kligler B. Integrative health in the Veterans Health Administration. *Med Acupunct.* 2017;29(4):187–188. [PMID: 28874918]

Misra SM, Guffey D, Tran X, et al. Survey of complementary and alternative medicine (CAM) services in freestanding US children's hospitals. *Clin Pediatr.* 2016;56:33–36. [PMID: 27130201]

Nahin RL, Barnes PM, Stussman BJ. Expenditures on complementary health approaches: United States, 2012. National Health Statistics Reports. Hyattsville, MD: National Center for Health Statistics; 2016.

National Institutes of Health. Complementary, alternative, or integrative health: what's in a name? https://nccih.nih.gov/health/integrative-health#term. Accessed November 25, 2019.

National Center for Complementary and Integrative Health. Fiscal Year 2017 Budget Request. http://nccam.nih.gov/about/budget/congressional/2017#Org. Accessed August 2, 2018.

Saper RB, Phillips RS, Sehgal A, et al. Lead, mercury and arsenic in US and Indian-manufactured Ayurvedic medicines sold via the Internet. *JAMA.* 2008;300(8):915–923. [PMID: 18728265]

Tindle HA, Davis RB, Phillips RS, et al. Trends in use of complementary and alternative medicine by US adults: 1997–2002. *Altern Ther Health Med.* 2005;11(1):42–49. [PMID: 15712765]

Wahner-Roedler DL, Vincent A, Elkin PL, et al. Physicians' attitudes toward complementary and alternative medicine and their knowledge of specific therapies: a survey at an academic medical center. *Evid Based Complement Alternat Med.* 2006;3(4):495–501. [PMID: 17173114]

Websites

Academic Consortium for Integrative Medicine and Health. Moving beyond medications. https://imconsortium.org/resourcesjournal/moving-beyond-medications/

National Center for Complementary and Integrative Health, National Institutes of Health. Fiscal Year 2008 Budget for the National Institutes of Health. http://nccam.nih.gov/about/offices/od/directortestimony/0607.htm

National Center for Complementary and Integrative Health, National Institutes of Health. Use of complementary health approaches in the U.S. https://nccih.nih.gov/research/statistics/NHIS/2012/multimedia

▶ Role of the Family Physician

What is the role of the family physician in the management of CAM and the delivery of appropriate integrative health care? The goal is to help patients make informed choices about CAM as they do in conventional medicine and implement evidence-based approaches to healing. Specifically, physicians must continue to apply the ethical principle of beneficence and autonomy and play the role of patient advocate—a professional should protect, permit, promote, and partner with patients about CAM and IM practices as appropriate.

A. Protecting Patients from Risks of CAM

Many practices, such as acupuncture, biofeedback, homeopathy, and meditation, are low-risk if delivered by competent practitioners. However, if used in place of more effective treatments, CAM may result in harm. The practitioners who apply these modalities should be qualified to help patients avoid inappropriate use. Many herbal preparations contain powerful pharmacologic substances with direct toxicity and herb-drug interactions. Contamination and poor quality control occur more often than with conventional drugs, especially if preparations are obtained from overseas. The family physician can help distinguish between CAM practices with little or no risk of direct toxicity (eg, homeopathy, acupuncture) and those with greater risk of toxicity (eg, megavitamins and herbal supplements). Physicians should be especially cautious about those products that can produce toxicity, work with patients to ensure that they do not abandon proven care, and alert patients to signs of possible fraud or abuse. "Secret" formulas, cures for multiple or life-threatening conditions, slick advertising for mail order or online products, pyramid marketing schemes, and any recommendation to abandon conventional medicine are "red flags" and should be suspect.

B. Permitting Use of Nonspecific Therapies

Spontaneous healing and placebo effects account for the improvement seen in many illnesses. The medical literature does contain essays and polemics that attempt to separate and often denigrate these factors (often calling them placebo effects) from those that are considered identifiable, tangible, specific aspects of a therapy. The clinician, however, is interested in how to combine both specific and nonspecific factors for maximum benefit. Many CAM systems emphasize high-touch, personalized approaches for the management of chronic disease and the crises associated with acute illness. The physician can permit the integration of selected CAM approaches that are not harmful or expensive and that may enhance these nonspecific, placebo factors.

C. Promoting CAM Use

Proven therapies that are safe and effective should be available to the public. As research continues, more CAM practices will be found to be effective. Gradually, physicians and patients will have more options for management of disease. In arthritis, for example, there are studies suggesting improvements with homeopathy, acupuncture, vitamin and nutritional supplements, botanical products, diet therapies, mind-body approaches, and manipulation. A similar collection of studies exists for other conditions such as heart disease, depression, asthma, pain, and addictions. The Cochrane Collaboration conducts systematic reviews (SRs) of randomized controlled trials (RCTs) on both conventional and complementary medicine and is an excellent source for evidence-based evaluation of such studies. Other groups such as RAND, the Agency for Healthcare Research and Quality, EPIC, and Samueli Institute also conduct such reviews. The Samueli Institute developed a streamlined but effective way to do these reviews called the *Systematic Evaluation of Research and Claims for Healing (SEaRCH)*. As research accumulates, rational therapeutic options can be developed in these areas.

As CAM information is presented in peer-reviewed professional journals, the challenge will be to implement its coordinated application via IM and integrative health strategies within clinical teams with effective models in hospitals, offices, clinics, and other care venues. The availability of pluralistic care delivery with onsite, certified, and licensed CAM practitioners will require the training of physicians who can guide the appropriate selection of modalities using evidenced-based evaluation methods on safety and efficacy. In fact, an increasing number of team-based care and group visits will be required to accomplish this. Although the physician may be the cornerstone of this team, optimal care will require collaboration among all members with honest communication, generous listening, a shared commitment to treating the whole person, integrated care plans, and appropriate referral when necessary.

D. Partnering with Patients About CAM Use

Over 60% of patients who use CAM practices do not reveal this information to their conventional physicians. Thus, there is a major communication gap between physicians and the public about CAM. Patients use alternative practices for various reasons: their culture or social network, dissatisfaction with the results of their conventional care, or an attraction to CAM philosophies and health beliefs. The overwhelming majority of patients use CAM practices as an *adjunct* to conventional medicine. Fewer than 5% use CAM *exclusively*. Patients who use alternative medicine do not foster antiscience or anti–conventional medicine sentiments or represent a disproportionate number of the uneducated, poor, seriously ill, or neurotic. Patients often do not understand the role of science in medicine and will accept anecdotal evidence or slick marketing as sufficient justification for use. The family physician can play a role in examining the research base of these medical claims and partner with patients to incorporate more evidence into their healthcare decisions. Quality research on CAM practices provide this evidence, and the physician can help bridge this gap with patients.

Other social factors have also influenced the emergence of CAM. These include rising rates of chronic disease, increasing access to health information, growing use of technology in medicine, declining faith that science will benefit personal health, and increasing interest in spirituality. In addition, both the public and health professionals are increasingly concerned about side effects, medical errors, and the escalating costs of conventional care. Physicians and scientists who ignore CAM only broaden the communication gap between the public and the profession that serves them. Thus, as patient advocates, physicians will best meet their patients' needs by learning about these practices and openly engaging in dialogue.

Chez RA, Jonas WB. The challenge of complementary and alternative medicine. *Am J Obstet Gynecol.* 1997;177(5):1156–1161. [PMID: 9396912].

Eisenberg DM, Kessler RC, Van Rompay MI, et al. Perceptions about complementary therapies relative to conventional therapies among adults who use both: results from a national survey. *Ann Intern Med.* 2001;135:344–351. [PMID: 11529698]

Jonas WB. *How Healing Works: Get Well and Stay Well Using Your Hidden Power to Heal.* Lorena Jones Books, 2018.

Jonas WB, Crawford C, Hilton L, Elfenbaum P. Scientific evaluation and review of claims in health care (SEaRCH): a streamlined, systematic, phased approach for determining "what works" in healthcare. *J Altern Complement Med.* 2017;23(1):18–25. [PMID: 28026968]

Lewith G, Jonas WB, Walach H, et al. *Clinical Research in Complementary Therapies: Principles, Problems and Solutions.* London, United Kingdom: Churchill Livingston; 2010.

Websites

Cochrane Collaboration. www.cochrane.org

Dr. Wayne Jonas. https://drwaynejonas.com/

▶ Evidence Hierarchy or Evidence House?

We all need good evidence to make medical decisions. Evidence comes in a variety of forms, and what may be good for one purpose may not be good for another. The term *evidence-based medicine* (EBM) has become a synonym for "good" medicine recently and is often used to support or deny the value of complementary medicine. EBM uses the "hierarchy of evidence" (Figure 50–3). In this hierarchy, SRs are seen as the "best" evidence, then individual RCTs, then nonrandomized trials, then observational studies, and finally case series. All efforts are focused on approximating evidence at the top of the pyramid, and lower levels are considered inferior. Clinical experiments on causal links between an intervention and outcomes become the gold standard when this model is used.

All family physicians have seen patients who recover from disease because of complex factors, many of which are not additive and cannot be isolated in controlled experiments. Under these circumstances, observational data from clinical practice may provide the best evidence rather than controlled trials. Patients' illnesses are the human experience of the disease—the manifestation of the patient's beliefs, fears, and expectations. As such, they are complex, and holistic phenomena cannot be reduced to single, objective measures. Often highly subjective judgments about life quality may be

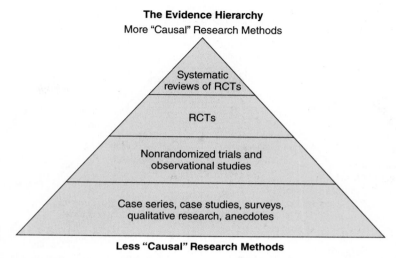

▲ Figure 50–3. The evidence hierarchy. RCTs, randomized controlled trials.

the best information with which to decide. Such experiences and beliefs may be captured only with qualitative research, not with scans or blood tests. Often the meaning that patients infer regarding their illness and recovery is the "best" evidence for medical decisions.

Sometimes the "best" evidence comes from laboratory tests. For example, the most crucial evidence for management of St. John's wort in patients on immunosuppressive medications originates from a laboratory finding that it accelerates drug metabolism via cytochrome P450. Arranging evidence in a hierarchy obscures the fact that the "best" evidence may be neither related to cause and effect, nor objective, nor clinical.

We suggest that family physicians not use an evidence hierarchy but rather build an evidence "house" (Figure 50–4). On the left side of this house is evidence for causal attributions, for mechanisms of action, and for "proof." If physicians confine themselves to the left side of the house, they will never know about the relevance of a treatment for patients or what happens in the real world of clinical practice. They will also not know whether proven treatments can be generalized to populations such as the ones they see or the healthcare delivery system in which they practice. The "rooms" on the right side of the house provide evidence about patient relevance and usefulness, in practices both proven and unproven.

How evidence is approached has ethical implications. Different groups prefer different types of evidence. Regulatory authorities are most interested in RCTs or SRs (left side), which may never be done because of the issues of time, cost, and access. Healthcare practitioners usually want to know the likelihood of benefit or harm from a treatment

(right side). Patients are intensely interested in stories and descriptions of cures (right side). Rationalists want to know how things work and so need laboratory evidence (left side). If one type of evidence is selected to the exclusion of others, science will not allow for full public input into clinical decisions. A livable house needs both a kitchen and a bathroom and places to sleep and play. Each type of evidence has different functions and value, and all types need to be of high quality.

Jonas WB. Evidence, ethics and evaluation of global medicine. In: Callahan D, ed. *Ethical Issues in Complementary and Alternative Medicine.* New York, NY: Hastings Center Report; 2001.
Lewith G, Walach H, Jonas W. *Clinical Research in Complementary Medicine,* 2nd ed. New York, NY: Elsevier; 2012.
Linde K, Jonas WB. Evaluating complementary and alternative medicine: the balance of rigor and relevance. In: Jonas WB, Levin J, eds. *Essentials of Complementary and Alternative Medicine.* Philadelphia, PA: Lippincott Williams & Wilkins; 1999.

▶ An Evidence-Based Approach

Fortunately, most treatment decisions need information only on whether a practice has a specific effect and on the magnitude of that effect in practice. This is evidence from RCTs and outcomes research, respectively. An evidence-based practice would then involve clinical expertise, informed patient communication, and quality research. This presumes that the physician has good clinical and communication skills. Medical training and experience address these, but evaluation of the CAM research evidence may not be something that physicians feel fully prepared to undertake. Obtaining research, selecting appropriate research for clinical situations, and

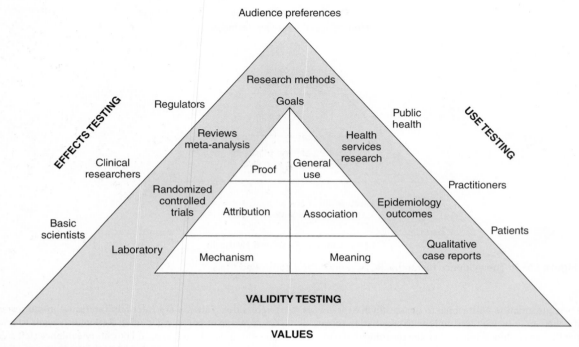

▲ **Figure 50–4.** The evidence house.

then evaluating the quality of that research in CAM are essential for a fully evidence-based practice that addresses these topics.

A. Finding and Selecting Good Information

Where can the family physician obtain research on CAM? A number of groups have collated and produced CAM-specific databases (Cochrane Collaboration, Evidence Based Medicine Reviews, Samueli Institute, and Natural Standard and search engines like Google). Table 50–2 lists some good sources of clinical information on CAM and what they provide. When searching these databases, look for the following key terms: (1) meta-analyses, (2) RCTs, and (3) observational or prospective outcomes data. Although there are many other types of studies, it is necessary to be cautious about using these for problem-oriented decision making in practice. If no research information is found from the databases or search engines listed, it is likely that there is little relevant evidence for the practice on that clinical condition. A search for this information need not take up a lot of time. A trained research assistant or librarian can often do the search, streamlining time spent on this process. Many librarians, especially those at health centers and hospitals, are now receiving training in literature searching methodology and growing awareness

and expertise in CAM databases. Increasingly, these searches are done directly online and by the physician at the point of care. After a literature search, the physician can be confident in knowing the quantity of evidence on the therapy (Figure 50–5). Patients are usually grateful for this effort as they will come to their physician in the hopes of obtaining science-based information they can trust.

B. Risks and Types of Evidence for Practice

If there are studies on a specific type of CAM practice, then the risk of toxicity and the cost of the therapy indicate which types of data are needed. Low-risk practices include over-the-counter homeopathic medications, acupuncture and gentle massage or manipulation, meditation, relaxation and biofeedback, other mind-body methods, and vitamin and mineral supplementation below toxic doses. Low-cost therapies involving self-care are also often low-risk. High-risk practices include herbal therapies, high-dose vitamins and minerals, colonics, and intravenous administration of substances or extreme diets. Some otherwise harmless therapies can produce considerable cost if they require major life-style changes. Herbal therapies can produce serious adverse effects secondary to their impact on cell function, including enzymatic reactions or contamination with toxic materials.

Table 50–2. Sources of CAM information for healthcare practitioners.

Source of CAM Information	Description	Where to Go
Cochrane Library	Database of Systematic Reviews: systematic reviews of RCTs of CAM and conventional therapies Controlled Trials Register: extensive bibliographic listing of controlled trials and conference proceedings	http://www.cochrane.org http://gateway.ovid.com
Natural Medicines Comprehensive Database	Comprehensive listing and cross-listing of natural and herbal therapies, separate "all known uses" and "effectiveness" sections, safety ratings, mechanisms of action, side effects, herb-drug interactions, and review of available evidence	https://naturalmedicines.therapeuticresearch.com/
National Library of Medicine	Powerful search engine that allows searches of PubMed and all government guidelines combined Includes "synonym and related terms" option	Search engine: https://www.nlm.nih.gov/ Individual guidelines at: https://www.ahrq.gov/gam/index.html http://www.cdc.gov/publications
Dr. Wayne Jonas	Evidence-based information oriented for rapid use in practice summarizing current evidence, extent of use, credentialing and licensing information and linked to patient and provider summaries free for downloading. Supported by an unrestricted grant from the Samueli Foundation	www.drwaynejonas.com
PubMed Clinical Queries Search Engine	The old standby has a clinical queries filter to limit your search results Click on "Clinical Queries" on the left blue banner to access the filter For the most comprehensive search, use the keywords "complementary medicine"	https://www.ncbi.nlm.nih.gov/pubmed
National Center for Complementary and Integrative Health (NCCIH)	Clinical Trials Section: listing of clinical trials indexed by treatment or by condition Crosslinked to http://www.clinicaltrials.gov and PubMed	https://nccih.nih.gov/
Agency for Healthcare Research and Quality (AHRQ)	For information on the quality, safety, efficiency, and effectiveness of health care for all Americans	http://www.ahrq.gov
Clinical Evidence	Promotes informed decision making by summarizing what is known, and not known, about >200 medical conditions and >2000 treatments	http://www.clinicalevidence.com/ceweb/condition/index.jsp
Turning Research into Practice (TRIP)	Allows health professionals to easily find the highest quality material available on the Internet	http://www.tripdatabase.com
Family Physicians Inquiries Network	Provides clinicians with answers to 80% of their clinical questions in 60 seconds	http://www.fpin.org

CAM, complementary and alternative medicine; RCT, randomized controlled trial.
Adapted with permission from Birrer RB, O'Connor FG: *Sports Medicine for the Primary Care Physician.* Boca Raton, FL: CRC Press; 2004.

Because patients frequently take herbal products along with calculated dose prescription medications, physicians should specifically inquire about their use. High-risk or high-cost practices and products require RCT data.

Under some circumstances, observational (outcomes) data are more important, and in other circumstances, RCT data are more important. Outcomes research provides the probability of an effect and the absolute magnitude of effects in the context of normal clinical care. It is more similar to clinical practice and usually involves a wide variety of patients and variations of care to fit the patient's circumstances. It does not provide information on whether a treatment is specific or better than another treatment.

With low-risk practices, the physician wants to know the probability of benefit from the therapy. Quality observational data from practices are preferable to RCT data if the data are collected from actual practice populations similar to those of the practitioner. This may be sufficient

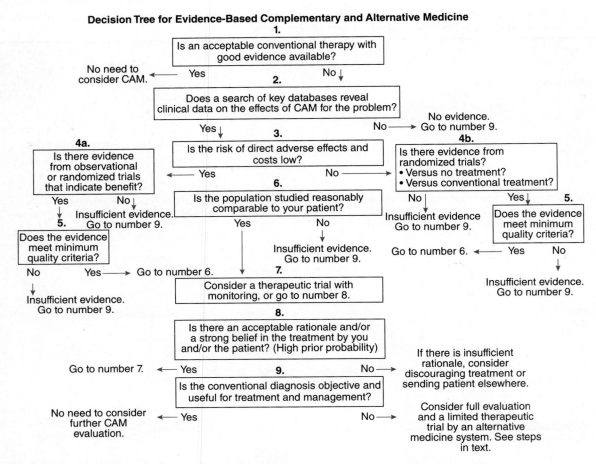

Decision Tree for Evidence-Based Complementary and Alternative Medicine

1. Is an acceptable conventional therapy with good evidence available?
— Yes → No need to consider CAM.
— No ↓

2. Does a search of key databases reveal clinical data on the effects of CAM for the problem?
— Yes ↓
— No → No evidence. Go to number 9.

3. Is the risk of direct adverse effects and costs low?
— Yes ← 4a.
— No →

4a. Is there evidence from observational or randomized trials that indicate benefit?
— Yes ↓
— No ↓ Insufficient evidence. Go to number 9.

5. Does the evidence meet minimum quality criteria?
— No ↓ Insufficient evidence. Go to number 9.
— Yes → Go to number 6.

4b. Is there evidence from randomized trials?
• Versus no treatment?
• Versus conventional treatment?
— No ↓ Insufficient evidence Go to number 9.
— Yes ↓

5. Does the evidence meet minimum quality criteria?
— Yes → Go to number 6.
— No ↓ Insufficient evidence. Go to number 9.

6. Is the population studied reasonably comparable to your patient?
— Yes ↓
— No ↓ Insufficient evidence. Go to number 9.

7. Consider a therapeutic trial with monitoring, or go to number 8.

8. Is there an acceptable rationale and/or a strong belief in the treatment by you and/or the patient? (High prior probability)
— Yes → Go to number 7.
— No → If there is insufficient rationale, consider discouraging treatment or sending patient elsewhere.

9. Is the conventional diagnosis objective and useful for treatment and management?
— Yes → No need to consider further CAM evaluation.
— No → Consider full evaluation and a limited therapeutic trial by an alternative medicine system. See steps in text.

▲ **Figure 50–5.** Decision tree for evidence-based complementary and alternative medicine (CAM).

evidence for making clinical decisions. Often, it will be the only useful information available for chronic conditions. For example, if quality outcome studies report a 75% probability of improving allergic rhinitis using a nontoxic, low-cost, homeopathic remedy, this information can assist in deciding on its use.

For high-risk, high-cost interventions, the physician should use RCTs (or meta-analyses of those trials). RCTs address the relative benefit of one therapy over another (or no therapy). RCTs can determine whether the treatment is the cause of improvement and how much the treatment adds to either no treatment or placebo treatment. RCTs provide relative (not absolute) information effects between a CAM and control practice. They are difficult to do properly for more than short periods and difficult if the therapy being tested is complex and individualized or if there are marked patient preferences. In addition, RCTs remove any choice about therapy and, if blinded, blunt expectations—both of which affect outcomes. Placebo-controlled RCT differences are dependent largely on the control group, which requires careful selection and management. Strong patient preferences for CAM, differing cultural groups, and informed consent may also alter RCT results. RCTs are more important if we need to know more about specific benefit-harm comparisons, such as with high-risk, high-cost interventions. Recently *comparative effectiveness research* (CER) has emerged as an important goal and set of methods. CER may be a valuable addition to CAM research, allowing whole systems of care to be compared to other different systems.

The more a CAM practice addresses chronic disease and depends on self-care (eg, meditation, yoga, biofeedback) or involves a complex system (eg, classical homeopathy, traditional Chinese medicine, Unani-Tibb), the more local, observational data are important. The more a CAM practice involves high-risk or high-cost interventions, the more essential RCT data become.

C. Evaluating Study Quality

Once data are found and the preferred type of study is selected, the practitioner should apply some minimum quality criteria to these studies. Three items can be quickly checked: (1) blind and random allocation of subjects to comparison groups (in RCTs) or blind outcome assessments (in observational research), (2) the clinical relevance and reliability of the outcome measures, and (3) the number of subjects that could be fully analyzed at the end of the study compared to the number entered. These same minimum quality criteria apply to RCTs or observational studies, except that blinded, random allocation to treatment and comparison groups does not apply in the latter. However, evaluation of effects before or after treatment can be blinded to the treatment given in any study. Detailed descriptions of patients, interventions, and dropouts are hallmarks of a quality outcomes trial.

Finally, one can ask if the probability of benefits reported in an outcomes study is worth the inconvenience, risk of side effects, and costs of the treatment and, in addition, whether confidence intervals were reported. *Confidence intervals* are the range of minimum to maximum effects expected in 95% of similar studies. If confidence intervals are narrow, the physician can be confident that similar results will occur with other patients. If confidence intervals are broad, the chance of obtaining those effects from treatment in other patients will be less predictable.

If the quality screening questions reveal marked quality flaws in the studies retrieved, the evidence in the study is insufficient and should not be used as a basis for clinical decisions.

D. The Population Studied

Even if good evidence is found for a practice, physicians should determine whether the population in the studies is similar to the patient being seen. Although this matching is largely subjective, the physician can compare five areas. Specifically, determine whether the study was done (1) in a primary, secondary, or tertiary referral center; (2) in a Western, Eastern, developing, or industrialized country; and (3) with diagnostic criteria similar to the patient (eg, the same criteria were used to diagnose osteoarthritis or congestive heart failure). Also, determine whether the age (4) and gender(s) (5) of the study population were similar. If the study population is not similar to the patient being seen, then the data, even though valid, cannot be applied to the situation. The study country may be especially important for some CAM practices. For example, data on use of acupuncture to treat chronic pain may come from China. Pain perception and reporting are different in China from those in the United States and Europe. Thus, results from a study done in one country may not be applicable in another. If the study and clinic population match, an appropriate body of evidence for moving forward with a therapeutic trial exists.

E. Balancing Beliefs

Belief in the treatment by the physician and the patient needs to be explicitly considered in CAM. In conventional medicine, both patient and physician usually accept the plausibility of treatment. Belief has long been known to affect outcome. Strong belief enhances positive outcomes, and weak or negative belief interferes with them. A physician may feel that a CAM practice has incredibly low plausibility, although the patient may have a strong belief in the therapy. This "prior probability" (or belief) by the physician and patient should be considered in the decision to allow or not allow the patient to use a treatment. If physician and patient have similar beliefs, then a decision is easily made. Sometimes, however, the patient has a strong belief in the therapy, but the physician finds it unbelievable or thinks it is harmful. In such situations, the physician should work with the patient to decide the best action, including referral elsewhere as an option.

F. Alternative Diagnoses

Some diagnoses are not very useful for management of a patient's illness. If the family physician's conventional diagnosis is not helping a patient, the clinician may want to consider an evaluation by an alternative system. Chinese medicine uses energy diagnosis, for example, and homeopathy has a unique remedy classification system. Sometimes, obtaining an assessment from a practitioner experienced in a CAM system may prove useful. For example, a 51-year-old woman with several years of idiopathic urticaria had obtained no relief from several conventional physicians. A homeopathic assessment showed that she might benefit from the remedy Mercurius 200C (*mercurius virax*). She was given several small doses, and the urticaria cleared. The effect may have been due to placebo, but the treatment was not harmful and she had exhausted conventional treatments.

The physician should also be alert to practitioners who pursue CAM diagnoses that are not useful. A complicated CAM evaluation and treatment with little effect might be managed simply and effectively by conventional medicine. For example, a 57-year-old man with cardiovascular disease and recurrent bouts of angina was treated by a CAM practitioner for 3 years with special diets and nutritional supplements without help. Consultation with a conventional practitioner showed that he had myxedema. A thyroid supplement cleared his angina rapidly. In cases in which the diagnostic approach of the medical system fails, a professional consultation may be needed. In situations in which the alternative system's diagnostic and treatment approach is clear, a limited therapeutic trial with specific treatment goals and follow-up can be attempted. Of course, quality products and qualified practitioners must be located. In situations of serious disease, such as cancer, desperate patients may seek out CAM treatments. Under these circumstances, good

Table 50–3. Questions for evidence-based complementary and alternative medicine therapy (CAMT) management.

A patient is using a CAMT or an alternative treatment is sought. The following questions should be answered.

1. Has the patient received proper conventional medical care?
2. Is the CAMT likely to produce direct toxic or adverse effects, or is it expensive?
3. Are there clinical data from randomized trials or outcomes research on the CAMT?
4. Do the studies meet minimum quality criteria?
5. Is the study population similar to the patient using or seeking the CAMT?
6. Is the plausibility of the therapy acceptable to both patient and physician?
7. Can a quality product or a qualified practitioner be accessed?
8. Can the patient be monitored while undergoing the CAMT?
9. Is a full diagnostic assessment by a conventional or CAM system in order?

training and clinical experience and protection of patients from harm (even from themselves) should prevail. The website www.drwaynejonas.com offers a guide to finding and selecting a qualified CAM provider to work with.

EBM can be applied to CAM. Table 50–3 summarizes questions and provides a stepwise decision tree for EBM-CAM management. Thus, appropriate data-driven clinical decisions can be made with CAM as with all medical care.

► Summary

American medicine continues to evolve in its focus, capabilities, technology, and demands. Our population is aging, and with that comes more chronic disease. By definition, chronic disease cannot be cured—patients may suffer with disability, diminished function, emotional challenges, economic burden, and overall challenges to quality of life. Conventional medicine is failing to provide the necessary and required care that these patients deserve. Although cure cannot always be the physician's primary goal, the provision of individualized, person-centered care suffused with empathy and compassion remains the foundation of all medical practice and should be provided for all patients. The knowledgeable use of integrative health, combining the best of CAM and conventional therapies and self-care, will empower patients to participate in a process of healing with their healthcare team by activating their inherent healing capacities and enhancing their expectation, hope, understanding, and belief, knowing that well-being can manifest.

Eisenberg DM. Advising patients who seek alternative medical therapies. *Ann Intern Med*. 1997;127:61–69. [PMID: 9214254]

Gatchel RJ, Maddrey AM. Clinical outcome research in complementary and alternative medicine: an overview of experimental design and analysis. *Alt Ther Health Med*. 1998;4(5):36–42. [PMID: 9737030]

Jonas WB. Clinical trials for chronic disease: randomized, controlled clinical trials are essential. *J NIH Res*. 1997;9:33. [No PMID]

Jonas W. *How Healing Works*. Oakland, CA: Ten Speed Press; 2018.

Jonas WB, Linde K, Walach H. How to practice evidence-based complementary and alternative medicine. In: Jonas WB, Levin JS, eds. *Essentials of Complementary and Alternative Medicine*. Philadelphia, PA: Lippincott Williams & Wilkins; 1999.

Kirsch I. *How Expectancies Shape Experience*. Washington, DC: American Psychological Association; 1999.

Websites

Dr. Wayne Jonas. www.drwaynejonas.com

National Center for Complementary and Integrative Health (NCCIH). https://nccih.nih.gov/

► Acknowledgment

Special thanks to Lexie Robinson, Cindy Crawford, and Viviane Enslein in helping collect background information and preparing the manuscript.

Chronic Pain Management

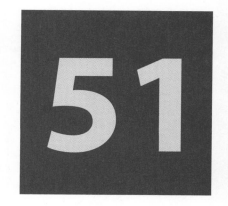

John N. Boll, Jr, DO, FAAFP
Ronald M. Glick, MD

▶ General Considerations

Pain is defined by the International Association for the Study of Pain as "an unpleasant sensory or emotional experience associated with actual or potential tissue damage or described in terms of such damage." This emphasizes that the pain experience is multidimensional and may include sensory, cognitive, and emotional components. Additionally, it allows for the possibility, as in chronic pain states, that overt tissue damage may no longer be present. Chronic pain is pain persisting for >3 months or beyond the time of normal tissue healing. Many of the secondary problems associated with chronic pain, such as deconditioning, depression, sleep disturbance, and disability, begin within the first few months of the onset of symptoms of pain. Early identification and treatment are essential to reduce chronicity and prevent further disability.

Chronic pain is one of the most common complaints in primary care. The subjective nature of pain makes quantifying the incidence and prevalence a challenging endeavor. A 2012 population study estimated that 11.2% of adults, or 25.3 million adults, experience chronic pain, whereas the Institute of Medicine noted that 100 million Americans experience chronic pain with estimated annual medical and indirect costs of approximately $600 billion. Low back pain is most common, followed closely by migraines, neck pain, and other arthritic joint pain complaints. Given the frequency of chronic pain in primary care and its multidimensional nature, family physicians are uniquely positioned to support patients in preventing, treating, and coping with chronic pain.

Committee on Advancing Pain Research Care and Education–Board on Health Sciences Policy. *Relieving Pain in America: A Blueprint for Transforming Prevention, Care, Education and Research*. Washington, DC: Institute of Medicine; 2011.

Nahin RL. Estimates of pain prevalence and severity in adults: United States, 2012. *J Pain*. 2015;16(8):769–780. [PMID: 26028573]

▶ Pathogenesis

The development of chronic pain is a complex interplay of modifiable and nonmodifiable risk factors unique to an individual. Studies performed on persistent postsurgical pain, persistent posttrauma pain, and postherpetic neuralgia assist in the understanding of the pathogenesis of chronic pain because of a defined mechanism and onset to the pain syndrome. Modifiable risk factors include such things as the nature and severity of the pain, predisposing mental health diagnoses, tobacco or alcohol exposure, physical activity and exercise, employment status, and occupational factors. Nonmodifiable risk factors include age, gender, cultural background, socioeconomic factors, epigenetics, and history of trauma, injury, or interpersonal violence.

The transition from acute to chronic pain involves a nociceptive and behavioral cascade with onset soon after the initial tissue injury. The noxious stimuli cause inflammatory changes leading to peripheral sensitization, which is known as *acute pain*. This stimulus is then transmitted via the spinal cord to the brainstem and cortical regions of the brain via afferent pathways. As this stimulus is processed, the individual characteristics of the patient will cause unique perception of the pain. When this process leads to central sensitization, essentially it turns on a switch, leading to the development of *chronic pain*. This transformation to chronicity impacts the patient at all levels of their functioning including behavioral, emotional, and physical.

McGreevy K, Bottros MM, Raja SN. Preventing chronic pain following acute pain: risk factors, preventive strategies, and their efficacy. *Eur J Pain Suppl*. 2011;5(2):365–372. [PMID: 22102847]

Van Hecke O, Torrance N, Smith BH. Chronic pain epidemiology: where do lifestyle factors fit in? *Br J Pain*. 2013;7(4):209–217. [PMID: 26516524]

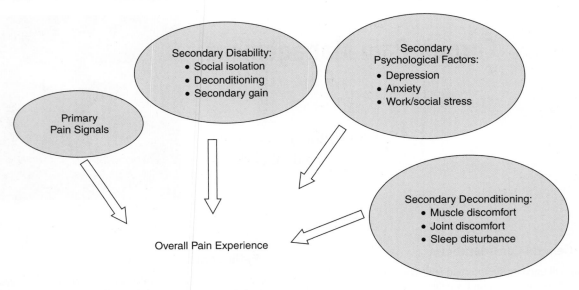

▲ **Figure 51–1.** Primary and secondary features of chronic pain.

▶ Clinical Findings

Given pain's subjective nature, the clinical findings of chronic pain vary depending upon the etiology. Common causes of chronic pain include migraine headaches, arthritis, fibromyalgia, low back pain, sickle cell disease, diabetic neuropathy, and cancer-related pain. Other contributors to chronic pain include chronic stress, psychological suffering, unrealistic expectations of pain relief, cognitive dysfunction, drug withdrawal, malingering, and psychiatric disease such as generalized anxiety disorder, major depressive disorder, somatic symptom disorder, and panic disorder. In many patients, multiple factors contribute to their pain presentation. To better understand patients' pain and suffering, primary care providers should perform a careful history and physical exam including the use of validated screens such as for assessing pain and function (PEG-3, Brief Pain Inventory [BPI]), anxiety (Beck's Anxiety Inventory), depression (Patient Health Questionnaire-9), personal trauma (Adverse Childhood Experience Questionnaire, Primary Care Posttraumatic Stress Disorder Screen), and substance use (Screening, Brief Intervention, Referral and Treatment). Patients identified as having a substance use disorder during the clinical assessment should be provided treatment or referral for their substance use disorder.

The overall pain experience includes primary pain-generating signals, along with common secondary problems that complicate management (Figure 51–1). Both physical (eg, joint restrictions and deconditioning) and psychological (eg, depression and anxiety) changes frequently accompany chronic pain. Psychological distress is common. In a survey of 500 patients with chronic low back, hip, or knee pain, depression or anxiety accompanied pain complaints in 46% of patients. Patients with pain plus the combination of depression and anxiety experienced significantly greater pain severity and disability (P <.0001 for each). Psychosocial stress may result from difficulties related to school or work, family, social isolation, and legal and financial areas. Although the possibility of secondary gain (eg, litigation) may increase complaints, true malingering and factitious disorders occur in only 1–10% of patients. The *Diagnostic and Statistical Manual of Mental Disorders*, 5th edition, recognizes that regardless of etiology, many individuals experience persistent thoughts, and high anxiety may be related to the pain problem. The diagnosis of *somatic symptom disorder with predominant pain* reflects an understanding that psychological factors may greatly compound distress and dysfunction. In addition, pain catastrophization and kinesiophobia are common concerns among individuals with chronic pain and can adversely affect functioning. Along with other psychological constructs, such as depression, anxiety, and pessimism, are areas that the family physician can address in medical counseling to impact the patient's cognitive precepts, which set the stage for cognitive and behavioral change.

American Psychiatric Association: *Desk Reference to the Diagnostic Criteria from DSM-5*. Arlington, VA: American Psychiatric Association; 2013.

Bair MJ, Wu J, Damush TM, et al. Association of depression and anxiety alone and in combination with chronic musculoskeletal pain in primary care patients. *Psychosom Med.* 2008;70:890–897. [PMID: 18799425]

Leung L. Pain catastrophizing: an updated review. *Ind J Psychol Med.* 2012;34(3):204–217. [PMID: 23441031]

Manhapra A, Becker WC. Pain and addiction: an integrative therapeutic approach. *Med Clin N Am.* 2018;102:745–763. [PMID: 29933827]

Uluğ N, Yakut Y, Alemdaroğlu İ, Yılmaz Ö. Comparison of pain, kinesiophobia and quality of life in patients with low back and neck pain. *J Physical Ther Sci.* 2016;28(2):665–670. [PMID: 27064399]

▶ Treatment

Treatment is best conceptualized the same as other chronic diseases such as diabetes, depression, or asthma using the *chronic disease management* model. Such a concept focuses on the relationship between the patient and the care team using an organized, proactive, multicomponent approach involving prevention, screening, multidimensional treatment, self-management goal setting, specialist support, and patient registries with electronic health record support (Figure 51–2). Prevention is crucial. *Primary* prevention is the prevention of acute pain by using strategies such as the shingles vaccine, seatbelts, avoidance of tobacco and illicit drugs, and practicing a healthy lifestyle. *Secondary* prevention involves the transition between acute and chronic pain. Acute pain should be viewed as *prechronic* and actively addressed to prevent progression to chronic pain, conceptually like a family physician would approach *prediabetes*. This requires aggressive management of prechronic pain by keeping patients active, limiting opioids, providing hope and empathy, treating substance use and psychiatric disease, and identifying patient goals (Table 51–1). Although not given the same attention in the literature as acute and chronic states, it is helpful to consider the development of subacute pain. As an example, an episode of acute low back pain going

Table 51–1. Strategies for primary and secondary prevention of pain.

Primary Prevention	Secondary Prevention
Injury prevention, eg, seatbelt and helmet use	Stay active and address barriers to activities
Vaccinations, eg, shingles vaccine	Identify goals and work to accomplish them
Healthy lifestyle, eg, regular exercise	Treat mental health disorders
Avoid tobacco, illicit drugs, and excessive alcohol use	Treat substance use disorder
Treat mental health disorders	Restore function with osteopathic manipulation, yoga, or physical therapy
Preemptive analgesia for surgeries	Avoid opioids except when immediately postsurgery, in severe pain (≥7), or when other treatments are ineffective

in the fourth week, associated with insomnia, alcohol use for sleep, extended time off work, and dysphoria, requires a different approach than pain in the first week.

As with other chronic diseases, it is important at all levels of chronic pain treatment to identify the goal of treatment regarding pain and function. Many studies look for 30% improvement to determine *clinically meaningful improvement*. This may contrast with the patient's expectations for something to "take the pain away" completely. Thus, chronic pain management focuses on reduction in symptoms and improvement of function rather than on cure. Both medication and nonpharmacologic modalities effectively decrease primary and secondary symptoms of chronic pain, with a range of treatments often provided through a treatment team

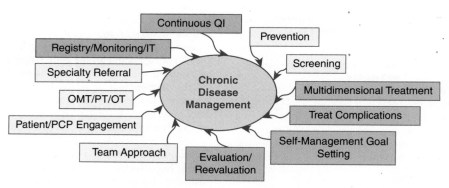

▲ **Figure 51–2.** Components of chronic disease management. IT, information technology; OMT, osteopathic manipulative treatment; OT, occupational therapy; PCP, primary care physician; PT, physical therapy; QI, quality improvement.

Table 51–2. Comprehensive treatment of chronic pain.

Specialist	Treatment Modalities
Physician	Analgesics, adjunctive medications, nerve blocks, medical counseling to foster self-management
Complementary/integrative therapist	Acupuncture, yoga/tai chi, meditation, manipulation therapy
Psychology/psychiatry	Address locus of control, depression therapy, anxiety therapy, mindfulness-based stress reduction
Physical/occupational therapist	Musculoskeletal dysfunction, deconditioning, work simplification, graded exercise
Spiritual counselor	Provide meaning and purpose to the suffering
Substance use disorder treatment	Provide counseling and medication-assisted treatment

(Table 51–2). Physicians and patients must accept that complete resolution may not be possible and work toward reducing symptoms and minimizing disability. The patient must shift from searching for a medical cure to engaging in collaborative rehabilitation, geared toward decreasing pain and optimizing function. Goals of chronic pain rehabilitation are improvement in both pain and secondary symptoms, including deconditioning, depression, and disability (Table 51–3). Early identification and treatment should reduce the severity of secondary symptoms.

Table 51–3. Appropriate treatment goals.

General Goal	Specific Treatment Target
Decreased pain	Pain reduction to moderate levels; reduced frequency and duration of flares
Improved function	Return to school or work; increased number of household chores; increased participation in leisure activities
Improved sleep	Reduced number of wake-ups; improved overall sleep to 5 hours per night
Improved mood	Increased participation in social activities; reduced time in bed/being inactive; improved nutrition intake
Reduced use of medical resources	Reduced emergency department visits; reduced use of excessive analgesics; decreased repeat consultations or studies

The effectiveness, benefits, and harms of specific treatments for chronic pain were reviewed by the Centers for Disease Control and Prevention (CDC) in a 2016 publication. Nonpharmacologic and nonopioid pharmacologic therapy are preferred for treatment of chronic pain. Treatment starts by establishing goals and using clinical findings to diagnose and treat the primary pain-generating signals. This treatment can involve interventional techniques, acupuncture, manipulative therapy (osteopathic or chiropractic), or mindfulness-based stress reduction. Through self-management goal setting, promote healthy behaviors such as exercise, tobacco cessation, or weight loss and restore sleep whether through behavioral changes or medication. An underlying sleep disorder can prevent effective engagement in a treatment plan and increase risk of opioid overdose if the patient has underlying obstructive sleep apnea. Based on the clinical findings, treat associated secondary complications such as a psychiatric disorder, since this can both cause chronic pain and prevent improvement if left untreated. If medications are used, maximize nonopioid and adjuvant pain medications while minimizing side effects. Only consider an opioid trial after maximizing the nonopioid options. Use the lowest possible opioid dose to minimize patient risk, and have a willingness to discontinue the medication if no benefit is obtained.

Dowell D, Haegerich TM, Chou R. CDC guideline for prescribing opioids for chronic pain: United States, 2016. *MMWR Recomm Rep.* 2016;65(1):1–50. [PMID: 26987082]
Henry JL. The need for knowledge translation in chronic pain. *Pain Res Manage.* 2008;13(6):465–476. [PMID: 2799315]

A. Psychological Approaches

Family physicians are uniquely positioned to provide behavioral and psychological care to their patients due to their long-term relationships with their patients and their understanding of their broader family and community support system. Focused counseling may be needed for mood, sleep, and other psychosocial factors. Severe symptoms of depression or anxiety or significant psychosocial stressors may necessitate a specialty referral for psychology or psychiatry. For all patients with chronic pain, family physicians should be assessing the patient's readiness to change and assisting the development of self-management goals. The Pain Stages of Change Questionnaire is one example of a validated survey for identifying a patient's readiness to change, but family physicians can assess this from a basic interview as well. *Precontemplation* indicates no desire to change. *Contemplation* indicates a readiness to make a behavioral change but reluctance to accept internal means to accomplish this change. *Active* stage accepts a self-management goal and seeks to accomplish this change. *Maintenance* is characterized by working to maintain these changes and an established self-management perspective. A patient's stage of change indirectly reflects the patient's level of medicalization, and patients in the active or maintenance stage will rely on less diagnostic tests and medications for pain care. Within the stages of change model, the family physician can help to move the patient toward greater readiness for change. As one example, consider a patient with degenerative disk disease with chronic discogenic and radicular pain after two back surgeries. The patient may not be aware of the impact of tobacco use on disk health and healing or the impact of obesity on fueling inflammation systemically and conceivably affecting spinal nerves as well. That education may not be sufficient to move the patient from precontemplation to contemplation, but it may start a dialogue between the patient and physician.

Self-management goal setting is best accomplished using cognitive behavioral therapy (CBT) methods. CBT is an effective psychological treatment technique that challenges dysfunctional precepts or perception of pain ("My pain must be cured. I can't do anything if I have pain") and replaces it with one that is more conducive to change ("Pain limits me from lifting 25 pounds, but I can still carry a bag of groceries"). CBT helps change patients' perceptions or locus of control from external (believing that pain is not controllable by the patient) to internal (believing that the patient can positively influence symptoms). Patients with an external locus of control see themselves as powerless victims of pain, similar to the precontemplation stage of change. This results in the expectation that only fate or the physician can help when pain becomes severe. When expectations are not met, patients may seek alternative evaluations and treatments (eg, another physician, a different diagnostic test, or surgical procedures) that may not be in their best interest. The clinician must help patients to move into a pain self-management–internal locus of control belief system. Greater perceived self-control of pain decreases both pain and secondary symptoms.

Coleman MT, Pasternak RH. Effective strategies for behavior change. *Prim Care*. 2012;39(2):281–305. [PMID: 22608867]

Habib S, Morrissey SA, Helmes E. Readiness to adopt a self-management approach to pain: evaluation of the pain stages of change model in a non-pain-clinic sample. *Pain*. 2003;104:283–290. [PMID: 12855339]

Jensen MP, Turner JA, Romano JM. Changes after multidisciplinary pain treatment in patient pain beliefs and coping are associated with concurrent changes in patient functioning. *Pain*. 2007;131:38–47. [PMID: 17250963]

B. Exercise Therapy

Restoration of function and overcoming the cycle of inactivity and disability require an active management plan incorporating exercise therapy. Identification and treatment of musculoskeletal dysfunctions and decisions concerning limitations on activity often require consultation with physical or occupational therapists but can also be part of an in-home self-management plan. Methods of exercise therapy include reconditioning, active stretching and strengthening exercises, and aquatic and graded activity programs. Physical therapists should instruct patients in a daily exercise routine as well as flare management techniques (eg, trigger point massage, oscillatory movements, and use of heat and ice). Occupational therapists address work simplification, body mechanics, and pacing skills. They can facilitate returning to a normal activity schedule (eg, work or school), even on a modified basis. Prolonged absence from normal activities increases the difficulty of reducing disability. Return to normal activity as soon as possible, however, should be the primary goal of pain management.

The greatest challenge, for individuals with chronic pain, is to help them to move to a higher level of regular aerobic physical activity. Aerobic exercise is analgesic, through its impact on endorphins and other neurochemical pathways. Additionally, it can benefit mood, sleep, anxiety, weight, and overall functioning. The challenge is that, almost by definition, individuals with chronic pain tend to self-limit activity and commonly indicate that exercise increases their pain. To the extent that we can help patients get back into aerobic activity, we can move them to more of a self-care model. One issue is the idea of a progressive exercise program and telling patients to start at a low level of intensity and short duration and gradually step things up. Another task is to help a patient find specific activities they can engage in without flaring their pain. Activities tolerated by most individuals with chronic pain include the use of a recumbent exercise bike and a gentle pool exercise/aerobic program.

C. Pharmacotherapy

Due to the opioid overdose epidemic in the United States, an obligatory paradigm shift has occurred in the management of chronic pain. Based on recommendations supporting opioid use for chronic pain published in the 1990s, opioid prescribing increased dramatically, especially in primary care. The dramatic increase in opioid overdoses and deaths led to the 2016 publication from the CDC of clear new recommendations for the initiation and ongoing management of opioids for chronic pain in primary care, excluding active cancer treatment, palliative care, or end-of-life care. However, for those previously on high opioid doses for chronic pain, the recommendations were less clear. One example is the decreased functioning and increased pain that some patients experience with long-term opioid therapy known as *opioid-induced hyperalgesia*. In this situation, appropriate patient-centered treatment is a taper of the opioids. This, plus avoidance of polypharmacy, may be the best therapeutic option in the care of certain patients, and nonpharmacologic and nonopioid options are always preferred.

Table 51–4. Medication management of chronic pain.

Symptom Treated	Medication Class	Examples
Pain	Analgesics	Acetaminophen NSAIDs
	Opioids—full or partial mu-receptor agonists	Sustained-release morphine, oxycodone, and transdermal fentanyl or buprenorphine
Neuropathic pain	Antidepressants Anticonvulsants	Duloxetine, 30–60 mg BID Gabapentin, 300–1200 mg TID Pregabalin, 75–200 mg TID
Muscle spasm	Muscle relaxants	Tizanidine, 2–8 mg at bedtime to TID
Sleep disturbance	Antidepressants	Nortriptyline, 25–75 mg at bedtime Trazodone, 50–150 mg at bedtime
Depression	Antidepressants	Bupropion, extended release, 150–300 mg daily Citalopram, 20–40 mg daily

BID, twice daily; NSAIDs, nonsteroidal anti-inflammatory drugs; TID, 3 times daily.

Other uses of pharmacotherapy for chronic pain can focus on treating underlying medical conditions (eg, disease-modifying medications in rheumatoid arthritis) or relieving not just symptoms of pain but also the secondary symptoms (eg, depression, anxiety, or sleep disturbance). Most medications used to treat chronic pain address the latter two factors (Table 51–4).

1. Nonopioid Analgesics—Well established for prechronic and chronic pain, nonopioid analgesics such as acetaminophen, nonsteroidal anti-inflammatory drugs (NSAIDs), and cyclooxygenase-2 (COX-2) inhibitors are generally well tolerated and recommended as first-line agents for osteoarthritis and low back pain. Given the number of over-the-counter products that contain acetaminophen and risk for overdose, McNeil PPC reduced the recommended adult, maximum dosage of acetaminophen to 3 g per 24 hours in 2011. Acetaminophen should be restricted in patients with significant alcohol intake or liver disease. Studies have shown an increased risk of elevated blood pressure and the potential to interact with other medications that have hepatic clearance.

NSAIDs can be very effective for pain and inflammation. Comparison studies between opioids and NSAIDs have shown in certain patients an equal analgesic affect with NSAIDs but also improved function, although patient response to different NSAIDs and COX-2 inhibitors may vary. Common NSAIDs used for pain include ibuprofen, naproxen, and diclofenac and the COX-2 inhibitor celecoxib. Topical NSAIDs, such as diclofenac gel, can be used for more localized pain complaints with less risk of systemic side effects including gastric ulcers, which occur in 15–30% of chronic NSAID users. Frequent use of NSAIDs has also been linked with increased risk of hypertension and renal insufficiency. NSAIDs must be used with caution in the elderly, as they reduce effectiveness of diuretics and double the risk for hospitalization from congestive heart failure. COX-2 inhibitors were initially used in patients with chronic pain to minimize costs from gastric toxicity; however, postmarketing identification of increased risk for myocardial infarction and stroke has restricted use, especially in older patients. NSAIDs and COX-2 inhibitors should be avoided in the first and third trimesters of pregnancy.

Vonkeman HE, van de Laar MA. Nonsteroidal anti-inflammatory drugs: adverse effects and their prevention. *Semin Arthritis Rheum.* 2010;39:294–312. [PMID: 18823646]
Welsch P, Sommer C, Schiltenwolf M, et al. Opioids in chronic noncancer pain: are opioids superior to nonopioid analgesic? A systematic review and meta-analysis of efficacy, tolerability and safety in randomized head-to-head comparisons of opioids versus nonopioid analgesics of at least 4 weeks duration. *Schmerz.* 2015;29(1):85–95. [PMID: 25376546]

2. Adjunctive medications—Adjunctive medications supplement the benefits from analgesics, treat neuropathic or central pain, and treat secondary complaints. In addition, effective use of adjunctive agents often reduces the need for primary analgesics. Adjunctive agents interact with the mechanism of neuropathic or central pain and chronic headache by reducing *nervous system windup*, the process by which the nervous system amplifies and eventually perpetuates pain signals in the absence of ongoing nociceptive input from the periphery. Before prescribing, physicians should be familiar with the dosing, side effects, and monitoring of these medications.

Among the antidepressants, the greatest analgesia is achieved by agents with dual effects on serotonin and norepinephrine. Evidence suggests that both tricyclic antidepressants (TCAs), such as amitriptyline, nortriptyline, and imipramine, and serotonin-norepinephrine reuptake inhibitors (SNRIs), such as duloxetine, milnacipran, and venlafaxine, relieve fibromyalgia, neuropathic pain, and chronic headaches. TCAs have also shown short-term improvement in chronic back pain. The TCA nortriptyline is often better tolerated, especially in older patients, than amitriptyline with comparable efficacy. The SNRI duloxetine has been approved by the US Food and Drug Administration (FDA) for painful diabetic neuropathy, fibromyalgia, and chronic musculoskeletal pain. Comorbid depression, anxiety symptoms, sleep disturbance, and loss of energy are commonly seen in individuals with chronic pain. Such individuals may prefer an agent that will also help with mood and associated symptoms. For example, a patient who has anergia and obesity with fibromyalgia may benefit from bupropion; alternatives to TCAs for a patient with depression and a sleep disturbance would include mirtazapine or trazodone.

Selective serotonin reuptake inhibitors (SSRIs) and bupropion have been associated with seizures in higher doses and should be used with caution in patients with a seizure history. Venlafaxine and milnacipran can have a cardiac stimulatory effect at higher doses, and blood pressure should be monitored. Duloxetine and milnacipran can cause hepatotoxicity and should be avoided in patients with liver disease. Antidepressants, particularly those with a prominent serotoninergic effect, have been associated with the potential for suicidality and should be monitored closely in patients at risk and in children or adolescents. Combining serotonergic agents has the potential to create a serotonin syndrome, characterized by tremors, irritability, and cardiac excitation. Caution should be exercised when combining agents such as a classical antidepressant, trazodone for sleep, and tramadol for pain. TCAs, typically prescribed in low to moderate doses for neuropathic pain, are still associated with a small risk for cardiac arrhythmia due to QTc and PR elongation. Older adults, individuals with a history of cardiac disease, or those prescribed other medications that impact QTc should be monitored with electrocardiograms when TCA doses approach the low therapeutic range. Most concerning in this regard is methadone, which is discussed in the opioid section.

Anticonvulsants, particularly pregabalin and gabapentin, have become a mainstay in the treatment of neuropathic pain. They also benefit chronic headaches and possibly fibromyalgia. Several other anticonvulsants, such as carbamazepine, valproate, and topiramate, are considered second line. Pregabalin and gabapentin are related anticonvulsants with indications for pain associated with diabetic peripheral neuropathy and postherpetic neuralgia. Pregabalin is approved for fibromyalgia as well. Carbamazepine is the drug of choice for trigeminal neuralgia. Anticonvulsants used as pain adjuvants are generally well tolerated. Pregabalin and gabapentin may cause dizziness, peripheral edema, and somnolence, and both need renal adjustment. Recent anecdotal evidence suggests potential abuse, which warrants monitoring by prescribing physicians. This has led to the reclassification of gabapentin as a controlled substance in some states. Carbamazepine's potential side effects include agranulocytosis, and patients will need blood count, kidney function, liver tests, and drug level monitoring periodically.

Most muscle relaxants, such as cyclobenzaprine, used to treat prechronic musculoskeletal pain are associated with significant sedation, reducing their usefulness as a treatment for chronic pain, for which the primary focus is on reducing disability and time spent in bedrest. Tizanidine, a unique muscle relaxant with both antispasticity and α-adrenergic effects, results in reduced spasticity and reduced pain perception with both acute and chronic use. In addition to reducing spasticity related to neurologic conditions (eg, multiple sclerosis, stroke, or spinal cord injury), tizanidine can also reduce symptoms associated with myofascial pain, fibromyalgia, and headaches, with some evidence of benefit for neuropathic pain. Tizanidine is mildly sedating, which can assist with associated sleep disturbance. Muscle relaxants have abuse potential. As an example, carisoprodol is not recommended given the metabolite meprobamate, which can cause dependence and a withdrawal syndrome.

Topical adjunctive agents for chronic pain such as lidocaine and capsaicin can be helpful for patients who want to avoid the systemic side effects of oral medications. The 5% lidocaine patch is FDA approved for postherpetic neuralgia but is often trialed when a patient has localized neuropathic pain. Capsaicin cream comes both over the counter and as a physician-prescribed high-concentration 8% patch. Capsaicin cream is used for several painful conditions and appears to have a greater role when other adjunctive agents have failed. Given the mechanism of action in depleting substance P, the cream needs to be applied 3–4 times per day to prevent burning and stinging during the application. The capsaicin patch is approved for postherpetic neuralgia.

Another class of adjuvant drugs includes cannabis/cannabinoids. Cannabinoids are gaining favor across the United States, but their use is still controversial. A recent systematic review and meta-analysis looking at 79 trials showed moderate-quality evidence to support cannabinoids for the treatment of chronic pain and spasticity. In addition, states with medical cannabis laws had a 24.8% lower mean annual opioid overdose mortality rate. However, a 4-year prospective, observational cohort study found no evidence that cannabinoids for chronic pain improved patient outcomes. Given the risk of abuse and adverse effects of cannabis such as anxiety and impairment of cognition and memory, mainstream use for chronic pain is still debatable. However, given the public's interest in this modality, family physicians will be asked about medical marijuana and should stay informed regarding this potential treatment option.

Bachhuber MA, Saloner B, Cunningham CO, et al. Medical cannabis laws and opioid analgesic overdose mortality in the United States, 1999-2010. *JAMA Inter Med.* 2014;174(10): 1668–1673. [PMID: 25154332]

Campbell G, Hall WD, Peacock A, et al. Effect of cannabis use in people with chronic non-cancer pain prescribed opioids: findings from a 4-year prospective cohort study. *Lancet Public Health.* 2018;3(7):e341–e350. [PMID: 29976328]

Kroenke K, Bair MJ, Damush TM. Optimized antidepressant therapy and pain self-management in primary care patients with depression and musculoskeletal pain: a randomized controlled trial. *JAMA.* 2009;301(20):2099–2110. [PMID: 19470987]

Mason L, Moore RA, Derry S, et al. Systemic review of topical capsaicin for the treatment of chronic pain. *BMJ*. 2004;328:991. [PMID: 15033881]

Saarto T, Wiffen PJ. Antidepressants for neuropathic pain: a Cochrane review. *J Neurol Neurosurg Psychiatry*. 2010;81: 1372–1373. [PMID: 20543189]

Whiting PF, Wolff RF, Deshpande S, et al. Cannabinoids for medical use: a systemic review and meta-analysis. *JAMA*. 2015;313(24):2456–2473. [PMID: 26103030]

3. Opioid analgesics—At the core of chronic pain treatment is patient functioning, which often dictates whether an opioid (eg, hydrocodone, oxycodone, fentanyl, methadone) is prescribed. However, this decision is much more complex when focusing on short- or long-term functioning and, in a broader sense, the ripple effects of the opioid epidemic. Evidence for opioids in long-term treatment of chronic pain is lacking. In a systematic review, the National Institutes of Health Pathways to Prevention Workshop found insufficient evidence for the effectiveness of long-term opioid therapy, but there was a dose-dependent risk for serious harms. In the 2016 CDC clinical evidence summary, a similar finding was identified with no long-term (≥1 year) benefit in pain or function. Patients initiating daily opioids risk developing tolerance after 5–6 weeks of therapy, which limits the long-term benefit. In addition, opioid use has other common side effects such as constipation, pruritis, nausea, dizziness, and fatigue. More serious risks include dose-dependent risk of overdose, substance use disorder with addiction, increased falls, opioid-induced hyperalgesia, and significant drug interactions. Tramadol, a weak mu-receptor agonist, also inhibits the reuptake of serotonin and norepinephrine and can cause serotonin syndrome when combined with other antidepressants. Tramadol also decreases the seizure threshold. Methadone has complex pharmacokinetics and can prolong the QTc interval, which leads to more deaths as compared to other prescribed opioids.

For patients with chronic pain, opioids should be considered only in the context of a structured plan of chronic disease management following a comprehensive assessment with the goals of providing clinically meaningful improvement, minimizing side effects and risks, and maximizing nonopioid and nonpharmacologic options. The 2016 CDC guidelines outline recommendations for prescribing opioids in that context (Table 51–5). In primary care, a study determined that 20% of outpatients presenting with noncancer pain or pain-related diagnoses received opioid prescriptions. Thus, many patients have prior opioid exposure, and some have high-dose chronic opioid use. While providing patient-centered care in this context, remember a few basic questions (Table 51–6): Have I treated the patient as a *person* and worked to enhance the relationship? Have I addressed the patient's *suffering*? What is the underlying *diagnosis*? Does the patient have a *substance use disorder*? Is this *palliative*

Table 51–5. Clinical reminders for opioid use in chronic pain: Centers for Disease Control and Prevention guidelines.

Determine when to initiate or continue opioids for chronic pain

1. Opioids are not first-line or routine therapy for chronic pain.
2. Establish and measure goals for pain.
3. Discuss benefits and risks and availability of nonopioid therapies with patient.

Opioid selection, dosage, duration, follow-up, and discontinuation

4. Use immediate-release opioids when starting.
5. Start low and go slow.
6. When opioids are needed for acute pain, prescribe no more than needed; do not prescribe extended-release/long-acting opioids for acute pain.
7. Follow-up and reevaluate risk of harm; reduce dose or taper and discontinue if needed.

Assessing risk and addressing harms of opioid use

8. Evaluate risk factors for opioid-related harms.
9. Check prescription drug monitoring program for high dosages and prescriptions from other providers.
10. Use urine drug testing to identify prescribed substances and undisclosed use.
11. Avoid concurrent benzodiazepine and opioid prescribing.
12. Arrange treatment for opioid use disorder if needed.

or *end-of-life* care? Is the patient undergoing *active cancer treatment*? Has *prevention* been addressed? Have *nonopioid options* been maximized? Is *risk mitigation* maximized? Did I *document* what is required? The answers provide guidance for management of patients in four general opioid categories seen in primary care: opioid naïve, high-dose chronic users, opioid-dependent seeking within health care, and opioid-dependent seeking outside of health care. For opioid-naïve patients, avoid opioids if possible, but if opioids are used, immediate-release opioids (eg, hydrocodone, oxycodone) for short durations are ideal to avoid tolerance and dependence. Avoid long-acting opioids (eg, transdermal fentanyl) in opioid-naïve patients. For high-dose chronic opioid users, also consider compassionately tapering to reduce complications of chronic opioid therapy. Those functioning well and experiencing no side effects can continue with no dose adjustment. Tapering is best for those with adverse side effects or who are not attaining their goals of self-management or clinically meaningful improvement. For opioid-dependent patients, address the dependency, or if a substance use disorder is diagnosed, provide access to standard-of-care therapy with medication-assisted treatment and counseling.

If prescribing opioids for chronic pain, physicians should not only be knowledgeable in their use, but also have office

Table 51–6. Questions for family physicians treating patients with pain.

Questions	Examples
Have I treated the patient as a person and worked to enhance the relationship?	Compassion, listening, involving the patient in his or her care
Have I addressed the patient's suffering?	Counseling, empathy, providing hope
What is the underlying diagnosis? Does the patient have a substance use disorder?	Migraine headache, anxiety disorder, drug withdrawal, addiction, rheumatoid arthritis
Is this palliative or end-of-life care? Does the patient have active cancer treatment?	The patient has end-stage disease and should be enrolled in palliative care as the next step in his or her treatment
Has prevention been addressed?	Depression, medication side effects, addiction
Have nonopioid options been maximized?	Physical therapy, trigger point injections, yoga
Is risk mitigation maximized?	Urine drug screening, prescription drug monitoring programs, controlled substance agreements, naloxone co-prescribing
Did I document what is required?	Clinical exam, diagnosis, screen for substance abuse

structures to enable monitoring and provide the patient with risk mitigation strategies. *Risk mitigation* is a process to reduce adverse effects. An example would be methods to decrease the likelihood of unintentional overdose, such as avoiding co-prescribing of benzodiazepines (eg, alprazolam and diazepam) with opioids. Risk mitigation steps are best incorporated into the electronic health system and managed by a team-based approach in an office setting. Strategies include education regarding the risk of overdose and addiction, adherence monitoring with urine drug screens and pill counts, using the state prescription drug monitoring program, co-prescribing naloxone to patients on >50 mg/d morphine equivalent dose (MED) or other risk factors for overdose, and routine visits at least every 3 months. Following a careful clinical assessment for the patient's chronic pain, including a PEG-3 or BPI and a screen for substance abuse, and prior to prescribing opioids, physicians and patients should discuss the risks and benefits, including overdose and addiction, and how the opioids will be discontinued. As a baseline, obtain a urine drug screen, review the state's prescription drug monitoring program, and sign a controlled substance agreement. In the 2016 CDC evidence

review, tools such as the Opioid Risk Tool (ORT) or Screener and Opioid Assessment for Patients with Pain-Revised (SOAPP-R) showed insufficient sensitivity and specificity to stratify patients' risk with opioids but still can give valuable information. Patients started on opioids should be seen 1–3 weeks after initiation and have a repeat PEG-3 or BPI performed to document clinically meaningful improvement. Avoid opioids if the patient is on another sedative-hypnotic drug such as a benzodiazepine, shows no clinically meaningful improvement, or has an adverse outcome, a current substance use disorder, or a history of opioid use disorder. Given the risk of overdose as the MED increases, it is recommended to carefully assess your patient before increasing the dose to 50 mg/d and avoid dosages of 90 mg/d MED or greater if possible. For patients who are not meeting their goals of treatment, compassionately taper the opioid and use other nonopioid options for pain treatment.

Agency Medical Directors' Group. Interagency guideline on prescribing opioids for pain. http://www.agencymeddirectors.wa.gov/Files/2015AMDGOpioidGuideline.pdf. Accessed November 25, 2019.

Chou R, Turner JA, Devine EB, et al. The effectiveness and risks of long-term opioid therapy for chronic pain: a systematic review for a National Institutes of Health Pathways to Prevention Workshop. *Ann Intern Med.* 2015;162:276–286. [PMID: 25581257]

Dowell D, Haegerich TM, Chou R. CDC guideline for prescribing opioids for chronic pain: United States, 2016. *JAMA.* 2016;315(15):1624–1645. [PMID: 26977696]

Martin L, Laderman M, Hyatt J, et al. *Addressing the Opioid Crisis in the United States.* IHI Innovation Report. Cambridge, MA: Institute for Healthcare Improvement; 2016.

D. Interventional Pain Management

Interventional techniques are considered for patients failing conservative therapy or when specific nervous system pathology has been identified. Lumbar epidural steroid injections are effective for treating herniated disks or spinal stenosis. Sympathetic blocks reduce the burning pain of complex regional pain syndrome or reflex sympathetic dystrophy that may develop after acute extremity injury or surgery. Trigger point injections are useful for localized muscle pain. The benefit from injections is often transient, so these techniques are generally used in conjunction with physical therapy and medication management. Radiofrequency treatment (including ablative therapy and pulsed treatment) may be considered for patients with recalcitrant musculoskeletal or nerve pain. Conventional radiofrequency ablation is used for lumbar zygapophyseal joint pain, whereas pulsed treatment is more effective for cervical radicular pain and shoulder joint pain. Pulsed treatment may also have a role for treating discogenic pain, chronic inguinal herniorrhaphy pain, and chronic testicular pain.

Implantable devices, including intrathecal pumps and dorsal column stimulators, can be used to treat individuals with cancer-related pain or severe incapacitating pain resulting from nonmalignant conditions. Intrathecal medications are considered for patients requiring high medication doses when side effects from oral medications become intolerable. Dorsal column stimulators are most commonly used for treating patients with persistent severe back pain after surgery (failed back syndrome) and complex regional pain syndrome. For the treatment of pain resulting from nonmalignant conditions, it is essential to obtain psychological consultation prior to the surgery.

Nerve blocks may be particularly beneficial for postherpetic neuralgia, which can be quite difficult to treat. Nerve blocks, particularly thoracic epidural local anesthetics or intercostal blocks, can be used in the acute or chronic stage. Early use of nerve blocks, especially within the first 2 months of onset of symptoms, greatly decreases the incidence and severity of postherpetic neuralgia.

Chua NH, Vissers KC, Sluijter ME. Pulsed radiofrequency treatment in interventional pain management mechanisms and potential indications—a review. *Acta Neurochir.* 2011;153: 763–771. [PMID: 21116663]

Manchikanti L, Boswell MV, Singh V, et al. Comprehensive evidence-based guidelines for interventional techniques in the management of chronic spinal pain. *Pain Physician.* 2009;12:699. [PMID: 19644537]

Patel VB, Manchikanti L, Singh V, et al. Systematic review of intrathecal infusion systems for long-term management of chronic non-cancer pain. *Pain Physician.* 2009;12:345–360. [PMID: 19305484]

Rainov NG, Heidecke V, Burkert W. Long-term intrathecal infusion of drug combinations for chronic back and leg pain. *J Pain Symptom Manage.* 2001;22:862. [PMID: 11576803]

Yampolsky C, Hem S, Bendersky D. Dorsal column stimulator applications. *Surg Neurol Int.* 2012;3(Suppl4):S275–S289. [PMID: 23230533]

E. Complementary and Alternative Therapies

Complementary and alternative treatments are used by 40% of chronic pain sufferers. As in the discussion of psychological approaches, the greatest emphasis is on active strategies that can enhance an individual's self-management skills. Mind-body approaches such as mindfulness meditation and movement approaches such as yoga and Tai Chi fall within this model and have shown efficacy for several pain conditions. A meta-analysis revealed benefit over placebo of acupuncture for chronic conditions, including back and neck pain, osteoarthritis, headache, and shoulder pain. Chiropractic treatment is recommended for acute spinal pain, but there is no clear consensus on the effectiveness of chiropractic manipulation for chronic pain, and controlled studies are under way to provide efficacy data. Among biologically based treatments, glucosamine sulfate and chondroitin sulfate have had mixed success in studies, but they may provide an alternative to chronic nonsteroidal treatment for some patients, particularly with knee osteoarthritis. Another agent that merits further study for possible analgesic and anti-inflammatory effects is fish oil, in a dose of 1–2 g/d.

Tai Chi Chuan (TC) is emerging as a potential clinically effective and cost-effective treatment for chronic pain conditions. A randomized controlled trial found comparable improvement in pain and function with TC and physical therapy, consistent with other studies showing benefit. The same group found significant benefit of TC over wellness education and exercise and for both knee osteoarthritis and fibromyalgia.

Clegg DO, Reda DJ, Harris CL, et al. Glucosamine, chondroitin sulfate, and the two in combination for painful knee osteoarthritis. *N Engl J Med.* 2006;354(8):795–808. [PMID: 16495392]

Posadzki P, Ernst E, Terry R, Lee MS. Is yoga effective for pain? A systematic review of randomized clinical trials. *Complement Ther Med.* 2011;19(5):281–287. [PMID: 21944658]

Santilli V, Beghi E, Finucci S, et al. Chiropractic manipulation in the treatment of acute back pain and sciatica with disc protrusion: a randomized double-blind clinical trial of active and simulated spinal manipulations. *Spine J.* 2006;6:131–137. [PMID: 16517383]

Vickers AJ, Cronin AM, Maschino AC, et al. Acupuncture for chronic pain: individual patient data meta-analysis. *Arch Intern Med.* 2012;172(19):1444–1453. [PMID: 22965186]

Walker BF, French SD, Grant W, Green S. A Cochrane review of combined chiropractic interventions for low-back pain. *Spine.* 2011;36(3):230–242. [PMID: 20393942]

Wang C, Schmid CH, Iversen MD, et al. Comparative effectiveness of Tai Chi versus physical therapy for knee osteoarthritis: a randomized trial. *Ann Intern Med.* 2016;165(2):77–86. [PMID: 27183035]

Wang C, Schmid CH, Rones R, et al. A randomized trial of tai chi for fibromyalgia. *N Engl J Med.* 2010;363(8):743–754. [PMID: 20818876]

Weiner DK, Ernst E. Complementary and alternative approaches to the treatment of persistent musculoskeletal pain. *Clin J Pain.* 2004;20(4):244–255. [PMID: 15218409]

Wong SY, Chan FW, Wong RL, et al. Comparing the effectiveness of mindfulness-based stress reduction and multidisciplinary intervention programs for chronic pain: a randomized comparative trial. *Clin J Pain.* 2011;27(8):724–734. [PMID: 21753729]

▶ Tying in Mechanism with Treatment Consideration

Patient care of congestive heart failure begins with basic mechanisms such as Frank-Starling dynamics. Similarly, it is helpful for the clinician to keep in mind the basic mechanisms involved with transmitting, amplifying, and dampening the pain signal. Considerations include gate control theory, endorphins and related peptides, serotonergic and noradrenergic pathways, wind-up and central sensitization, and inflammation. Briefly reviewing these systems can help with pragmatic considerations of patient treatment options when approaching patients in the exam room.

A. Gate Control Theory

Presented in *Science*, in 1965, Melzack and Wall are the Watson and Crick of a modern understanding of pain mechanisms. In modern parlance, the central processing unit was identified as a "T cell," which we recognize as a spinal-thalamic tract cell in the middle of Rexed's laminae. This cell responds to excitatory or inhibitory stimulation coming from the periphery, as well as through descending pathways. Within this system, "rubbing it where it hurts" or engaging in relaxation techniques are not just distractions; they tone down the pain at its source before it enters conscious awareness.

B. Endogenous Inhibitory Neuropeptides

Close to a decade later, filling in the blanks within the backdrop of gate control theory, Basbaum and Fields elucidated descending inhibitory pathways, with a focus on endorphins. Research quickly extended to enkephalins, dynorphins, monoamines, and other inhibitory neurochemicals. This led to our current understanding of diffuse noxious inhibitory control, that nociceptive stimulation leads to a dampening response. This partly accounts for the mechanism of acupuncture. In addition, it explains much of the benefit for an activity and rehabilitation-based approach to chronic pain management. Conversely, blockade of this system is a purported mechanism for the central sensitization that may occur with chronic opioid therapy.

C. Serotonergic and Noradrenergic Descending Inhibitory Pathways

Among the systems involved with pain inhibition are key monoaminergic brain centers such as the locus coeruleus and nucleus raphe magnus. Through these mechanisms, it is not surprising that depression and pain are common comorbid conditions and that dual serotonin/norepinephrine agents have analgesic properties.

D. Wind-Up and Central Sensitization

In animal models of the genesis of chronic pain, repetitive nociceptive stimulation results in a similar array of symptoms seen in chronic pain states, particularly neuropathic pain. These include *hyperalgesia*, augmented pain perception and response to subsequent stimuli; and *allodynia*, a pain response to normally nonnociceptive stimuli such as light touch and spread of the region of sensitivity to adjacent dermatomes. Although multiple mechanisms are involved, *N*-methyl-D-aspartate (NMDA) and glutamate are central to these effects and potential pharmacologic targets, addressed by anticonvulsants and most dramatically using ketamine infusions.

E. Inflammation

The role of inflammation in chronic pain is universally recognized where prostaglandins and other inflammatory chemicals directly stimulate nociceptors. Historically, osteoarthritis was termed *osteoarthrosis* in Britain, with the understanding that the primary process was degeneration, but our current understanding reflects the role of inflammatory mediators in osteoarthritis. This is compounded in the case of degenerative disk disease, with the nucleus pulposus being proinflammatory with a direct effect on spinal nerves as they exit neuroforamina. In addition to nonsteroidal agents, lifestyle-oriented approaches may have the same importance in management of chronic pain as with heart disease.

How does one implement strategies for pain management based on this understanding of physiologic pathways? Considerations may include the following:

- Physical modalities, such as heat or ice, may impact the balance of small and large fiber activation, limiting the ascending pain message coming from the wide dynamic range neuron.

- SNRIs such as duloxetine: It may be helpful for a patient to hear that although this is chemically an antidepressant, we are taking advantage of its pain-inhibitory properties.

- Stretching of tight muscles may prevent the development of muscle spasms when a sedentary individual starts to step up activity.

- Aerobic conditioning directly stimulates endorphin production. Individuals with chronic pain and deconditioning may feel that their body does not make endorphins because they experience flares with attempts to increase activity and may need guidance from a physical therapist or athletic trainer.

- Lifestyle-oriented approaches targeting smoking cessation, dietary modification, and progressive exercise can benefit pain through multiple mechanisms. The exercise itself is therapeutic. Shifting to an anti-inflammatory diet and quitting smoking may decrease systemic inflammation with potential impact on nociception. To the extent that a patient is successful advancing such a program and reduces weight, decreased load on the spine and weight-bearing joints can go a long way to reduce pain.

- Acupuncture stimulates endorphins, monoamines, and other inhibitory neuropeptides. Presumably, acupuncture has other mechanisms of action, and the lasting benefit from a course of treatment suggests that it may "wind down" central sensitization.

- Mind-body approaches, such as biofeedback or mindfulness meditation, may help "close the gate" in gate control theory by stimulating or augmenting descending inhibitory pathways. Additionally, these may have salient benefit for associated psychological distress and constructs such as catastrophization and kinesiophobia.

For more detailed discussion of pain management in specific conditions, please see Chapter 25 for low back pain, Chapter 26 for neck pain, and other sections under the disease entity.

Basbaum AI, Fields HL. Endogenous pain control systems: brainstem spinal pathways and endorphin circuitry. *Annu Rev Neurosci.* 1984;7:309–338. [PMID: 6143527]

Katz J, Rosenbloom BN. The golden anniversary of Melzack and Wall's gate control theory of pain: celebrating 50 years of pain research and management. *Pain Res Man.* 2015;20(6):285–286. [PMID: 26642069]

Melzack R, Wall PD. Pain mechanisms: a new theory. *Science.* 1965;150:971–979. [PMID: 5320816]

Travel Medicine

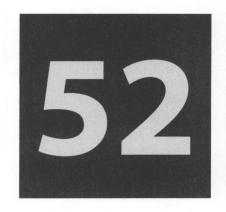

Deepa Burman, MD, FAASM

Timothy Scott Prince, MD, MSPH, FACOEM, FACPM

In 2012, the United Nations World Tourism Organization reported that international arrivals across boundaries surpassed the 1 billion mark for the first time in history, and this number continues to increase steadily, with >1.3 billion in 2017. Unfortunately, travel can lead to health problems that range from unpleasant inconveniences to life-threatening injuries and illnesses.

It is estimated that fewer than half of travelers seek any kind of pretravel advice. Many people ask their family physicians for recommendations, and the challenge is providing recommendations that are current, complete, and itinerary specific. Individuals returning to their country of origin are less likely to consult a physician before travel, and preventable systemic illness is seen more commonly in this group than other tourists. It is important that all primary care physicians give accurate advice to travelers about both pretravel preparation and how to deal with illnesses contracted abroad. Sometimes there is not enough time to obtain the required immunizations, and priorities must be established. The goal of this chapter is to enable the family physician to provide guidance to patients wishing to be prepared before travel and address common posttravel conditions.

Jong EC, Sanford C. *The Travel and Tropical Medicine Manual*, 5th ed. Philadelphia, PA: Saunders Elsevier; 2017.

Leder K, Tong S, Weld L, et al. Illness in travelers visiting friends and relatives: a review of the GeoSentinel Surveillance Network. *Clin Infect Dis.* 2006;43:1185–1193. [PMID: 17029140]

World Tourism Organization. 2017 International Tourism Results, 2018. http://mediaunwto.org/press-release/208-01-15/2017. Accessed May 4, 2018.

PRETRAVEL PREPARATION & CONCERNS

▶ Example Case

A 28-year-old man in good health is planning a 2-month trip to Kenya. He will be working in Nairobi but also plans to visit game parks and participate in outdoor activities.

- What medical history is important?
- What specific health advice should be given?
- What immunizations are needed?
- Are any prophylactic medications recommended?
- Where can the physician find the answers to these questions?

The first step is to obtain a thorough history—including any preexisting medical conditions and use of medications—and to perform a focused physical examination for conditions that might impact travel risk. What is the specific itinerary, including stops en route? What accommodations will he have? Will he remain in urban areas or visit some rural regions? What is his immunization history? This information will help determine necessary immunizations and prophylaxis. The physician can also recommend important items to take on the trip, such as insect repellent. If the patient has a chronic illness, he should be given pertinent portions of his record, including list of medications and allergies, to take in case he needs medical care abroad.

Several websites provide information about travel and health requirements (see listing at the end of this chapter).

After reviewing, this patient faces several risks to be discussed, including the following:

- Malaria, yellow fever, Zika, and other insect-borne diseases
- Diarrhea, caused by parasites, viruses, or bacteria such as *Escherichia coli* or *Shigella*
- Typhoid fever and other salmonelloses
- Hepatitis
- Schistosomiasis, especially if swimming or wading in local bodies of water
- Violence and theft, especially in urban areas such as Nairobi
- Human immunodeficiency virus (HIV)/acquired immunodeficiency syndrome (AIDS) and other sexually transmitted diseases
- Poor emergency response infrastructure, especially outside of urban areas

In the United States, as more baby boomers reach retirement age, increasing numbers of older adults will plan for international travel. They will require these same steps, but since they are more likely to have chronic conditions, they may need some additional preparation.

Centers for Disease Control and Prevention. *CDC Yellow Book 2018, Health Information for the International Traveler.* New York, NY: Oxford University Press; 2017.

Schlaudecker JD, Moushey EN, Schlaudecker EP. Keeping older patients healthy and safe as they travel. *J Fam Practice.* 2013; 62(1):16–23. [PMID: 23326818]

▶ Travelers' Medical Kit

Every traveler should carry a medical kit that addresses basic care for common illnesses and injuries. Some common components include emergency information, skin cleaning wipes/sanitizer, insect repellent, sunscreen, and any prophylactic or self-treatment medications recommended for the trip, such as acetazolamide for travel to elevations >2500 m above sea level, malaria medication, and treatment for traveler's diarrhea. The Centers for Disease Control and Prevention (CDC) travel information webpages include a "Healthy Travel Packing List" specific to the destination country, but these should be adjusted depending on specific needs and itinerary. The traveler should pack a supply of their usual medication to last for the entire trip and enough extra allow for changes in travel plans, with a small, labeled supply in carry-on bags in case checked luggage is lost or delayed. All airline and destination countries' regulation and laws regarding medication must be observed to avoid confiscation or legal entanglements. If a prescribed controlled substance is permitted in the destination countries, travelers should carry a letter from their physician, which can also be considered for any needles or autoinjectors to address potential concerns from authorities. Travelers should not forget to bring spare eyeglasses or contact lenses, contact lens solution, and their ophthalmologic prescriptions in case of loss or breakage.

For longer stays, the physician may assist in arranging for an ongoing supply of medication and source for local medical care. Travelers should use reliable sources and carefully examine any medications bought overseas, because ingredients may differ from those in the US products.

Sanford C, Pottinger P, Jong E. *The Travel and Tropical Medicine Manual,* 5th ed. Philadelphia, PA: Saunders Elsevier; 2017.

▶ Insurance

Travelers should check their health insurance policies to determine whether they include coverage for medical expenses incurred abroad. If coverage is provided, they should carry or have access to a blank insurance form. Term travel health insurance policies are also available. For many itineraries, evacuation insurance is essential in the event of a serious accident or medical problem. Some policies will return travelers to their home cities; others will evacuate them to the nearest location where they can receive medical care comparable to that available in their home country. The traveler may wish to purchase more comprehensive trip insurance. This type of insurance can cover a variety of contingencies, including reimbursement for trip cancellation for medical or other reasons beyond the traveler's control. This insurance is especially attractive for older travelers, who are more likely to have a medical emergency that prevents them from traveling. The US Department of State answers questions about medical coverage on their website (https://travel.state.gov/content/travel/en/international-travel/before-you-go/your-health-abroad/insurance-providers-overseas.html; accessed May 14, 2018).

▶ Air Travel Concerns

Several medical conditions require special attention during air travel. These conditions include many common illnesses: anemia, clotting disorders, disfiguring dermatoses, dyspnea at rest, incontinence, otitis media, pulmonary or acute upper respiratory infections, and sickle cell hemoglobinopathies. Medical contraindications to air travel are listed in Table 52–1, but travelers with significant diagnoses should also check their airline's regulations (and entry requirements of their destination countries). A physician should clear any traveler with an acute or chronic infectious disease before traveling. If there is any question about the diagnosis or stability of a condition, the individual should not travel until the risk is clarified. Ill travelers or those with mobility issues should notify their airlines 72 hours before departure to ensure that the plane is properly equipped. Services such as a wheelchair, oxygen, stretcher, and other common

Table 52–1. Contraindications to air travel.

Unstable angina
Myocardial infarction in past 2 weeks (or 6 weeks if complicated)
Active bronchospasm
Neurosurgery or skull fracture in the past 2 weeks
Uncontrolled cardiac disease (congestive heart failure or arrhythmia)
Percutaneous coronary intervention in past 5 days (or 2 weeks if complicated)
Cerebral infarction in past 2 weeks
Pneumothorax in past 2–3 weeks
Colonoscopy with polypectomy in past 24 hours
Late pregnancy after 36 weeks' gestation (long flights)
Highly contagious diseases, including active tuberculosis
Major uncontrolled psychiatric disorders
Cyanosis
Pulmonary hypertension
Recent middle ear or sinus surgery
Scuba diving in past 24 hours
Hemoglobin <7.5 g/dL
Heart, lung, or gastrointestinal surgery in past 3 weeks
Noncommunicating lung cysts
Tooth or gum disease with trapped air

equipment can often be provided or accommodated with advance notice.

A. Use of Respiratory Assistive Devices on Aircraft

Patients with sleep apnea or requiring oxygen should carry their portable machines with them especially during long travels. In May 2009, the US Department of Transportation issued a final ruling that all air carriers conducting passenger service (on aircraft originally designed for a passenger capacity of ≥19 seats) must permit someone with a disability to use a ventilator, respirator, continuous positive airway pressure machine, or a Federal Aviation Administration (FAA)–approved portable oxygen concentrator (POC), unless the device fails to meet applicable FAA requirements for medical portable electronic devices (M-PEDs) and does not display a manufacturer's label indicating that the device meets those FAA requirements. Currently, all FAA-approved POCs meet FAA requirements for M-PEDs.

US Department of Transportation. *Info for Operators*. Washington, DC: Federal Aviation Administration; 2009. http://www.faa.gov/other_visit/aviation_industry/airline_operators/airline_safety/info/all_infos/media/2009/info09006.pdf. Accessed May 8, 2018.

Travel Health at Sea or on Cruise Ships

The sea has drawn adventurers, explorers, and settlers, as well as recreational travelers, to its shores and beyond for centuries. In 2017, approximately 26 million passengers took cruises, up from 19 million in 2010. Most cruise ships offer at least some form of on-board clinic or other medical assistance. Exposure to dry, recirculated air, unfamiliar viral and bacterial pathogens, and new environmental allergens make respiratory illness the most common diagnosis in a ship's infirmary. Most cases are self-limited and should be treated symptomatically. Seasickness and isolated cases of gastrointestinal illness aboard cruise ships are common, representing 10–25% and 9–10% of sickbay visits, respectively. Fortunately, outbreaks of food- and waterborne illness are rare. As with shoreside outbreaks, more than half are due to the Norwalk (or related) viruses or undetermined agents. The rest are due to various bacterial agents, most notably enterotoxigenic *E coli*, *Salmonella*, *Shigella*, *Staphylococcus aureus, Clostridium perfringens*, and campylobacter. The Vessel Sanitation Program, developed and administered by the CDC, has been instrumental in the steady decline of gastrointestinal outbreaks aboard cruise ships.

Regan J, Tardivel K, Lippold S, Duong K. *Cruise Ship Travel*. Atlanta, GA: Centers for Disease Control and Prevention; 2018. https://wwwnc.cdc.gov/travel/yellowbook/2018/conveyance-transportation-issues/cruise-ship-travel. Accessed November 25, 2019.

Food and Water Sanitation

Many infectious diseases can be prevented by attention to food and water sanitation and good hygiene. Travelers should avoid eating food that has not been cooked adequately or peeled by them. If fish are eaten, they should be fresh, not dried or old-looking. Cans should be inspected for bulging or gas formation. Only pasteurized dairy products should be consumed, and those ultrapasteurized by the ultraheat treatment method are preferred. Avoid raw vegetables and unpeeled fruits. Fruits and vegetables should be peeled by the traveler before consumption. Clean silverware and plates should be used; these can be rinsed in boiling water or bleach rinse to sterilize them.

Bottled or canned drinks are generally safe as long as the seal is intact and area around opening is clean. Iced and lukewarm drinks should not be trusted, but hot drinks such as coffee or tea are generally safe if prepared recently and still hot when served. Tap water can be disinfected by boiling, treatment with iodine or chlorine, or using an ultrafilter water purification system:

- Bring water to a rolling boil for 1 minute. Although the actual temperature reached will be slightly lower at higher elevation, this does not seem to have clinical relevance.

- Treat the water with iodine (10 drops of tincture per liter), or chlorine (1–2 drops of 5% chlorine bleach per liter of water). Let stand for 30 minutes. Although chlorine may not kill all parasitic cysts or viruses, water treated with chlorine has a better taste than iodized water; furthermore, chlorine does not affect thyroid function over long periods of use.

- Reliable water filtration systems are available through various sources. A pore size of 0.2 µm is needed to filter out all enteric bacteria and parasites. If the water is cloudy or especially dirty looking, some gross filtration or sedimentation must be done first before using a small-pore filter. Adding iodine resins to the filter will kill viruses if contact is sufficient.

Backer HD. Field water disinfection. In: Auerbach PS, ed. *Wilderness Medicine*, 6th ed. Philadelphia, PA: Mosby; 2011:1324–1359.

Injury Prevention & Personal Security

The leading cause of mortality in travelers is motor vehicle accidents. Drivers should be aware of local motor vehicle laws and never mix alcohol with driving or any activity that requires mental alertness. Other common accidents that occur during travel include drowning, carbon monoxide poisoning, electric shock, and drug reactions. Travelers should be aware that jet lag and other causes of drowsiness while traveling (eg, medications to alleviate motion sickness) may heighten the risk of injury. If a traumatic injury occurs, travelers should be cautioned not to agree to blood transfusions unless absolutely necessary.

Although the risks to personal security in many parts of the world may be similar to those encountered in many urban areas of the United States, travelers may be at greater risk in areas where they are obviously foreigners or tourists. Most commonly, the risks to personal security are related to theft of personal belongings and the occasional violent methods used.

Another rarely discussed but important area of personal security is that of sexual activity while traveling. The freedom from a daily schedule and uniqueness of the situation may cause travelers to let down their normal guard. The incidence of sexually transmitted diseases, especially HIV, is quite high in many popular tourist destinations. Travelers should be cautioned to use good judgment (especially in situations involving alcohol use), barrier protection such as condoms, and caution with oral-genital contact.

Sanford C. Urban medicine: threats to health of travelers to developing world cities. *J Travel Med*. 2004;11:313–327. [PMID: 15544716]

Obtaining Medical Care Abroad

Obtaining reliable medical care abroad can be difficult. Some international insurance plans included assistance in obtaining care. Frequent travelers may wish to become members of the International Association for Medical Assistance to Travelers, which provides up-to-date advice on where to seek competent medical care for virtually any area of the world (www.iamat.org). The International Society of Travel Medicine (www.istm.org) and the American Society of Tropical Medicine and Hygiene (www.astmh.org) are also excellent resources for those seeking to find travel clinics.

Immunizations

At present, the only vaccine *required* for routine travel is yellow fever if travel is planned through an endemic area, although Saudi Arabia now requires that Hajj visitors be vaccinated with a tetravalent meningococcal vaccine before entering. However, all travelers should be up to date on routine immunizations, including diphtheria, pertussis, tetanus, measles, mumps, varicella-zoster, rubella, influenza, pneumonia, and, for children, *Haemophilus influenzae* type b. For adults previously immunized as children, a single dose of polio vaccine is recommended for travel to the few remaining areas with a risk of polio. Check the CDC or similar source for up-to-date risk information. Currently, Europe, Australia, the Western Pacific, and the Western Hemisphere have been certified as polio free.

Yellow fever vaccine is recommended for travelers to certain areas of Africa and equatorial South America to the canal zone. If there is a definite risk, the vaccine is recommended for all travelers at least 9 months of age. In some areas, it is not generally recommended unless the person is at high risk (prolonged travel, heavy exposure to mosquitoes, or inability to avoid mosquito bites). In areas without transmission, the vaccine is not medically recommended but may be required for travel due to order of itinerary. A waiver letter may be provided for the immunosuppressed or other travelers legally required to have the vaccine but for whom the risk of vaccination outweighs the benefits.

Typhoid and hepatitis A vaccines are recommended for travelers to most areas of the world. Two typhoid vaccines are currently available in the United States: Ty21a and Vi. Efficacy of both vaccines is 50–80%. Ty21a is a live oral vaccine that conveys protection for 5 years. It is taken as a series of four tablets, one every other day. The tablets must be refrigerated until ingested. Vi is a parenteral vaccine that provides protection for 2 years. Persons receiving this vaccine have a higher incidence of systemic reactions such as fever or malaise for the first 2–3 days after administration than those who receive the oral vaccine, and they may also develop injection site soreness.

Meningococcal vaccine is indicated for travelers to areas of sub-Saharan Africa and any area where meningococcal disease is endemic or epidemic. Duration of immunity is at least 5 years, and adverse reactions are generally mild. Japanese encephalitis vaccine is recommended for travelers to endemic areas of rural Asia during periods of transmission, especially if the traveler plans to live there or stay for >30 days.

An oral cholera vaccine (Vaxchora) was approved for use by the US Food and Drug Administration (FDA) in 2016. It is recommended as a single dose for adults up to 64 years old traveling to an area with significant risk for

Vibrio cholerae. Another oral vaccine, *V cholerae* whole-cell/B subunit vaccine (Dukoral), is available abroad. This vaccine also provides limited protection against infection with enterotoxic *E coli*. No country now requires cholera vaccination; however, some local authorities may ask for this documentation. A single dose of the oral vaccine is sufficient, or a medical waiver written on physician letterhead will satisfy this request.

Rabies vaccine is recommended for travelers to high-risk developing countries and countries where rabies immune globulin is not available. Long-term travelers or those who may have extensive outdoor or nighttime exposure and those whose occupations place them at risk should consider this vaccine. Postexposure vaccination is still required.

Hepatitis B vaccine is recommended for travelers to high-risk areas, especially long-term travelers and those engaging in high-risk sexual behaviors. Medical workers must be vaccinated, as should the future adoptive parents of children from a developing country.

All travelers are at a risk of pertussis, and all adults age >19 years who have not received a prior Tdap (tetanus, diphtheria, and pertussis) or are in close contact with infants should receive a single dose of Tdap even if a Td booster has been administered recently.

Up-to-date immunization information can be obtained from the CDC (www.cdc.gov/travel).

Brunette GW, ed. *CDC Yellow Book 2018, Health Information for the International Traveler*. New York, NY: Oxford University Press; 2017.

TREATMENT & PREVENTION OF TRAVEL-RELATED ILLNESSES

Acute Traveler's Diarrhea

ESSENTIALS OF DIAGNOSIS

- ▶ Twofold increase in frequency of unformed bowel movements, usually more than four to five per day.
- ▶ Abrupt onset while traveling or soon after returning home.
- ▶ Usually associated with abdominal cramps, rectal urgency, bloating, and malaise.
- ▶ Generally is self-limiting after 3–4 days.

▶ General Considerations

Traveler's diarrhea occurs in a significant number of people who travel to foreign countries, and up to 50% of travelers with high-risk itineraries will develop diarrhea during a 2-week stay. It is caused by fecal-oral contamination of food or water by bacteria, parasites, and viruses. The condition is more common in young adults, and the best chance for prevention involves strict attention to hygiene, sanitation, and food preparation, as outlined earlier. It is extremely difficult to avoid all dangers in food and drink, and multiple studies have shown no correlation between personal hygiene measures and traveler's diarrhea. Nevertheless, it is prudent to follow basic hygiene measures while abroad.

In contrast to the developed world, where viruses are the most common cause of diarrhea, enterotoxigenic *E coli* and other bacteria such as *Shigella, Salmonella, Vibrio*, and *Campylobacter* species are the most common causes of diarrhea in most parts of the developing world, with significant regional differences.

▶ Clinical Findings

Traveler's diarrhea is characterized by the abrupt onset of loose stools, usually 4–14 days after arrival or sooner if the concentration of bacteria ingested is sufficiently high. Common signs and symptoms include watery stool, abdominal cramping, bloating, urgency, malaise, and nausea. Vomiting occurs in ≤15% of those affected. Symptoms usually resolve in 3–4 days if not treated but can last longer (see later discussion regarding prolonged diarrhea). Depending on the cause, fever, bloody stool, and painful defecation may occur, but these symptoms are not common. Physical findings include a benign abdomen with diffuse tenderness but no rigidity and increased bowel sounds. Patients may appear dehydrated depending on the severity of the diarrhea. Although traveler's diarrhea is not life threatening, it can result in significant morbidity; one in five travelers with diarrhea is bedridden for a day, and >33.3% have to alter their activities. Stool examination, testing, and culture may yield a causative agent, but in roughly half of the cases, no pathogen is identified.

▶ Treatment

Treatment for traveler's diarrhea includes fluid replacement and, in mild cases that do not interrupt travel activities, loperamide or bismuth subsalicylate. Treatment for moderate to severe cases often includes antibiotics, although if no bloody stools are present and symptoms are not incapacitating, loperamide can be considered for monotherapy (or as adjunct with antibiotics). Trimethoprim-sulfamethoxazole and doxycycline are no longer recommended because of the development of widespread resistance. Azithromycin is becoming the preferred treatment in severe cases as resistance to fluoroquinolones is becoming more common. Fluoroquinolones and rifaximin, which have the advantage of not being absorbed systemically, can also be used to treat moderate traveler's diarrhea, but current resistance patterns and risk of invasive pathogens should be considered. Although a 3-day course is often recommended, a single day of antibiotic treatment has been shown to be effective for azithromycin and the fluoroquinolones.

Bismuth subsalicylate can be used by chewing two tablets (or taking 1 oz of liquid) every 30 minutes in up to eight doses. The potential for toxicity should be considered in patients taking aspirin, pregnant women, or children. Loperamide may be used for adults but never in the presence of high fever or bloody stool.

Fluid replacement using World Health Organization (WHO) oral rehydration salts is available in most countries. A simple rehydration solution can be prepared at home using ½ teaspoon of table salt, ½ teaspoon of baking soda, and 4 tablespoons of sugar in 1 L of water; orange juice can be added to provide potassium. Adults should drink 8 oz after every diarrheal stool. Children age <2 years should be given 2–4 oz and those age 2–10 years, 4–7 oz.

▶ Prevention

Although, as mentioned earlier, dietary precautions have not been conclusively proven to prevent traveler's diarrhea, it is important to observe good hygiene and sanitation and pay strict attention to food preparation and avoid high-risk foods. Bismuth subsalicylate (dosed as detailed earlier, but for up to 2 weeks) provides >60% protection.

The CDC does not recommend antibiotic prophylaxis for most travelers; however, it may be considered indicated in patients with active inflammatory bowel disease, brittle diabetes mellitus type 1, AIDS and other immunosuppressive disorders, unstable heart disease, and others with high risk of complications from diarrhea. Travelers planning an exceptionally critical short trip, where even 1 day of illness could impact the purpose of the trip, may wish to use a prophylactic medication. Rifaximin is preferred if antibiotic prophylaxis is needed. Bismuth subsalicylate (Pepto-Bismol up to two tablets 4 times a day) in adults without risk for toxicity provides >60% protection against traveler's diarrhea,

Brunette GW, ed. *CDC Health Information for International Travel 2018*. US Department of Health and Human Services, Public Health Service, Centers for Disease Control and Prevention. New York, NY: Oxford University Press; 2017.

Dupont HL, Jiang ZD, Okhuysen PC, et al. A randomized, double-blind, placebo-controlled trial of rifaximin to prevent travelers' diarrhea. *Ann Intern Med*. 2005;142:805–812. [PMID: 15897530]

Riddle MS, Connor BA, Beeching NJ, et al. Guidelines for the prevention and treatment of travelers' diarrhea: a graded expert panel report. *J Trav Med*. 2017;24(Suppl 1):S63–S80. [PMID: 28521004]

Malaria

ESSENTIALS OF DIAGNOSIS

▶ Abrupt onset of fever, headache, chills, myalgias, and malaise during or after returning from an area in which malaria is endemic.

▶ Recurrence of symptoms every 1–2 days (highly variable).

▶ Thick and thin Giemsa-stained blood smears showing *Plasmodium* (diagnostic gold standard) or confirmation by rapid diagnostic testing for malaria.

▶ General Considerations

Despite recent progress in control measures, malaria remains a major international public health problem, responsible for >500,000 deaths per year. Although 90% of cases occur in sub-Saharan Africa, the disease is found throughout the tropics. In most countries, the distribution is spotty. Few Americans know much about the disease because it was eradicated in the United States in the 1940s, but there are approximately 2000 cases of malaria seen each year.

Malaria is caused by infection with *Plasmodium falciparum, P vivax, P malariae, P ovale,* or *P knowlesi.* The first two species account for the majority of infections, and most cases of severe infection and death are due to *P falciparum.* The vector for transmission to humans is the female *Anopheles* mosquito. With the exception of Central America and parts of the Middle East, most *P falciparum* infections are resistant to chloroquine, and some strains of *P vivax* are also resistant to chloroquine. Travelers to the tropics should receive prophylaxis based on the latest CDC recommendations.

Incubation periods differ among the *Plasmodium* species, and at times, they may be much longer than those usually reported. *P falciparum, P malariae,* and *P. knowlesi* do not form hypnozoites in the liver, and infected patients should not relapse if treatment is adequate. However, with *P vivax* and *P ovale,* reactivation of dormant hypnozoites in the liver can occur, leading to relapse—sometimes decades after the original infection.

▶ Clinical Findings and Diagnosis

A. Symptoms and Signs

Classical symptoms of malaria in a nonimmune person are fever, chills and sweats, headache, and muscle and joint pains. Nausea, vomiting, abdominal pain, and diarrhea can also occur. Symptoms usually begin 10 days to 4 weeks after infection; however, depending on the species, they may develop as early as 1 week or as late as 1 year. Physical findings include fever, tachycardia, and flushed skin; mental confusion and jaundice may be present. The spleen and liver are often palpable, especially in persons who have had repeated infections. Symptoms may be much milder in a semi-immune person and may be only a headache or general body aches.

Severe malarial infection, usually due to *P falciparum*, causes a multitude of complications, including cerebral malaria (with seizures, coma, or death), renal failure, hemoglobinuria (also called "black water fever"), hemolytic anemia, acute respiratory failure, shock, and hypoglycemia. Long-term complications include hypersplenism, nephrotic syndrome, and a seizure disorder.

B. Laboratory Findings

The gold standard for diagnosis remains detection of parasites by Giemsa-stained thick and thin blood smears. Thick films are more sensitive for picking up infections and for measuring parasite density, and thin films are more accurate for identification of species. Multiple smears, up to one every 8 hours for 2 days, increase the sensitivity of the testing. Properly preparing and interpreting the slides requires experience, and reliable laboratories can be difficult to identify by a traveler abroad. Also, where malaria is no longer endemic (ie, the United States), healthcare providers may not be familiar with the disease, and laboratory workers may lack the experience to reliably detect the parasites when examining blood smears.

Over the past few years, rapid diagnostic tests (RDTs) for diagnosis of malaria in endemic areas have become accepted as the standard of care. Thus far, only one RDT has been approved by the FDA: the BinaxNOW malaria test kit. It tests for the histidine-rich protein II (HRP2) antigen specific for *P falciparum* plus a panmalarial antigen specific for all human plasmodia. Sensitivity and specificity to *P falciparum* are 95% and 94%, respectively. *P vivax* sensitivity and specificity are 69% and 100%, respectively.

Limitations of the BinaxNOW malaria test kit include the following: samples containing *P falciparum* are needed as positive controls, negative results require confirmation by thick and thin smears, and smears should also be obtained in positive BinaxNOW results to determine the specific species. Complete information about RDTs is available from the WHO website at https://www.who.int/malaria/areas/diagnosis/rapid-diagnostic-tests/en/, with specifics related to use of BinaxNOW available at https://www.cdc.gov/malaria/diagnosis_treatment/diagnostic_tools.html.

McCutchan TF, Piper RC, Makler MT. Use of malaria rapid diagnostic test to identify *Plasmodium knowlesi* infection. *Emerg Infect Dis*. 2008;14(11):1750–1752. [PMID: 18976561]

C. Differential Diagnosis

The differential diagnosis of malaria includes most febrile tropical illnesses prevalent in the area that the traveler has visited (see section on fever in returning traveler, later in this chapter). The illnesses most often confused with malaria include influenza and viral infections, dengue fever, babesiosis, relapsing fever, yellow fever, hepatitis, typhoid fever, kala-azar, urinary tract infections, tuberculosis, endocarditis, and meningitis (especially with cerebral symptoms).

▶ Treatment

The medications used for the treatment of malaria vary and are frequently used in combinations. Ideally, determination of the correct treatment involves identification of the species of malaria, knowledge of where the traveler has been, and the medical history of the patient. No one drug acts on all stages of the disease, and different species of parasites show different responses. Full discussion of the treatment of malaria is beyond the scope of this chapter and may be found at www.cdc.gov/malaria/diagnosis_treatment/treatment.html.

A traveler who plans to visit a remote area without adequate medical facilities may wish to take along a reliable supply of medication for a full course of presumptive treatment if symptoms of malaria develop. Presumptive self-treatment should never take the place of being evaluated at a medical facility; however, it could be lifesaving if there is no nearby help. Table 52–2 includes two suggestions for presumptive self-treatment: atovaquone-proguanil (Malarone) or artemether-lumefantrine (Coartem). Malarone should not be used if the patient is taking this as prophylaxis, and Coartem should not be used in patients taking mefloquine prophylaxis.

Artemisinin derivatives such as artemether and artesunate are well tolerated and are given in combination with another drug such as amodiaquine, sulfadoxine-pyrimethamine, mefloquine, or lumefantrine. Artemether-lumefantrine is the only artemisinin-based combination therapy currently available in the United States, but others are available abroad. There have been a few reports of resistance to artemisinin. Combination therapy has the advantages of slowing the development of resistance, reducing the length of the required treatment course, and greater effectiveness.

CDC clinicians are also on-call to provide advice to clinicians on the diagnosis and treatment of malaria and can be reached through the Malaria Hotline 770-488-7788 (or toll-free at 855-856-4713) 9 AM to 5 PM Eastern Standard Time or 770-488-7100 for emergencies during other hours.

▶ Prevention

A common approach to malaria prevention is to follow the "ABCD" rule (**a**wareness of risk, **b**ite avoidance, **c**ompliance with chemoprophylaxis, and prompt **d**iagnosis in case of fever).

A. General Measures

Travelers to endemic areas should be advised about basic measures to prevent mosquito bites, including wearing

Table 52–2. Prophylaxis and presumptive treatment dosages for malaria.

Drug	Adult Dosage	Dosage in Children
Malaria Presumptive Treatment Atovaquone-proguanil[a,b] Adult tabs = 250 mg atovaquone + 100 mg proguanil Pediatric tabs = 62.5 mg atovaquone + 25 mg proguanil	4 adult tabs once daily for 3 days	5–8 kg: 2 pediatric tabs/d for 3 days 9–10 kg: 3 pediatric tabs/d for 3 days 11–20 kg: 1 adult tab/d for 3 days 21–30 kg: 2 adult tabs/d for 3 days 31–40 kg: 3 adult tabs/d for 3 days >40 kg: use adult dose
Artemether-lumefantrine[b,c] 20 mg artemether + 120 mg lumefantrine per tablet	Adult and pediatric doses based on weight 5–14 kg: 1 tablet per dose 15–24 kg: 2 tablets per dose 25–34 kg: 3 tablets per dose ≥35 kg: 4 tablets per dose Second dose given 8 hours after first dose, then a dose is given twice a day for next 2 days for a total of 6 doses over 3 days	Pediatric doses based on weight as in adult dose
Malaria Prophylaxis Chloroquine phosphate	300 mg base (500 mg salt) per week; start 1–2 weeks before travel and continue for 4 weeks after last exposure	5 mg base/kg per week (8.3 mg salt/kg) to maximum of adult dose
Hydroxychloroquine sulfate	310 mg base (400 mg salt) per week Start 1–2 weeks before travel and continue for 4 weeks after last exposure	5 mg base/kg per week (6.5 mg salt/kg) to maximum of adult dose
Mefloquine[d]	228 mg base (250 mg salt) per week Start 2–3 weeks before travel and continue for 4 weeks after last exposure	4.6 mg base/kg per week (5 mg salt/kg) per week: 9–19 kg: ¼ adult tablet per week 20–30 kg: ½ adult tablet per week 31–45 kg: ¾ adult tablet per week >45 kg: 1 adult tablet per week
Atovaquone-proguanil[a,b]	1 adult tablet (250 mg atovaquone + 100 mg proguanil) per day; start 1–2 days before travel and continue for 7 days after last exposure	Pediatric tabs contain 62.5 mg atovaquone + 25 mg proguanil; dosages based on child's weight: 5–8 kg: ½ pediatric tab daily 9–10 kg: ¾ pediatric tab daily 11–20 kg: 1 pediatric tab daily 21–30 kg: 2 pediatric tabs daily 31–40 kg: 3 pediatric tabs daily >40 kg: 1 adult tab daily
Doxycycline[e]	100 mg/d Start 1–2 days before travel and continue for 4 weeks after last exposure	Children ≥8 years: 2.2 mg/kg daily up to max of adult dose
Primaquine[f,g] For short-duration exposure in areas with primarily *Plasmodium vivax*	30 mg base (52.6 mg salt) daily Start 1–2 days before travel and continue for 7 days after return	0.5 mg base/kg (0.8 mg/kg salt) up to adult dose daily
For terminal prophylaxis in people with prolonged exposure to or infection with *P vivax* and/or *Plasmodium ovale*	30 mg base (52.6 mg salt) daily for 14 days after leaving area	0.5 mg base/kg (0.8 mg/kg salt) daily up to adult dose for 14 days after leaving area

[a]Contraindicated with severe renal impairment.
[b]Not for use in children <5 kg, pregnant women, or lactating women breastfeeding an infant <5 kg.
[c]Do not use if taking mefloquine prophylaxis.
[d]Cautious use in pregnancy.
[e]Contraindicated in pregnant or lactating women and in children younger than 8 years.
[f]Contraindicated with glucose-6-phosphate dehydrogenase deficiency (G6PD) deficiency and in pregnancy and lactation unless the infant has a documented normal G6PD level.
[g]All patients should have a documented normal G6PD level before taking primaquine.
Tab, tablet.

long sleeves, long pants, and light-colored clothing at dusk; avoiding perfumes that might attract mosquitoes; and treating bed nets and/or clothing with permethrin. A mosquito repellent containing 30–50% DEET or 20% of picaridin is recommended.

B. Malaria Prophylaxis

Chemoprophylaxis is a strategy that uses medications before, during, and after the exposure period to prevent the disease caused by malaria parasites. The aim of prophylaxis is to prevent or suppress symptoms caused by blood-stage parasites. In addition, presumptive antirelapse therapy (also known as *terminal prophylaxis*) uses a medication (primaquine) toward the end of the exposure period (or immediately thereafter) to prevent relapses or delayed-onset clinical presentations of malaria caused by dormant liver stages of *P vivax* or *P ovale*.

In choosing an appropriate chemoprophylactic regimen, the traveler and the healthcare provider should consider several factors. The travel itinerary should be reviewed in detail to determine whether the traveler is actually at risk for acquiring malaria. The next step is to determine whether significant antimalarial drug resistance has been reported in that location. Resistance to antimalarial drugs has developed in many regions of the world. Healthcare providers should consult the latest information on resistance patterns before prescribing prophylaxis for their patients.

Five medications are currently available and approved in the United States for malaria prophylaxis: chloroquine, mefloquine, doxycycline, atovaquone-proguanil, and primaquine. See Table 52–2 for prophylactic dosages in adults and children.

1. Chloroquine (or hydroxychloroquine)—This drug is still effective for prophylaxis in Central America above the Panama Canal and in some areas of the Middle East, but should not be used for prophylaxis in other areas. Side effects include pruritus, headache, blurred vision, myalgia, alopecia, and spotty depigmentation. It can cause exacerbations of psoriasis, eczema, and dermatitis. Retinal injury may occur with lifetime doses of >100 g. Chloroquine is safe in pregnancy and breastfeeding. Prophylaxis should begin 1–2 weeks before arrival in a malaria-endemic area and should continue for 4 weeks after departure.

2. Mefloquine—This agent is effective for prophylaxis in most of the world, although *P falciparum* shows a patchy, but increasing, resistance to the drug in some areas. It is considered safe to use in pregnancy and breastfeeding, although small amounts are passed in breast milk. The most serious side effects are neuropsychiatric, such as bad dreams, paresthesias, hallucinations, and even psychotic reactions, which have reduced its use a first-choice agent. Other side effects include vertigo, seizures, hepatotoxicity,

headache, confusion, gastrointestinal upset, pruritus, and depression. It is contraindicated with psychiatric disorders or seizures. Caution is advised in patients with cardiac conduction abnormalities. Prophylaxis should begin 2 weeks before arrival in a malaria area and continue for 4 weeks after departure.

3. Atovaquone/proguanil—This drug is effective and safe for children, but there is insufficient evidence to recommend it for use in pregnant women, children weighing <5 kg, or women breastfeeding infants weighing <5 kg. It is contraindicated in patients with severe renal impairment (creatinine clearance <30 mL/min). Side effects are generally mild and include abdominal pain, vomiting, and headache. Prophylaxis should begin 1–2 days before arrival in a malaria-endemic area and continue for 7 days after departure.

4. Doxycycline—This agent is efficacious, safe, and the least expensive choice for prophylaxis. Its use is contraindicated in pregnancy, breastfeeding, and in children age <8 years. Side effects include gastrointestinal upset, esophagitis, vaginal yeast infection, phototoxicity, hepatic toxicity, pseudomembranous colitis, and increased intracranial pressure. Prophylaxis should begin 1 day before arrival in a malaria-endemic area and continue for 4 weeks after departure.

5. Primaquine—Primaquine may be used as primary prophylaxis in areas with primarily *P vivax*. It is taken 1–2 days before travel to a malarial area and daily for 7 days after return. Terminal prophylaxis is not needed if primaquine is used as primary prophylaxis. When used as terminal prophylaxis, it is taken daily for 14 days after leaving the malarial area. It should be used only in those with documented evidence of a normal glucose-6-phosphate dehydrogenase (G6PD) level, as patients with G6PD can have sever hemolysis. Adverse effects include gastrointestinal upset.

Brunette GW, ed. *CDC Health Information for International Travel 2018*. US Department of Health and Human Services, Public Health Service, Centers for Disease Control and Prevention. New York, NY: Oxford University Press; 2017.

Freedman DO. Malaria prevention in short-term travelers. *N Engl J Med*, 2008;359(6):603–612. [PMID: 18687641]

Hahn WO, Pottinger PS. Malaria in the traveler: how to manage before departure and evaluate upon return. *Med Clin North Am.* 2016;100(2):289–302. [PMID: 26900114]

TREATMENT OF THE RETURNING TRAVELER

Despite the best preparations, travelers may become sick while abroad or are ill on their return home. Of the 50 million travelers to the developing world each year, approximately half will have a travel-related health impairment, and 5–10% will consult a physician due to a travel-related illness. This section describes three common problems faced by the family physician—fever, diarrhea, and eosinophilia—with the goal of assisting the physician in making the diagnosis and providing appropriate treatment. The differential diagnosis depends on the traveler's itinerary and other factors, and all the possibilities cannot be covered here. Fever and eosinophilia, in particular, may occur as symptoms in a wide range of infectious and inflammatory conditions.

Fever in a Returning Traveler

Fever in a returning traveler requires a thorough history (including immunizations and any use of prophylactic medications, illness in companions, sexual activities, and any nonprescribed drug use) and physical examination. Often, localized symptoms or signs (eg, respiratory symptoms, jaundice) help narrow the diagnosis. If the diagnosis is not immediately obvious, consider common diseases endemic to the area(s) visited. If Zika is suspected, counsel regarding reproductive risks and precautions; update when testing is complete. In posttravel patients reported to the GeoSentinel Network from 2007 to 2011, fever was reported in 23% of patients, with 29% of those found to have malaria—primarily from travelers to Africa—and 15% to have dengue fever. In 40%, the cause of fever was not determined. Seriously ill patients should be hospitalized, and any patient suspected of having a contagious serious condition must be isolated, with appropriate reporting to the health department and CDC. Stable patients not at risk for transmitting a serious disease may be observed for a few days, and most fevers will resolve spontaneously.

If fever persists or the patient is unstable or has other serious symptoms or findings, laboratory investigation becomes the key to the diagnosis. Although detailing the potential permutations of itinerary and presentation are beyond the scope of this chapter, appropriate studies may include complete blood count; smears for malaria, *Borrelia*, *Babesia*, and filariasis; rapid diagnostic tests; typhoid culture or antigen test; urinalysis; liver function tests; cultures of blood, urine, and possibly cerebrospinal fluid; stool examination; biopsy of skin lesions, lymph nodes, or other masses; bone marrow aspirate; hepatitis and other serologies tests depending on the patient's possible exposures; and acute and convalescent sera when appropriate. Chest radiographs should generally be done in febrile patients with respiratory symptoms or findings; other scans may be appropriate for fever with localizing symptoms. Fever usually has an infectious cause, but occult malignancies and rheumatologic conditions should be considered in the differential diagnosis.

It is important to remember that "the common is still common," and in fact, many common causes of fever in returned travelers are routine illnesses such as upper and lower respiratory tract infections, sinusitis, urinary tract

Table 52–3. Possible diagnoses with certain physical findings in febrile travelers.

Finding	Possible Associated Diseases
Rash	Dengue, typhoid, rickettsial infections, syphilis, gonorrhea, brucellosis, hemorrhagic fever viruses, Chikungunya and other viral illnesses including arboviruses, acute human immuno-deficiency virus (HIV) infection, measles
Jaundice	Hepatitis, malaria, yellow fever, leptospirosis, relapsing fever
Lymphadenopathy	Mononucleosis and other viruses, rickettsial infections, brucellosis. dengue, acute HIV, visceral leishmaniasis, Lassa fever, toxoplasmosis
Hepatomegaly	Amebiasis, malaria, hepatitis, leptospirosis
Splenomegaly	Malaria, relapsing fever, trypanosomiasis, typhoid, brucellosis, visceral leishmaniasis, typhus, and dengue
Eschar	Rickettsial infections (especially Tsutsugamushi disease), *Borrelia*, Crimean-Congo hemorrhagic fever
Hemorrhage	Dengue, meningococcemia, leptospirosis, Lassa fever, Marburg and Ebola fever, Crimean-Congo fever, Rift Valley fever, yellow fever, rickettsial infections (Rocky Mountain spotted fever, louseborne typhus).

Data from Leggat PA. Assessment of febrile illness in the returned traveler. *Aust Fam Physician.* 2007 May;36(5):328-332 and Wilson ME. *Fever in Returning Travelers.* Atlanta, GA: CDC, 2011.

infections, and influenza. An extensive list of potentially travel-related etiologies is provided in Tables 52–3 and 52–4, but these should be considered only if a more common cause is not apparent.

In a seriously ill febrile traveler without a readily apparent diagnosis, empirical treatment should be considered for malaria, if possible from the history or itinerary, and other causes of sepsis or serious infection. Empirical treatment may also be considered in less severe cases, particularly if fever persists past 7 days or if rickettsia/leptospirosis is a consideration.

Leder K, Torresi J, Libman MD, et al. GeoSentinel surveillance of illness in returned travelers, 2007-2011. *Ann Intern Med.* 2013; 158(6):456–468. [PMID: 23552375]

Leggat PA. Assessment of febrile illness in the returned traveler. *Austral Fam Phys.* 2007;36(6):328–333. [PMID: 17492066]

Thwaites G, Day N. Approach to fever in the returning traveler. *N Engl J Med.* 2017;376:548–560. [PMID: 28177860]

Table 52–4. Selected causes of fever in a traveler returning from the tropics (not in order of frequency).

Short Incubation (<28 days)	Long Incubation (>28 days)
Arboviruses such as chikungunya	Brucellosis (some cases)
Babesiosis	Filariasis
Bacterial diarrhea	Fungal diseases
Bartonellosis	Hepatitis B, C, E, and A (some cases)
Borreliosis	Leishmaniasis
Brucellosis (some cases)	Human immunodeficiency virus
Cytomegalovirus and other viruses	infection
Dengue fever, yellow fever, and	Liver abscess (amoebic)
hemorrhagic fever viruses	Malaria (some cases)
Endocarditis	Melioidosis
Hepatitis A (some cases)	Schistosomiasis
Histoplasmosis and other fungal	Syphilis
diseases	Trypanosomiasis (American and
Influenza and other acute respiratory	African)
infections	Tuberculosis
Leptospirosis	
Listeriosis	
Malaria (some cases)	
Meningococcemia	
Plague	
Rickettsial diseases	
Sepsis	
Toxoplasmosis	
Typhoid or paratyphoid fever and	
enteric fever	
Zika	

Persistent Diarrhea in a Returning Traveler

Although most traveler's diarrhea resolves within 2 weeks, some travelers develop persistent diarrhea or other gastrointestinal (GI) symptoms that can be difficult to diagnose and treat. In fact, a recent study showed diarrhea and other GI symptoms constitute 35% of all problems in travelers presenting to their family physicians. Some travelers will have a transient lactase deficiency, which usually responds to lactose restriction for 7–10 days. Some travelers, especially those not careful with their diet, may develop a small bowel bacterial overgrowth, which may require antibiotic treatment. In some travelers, just a change from their usual diet or the consumption of treated or boiled water or unpasteurized milk can cause a lingering diarrhea termed *Brainerd diarrhea*.

Causes of persistent diarrhea in a returning traveler include bacterial and parasitic infection, and if a patient's diarrhea persists for >7 days, a stool examination should be performed, preferably with three samples examined to increase sensitivity. In addition to ova and parasites, an evaluation for antigens and bacterial cultures should also be performed. If symptoms of rectal disease are present, anoscopic and sigmoidoscopic examination should be done with biopsies as needed. If the results of these tests are negative, the physician should consider an empiric trial of metronidazole for the treatment of a possible *Giardia* or other protozoan infection. Irritable bowel syndrome (IBS) and, less commonly, inflammatory bowel disease may develop after travel in those who experience a bout of bacterial or viral diarrhea. One study showed that 63% of a group of 97 healthy student travelers to Mexico developed diarrhea compatible with traveler's diarrhea. Six months later, 18% still reported loose stools, 18% reported abdominal pain, and 9% had fecal urgency. Even after 6 months, 11.7% met the criteria for IBS. Finally, sometimes underlying GI pathology, such as celiac sprue and other malabsorption disorders and even GI malignancy, can be unmasked after a bout of diarrhea.

Bhatti M, Enzler M. Approach to diarrhea in returned travelers. In: Sanford C, Pottinger P, Jong E, eds. *The Travel and Tropical Medicine Manual*, 5th ed. Philadelphia, PA: Saunders Elsevier; 2017.

Caumes E, Legros F, Duhot D, et al. Health problems in returning travelers consulting general practitioners. *J Trav Med*. 2008; 15(6):457–459. [PMID: 19090803]

Okhuysen PC, Jiang ZD, Carlin L, et al. Post-diarrhea chronic intestinal symptoms and irritable bowel syndrome in North American travelers to Mexico. *Am J Gastroenterol*. 2004;99: 1774–1778. [PMID: 15330917]

Eosinophilia in a Returned Traveler

While there are many causes of eosinophilia, including allergic and inflammatory disorders, a high level of eosinophilia (>450 eosinophils/μL) in a returning traveler is indicative of a parasitic infection and is characteristic of helminthic infections, particularly those with an extraintestinal migration phase or tissue infection. Strongyloides and filariasis cause some of the highest levels, and infection in humans can persist for many years if not treated. Common protozoans, such as *Giardia* and *Plasmodium* species, rarely cause eosinophilia, with the exceptions of *Blastocystis hominis*, *Dientamoeba fragilis*, and *Isospora belli*. Schistosomiasis has become a serious problem for people swimming or rafting in freshwater in Africa. In one study from Israel, 82 of 995 travelers (8.2%) were found to have significant eosinophilia. Of these, 44 (53.7%) were found to have schistosomiasis mostly acquired in sub-Saharan Africa. Of the remaining 38 cases, a definitive parasitologic diagnosis could be made in only 9 (23.7%) travelers. This is compatible with other studies. A therapeutic trial of albendazole was given to most of the cases without a specific diagnosis, and approximately 90% reported a favorable response with resolution of symptoms and a significant decrease in the eosinophil count after 2 months.

The workup for a traveler with eosinophilia must include multiple stool examinations. If schistosomiasis is suspected due to travel to Africa, include stool concentration and terminal urine microscopy. If present, biopsy specimens of skin lesions (onchocerciasis) or swollen lymph nodes (filariasis) can be examined for definitive diagnosis. Serologic tests are available from the CDC and other specialized laboratories, but be aware of any cross-reactivity and possible need for convalescent samples due to delay in antibody response. Other infectious causes of eosinophilia such as hepatitis B, HIV, and fungal infections should be considered. A therapeutic trial of albendazole is probably warranted if no diagnosis is found. The workup, including *Strongyloides* stool culture, should be repeated at 3 month if eosinophilia persists.

Meltzer E, Percik R, Shatzkes J, et al. Eosinophilia among returning travelers: a practical approach. *Am J Trop Med Hyg*. 2008; 78(5):702–709. [PMID: 18458300]

Ustianowski A, Zumla A. Eosinophilia in the returning traveler. *Infect Dis Clin N Am*. 2012;26:781–789. [PMID: 22963783]

Websites

Centers for Disease Control and Prevention. Current information on wide range of topics, including special needs, children, vaccines, medical kits, cruise ships, prophylactic medication and disease outbreaks. http://www.cdc.gov/travel

Pan-American Health Organization. Information on countries in the Western hemisphere. http://www.paho.org

ProMED. A listserv monitoring emerging diseases worldwide. http://www.promedmail.org

Travel Medicine. General information on travel medicine with links to many other sites. https://www.travmed.com

World Health Organization. The World Health Organization website has much useful information, including worldwide disease surveillance. http://www.who.int

Tickborne Disease

Niladri Das, MD

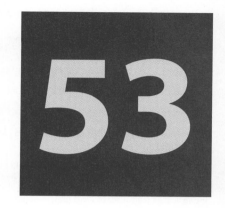

53

ESSENTIALS OF DIAGNOSIS

▶ Tick bites are typically painless, and <50% of patients with tickborne disease present with a known bite.

▶ Consider tickborne diseases (TBDs) in the summer months for patients who present with fever, myalgias, and headaches but without gastrointestinal (GI) or upper respiratory symptoms who live in tick-endemic regions of the United States.

▶ Diagnosis can be difficult because of nonspecific symptoms and difficulty in timely confirmatory testing.

▶ Treatment with doxycycline should be initiated when Rocky Mountain spotted fever, human granulocytic anaplasmosis, and/or ehrlichiosis is included in the differential diagnosis.

General Considerations

TBDs continue to be on the rise in the United States. Several factors contribute to this surge, including suburban development, climate change, a rise in human outdoor activities, and an increase in vector hosts such as the white-tailed deer. Lyme disease is the most widely known tickborne illness to the public, as well as the most common. During 2000–2010, there were 250,000 reported cases of Lyme disease in the United States, and from 2011–2017, the number of cases surpassed that number. The incidence of reported cases of almost all TBDs have increased over that period of time, as well as the recognition of new illnesses that were not even identified when this chapter was originally written. As of this writing, 14 bacterial, 1 protozoal, and 4 viral TBDs have been identified in the United States. The tickborne illnesses we focus on in this chapter are Lyme disease, Rocky Mountain spotted fever (RMSF), ehrlichiosis, human granulocytic

anaplasmosis (HGA), and babesiosis. Numerous other diseases associated with ticks should be considered in certain locations during summer months. For more information regarding these illnesses, visit the following Centers for Disease Control and Prevention (CDC) webpage: http://www.cdc.gov/ticks.

Essential to the diagnosis and treatment of TBD is the geographic distribution of the particular disease and the ticks that transmit them. Lyme disease, RMSF, ehrlichiosis, HGA, and babesiosis are all associated with particular species of ticks. Table 53–1 lists the six tick species of significance for this chapter, including their distribution and primary hosts. However, the patient rarely presents with the actual tick attached, and therefore, visual identification of species is typically unnecessary. Tick bites are typically painless, and <50% of patients with TBD present with a known bite.

Centers for Disease Control and Prevention. *Tickborne Diseases of the United States: A Reference Manual for Health Care Providers.* 5th ed. 2018. https://www.cdc.gov/ticks/tickbornediseases/Tickborne-Diseases-P.pdf. Accessed December 2, 2019.

Decker CF. Tick-borne illnesses: an overview *Dis Mon.* 2012;58(6): 327–329 [PMID: 22608118]

Pujalte GGA, Marberry ST, Libertin CR. Tick-borne illnesses in the United States. *Prim Care Clin Office Pract.* 2018;45:379–391 [PMID: 30115329]

Pathogenesis

As is the case in any vector-borne disease, ticks require hosts to survive and to transmit pathogens. Their lifecycle consists of egg, larval, nymph, and adult stages. Only ticks in the nymph and adult stages attach to humans. These stages are most active during the summer months, hence the seasonality of most TBDs. Humans are incidental, not primary, hosts. Primary hosts (mice, deer, dogs) serve as reservoirs for the diseases and ticks attach to any host from outdoor contact with grasses, shrubs, and foliage. Ticks feed on blood, and

CHAPTER 53

Table 53–1. Tick species.

Tick (Common Name/Species Name)	Primary Range	Transmits	Additional Facts
Black-legged tick/deer tick (*Ixodes scapularis*)	Northeastern United States, Great Lakes region	Lyme, HGA, babesiosis	Can remain active in warmer winters
Western black-legged tick (*Ixodes pacificus*)	Pacific Coast, particularly northern California	Lyme, HGA	Rates of infection are low
American dog tick (*Dermacentor variabilis*)	East of Rockies	RMSF	Also known as wood tick
Rocky Mountain wood tick (*Dermacentor andersoni*)	Rocky Mountain states	RMSF	Live in elevations 4000–10,500 feet
Lone Star tick (*Amblyomma americanum*)	Southeast United States, but can be found from Texas to Maine	Ehrlichiosis	Bites can be particularly irritating
Brown dog tick (*Rhipicephalus sanguineus*)	Throughout United States	RMSF	Primary host: dogs

HGA, human granulocytic anaplasmosis; RMSF, Rocky Mountain spotted fever.

in order to do so, they extend a mouthpiece into the host, secreting saliva with anesthetic properties. This saliva is where TBD pathogens are contained. In cases where saliva and blood contact is made, transmission can occur.

The pathogens themselves complicate the diagnosis of TBD. In the United States, the causative organism of Lyme disease (*Borrelia burgdorferi*) is a spirochete, RSMF (*Rickettsia rickettsii*) is a gram-negative intracellular bacillus, ehrlichiosis (*Ehrlichia chaffeensis/ewingii*) and HGA (*Anaplasma phagocytophilum*) are intracellular gram-negative coccobacilli, and babesiosis (*Babesia microti*) is an intraerythrocyte protozoa. The atypical nature of these organisms makes for complicated pathophysiology in disease, but also complicates diagnosis and treatment.

Centers for Disease Control and Prevention. Tick life cycle and hosts. https://www.cdc.gov/ticks/life_cycle_and_hosts.html. Accessed December 2, 2019.
Salinas LJ, Greenfield RA, Little SE, et al. Tickborne Infections in the southern United States. *Am J Med Sci*. 2010;340(3):194–201. [PMID: 20697259]

▶ Prevention

Primary prevention of TBD is achieved through a reduction of bites. Wearing light-colored clothing to facilitate tick visualization, as well as decreasing exposed skin area, has been demonstrated to be effective. Skin examination and showering within 2 hours after spending extended periods outdoors is recommended in tick-endemic areas. If a tick is discovered, forceps (Figure 53–1) or a commercial tick removal device should be used to mechanically remove the arthropod. No chemical means of removal are recommended.

Environmental alterations such as cutting tall grass and reducing brush and leaf piles will reduce outdoor areas where people would likely be affected by ticks. These measures

also prevent attracting native hosts such as deer and mice. An environmental pesticide can also be extremely useful in endemic areas for total tick population reduction. At present, there are no TBD vaccines available on the market for humans. A previously available Lyme disease vaccine has been off the market for many years. Those who were inoculated using this product should no longer consider themselves immunized against Lyme disease. Of the personal

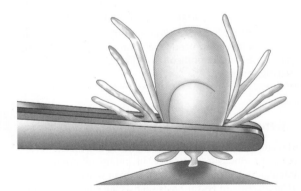

▲ **Figure 53–1.** (1) Use fine-tipped tweezers to grasp the tick as close to the skin's surface as possible; (2) pull upward with steady, even pressure—do not twist or jerk the tick, as this can cause the mouthparts to break off and remain in the skin (if this happens, remove the mouthparts with tweezers; if you are unable to remove the mouthparts easily with clean tweezers, leave it alone and let the skin heal); (3) after removing the tick, thoroughly clean the bite area and your hands with rubbing alcohol, an iodine scrub, or soap and water. (Reproduced with permission from Centers for Disease Control and Prevention. Tick removal. https://www.cdc.gov/ticks/removing_a_tick.html.)

repellents, products with *N,N*-diethyl-3-metylbenzamide (DEET) are the most effective. DEET product concentration ranges from 5% to 100%. The American Academy of Pediatrics advises against using any concentration that is >30%, although the CDC specifically recommends concentrations >20% for tick bite prevention. Children age >2 months can use DEET. Its efficacy in patients of all ages lasts between 1 and 5 hours depending on the concentration, and extended periods outdoors merit reapplication to skin and clothing. The same rule applies for picaridin, which is effective for ≤3 hours and can been applied to the skin as well as clothing. No other repellents can be safely applied to the skin, but clothing immersed in permethrin solutions has been shown to be effective tick repellents.

Lyme disease is the only TBD for which antibiotic prophylaxis is recommended. If a patient presents with the history of tick attachment for >36 hours, antibiotic prophylaxis may be given within 72 hours after the removal. Doxycycline is the only antibiotic indicated for this: 200 mg by mouth (PO) once or ≤200 mg per 8 mg/kg for children age >8 years. Prophylaxis with doxycycline is recommended only in the Lyme-endemic areas, which include locations with a tick infection rate of >20%. In order to determine the prevalence rate of Lyme-infected ticks in your area, contact your local health department or the CDC.

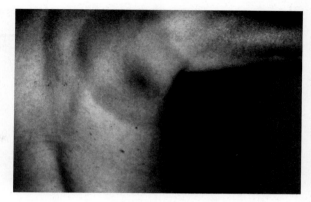

▲ **Figure 53–2. Erythema migrans.** (Reproduced with permission from CDC Public Health Image Library.)

reactions and not indicative of TBD. EM is diagnostic of Lyme disease, and its presence is the only instance in which confirmatory testing is not necessary. This Lyme rash can present alternatively as a nontargetoid bluish lesion, as a rash with central crusting and no clearing, or as multiple red lesions with dusky centers known collectively as *disseminated EM*, which is indicative of disease spread. Seventy to 80% of patients with Lyme disease present with EM, which typically resolves within 3–4 weeks without treatment. Along with EM, the most common presenting symptoms of Lyme are fever, headache, myalgias, malaise, and fatigue, which are mostly consistent with a flulike illness but lack upper respiratory or GI symptoms (Table 53–2).

The disseminated stage of Lyme disease typically occurs weeks after the initial infection. This can be manifested as disseminated EM as well as the persistence of flulike symptoms. Disseminated Lyme should be suspected in patients presenting in late summer/fall with aseptic meningitis, cranial nerve palsies (particularly Bell palsy), atrioventricular block, myocarditis/pericarditis, migratory joint pain, and large-joint monoarthritis or oligoarthritis. Late- stage Lyme can manifest with one or more of these symptoms, and in endemic areas, it is important to include TBD in the differential for any of these symptoms so that proper laboratory workup can be performed (Table 53–2).

B. Laboratory Findings

Laboratory evaluation in localized Lyme is often nonspecific. An elevated erythrocyte sedimentation rate, elevated liver enzymes, and hematuria or proteinuria can be seen. If a patient is suspected to have aseptic meningitis presenting with fever and headache, the cerebrospinal fluid (CSF) can demonstrate elevated lymphocytes/lymphocytic predominance, mild increase in protein, and normal glucose. The CDC has two accepted diagnosis methodologies for Lyme disease: EM

Centers for Disease Control and Prevention. CDC features: DEET, showers, and tick checks can stop ticks. https://www.cdc.gov/features/stopticks/index.html. Accessed December 2, 2019.
Clark RP, Hu LT. Prevention of Lyme disease and other tickborne infections. *Infect Dis Clin North Am.* 2008;22(3):381–396. [PMID: 18755380]

LYME DISEASE

▶ General Considerations

A. Symptoms and Signs

Connecticut, Delaware, Maine, Maryland, Massachusetts, Minnesota, New Jersey, New Hampshire, New York, Pennsylvania, Virginia, and Wisconsin account for 95% of reported cases of Lyme disease. Despite being the most common vector-borne disease in the United States, the diagnosis of Lyme is complicated by two potential stages of illness with variable presentations involving dermatologic, musculoskeletal, neurologic, and cardiac findings.

The localized stage of Lyme disease is most likely to present in the summer months 3–30 days after a tick bite. The hallmark of localized Lyme disease is erythema migrans (EM) (Figure 53–2). EM is typically at the site of prior tick attachment, often presenting for 7 days after the initial bite. It is characterized by an erythematous, ring or target macular lesion, typically measuring ≥5 cm. Rashes at the site of tick bites in the first 48 hours after a bite are typically local

Table 53–2. Diagnosis of tickborne diseases.

Disease	Incubation	Signs and Symptoms	General Labs	Confirmatory Labs
Localized Lyme disease	3–30 days	EM, flulike illness	Elevated ESR (typically <80), mild LFT elevation	Not typically applicable; see below; EM diagnostic
Disseminated Lyme disease	Month(s) after bite	Disseminated EM, large-joint arthritis, CN palsies, meningitis	CSF lymphocytic pleocytosis, elevated ESR/CRP	IgG/IgM; if + antibodies, then Western blot confirmation
RMSF	2–14 days	Fever, maculopapular rash 2–5 days after fever, petechiae after day 6, severe headache, AMS, meningismus	Thrombocytopenia, mild LFT elevation, hyponatremia	IgG + 7–10 days after onset of illness, fourfold increase after 2–4 weeks; IgM false + common, early disease seronegative
Ehrlichiosis	7–14 days	Fever, headache, malaise, rash in 60% of children	Mild anemia, thrombocytopenia, leukopenia, elevated LFTs	*Ehrlichia* IgG + 1 week after onset of illness, fourfold increase after 2–4 weeks + PCR before abx
HGA	7–14 days	Fever, headache, myalgias	Mild anemia, thrombocytopenia, leukopenia, elevated LFTs	IgG + 1 week after onset of illness, fourfold increase after 2–4 weeks + PCR before abx
Babesiosis	7 days–2+ months	Fever, malaise, dark urine, nausea	Hemolytic anemia, thrombocytopenia, elevated BUN/Cr	Blood smear ID of protozoa, + PCR, antibody testing

abx, antibiotics; AMS, altered mental status; BUN/Cr, blood urea nitrogen/creatinine; CN, cranial nerve; CRP, C-reactive protein; CSF, cerebrospinal fluid; EM, erythema migrans; ESR, erythrocyte sedimentation rate; HGA, human granulocytic anaplasmosis; ID, identification; LFT, liver function test(s); PCR, polymerase chain reaction; RMSF, Rocky Mountain spotted fever.

and the presence of at least one sequela of late-stage disease and confirmatory testing. Serologic antibody testing is the laboratory diagnostic test of choice. However, antibody testing is not helpful for early disease, as immunoglobulin (Ig) M does not develop until 2–4 weeks after initial disease and IgG typically takes longer than 4 weeks to develop. When enzyme-linked immunosorbent assay (ELISA) testing is ordered, positive or indeterminate tests are typically followed by Western blot confirmation as false positives are common. Lyme disease–specific antibodies from CSF may be helpful in diagnosing cases of meningitis (Table 53–2).

C. Other Considerations

Imaging studies may be useful in ruling out other etiologies when considering Lyme disease. The differential diagnosis should include other TBDs, especially HGA, babesiosis, and *Borrelia miyamotoi* disease. *Borrelia miyamotoi* disease is similar in presentation to early Lyme, but rarely has a rash and is known to occur in the upper Midwest, Northeast, and mid-Atlantic states. At present, the CDC recommends using the same antibiotics to treat *Borrelia miyamotoi* disease that are used to treat Lyme.

Non–tick-related differentials for EM include local tick bite reaction, cellulitis, erythema multiforme, nummular eczema, granuloma annulare, contact dermatitis, and alternative arthropod bites. For late stage Lyme, the differential includes juvenile idiopathic arthritis, rheumatoid arthritis, septic arthritis, gout, pseudogout, viral meningitis, multiple sclerosis, other etiologies of Bell palsy, and lymphoma.

▶ Treatment

The treatment of Lyme disease is complicated by the local and disseminated stages. Treatment options for those presenting with EM are doxycycline, cefuroxime, and amoxicillin for a ≥14-day course. There is some evidence supporting doxycycline use for only 10 days. Intravenous dosing with ceftriaxone, cefotaxime, and penicillin G is indicated in patients with central nervous system (CNS) and cardiac manifestations. Arthritis manifestations without CNS manifestations can be treated with the aforementioned oral medications for 28 days (Table 53–3).

▶ Prognosis

Prognosis for Lyme is good, especially with early treatment. Even if disease progresses to disseminated stage, disability is uncommon. Treatment at any stage portends a high likelihood of symptom resolution, but lasting symptoms typically consist of arthralgias and/or sensory deficits (cranial nerve VII). Chronic Lyme disease is a separate entity with symptoms typically consisting of musculoskeletal pain and fatigue. Chronic or posttreatment Lyme continues to be an area of

Table 53–3. Treatment of tickborne diseases.

Disease	First-Line Antibiotics (Adults)	First-Line Antibiotics (Children)	Duration	Alternative Regimens/Comments
Localized Lyme disease[a]	Doxycycline 100 mg PO BID, amoxicillin 500 mg PO TID Cefuroxime 500 mg PO BID	Doxycycline 4 mg/kg in divided doses BID, amoxicillin 50 mg/kg in divided doses TID, cefuroxime 30 mg/kg in divided doses BID	14 days, although can be extended to 21 days depending on case presentation	Macrolides can be used for patients who are intolerant of antibiotics listed; they are less effective; doxycycline 200 mg can be given as single-dose prophylaxis
Disseminated Lyme disease	CNS/carditis: Ceftriaxone 2 g IV once daily Cefotaxime 2 g IV every 8 hours Penicillin G 18–24 million units/d in 6 divided doses Arthritis without CNS: treat with antibiotics for localized disease	CNS/carditis: ceftriaxone 50–75 mg/kg IV Arthritis without CNS: treat with antibiotics for localized disease	CNS/carditis: 14–28 days Arthritis without CNS: 28 days	Doxycycline 200–400 mg/d orally in 2 divided doses if unable to tolerate β-lactam antibiotics Carditis patients should preferentially be treated with ceftriaxone
RMSF	Doxycycline 100 mg PO or IV BID	Doxycycline 2.2 mg/kg per dose PO or IV BID	At minimum 3 days after resolution of fever; minimum 5–7 days	Use doxycycline if RMSF suspected in all cases, including children; other antibiotics increase likelihood of mortality
Ehrlichiosis/HGA	Doxycycline 100 mg PO or IV BID		At minimum 3 days after resolution of fever; minimum 5–7 days	Rifampin is an alternative in special circumstances
Babesiosis	(1) Atovaquone 750 mg PO every 12 hours + azithromycin 500–1000 mg PO on day 1 and 250 mg once daily thereafter (2) Clindamycin 300–600 mg IV every 6 hours or 600 mg PO every 8 hours + quinine 650 mg PO every 6–8 hours	(1) Atovaquone 20 mg/kg PO every 12 hours + azithromycin 10 mg/kg PO on day 1 and 5 mg/kg once daily thereafter (2) Clindamycin 7–10 mg/kg IV or PO every 6–8 hours + quinine 8 mg/kg PO every 8 hours	Treat for at least 7–10 days	Clindamycin plus quinine is the standard for severe babesiosis, but not as well tolerated Treatment not recommended for asymptomatic patients

[a]The treatment recommendations for southern tick-associated rash illness at present are to use the same antibiotics indicated for localized Lyme disease.

BID, twice a day; CNS, central nervous system; HGA, human granulocytic anaplasmosis; IV, intravenous; PO, oral; RMSF, Rocky Mountain spotted fever; TID, 3 times a day.

controversy. Studies are ongoing as to potential etiologies, but continued antibiotic treatment after resolution of active disease is not indicated.

Centers for Disease Control and Prevention. *Tickborne Diseases of the United States: A Reference Manual for Health Care Providers.* 5th ed. 2018. https://www.cdc.gov/ticks/tickbornediseases/TickborneDiseases-P.pdf. Accessed December 2, 2019.

Graham J, Stockley K, Goldman RD. Tick-borne illness: a CME update. *Pediatr Emerg Care.* 2011;27(2):141–147. [PMID: 21293226]

Wormser GP, Dattwyler RJ, Shapiro ED, et al. The clinical assessment, treatment and prevention of Lyme disease, human granulocytic anaplasmosis, and babesiosis: clinical practice guidelines by the Infectious Diseases Society of America. *Clin Infect Dis.* 2006;43:1089–1134. [PMID: 17029130]

ROCKY MOUNTAIN SPOTTED FEVER (RSMF)

▶ General Considerations

A. Symptoms and Signs

RMSF cases have been reported in most US states. It is a medical misnomer because 60% of cases occur in North Carolina, Oklahoma, Arkansas, Tennessee, and Missouri. RMSF is considered to be the most severe tickborne illness in the United States because it causes a systemic, small-vessel vasculitis and has a mortality rate of ≥25% without treatment. The classic presentation of RMSF is fever, rash, and headache 2–14 days after a tick bite. However, myalgias, nausea, and changes in mental status are common on acute presentation. The hallmark rash of RMSF is maculopapular

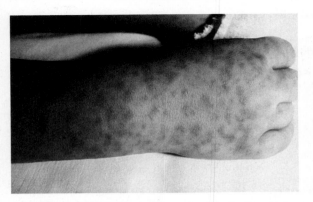

▲ **Figure 53–3.** Maculopapular rash of Rocky Mountain spotted fever. (Reproduced with permission from CDC Public Health Image Library.)

and occurs in ≤90% of patients, typically 2–5 days after the fever presents. The rash classically first appears as discrete, blanchable lesions on the wrists, ankles, and forearms that spread to the trunk, palms, and soles (Figure 53–3). However, diagnosis should not be based on the appearance of a rash, as this can delay treatment (Table 53–2).

Because of the vasculitic nature of the disease, petechiae can occur after 6 days of symptoms. Development of petechiae often occurs in untreated disease and is a poor prognostic sign. Another poor prognostic sign is CNS involvement with meningismus and altered mental status. Clinical diagnosis is imperative to initiating proper treatment, which significantly reduces morbidity.

B. Laboratory Findings

Early disease is associated with thrombocytopenia (most common), a mild elevation in liver enzymes, anemia, and hyponatremia. Again, RMSF is a clinical diagnosis because antibodies are detectable only 7–10 days after illness onset. In the event of a positive IgG antibody test, repeat testing 2–4 weeks following the initial testing is recommended. If the follow-up IgG testing demonstrates a fourfold titer increase, RMSF is confirmed. For patients presenting with CNS symptoms, CSF analysis is typically unremarkable (Table 53–2).

C. Other Considerations

Twenty percent of RMSF cases occur in children, making the diagnosis even more difficult given initial symptom overlap with other viral illnesses as well as other TBDs. It is important to bear in mind that 90% of cases are reported between April and September. In patients who are acutely ill, it is important to obtain infectious disease consultation early in the course of the evaluation and treatment.

Rickettsia parkeri rickettsiosis is a TBD closely related to RMSF. It is found in Gulf Coast ticks in the southeastern and mid-Atlantic states, as well as Arizona. *R parkeri* rickettsiosis is typically less severe than RMSF but often associated with an eschar at the site of the tick bite, which is not found in RMSF. Treatment is the same as that for RMSF.

▶ Treatment

The key treatment decision when RMSF is considered in the differential is to select doxycycline as the antibiotic of choice. Clinical suspicion merits treatment. Doxycycline is first-line therapy for patients of all ages, including children. There is no evidence to show permanent teeth discoloration with limited dosing, and unfortunately, the use of other antibiotics has been shown to increase mortality (Table 53–3).

▶ Prognosis

In patients who receive early antibiotics, the mortality rate with RMSF is approximately 2–3%. A delay in antibiotic treatment to >5 days increases that rate to >20%. Although most patients who are treated with antibiotics recover without long-term complications, some patients have persistent neurologic symptoms such as gait abnormalities, speech difficulty, dysphagia, and/or encephalopathy. These symptoms may resolve over time but reinforce the critical nature of early treatment with doxycycline.

Centers for Disease Control and Prevention. *Tickborne Diseases of the United States: A Reference Manual for Health Care Providers.* 5th ed. 2018. https://www.cdc.gov/ticks/tickbornediseases/TickborneDiseases-P.pdf. Accessed December 2, 2019.

Decker CF. When to suspect tick-borne illness. *Dis Mon.* 2012; 58(6):330–334. [PMID: 22608119]

Salinas LJ, Greenfield RA, Little SE, et al. Tickborne infections in the southern United States. *Am J Med Sci.* 2010;340(3):194–201. [PMID: 20697259]

Woods CR. Rocky Mountain spotted fever in children. *Pediatr Clin North Am.* 2013;60(2):455–470. [PMID: 23481111]

HUMAN GRANULOCYTIC ANAPLASMOSIS AND EHRLICHIOSIS

▶ General Considerations

A. Symptoms and Signs

Ehrlichiosis and HGA have similar clinical manifestations but are associated with two different species of ticks. HGA, commonly known as *anaplasmosis*, is associated with the *Ixodes* species and is also the tick that carries Lyme disease. Therefore, coinfection is possible as HGA is found in the same primary range of the Great Lakes and northeastern United States. Ehrlichiosis is reported most frequently in the southeastern United States. Both diseases present with fever, headache, malaise, and myalgias 1–2 weeks after tick bite. These nonspecific symptoms make the diagnosis difficult, and occasionally nausea, vomiting, and a maculopapular rash (particularly in children) complicate the diagnostic picture, due to a clinical presentation similarity to RSMF or Lyme disease.

Laboratory Findings

Nonspecific findings for both HGA and ehrlichiosis include mild anemia, thrombocytopenia, leukopenia, and liver enzyme elevation. During the early phase of illness, morulae, or HGA/ehrlichial inclusion bodies, may be visualized in leukocytes and are highly indicative of acute infection. However, the absence of morulae on peripheral smears does not exclude either diagnosis. Similar to RMSF, antibody testing is the gold standard for confirmation of disease. Initial IgG antibody titers positive for HGA or ehrlichiosis occur 7–10 days after symptoms start. Confirmation of disease is made by repeating IgG testing in 2–4 weeks and noting a fourfold increase in titers. Unlike RMSF, early polymerase chain reaction (PCR) testing is available, but most sensitive in the first week of illness, particularly before the administration of antibiotics.

Treatment

Despite the complexity in diagnosis plus overlapping range and symptoms with other TBDs, ehrlichiosis, HGA, Lyme, and RMSF can all be treated with doxycycline (Table 53–3). The rule of thumb should be that if a serious TBD is considered in the differential, use doxycycline for treatment. It can easily be discontinued or treatment refined if an alternative diagnosis is made. However, as with RMSF, doxycycline is the only antibiotic that is highly effective against HGA and ehrlichiosis. As in the case with all TBDs and pregnancy, consider an infectious disease consultation.

Prognosis

Mortality rates with HGA and ehrlichiosis are between 1% and 3% of those with known infections. Although 35–50% of patients will require hospitalization, a majority of those will recover completely with no long-term effects. The elderly and immunocompromised patients are at higher risk.

Centers for Disease Control and Prevention. *Tickborne Diseases of the United States: A Reference Manual for Health Care Providers.* 5th ed. 2018. https://www.cdc.gov/ticks/tickbornediseases/TickborneDiseases-P.pdf. Accessed December 2, 2019.

Qasba N. A case report of human granulocytic anaplasmosis (ehrlichiosis) in pregnancy and a literature review of tick-borne diseases in the United States during pregnancy. *Obstet Gynecol Surv.* 2011;66(12):788–796.

Salinas LJ, Greenfield RA, Little SE, et al. Tickborne infections in the southern United States. *Am J Med Sci.* 2010;340(3):194–201. [PMID: 20697259]

Wormser GP, Dattwyler RJ, Shapiro ED, et al. The clinical assessment, treatment and prevention of Lyme disease, human granulocytic anaplasmosis, and babesiosis: clinical practice guidelines by the Infectious Diseases Society of America. *Clin Infect Dis.* 2006;43:1089–1134. [PMID: 17029130]

BABESIOSIS

General Considerations

A. Symptoms and Signs

Unlike the TBDs described earlier, babesiosis is a protozoan-induced infection. It is reported in the northeastern United States and Great Lakes region, but sporadic cases have been noted across the country, and its incubation period ranges from 1 week to >2 months. The geographic variability and delayed presentation also confirm that babesiosis can be contracted via blood transfusion, which is unique among TBDs. There are approximately 10 such case reports a year.

Babesiosis can be asymptomatic, with only 60% of children and 80% of adults presenting with signs of infection. Typical symptoms include fever, chills, malaise, arthralgias, anorexia, nausea, and dark urine. The physical exam may demonstrate hepatosplenomegaly and jaundice secondary to hemolysis. Patients with hemolysis can have fulminant disease.

B. Laboratory Findings

Anemia secondary to this hemolysis is often noted in babesiosis, as is elevated blood urea nitrogen (BUN) and serum creatinine. Acutely, elevated liver enzymes and thrombocytopenia may also be noted. Microscopic identification of *Babesia* in the erythrocytes by peripheral blood smear is diagnostic, but the sensitivity is low. PCR analysis positive for *Babesia* is confirmatory, and IgG testing can be supportive but does not distinguish between acute and past infection.

Treatment

Similar to malaria, babesiosis requires the use of antiprotozoals. Two combination therapies are recommended: atovaquone plus azithromycin or quinine plus clindamycin. The latter combination is recommended in cases of serious infection. Treatment duration of 7–10 days is usually adequate.

Prognosis

Symptoms of fatigue may persist weeks to months after successful treatment, but complete resolution is common without persisting disability. Recurrence of infection, particularly in the elderly, immunocompromised, and asplenic requires extended treatment.

Cable RG, Leiby D. Risk and prevention of transfusion-transmitted babesiosis and other tick-borne diseases. *Curr Opin Hematol.* 2003;10(6):405–411. [PMID: 14564169]

Vannier E, Krause PJ. Human babesiosis. *N Engl J Med.* 2012;366(25):2397–2407 [PMID: 22716978]

Wormser GP, Dattwyler RJ, Shapiro ED, et al. The clinical assessment, treatment and prevention of Lyme disease, human granulocytic anaplasmosis, and babesiosis: clinical practice guidelines by the Infectious Diseases Society of America. *Clin Infect Dis.* 2006;43:1089–1134. [PMID: 17029130]

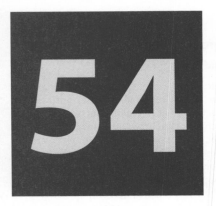

Tuberculosis

N. Randall Kolb, MD

Gordon Liu, MD, AAHIVS

Tuberculosis (TB) remains an important infectious disease for primary care physicians. In some parts of the world, significant problems exist in recognizing and diagnosing active TB and in using correct treatment to prevent the development of multidrug-resistant TB (MDR-TB). People infected with TB bacteria have a 5–15% lifetime risk of falling ill with TB. However, persons with compromised immune systems, such as people living with human immunodeficiency virus (HIV), malnutrition, or diabetes or people who use tobacco, have a higher risk of falling ill.

When a person develops active TB disease, the symptoms (eg, cough, fever, night sweats, or weight loss) may be mild for many months. This can lead to delays in seeking care and results in transmission of the bacteria to others. People with active TB can infect 10–15 other people through close contact over the course of a year. Without proper treatment, active TB will lead to death in about 45% of HIV-negative people and nearly all HIV-positive people. In the United States, nearly all people diagnosed with TB complete therapy, which limits the risk for further spread and prevents development of MDR-TB. Identification and treatment of people with latent TB infections (LTBI) will prevent active disease and is a public health priority in the United States.

Pennell PB, French JA, Harden CL, et al. Fertility and birth outcomes in women with epilepsy seeking pregnancy. *JAMA Neurol.* 2016;316(9):962–969. [PMID: 29710218]

World Health Organization. Tuberculosis data. www.who.int/tb/data. Accessed December 2, 2019.

▶ Definitions

TB infection is caused by *Mycobacterium tuberculosis*, which generally affects the lungs but can occur at many locations in body.

LTBI is exposure to *M tuberculosis* without active disease on clinical evaluation.

Primary TB is infection occurring shortly after exposure to *M tuberculosis*, which typically evolves to LTBI as immunity develops but can progress to active TB.

Postprimary TB is TB infection in patients previously sensitized to *M tuberculosis* that usually occurs as reactivation TB, but may occur with reinfection with a new strain of *M tuberculosis* (usually identified by genotype testing).

Extrapulmonary TB is localized infection at a site other than lungs such as lymph nodes, pleura, kidneys, genitalia, bones or joints, heart, nervous system (particularly meninges), any intra-abdominal organ (particularly at terminal ileum and cecum), peritoneum, and pericardium.

MDR-TB is defined as *M tuberculosis* resistant to isoniazid and rifampin.

Extensively drug-resistant (XDR) TB is defined as *M tuberculosis* isolates resistant to isoniazid, rifampin, any fluoroquinolone, and at least one of three injectable second-line drugs (amikacin, kanamycin, or capreomycin).

Treatment failure is defined as lack of symptom resolution or worsening symptoms, continued weight loss, or positive sputum smear after 2 months of treatment with anti-TB medication. Patients with advanced disease (ie, cavitary TB disease) may take longer to convert sputum cultures to negative but should be considered a treatment failure after 4 months of therapy.

Centers for Disease Control and Prevention. Progress toward elimination of rubella and congenital rubella syndrome–the Americas, 2003-2008. *MMWR Morb Mortal Wkly Rep.* 2006; 55(43):1176–1179. [PMID: 18971920]

World Health Organization. Treatment of tuberculosis: guidelines. 4th ed. https://www.ncbi.nlm.nih.gov/books/NBK138748/. Accessed December 2, 2019.

General Considerations

Globally, TB incidence is decreasing by about 2% per year, but TB remains one of the top 10 causes of death. In 2017, approximately 10 million people contracted TB, and 1.6 million died from the disease, including an estimated 1 million children who contracted the disease, of whom 230,000 died. It remains the leading cause of death and morbidity among people living with HIV, with 390,000 deaths in 2014.

In the United States, 9105 cases of TB were reported in 2017 and 528 deaths were attributed to TB in 2016. TB occurs in every part of the world, but there are wide variations in the incidence among countries. In 2017, the largest number of new TB cases occurred in the Southeast Asia and Western Pacific regions, with 62% of new cases, followed by the African region, with 25% of new cases. Ending the TB epidemic by 2030 is among the health targets of the newly adopted Sustainable Development Goals. The World Health Organization (WHO) has gone one step further and set a 2035 target of 95% reduction in deaths and a 90% decline in TB incidence, a rate similar to current levels in countries with low TB incidence.

MDR-TB remains a public health crisis and a health security threat. WHO estimates that there were 558,000 new cases with resistance to rifampicin, which is the most effective first-line drug. Eighty-two percent of these cases had MDR-TB. China, India, and the Russian Federation has the greatest burden of MDR-TB. Globally, about 8.5% of the MDR-TB cases are extensively resistant. The rate of MDR-TB has remained steady in the United States for the past 20 years at about 2% of cases, and XDR-TB occurred in two patients in 2017.

A total of 9105 TB cases (a rate of 2.8 cases per 100,000 persons) were reported in the United States in 2017, the lowest incidence of cases on record. The TB rate varies by race/ethnicity in the United States. Rates per 100,000 in 2017 were 19.1 in Native Hawaiians and other Pacific Islanders, 17.7 in Asians, 4.7 in blacks, 4.4 in Latinos, 3.9 in American Indians or Alaska Natives, and 0.5 in whites. The Centers for Disease Control and Prevention (CDC) estimates that only 13% of US TB cases are from recent transmission, with most cases resulting from reactivation of untreated LTBI.

The people most commonly affected in the United States are persons who were born in or travel to countries with high incidence of TB (70% of cases in US were among foreign-born persons in 2017), persons infected with HIV, homeless persons, and those who are incarcerated. Additional risk factors for TB are diabetes, excessive alcohol use, and intravenous (IV) drug use.

Centers for Disease Control and Prevention. Trends in Tuberculosis, 2018. www.cdc.gov/tb/publications/factsheets/statistics/tbtrends.htm. Accessed December 2, 2019.

World Health Organization. Global tuberculosis report. WHO/CDS/TB/2018.25. https://www.who.int/tb/publications/global_report/tb18_ExecSum_web_4Oct18.pdf. Accessed December 2, 2019.

Prevention

Adults with active TB are the most common source of TB, so prevention depends on timely diagnosis of active TB and prevention of active TB by treating LTBI in persons likely to develop active TB. Public health programs with intensive screening, treatment, and preventative therapy for household contacts of active TB cases may modestly decrease TB incidence rates by effectively preventing new cases of active TB. In countries with a high incidence of TB, WHO guidance issued in 2018 includes a new recommendation to consider testing and treatment for people age 5 years or older who are household contacts of bacteriologically confirmed pulmonary TB cases even in low-resource countries.

Tuberculin skin testing (TST) or interferon-γ release assays (IGRAs) are the primary screening methods in the United States for LTBI. These tests are not accurate in testing for active TB. The lack of a gold standard for diagnosis of LTBI prevents direct comparison of TST and IGRA, but latent class analysis provides estimates of test performance. The TST has low specificity among foreign-born children and adults, and the IGRA is the better test. In US-born, HIV-seropositive persons, the QuantiFERON-TB Gold had a low positive predictive value (relatively frequent false-positive results).

The method of administering the TST (previously referred to as a purified protein derivative [PPD]) is as follows:

- Inject 0.1 mL of PPD intradermally.
- This should produce a wheal of 6–10 mm.
- Read 48–72 hours after placement; do not let healthcare workers read their own results.
- Find and measure induration; do not measure redness.
- Sokal ballpoint pen method is as follows:
  - Place tip of ballpoint pen 1–2 cm away from margin of skin test reaction.
  - Move pen slowly toward center of reaction while applying moderate pressure.
  - Maintain skin tension if necessary by applying slight traction on skin behind pen in direction opposite pen movement.
  - When ballpoint reaches margin of induration and definite resistance to further movement is noted, lift pen.
  - Repeat procedure from opposite side of reaction.
  - Measure distance between margins of induration and record result.

If the TST reaction is read as ≥15 mm up to 7 days after placement, the result can be considered positive. Pregnant patients require no modification in testing or interpretation of results.

Persons at high priority for treatment of LTBI include the following:

1. Those with a positive TB blood test (IGRA).

2. TST induration ≥15 mm in persons with no risk factors for TB. Targeted TB testing programs should only be conducted among high-risk groups.

3. TST induration ≥10 mm in the following:

   - Persons from countries where TB is common, including Mexico, the Philippines, Vietnam, India, China, Haiti, and Guatemala, or other countries with high rates of TB (Of note, people born in Canada, Australia, New Zealand, or western and northern European countries are not considered at high risk for TB infection, unless they spent time in a country with a high rate of TB.)

   - Injection drug users

   - Residents and employees of high-risk congregate settings (eg, correctional facilities, nursing homes, homeless shelters, hospitals, and other healthcare facilities)

   - Mycobacteriology laboratory personnel

   - Children under 4 years of age or children and adolescents exposed to adults in high-risk categories

4. TST induration ≥5 mm in the following:

   - HIV-infected persons

   - Recent contacts of a patient with active TB disease

   - Persons with fibrotic changes on chest radiograph consistent with old TB

   - Organ transplant recipients

   - Persons who are immunosuppressed for other reasons (eg, taking the equivalent of >15 mg/d of prednisone for 1 month or longer, taking tumor necrosis factor-α antagonists)

Interpretation of the TST should not be affected by patient history of bacille Calmette-Guérin (BCG) vaccination, although the IGRA is the preferred test in this population

IGRA or TST is recommended before treatment with tumor necrosis factor-α inhibitors, such as infliximab (Remicade), etanercept (Enbrel), and adalimumab (Humira) See Table 54–1 for treatment of LTBI.

TST boosting is an issue in populations that will have repeated TST over time. Boosting occurs when a person with LTBI has a negative TST reaction when tested many years after the initial infection. The initial TST may stimulate (boost) T-cell ability to react, and then positive reactions to subsequent TSTs could be misinterpreted as recent conversions indicating recent infection. This problem is avoided by using the two-step testing for the initial TST. Testing with a blood assay for *M tuberculosis* such as QuantiFERON-TB Gold does not produce a boost, so a single baseline test is adequate.

Stout JE, Wu Y, Ho CS, et al. Evaluating latent tuberculosis infection diagnostics using latent class analysis. *Thorax.* 2018;73:1062–1070. [PMID: 29982223]

A. TST Two-Step Testing

Used for initial baseline *M tuberculosis* testing for those who will be given TST periodically (eg, healthcare workers or staff in homeless shelters). The two-step testing process is as follows:

- No previous TST: do two-step test

- First test positive: consider TB infected

- First test negative: retest in 1–3 weeks (after first TST result was read)

- Second test positive: consider TB infected

- Second test negative: consider not infected

When serial testing identifies a staff member who converts to a positive TST (≥10 mm increase in TST) or has a new positive blood assay for *M tuberculosis*, do a problem evaluation with contact investigation. This includes determining the likelihood and extent that *M tuberculosis* transmission occurred. Identify persons exposed and, if possible, the source of potential transmission. Identify factors that could have contributed to transmission (eg, failure of isolation procedures) and ensure that exposure to *M tuberculosis* has been terminated and conditions leading to exposure have been eliminated.

B. Screening for TB in Healthcare Providers

Baseline or preplacement TB screening of all healthcare providers (without documented prior TB disease or LTBI) should include both a symptom evaluation and a test (IGRA or TST). Serial screening is not recommended routinely, although healthcare facilities may screen annually certain groups identified to be at higher risk (eg, pulmonologists or respiratory therapists). All healthcare providers with LTBI should be offered treatment unless a contraindication exists. Healthcare personnel who do not complete LTBI treatment should be monitored with annual symptom evaluation to detect early evidence of TB disease.

Sosa LE, Njie GJ, Lobato MN, et al. Tuberculosis screening, testing, and treatment of U.S. health care personnel: recommendations from the national tuberculosis controllers association and CDC, 2019. *MMWR Morb Mortal Wkly Rep.* 2019;68:439–443. [PMID: 31099768]

C. Preventing TB in HIV-Positive Patients

In the United States, the most common predisposing factor for TB infection is birth or residence outside of the

Table 54–1. Latent tuberculosis infection treatment regimens.

Drug(s)	Duration	Dose	Frequency	Total Doses	
Isoniazid (INH)[a] and rifapentine (RPT)[b]	3 months	**Adults and children age 12 years and older:** INH: 15 mg/kg rounded up to the nearest 50 or 100 mg; 900 mg maximum RPT: 10–14.0 kg: 300 mg 14.1–25.0 kg: 450 mg 25.1–32.0 kg: 600 mg 32.1–49.9 kg: 750 mg ≥50.0 kg: 900 mg maximum **Children age 2–11 years:** INH[a]: 25 mg/kg; 900 mg maximum RPT[b]: as above	Once weekly[c]	12	
Rifampin[d]	4 months	Adult: 10 mg/kg Children: 15–20 mg/kg[e] Maximum dose: 600 mg	Daily	120	
INH	9 months	Adult: 5 mg/kg Children: 10–20 mg/kg[f] Maximum dose: 300 mg	Daily	270	
		Adult: 15 mg/kg Children: 20–40 mg/kg[f] Maximum dose: 900 mg	Twice weekly[c]	76	
	6 months	Adult: 5 mg/kg Children: Not recommended Maximum dose: 300 mg	Daily	180	
		Adult: 15 mg/kg Children: Not recommended Maximum dose: 900 mg	Twice weekly[c]	52	

[a]INH is formulated as 100-mg and 300-mg tablets.
[b]RPT is formulated as 150-mg tablets in blister packs that should be kept sealed until use.
[c]Intermittent regimens must be provided via directly observed therapy; that is, a healthcare worker observes the ingestion of medication.
[d]Rifampin (rifampicin) is formulated as 150-mg and 300-mg capsules.

United States. Therefore, patients with HIV infection who travel or work internationally in settings with a high prevalence of TB should be counseled about the risk of TB acquisition and the advisability of getting tested for LTBI upon return. Although there are risks for TB exposure in some healthcare and correctional settings in the United States, there is no need for precautions for persons with HIV infection beyond those taken for all persons in those settings. The estimated annual risk for active TB among untreated HIV-infected persons with LTBI is 3–16% per year. Annual testing for LTBI using TST is recommended for HIV-infected persons who are at high risk for repeated or ongoing exposure to persons with active TB. All patients with a positive TST or IGRA must be evaluated for active TB disease. The presence of cough (of any duration), fever, night sweats, weight loss, or lymphadenopathy or an abnormal chest radiograph requires obtaining a sputum culture.

After active TB is excluded, drug treatment of LTBI in patients with HIV infection is indicated for patients with a history of TST ≥5 mm, a positive result. Because the tests for LTBI depend on immune response, persons with negative diagnostic tests, with advanced HIV infection (CD4 cell count <200 cells/mm³), and without indications for initiating empiric LTBI treatment (ie, no recent exposure to a culture-confirmed TB case) should be retested for LTBI once they start antiretroviral therapy (ART) and attain a CD4 count ≥200 cells/mm³ to ensure the initial test was a true-negative result. HIV-infected close contacts of a case of infectious TB should be treated regardless of a negative TST or IGRA.

The preferred regimen is isoniazid (INH) 300 mg orally once daily and pyridoxine 50 mg orally once daily for 9 months. Alternative regimens include rifampin 600 mg orally once daily for 4 months (10–20 mg/kg/d for 6 months in children) or INH 15 mg/kg (maximum 900 mg) plus rifapentine 900 mg (reduced dose if <50 kg) once weekly under direct observation for 12 weeks. Despite the lack of clinical trial outcome data, once-weekly rifapentine/INH can be used with efavirenz or raltegravir without dose adjustment based on available pharmacokinetic data. Increased clinical monitoring is not recommended but should be based on clinical judgment. When using rifampin-containing regimens, either dose adjustment or substitution of key ART drugs may be needed. For persons exposed to drug-resistant TB, select treatment after consultation with experts or public health authorities.

> National Institutes of Health. Guidelines for the prevention and treatment of opportunistic infections in adults and adolescents with HIV. http://aidsinfo.nih.gov/contentfiles/lvguidelines/adult_oi.pdf. Accessed April 2019.

D. Monitoring Response to Treatment of LTBI

Individuals receiving self-administered LTBI treatment should be seen monthly to assess adherence and monitor for drug toxicity. If baseline serum aspartate aminotransferase or alanine aminotransferase and total bilirubin are abnormal, then they should be repeated monthly. If the liver enzymes increase by >5 times the upper limit of normal (or 3 times the upper limit of normal with symptoms), then treatment should be stopped. The risk of clinical hepatitis increases with daily alcohol consumption, underlying liver disease, and concurrent treatment with other hepatotoxic drugs. Patients should be reminded each visit about adverse side effects (unexplained anorexia, nausea, vomiting, dark urine, icterus, rash, persistent paresthesia of the hands and feet, persistent fatigue, weakness or fever lasting 3 or more days, abdominal tenderness, easy bruising or bleeding, and arthralgia) and be told to stop INH and go to the clinic for evaluation should any of these occur.

E. BCG Vaccination: CDC Guidelines

1. Children—BCG vaccination should only be considered for children who have a negative TST and who are continually exposed to, and cannot be separated from, adults who:

- Are untreated or ineffectively treated for TB disease (if the child cannot be given long-term treatment for infection); or
- Have TB caused by strains resistant to INH and rifampin.

2. Healthcare workers—BCG vaccination of healthcare workers should be considered on an individual basis in settings in which:

- A high percentage of TB patients are infected with *M tuberculosis* strains resistant to both INH and rifampin;
- There is ongoing transmission of such drug-resistant *M tuberculosis* strains to healthcare workers and subsequent infection is likely; or

- Comprehensive TB infection control precautions have been implemented but have not been successful.

Healthcare workers considered for BCG vaccination should be counseled regarding the risks and benefits associated with both BCG vaccination and treatment of LTBI.

3. Contraindications—BCG vaccination should not be given to persons who are immunosuppressed (eg, persons who are HIV infected) or who are likely to become immunocompromised (eg, persons who are candidates for organ transplant).

BCG vaccination should not be given during pregnancy. Even though no harmful effects of BCG vaccination on the fetus have been observed, further studies are needed to prove its safety.

Current evaluation is ongoing regarding whether BCG is helpful in persons who will have extended travel to endemic areas (eg, US active military personnel and US diplomatic corps); the published risk of infection is 4–8% for such travelers.

> The role of BCG vaccine in the prevention and control of tuberculosis in the United States. A joint statement by the Advisory Council for the Elimination of Tuberculosis and the Advisory Committee on Immunization Practices. *MMWR Recomm Rep.* 1996;45(RR-4):1–18. [PMID: 8602127]

▶ Preventing Transmission

Isolation and quarantine are components of preventing the spread of TB. Federal air travel restrictions allow health officers to notify the CDC and place a person with active TB on the "Do Not Board" list, which prevents people from boarding commercial aircraft in the United States. Patients with active TB are considered noninfectious and can board aircraft if they are on adequate drug therapy, show clinical response, and have two negative smears. Patients with MDR-TB represent a greater public health risk, and two negative cultures are recommended before removing them from the "Do Not Board" list.

While they are hospitalized, patients with confirmed or suspected active TB should be placed in respiratory isolation using the following standards:

- Place in an airborne infection isolation room. In existing healthcare settings, airborne infection isolation rooms should have airflow of six or more air changes per hour; 12 air changes per hour are recommended in new or renovated rooms.
- Healthcare workers should wear N95 disposable filtering face piece respirators, which must be fitted properly. Healthcare workers with significant facial hair should wear powered air purifying respirators with high-efficiency filters.
- The N95 respirator is designed to filter out droplet nuclei; it is *not* to be worn by the patient.

- Patients should be in a single room with a separate bathroom.
- Infectious patients should wear a surgical mask to stop droplet nuclei from being exhaled; surgical masks are *not* to be worn by healthcare workers or visitors.

Patients can be removed from respiratory isolation when infectious TB is unlikely and another diagnosis is made that explains the syndrome or the patient has three consecutive negative acid-fast bacillus (AFB) sputum smear results obtained at least 8 hours apart, has received standard anti-TB treatment (minimum of 2 weeks), and has demonstrated clinical improvement. For patients with MDR-TB, maintain isolation until they have a negative culture. Hospitalization for respiratory isolation is *not* required for newly diagnosed patients who can be treated as outpatients when directly observed therapy (DOT) has been arranged and the patient is willing to remain inside until noninfectious. In situations where household contacts are at high risk of contracting TB (immunocompromised person or those <4 years old), strongly consider alternate housing until the index patient is noninfectious.

World Health Organization. Tuberculosis and air travel. http://www.who.int/tb/publications/2008/WHO_HTM_TB_2008.399_eng.pdf. Accessed December 2, 2019.

▶ Clinical Findings of Active Tuberculosis

A. History

- Pulmonary TB
  - Cough may be productive or nonproductive but is often not present in patients with acquired immunodeficiency syndrome (AIDS)
  - Unexplained productive cough of >2 weeks in duration is common
  - Hemoptysis possible (but is a sign of advanced infection)
- Pulmonary and extrapulmonary TB symptoms
  - Fever
  - Loss of appetite
  - Weight loss
  - Weakness
  - Night sweats
  - Malaise
- Symptoms in extrapulmonary TB are often slight or absent until the disease is advanced and depend on the system/organ involved, but may include:
  - Lymphadenopathy
  - Painful urination, blood in urine, or frequent urination in genitourinary infection

  - Pelvic pain, menstrual irregularities (genitourinary TB in women)
  - Painless scrotal mass (genitourinary TB in men)
  - Pain in bones or joints
  - Headache, neck stiffness, decreased level of consciousness (TB meningitis)
  - Abdominal pain (gastrointestinal TB)
  - Chest pain (pericardial TB)
- Common symptoms in children
  - Cough >21 days
  - Fever >38°C (100.4°F) for 14 days
  - Weight loss
  - Pain is usual presenting symptom in skeletal TB; additional findings can include
    - Joint swelling
    - Limited range of motion
    - Bone tenderness
    - Limping

Symptom combination may be used to predict pulmonary TB in children in resource-poor settings. The combination of persistent cough for >2 weeks, documented failure to thrive (weight loss or deviation from growth percentiles) in prior 3 months, and fatigue had 82% sensitivity, 90% specificity, and 82% positive predictive value (PPV) in children age 3 years and older without HIV infection. In children <3 years old without HIV infection, the combination had 52% sensitivity, 92.5% specificity, and 90% PPV.

Marais BJ, Gie RP, Hesseling AC, et al. A refined symptom-based approach to diagnose pulmonary tuberculosis in children. *Pediatrics*. 2006;118(5):e1350–1359. [PMID: 17079536]
World Health Organization. Guidance for national tuberculosis programmes on the management of tuberculosis in children. WHO/HTM/TB/2006.371. https://www.who.int/tb/publications/childtb_guidelines/en/. Accessed December 2, 2019.

B. Physical Exam Findings

- Fever
- Weight loss
- Children may show poor weight gain or fall off growth curve

Head, eyes, ears, nose, and throat

- Choroidal tubercle (granuloma in choroid of retina) strongly suggestive of disseminated TB

Neck

- Lymphadenopathy
- Extrapulmonary TB in children is associated with nontender cervical lymphadenopathy with fistula formation

Chest

- Physical findings generally not helpful in diagnosis of pulmonary TB
  - Assess for rales, wheezes, or decreased breath sounds
  - Assess for tachycardia or friction rub

Abdomen

- With disseminated or abdominal TB
  - Hepatomegaly
  - Splenomegaly
  - Abdominal tenderness
  - Palpable mass
- Flank pain may be seen with genitourinary involvement

Back

- Extrapulmonary TB in children associated with gibbus (sharply angled kyphosis), especially of recent onset

C. Laboratory Testing Overview

When pulmonary TB is suspected, proceed with the following tests: (1) chest x-ray (may be omitted in resource-poor situations), (2) collect an initial sputum specimen and two subsequent morning samples to be tested for *M tuberculosis* identification using microscopy, including AFB smear (often negative in persons with HIV and active TB) or nucleic acid amplification testing (NAAT), which helps identify nontuberculous *Mycobacterium* in AFB-positive patients; and (3) send a culture, which is the gold standard for diagnosing TB (Table 54–2). The Xpert MTB/RIF test provides a rapid NAAT for diagnosis and detection of rifampin resistance. Sputum collection may require additional approaches in children who cannot produce a specimen. Gastric lavage may have higher yield than bronchoscopy, although nasopharyngeal aspiration may be preferable to gastric aspiration in children.

The NAAT can identify TB in smear-negative cases weeks earlier than culture and identify nontuberculous *Mycobacterium* in smear-positive cases, which helps accurately target contact investigations. CDC recommendations on use of smear and NAAT to direct therapy are as follows:

1. If the NAAT result is positive and the AFB smear result is positive, presume the patient has TB and begin anti-TB treatment while awaiting culture results.

2. If the NAAT result is positive and the AFB smear result is negative, use clinical judgment whether to begin anti-TB treatment while awaiting culture results and determine if additional diagnostic testing is needed. Consider testing an additional specimen using NAAT to confirm the NAAT result. A patient can be presumed to have TB, pending culture results, if two or more specimens are NAAT positive.

3. If the NAAT result is negative and the AFB smear result is positive, a test for inhibitors should be performed and an additional specimen should be tested with NAAT. Sputum specimens (3–7%) might contain inhibitors that prevent or reduce amplification and cause false-negative NAAT results.

   A. If inhibitors are detected, the NAAT test is of no diagnostic help for this specimen. Use clinical judgment to determine whether to begin anti-TB treatment while awaiting results of culture and additional diagnostic testing.

   B. If inhibitors are not detected, use clinical judgment to determine whether to begin anti-TB treatment while awaiting culture results and determine if additional diagnostic testing is needed. A patient can be presumed to have an infection with nontuberculous mycobacteria if a second specimen is smear positive and NAAT negative and has no inhibitors detected.

4. If the NAAT result is negative and the AFB smear result is negative, use clinical judgment to determine whether to begin anti-TB treatment while awaiting results of culture and additional diagnostic tests. Currently available NAAT tests are not sufficiently sensitive (detecting 50–80% of AFB smear-negative, culture-positive pulmonary TB cases) to exclude the diagnosis of TB in AFB smear-negative patients suspected to have TB.

Bronchoscopy is useful if active TB is suspected and smear is negative.

When extrapulmonary TB is suspected, collect fluid or tissue to test for *M tuberculosis* identification. A urinalysis should be sent if genitourinary infection is suspected, which may show pyuria or hematuria. Biopsy, needle aspiration, or imaging may be done as appropriate to site of suspected infection. Tests for protein, glucose, cell count, and differential are done on pleural, peritoneal, cerebrospinal or pericardial fluids of suspected infection site. For patients with HIV infection with no obvious localized infection but with fever, obtain blood or bone marrow culture for *M tuberculosis*. TST is not generally useful in the diagnosis of active TB but may be helpful in children and can support diagnosis in culture-negative cases. IGRAs do not appear to be accurate for diagnosing or ruling out active pulmonary or extrapulmonary TB, although they may help in diagnosis of pleural TB.

When TB is diagnosed, obtain baseline testing for management, including complete blood count, electrolytes, liver enzyme assay, creatinine, HIV test, and visual acuity and red-green color discrimination if ethambutol is used.

▶ Differential Diagnosis

See Table 54–3 for the differential diagnosis of TB.

Table 54–2. Diagnostic tests for tuberculosis (TB).

Test	Sensitivity (%)	Specificity (%)	Notes
Chest radiograph			May be normal with primary infection. Reactivation classic appearance is lesions in the apical-posterior segments of upper lung and superior segments of lower lobe. Cavitary lesions are associated with infectivity. In children, most common finding is opacification in the lung together with enlarged hilar or subcarinal lymph glands. HIV-positive patients have atypical radiographic changes more often than the classical findings.
Tuberculin skin test	59–100	44–100	Sensitivity and specificity vary with risk factors and size of induration. Generally positive 2–3 weeks after infection but can be as late as 12 weeks after exposure. Skin test is negative in about 25% of active TB patients. Most useful in diagnosing latent TB infection (LTBI).
Interferon-γ release assays: T-SPOT.TB or QuantiFERON-TB Gold	78	99	For diagnosis of LTBI.
Acid-fast bacillus smear	20–80		Early morning sputum or gastric aspirate (especially useful in children). Sensitivity increases to >90% with multiple specimens. False positive with nontuberculous mycobacteria. Specificity highest in endemic countries; sensitivity varies widely by laboratory. Sensitivity lower in HIV co-infection cohorts, so negative smear has low ability to rule out TB.
Solid media culture (Lowenstein-Jensen media)	67–82	99–100	Gold standard for diagnosis.
Liquid culture media (7H-12 BACTEC)	93–97	98	Can be used on specimen from any site. Can be positive in 2 weeks.
Nucleic acid amplification test	96 66	85 98	Smear-positive sample: positive predictive value >95% Smear-negative sample
Xpert MTB/RIF automated molecular test identification TB	90 82	98 98	HIV co-infection cohort
Xpert MTB/RIF automated molecular test for rifampin resistance	89 80	99 97	HIV negative HIV positive

▶ Treatment

CDC-recommended treatment regimens for adults and children include an initial phase treatment with INH, rifampin, pyrazinamide, and ethambutol, and then continuation phase treatment based on chest x-ray and sputum culture results (Table 54–4). In children whose visual acuity cannot be monitored, ethambutol is usually not recommended unless there is an increased likelihood of disease caused by INH-resistant organisms or the child has "adult-type" (upper lobe infiltration, cavity formation) TB. Extrapulmonary TB requires 6 months of therapy, except bone and joint disease, which requires 6–9 months, and neurotuberculosis requires 9–12 months. Corticosteroids are generally *not*

recommended but are strongly recommended in cases of TB pericarditis and neurotuberculosis.

- Initial empiric therapy usually includes four drugs daily for 2 months.
  - INH orally, IV, or intramuscularly: adult, 5 mg/kg/d (maximum 300 mg/d); children, 10–15 mg/kg/d (maximum 300 mg/d); weekly adult dose, 15 mg/kg (maximum 900 mg); twice weekly adult dose, 15 mg/kg (maximum 900 mg); children, 20–30 mg/kg (maximum 900 mg)
  - Rifampin orally or IV: adult, 10 mg/kg/d (maximum 600 mg/d); children, 10–20 mg/kg/d (maximum 600 mg/d)

Table 54–3. Differential diagnosis of tuberculosis (TB).

Disease	Characteristics
Nontuberculous *Mycobacterium*	Signs and symptoms may be the same as for *Mycobacterium tuberculosis*. Typically has less fever and weight loss.
Sarcoidosis	Dyspnea and cough. Chest x-ray: diffuse infiltrative lung disease with bilateral hilar adenopathy. Noncaseating granulomas on biopsy.
Aspiration pneumonia	May have indolent course. Radiologic infiltrates are more common in dependent areas. Look for risk factors such as loss of gag reflex and loss of consciousness.
Lung abscess	Frequently in posterior upper segment of upper lobes. May be acute or indolent. Patient usually has very foul-smelling sputum. Obtain specimen for culture.
Pulmonary fungal infections, such as histoplasmosis or coccidioidomycosis	Patient may have fever, cough, night sweats. These diseases are usually geographically specific. Chest x-rays may be miliary or can be cavitary. Obtain specimen for fungal stain and culture.
Granulomatosis with polyangiitis (Wegener)	Patients have fever and cough. Necrotizing granulomas in the lung and necrotizing glomerulonephritis. Chest x-ray often shows a cavitary lesion.
Actinomycosis	Cough, hemoptysis, and eventually draining sinuses with sulfur granules seen on stain are characteristic. Indolent course is common.
Neoplasm	Patients may have weight loss and cough similar to TB findings. Primary lung cancer, lymphoma, metastasis. Obtain specimen for cytology or biopsy.

- Pyrazinamide orally: adult, 25 mg/kg/d (maximum 2 g/d); children, 15–30 mg/kg/d
- Ethambutol orally: adult, 15 mg/kg/d (maximum 1.6 g/d); children, 20 mg/kg/d
- Streptomycin 15 mg/kg/d may be additional drug or substituted for ethambutol in some patients.
- Regardless of initial regimen, continuation phase typically is 4 months with INH and rifampin.

CDC-recommended number of doses to complete therapy is defined by completion of the recommended total number of doses, not necessarily the expected duration of therapy. If the specified number of doses cannot be administered in the expected time frame, the initial phase can be extended to 3 months, and doses for 18-week continuation phase can be extended for 6 months; if longer time frame cannot be met, consider as interrupted therapy. Treatment with DOT 5 days a week is considered equivalent to 7 days per week treatment.

WHO recommendations for dosing frequency in treatment of pulmonary TB in adults include DOT as the preferred initial management, and all patients receiving drugs for <7 days a week must receive DOT. New patients with pulmonary TB may receive 3 times weekly dosing throughout therapy, provided that every dose is directly observed and the patient is *not* HIV positive or living in an HIV-prevalent setting.

The standard regimen for new patients with TB is INH, rifampin, pyrazinamide, and ethambutol orally daily for 2 months, followed by INH and rifampin for 4 months. In countries with high levels of INH resistance in new patients and where INH drug susceptibility testing results are unavailable before the continuation phase begins, add ethambutol to 4-month INH and rifampin continuation phase (recommendation based on expert opinion not evidence).

WHO recommendations for treatment of TB in children are as follows (note higher dose of pyrazinamide compared to CDC):

- Recommended doses of anti-TB medications
  - INH: 10 mg/kg (range 7–15 mg/kg); maximum dose 300 mg/d
  - Rifampicin: 15 mg/kg (range 10–20 mg/kg); maximum dose 600 mg/d
  - Pyrazinamide: 35 mg/kg (30–40 mg/kg)
  - Ethambutol: 20 mg/kg (15–25 mg/kg)

World Health Organization. Treatment of tuberculosis guidelines. http://whqlibdoc.who.int/publications/2010/9789241547833_eng.pdf. Accessed December 2, 2019.

A. Treatment of Active TB in Patients With HIV

Initiation of ART during anti-TB therapy is associated with increased survival but also an increase in the risk of immune reconstitution inflammatory syndrome (IRIS). This paradoxical response as the patient is responding to the ART is presumed to be from the stronger immune response to TB

Table 54–4. Treatment regimens for patients with culture-positive pulmonary tuberculosis caused by drug-susceptible organisms: CDC guidelines.

Initiation Phase		Continuation Phase			Notes
Agents	Dosage and Minimal Duration	Agents	Dosage and Minimal Duration	Length of Therapy (total doses)	Notes
Isoniazid (INH), rifampin (RIF), pyrazinamide, ethambutol	Once daily for 8 weeks (56 doses) *or* 5 times per week for 8 weeks (40 doses DOT)	INH and RIF	Once daily for 18 weeks (126 doses) *or* 5 times per week for 18 weeks (90 doses DOT)	26 weeks (130–182)	Preferred regimen directly observed therapy (DOT) required for <7 times a week dosing. Daily regimen is required if HIV positive. When susceptibility testing shows sensitivity to INH and RIF, then ethambutol may be discontinued. If sputum smear positive at 2 months, repeat smear at 3 months.
		INH and RIF	Twice weekly for 18 weeks (36 doses DOT)	26 weeks (76–92)	Intermittent dosing not recommended for HIV-positive patients.
		INH and RIF	Once weekly for 18 weeks (18 doses DOT)	26 weeks (58–74)	Only for HIV-negative patients with no cavity on CXR and negative sputum at 2 months.
		INH and RIF	Daily for 31 weeks (217 doses, 155 DOT)	39 weeks (195–273)	If cavity on CXR and sputum positive at 2 months, maintain continuation phase for 31 weeks.
		INH and RIF	Twice weekly for 31 weeks (62 doses DOT)	39 weeks (102–118)	
INH, RIF, pyrazinamide, ethambutol	Once daily for 2 weeks, then twice weekly for 6 weeks (26 doses DOT) *or* 5 times per week for 2 weeks, then twice weekly for 6 weeks (22 doses DOT)	INH and RIF	Twice weekly for 18 weeks (36 doses DOT)	26 weeks (58–62)	Intermittent dosing not recommended for HIV-positive patients.
		INH and rifapentine	Once weekly for 18 weeks (18 doses DOT)	26 weeks (40–44)	Only for HIV-negative patients with no cavity on CXR and negative sputum at 2 months.
INH, RIF, pyrazinamide, ethambutol	3 times per week for 8 weeks (24 doses DOT)	INH and RIF	3 times per week for 18 weeks (54 doses DOT)	26 weeks (78)	
INH, RIF, ethambutol	Once daily for 8 weeks (56 doses) *or* 5 times per week for 8 weeks (40 doses DOT)	INH and RIF	Once daily for 31 weeks (217 doses) *or* 5 times per week for 31 weeks (155 doses DOT)	39 weeks (195–273)	May withhold pyrazinamide if pregnant, severe liver disease, or gout with extended continuation phase.
		INH and RIF	Twice weekly for 31 weeks (62 doses DOT)	39 weeks (102–118)	

CXR, chest x-ray; HIV, human immunodeficiency virus.

and includes fever, worsening pulmonary infiltrates and lymphadenopathy, and rarely, death.

US Department of Health and Human Services recommendations for timing of ART in patients with HIV and *M tuberculosis* coinfection are as follows:

- Start TB treatment immediately in patients with HIV infection and active TB
- All patients with HIV infection and active TB should be given ART.
  - For patients with CD4 counts <50 cells/mm³, start ART within 2 weeks of starting TB treatment to improve survival.
  - In patients with CD4 counts ≥50 cells/mm³ and no severe clinical disease, there is less evidence that early ART improves survival with treatment of active TB. ART can be delayed to 8 weeks to reduce the risk of IRIS.
  - In pregnant women, start ART as early as possible, both for maternal health and prevention of mother-to-child transmission.
  - In patients with documented MDR-TB and XDR-TB, start ART within 2–4 weeks of confirmation of TB drug resistance and initiation of second-line TB therapy.
- For patients on ART who develop TB, treatment should begin immediately and ART modified to reduce the risk of drug interaction and maintain viral suppression.

The cotreatment of HIV-related TB disease is rifampin-based therapy with an antiretroviral regimen of efavirenz plus two nucleoside(tide) analogs. Standard-dose efavirenz (600 mg) is the US public health recommendation. Other guidelines recommend the combination of raltegravir-based ART using 400 or 800 mg twice daily with the standard rifampin dosing. The recommended initial TB treatment is four drugs for 2 months consisting of INH plus rifampicin (or rifampin) plus pyrazinamide plus ethambutol; rifabutin is substituted for rifampin in patients taking protease inhibitors or maraviroc. The preferred continuation therapy is INH plus rifampicin for 4 months, given once daily or 2–3 times weekly (but not twice weekly if CD4 counts <100 cells/mm³). Duration of therapy is 6 months, except for patients with cavitary lung disease, delayed response to therapy, or extrapulmonary TB, in which case duration of therapy is 9 months. Extending treatment from 6 months to 12 months in patients with HIV infection with pulmonary TB may reduce relapse rates. Long-term INH plus sulfadoxine/pyrimethamine may reduce recurrence and sick days after recovery from pulmonary TB in patients with HIV infection. Because of significant drug interactions, the following should not be used with rifampin: rilpivirine, etravirine, and elvitegravir coformulated with cobicistat. Tenofovir alafenamide should not be used with any of the rifamycins.

Trimethoprim/sulfamethoxazole (cotrimoxazole) reduces mortality in patients with HIV infection treated for pulmonary TB. Add corticosteroids when treating central nervous system and pericardial disease. Adjunctive prednisolone therapy may reduce mortality in patients with tuberculous pericarditis. Recommended doses are dexamethasone 0.3–0.4 mg/kg/d tapered over 6–8 weeks or prednisone 1 mg/kg/d for 3 weeks then tapered for 3–5 weeks.

The WHO proposes the following approach that is useful in resource-limited environments for the diagnosis and treatment of TB in HIV-prevalent settings. For ambulatory patients with cough for 2–3 weeks and no danger signs (ie, respiratory rate >30/min, fever >39°C [102.2°F], pulse rate >120 bpm, unable to walk unaided), obtain an AFB and HIV test at the first visit. Treat patients who are HIV positive or whose status remains unknown as follows:

- If AFB positive: treat for TB, cotrimoxazole, HIV assessment
- If AFB-negative: chest x-ray, sputum AFB and culture, clinical assessment (all at same time wherever possible to decrease visits and time to diagnosis)
  - If TB likely: treat for TB, cotrimoxazole, HIV assessment
  - If TB unlikely: HIV assessment and one of the following
    - Treat for bacterial infection plus cotrimoxazole
    - Treat for *Pneumocystis jirovecii* pneumonia, especially if hypoxic
      - If response: advise to return if symptoms recur
      - If no or partial response: reassess for TB

WHO recommendations for dosing regimens in children with and without HIV are as follows:

- Four-drug regimen of INH, rifampin, pyrazinamide, and ethambutol for 4 months, followed by INH and rifampin regimen for 4 months, should be given in any of following cases:
  - Children with extensive pulmonary disease
  - Children living in places with high INH resistance or high HIV prevalence (≥1% in adult pregnant women or ≥5% in patients with TB) who have suspected or confirmed:
    - Pulmonary TB, or
    - Tuberculous peripheral lymphadenitis
- Three-drug regimen (INH, rifampin, pyrazinamide) for 2 months followed by a two-drug regimen of INH and rifampin for 4 months can be given to children without HIV infection living in places with low HIV prevalence and INH who have suspected or confirmed:
  - Pulmonary TB, or
  - Tuberculous peripheral lymphadenitis

- Avoid intermittent (2 times weekly or 3 times weekly) dosing regimens in children with HIV infection or in any children living in high HIV prevalence areas with suspected/confirmed pulmonary TB or tuberculous peripheral lymphadenitis.

- Treat children with suspected or confirmed tuberculous meningitis or osteoarticular TB with standard four-drug regimen of INH, rifampin, pyrazinamide, and ethambutol for 2 months, followed by standard two-drug regimen of INH and rifampin for 10 months, for total duration of treatment of 12 months.

WHO recommendations for dosing frequency in patients with HIV are as follows: TB patients with known positive HIV status and all TB patients living in HIV-prevalent settings should receive daily TB treatment during the intensive and continuation phase.

Guidelines for treatment of drug-susceptible tuberculosis and patient care: 2017 update. Geneva: World Health Organization; 2017 (WHO/HTM/TB/2017.05; http://apps.who.int/iris/bitstream/10665/255052/1/9789241550000-eng.pdf?ua=1, accessed 1 May 2018).

B. Treatment of MDR-TB

The most effective way to prevent MDR-TB is to implement quality TB programs. Availability of appropriate medications and adherence to TB treatment and care help prevent the development of MDR-TB; availability of and adherence to MDR-TB treatment, in turn, help prevent the development of XDR-TB.

CDC recommendations for treatment of MDR-TB are as follows: Never add only one new drug to an ineffective regimen. When starting or changing treatment, use three or more previously unused drugs that have demonstrated in vitro susceptibility. Use more than three agents if other previously unused drugs likely to be active are available. Bedaquiline may be used if other agents are not available and the benefit is considered greater than the risk. If this agent is used with drugs that induce or suppress CYP3A4, contact the CDC for specific information on risks and monitoring. In patients with MDR-TB resistant to INH, rifampin, and

another first-line agent, consider regimens with four to six medications, and institute hospital-based or home-based DOT for oral medications.

The duration of therapy to cure TB patients can range from 6 months for drug-susceptible TB to >2 years for XDR-TB. During treatment, some patients may travel or move to another country without plans for continuing their treatment in their destination.

WHO principles of treatment of MDR-TB have been revised and are evolving. The guidelines include extensive information on treatment length and monitoring for effectiveness and side effects. The basic treatment involves medications from three groups and focuses on oral medications.

Group A: Fluoroquinolones (levofloxacin and moxifloxacin), bedaquiline, and linezolid were considered highly effective and strongly recommended to be included in all regimens unless contraindicated; include three drugs from this group.

Group B: Clofazimine and cycloserine or terizidone were conditionally recommended as agents of second choice; one or both added to the group A medications.

Group C: Included all other medicines that can be used when a regimen cannot be composed with group A and B agents. The medicines in group C are ranked by the relative balance of benefit to harm usually expected of each. These include the following:

Ethambutol

Delamanid

Pyrazinamide

Imipenem-cilastatin *or* meropenem

Amikacin (*or* streptomycin)

Ethionamide *or* prothionamide

p-Aminosalicylic acid

World Health Organization. WHO treatment guidelines for multidrug- and rifampicin-resistant tuberculosis, 2018 update. https://www.who.int/tb/areas-of-work/drug-resistant-tb/guideline-update2018/en/. Accessed December 2, 2019.

HIV Primary Care

Ramakrishna Prasad, MD, MPH
Praneeth Pillala, MBBS
Gordon Liu, MD, AAHIVS

 ESSENTIALS OF DIAGNOSIS AND TREATMENT

▶ In the United States of America, the Human Immunodeficiency Virus (HIV) Laboratory Diagnostic Testing Algorithm (Centers for Disease Control and Prevention [CDC]) is used. This algorithm recommends initial testing with an HIV-1/2 antigen/antibody immunoassay (step 1). A single HIV test result cannot provide a definitive HIV-positive diagnosis. If the initial test is *reactive*, specimens should be tested with an HIV-1/HIV-2 antibody differentiation assay (step 2). In case of *negative or indeterminate* results at step 2, HIV-1 nucleic acid amplification test (NAAT) is recommended. Globally, the World Health Organization (WHO)–recommended testing algorithms are widely used. The HIV prevalence of the population—either high (≥5%) HIV prevalence or low (<5%) HIV prevalence—is used to inform national HIV testing algorithms (which may vary from country to country).

▶ HIV RNA level (viral load) should be ideally used to monitor response to antiretroviral therapy. In resource-limited settings where access to viral load monitoring is limited, CD4 measurements along with clinical assessments may be used to monitor therapy.

▶ Absolute CD4 lymphocyte count is widely used for staging HIV disease. *Acquired immunodeficiency syndrome* (AIDS) is defined as a CD4 <200 cells/mm³. AIDS represents advanced HIV disease that is associated with opportunistic infections or malignancy in the absence of treatment.

▶ Although HIV infection cannot be cured currently, antiretroviral drugs are highly effective in suppressing viral replication and enable people living with HIV to enjoy

healthy, long, and productive lives. Additionally, they prevent transmission to others.

▶ One of the landmark recent advances with the potential to combat stigma has been the recognition of "U = U" (undetectable = untransmittable). There is now evidence-based confirmation that the risk of HIV transmission from people living with HIV, who are on antiretroviral therapy (ART) and have achieved an undetectable viral load in their blood for at least 6 months, is negligible.

▶ General Considerations

As we approach the conclusion of the fourth decade of the HIV/AIDS epidemic, major shifts in the epidemiology and prognosis of HIV disease have occurred. Significant advances in treatment of HIV infection have transformed this fatal disease into a chronic multisystem disease characterized by multiple comorbidities, with noninfectious complications. A major achievement in the past decade has been the scale-up of access to ART globally. In 2017, 21.7 million people living with HIV were receiving ART, with 59% of adults and 52% of children living with HIV receiving lifelong ART. The global ART coverage for pregnant and breastfeeding women living with HIV is high, at 80%. Between 2000 and 2017, new HIV infections fell by 36%, and HIV-related deaths fell by 38%, with 11.4 million lives saved due to ART in the same period. In July 2017, the CDC published a comprehensive analysis of the US HIV care continuum showing that, in 2014, of the estimated 1.1 million people living with HIV in the United States, 85% knew they were infected, and about half (49%) were virally suppressed.

HIV continues to be a major global public health issue. In 2017, nearly a million people died from HIV-related causes globally. There were approximately 36.9 million people living with HIV at the end of 2017 with 1.8 million people

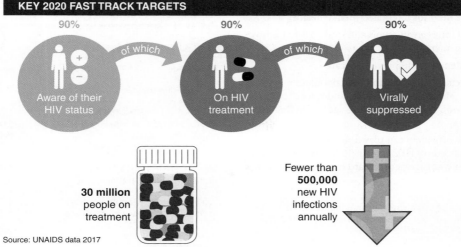

90-90-90 treatment targets:

Source: UNAIDS data 2017

▲ **Figure 55–1.** Global 90-90-90 Targets set by the United Nations Program on AIDS/HIV (UNAIDS) to help end the AIDS epidemic.

becoming newly infected in 2017 globally. The WHO African region is the most affected region, with 25.7 million people living with HIV in 2017. The African region also accounts for over two-thirds of the global total of new HIV infections.

The HIV epidemic continues to be particularly devastating among key populations. Key populations are groups who are at increased risk of HIV irrespective of epidemic type or local context. They include men who have sex with men, people who inject drugs, people in prisons and other closed settings, sex workers and their clients, and transgender people. In 2017, an estimated 47% of new infections occurred among key populations and their partners. Key populations often have legal and social issues that increase vulnerability to HIV and reduce access to testing and treatment programs.

Nearly 80% of new HIV transmissions are from persons who do not know they have HIV infection or are not receiving regular care. This not only impedes their linkage to care but also establishes a reservoir for the spread of HIV within populations.

Previous AIDS targets sought to achieve incremental progress. However, the aim now is to put an end to the AIDS epidemic by 2030. Momentum is now being built toward this final and ambitious target with confidence that it is achievable through global concerted action. The goals are as follows:

- By 2020, 90% of all people living with HIV will know their HIV status.

- By 2020, 90% of all people with diagnosed HIV infection will receive sustained ART.

- By 2020, 90% of all people receiving ART will have viral suppression.

The Global 90-90-90 Targets set by the United Nations Program on AIDS/HIV (UNAIDS) to help end the AIDS epidemic are shown in Figure 55–1.

Li Z, Purcell DW, Sansom SL, et al: Vital Signs: HIV transmission along the continuum of care—United States, 2016. https://www.cdc.gov/mmwr/volumes/68/wr/mm6811e1.htm. Accessed on May 10, 2019.

UNAIDS. 90-90-90: An ambitious treatment target to help end the AIDS epidemic; 2017. http://www.unaids.org/en/resources/909090. Accessed May 7, 2019.

▶ **Intended Audience of This Chapter**

This chapter is intended for primary care providers, including family physicians, internists, nurse practitioners, and physician assistants. It is also geared to the needs of medical students and postgraduate trainees in family medicine, internal medicine, and other fields.

The aspects of HIV care discussed in this chapter are as follows:

- Risk factors and transmission

- Natural history and staging of HIV disease

- Screening and diagnosis of HIV infection

- Initial evaluation and management of an HIV-infected individual, including medical history and physical examination, laboratory assessments, and diagnostic testing

- Principles of treatment of HIV infection, including prevention of opportunistic infections

- Overview of comorbidities, complications, and end-organ dysfunction associated with chronic HIV infection including the need for integrated mental health

- Motivational interviewing tools and strategies to improve patient engagement

- Health maintenance and preventive care

- Unique aspects of HIV care in special populations such as lesbian, gay, bisexual, transgender, and queer (LGBTQ) groups and women of childbearing age (including pregnant women)

Primary care providers can play a major role in improving the overall cascade of HIV care, including detection, linkage, retention, and engagement toward improving outcomes of treatment.

Chu C, Selwyn PA. An epidemic in evolution: the need for new models of HIV care in the chronic disease era. *J Urban Health*. 2011;88(3):556–566. [PMID: 21360244]

▶ Risk Factors & Transmission

HIV is a retrovirus transmitted by (1) unprotected sexual contact, (2) exposure to infected blood through sharing of injection drug use paraphernalia or receipt of contaminated blood products, and (3) perinatal transmission. Studies have yielded estimates of the probability of HIV transmission by various routes in adults and adolescents (Table 55–1). Factors such as plasma HIV RNA levels in the source patient; presence of sexually transmitted infections (STIs), including syphilis, gonorrhea, herpes simplex, chlamydial infection, and human papillomavirus infection; and the quantity of infectious blood transferred influence per-exposure probabilities of transmission.

There is now evidence-based confirmation that the risk of HIV transmission from a person living with HIV who is on ART and has achieved an undetectable viral load in his or her blood for at least 6 months is negligible to nonexistent. Thus, regular monitoring of patients on ART through a viral load test not only has benefits of early detection of drug resistance, but also has the positive benefit of empowering HIV-positive individuals to commit to initiating and adhering to a successful treatment regimen. The "U = U" (undetectable = untransmittable) principle allows serodiscordant couples to enter into a sexual relationship, marry, and conceive an HIV-negative child.

UNAIDS. Undetectable = Untransmittable, 2018. http://www .unaids.org/sites/default/files/media_asset/undetectable-untransmittable_en.pdf. Accessed May 7, 2019.

▶ HIV Subtype Diversity & the Increasing Challenge of Drug-Resistant HIV

The dominant strains of HIV differ in different parts of the world. Figure 55–2 shows the distribution of HIV-1 subtypes

Table 55–1. Per exposure probabilities of HIV transmission by route.

Manner of HIV Exposure	Per-Exposure HIV Acquisition Risk
Blood transfusion	90–95 in 100
Mother-to-child transmission (without ART)	15–40 in 100
Injection drug use (needle sharing) Percutaneous needlestick (healthcare setting, known HIV-infected blood) Needlestick in community setting	6.7 in 1000 3 in 1000 Not reported to date
Unprotected receptive anal intercourse Unprotected insertive anal intercourse	5–32 in 1000 6.5 in 10,000
Unprotected receptive vaginal intercourse Unprotected insertive vaginal intercourse	1–3 in 1000 3–9 in 10,000
Receptive oral intercourse Insertive oral intercourse	1 in 10,000 5 in 100,000
Mucous membrane exposure (healthcare setting, known HIV-infected blood)	9 in 10,000

ART, antiretroviral therapy.
Modified with permission from Tolle MA, Schwarzwald HL: Postexposure prophylaxis against human immunodeficiency virus. *Am Fam Physician*. 2010 Jul 15;82(2):161–166.

and circulating recombinant forms (CRFs). Clades and CRFs are important because of differences in transmission, rates of disease progression, drug susceptibilities, and potential efficacy issues with a vaccine. For instance, studies have shown that subtype D, found in Kenya, results in higher mortality rates and faster CD4 T-cell declines than subtypes A or C.

Minimizing the emergence and transmission of HIV drug resistance (HIVDR) is a critical aspect of the broader response required to achieve the Global 90-90-90 Targets for treatment. The human costs of HIVDR are significant: people with nonnucleoside reverse transcriptase inhibitor (NNRTI) resistance are less likely to achieve viral suppression; more likely to experience virologic failure or death; more likely to discontinue treatment; and more likely to acquire new HIVDR mutations. Preventing, monitoring, and responding to HIVDR are therefore critical to maintaining current achievements, improving treatment outcomes for people living with HIV, protecting investments, and guaranteeing the long-term sustainability of care and treatment programs.

Drug resistance in HIV is typically characterized as (1) primary or transmitted or pretreatment drug resistance or (2) secondary or acquired or posttreatment drug resistance. Primary drug resistance is when a drug-resistant HIV (DR-HIV) strain is transmitted to a previously uninfected individual, such that the recipient now has pretreatment DR-HIV.

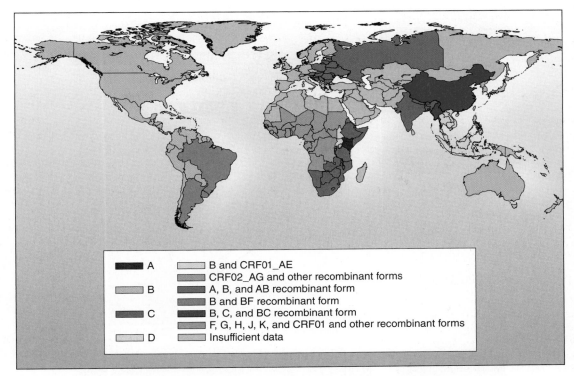

▲ Figure 55–2. Current global distribution of HIV-1 subtypes and recombinant forms.

Pretreatment drug resistance is more than twofold higher among people starting first-line ART with prior antiretroviral drug exposure, compared to antiretroviral drug–naive individuals. With continued ART scale-up, this group is likely to represent an increasing proportion of people initiating treatment who may not be receiving effective treatment.

Secondary DR-HIV is the more common type of HIVDR. It arises in an individual on therapy. This happens when the concentration of ART is not sufficient to suppress the virus but is high enough to exert a positive selective pressure on the virus to become resistant. Factors that influence secondary DR-HIV include lack of adequate and regular adherence counseling, lack of sufficient social support networks for the patient, irregular supply of ART, or other reasons that lead to a less than optimal drug dosage within the patient. Acquired DR-HIV is associated with increased risk of mortality.

A genotypic resistance test is used to determine whether the patient was infected with drug-resistant virus, which could affect the choice of initial therapy. In settings where access to resistance testing exists, it should always be performed at baseline, regardless of the need for ART. Resistance testing is also used at the time of virologic failure to choose the subsequent antiretroviral regimen.

It is important for healthcare professionals to be aware of the rising burden of HIVDR. In the coming decade, the issue of HIVDR is anticipated to increase in importance and, if not addressed adequately and in a concerted manner, threatens to derail the accomplishment of the 90-90-90 targets.

Taylor BS, Hammer SM. The challenge of HIV-1 subtype diversity. *N Engl J Med*. 2008;359(18):1965–1966. [PMID: 18971501]

World Health Organization. HIV drug resistance report, 2017. https://www.who.int/hiv/pub/drugresistance/hivdr-report-2017/en/. Accessed May 7, 2019.

PROGRESSION OF HIV INFECTION

The progression of HIV disease is well established. On infection, and in the absence of treatment, viral replication progressively depletes the immune system and results in immunodeficiency, which renders the infected individual susceptible to a multitude of opportunistic infections and malignancies (Figure 55–3). The stages of HIV infection are shown in Table 55–2. Table 55–3 lists opportunistic infections by CD4 counts. The rate of progression is variable, and

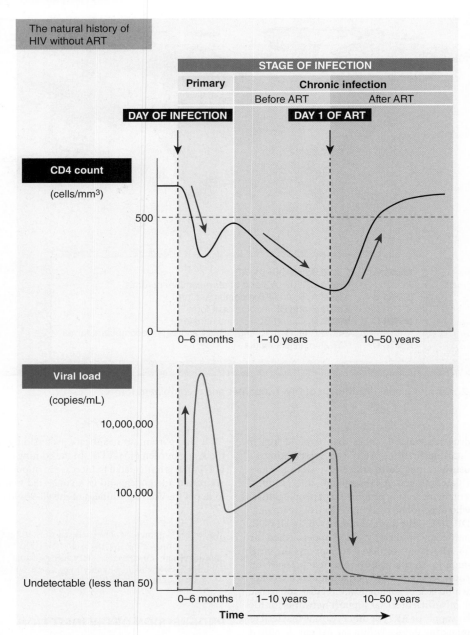

▲ **Figure 55–3.** Progression of HIV disease. (Reproduced with permission from HIV i-Base. http://i-base.info/guides/art-in-pictures/the-natural-history-of-hiv-without-art.)

Table 55–2. Clinical stages of HIV/AIDS.

Acute infection or seroconversion	1. Presents as a flulike illness. 2. Usually within *2–4 weeks* after infection with HIV. 3. Infected individuals may experience fever (80–95%), sore throat (70–80%), lymphadenopathy (40–80%), rash (40–70%), and other symptoms including diarrhea, malaise, thrush, weight loss, or hepatosplenomegaly. 4. Because of extremely high viral loads and lack of awareness of one's serostatus, this is a highly infectious period.
Clinical latency	1. This is a prolonged period of usually asymptomatic infection that ensues. 2. During this phase, HIV reproduces at relatively lower levels. While CD4 T-cell destruction is ongoing, their levels are high enough that the patient may remain asymptomatic and without any *opportunistic infections*. 3. This period may last up to *8 years* or longer.
AIDS	1. Over the course of many years of lymphocyte depletion, eventually the absolute CD4 cell count falls below *200 cells/μL* (normal CD4 counts are 500–1600 cells/mm³). 2. This stage is characterized by numerous opportunistic infections and malignancies. 3. Without treatment, individuals with AIDS have a life expectancy of 1–3 years.

Table 55–3. Common opportunistic infections (OIs) by CD4 count.

Absolute CD4 Count	Opportunistic Infection/ Malignancy	Specific OI Prophylaxis Recommended
>300	Vaginal candidiasis Tuberculosis Skin disease Fatigue Bacterial pneumonia Herpes zoster	No specific OI prophylaxis
<300	Oral hairy leukoplakia Thrush, Fever, diarrhea, weight loss	
<200	Kaposi sarcoma Non-Hodgkin lymphoma *Pneumocystis carinii* pneumonia Central nervous system (CNS) lymphoma	Pneumocystis prophylaxis with Bactrim (sulfamethoxazole/trimethoprim; 1 tablet daily) [Stop primary or secondary prophylaxis in individuals with CD4 counts of 100 cells/mm³ to 200 cells/mm³ if HIV plasma RNA levels remain below limits of detection for ≥3 months to 6 months]
<100	Toxoplasmosis Esophageal candidiasis Cryptococcosis	Toxoplasma prophylaxis with Bactrim DS (1 tablet daily)
<50	Cytomegalovirus *Mycobacterium avium* complex (MAC) CNS lymphoma	MAC prophylaxis with azithromycin (1200 mg weekly) [In individuals who immediately initiate antiretroviral therapy, it is no longer recommended, regardless of CD4 cell count]

in a small number of individuals, disease progression may be significantly slower.

▶ Screening

It is important to recognize that risk factor–based HIV testing has not been successful. The CDC has recommended **universal screening** for HIV infection since 2006. In 2012, the US Preventive Services Task Force (USPSTF) also updated its recommendations and now endorses screening all individuals age 15–65 years for HIV infection, **irrespective of risk factors**. Thereafter, screening should be repeated upon risk assessment. All pregnant women should also be screened for HIV. **Testing should be performed on an "opt-out" basis, meaning that unless patients decline, they should be tested.** It is critical to recognize that unless an infected individual is tested and detected to be HIV infected, they have no opportunity to access treatment.

Association of Public Health Laboratories. Suggested reporting language for the HIV laboratory diagnostic testing algorithm, 2019. https://www.aphl.org/aboutAPHL/publications/Documents/ID-2019Jan-HIV-Lab-Test-Suggested-Reporting-Language.pdf. Accessed May 7, 2019.

Centers for Disease Control and Prevention. New CDC recommendations for HIV testing in laboratories, 2014. https://www.cdc.gov/nchhstp/newsroom/docs/2014/HIV-testing-Labs-Flowchart.pdf. Accessed May 7, 2019.

US Preventive Services Task Force. Human immunodeficiency virus (HIV) infection: screening. 2013. https://www.uspreventiveservicestaskforce.org/Page/Document/UpdateSummaryFinal/human-immunodeficiency-virus-hiv-infection-screening. Accessed April 19, 2019.

World Health Organization. Quality of HIV testing and prevention of misdiagnosis, 2017. https://www.who.int/hiv/mediacentre/news/hiv-misdiagnosis-qa/en/index2.html. Accessed April 24, 2019.

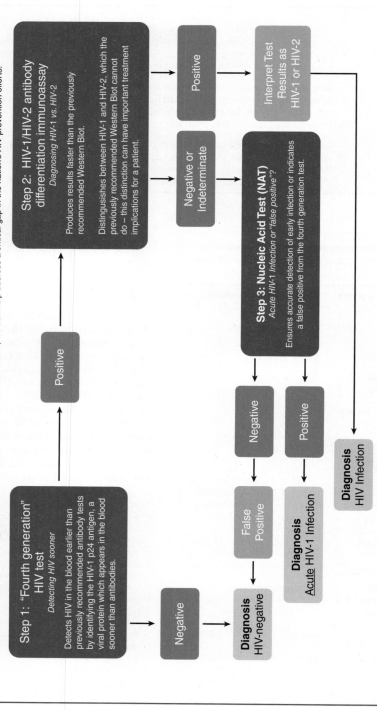

▲ **Figure 55–4.** Centers for Disease Control and Prevention (CDC) recommendations for HIV testing in laboratories. (Reproduced with permission of the Centers for Disease Control and Prevention (CDC).)

Postexposure Prophylaxis Against HIV

PEP stands for *postexposure prophylaxis*. The word *prophylaxis* means to prevent or protect from an infection or disease. PEP must be started within 72 hours (3 days) after a possible exposure to HIV. The sooner you start PEP after a possible HIV exposure, the better. PEP involves taking HIV medicines every day for 28 days.

National Institutes of Health. AIDS info: Postexposure prophylaxis, 2018. https://aidsinfo.nih.gov/understanding-hiv-aids/fact-sheets/20/87/post-exposure-prophylaxis–pep-. Accessed May 7, 2019.

The Window Period

The time between when a patient gets infected with HIV and when a test can reliably detect HIV is called the *window period*. The window period differs from individual to individual as well as by type of HIV test. Figure 55–5 shows the different types of window periods for various tests.

Preexposure Prophylaxis Against HIV

Preexposure prophylaxis (or PrEP) is for people at high risk of contracting HIV. As a part of PrEP, they can take HIV medicines daily (or episodically in some situations) to lower their risk of getting infected. It is highly effective for preventing HIV if used as prescribed, but it is much less effective when not taken consistently.

Daily PrEP reduces the risk of getting HIV from sex by >90%. Among people who inject drugs, it reduces the risk by >70%. A person's risk of getting HIV from sex can be even lower if PrEP is used in combination with condoms and other prevention methods.

Additionally, particularly among men who have sex with men, PrEP (a combination pill of tenofovir disoproxil fumarate and emtricitabine) has been used in an on-demand basis to decrease HIV-1 infection rates. The risk reduction in this study (86%) was much better than the 44% seen in the prior study that used daily PrEP in this population. The higher benefit of on-demand PrEP is likely due to increased compliance with medication use. However, this practice is limited to a small number of countries, with most countries offering PrEP on a daily basis. It is advisable to refer to one's local/national guidelines before prescribing.

It is important for practitioners to be aware of PrEP as a potential preventive strategy. Adherence is important to maintain protection. The cost of therapy may limit access; it is important that one select and offer this option judiciously with close monitoring.

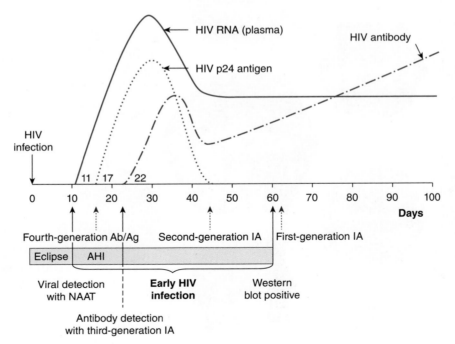

▲ **Figure 55–5.** Window periods of different tests for HIV screening. Ab, antibody; Ag, antigen; AHI, acute HIV infection; IA, immunoassay; NAAT, nucleic acid amplification test.

Centers for Disease Control and Prevention. PrEP. https://www
.cdc.gov/hiv/basics/prep.html. Accessed May 7, 2019.

Justesen K, Prasad S. PURLs: On-demand pill protocol protects
against HIV. *J Fam Pract.* 2016;65(8):556–558. [PMID: 27660840]

> ### Initial Evaluation of HIV-Infected Individuals in the Outpatient Setting

The initial evaluation of an HIV-infected individual represents one of the most significant encounters between the patient and the healthcare provider. The diagnosis of HIV infection is often a profound life-altering experience for individuals. The main goals of this visit are to (1) lay the foundation for fostering a strong and empathic physician-patient relationship; (2) develop and document a comprehensive understanding of the patient's history, stage of disease, and physical findings; and (3) address psychosocial elements that play a major role in treatment success, including stigma, coping mechanisms, social support, social work needs, and housing (Figure 55–6).

Often several visits may be needed to achieve these goals. The initial evaluation is discussed in detail in the HIV primary care guidelines from the HIV Medicine Association (HIVMA) and the Infectious Diseases Society of America (IDSA). Table 55–4 lists the various elements of the initial evaluation.

Infectious Diseases Society of America. Primary care guidelines
for the management of persons infected with HIV 2013. https://
www.idsociety.org/globalassets/idsa/practice-guidelines/
primary-care-guidelines-for-the-management-of-persons-
infected-with-hiv-2013-update-by-the-hiv-medicine-
association-of-the-infectious-diseases-society-of-america.pdf.
Accessed May 7, 2019.

A. History and Physical Examination

Individuals presenting for evaluation with HIV infection may be at any stage of the infection. This can range from asymptomatic individuals to those presenting with full-blown AIDS involving virtually every organ system. In order to

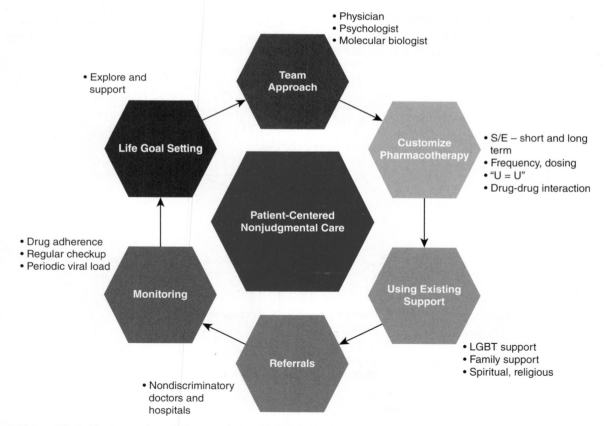

▲ **Figure 55–6.** Elements of nonjudgmental patient centered care. LGBT, lesbian, gay, bisexual, and transgender; S/E, side effects; U = U.

Table 55–4. Elements of the initial evaluation.

Initial Evaluation and Preventive Care	
Psychosocial assessment	Emotional response to illness Support networks Durable power of attorney for health care, advance directives
History	Illnesses High-risk behaviors Travel Drug allergies Medications Cigarette, alcohol, recreational drug use Review of systems
Physical examinations	Complete physical examination Cervical Pap smear for women Consider anal Pap screening for dysplasia
Skin testing and treatment of latent TB infection (LTBI)	PPD and baseline CXR If (+) PPD (>5 mm) and no evidence of old infection on CXR, LTBI should be treated Interferon-γ release assay (IGRA)
Vaccines	Pneumococcal vaccine (conjugate and polysaccharide) Hepatitis A vaccine if hepatitis A IgG negative Hepatitis B vaccine if seronegative Flu vaccine if at risk for exposure Tetanus, MMR, HPV, meningococcal vaccine, inactivated polio if indicated per usual guidelines
Laboratory data	CD4 count HIV viral load by PCR, genotype Complete blood count Electrolytes, creatinine AST, alkaline phosphatase Urine routine Hepatitis A, B, and C serologies RPR/VDRL, treponemal antibody *Toxoplasma gondii* IgG G6PD before dapsone Baseline CXR
Counseling	Safer sex and birth control Smoking cessation Alcohol and drug use Nutrition and exercise
Referrals	Registered dietician with HIV expertise Ophthalmologist if CD4 <50 (especially if visual symptoms) Dentist Psychotherapist/drug treatment

AST, aspartate aminotransferase; CXR, chest radiograph; G6PD, glucose-6-phosphate dehydrogenase; HPV, human papillomavirus; IgG, immunoglobulin G; MMR, measles-mumps-rubella; PCR, polymerase chain reaction; PPD, purified protein derivative; RPR, rapid plasma reagin; TB, tuberculosis; VDRL, Venereal Disease Research Laboratory.

establish a timeline for infection in the individual, the initial evaluation should include inquiries about any previous HIV testing, prior negative test results, occurrence of symptoms, and timing of high-risk activities. In individuals who have an established diagnosis, the lowest CD4 cell count and highest HIV load should be ascertained, if possible. Individuals should be asked about any prior HIV-associated complications and comorbidities, including opportunistic infections, malignancies, and cardiovascular disease history and risk. Efforts should be made to obtain previous medical records.

1. Past medical history—Information about chronic medical conditions, such as peripheral neuropathy, gastrointestinal disease, chronic viral hepatitis, psychiatric illness, hyperlipidemia, diabetes mellitus, or renal insufficiency may affect the choice of therapy or response to therapy and hence should be collected. Other medical conditions of significance in HIV-infected individuals include a history of chickenpox or shingles, tuberculosis or tuberculosis exposure, STIs, and gynecologic or perianal problems.

2. Medications—It is also critical to obtain a thorough medication history. This is particularly important for individuals who have already received ART. Details including drug combinations taken, response to each regimen, CD4 cell count and viral load, duration of treatment, reasons for treatment changes, any drug toxicities, adherence, and prior drug resistance test results should be sought. Patients should be asked about any medications they take, including prescription and over-the-counter drugs, methadone, antacids, intranasal or intravenous steroids, and dietary or herbal supplements, some of which have been shown to interact with antiretroviral drugs. A discussion of allergies should include questions about hypersensitivity reactions to prior therapies, especially sulfa drugs and any antiretroviral agents.

3. Travel and immunizations—It is important to ask patients about travel and where they have lived. For example, patients living in areas endemic for histoplasmosis (eg, Ohio and Mississippi River Valleys in the United States) may be at risk for reactivation disease, even after moving to areas in which these infections are not endemic. The status of immunizations, including tetanus toxoid, pneumococcal vaccine, and hepatitis A and B vaccines, should be elicited. A full birth history and review of maternal history and risk factors should be obtained for all children.

4. Social history—The social history should include a discussion of the use of tobacco, alcohol, heroin, and recreational drugs, including marijuana, cocaine, 3,4-methylenedioxymethamphetamine (ie, MDMA or "ecstasy"), ketamine, methamphetamine, and bath salts. Active injection drug users should be asked about their drug use practices, the source of their needles, and whether they share needles. It is of paramount importance to obtain sexual history in an open, nonjudgmental manner. Patients should be asked about their partners, sexual practices (including condom and contraceptive use), and whether their partner(s) have been informed of their HIV status. Patients may also be asked if they are aware of whether any of their sexual contacts is on ART. Laws vary from state to state regarding the obligation of healthcare providers to notify sex partners, and clinicians should be aware of laws in their own jurisdiction.

5. Social support—Patients should also be specifically asked whom they have informed of their HIV status, how they have been coping with the diagnosis of HIV infection, and what kinds of support they have been receiving. It is important to know about the patient's family, living situation, and work environment and how the patient has been affected by the diagnosis of HIV infection. Other pertinent information includes housing issues, employment, and plans for having children.

6. Family history—As HIV-infected individuals live longer and age, family history may help in assessing their risk of developing certain malignancies, neurologic diseases, and atherosclerotic disease.

7. Review of systems—The review of systems should be comprehensive. Fever, night sweats, weight loss, headaches, visual changes, oral thrush or ulceration, swallowing difficulties, respiratory symptoms, diarrhea, skin rashes or lesions, and changes in neurologic function or mental status may be noted in patients with advanced or uncontrolled HIV infection. For women, a menstrual and obstetric history should be obtained.

8. Depression screening—Depression is common among HIV-infected patients, and the review of systems should include questions focusing on changes in mood, libido, sleeping patterns, appetite, concentration, and memory. Women with HIV infection have high rates of adult sexual and physical abuse and of childhood sexual abuse. The prevalence of depression among those with HIV infection is particularly high in the setting of violence or victimization. As part of the initial evaluation and at periodic intervals thereafter, providers should assess the presence of depression and domestic violence by means of direct questions or validated screening tools such as the Patient Health Questionnaire (PHQ)-2 or PHQ-9.

9. Physical examination—A complete physical examination should be performed at the initial encounter. Vital signs should be obtained. The height and weight for all patients should be measured. For children age <3 years, head circumference should also be measured and plotted against standard growth curves. Abnormal measurements should be followed up.

The overall body habitus may reveal cachexia (especially seen in AIDS) or lipodystrophy (especially in patients with a history of receiving older antiretroviral medications). Lipodystrophy may present either as lipoatrophy (eg, loss of subcutaneous fat in the face, extremities, or buttocks) or lipohypertrophy (eg, increased dorsocervical fat pad, gynecomastia, or abdominal protuberance from visceral fat). See Table 55–5 for a listing of common physical findings organized by organ system.

Table 55–5. Physical examination findings in HIV-infected individuals (by organ system).

System	Findings
Skin	Common findings include folliculitis, seborrheic dermatitis, Kaposi sarcoma, superficial fungal infections, psoriasis, and herpes zoster.
Eye	A dilated fundoscopic examination should be performed by an ophthalmologist in patients with advanced HIV disease (CD4 cell count <50 cells/mm³). Patients with advanced disease or ocular symptoms may have evidence of cytomegalovirus (CMV) retinitis and other ocular manifestations of HIV infection.
Oral cavity	The oropharynx should be carefully examined for evidence of candidiasis, aphthous ulceration, oral hairy leukoplakia, mucosal Kaposi sarcoma, and periodontal disease.
Lymph nodes	Persistent generalized lymphadenopathy is common among HIV-infected patients. However, it does not correlate with prognosis or disease progression. Localized lymphadenopathy, hepatomegaly, or splenomegaly may be a sign of infection or malignancy and should be evaluated further.
Cardiopulmonary	Examination may reveal evidence of pneumonia (including *Pneumocystis jirovecii* pneumonia), chronic obstructive pulmonary disease, tuberculosis, and peripheral vascular disease.
Anogenital	It is important to perform a careful examination for evidence of rectal lesions (including cancer) and sexually transmitted diseases, including condylomata and herpes simplex infection. HIV-infected women should have a pelvic examination. The pelvic examination should include visual inspection of the vulva and perineum for evidence of genital ulcers, warts, or other lesions. Speculum examination is used to assess the presence of abnormal vaginal discharge or vaginal or cervical lesions.
Neurologic	The neurologic examination should include a general assessment of cognitive function, as well as motor and sensory testing. Patients with suspected cognitive dysfunction may need formal neuropsychological testing. Developmental assessment is important in infants and children.

B. Baseline Laboratory Evaluation

A number of initial laboratory studies are indicated for patients presenting with HIV infection (Tables 55–6). The tests are used for determining HIV disease status, assessing baseline organ function, and screening for co-infections and comorbidities. From an HIV disease-specific perspective, the three most important initial laboratory studies are the plasma quantitative HIV RNA level (viral load), CD4 cell count, and drug resistance genotype test.

The CD4 cell count measures the degree of HIV-associated immunodeficiency. Since the universal test and treat policy, it has become irrelevant for the initiation of ART. However, it is the most important criterion for initiation of opportunistic infection prophylaxis.

The viral load measures the amount of viral activity and replication. It is typically reported as copies of HIV RNA/mL. There are differences between viral load tests in their lowest limit of detection: some viral load tests measure viral loads

Table 55–6. Laboratory studies and other investigations indicated in HIV-infected patients at baseline evaluation.

Investigations/Studies	Common Findings
Complete blood count with differential	May reveal cytopenias such as anemia, neutropenia, and thrombocytopenia that are often associated with HIV disease.
Comprehensive chemistry panel	Allows assessment of transaminases for hepatitis, creatinine for kidney function, and albumin for nutritional status. Kidney function should be further measured by calculation of creatinine clearance.
Urinalysis	May detect proteinuria, a common manifestation of HIV-associated nephropathy (noted particularly in patients of African ancestry or those on tenofovir)
Hepatitis serologies	Hepatitis B surface antigen test and anti–hepatitis C antibody test generally rule out chronic hepatitis B and C, respectively. Seronegative patients with unexplained transaminase elevations may need hepatitis B DNA and/or hepatitis C RNA to rule out seronegative hepatitis, especially for those at high risk or with low CD4 counts. Hepatitis B surface antibody and total hepatitis A antibody are also used to assess the need for vaccination.
Testing for sexually transmitted infections	Serologic testing for syphilis is indicated in all patients at baseline. Assessment for gonorrhea (GC) and *Chlamydia* using urine, vaginal, or rectal swabs cultures (GC and *Chlamydia*) should be done. In patients at risk, throat cultures (GC) may also be useful.
Fasting lipid panel	Helps establish a baseline before starting antiretroviral therapy because many antiretroviral agents alter lipid levels.
Screening for latent *Toxoplasma* infection (anti–*Toxoplasma* immunoglobulin G, or IgG)	Determines the need for primary prophylaxis. Those with negative tests should be counseled about the prevention of infection with proper preparation of meat and avoidance of cat feces.
Glucose-6-phosphate dehydrogenase (G6PD) level	If pneumocystis prophylaxis with dapsone is being considered, G6PD level testing helps determine risk of developing hemolytic anemia (this is particularly useful in patients of Mediterranean or African descent).
Tuberculin skin test	Useful to diagnose latent *Mycobacterium tuberculosis* infection (LTBI). The criterion for positivity is 5 mm of induration in HIV-infected patients. LTBI treatment should be offered regardless of age after active tuberculosis has been ruled out.
Pap smears	A cervical Pap smear is recommended at baseline and on a regular basis thereafter in all HIV-infected women. Abnormal results should be followed up with colposcopy. Anal pap smears (with follow-up high-resolution anoscopy as indicated) are increasingly being recommended in HIV-infected men and women, especially those who have had receptive anal intercourse, to screen for human papillomavirus–associated anal dysplasia.
Baseline chest x-ray (CXR)	Pulmonary tuberculosis is commonly found among HIV-infected individuals, especially those who are undiagnosed or not on treatment. In this context, a baseline CXR is particularly useful. Additionally, it can be suggestive of pneumocystis pneumonia and interstitial pneumonitis.
Pregnancy Test	All women of childbearing age should be offered a pregnancy test. The management of HIV-infected pregnant women takes into account a number of additional considerations related to antiretroviral medication dosing, safety to the unborn child, and other elements.

of 400 copies/mL and above; many measure levels of virus between 20 and 50 copies/mL. Viral load is correlated with the risk of transmission and progression of disease and is the most important indicator of the success of ART.

Other baseline studies and interventions that are indicated in HIV-infected patients are listed in Table 55–6.

PRINCIPLES OF ANTIRETROVIRAL THERAPY: WHEN TO START & WHAT TO START

The primary goals for initiating ART are to reduce HIV-associated morbidity and prolong the duration and quality of survival, restore and preserve immunologic function, durably suppress plasma HIV viral load to below the detection limit, and prevent HIV transmission. In recent years, ART has become simpler for patients with respect to pill burden, dosing frequency, and tolerability. In order to prescribe ART safely and effectively, clinicians require an understanding of preferred regimens, drug resistance, drug-drug interactions, medication-associated toxicities, and how comorbidities influence treatment choices. ART recommendations change frequently as new data and drugs become available. The US Department of Health and Human Services publishes updated guidelines for reference.

▶ When to Start ART

The question of when to start ART has been a moving target. In settings where access to ART exists, all individuals who are motivated and ready to start therapy (acceptance by HIV individual; please check five-stage grief model Kubler-Ross

cycle [Figure 55–7]) should start regardless of CD4 count or viral load ("test and treat" policy).

The rationale for this is as follows: HIV infection is now known to cause heightened levels of immune activation and inflammation, which may increase the incidence of myocardial infarction and malignancy independent of CD4 count. There is increasing evidence to support the theory that untreated HIV infection may lead to accelerated aging, with premature loss of bone density and neurocognitive decline. In addition, recent studies such as the HPTN-052 study showed a 96% decrease in HIV transmission validating "treatment as prevention." Successful suppression of viral replication by ART mitigates these consequences significantly.

▶ What to Start in Terms of ART

The goal of ART is suppression of the viral load to undetectable levels (<50 copies/mL). Initial antiretroviral regimens typically consist of a "backbone" of two nucleoside analog reverse transcriptase inhibitors plus a third agent, typically an NNRTI, a protease inhibitor (PI), or an integrase inhibitor. PIs are usually combined with a low dose of ritonavir (RTV), a potent inhibitor of CYP3A4-mediated PI metabolism. RTV "boosting" increases PI drug concentrations, prolongs half-life, simplifies dosing, and helps to prevent the emergence of PI resistance. The preferred first-line regimens and alternatives are listed in Table 55–7.

Having a visual chart of available antiretroviral agents is a helpful tool for counseling. One such chart can be found at https://www.poz.com/article/2018-hiv-drug-chart. This also

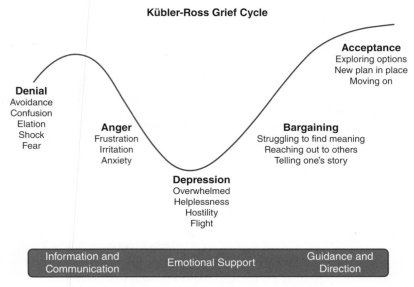

Kübler-Ross Grief Cycle

Denial
Avoidance
Confusion
Elation
Shock
Fear

Anger
Frustration
Irritation
Anxiety

Depression
Overwhelmed
Helplessness
Hostility
Flight

Bargaining
Struggling to find meaning
Reaching out to others
Telling one's story

Acceptance
Exploring options
New plan in place
Moving on

Information and Communication　　Emotional Support　　Guidance and Direction

▲ **Figure 55–7.** Kübler-Ross grief cycle.

Table 55–7. Recommended ART-naïve regimen.

Formula: 2 NRTIs + third active ARV drug from one of three drug classes INSTI, NNRTI, or PI with a pharmacokinetic enhancer (also known as a booster)			Formula: 2 NRTIs plus ritonavir-boosted PI or INSTI	
Initial regimen	INSTI plus 2NRTIs	• BIC/TAF/FTC • DTG/ABC/3TC if HLA-B*5701 negative • DTG plus TDF or TAF/FTC • RAL plus TDF or TAF/FTC	Preferred Two NRTI backbones	ABC/3TC TDF/FTC or TDF/3TC
			Alternative Two NRTI backbones	ZDV/3TC
Alternative regimens	INSTI plus 2NRTIs	• EVG/cobi/TDF or TAF/FTC • RAL plus ABC/3TC if HLA-B*5701 negative	Preferred NNRTI backbones	None
			Alternative NNRTI	EFV RPV
	Boosted PI plus 2 NRTIs	• (DRV/cobi or DRV/r) plus TDF or TAF/FTC • (ATV/cobi or ATV/r) plus TDF or TAF/FTC • (DRV/cobi or DRV/r) plus ABC/3TC	Preferred PI	ATV/r DRV/r
			Alternative PI	LPV/r
			Preferred INSTI	RAL
			Alternative INSTI	DTG
			Special clinical scenario considerations	
	NNRTI plus 2 NRTIs	DOR/TDF or TAF/3TC or DOR plus TDF or TAF/FTC EFV plus TDF or TAF/FTC or EFV/TDF or TAF/3TC RPV/TDF or TAF/FTC	CD4 cell count <200 cells/mm³	Do not use: RPV-based regimens DRV/r plus RAL
			HIV RNA >100,000 copies/mL	Do not use: RPV-based regimens ABC/3TC with EFV or ATV/r DRV/r plus RAL
Recommended ART in pregnant women or women of reproductive age			HLA-B*5701 positive or result unknown	Do not use ABC

Abbreviations: 3TC, lamivudine; ABC, abacavir; ART, antiretroviral therapy; ARV, antiretroviral; ATV, atazanavir; ATV/cobi, atazanavir/cobicistat; ATV/r, atazanavir/ritonavir; BIC, bictegravir; CD4, CD4 T lymphocyte; DOR, doravirine; DRV, darunavir; DRV/cobi, darunavir/cobicistat; DRV/r, darunavir/ritonavir; DTG, dolutegravir; EFV, efavirenz; EVG, elvitegravir; EVG/cobi, elvitegravir/cobicistat; FTC, emtricitabine; HLA, human leukocyte antigen; INSTI, integrase strand transfer inhibitor; NNRTI, nonnucleoside reverse transcriptase inhibitor; NRTI, nucleoside reverse transcriptase inhibitor; PI, protease inhibitor; RAL, raltegravir; RPV, rilpivirine; TAF, tenofovir alafenamide; TDF, tenofovir disoproxil fumarate.
Data from National Institutes of Health. Preferred and alternative antiretroviral regimens for antiretroviral therapy-naive patients. https://aidsinfo.nih.gov/contentfiles/lvguidelines/AA_Tables.pdf.

promotes collaborative decision making between the health-care provider and the patient. Readers are referred to the Department of Health and Human Services (DHHS) guidelines for updated information and a more detailed discussion of all available antiretrovirals.

▶ Monitoring Response to ART

Suppression of viral load should be achieved within 3–6 months, depending on the baseline viral load. Viral suppression is usually accompanied by an increase in the CD4 cell count, with the greatest increase occurring during the first months of therapy, followed by a slower rise that typically continues for several years. Successful ART often leads to weight gain and improvement in overall health, including reversal or resolution of a number of HIV-associated conditions.

An increase in viral load to detectable levels after achieving suppression may indicate early treatment failure (often because of nonadherence). The management of treatment failure is complex and should be directed by an expert. Various forms of resistance testing are usually required, as well as a thorough review of the patient's antiretroviral history in designing salvage therapy. Clinicians may consider consulting an HIV specialist in these situations. See Table 55–8 for laboratory monitoring schedules for patients before and during initiation of ART.

▶ Side Effects

Clinicians managing HIV-infected individuals should be able to recognize common adverse effects of these agents. These include hepatotoxicity, nephrotoxicity, rash

Table 55–8. Monitoring schedule on antiretroviral therapy (ART).

Test	Prior to Initiating ART (Pre-ART Phase)		After Initiating ART (ART Phase)						
	Entry into Care	Follow-Up Before ART	ART Initiation or Modification[a]	2–8 Weeks After ART Initiation or Modification	Every 3–6 Months	Every 6 Months	Every 12 Months	Treatment Failure	Clinically Indicated
CD4 count	✓	Every 3–6 months	✓		✓	In clinically stable patients with suppressed viral load, CD4 count can be monitored every 6–12 months		✓	✓
Viral load	✓	Every 3–6 months	✓	✓[b]	✓[c]			✓	✓
Resistance testing	✓		✓[d]					✓	✓
HLA-B*5701 testing			If considering ABC						
Tropism testing			✓ If considering a CCR5 antagonist					If considering a CCR5 antagonist or for failure of CCR5 antagonist-based regimen	✓
Hepatitis B serology[e]	✓		✓ May repeat if HBsAg (−) and anti-HBs (−) at baseline						
Basic chemistry[f]	✓	Every 6–12 months	✓	✓	✓				✓
ALT, AST, total bilirubin	✓	Every 6–12 months	✓	✓	✓				✓
CBC with differential	✓	Every 3–6 months	✓	If on ZDV	✓				✓

Fasting lipid profile	✓	✓ If normal, annually	✓	✓ Consider 4–8 weeks after starting new ART	If abnormal at last measurement	✓ If abnormal at last measurement	✓ If normal at last measurement
Fasting glucose	✓	✓ If normal, annually	✓		✓ If abnormal at last measurement	✓ If normal at last measurement	✓ If normal at last measurement
Urinalysis	✓	✓	✓			✓ If on TDF[g]	✓
Pregnancy test	✓	✓	✓				✓

[a] Antiretroviral modification may be done for treatment failure, adverse effects, or simplification.

[b] If HIV RNA is detectable in 2–8 weeks, repeat every 4–8 weeks until suppression to <200 copies/mL, then every 3–6 months.

[c] For adherent patients with suppressed viral load and stable clinical and immunologic status for >2–3 years, some experts may extend the interval for HIV RNA monitoring to every 6 months.

[d] For ART-naive patients, if resistance testing was performed at entry into care, repeat testing is optional; for patients with viral suppression who are switching therapy for toxicity or convenience, resistance testing will not be possible and, therefore, not necessary.

[e] If HBsAg is positive at baseline or prior to initiation of ART, TDF plus either FTC or 3TC should be used as part of ART regimen to treat both HBV and HIV infections. If HBsAg and anti-HBs are negative at baseline, hepatitis B vaccine series should be administered.

[f] Serum Na, HCO_3, chloride, blood urea nitrogen, creatinine, glucose (preferably fasting); some experts suggest monitoring phosphorus while on TDF; determination of renal function should include estimation of creatinine clearance using Cockcroft-Gault equation or estimation of glomerular filtration rate based on MDRD equation. For patients with renal disease, consult *Guidelines for the Management of Chronic Kidney Disease in HIV-Infected Patients: Recommendations of the HIV Medicine Association of the Infectious Diseases Society of America.*

[g] More frequent monitoring may be indicated for patients with increased risk of renal insufficiency, such as patients with diabetes.

3TC, lamivudine; ABC, abacavir; ALT, alanine aminotransferase; ART, antiretroviral therapy; AST, aspartate aminotransferase; CBC, complete blood count; EFC, efavirenz; FTC, emtricitabine; HBs, hepatitis B surface antibody; HBsAg, hepatitis B surface antigen; HBV, hepatitis B virus; MDRD, Modification of Diet in Renal Disease (equation); TDF, tenofovir; ZDV, zidovudine.

Data from National Institutes of Health. Preferred and alternative antiretroviral regimens for antiretroviral therapy-naive patients. https://aidsinfo.nih.gov/contentfiles/lvguidelines/AA_Tables.pdf.

(including potentially life-threatening efavirenz- or abacavir-related hypersensitivity rash), lipodystrophy, and pancreatitis.

In addition to the potentially serious toxicities, antiretroviral agents can also cause several side effects that can adversely affect adherence or quality of life. These include gastrointestinal side effects such as nausea, diarrhea, and flatulence and central nervous system effects such as vivid dreams, dizziness, insomnia, difficulty concentrating, headache, and sometimes mood changes. These side effects may improve with continued dosing, but patients who have severe or persistent side effects may need to switch agents. Readers are referred to the DHHS guidelines for a more detailed discussion of common adverse effects encountered with individual antiretroviral medications.

▶ Immune Reconstitution Inflammatory Syndrome

It is important for practitioners to be aware of the phenomenon of immune reconstitution inflammatory syndrome (IRIS), which is an exaggerated inflammatory reaction that occurs once the immune system begins to recover following initiation of ART. Two forms of IRIS occur: (1) unmasking IRIS due to the flare-up of an underlying, previously undiagnosed infection soon after ART is started and (2) paradoxical IRIS where worsening of a previously treated infection occurs after ART is started.

IRIS can be mild or life threatening. It is managed with anticipatory counseling, antipyretics, nonsteroidal anti-inflammatory drugs, occasionally steroids, and rarely ART discontinuation. Occasionally, IRIS presents a complex diagnostic or management dilemma. At such times, it may be valuable to seek the advice of an experienced HIV specialist.

New York State Department of Health AIDS Institute. Management of IRIS, 2017. https://www.hivguidelines.org/antiretroviral-therapy/iris/. Accessed May 7, 2019.

▶ Drug Interactions

The NNRTIs, PIs, and CCR5 antagonists are especially prone to drug-drug interactions because they are metabolized through the CYP3A4 enzyme system. Before prescribing medications to HIV-infected individuals, general practitioners should be aware of common interactions between antiretroviral agents and other medications. Clinicians should be particularly cautious when prescribing warfarin, rifamycins, oral contraceptives, anticonvulsants, statins, clarithromycin, calcium channel blockers, antiarrhythmics, inhaled/intranasal/intra-articular steroids, hepatitis C antivirals, metformin, midazolam, certain benzodiazepines and opiates, and drugs for erectile dysfunction to patients taking ART regimens that include NNRTIs, PIs, or CCR5 antagonists.

The Liverpool drug interaction charts (http://www.hiv-druginteractions.org/), Johns Hopkins HIV Guide (http://www.hopkins-hivguide.org), and the Clinical Care Options website (https://www.clinicaloptions.com) are well-regarded and easy to use resources that can be used at the point of care.

National Institutes of Health. AIDS info: Table 3. Laboratory monitoring schedule for patients before and after initiation of antiretroviral therapy. http://aidsinfo.nih.gov/contentfiles/lvguidelines/AA_Tables.pdf. Accessed May 7, 2019.

PATIENT ADHERENCE TO HIV THERAPY

In the long-term management of HIV-infected individuals, it is critical to realize that suppression of the HIV RNA viral load cannot be fully realized if patients do not adhere to the prescribed regimens. Inadequate adherence to medication regimens remains a major problem worldwide. In the context of HIV management, adherence is of particular concern as patients must consume at least 95% of their medications to avoid problems with viral resistance and therapeutic failure.

Persistent viremia is often due to nonadherence and should be addressed and assessed by the primary care physician before changing medication regimen. Factors that contribute to patient nonadherence to antiretroviral regimens include poor health literacy, depression, substance abuse, increased pill burden, adverse effects of medications, poor patient-physician relationships, and lack of socioeconomic support systems. Currently, some methods used for assessing patient adherence include pill counts, direct observation of therapy by a trusted family member or friend, and pharmacy refill data via the electronic medical record. Technologies such as the use of electronic medication event monitoring systems caps, in which a computer chip is embedded in a specially designed pill bottle cap, may be a valuable tool in the future. To facilitate adherence and to assist patients in achieving therapeutic goals, physicians should establish open lines of communication with patients to use every visit to stress the value of therapy adherence. The serious potential consequences of DR-HIV underscore the importance of regular adherence counseling, supply of ART medications, and monitoring by viral load testing.

▶ COMORBIDITIES & COMPLICATIONS OF CHRONIC HIV INFECTION

Patients with HIV infection often develop multiple complications and comorbidities. A limited account is provided here. Comorbidities and complications could be directly related to HIV infection. However, they could also be completely unrelated to HIV infection and finally arise as a result of HIV drug therapy. Hence, it is important for the clinician providing care to HIV-infected individuals to consider a relatively broad differential diagnosis. Table 55–9 provides a list of

Table 55–9. Comorbidities and complications by organ system in patients with HIV/AIDS.

	Complications in Patients with HIV/AIDS		
System	Comorbidities and Complications	Important Opportunistic Infections/Malignancies	Antiretroviral Treatment–Related Adverse Effects
Neuropsychiatric	1. HIV-associated neurocognitive disorders 2. Neuropathy, radiculopathy, myelopathy 3. Chronic psychiatric disorders	a. Cryptococcal meningitis b. Cerebral toxoplasmosis c. Cytomegalovirus (CMV) encephalitis d. JC virus–related progressive multifocal leukoencephalopathy (PML) e. Primary CNS lymphoma	1. Efavirenz (Sustiva): vivid dreams, sedation 2. NRTIs: peripheral neuropathy
Head and neck	1. HIV-associated retinopathy 2. Gingivitis, dental and salivary gland disease	a. CMV and toxoplasma retinitis b. Acute retinal necrosis and progressive outer retinal necrosis due to varicella-zoster virus c. Otitis, sinusitis due to invasive fungi	
Cardiovascular	1. HIV-associated cardiomyopathy 2. Atherosclerosis	a. Pericarditis/myocarditis due to CMV, invasive fungi, *Mycobacterium* species, *Toxoplasma gondii*	1. Abacavir-related cardiotoxicity 2. Protease inhibitor–associated dyslipidemia
Pulmonary	1. HIV-associated pulmonary hypertension 2. Chronic obstructive pulmonary disease 3. Lung cancer	a. Pulmonary tuberculosis: *Mycobacterium tuberculosis* b. Kaposi sarcoma c. Lymphoma d. Pneumonia/pneumonitis due to CMV, invasive fungi, *Pneumocystis jirovecii* (formerly *Pneumocystis carinii*)	
Gastrointestinal	1. HIV-induced enteropathy 2. Viral hepatitis (especially hepatitis B and C) 3. Nonalcoholic fatty liver disease 4. HPV-related malignancies	a. Chronic diarrhea due to *Cryptosporidium, Isospora, Microsporidium, Cyclospora,* and *Giardia* b. Lymphoma, Kaposi sarcoma c. Oral/esophageal candidiasis d. Esophagitis due to CMV and HSV	1. NRTI-associated pancreatitis 2. Protease inhibitor–associated diarrhea, fatty liver
Renal/genitourinary	1. HIV-associated nephropathy 2. Chronic kidney disease not caused by HIV-associated nephropathy 3. Sexually transmitted infections		1. Protease inhibitor–related nephrolithiasis 2. Tenofovir-associated nephrotoxicity
Endocrine	1. Impaired lipid and glucose metabolism 2. HIV-associated wasting 3. Hypogonadism	a. Adrenal gland infiltration by CMV, invasive fungi, and *Mycobacterium* species	1. Protease inhibitor–associated lipid or glucose disorders and lipodystrophy
Musculoskeletal	1. Myopathy/myositis 2. Osteopenia, osteoporosis 3. Avascular necrosis		1. NRTI or NNRTIs associated with osteomalacia 2. Protease inhibitors with statins increase risk of myopathy
Hematologic or oncologic	1. Anemia of chronic disease 2. Coagulation disorders 3. Multiple myeloma	a. Lymphoma b. Parvovirus B19–related pure red cell aplasia (PRCA) c. Bone marrow infiltration (leading to pancytopenia) by CMV, invasive fungi, and *Mycobacterium* species	1. Zidovudine and trimethoprim/sulfamethoxazole-related anemia
Dermatologic	1. Eosinophilic folliculitis 2. Papulosquamous disorders (eg, eczema, seborrheic dermatitis, psoriasis) 3. Molluscum contagiosum	a. Kaposi sarcoma b. Fungal dermatoses, varicella-zoster virus	

CNS, central nervous system; HPV, human papillomavirus; HSV, herpes simplex virus; NNRTI, nonnucleoside reverse transcriptase inhibitor; NRTI, nucleoside reverse transcriptase inhibitor.
Adapted with permission from Chu C, Selwyn PA. Complications of HIV infection: a systems-based approach. *Am Fam Physician.* 2011 Feb 15; 83(4):395–406.

comorbidities, opportunistic infections, and antiretroviral-related adverse effects by organ system.

Chu C, Selwyn PA. Complications of HIV infection: a systems-based approach. *Am Fam Physician.* 2011;83(4):395–406. [PMID: 21322514]

▶ Prevention of Opportunistic Infections

The effectiveness of ART has decreased the emphasis on the prevention and management of opportunistic infections. However, patients with CD4 cell counts of <200 cells/mm^3 remain at risk for opportunistic infections and require primary prophylaxis. Table 55–3 lists the common opportunistic infections and the prophylaxis of select infections that are frequently encountered in HIV primary care. Patients who have been treated for opportunistic infections often require secondary prophylaxis or maintenance therapy. The diagnosis and management of HIV-related opportunistic infections are beyond the scope of this chapter. Details can be found in the opportunistic infection treatment and prevention guidelines.

National Institutes of Health. AIDS info: guidelines for the prevention and treatment of opportunistic infections in HIV-infected adults and adolescents, 2019. https://aidsinfo.nih.gov/content-files/lvguidelines/adult_oi.pdf. Accessed May 7, 2019.

HEALTH MAINTENANCE & OTHER PRIMARY CARE ISSUES

Many HIV-infected individuals develop multiple complications and comorbidities. Some complications of HIV infection are the direct result of long-term infection, whereas others are the indirect result of aging, ART, or other patient factors. Primary care providers of HIV-infected individuals should screen patients with routine laboratory monitoring (eg, comprehensive metabolic and lipid panels) and validated tools (eg, the HIV Dementia Scale). Treatment of many chronic complications is similar for patients with and without HIV infection. Many HIV-associated complications, such as dyslipidemia, diabetes, depression, and obesity, are familiar to primary care providers. However, special attention should be given to patients taking antiretroviral drugs because of potential drug interactions. Preventive care, health promotion (eg, safe sex education, smoking cessation, healthy lifestyles), and psychosocial assessments are central to the HIV primary care.

▶ Screening for Other Diseases

A. Cervical Cancer Screening

Cervical cancer screening should be performed as part of the initial evaluation in all HIV-infected women. Management in women with abnormal Papanicolaou (Pap) tests is based on cytologic findings. Please refer to American College of Obstetricians and Gynecologists screening guidelines.

B. Anal Cancer Screening

HIV infection is associated with an increased risk for anal cancer in both men and women. In several HIV clinics, anal Pap screening for HPV-associated dysplasia is considered the standard of care among HIV-infected adults. Patients with any abnormality on the anal Pap test should be referred for high-resolution anoscopy and biopsy.

C. Screening for Other STIs

Patients with HIV infection should be screened for other STIs at the initial evaluation. Discussion of sexual practices along with prevention counseling should be incorporated regularly into visits. Periodic screening for STIs should be performed in persons at continued risk. Please refer to the chapter on STIs in this book for a more detailed discussion.

D. Tuberculosis Screening

Prophylaxis against *Mycobacterium tuberculosis* infection is recommended for HIV-infected patients with a positive purified protein derivative (PPD; ≥5 mm induration) or positive interferon-γ test, history of a positive PPD without prior treatment, or contact with a person with active pulmonary tuberculosis (TB). The WHO recommends isoniazid preventive therapy for at least 6 months for all people living with HIV. A chest x-ray and clinical evaluation should be performed in all patients with a positive TB screening test to exclude active disease prior to the initiation of prophylaxis.

World Health Organization. The three I's for TB/HIV: isoniazid preventive therapy (IPT). https://www.who.int/hiv/topics/tb/3is_ipt/en/. Accessed May 7, 2019.

E. Co-infection with Hepatitis B and/or Hepatitis C

Hepatitis B virus (HBV) and HIV are bloodborne viruses transmitted primarily through sexual contact and injection drug use. Because of these shared modes of transmission, people at risk for HIV infection are also at risk for HBV infection. Hepatitis C virus (HCV) is a bloodborne virus transmitted through direct contact with the blood of an infected person. It is estimated that HCV affects 2–15% of people living with HIV worldwide (and up to 90% of those are people who inject drugs [PWID]) and that chronic HBV infection affects an estimated 5–20% of people living with HIV.

The global estimate of burden of HIV/HCV co-infection is 2.75 million, of whom 1.3 million are PWID, and the global estimate of burden of HBV/HCV co-infection is 2.6 million. The burden of these co-infections is greatest in the African and Southeast Asia regions. HIV-positive persons who become infected with HBV or HCV are at increased risk for developing chronic hepatitis. In addition, persons who are co-infected with HIV and hepatitis can have serious medical complications, including an increased risk for liver-related morbidity and mortality. WHO recommends that HIV-positive individuals are vaccinated as early as possible with the HBV vaccine. Postvaccination testing of people living with HIV is recommended 1–2 months after administration of the last dose of the vaccine series.

HIV/HCV co-infection is common due to shared routes or risk factors for acquisition and has been associated with more rapid HCV-induced fibrosis progression and lower odds of successful treatment outcome with interferon-based therapy. With the development of interferon-free direct-acting antiviral therapy, efficacy in HIV/HCV co-infected persons has received significant recent attention. Eradicating HCV in HIV co-infected persons is now medically achievable in most cases, when access to medication is possible.

HIV patients should be evaluated for viral hepatitis. Those who do not have evidence of immunity should be vaccinated and monitored for response. Those who have HIV/HBV should have additional serologies checked to evaluate for hepatitis B e antigen status and level of viremia. All HIV/HBV coinfected patients should be started on ART with tenofovir-based regimens. Those with HIV/HBV and cirrhosis should be screened for hepatocellular cancer every 6 months.

World Health Organization. HIV and hepatitis co-infections. https://www.who.int/hiv/topics/hepatitis/hepatitisinfo/en/. Accessed May 7, 2019.

F. Screening for Other Conditions

Age-appropriate screening for breast, colon, and prostate cancer should be performed in HIV-infected patients according to recommendations used for the general population. Please refer to the USPSTF guidelines for more information on these.

▶ Immunizations

Immunizations are an important part of preventive care for HIV-infected individuals. The pneumococcal conjugate and polysaccharide vaccine, influenza vaccine, meningococcal vaccine, and tetanus toxoid are indicated in all HIV-infected individuals. Revaccination with pneumococcal polysaccharide vaccine should be considered 5 years after the initial vaccination or sooner if it was initially administered when the CD4 count was <200 cells/mm^3 and if subsequently the CD4 count has increased to >200 cells/mm^3 on ART. All HIV-infected individuals should receive influenza vaccination annually. This is especially important in those who smoke cigarettes or have underlying lung disease. Patients without immunity to hepatitis B or A should be vaccinated against both viruses. This is particularly important if they are co-infected with hepatitis C. All inactivated vaccines are considered safe in this setting, but live attenuated vaccines should be avoided in patients with advanced HIV disease (CD4 <200/mm^3). The HPV vaccine is recommended for HIV-infected males and females between 13 and 26 years of age.

National Institutes of Health. AIDS info: recommended immunization schedule for adults and adolescents with HIV infection. https://aidsinfo.nih.gov/guidelines/html/4/adult-and-adolescent-opportunistic-infection/365/figure–immunization. Accessed May 8, 2019.

▶ Psychiatric Disorders & Behavioral Risk Reduction Counseling

Studies estimate that up to 50% of patients with HIV infection have concurrent chronic psychiatric and substance use disorders. Depression, anxiety, and substance abuse are highly prevalent among HIV-infected individuals. Psychiatric symptoms may also be manifestations of HIV-related neurocognitive dysfunction. Prompt recognition and treatment of psychiatric comorbidities are central to the effective management of HIV-infected individuals.

Behavioral risk reduction counseling is also a cornerstone of HIV primary care. Each visit presents an opportunity to review the patient's sexual and drug use activities. Discussion should focus on risk reduction interventions tailored to the individual's behaviors. Counseling to limit the number of sexual partners, engage in lower risk sexual activities, and consistently use latex condoms during sexual intercourse should be provided. Patients should also be strongly encouraged to disclose their sero-status to all sexual partners. The potential for acquiring different and potentially drug-resistant strains of HIV, resulting in treatment failure, should be discussed.

Patients who use injection drugs should be counseled about the risks of continued use, including acquisition of other bloodborne pathogens such as HBV, HCV, and new strains of HIV. Patients who are unable to stop injecting drugs should be told not to reuse or share needles. The entry of patients into substance abuse treatment program may need to be facilitated.

CARE OF SPECIAL POPULATIONS

▶ Gay, Bisexual, & Other Men Who Have Sex with Men

Men who have sex with men (MSM) are the only group in which new HIV infections have been increasing since the early 1990s. Homophobia, stigma, and discrimination put

MSM at risk for multiple physical and mental health problems and affect whether MSM seek and are able to obtain high-quality health services. The care of HIV-infected MSM requires particular attention to a sensitive and inclusive approach with an emphasis on risk reduction counseling. Special attention is needed for STIs, anal cancer screening, alcohol and tobacco use, psychological health, domestic violence, and stigma. Physicians should also inquire about "club drugs," such as methamphetamines, the use of which has been associated with high-risk sexual behaviors.

HIV Infection in Women

Worldwide, almost an equal number of women are infected with HIV compared with men. In some parts of the world (eg, sub-Saharan Africa), they constitute the majority of infected individuals. The burden of HIV in women is significantly complicated by gender inequality and stigma.

Primary care of the HIV-infected woman requires special attention to issues such as drug toxicities, contraception, and family planning. A baseline pregnancy test should be performed in women prior to initiation of ART. Certain antiretroviral agents (eg, efavirenz, dolutegravir) should be used with caution in women of childbearing age because of teratogenicity-related concerns. Contraceptive methods should be recommended following due consideration of potential interactions between antiretroviral drugs and hormonal contraceptives.

The significant reduction of perinatal transmission due to antenatal treatment of HIV infection with ART has been a great public health success story. In the absence of treatment, the risk of vertical transmission of HIV is as high as 25–30%. In women on ART with undetectable viral load or HIV RNA level ≤1000 copies/mL, vaginal delivery is recommended.

In terms of breastfeeding, the WHO recommends breastfeeding by HIV-infected mothers in resource-limited settings. However, in more economically developed countries, the norm is to avoid breastfeeding. Given the profound personal and cultural importance of breastfeeding, women should be offered the evidence and provided support to choose whether to breastfeed or not.

National Institutes of Health. AIDS info: recommendations for the use of antiretroviral drugs in pregnant women with HIV infection and interventions to reduce perinatal HIV transmission in the United States, 2018. http://www.aidsinfo.nih.gov/guidelines/html/3/perinatal-guidelines/0/. Accessed May 7, 2019.
World Health Organization. Updates on HIV and infant feeding, 2016. https://apps.who.int/iris/bitstream/handle/10665/246260/9789241549707-eng.pdf?sequence=1. Accessed May 7, 2019.

HIV Infection in Children

Although in the developed world, the number of children living with HIV infection is small, worldwide, an estimated 3.4 million children were living with HIV at the end of 2011. More than 90% of these children were in sub-Saharan Africa. Most children acquire HIV from their HIV-infected mothers during pregnancy, birth, or breastfeeding. Pediatric HIV infection may affect normal neurologic and immunologic development at critical phases and present unique management challenges. Some clinical features uniquely seen in HIV-infected children are growth failure/short stature, developmental delay/mental retardation, aspiration and swallowing problems, recurrent ear infections, and delayed puberty. A detailed description of pediatric HIV/AIDS and its management may be found in the *Red Book* published by the American Academy of Pediatrics.

HIV Infection in Older Adults

The prevalence and incidence of HIV infection in patients age >50 are increasing because of the success of potent ART, as well as the occurrence of new primary infections. Treatment of HIV infection in this population is often complicated by comorbidities and an increased potential for drug toxicity and drug-drug interactions. The help of a clinical pharmacist is valuable in these circumstances.

National Institutes of Health. AIDS info: considerations for antiretroviral use in special patient populations—HIV and the older patient. https://aidsinfo.nih.gov/guidelines/html/1/adult-and-adolescent-arv/277/hiv-and-the-older-patient. Accessed May 8, 2019.
Sangaralangkam A, Appelbaum JS. Caring for older adults with the human immunodeficiency virus. *J Am Geriatr Soc*. 2016;64(11):2322–2329. [PMID: 27682476]

COMPLEMENTARY & ALTERNATIVE THERAPIES IN HIV/AIDS

No alternative and complementary modalities have proven beneficial in HIV treatment or control of infection. However, acupuncture, plant products (eg, herbal supplements), massage, aromatherapy, and meditation are frequently used complementary and alternative medicine (CAM) modalities by HIV-infected individuals to improve general health, energy, and overall sense of well-being. They also use these modalities to alleviate ART-related side effects.

Some studies have reported rates of usage to be as high as 74%, particularly among patients with lipodystrophy. Patients seldom disclose their use to their providers. Hence, it is important for providers to ask about the use of herbal supplements. Although some CAM therapies, such as meditation, might help to improve the sense of well-being and quality of life, caution should be exercised with the use of herbal supplements. Drug-drug interactions with antiretroviral medications are a significant concern with the use of herbal products. For example, St. John's wort is known to have drug-drug interactions with PIs and may increase the risk of virologic failure. In order to promote health and diminish the risk of treatment failure, it is extremely important for providers to have an open and ongoing discussion with HIV-infected individuals regarding the use of these therapies.

MOTIVATIONAL INTERVIEWING TO ENHANCE PATIENT ENGAGEMENT

Facilitating and supporting behavior change lies at the heart of providing care to HIV-infected individuals. Healthier behaviors allow people living with HIV to experience better outcomes. Motivational interviewing (MI) is a patient-centered and relationship-based communication approach that aims to facilitate exploration and resolution of ambivalence toward reducing unhealthy or problematic behaviors and adopting healthier ones. At the heart of MI is a spirit of empathy, acceptance, respect, honesty, and caring.

▶ Tools & Strategies of Motivational Interviewing

Several strategies are used during MI including open questions, affirmation, empathy through reflective listening, gently identifying and enabling a realization in the patient of a discrepancy between the patient's goals or values and the patient's current behavior, avoiding argument and direct confrontation, rolling with resistance, and supporting self-efficacy and autonomy.

OARS (open-ended questions, affirmative statements, reflective statements, and summarizing) and LURE (listening, understanding the patient's motivations, resisting the urge to correct the patient, and empowering the patient) are two practical guiding tools for MI that providers can use in practice.

▶ Matching Your Responses to the Patient's Readiness for Change

Assessment and choosing an appropriate response that matches the patient's readiness for change are some of the most important skills involved in effective MI. The Stages of Change Model provides a framework providers can use to help patients make positive health changes at every stage of readiness.

▶ Conclusion & Take-Home Points

1. Active listening with genuineness and empathy enables a deeper and more connected understanding of your patient's motivations. It also powerfully demonstrates that you care about your patients, which by itself can have a strong therapeutic impact.

2. The patient's reasons, rather than the provider's, are more likely to hold the key to behavior change.

3. Care providers have a powerful desire to heal, prevent harm, and "set the patient straight," but this can have a paradoxical effect because people do not like to be told what to do. The practitioner of MI avoids the righting reflex by replacing it with reflective listening (eg, "If I understand, do you feel like by telling your boyfriend that you don't want to have sex whenever he wants, he might react with violence?").

4. Options and solutions generated by the patient are more likely to be successful than options generated by the provider. You can empower your patients by soliciting options from the patient and stewarding the decision-making process in a patient-centered manner where the patient feels a sense of ownership for the decisions taken.

Cook PF, Corwin MA, Bradley-Springer L. *Motivational Interviewing and HIV: Reducing Risk, Inspiring Change.* HIV Provider Reference Series. A Publication of the Mountain Plains AETC. https://aidsetc.org/sites/default/files/resources_files/etres-441.pdf. Accessed May 2018.

Depression in Diverse Populations & Older Adults

Poh Choo How, MD, PhD
Ruth S. Shim, MD, MPH
Annelle B. Primm, MD, MPH

ESSENTIALS OF DIAGNOSIS

Depression is a clinical diagnosis characterized by ≥2 weeks of depressed mood and/or anhedonia (lack of interest in pleasure) and multiple additional symptoms:

► Change in appetite (or weight change)
► Change in sleep pattern
► Change in activity
► Fatigue and/or loss of energy
► Guilt and/or feeling of worthlessness
► Diminished concentration
► Suicidal thoughts

Anxiety symptoms are common among depressed individuals. Among older adults, cognitive impairment may be associated with depression. Within various cultures, depression can manifest with more somatic symptoms rather than mood symptoms.

GENERAL CONSIDERATIONS

Mental health is essential and integral to overall health. Due to stigma of mental illness, the perceived gap between physical and mental health has increased. As a result, individuals are reluctant to report mental health symptoms and seek specialized treatment. In addition, some demographic groups are also at higher risk for having unmet mental health needs, including children and youth, older adults, and members of medically underserved ethnic and racial groups. Because these groups are most likely to be evaluated in primary care settings, it is essential that primary care physicians and other allied health practitioners are equipped to provide high-quality mental health services.

Depression is one of the leading causes of disability worldwide. By the year 2030, it is projected to be the leading cause of overall disease burden in high-income countries. It is a highly prevalent condition, affecting 35% of patients seen in primary care settings, and its prevalence in all age groups has been increasing in recent years. The most common age of onset is between 25 and 35 years old, and an earlier age of onset of depression is associated with worse prognosis and functional impairment over time. Depression is twice as common among women as men, and black and Hispanic individuals with a diagnosis of depression are less likely to receive mental health services compared to their white counterparts. In addition, older adults are less likely to receive mental health services compared to younger adults.

Depression is a highly comorbid condition, particularly in later life. Medical illness and disability, which are more common in the elderly, are risk factors for depression. Depression diminishes quality of life, leads to nonadherence with self-care and treatment recommendations, increases the use of medical services, and is associated with cognitive impairment in adults. Furthermore, depression is often associated with medical and social complexity; patients with depression often have multiple chronic conditions, poor socioeconomic status, and poor social support, which in turn increase the risk of developing depression. Additionally, major psychosocial risk factors for depression include bereavement, caregiver strain, social isolation, disability, chronic medical illness, and role transitions.

Agency for Healthcare Research and Quality. *2016 National Healthcare Quality and Disparities Report.* Rockville, MD: Agendcy for Healthcare Research and Quality; 2017.

González HM, Vega WA, Williams DR, Tarraf W, West BT, Neighbors HW. Depression care in the United States: too little for too few. *Arch Gen Psychiatr.* 2010;67(1):37–46. [PMID: 20048221]

Haugen PT, McCrillis AM, Smid GE, Nijdam MJ. Mental health stigma and barriers to mental health care for first responders: a systematic review and meta-analysis. *J Psychiatr Res.* 2017;94: 218–229. [PMID: 28800529]

Martin D, Martin JL, Guthrie B, Gunn J, Mercer SW. Depression and multimorbidity: a cross-sectional study of 1,751,841 patients in primary care. *J Clin Psychiatry.* 2014;75(11):1202–1208. [PMID: 25470083]

Roca M, Gili M, Garcia-Garcia M, et al. Prevalence and comorbidity of common mental disorders in primary care. *J Affect Disord.* 2009;119(1):52–58. [PMID: 19361865]

Vos T, Abajobir AA, Abate KH, et al. Global, regional, and national incidence, prevalence, and years lived with disability for 328 diseases and injuries for 195 countries, 1990–2016: a systematic analysis for the Global Burden of Disease Study 2016. *Lancet.* 2017;390(10100):1211–1259. [PMID: 28919117]

World Health Organization. *The Global Burden of Disease: 2004 Update.* Geneva, Switzerland: WHO Press; 2008.

Prevention

Preventive interventions that target individuals at higher risk for depression (or the adverse effects of depression) can allow primary care providers to focus their efforts on promoting whole-person health. Effective primary prevention efforts that decrease the incidence of depression often require a multifactorial, interdisciplinary approach that targets multiple risk factors across various sectors. Interventions may include education about stress-coping techniques; facilitating healthy relationships with friends, family, and support groups; promoting physical activity; and protecting sleep quality through better sleep hygiene. Primary prevention is especially crucial in groups that are at higher risk of developing depression such as those with chronic illnesses and older adults who carry a higher burden of medical comorbidity and bereavement and have lower remission rates relative to younger adults.

Secondary prevention strategies include screening tools to enhance detection and treatment of depression. Universal screening in primary care settings, when coupled with effective treatment, can be an important tool in the prevention of depression. Finally, tertiary prevention efforts, which include antidepressant treatment and psychotherapy, have been shown to reduce relapse rates and morbidity associated with depression. Universal, selective, and indicated preventive interventions target the general public or specific individuals at highest risk for developing depression in the future.

Conejo-Cerón S, Moreno-Peral P, Rodríguez-Morejón A, et al. Effectiveness of psychological and educational interventions to prevent depression in primary care: a systematic review and meta-analysis. *Ann Fam Med.* 2017;15(3):262–271. [PMID: 28483893]

Hall CA, Reynolds CF III. Late-life depression in the primary care setting: challenges, collaborative care, and prevention. *Maturitas.* 2014;79(2):147–152. [PMID: 24996484]

Mammen G, Faulkner G. Physical activity and the prevention of depression: a systematic review of prospective studies. *Am J Prevent Med.* 2013;45(5):649–657. [PMID: 24139780]

Primm AB, Vasquez MJ, Mays RA, et al. The role of public health in addressing racial and ethnic disparities in mental health and mental illness. *Prev Chronic Dis.* 2017;7(1):A20. [PMID: 20040235]

Clinical Findings

The type and severity of depression run along a spectrum, ranging from subclinical varieties (eg, dysthymia, unspecified depressive disorder) to major depressive disorder (with mild, moderate, or severe episodes). Major depression typically occurs in discrete episodes, each with a clear beginning and end. After an initial episode, >50% of individuals will have additional episodes in their lifetime. Among older adults with depression, about half had experienced depression earlier in their lives, and the other half experienced it for the first time after the age of 60. A kindling effect is seen in that the likelihood of a recurrent episode of major depression increases with each untreated major depressive episode. At the same time, recent data suggest discordance between patients presenting with symptoms of depression and physicians' appraisal of depression symptoms during primary care visits. The prevalence of major depression in primary care settings is about 12%; yet, it is recognized in only about 50% of primary care patients with the disorder. This highlights the importance of screening and assessing for major depression in primary care settings.

Henry SG, Feng B, Franks P, et al. Methods for assessing patient–clinician communication about depression in primary care: what you see depends on how you look. *Health Serv Res.* 2014;49(5):1684–1700. [PMID: 24837881]

Mitchell AJ, Vaze A, Rao S. Clinical diagnosis of depression in primary care: a meta-analysis. *Lancet.* 2009;374(9690):609–619. [PMID: 19640579]

Initial Assessment

Many individuals are reluctant to seek care for mental health problems. Only 20–30% of patients with emotional or psychological issues report their concerns to their primary care physicians. Rather, patients with depression more commonly present with somatic complaints. The most common somatic symptom reported by more than half of patients with major depression was "feeling fatigued, weak, or tired all over." Depression has also been found to be related to previous complaints of sleep disturbance and other medically unexplained symptoms.

Initial assessment should include a focused psychiatric history and examination and, for older adults, a brief clinical cognitive examination with the Mini-Mental State Examination (MMSE) or Montreal Cognitive Assessment (MoCA). In addition, a medical history, physical examination, focused neurologic examination, and laboratory studies to rule out physical conditions with similar symptoms are preferred as part of the assessment. It is also important to assess other domains, particularly for older adults, including level of functioning or disability, loss or grief concerns, the physical environment, and psychosocial stressors.

Bell RA, Franks P, Duberstein PR, et al. Suffering in silence: reasons for not disclosing depression in primary care. *Ann Fam Med.* 2011;9(5):439–446. [PMID: 21911763]

Flyckt L, Hassler E, Lotfi L, Krakau I, Nilsson GH. Clinical cues for detection of people with undiscovered depression in primary health care: a case–control study. *Prim Health Care Res Dev.* 2014;15(3):324–330. [PMID: 23953229]

van der Sluijs JvE, Ten Have M, Rijnders C, van Marwijk H, de Graaf R, van der Feltz-Cornelis C. Medically unexplained and explained physical symptoms in the general population: association with prevalent and incident mental disorders. *PloS One.* 2015;10(4):e0123274. [PMID: 25853676]

A. Symptoms and Signs

Specific features associated with depressive disorders are described as follows:

- **Depressed mood:** Feeling sad, low, empty, hopeless, gloomy, or down in the dumps, different from a normal sense of sadness or grief.

- **Anhedonia:** Inability to enjoy usually pleasurable activities (eg, sex, hobbies, daily routines).

- **Changes in appetite or weight:** A decrease in appetite (most patients) or an increase in appetite associated with craving specific foods.

- **Changes in sleep patterns:** Insomnia (difficulty falling asleep or staying asleep or early morning awakening) in most patients; hypersomnia in some patients.

- **Changes in activity:** Psychomotor retardation (speech, thinking, movement) or psychomotor agitation (cannot sit still, pacing, hand wringing).

- **Loss of energy:** Decreased energy, tiredness, fatigue.

- **Cognitive changes:** Inability to think, concentrate, or make decisions.

- **Sense of worthlessness or guilt:** Excessive feelings of low self-esteem, self-blame, and lack of self-worth.

- **Suicidal ideation:** Thoughts of death or suicide, with and without a plan, or suicide attempts.

A total of five of the nine features, including either depressed mood or anhedonia, must be present during the same 2-week period for the patient to be diagnosed with major depressive disorder. Among older adults, special consideration should be given to symptom presentation, which may differ considerably from younger adults. Older adults are less likely to present with affective symptoms than younger adults. As a result, primary care providers should focus on cognitive difficulty, sleep disturbance, psychomotor retardation, and feelings of hopelessness.

Park M, Unützer J. Geriatric depression in primary care. *Psychiatr Clin.* 2011;34(2):469–487. [PMID: 21536169]

B. Screening Measures

The US Preventive Services Task Force recommends screening for depression in primary care settings where diagnosis, treatment, and follow-up for depression are available. Many validated screening instruments exist for screening depression in diverse populations. In the primary care setting, screening can be initiated using a two-question initial screening test to detect the presence of depressed mood and anhedonia: "Over the past 2 weeks, have you felt down, depressed, or hopeless?" and "Over the past 2 weeks, have you felt little interest or pleasure in doing things?" This short screening test is often referred to as the Patient Health Questionnaire-2 (PHQ-2). PHQ-2 scores ≥ 3 are 83% sensitive and 92% specific for diagnosing major depression when used in primary care settings. Patients who screen positive on the PHQ-2 can be further evaluated with the PHQ-9, which has been validated in multiple culturally diverse populations, including African Americans, Africans, Chinese Americans, Latinos, and others, as well as in older adults.

Among older adults, the Geriatric Depression Scale (GDS) has several versions, including an original 30-item version. The GDS-15 has been shown to have greater sensitivity and specificity for depression than the 30-item scale. The Hospital Anxiety and Depression Scale (HADS) is a 14-item self-report scale specifically designed for evaluation of psychiatric symptoms with medical comorbidities and does not cover somatic symptoms. The Beck Depression Inventory II has 21 items and is widely used for measuring the severity of depression.

The PHQ-9 and GDS-15 have been proven effective in detecting suicidal ideation. Risk factors for attempting suicide include mood disorders and other mental disorders, substance use disorders, history of deliberate self-harm, becoming disabled, and a history of suicide attempts. A majority of individuals who have completed suicide will have seen their primary care physician in the month before their death, which signals an opportunity for primary care providers to provide lifesaving interventions. Once a patient has been deemed to be at higher risk of suicide, immediate referral to specialty mental health services is indicated. Table 56–1 lists several screening instruments for depression.

Table 56–1. Depression and suicide screening instruments.

Screening Tool	Cutoff Score for Depression
Patient Health Questionnaire-2 (PHQ-2)[a]	3/6
Patient Health Questionnaire-9 (PHQ-9)[a]	10/21
Geriatric Depression Scale-15 (GDS-15)[a]	6/15
Beck Depression Inventory II (BDI-II)	20/63
Hospital Anxiety and Depression Scale (HADS)[a]	8/21

[a]Free for clinical use.

Arroll B, Goodyear-Smith F, Crengle S, et al. Validation of PHQ-2 and PHQ-9 to screen for major depression in the primary care population. *Ann Fam Med* 2010;8(4):348–353. [PMID: 20644190]

Mitchell AJ, Bird V, Rizzo M, Meader N. Diagnostic validity and added value of the Geriatric Depression Scale for depression in primary care: a meta-analysis of GDS30 and GDS15. *J Affect Disord*. 2010;125(1):10–17. [PMID: 19800132]

Smarr KL, Keefer AL. Measures of depression and depressive symptoms: Beck Depression Inventory-II (BDI-II), Center for Epidemiologic Studies Depression Scale (CES-D), Geriatric Depression Scale (GDS), Hospital Anxiety and Depression Scale (HADS), and Patient Health Questionnaire-9 (PHQ-9). *Arthritis Care Res*. 2011;63(Suppl 11) S454–S466. [PMID: 22588766]

► Differential Diagnosis

The most critical comorbid health conditions to consider in persons with depression include alcohol and substance use disorders and the use of medications that can cause depressive symptoms (eg, treatment with interferon-α, chronic use of opioid pain medications and benzodiazepines). Late-life depression often coexists with cognitive impairment and other illnesses of the central nervous system, and the co-occurrence increases the risk of developing dementia compared with those with cognitive impairments without depression. Bipolar depression must also be ruled out in patients presenting with depressive symptoms. All patients with depressive symptoms should be screened for a history of manic or hypomanic symptoms. This is important in order to determine the appropriate course of treatment as treatment of bipolar depression with an antidepressant increases the risk of conversion to a manic or hypomanic episode.

Depending on the clinical presentation, physicians should also assess the patient for a variety of general medical problems that could be contributing to mood symptoms, including pain, cardiac disease, diabetes, and certain types of cancer and inflammatory diseases. Among older adults, the potential of accidental misuse of medications and the possibility of physical, verbal, or emotional abuse by caregivers or relatives should also be evaluated. Psychosocial factors such as financial strain, unemployment, housing instability, or food insecurity, as well as experience of discrimination, should also be considered in the evaluation of secondary causes of depression.

Ismail Z, Elbayoumi H, Fischer CE, et al. Prevalence of depression in patients with mild cognitive impairment: a systematic review and meta-analysis. *JAMA Psychiatr*. 2017;74(1):58–67. [PMID: 27893026]

► Complications

If untreated, depression can lead to multiple complications, including more serious, treatment-resistant forms of the illness, worsening physical health, and suicide. Individuals with untreated depression are at greater risk for complications from general medical problems, alcohol and substance use disorders, and relationship problems. Impairment in social and occupational functioning can lead to further disability.

► Treatment

Treatment of mental disorders has increased substantially over the past decades. Primary care physicians prescribe the majority of antidepressant medication in the United States. Yet a majority of adults with mental disorders do not receive treatment at all or do not receive treatment in accordance with accepted standards of care. Within a year of diagnosis, only about 24% of patients with major depression receive any form of treatment, and only 9% receive adequate treatment, with 6% achieving remission. Patient preference may contribute to these low numbers as approximately 40% of patients with major depression do not want or perceive the need for treatment. For racially and ethnically diverse populations, rates of quality mental health treatment are even lower.

Selection of an initial treatment modality should be influenced by both clinical factors (eg, severity of symptoms, avoiding drug-drug interactions and adverse drug events) and patient preference. In general, evidence-based recommendations for treatment of moderate to severe depression in the primary care setting involves a combination of pharmacotherapy and psychotherapy, and for the treatment of mild depression, psychotherapy or pharmacotherapy alone.

Although the majority of depressed patients are treated in primary care settings, some cases are especially difficult to manage in general medical clinics without specialized services. Specialized psychiatric care is strongly indicated if clinical findings support a diagnosis of depression with psychotic symptoms, bipolar disorder, active suicidal ideation, depression with comorbid substance use disorder, depression with comorbid dementia, and other clinical scenarios requiring more specialized assessment.

Mark TL, Levit KR, Buck JA. Datapoints: psychotropic drug prescriptions by medical specialty. *Psychiatr Serv*. 2009;60(9):1167. [PMID: 19723729]

Pence BW, O'Donnell JK, Gaynes BN. The depression treatment cascade in primary care: a public health perspective. *Curr Psychiatry Rep*. 2012;14(4):328–335. [PMID: 22580833]

A. Psychotherapeutic Interventions

For patients with mild symptoms of major depressive disorder, psychotherapy alone may be appropriate. Cognitive behavioral therapy (CBT) and interpersonal therapy are evidence-based psychotherapeutic approaches used in the treatment of patients with major depressive disorder. Factors to consider when determining how often to see an individual patient include the goals of the psychotherapy, the frequency necessary to create and maintain a therapeutic alliance, the frequency required to ensure treatment adherence, and the frequency necessary to monitor and address suicidality. Many times, if there is not a skilled therapist available in the primary care setting, referral to a mental health specialist may be indicated (eg, psychiatric nurses, licensed clinical social workers, psychologists, or psychiatrists). Studies show that patients often prefer psychotherapy to pharmacotherapy, particularly individuals from diverse racial or ethnic groups. Physicians should ensure that patients are made aware of psychotherapy as an option and that they are assisted in accessing psychotherapeutic interventions.

B. Pharmacotherapy

Patients with mild symptoms of depression may choose between treatment with pharmacotherapy or psychotherapy. However, pharmacotherapy is recommended as the standard of care for all patients with moderate to severe depressive episodes. The goal of antidepressant therapy is to achieve full remission of depressive symptoms. In general, improvement should be noted within 6–8 weeks of initiating therapy. Ongoing antidepressant treatment is recommended up to 6 months after full remission is first achieved. Thereafter, maintenance antidepressant therapy is suggested in patients with a mild or a single episode of major depression, whereas it is strongly recommended for those with recurrent episodes of major depression or with moderate or severe episodes, to preserve improvements and prevent recurrence.

The most commonly used antidepressant mediations are listed in Table 56–2. Selective serotonin reuptake inhibitors (SSRIs) and serotonin-norepinephrine reuptake inhibitors (SNRIs) are usually first-line therapy, due to greater tolerability and equal efficacy compared to other antidepressants. Other medications likely to be optimal for most patients include bupropion and mirtazapine. Because of their potential to cause serious side effects and the need for dietary restrictions, tricyclic antidepressants (TCAs) and monoamine oxidase inhibitors (MAOIs) are typically reserved for patients with treatment-resistant depression.

Numerous factors can influence how an individual responds to a particular antidepressant medication, including a person's racial or ethnic origins and age. Due to pharmacokinetic and pharmacodynamic changes with age, antidepressants should be initiated at a lower starting dose and slower titration rate in older adults to prevent adverse effects. Antidepressants that should be avoided in the older adults because of cardiotoxic side effects and other safety concerns include TCAs, such as amitriptyline, imipramine, nortriptyline, and doxepin. Additional caution is recommended for those taking multiple medications because polypharmacy increases the risk of adverse drug events.

Patients prescribed antidepressant medication should be monitored to assess their response to pharmacotherapy as well as side effects and adverse reactions. After dosing antidepressant medication at the recommended starting dose, it is important to increase the medication over time to an efficacious dose. Few patients treated for depression in primary care reach the recommended therapeutic dosage of the medicine. Screening tests can be used to objectively monitor a patient's progress throughout treatment. To maintain consistency with clinical practice guidelines, patients should be seen for follow-up within 1 month after initiating pharmacologic treatment. If no response is seen within the initial 6- to 8-week period of adequate pharmacotherapy, switching to another first-line antidepressant is recommended. Several trials may be needed because there is only an approximate 30% probability that patients will achieve remission with the first antidepressant that they try. Referral for specialty mental health care may be considered with failure of two or more antidepressants.

Stepped care models have been used in primary care settings to manage diverse conditions such as hypertension and have been proven effective in improving the quality of depression care for patients in primary care settings, especially in those with medical comorbidities.[24] Stepped care models are systematic procedures based on using the most effective, but least intensive, treatment for patients, and include detailed monitoring and tracking of patients' response to interventions. An example of a stepped care model for depression treatment is shown in Table 56–3.

National Collaborating Centre for Mental Health. Depression in adults: recognition and management. https://www.nice.org.uk/guidance/cg90/chapter/1-Guidance#stepped-care. Accessed April 2018.

Stoop C, Nefs G, Pommer A, Pop V, Pouwer F. Effectiveness of a stepped care intervention for anxiety and depression in people with diabetes, asthma or COPD in primary care: a randomized controlled trial. *J Affect Disord.* 2015;184:269–276. [PMID: 26118755]

C. Complementary and Alternative Therapies

Complementary and alternative therapies may be considered in treating mild episodes of depression or as adjunctive treatments in moderate to severe depression. Exercise has been shown to have some beneficial effects in the treatment of depression compared to antidepressant medication alone. Mindfulness-based cognitive therapies have been shown to prevent relapse and recurrence of depressive episodes. Other meditative activities such as yoga, tai chi, music, and massage therapy have demonstrated benefit in older adults. A variety of coping and self-management strategies can also be helpful, such as peer support, good nutrition, progressive muscle relaxation, setting aside time for pleasurable activities, and setting small, achievable goals. Furthermore, increasing evidence in the medical literature supports the beneficial role of spirituality in the health of patients.

St. John's wort is a popular supplement used by patients who wish to avoid prescription antidepressants. Multiple

Table 56–2. Medications used in treatment of depression.[a]

Drug Type: Brand (generic)	Typical Daily[b] Dosage (mg)	Indications/Caution/Side Effects
Selective serotonin reuptake inhibitors (SSRIs)		SSRIs have a black box warning for increasing the risk of suicidal ideation in adolescents and young adults. This risk should be discussed with patients and their parents before prescribing, and patients should be educated to monitor for this side effect and contact the prescriber or seek medical attention and/or emergency services should it arise. Common side effects: gastrointestinal upset, sexual dysfunction
Celexa (citalopram)	20–40	Increased risk of QTc prolongation; monitor or avoid in cardiac disease
Lexapro (escitalopram)	10–20	
Paxil (paroxetine)	20–50	Short half-life; choose controlled-release formulation to avoid discontinuation syndrome
Paxil CR (paroxetine, controlled-release)	12.5–62.5	
Prozac (fluoxetine)	20–60	Many CYP450 interactions; check for drug-drug interactions in patients taking multiple prescription drugs
Prozac Weekly (fluoxetine)	90	
Zoloft (sertraline)	50–200	
Serotonin-norepinephrine reuptake inhibitors (SNRIs)		SNRIs also have a black box warning for increasing the risk of suicidal ideation in adolescents and young adults. Common side effects: nausea, dizziness, diaphoresis. May cause sexual dysfunction. Dose-dependent increase in blood pressure.
Cymbalta (duloxetine)	60–120	Efficacious with comorbid fibromyalgia and neuropathic pain
Effexor (venlafaxine)	75–375	Efficacious with comorbid anxiety
Effexor XR (venlafaxine, extended-release)	75–225	
Pristiq (desvenlafaxine)	50–100	
Other		
Remeron (mirtazapine)	15–45	Common side effects: increased appetite, weight gain, drowsiness
Desyrel (trazodone)	150–400	Common side effects: drowsiness
Wellbutrin, Wellbutrin XL (bupropion)	150–450	Decreases seizure threshold; avoid in patients with a history of bulimia, seizures, or electrolyte abnormalities. Also indicated for smoking cessation.
Wellbutrin SR (bupropion, sustained-release)	150–400	Common side effects: weight loss, insomnia.
Tricyclic antidepressants (TCAs)		
Elavil (amitriptyline)	150–300	TCAs can cause cardiac arrhythmias and should be avoided in those with cardiac disease and in the elderly.
Aventyl, Pamelor (nortriptyline)	75–150	Common side effects: anticholinergic side effects (dry mouth, urinary retention, constipation, blurry vision)
Norpamin (desipramine)	150–300	
Sinequan (doxepin)	25–300	
Tofranil (imipramine)	150–200	
Monoamine oxidase inhibitors (MAOIs)		
Emsam skin patch (selegiline)	6–12	Avoid foods high in tyramine (fermented foods and beverages; eg, cheese, alcohol) to avoid hypertensive crises. Increased risk of serotonin syndrome when combined with SSRIs and SNRIs. Many drug-drug interactions.
Marplan (isocarboxazid)	30–60	
Nardil (phenelzine)	45–90	
Parnate (tranylcypromine)	10–60	

[a]This list represents the most commonly prescribed antidepressants.
[b]These dosages represent an average range for the treatment of depression. The precise effective dosage varies from patient to patient and depends on many factors. *Starting dosages tend to be lower for older adults, children, and adolescents.*
Data from Schatzberg AF, DeBattista C: *Manual of Clinical Psychopharmacology.* 8th ed. Washington, DC: American Psychiatric Publishing; 2015.

Table 56–3. Stepped care model of depression treatment.

Step 1: All known and suspected presentations of depression	Assessment, support, psychoeducation, active monitoring, and referral for further assessment and interventions
Step 2: Persistent subthreshold depressive symptoms, mild to moderate depression	Low-intensity psychological and psychosocial interventions, medication, and referral for further assessment and interventions
Step 3: Persistent subthreshold depressive symptoms or mild to moderate depression with inadequate response to initial interventions; moderate and severe depression	Medication, high-intensity psychological interventions, combined treatment, collaborative care, and referral for further assessment and interventions
Step 4: Severe and complex depression; risk to life; severe self-neglect	Medication, high-intensity psychological interventions, electroconvulsive therapy, crisis service, combined treatments, multiprofessional and inpatient care

Reproduced with permission from National Collaborating Centre for Mental Health. *Depression: Quick Reference Guide.* NICE Clinical Guidelines; 2009. https://www.nice.org.uk/guidance/cg90/chapter/1-Guidance#stepped-care. Accessed December 3, 2019.

randomized clinical trials have demonstrated its modest efficacy in treating mild to moderate depression. However, the long-term safety and efficacy of St. John's wort is not well studied. Providers should screen for its use because patients are often less likely to share information about their use of herbal supplements. This is important because St. John's wort has increased medication interactions, particularly in older adults, and is generally not recommended for treatment of depression in most populations. Other alternative medication therapies have conflicting reports about efficacy but include *S*-adenosyl methionine (SAM-e), omega-3 fatty acids, and folic acid supplementation; however, further research is needed to determine their efficacy in the treatment of depression.

Fava M. Using complementary and alternative medicines for depression. *J Clin Psychiatry.* 2010;71(9):e24. [PMID: 20923617]

Huijbers M, Speckens A. Mindfulness-based cognitive therapy as an alternative to maintenance antidepressant medication to prevent relapse and recurrence in depression. *Evid Based Ment Health.* 2015;8(4):126. [PMID: 26337984]

Ng QX, Venkatanarayanan N, Ho CYX. Clinical use of *Hypericum perforatum* (St John's wort) in depression: a meta-analysis. *J Affect Disord.* 2017;210:211–221. [PMID: 28064110]

Nyer M, Doorley J, Durham K, Yeung AS, Freeman MP, Mischoulon D. What is the role of alternative treatments in late-life depression? *Psychiatr Clin.* 2013;36(4):577–596. [PMID: 24229658]

Rasic D, Robinson JA, Bolton J, Bienvenu OJ, Sareen J. Longitudinal relationships of religious worship attendance and spirituality with major depression, anxiety disorders, and suicidal ideation and attempts: findings from the Baltimore epidemiologic catchment area study. *J Psychiatr Res.* 2011;45(6):848–854. [PMID: 21215973]

D. Combination Therapy

A combination of psychotherapy and medication is recommended for patients with moderate to severe depression. Patients who have a history of only partial response to adequate trials of either treatment modality alone may benefit from combined treatment. Sequential treatment of psychotherapy and pharmacotherapy may also be beneficial. Patients with poor adherence to individual treatments may also benefit from combined treatment of any form. Most studies of CBT support its use either alone or in addition to pharmacotherapy in decreasing the recurrence of depression.

E. Electroconvulsive Therapy

Although electroconvulsive therapy (ECT) remains a highly stigmatized treatment modality, it is also a very effective therapy for depression, particularly among older adults and patients with psychotic or treatment-resistant depression. ECT is administered under general anesthesia using electrodes that induce a seizure. Patients often have rapid improvement of symptoms of depression and usually receive two to three treatments per week for 3–6 weeks. Side effects include headache, muscle aches, and memory problems, which are more commonly associated with bilateral electrode placement on the head compared with unilateral electrode placement. Primary care providers should consider a referral to a mental health specialist for evaluation for ECT in patients who have not responded to multiple trials of medication and psychotherapy.

F. Integrated Care and Collaborative Care Models

Integrated care and collaborative care models have effectively improved the treatment of depression in primary care settings. An extremely well-studied model of using integrated care to treat depression in older adults is the Improving Mood–Promoting Access to Collaborative Treatment (IMPACT) collaborative care management program for late-life depression. The IMPACT model has shown significantly better outcomes for treatment of depression in older adults compared to usual care. The model embeds a depression care manager (supervised by a psychiatrist and primary care expert) in a primary care setting to provide comprehensive services to older adults with depression.

Integrated care models have shown particular efficacy among older adults, who are more likely to accept treatment for depression in primary care settings rather than in specialty mental health settings. Within diverse populations, integrated care/collaborative care models have also shown efficacy in African American and Latino populations. A recent study demonstrated improvement in outcome disparities of minority patients with depression with the implementation of collaborative care in the primary care setting.

Angstman KB, Phelan S, Myszkowski MR, et al. Minority primary care patients with depression: outcome disparities improve with collaborative care management. *Med Care.* 2015;53(1):32–37. [PMID: 25464162]

Hunkeler EM, Katon W, Tang L, et al. Long term outcomes from the IMPACT randomised trial for depressed elderly patients in primary care. *BMJ.* 2006;332(7536):259–263. [PMID: 16428253]

Katon W. Collaborative depression care models: from development to dissemination. *Am J Prevent Med.* 2012;42(5):550–552. [PMID: 22516497]

Woltmann E, Grogan-Kaylor A, Perron B, Georges H, Kilbourne AM, Bauer MS. Comparative effectiveness of collaborative chronic care models for mental health conditions across primary, specialty, and behavioral health care settings: systematic review and meta-analysis. *Am J Psychiatry.* 2012;169(8):790–804. [PMID: 22772364]

G. Addressing Disparities and Cultural Differences in Depression Care

Studies have shown that different racial and ethnic groups, as well as age and gender groups, experience and communicate symptoms of depression differently and prefer different forms of treatment. If the provider does not speak the patient's native language, a well-trained healthcare interpreter should be used to ensure that accurate information is exchanged. In general, some populations are more receptive to psychotherapy than pharmacotherapy, and patient preferences should be explored in order to practice cultural competence. Because stigma continues to be a pervasive barrier to seeking appropriate mental health treatment, primary care providers should encourage open dialogue and help correct any false assumptions about the origins of mental health problems and judgments about individuals with mental health problems.

Patient-provider communication is critical to diagnosis and treatment. The physician should elicit patients' explanatory models (what patients believe is causing their illness) and agendas (what patients seek from treatment), the role of family members in their lives, how those family members will react to the patient being treated, and how patients perceive treatment. For some people, experiences of racism and prejudice may leave people suspicious of diagnoses that do not require radiologic or laboratory examinations. The provider must use excellent communication skills to convey humility, empathy, respect, and compassion, as these are important factors in securing an accurate diagnosis and effective treatment of depression in racially, ethnically, and culturally diverse populations (Table 56–4).

Table 56–4. Factors affecting cultural competence in assessment, diagnosis, and treatment of depression.

Recognition of language differences
Health literacy barriers
Somatic presentation
Use of cultural idioms of distress
Treatment preferences
Non-Western context of mental illness and treatment
Individually tailored treatment plans

Spirituality is often an important determinant of mental health. The mere presence of a religious affiliation and the saliency of a person's religion have been shown to be strong protective factors for depression and suicide, particularly in older adults with medical illnesses or disability. This is important for providers not only because it may largely influence how patients cope with their illnesses, but also because studies have shown that validating this aspect of a patient's life and incorporating it into treatment plans can positively affect the patient's adherence to treatment and even accelerate rates of remission.

Rasic D, Robinson JA, Bolton J, Bienvenu OJ, Sareen J. Longitudinal relationships of religious worship attendance and spirituality with major depression, anxiety disorders, and suicidal ideation and attempts: findings from the Baltimore epidemiologic catchment area study. *J Psychiatr Res.* 2011;45(6):848–854. [PMID: 21215973]

van Loon A, van Schaik A, Dekker J, Beekman A. Bridging the gap for ethnic minority adult outpatients with depression and anxiety disorders by culturally adapted treatments. *J Affect Disord.* 2013;147(1):9–16. [PMID: 23351566]

▶ Prognosis

Primary care practitioners are the sole contacts for >50% of patients with mental illness and therefore are important in ensuring recognition and treatment of depression. The good news is that most patients can be treated to remission, especially if medication and psychotherapy are combined. Depression is generally a chronic, relapsing illness; however, treatment works not only to make patients well, but also to keep them well. Treatment provides symptomatic relief, facilitates functional improvements, and prevents relapse and recurrence.

Roca M, Gili M, Garcia-Garcia M, et al. Prevalence and comorbidity of common mental disorders in primary care. *J Affect Disord.* 2009;119(1):52–58. [PMID: 19361865]

Anxiety Disorders

57

Philip J. Michels, PhD

▶ General Considerations

Anxiety is a diffuse, unpleasant, and often vague subjective feeling of apprehension accompanied by objective symptoms of autonomic nervous system (ANS) arousal. The experience of anxiety is associated with a sense of danger or a lack of control over events. The psychological component varies from individual to individual and is strongly influenced by personality and coping mechanisms.

Many factors contribute to the experience of anxiety by individuals in our society. We live in a rapidly changing culture characterized by continuous technologic advancements, proliferation of increasingly refined information, and a mass media and entertainment industry saturated with violence and sexuality, all of which promote feelings of insecurity. In the workplace, downsizing, restructuring, mergers, and specialization are commonplace; transient work relationships and the elimination of benefits such as health insurance and retirement provisions increase the sense of insecurity.

Anxiety is pathologic when it occurs in situations that do not call for fear or when the degree of anxiety is excessive for the situation. Anxiety may occur as a result of life events, as a symptom of a primary anxiety disorder, as a secondary response to another psychiatric disorder or medical illness, or as a side effect of a medication.

The majority of individuals with mental disorders receive psychiatric care from primary care settings, whereas <20% receive care in specialized mental health settings. Anxiety disorder increases the risk of mortality (relative risk [RR] = 1.43; 95% confidence interval [CI], 1.24–1.64) with approximately 2.41 million deaths attributable to anxiety disorder per year. Even though their relative risk is significantly lower compared to psychosis (RR = 2.54; 95% CI, 2.35–2.75), the prevalence of anxiety disorder is high, and therefore, the emphasis on screening these patients in primary care is essential. There is some controversy that comorbid depression in patients with anxiety attributes to increased mortality, but patients with anxiety disorders are at increased risk of other medical comorbidities, contributing to around 26,500 disability-adjusted life-years (DALYs), accounting for approximately 15% of DALYs among mental disorders.

Combs H, Markman J. Anxiety disorders in primary care. *Med Clin North Am.* 2014;98(5):1007–1023. [PMID: 25134870]

Miloyan B, Bulley A, Bandeen-Roche K, et al. Anxiety disorders and all-cause mortality: systematic review and meta-analysis. *Soc Psychiatry Psychiatr Epidemiol.* 2016;51(11):1467–1475. [PMID: 27628244]

Walker ER, McGee RE, Druss BG. Mortality in mental disorders and global disease burden implications: a systematic review and meta-analysis. *JAMA Psychiatry.* 2015;72(4):334–341. [PMID: 25671328]

Whiteford HA, Degenhardt L, Rehm J, et al. Global burden of disease attributable to mental and substance use disorders: findings from the Global Burden of Disease Study 2010. *Lancet.* 2013;382(9904):1575–1586. [PMID: 23993280]

▶ Pathogenesis

A. Biomedical Influences

Because the symptoms of anxiety are so varied and prevalent, several etiologies exist to explain them. Functional magnetic resonance imaging (MRI) shows hypofunction of cortical areas leading to a dysfunctional inhibition of the amygdala resulting in emotional dysregulation.

Risk factors for generalized anxiety disorder (GAD) include stressful life events during childhood, parental history of mental disorders, low socioeconomic status, and marital difficulties including being widowed or divorced. Hispanics, compared with blacks and non-Hispanics, have little risk of GAD. Tobacco dependence and alcohol binge drinking are associated with an increased incidence of panic disorders. There is less evidence to show a consistent pattern of γ-aminobutyric acid (GABA) deficits in anxiety disorder as initially thought.

B. Psychological and Social Influences

Family dysfunction and parental psychopathology are involved in the development and maintenance of anxiety. Families of anxious children are more involved, controlling, and rejecting, and less intimate than are families who do not manifest anxiety. Parents of anxious children promote cautious and avoidant child behavior.

Behavioral and cognitive explanations define anxiety as a learned response. Anxiety develops in response to neutral or positive stimuli that become associated with a noxious or aversive event. Fearful associations develop from the situational context and the physical sensations present at the time. The patient may generalize (ie, classify objects and events in terms of a common characteristic) and thereby establish new cues to trigger anxiety. Previously neutral situations become feared and avoided. By avoiding anxiety-arousing stimuli, anxiety is diminished.

As panic and avoidance become more chronic, the behaviors involved become more habitual, and awareness of one's thoughts in relation to these anxiety states diminishes. Information-processing prejudices such as selectively attending to threatening stimuli become involuntary and unconscious. A person's appraisal of an event, rather than intrinsic characteristics of that event, defines stress, evokes anxiety, and influences the ability to cope. Failure to cope elicits fear and vulnerability.

Goddard AW. Cortical and subcortical gamma amino acid butyric acid deficits in anxiety and stress disorders: clinical implications. *World J Psychiatry*. 2016;6(1):43–53. [PMID: 27014597]

Kagan J, Snidman N. Early childhood predictors of adult anxiety disorders. *Biol Psychiatr*. 1999;46:1536. [PMID: 10599481]

Mochcovitch MD, da Rocha Freire RC, Garcia RF, et al. A systematic review of fMRI studies in generalized anxiety disorder: evaluating its neural and cognitive basis. *J Affect Disord*. 2014;167:336–342. [PMID: 23993280]

Moreno-Peral P, Conejo-Cerón S, Motrico E, et al. Risk factors for the onset of panic and generalized anxiety disorders in the general adult population: a systematic review of cohort studies. *J Affect Disord*. 2014;168:337–348. [PMID: 25089514]

▶ Prevention

Training in stress inoculation, relaxation training, and cognitive behavioral therapy (CBT) can be implemented through an integrated curriculum in public education during the early and middle years. School settings provide furtive environments for group modeling and an opportunity to reach large numbers of people. The work of Dr. Martin Seligman (see Gillham et al, 1995) demonstrates the sizable advantages of such school-based programs.

Gillham JR, Reivich KJ, Jaycox LH, et al. Prevention of depressive symptoms in school-children: two-year follow-up. *Psychol Sci*. 1995;6:343–351. [PMID: 16643843]

▶ Clinical Findings

A. Symptoms and Signs

Examination of the patient usually yields few clues to assist in establishing the diagnosis of an anxiety disorder. Diagnosis is complicated by the number of symptoms and their overlap with other disease states; thus, anxiety often becomes a diagnosis of exclusion. Table 57–1 lists various symptoms of anxiety by organ system.

Despite the variety and diffuse nature of many of these symptoms, anxiety disorders can often be identified by exploration of the patient's history, along with a few laboratory values. The symptoms of each anxiety disorder are sufficiently specific to arrive at the diagnosis by taking a thorough history from the patient, including pertinent past, social, and family information. Recognition of anxiety subtypes is often based on history alone.

B. Diagnostic Criteria

The *Diagnostic and Statistical Manual of Mental Disorders,* 5th edition (*DSM-5*) differentiates several anxiety disorders. Diagnostic criteria for each disorder are presented below.

1. Separation anxiety disorder—This disorder involves excessive anxiety or fear concerning separation from those to whom the individual is attached.

2. Selective mutism—This disorder involves a consistent failure to speak in specific social situations where there is an expectation to speak despite speaking in other situations.

Table 57–1. Somatic symptoms of anxiety.

System	Symptoms
Musculoskeletal	Muscle tightness, spasms, back pain, headache, weakness, tremors, fatigue, restlessness, exaggerated startle response, jitters
Cardiovascular	Palpitations, rapid heartbeat, hot and cold spells, flushing, pallor
Gastrointestinal	Dry mouth, diarrhea, upset stomach, lump in throat, nausea, vomiting
Bladder	Frequent urination
Central nervous	Dizziness, paresthesias, lightheadedness
Respiratory	Hyperventilation, shortness of breath, constriction in chest
Miscellaneous	Sweating, clammy hands

Data from Flauherty JA: *Psychiatry: Diagnosis and Treatment.* Philadelphia, PA. Appleton & Lange; 1993.

3. Specific phobias—These phobias involve marked fear or anxiety about a specific object or situation (eg, flying, heights, receiving an injection).

4. Social anxiety disorder—This condition is characterized by marked fear or anxiety about one or more social situations where the individual is exposed to possible scrutiny by others. The individual fears that she or he will act in a certain way or show anxiety that will be negatively evaluated and avoids these social situations or endures them with intense fear or anxiety, out of proportion to the actual threat.

5. Panic disorder—The attack involves an abrupt surge of intense fear or discomfort that reaches a peak within minutes and can be recurrent and unexpected. Symptoms include nausea, dizziness, lightheadedness, tingling sensations, feelings of unreality or being detached from oneself, fear of going crazy, and fear of dying. The Patient Health Questionnaire for panic disorder has a positive likelihood ratio of 78 (95% CI, 29–210) and a negative likelihood ratio of 0.20 (95% CI, 0.11–0.37) and is feasible for use in primary care.

6. Agoraphobia—This is a marked fear or anxiety about using public transportation, being in open or enclosed spaces, being in a crowd, or being outside alone.

7. GAD—GAD is defined as at least 6 months of persistent and excessive anxiety and worry occur on most days, with difficulty controlling the worry. Symptoms include restlessness, being on edge, being easily fatigued, difficulty concentrating, irritability, muscle tension, and sleep disturbance. Several validated tools have been developed to screen for GAD, including the two-item and seven-item Generalized Anxiety Disorder scales (GAD-2, GAD-7). The GAD-7 scale has a positive likelihood ratio of 5.1 (95% CI, 4.3–6.0) and a negative likelihood ratio of 0.13 (95% CI, 0.07–0.25). These self-report questionnaires are easy to use and can assist primary care physicians in assessing the severity of GAD as well.

8. Substance/medication-induced anxiety disorder— Anxiety is a direct physiologic consequence of a drug of abuse, medication, or exposure to a toxin.

9. Anxiety disorder due to another medical condition— Panic attacks or anxiety predominate, and there is evidence that the disturbance is the direct pathophysiologic consequence of another medical condition.

10. Adjustment disorder with anxious mood—Clinically significant symptoms of anxiety occur in response to an identifiable stressor within 3 months after onset of the stressor and resolve within 6 months after termination of the stressor. However, symptoms may persist longer if they occur in response to a chronic stressor (eg, a disabling chronic medical condition) or to a stressor that has enduring consequences (eg, financial effects of a divorce).

Herr NR, Williams JW Jr, Benjamin S, et al. Does this patient have generalized anxiety or panic disorder? The Rational Clinical Examination systematic review. *JAMA*. 2014;312(1):78–84. [PMID: 25058220]

Spitzer RL, Kroenke K, Williams JB, et al. A brief measure for assessing generalized anxiety disorder: the GAD-7. *Arch Intern Med*. 2006;166(10):1092–1097. [PMID: 16717171]

C. Laboratory Findings

There are no gold standard laboratory studies on diagnosing anxiety disorders. It is reasonable to perform a limited empiric evaluation to identify the etiology of the symptoms as well as evaluate for comorbid medical problems that may complicate the treatment. This evaluation may include a complete blood count, electrolytes, glucose, creatinine, calcium, liver panel, and thyroid function tests. Further testing should be tailored on an individual basis, depending on the clinical circumstances. Urine drug screening should be considered, because illicit drug use and withdrawal may be a possible differential diagnosis and patients with anxiety may self-medicate with drugs of abuse.

Fricchione G. Clinical practice. Generalized anxiety disorder. *N Engl J Med*. 2004;351:675–682. [PMID: 15306669]

D. Imaging Studies

Imaging studies are completed only to preclude any laboratory abnormalities or organic disease that may mimic anxiety or panic. Such studies include, but are not limited to, thyroid scan and cardiac diagnostics. Functional MRI is a technique that enables one to map cognitive, affective, and experiential processes onto brain substrates. It is a proxy measure of how complex processes are implemented in different neural systems. Magnetic resonance spectroscopy is a noninvasive in vivo method used to quantify metabolites that are relevant to a wide range of brain processes. Previous studies have shown that there are significant metabolic differences in various regions of the brain between patients with anxiety disorders and healthy controls.

Paulus MP. The role of neuroimaging for the diagnosis and treatment of anxiety disorders. *Depress Anxiety*. 2008;25:348–356. [PMID: 18412061]

Trzesniak C, Araujo D. Magnetic resonance spectroscopy in anxiety disorders. *Acta Neuropsychiatr*. 2008;20:56–71. [PMID: 26953102]

E. Special Tests

Psychological tests resort to self-report of symptoms and are major assessment tools for anxiety. This is unfortunate as most other medical diagnoses (eg, diabetes mellitus) rely on both symptom self-report and systematic biomedical measurements (eg, the glucose tolerance test).

The State-Trait Anxiety Inventory (STAI) measures the frequency and intensity of transient anxiety processes and anxiety proneness as a character trait, whereas the Beck Anxiety Inventory-Trait (BAIT) is specific to measuring trait anxiety. Both self-report tests have excellent reliability and validity.

Other validated measures are the Endler Multidimensional Anxiety Scales (EMAS), which specifically measure responses to social evaluation, physical danger, and ambiguous and daily routines, and the Three Systems Anxiety Questionnaire (TSAQ), which assesses the behavioral, cognitive, and somatic components of anxiety. Comorbidity can comprehensively be assessed by the Minnesota Multiphasic Personality Inventory-II (MMPI-II), a test composed of 567 true/false test items that can be completed in approximately 2 hours. The Profile of Mood States (POMS) primarily measures mood states in psychiatric outpatients. Its advantage over the MMPI-II is a completion time of approximately 10 minutes.

Elwood LS, Wolitzky-Taylor K, Olatunji BO. Measurement of anxious traits: a contemporary review and synthesis. *Anxiety Stress Coping.* 2012;25(6):647–666. [PMID: 21644113]

Hathaway SR, McKinley C. *Minnesota Multiphasic Personality Inventory-2.* Minneapolis, MN: National Computer Systems, University of Minnesota; 1989.

McNair DM, Lorr M, Droppleman LF. *Profile of Mood States, Revised.* San Diego, CA: Educational and Industrial Testing Service; 1992.

Spielberger CD. *State-Trait Anxiety Inventory.* Palo Alto, CA: Consulting Psychologists Press; 1983.

▶ Differential Diagnosis

Because anxiety is a ubiquitous symptom of numerous conditions, family physicians must be alert to the possibility of alternative medical causes.

The first step in planning a diagnostic evaluation is to perform a thorough history and physical examination. Table 57–2 presents the differential diagnosis of other medical conditions that may present with anxiety-like symptoms. If anxiety did not predate a medical illness, subsequent anxiety may represent an adjustment disorder with anxious mood. The most likely organic cause of anxiety is alcohol and drug use (withdrawal or intoxication). Caffeine toxicity and increased sensitivity to caffeine also commonly mimic symptoms of anxiety.

Symptoms of cardiovascular abnormalities such as chest discomfort, shortness of breath, and palpitations are also cardinal symptoms of anxiety. Many anxious patients function poorly because they believe that they have heart disease. The electrocardiogram can be a useful tool to differentiate anxiety from a significant cardiac abnormality. Further evaluation should be considered according to the patient's symptoms and risk profile.

Table 57–2. Differential diagnosis of anxiety disorders.

Cardiovascular:
  Acute coronary syndrome, congestive heart failure, mitral valve prolapse, dysrhythmia, syncope, hypertension
Drugs:
  β-Agonists, caffeine, digoxin toxicity, levodopa, nicotinic acid, pseudoephedrine, selective serotonin reuptake inhibitors, steroids, stimulants (methylphenidate, dextroamphetamine), theophylline preparations, thyroid preparations
Endocrine disorders:
  Hyper-/hypothyroidism, hyperadrenalism
Neoplastic:
  Carcinoid syndrome, pheochromocytoma, insulinoma
Neurologic disorders:
  Parkinsonism, encephalopathy, restless leg syndrome, seizure, vertigo, brain tumor
Pulmonary:
  Asthma (acute), chronic obstructive pulmonary disease, hyperventilation, pneumonia, pneumothorax, pulmonary edema, pulmonary embolus
Psychiatric:
  Affective disorders, drug abuse and dependence/withdrawal syndromes
Other conditions:
  Anaphylaxis, anemia, electrolyte abnormalities, porphyria, menopause

A careful auscultatory examination of the heart may reveal evidence of mitral valve prolapse, the most common valvular abnormality in adults. Long-term studies have shown that complications from mitral valve prolapse are rare, but often these patients present with palpitations and a generalized sense of being unwell that may mimic anxiety.

Musculoskeletal pain syndromes and esophageal disorders, including esophageal motility disorders and gastroesophageal reflux disease (commonly known as "heartburn"), are the most common noncardiac explanations of chest pain. Anxiety exacerbates gastrointestinal conditions such as colitis, ulcers, and irritable bowel syndrome. Treating anxiety often resolves or improves gastrointestinal symptoms and its associated chest pain.

Most patients with chronic unexplained chest pain have concomitant psychiatric diagnoses, especially anxiety. When further cardiac evaluation yields normal results, the anxious patient is more effectively reassured.

The primary care physician must be alert to acute medical conditions that can present with hyperventilation or dyspnea such as pulmonary conditions. The differentiation between these entities can be as simple as checking a pulse oxygen saturation but will often require more advanced diagnostic studies such as chest radiography, computed tomography, or pulmonary angiography. Anxiety, hyperventilation, and dyspnea may accompany recurrent pulmonary emboli with few reliable physical signs. Anxiety has been shown to have a negative impact on quality of life in patients with asthma.

Hyperthyroidism and hypoglycemia may be mistaken for anxiety. Hypoparathyroidism, hyperkalemia, hyperthermia, hyponatremia, hypothyroidism, menopause, porphyria, and carcinoid tumors are less common causes of organic anxiety syndromes.

Depression is the most common psychiatric disorder associated with anxiety. Symptoms that discriminate clinical depression from anxiety include depressed mood, lack of energy, and loss of interest and pleasure.

Ingested substances such as medications or alcohol can elicit anxiety symptoms. Patients with anxiety disorders commonly drink to excess. Alcohol and drug problems involving dependence rather than abuse are most strongly associated with problems involving anxiety. Anxiety disorder and alcohol disorder can each initiate the other, especially in cases of alcohol dependence. Although many alcoholic patients present with anxiety, these symptoms decrease rapidly when the patient stops drinking. Only a small percentage of patients (perhaps 10%) has persistent symptoms of anxiety.

Since depression and substance abuse coexist with GAD, it is paramount to screen for these in primary care.

Kushner MG, Abrams K, Borchardt C. The relationship between anxiety disorders and alcohol use disorders: a review of major perspectives and findings. *Clin Psychol Rev.* 2000;20:149–171. [PMID: 10721495]

Lavoie KL, Bacon SL, Barone S, et al. What is worse for asthma control and quality of life: depressive disorders, anxiety disorders, or both? *Chest.* 2006;130:1039–1047. [PMID: 17035436]

▶ **Treatment**

The continuity of care and established physician-patient relationship characteristic of the primary care setting offer treatment advantages for patients with an anxiety disorder. However, physicians often miss signs of psychiatric problems in their patients because of a biomedical orientation. The result is excessive diagnostic testing, increased costs, frustrated patients, and cynical physicians.

Positive patient expectations and trust have a formidable impact on prognosis. By increasing their familiarity with standard CBT techniques and psychotropic medications, family physicians can enhance outcomes for patients with anxiety disorders. Several of the CBTs described later can easily be implemented by a busy family physician as supplemental treatment to psychopharmacology. Seeing patients more frequently while maintaining the time constraints of a 15-minute office visit can improve patient functioning without overwhelming the busy family physician. Other interventions can be offered through referral to mental health specialists. If the patient remains unimproved or nonadherent after several 15-minute office visits, referral or consultation is also appropriate.

Other characteristics have also been shown to facilitate the treatment of anxiety disorders. These include female gender, more years of practitioner experience, and social support. Positive characteristics of the organization such as level of expertise, time availability, financial resources, and administrative support are also helpful. A conducive reimbursement system has obvious positive consequences.

A. Pharmacotherapy

Medications are divided into two categories. The first category of medications includes the selective serotonin reuptake inhibitors (SSRIs), serotonin-norepinephrine reuptake inhibitors (SNRIs), and tricyclic antidepressants (TCAs). These agents work to prevent future anxiety. However, they take 4–8 weeks to show efficacy. Withdrawal reactions may occur with stopping the SSRI or SNRI abruptly, especially with medications with short half-lives.

The second category of medications includes benzodiazepines and nonbenzodiazepines; these medications do little to prevent future recurrence, and their primary purpose is to abort acute symptoms of anxiety. In contrast to SSRIs and SNRIs, benzodiazepines do not treat depression, which is a common comorbid condition in anxiety disorders, and therefore, benzodiazepines should be used with caution.

The decision to prescribe medications should be based on the patient's degree of emotional distress, the level of functional disability, and the side effects of the medication. Table 57–3 provides a summary of the dosage range, indications, and financial costs associated with psychotherapeutic agents commonly used in the treatment of anxiety disorders.

1. SSRIs—SSRIs are now considered the first line of medication treatment for most anxiety disorders, with the exception of situational anxiety. SSRIs are well tolerated, have low potential for overdose, and are not associated with psychological or physical dependence. Relative to benzodiazepines, SSRIs do not impair learning or memory.

Recommendations on dosing have been to start low and titrate slowly upward to therapeutic levels in order to minimize jitteriness and insomnia that may occur with higher initial doses. Exceptions would be the treatment of obsessive-compulsive disorder (OCD) and panic disorder with or without agoraphobia, which often requires higher than usual dosing. When a patient exhibits both depression and anxiety, SSRIs are strongly recommended. Common side effects include nausea, diarrhea, headache, and sexual dysfunction. Interestingly, a recent review of these second-generation antidepressants revealed mild to moderate strength in treating anxiety.

2. SNRIs—Venlafaxine (Effexor, Effexor XR) and duloxetine (Cymbalta) are both approved for treatment of GAD. Duloxetine is also approved for treatment of peripheral neuropathy and fibromyalgia. Side effects include headache, elevated blood pressure, and increased heart rate. Sexual dysfunction and gastrointestinal intolerance occur less often than with SSRIs.

3. TCAs—These may be considered after failed trials of SSRIs when other agents are not an option because of side effects or concerns of addiction or dependence. They are more

Table 57–3. Pharmacotherapy for anxiety disorders.

Drug Name	Usual Dosage Range	FDA-Approved Indications	Comments
Benzodiazepines[a] Alprazolam[b] (Xanax, Xanax XR, Niravam)	0.5–4 mg (3–6 , ≤10 mg daily for panic) divided into 3 doses	Short-term relief of anxiety Panic disorder	XR dosed once daily Reduce doses for elderly or patients with hepatic disease Physical dependence can occur with relatively short-term use Abrupt discontinuation can result in rebound anxiety or withdrawal symptoms Rapid-dissolve tablet available
Clorazepate[b] (Tranxene)	15–60 mg in divided doses	Short-term relief of anxiety	Reduce doses for elderly or patients with hepatic disease Physical dependence can occur with relatively short-term use
Clonazepam[b] (Klonopin)	0.25–0.5 mg twice daily (max dose 4 mg/d)	Panic disorder	Long duration of effect results in smoother control Rapid-dissolve tablet available
Diazepam[b] (Valium)	2–10 mg 2–4 times daily (max dose 40 mg/d)	Anxiety disorders Short-term relief of anxiety	Reduce doses for elderly or patients with hepatic disease Physical and psychological dependence can occur with continuous use
Lorazepam[b] (Ativan)	2–6 mg in divided doses	Short-term relief of anxiety Anxiety associated with depression	Effective when given orally or by IM/IV injection Preferred in patients with hepatic insufficiency because of no active metabolites
Selective Serotonin Reuptake Inhibitors (SSRIs) Escitalopram (Lexapro)	10 mg once daily	GAD	No significant additional benefit if dose increased to 20 mg
Fluoxetine[b] (Prozac)	10–60 mg once daily	GAD Panic disorder OCD PMDD	Doses should be taken in the morning Start with low dose and titrate to effective dose
Paroxetine[b] (Paxil, Paxil CR)	10–60 mg (12.5–62.5 mg CR) once daily	Panic disorder Social anxiety disorder GAD PTSD OCD PMDD	Start with low dose and titrate to effective dose Abrupt discontinuation can result in rebound anxiety or withdrawal symptoms CR formulation has lower gastric intolerance
Sertraline (Zoloft)	25–200 mg once daily	Panic disorder Social anxiety disorder OCD PTSD Pediatric OCD	Start with low dose and titrate to effective dose Abrupt discontinuation can result in rebound anxiety or withdrawal symptoms
Miscellaneous Venlafaxine (Effexor, Effexor XR)	75–225 mg in 2–3 divided doses	GAD Social anxiety disorder	Initiate with 37.5 mg daily and titrate up to effective dose XR formulation dosed once daily Taper dose on discontinuation to avoid rebound or withdrawal symptoms
Buspirone[b] (BuSpar)	10–60 mg in divided doses	GAD	Not for situational anxiety; therapeutic benefit may not be achieved for ≤1 month No risk of physical or psychological dependence Avoid in patients with severe renal or hepatic impairment

[a]All benzodiazepines are Schedule IV controlled substances.
[b]Generic formulations are available.
CR, controlled release; FDA, US Food and Drug Administration; GAD, generalized anxiety disorder; IM, intramuscular; IV, intravenous; OCD, obsessive-compulsive disorder; PMDD, premenstrual dysphoric disorder; PTSD, posttraumatic stress disorder; XR, extended release.

commonly used as adjunctive therapy when the patient also has insomnia or chronic pain, although the evidence for insomnia is limited. Adherence is low secondary to the high incidence of intolerable side effects such as dry mouth, constipation, and urinary retention and concerns about toxicity.

4. Benzodiazepines—These agents remain the treatment of choice for panic attacks, anticipatory anxiety, phobic avoidance, and transient situational stress reactions. They may be used as short-term therapy of panic disorder until concurrent SSRIs become effective. Use of benzodiazepines should be limited to 2–4 months of continuous therapy to limit the potential for psychological or physical dependence. Common side effects include anterograde amnesia, difficulty in balance, impairment of driving ability, and additive effects with alcohol. Use in elderly patients has been associated with paradoxical excitement and an increased risk of falls and hip fractures, especially with longer-acting agents.

Tolerance to the antianxiety effects is uncommon. The abrupt discontinuation of benzodiazepines, especially those with short half-lives, is associated with withdrawal syndromes of relatively rapid onset. A rebound syndrome, similar to but more transiently intense than the original disorder, may begin over a few days. Abrupt discontinuation of high doses of alprazolam may result in psychotic behaviors or seizures; a slow taper is essential.

Usual treatment initially combines an SSRI and a benzodiazepine. Studies have shown that patients who received combined treatment demonstrated more rapid improvement than those receiving either class of drug alone. There appears to be no additional benefit from taking a benzodiazepine after the first 5 or 6 weeks.

5. Buspirone (BuSpar)—Buspirone has an unknown mechanism of action but appears to affect neurotransmitters differently than benzodiazepines. Because of delayed onset of action of ≥2 weeks, it is indicated only in the treatment of GAD. Although studies have found buspirone to be as effective as benzodiazepines for GAD, many patients who previously received benzodiazepines do not perceive it to be as effective because they do not experience the "buzz" they had with benzodiazepines. Buspirone does not impair driving or cognition and is not additive with alcohol. The most common side effects are restlessness, dizziness, and headache. Recent studies suggest that buspirone may be useful as adjunctive therapy in the treatment of resistant anxiety.

6. β-Blockers—These are used primarily to reduce the autonomic symptoms (rapid heart rate, flushing, sweating) associated with performance or social anxiety. The medication is usually taken only when needed approximately 30 minutes before an anxiety-inducing situation. Dizziness, drowsiness, and lightheadedness are the most common side effects.

7. Hydroxyzine—Hydroxyzine is a sedating antihistamine (H_1 blocker) that is used by many clinicians for GAD.

Compared to other anxiolytic agents such as benzodiazepines and buspirone, hydroxyzine was equivalent regarding efficacy, acceptability, and tolerability. However, the evidence is limited due to a large amount of bias in the included studies. It seems to be an alternative in patients for whom benzodiazepines are contraindicated but never used as first-line treatment for GAD.

8. Atypical anticonvulsants—These agents are being used frequently as adjunctive therapy to augment the activity of SSRIs in patients with refractory symptoms of anxiety. Gabapentin (Neurontin) has been shown to augment SSRI activity in the treatment of panic disorder and OCD and to reduce anxiety associated with chronic pain syndrome. Pregabalin (Lyrica) has also been used for GAD but is approved only for fibromyalgia and peripheral neuropathy. Clinical studies have also demonstrated the effectiveness of other atypical anticonvulsants such as carbamazepine, valproic acid, and lamotrigine. Doses should start low and be titrated to effective dose to minimize side effects. The most common side effects are drowsiness, dizziness, and blurred vision.

Bandelow B, Michaelis S, Wedekind D. Treatment of anxiety disorders. *Dialogues Clin Neurosci.* 2017;19(2):93–107. [PMID: 28867934]

Combs H, Markman J. Anxiety disorders in primary care. *Med Clin North Am.* 2014;98(5):1007–1023. [PMID: 25134870]

Guaiana G, Barbui C, Cipriani A. Hydroxyzine for generalised anxiety disorder. *Cochrane Database Syst Rev.* 2010;12:CD006815. [PMID: 21154375]

Thaler KJ, Morgan LC, Van Noord M, et al. Comparative effectiveness of second-generation antidepressants for accompanying anxiety, insomnia, and pain in depressed patients: a systematic review. *Depress Anxiety.* 2012;29:495–505. [PMID: 28859190]

B. Psychotherapeutic Interventions

1. Behavioral therapy—This form of therapy focuses on overt behavior, with an emphasis on "how to" improve rather than "why" the problem exists. Several forms of behavioral therapy are available to assist patients in managing anxiety. The family physician's role involves explaining a behavioral procedure and prescribing homework. Time management need not suffer; 15-minute office visits sequenced about 1–2 weeks apart are usually adequate to provide therapy.

During *exposure therapy* the patient is repeatedly brought into contact with what is feared until discomfort subsides. The longer the exposure interval and the more intensive the exposure experience (massed trials) are, the better. To enhance adherence initially, often a significant other is present or a benzodiazepine is used; as therapy proceeds, both are gradually eliminated.

Although few people are formally educated in stress management, a large repertoire of coping skills is available. Table 57–4 offers a partial list of such strategies that can be given as a patient handout.

Table 57–4. Effective coping strategies.

Talk or write about stressful problems
Do enjoyable activities
Get enough rest and relaxation
Exercise regularly
Eat properly (beware of caffeine, chocolate, and alcohol)
Plan your time and set priorities
Accept responsibility for your role in a problem
Make expectations realistic
Get involved with others
Build in self-rewards
Utilize a sense of humor
Learn assertiveness
Attend support groups

Numerous types of relaxation training are useful in the treatment of all anxiety disorders and also have been shown to assist in anger management. Learning to relax is an inexpensive and easily accessible strategy. Reductions in the body's consumption of oxygen, blood lactate level (associated with muscle tension), metabolism, and heart and respiration rates occur during practice. Home practice for ≥20 minutes twice each day in a quiet place produces significant effects. Commercialized relaxation tapes are available for eidetic imagery and progressive muscle relaxation.

Panic attacks can be mediated by a highly effective technique, *breathing retraining*, which involves slow, deep (diaphragmatic) breathing. Slow inhalation, holding the breath, and slow exhalation are repeated for ≥10 sequences. During slow, deep breathing, the patient is told to substitute realistic thoughts ("I'm having a panic attack and I'm not in any danger") for panic-inducing thoughts ("I'm having a heart attack and I'll die soon"). This provides a sense of self-mastery and restores oxygen–carbon dioxide balance to the body. *Interoceptive exposure*, in which patients go through the symptoms of a panic attack (eg, elevated heart rate, hot flashes, sweating) in a controlled setting, can also be beneficial, by reinforcing for patients that these symptoms need not develop into a full-blown attack.

In the *worry exposure technique*, the patient is asked to do the following:

1. Identify (perhaps write down) and distinguish worrisome thoughts from pleasant thoughts.

2. Establish a 30-minute worry period at the same place and time each day.

3. Use the 30-minute period to worry about concerns and to engage in problem solving.

4. Postpone worries outside the 30-minute worry period with reminders that they can be considered during the next worry period (the patient may choose to write down new worries to avoid worrying about forgetting them).

5. During intrusions, replace worries with attention to present-moment experiences, activities, or pleasant memories.

This strategy challenges dysfunctional beliefs about the uncontrollability of thoughts and the dangerous consequences of failing to worry. Delusional jealousy also can be mediated by this approach.

In *mismatch strategy*, the physician asks the patient to write a detailed account of the content of the worry (eg, exposure to a particular situation normally avoided) and then asks the patient to worry about what could happen in that situation. Finally, the patient is instructed to enter the situation and observe what really happens to assess the validity of the worry thoughts.

Finally, the family physician can ask the patient to practice alternative endings for worry sequences. Rather than rehearsing catastrophic outcomes, the patient contemplates positive scenarios in response to worry triggers.

2. Cognitive therapy—Cognitive therapy is behavioral therapy of the mind. Based on the theory that thoughts, images, and assumptions usually account for the onset and persistence of anxiety, cognitive therapy assumes that the way patients perceive and appraise events and interpret arousal-related body sensations as dangerous (anxiety sensitivity) provokes symptoms of anxiety. Patients with social phobia demonstrate overestimation of the probability of negative outcomes in social situations, and they also exaggerate the costs of negative social events. Cognitive changes are the best predictors of treatment outcome for the anxiety disorders.

Achieving thought control is of central importance to mental health. Patients with OCD and GAD are especially prone to poor thought control. These patients devalue their ability to adequately deal with threats. Homework involving "self-talk" must be considered useful by the patient because alternative interpretations and explanations (*cognitive restructuring*) are always available for upsetting events; patients can assume more control of and accept more responsibility for their adaptation. Acceptance of these assumptions empowers the patient. Documented durable improvement results from cognitive restructuring (substituting rational assumptions and perspectives and transforming the meaning of events and physiologic arousal cues).

Although it is not possible to control all outside events, it is possible to control one's reaction to any event. Patients are advised that as soon as they are aware of being upset, they should pause and reflect on the following:

1. The event

2. Thoughts about the event

3. Associated feelings

4. Another way to perceive the event (another meaning) that is also true and makes sense but is not upsetting

When time permits, patients may enter this information in a small notebook for review with the family physician at a subsequent office visit.

Halm MA. Relaxation: a self-care healing modality reduces harmful effects of anxiety. *Am J Crit Care.* 2009;18:169–172. [PMID: 19255107]

Mobini SR, Mackintosh S, Reynolds SA, et al. Clinical implications of cognitive bias modification for interpretative biases in social anxiety: an integrative literature review. *Cogn Ther Res.* 2013;37(1):173–182. [No PMID]

C. Complementary and Alternative Therapies

Use of alternative therapies is more common among people with psychiatric problems and especially people with self-defined anxiety than among the rest of the population. Most alternative therapies are used without supervision. Because there are so few data on the relative effectiveness of these therapies, most people tend to try a therapist who has been recommended and, by trial and error, find a preferred therapy.

Massage therapies can be classified as energy methods, manipulative therapies, and combinations of each. Swedish massage is the most common form of massage and is usually given with oil. Movements called *effleurage* (smooth stroking) and *pétrissage* (kneading-type movements) are done up and down the back and across many tissues of the body. The Trager method, similar to many other types of massage therapy, involves gentle holding and rocking of different body parts. *Reflexology*, an energy method, could be classified as massage therapy because it involves kneading, stroking, rubbing, and other massage procedures. These procedures are centered on particular points of the feet, hands, or ears. Although few controlled studies exist using massage therapy, most people report anxiety reduction benefits. There are no empiric data on the efficacy of reflexology.

Acupuncture has been demonstrated to reduce anxiety across various populations and presenting problems. However, additional double-blind, placebo-controlled studies are needed.

Research indicates the benefits of *yoga* to quality of life and improved health. Yoga, which involves body postures and *asanas* (body maneuvers), appears to exercise various tissues, organs, and organ systems and provides an avenue to address character armors, attitudes, and tensions. Specific application to stress management is widespread with generally significant positive results. As is the case with acupuncture, however, better controlled research is needed.

Herbal therapies for anxiety include kava-kava, inositol, and melatonin. Several clinical studies have demonstrated the effectiveness of short-term use of kava-kava, which has a mechanism of action similar to that of the benzodiazepines. However, long-term use or high doses are associated with development of peripheral neuropathy. The US Food and Drug Administration (FDA) has issued a warning regarding the potential for kava-kava to cause hepatotoxicity, and this product has been removed from the market in several European countries. Inositol has been shown to be effective in the treatment of panic disorder and OCD but should not be used in combination with SSRIs. Melatonin has been promoted primarily to reduce the symptoms of jet lag and sleep-cycle disturbances.

Because of the inconsistent effects shown in only small studies, valerian, St. John's wort, and passionflower are not routinely recommended, although their side effect profiles are benign. Limited data support the role of valerian in relieving anxiety and insomnia, but it has additive effects with other central nervous system depressants and alcohol disturbances.

Kessler RC, Soukup J, Davis RB, et al. The use of complementary and alternative therapies to treat anxiety and depression in the United States. *Am J Psychiatr.* 2001;158:289–294. [PMID: 11156813]

Saeed SA, Bloch RM, Antonacci DJ. Herbal and dietary supplements for treatment of anxiety disorders. *Am Fam Physician.* 2007;76:549–556. [PMID: 17853630]

D. Consultation or Referral

Attempting the previously discussed treatment recommendations during multiple 15-minute continuity office visits often renders referral unnecessary. However, referral may be necessary when symptoms recur or when tapering a medication is difficult. Referral is appropriate when the family physician is uncomfortable with an indicated therapy, when patients are potentially suicidal or are actively abusing drugs, when noncompliance is suspected, or when psychopathology is severe. Referral of patients with OCD and post-traumatic stress disorder is mandatory. Given the expected need to individualize treatment and provide novel treatment options, the busy family physician has neither the time nor the expertise to engage in the comprehensive interventions required.

If psychotherapy is the preferred method of managing symptoms, the specialized training of a clinical or a counseling psychologist is recommended. When psychopharmacology is warranted, the expertise of a psychiatrist is unmatched. Sound treatment is based on specific and accurate diagnosis and relies on empirically validated procedures that take into account the personality of the patient.

Table 57–5 provides several referral treatments and their indications for the effective nonpharmacologic management of anxiety disorders.

E. Management of Specific Anxiety Disorders

1. Panic disorder—Recommended treatment includes breathing retraining, cognitive restructuring, interoceptive exposure, and relaxation training. If anxiety is short term, benzodiazepines should be used; if anxiety is chronic,

Table 57–5. Referral interventions and indications for use.

Type of Intervention	Description	Indications
Psychotherapy		
Individual	Insight, empowerment, support	Privacy, complicated patient
Group	Interactive, common interest	Social skills, support, vicarious learning
Family	Therapeutic environment and patient	Enabling, dysfunctional family
Eye movement desensitization and reprocessing (EMDR)	Follow oscillation movement of object (pencil) thinking of trauma Mixed results	Posttraumatic stress disorder
Hypnosis	Relaxation induction; suggestions	Suggestible patient
Biofeedback	EMG, ECG, EEG monitoring of physiologic parameters to alter activity; cost is a limiting factor	Headaches, tension, blood flow, etc
Stress inoculation/anxiety management	Multifaceted, comprehensive cognitive behavioral therapy	All anxiety disorders
Assertiveness training	Learn skills to be firm, not nasty	Dependent, unassertive, aggressive patients
Transcranial magnetic stimulation (TMS)	Noninvasive, painless method of brain stimulation via electrical current using changing magnetic fields	Applications are in their infancy

ECG, electrocardiogram; EEG, electroencephalogram; EMG, electromyogram.

paroxetine, citalopram, fluoxetine, sertraline, and venlafaxine should be used. TCAs have a role in panic disorder, but SSRIs and SNRIs are better tolerated. Additionally, because of the high rates of depression comorbidity associated with panic attacks, SSRIs are the pharmacologic treatment of choice.

Although current treatments allow control of panic disorder, full recovery is questionable. Psychological treatments involve lower relapse rates, higher levels of acceptability, and lower attrition rates and are better tolerated than many pharmacologic treatments. Among all anxiety disorders, meta-analysis shows greater treatment effect with CBT in panic disorders compared to other anxiety disorders. Exposure and deep breathing are especially effective for patients with panic attacks and agoraphobia.

Benzodiazepines are best used for acute management and should be used with caution. If a panic attack lasts <20 minutes, short-acting benzodiazepines have a limited role because the attack would have been resolved before the onset of the drug action.

Among psychotherapies, CBT is the most extensively studied in panic disorder and is slightly superior to other therapies. CBT plays a pivotal role in the treatment of panic disorder, and meta-analyses have shown better outcomes than in other anxiety disorders. CBT is as effective as pharmacotherapy and, at times, superior to medication.

2. Simple phobias—Recommended treatment includes exposure therapy, deep breathing, relaxation training, and cognitive restructuring, as well as short-term use of benzodiazepines.

3. Social phobia—Recommended treatment includes exposure therapy, cognitive restructuring, relaxation training, social skills training, and group therapy; medications that may be helpful include paroxetine, sertraline, clonazepam, and β-blockers.

When fearing negative evaluation, patients narrow their attention to social threat cues. Cognitive therapy corrects these distortions, whereas exposure therapy reduces anticipatory fear. In cognitive behavioral group settings, 81% of patients had significant improvement that was maintained 5.5 years later.

The SSRIs sertraline and paroxetine are both approved by the FDA for treatment of social anxiety disorder. β-Blockers on an as-needed basis may be helpful in patients who experience performance anxiety, even though published data supporting their benefit are limited. These agents can reduce hand tremor and tachycardia symptoms without causing cognitive impairment.

4. OCD—Recommended treatment includes referral as well as exposure therapy, response prevention, cognitive restructuring, and pharmacotherapy with fluoxetine, fluvoxamine, sertraline, or clomipramine. Behavior therapy and SSRIs are primarily recommended. Homework assignments expose patients to stimuli associated with their obsessions. During *response prevention*, patients refrain from rituals (fixed behaviors that reduce anxiety) for progressively longer intervals until discomfort diminishes.

SSRIs have a number needed to treat of 5. Studies have noted that effective dosages are usually significantly higher than those required for depression or other anxiety disorders (eg, fluoxetine ≤80 mg/d). Clomipramine is the only TCA that is most effective for OCD, and its efficacy is similar to SSRIs or slightly superior in some randomized controlled trials. However, given the anticholinergic side effects and increased risk of arrhythmia and seizures with TCAs, they are considered only as a second-line treatment or as an augmentation in a slightly lower dose.

5. Posttraumatic stress disorder (PTSD)—Recommended treatment involves referral for individual or group psychotherapy, stress management, relaxation training, cognitive restructuring, and/or eye movement desensitization and reprocessing, which includes brief exposure to trauma-related images while patients visually track the therapist's rapid finger movements or receive other bilateral stimulation and cognitive interventions. Psychological treatments lead, on average, to large improvements in PTSD symptoms. Trauma-focused CBT, including focus on exposure and cognitive restructuring, has proved superior to other therapies. Some form of exposure or desensitization is essential. Patients put frightening memories into words while receiving new and incompatible information. Systematic exposure to the traumatic memory in a safe environment allows a reevaluation of and habituation to threat cues.

Pharmacotherapy plays a key role in reduction of PTSD symptoms. Among the SSRIs and SNRIs, fluoxetine, paroxetine, and venlafaxine have moderate strength of evidence in reduction of PTSD symptoms, and sertraline has low strength of evidence. Other medications, including prazosin, topiramate, olanzapine, and risperidone, may also have some benefit for reduction of symptoms. Prazosin has been helpful in the reduction of nightmares associated with PTSD and providers should counsel patients about their side effects such as dizziness and orthostatic hypotension.

Like OCD, PTSD is especially difficult to treat. Early intervention reduces tendencies for substance abuse, secondary gain, litigation, and malingering. Referral is mandatory.

6. GAD—Recommended treatment includes worry exposure, thought control techniques (mismatch, cognitive restructuring), and relaxation training. Pharmacotherapy may include venlafaxine, sertraline, escitalopram, paroxetine, buspirone, and benzodiazepines.

No treatment is convincingly effective for GAD. Although CBT appears to produce superior results, effects remain variable. Cognitive psychotherapy decreases probability overestimation (ie, overestimating the likelihood of negative events) and catastrophic thinking and has been shown to improve sleep quality.

Nonvalidated coping strategies such as physical action, thought replacement, analysis, counterpropaganda, and talking to a friend have been used, with varying success. No one strategy is more efficient, and none is rated "very efficient" by patients. Talking to a friend may be more efficient when thoughts are intense, whereas thought replacement may work well when intensity is low.

Antidepressants are often considered first-line therapy for GAD, in part because of the frequent association of GAD with depression. Although the TCAs are effective for GAD, the SSRIs are more frequently prescribed because of a more favorable side effect profile. The SSRIs are well-demonstrated medications of choice for most anxiety disorders, notably escitalopram (Lexapro), sertraline (Zoloft), and paroxetine (Paxil). The SNRIs, venlafaxine (Effexor), and duloxetine (Cymbalta) also have demonstrated effectiveness in the treatment of GAD. The atypical anticonvulsants gabapentin (Neurontin) and pregabalin (Lyrica) have off-label use in GAD, especially in patients with neuropathy or chronic pain syndromes, although there are no studies to demonstrate their efficacy in GAD. Benzodiazepines should be reserved for initial short-term overlap with the SSRIs since SSRIs have a delayed onset of effectiveness. When conspicuous worry, apprehension, irritability, and depression exist, buspirone has been especially effective and has been shown to be comparable to benzodiazepines in multiple studies of GAD.

7. Other anxiety disorders—Treatment of patients with substance-induced anxiety disorder consists of eliminating the drug of abuse, medication, or toxin exposure that is the cause of the disorder. Alcohol use commonly co-occurs with anxiety disorders and is associated with poorer outcomes. Evidence for effectiveness of medication in treatment of anxiety disorder with comorbid alcohol use is inconclusive, but studies have shown that SSRIs are well tolerated. It should be kept in mind that sodium abnormalities exist in alcohol abuse patient, and therefore, monitoring sodium in patients taking SSRIs is of paramount importance.

In patients with persistent symptoms of adjustment disorder with anxious mood, referral for psychotherapy is recommended.

When antidepressants are used in anxiety disorders, the practitioners should keep in the mind the higher risk of relapse after discontinuation of medication within 1 year of treatment (odds ratio = 3.11; 95% CI, 2.48–3.89). Therefore, it is recommended to continue the medication for at least a year after the symptoms have improved, although there is lack of evidence to suggest decreased risk of relapse after 1 year of treatment.

Bandelow B, Reitt M, Röver C, et al. Efficacy of treatments for anxiety disorders: a meta-analysis. *Int Clin Psychopharmacol.* 2015;30(4):183–192. [PMID: 25932596]

Batelaan NM, Bosman RC, Muntingh A, et al. Risk of relapse after antidepressant discontinuation in anxiety disorders, obsessive-compulsive disorder, and post-traumatic stress disorder: systematic review and meta-analysis of relapse prevention trials. *BMJ.* 2017;358: j3927. [PMID: 28903922]

Berlin RK, Butler PM, Perloff MD. Gabapentin therapy in psychiatric disorders: a systematic review. *Prim Care Companion CNS Disord.* 2015;17(5). [PMID: 26835178]

Cuijpers P, Gentili C, Banos RM, et al. Relative effects of cognitive and behavioral therapies on generalized anxiety disorder, social anxiety disorder and panic disorder: a meta-analysis. *J Anxiety Disord.* 2016;43:79–89. [PMID: 27637075]

Hirschtritt ME, Bloch MH, Mathews CA. Obsessive-compulsive disorder: advances in diagnosis and treatment. *JAMA.* 2017;317(13):1358–1367. [PMID: 28384832]

Hoffman V, Middleton JC, Feltner C, et al. Psychological and pharmacological treatments for adults with posttraumatic stress disorder: a systematic review update. Comparative Effectiveness Review No. 207. AHRQ Publication No. 18-EHC011-EF. PCORI Publication No. 2018-SR-01. Rockville, MD: Agency for Healthcare Research and Quality; May 2018.

Ipser JC, Wilson D, Akindipe TO, et al. Pharmacotherapy for anxiety and comorbid alcohol use disorders. *Cochrane Database Syst Rev.* 2015;1:CD007505. [PMID: 25601826]

Kapczinski F, Lima MS, Souza JS, et al. Antidepressants for generalized anxiety disorder. *Cochrane Database Syst Rev.* 2003;2:CD003592. [PMID: 12804478]

Kung S, Espinel Z, Lapid MI. Treatment of nightmares with prazosin: a systematic review. *Mayo Clin Proc.* 2012;87(9):890–900. [PMID: 22883741]

Pompoli A, Furukawa TA, Imai H, et al. Psychological therapies for panic disorder with or without agoraphobia in adults: a network meta-analysis. *Cochrane Database Syst Rev.* 2016;4:CD011004. [PMID: 27071857]

Raj BA, Sheehan DV. Social anxiety disorder. *Med Clin North Am.* 2001;85:711–733. [PMID: 11349481]

Shalev AY. Acute stress reactions in adults. *Biol Psychiatr.* 2002;51:532–543. [PMID: 11950455]

F. Special Populations

1. Children and youth—Transient fears are common in children of all ages and represent part of the normal developmental process. Normal fears need to be distinguished from the anxiety disorders of adulthood, which are more prevalent among children and adolescents than any other mental problem. Children with anxiety disorders exhibit a high rate of comorbidity, especially with other, secondary anxiety disorders.

Anxiety is often manifested among children by avoidance behavior, distorted thinking, or subjective distress. The *DSM-5* anxiety designations of childhood and adolescence include *separation anxiety disorder* (excessive anxiety concerning separation from home or from those to whom the child is attached). Separation anxiety disorder is treated by exposure to the feared event (eg, the child attends school despite discomfort). Psychotherapy is the treatment of choice.

CBT for children with anxiety disorders is the first-line treatment recommended and has been found superior to SSRIs/SNRIs in trials.

Targeted use of medication to lower agitation, improve energy, decrease psychotic symptoms, or improve concentration might make certain patients more accessible to psychotherapy. Despite these advantages, caution remains in effect regarding the prominent prescribing of medication for the treatment of childhood anxiety disorders because of the increased risk of suicidality, suicidal ideation, and suicide attempts. However, until now, the studies that have looked at the risk of suicidality have been too small or too short to assess the risk, and therefore, the suicidality risk is still under speculation. Therefore, earlier follow-up is recommended when children are treated with SSRIs/SNRIs. Despite this caution, FDA indications for adults with anxiety disorders are often used in children and adolescents. The combination of CBT and medications is likely more effective than either treatment alone.

Locher C, Koechlin H, Zion SR, et al. Efficacy and safety of selective serotonin reuptake inhibitors, serotonin-norepinephrine reuptake inhibitors, and placebo for common psychiatric disorders among children and adolescents: a systematic review and meta-analysis. *JAMA Psychiatry.* 2017;74(10):1011–1020. [PMID: 28854296]

Wang Z, Whiteside S, Sim L, et al. Anxiety in children. Comparative Effectiveness Review No. 192. Report No.: 17-EHC023-EF. Rockville, MD: Agency for Healthcare Research and Quality; 2017.

Wang Z, Whiteside SPH, Sim L, et al. Comparative effectiveness and safety of cognitive behavioral therapy and pharmacotherapy for childhood anxiety disorders: a systematic review and meta-analysis. *JAMA Pediatr.* 2017;171(11):1049–1056. [PMID: 28859190]

2. The elderly—Although the most common form of psychiatric condition in the elderly, anxiety disorders are still underdiagnosed. Polypharmacy is often present. Altered pharmacokinetics and pharmacodynamics in the geriatric population lead to greater sensitivity to and prolonged half-life of the medication due to decreased clearance of the drugs. Because of these drug complications, psychotherapy is attractive.

G. Patients with Related Conditions

1. Personality disorders—Personality disorders are lifelong characterological problems that significantly complicate treatment and outcome. Poor compliance, medication abuse, interpersonal agitation, and poor insight characterize patients with personality disorders. These patients suffer more from anxiety than patients without personality disorders. Prescribing of benzodiazepines is contraindicated. (For further discussion of personality disorders, see Chapter 58.)

2. Hyperventilation—During hyperventilation, excessive rate and depth of breathing produce a marked drop in carbon dioxide and blood alkalinity. These changes can be subtle. A person may slightly overbreathe for a long time. Even a yawn may trigger symptoms, accounting for the sudden nature of panic attacks during sleep. Breathing retraining is recommended.

3. Insomnia—Patients with anxiety disorders commonly have sleep problems that worsen anxiety. Sympathomimetic amines may cause sleep-onset insomnia, whereas alcohol abuse produces sleep-termination insomnia. Benzodiazepines are frequently prescribed as sedative-hypnotics. For sleep-onset insomnia, triazolam and zolpidem are rapidly acting compounds with short half-lives. For sleep maintenance, longer-acting drugs such as flurazepam and quazepam are more effective. Tolerance for the sedative effects, alteration of sleep topography, suppression of rapid eye movement (REM; dream sleep), impaired cognitive function, the occurrence of falls, and REM rebound following discontinuation are contraindications to the use of benzodiazepines in treatment of chronic insomnia. Few studies have shown improvement of sleep quality with low-dose doxepin and trazadone. There was no evidence for use of amitriptyline for insomnia despite its common use in clinical practice.

Sleep hygiene suggestions provide an effective initial treatment option. Patients are asked to review and alter lifestyle patterns that interfere with sleep. Table 57–6 outlines these suggestions for patient use. Adherence with recommendations and shift work are limiting factors.

Labellarte MJ, Ginsburg GS, Walkup JT, et al. The treatment of anxiety disorders in children and adolescents. *Biol Psychiatr.* 1999;46:1567–1578. [PMID: 10599484]

Lichstein KL, Riedel BW, Wilson NM, et al. Relaxation and sleep compression for late-life insomnia: a placebo-controlled trial. *J Consult Clin Psychol.* 2001;69:227–239. [PMID: 11393600]

Everitt H, Baldwin DS, Stuart B, et al. Antidepressants for insomnia in adults. *Cochrane Database Syst Rev.* 2018;5:CD010753. [PMID: 29761479]

Sheikh JI, Cassidy EL. Treatment of anxiety disorders in the elderly: issues and strategies. *J Anxiety Disord.* 2000;14:173–190. [PMID: 10864384]

▶ Prognosis

As recently as the early 1980s, it was estimated that 80% of patients with anxiety disorders would not significantly

Table 57–6. Sleep hygiene recommendations.

Keep a sleep diary for a few weeks and monitor sleep-related activities
Establish a regular sleep-wake cycle (go to bed at about the same time and get up at about the same time)
Get regular exercise
Reduce noise
Avoid all naps
Eat dinner at a reasonable hour to allow time to digest food
Avoid excessive amounts of caffeine (chocolates, soft drinks, coffee, tea), especially before bedtime
Avoid excessive fluid intake before bed
Avoid in-bed activities such as reading, eating, or watching TV
Avoid clock watching while trying to sleep
If not asleep within 10–15 minutes after going to bed, get up:
If you still want to lie down, do so in another room
When sleepy, go back to bed
If not asleep in 10–15 minutes, repeat these steps

benefit from available treatment. Today the opposite is true. For the majority of patients with anxiety disorders—especially panic disorder, specific phobias, and social phobia—treatment with a combination of CBT and an SSRI carries an excellent prognosis Although these treatments show promise in the treatment of OCD, GAD, and PTSD, efficacy is more variable.

Websites

Anxiety and Depression Association of America. http://www.adaa .org/

Internet Mental Health. http://www.mentalhealth.com/

58

Personality Disorders

William G. Elder, PhD

General Considerations

Personality disorders (PDs) are a heterogeneous group of deeply ingrained and enduring behavioral patterns characterized by inflexible and extreme responses to a broad range of situations, manifesting in cognition (ways of perceiving and interpreting self, others, and events), affectivity (range, intensity, lability, and appropriateness of response), interpersonal functioning, and impulse control. PDs impinge on medical practice in multiple ways, including self-destructive behaviors, interpersonal disturbances, and nonadherence. Appropriate physician responses and effective treatments exist for many PDs. Correct diagnosis and proper intervention will help to improve patient outcomes. Borderline personality disorder (BPD) is an extremely debilitating disorder that can significantly interfere with the physician-patient relationship. BPD will receive extra focus in several sections of this chapter.

Significant deliberation on PDs preceded the publication of the fifth edition of the *Diagnostic and Statistical Manual of Mental Disorders* (*DSM-5*) in May 2013. *DSM-5* continues to distinguish 10 PDs clinically, while also formulating an alternative model that emphasizes core impairments in personality functioning and pathologic traits. For *Currents*, we have chosen to retain description of all 10 PDs as it seems certain that clinicians will continue to use their labels (eg, histrionic personality) for years to come. Table 58–1 summarizes the 10 PDs.

PDs are relatively common, with a prevalence of 7.6% in the general US population. Patients with PDs may seek help from family physicians for physical complaints, rather than psychiatric help. Higher rates for all types of PDs are found in medical settings. Prevalence of BPD in the general community is 1.7%.

PDs have a pervasive impact because they are central to the person's identity. They are major sources of long-term disability and are associated with greatly increased mortality and extensive service utilization. Patients with PDs have fewer coping skills and during stressful situations may have greater difficulties, which are worsened by poor social

competency, impulse control, and social support. Patients with BPD are frequently maltreated in the forms of sexual, physical, and emotional abuse; physical neglect; and witnessing violence. PDs are identified in 70–85% of persons identified as criminal, 60–70% of persons with alcohol dependence, and 70–90% of persons who are drug dependent.

Borderline, schizoid, schizotypal, and dependent PDs are associated with high degrees of functional impairments and greater risk for depression and alcohol abuse. Obsessive-compulsive and narcissistic PDs may not result in appreciable degrees of impairment. Dependent PD is associated with a marked increase in healthcare utilization.

Bateman AW Gundeson J, Mulder R. Treatment of personality disorder. *Lancet.* 2015;385(9969);735–743. [PMID: 25706219]
Leichsenring F, Leibing E, Kruse J, et al. Borderline personality disorder. *Lancet.* 2011;377(9759):74–84. [PMID: 21195251]
Meuldijk D, McCarthy A, Bourke ME, Grenyer BF. The value of psychological treatment for borderline personality disorder: systematic review and cost offset analysis of economic evaluations. *PLoS One.* 2017;12:e0171592. [PMID: 28249032]
Skodol AE, Bender DS, Morey LC, et al. Personality disorder types proposed for DSM-5. *J Pers Disord.* 2011;25(2):136–169. [PMID: 21466247]

Pathogenesis

A. Personality Disorders

PDs are syndromes rather than diseases. Avoidant, dependent, and schizoid PDs appear to be heritable. Similarly, schizotypal disorder is considered to be heritable, as one end of a schizotypal-schizophrenia spectrum. Twin and adoption studies suggest a genetic predisposition for antisocial PD, as well as environmental influences, via poor parenting and role modeling. Histrionic PD may be related to indulged tendencies toward emotional expressiveness.

BPD may result from both constitutional and environmental factors. Neuroimaging studies demonstrate

Table 58–1. Clinical features and clusters of 10 *DSM-5* personality disorders.

Cluster	Personality Disorder	Clinical Features
Cluster A: odd, eccentric	Paranoid Schizotypal Schizoid	Suspicious; overly sensitive; misinterpretations Detached; perceptual and cognitive distortions; eccentric behavior Detached; introverted, constricted affect
Cluster B: dramatic, emotional, erratic	Antisocial Borderline Histrionic Narcissistic	Manipulative; selfish, lacks empathy; explosive anger; legal problems since adolescence Dependent and demanding; unstable interpersonal relationships, self-image, and affects; impulsivity; micropsychotic symptoms Dramatic; attention seeking and emotionality; superficial, ie, vague and focused on appearances Self-important; arrogance and grandiosity; need for admiration; lacks empathy; rages
Cluster C: anxious, fearful	Avoidant Dependent Obsessive-compulsive	Anxiously detached; feels inadequate; hypersensitive to negative evaluation Clinging, submissive, and self-sacrificing; needs to be taken care of; hypersensitive to negative evaluation Preoccupied with orderliness, perfectionism, and control

Data from American Psychiatric Association: *Diagnostic and Statistical Manual of Mental Disorders*, Fifth Edition. Arlington, VA, American Psychiatric Association, 2013.

hypoactivation in prefrontal and cingulate regions. BPD is 5 times more common among first-degree relatives with the disorder, but to say to what degree BPD is heritable is difficult, given the reciprocity between family and child that occurs during development. BPD has been attributed to highly pathologic and conflicted early interactions between parent and child. The conflict brings great ambivalence about relationships and affects ability to regulate affect. Previously BPD was attributed to child sexual abuse, but a recent meta-analysis did not support this hypothesis. It is certainly the case that traumatic childhood experiences are common in patients with BPD. As a group, patients with antisocial and borderline PDs report higher frequencies of perinatal brain injury, head trauma, and encephalitis.

B. Common Comorbid Conditions

Substance abuse disorders frequently occur comorbidly in community and clinical populations, particularly with antisocial, borderline, avoidant, and paranoid PDs. Anorexia nervosa, bulimia nervosa, and binge eating may be seen in patients who are obsessional, borderline, and avoidant, respectively. Self-injurious skin picking can be conceptualized as an impulse control disorder and has been found with significant frequency in patients with obsessive-compulsive PD and BPD. Up to 50% of patients with BPD have major depressive disorders or bipolar disorders.

American Psychiatric Association. *Diagnostic and Statistical Manual of Mental Disorders*, 5th ed. Washington, DC: American Psychiatric Association; 2013. http://dx.doi.org/10.1176/appi.books.9780890425596.910646.

Goodman M, New AS, Triebwasser J, et al. Phenotype, endophenotype, and genotype comparisons between borderline personality disorder and major depressive disorder. *J Pers Disord*. 2010;24(1):38–59. [PMID: 20205498]

Lobbestael J, Arntz A, Bernstein DP. Disentangling the relationship between different types of childhood maltreatment and personality disorders. *J Pers Disord*. 2010;24(3):285–295. [PMID: 20545495]

Ruocco AC, Amirthavasagam S, Zakzanis KK. Amygdala and hippocampal volume reductions as candidate endophenotypes for borderline personality disorder: A meta-analysis of magnetic resonance imaging studies. *Psychiatr Res*. 2012;201(3):245–252. [PMID: 22507760]

▶ Prevention

Except for efforts to address the roots of criminal behaviors that are common in antisocial PD, there is no literature on prevention of PDs. Primary prevention could consist of better treatment of parental mental illnesses that have a negative impact on parent-child interactions and public health interventions to reduce prenatal brain insults. Both primary and secondary prevention could occur with increased interventions in family functioning and parenting skills. There is a demonstrated relationship between adverse childhood experiences (ACEs) and PDs as well as brain morphology described earlier. Family interventions to prevent ACEs associated with household substance misuse; parental imprisonment; sexual, physical, and emotional traumas; domestic violence; and emotional and physical neglect have population health–level potential to reduce PDs.

▶ Clinical Findings

PDs were once referred to as *character disorders*. Various descriptive labels have appeared in the literature, such as the oral-fixated character, the impulsive personality, and the introverted personality type. Each of these represents a theory of personality (psychoanalytic, developmental, and analytical, respectively). Currently, there are few points of correspondence between personality theory and diagnosis of PDs with a relatively atheoretical, categorical perspective dominating clinical practice in the United States.

A. Symptoms and Signs

1. Personality disorder—Clinical lore about PD presentations exists. Anything extreme in appearance that is not ethnically appropriate or currently fashionable suggests a PD. Examples include flamboyant jewelry, particularly in men; tattoos and piercing in older patients; steel-toed boots in men; and excessive cosmetics and large hair ribbons in women.

The patient's style of interacting with the physician can be revealing about personality difficulties. For example, the dependent patient will seek much advice and be unable to make an independent decision. The antisocial patient may be "smooth talking" or threatening. Interactions with patients with BPD can be very difficult, with the patient switching from extreme idealization to devaluation of the physician. The patient may "split" the staff, which becomes evident when some side with the patient while others are angry with the patient. Table 58–2 describes problem behaviors associated with various PDs, as well as helpful responses and management strategies.

Physician reactions may be a sign of patient PD. Reactions such as anger, guilt, desire to punish, desire to reject, desire to please, sexual fantasies, and a sense that the physician is the "one person" capable of helping the patient are all examples of countertransference responses. Self-reflection about the encounter will help manage the strong feelings and interpersonal conflict encountered in care of PDs.

2. Borderline personality disorder—Physicians may over- or underattribute patient difficulties to BPD; therefore, it is important to be sensitive to BPD phenomena and to ascertain whether patient difficulties and symptoms represent BPD. Extreme sensitivity to perceived slights by the physician or staff is a red flag for BPD. BPD diagnostic criteria call for a pervasive pattern of instability in interpersonal relationships, self-image, and affect, and marked impulsivity beginning by early adulthood and present in a variety of contexts as indicated by at least five of the following:

1. Frantic efforts to avoid real or imagined abandonment (not including suicidal behaviors).

2. A pattern of unstable and intense interpersonal relationships characterized by alternating extremes of idealization and devaluation.

3. Identity disturbance: a markedly and persistently unstable self-image or sense of self.

4. Impulsivity in at least two areas that are potentially self-damaging (not including suicidal behaviors).

5. Recurrent suicidal behavior, gestures, threats, or self-mutilating behavior.

6. Affective instability due to a marked reactivity of mood (eg, intense episodic dysphoria, irritability, or anxiety usually lasting a few hours and only rarely more than a few days).

7. Chronic feelings of emptiness.

8. Inappropriate intense anger or difficulty controlling anger.

9. Transient, stress-related paranoid ideation or severe dissociative symptoms.

BPD involves subgroups of patients differing in affective, impulsive, and micropsychotic symptoms. These differences suggest different treatments, discussed later. Patients with BPD have significantly higher rates of suicidal ideation; 70–80% exhibit self-harming behavior at least once. While suicide attempts may be regarded as manipulative gestures, suicide rates are very high: 3–9.5% of patients with BPD receiving inpatient care eventually kill themselves. Self-harm in the form of self-mutilation, such as wrist scratching, is symptomatic. Nausea and vomiting may be a primary care analog of self-mutilation in some patients and a common chief complaint. Obtaining a history suggesting BPD may mitigate the need for extensive gastrointestinal symptom evaluations with more efficacious treatments directed to personality functioning.

B. Special Tests

No laboratory tests exist for PDs. Structured clinical interviews and personality inventories may be helpful in differentiating PDs and tracking treatment response. Interpretation by a psychologist enhances the value of the results. A consult should be considered in cases of diagnostic uncertainty.

Dubovsky AN, Kiefer MM. Borderline personality disorder in the primary care setting. *Med Clin North Am*. 2014 Sep;98(5): 1049–64. doi: 10.1016/j.mcna.2014.06.005.

Skodol A, Gunderson JG, McGlashan TH, et al. Functional impairment in patients with schizotypal, borderline, avoidant, or obsessive-compulsive personality disorder. *Am J Psychiatr*. 2002;159:276–283. [PMID: 11823271]

▶ Differential Diagnosis

A. Personality Disorders

Accurate diagnosis is essential for proper response to and treatment of PDs. The following comparisons may help avoid misattribution of BPD to other PDs:

- Histrionic PD patients are dramatic and manipulative but lack the affective instability of BPD. Impulsivity, when seen, is related to attention seeking and sexual acting out.

- Dependent PD patients fear abandonment, but patients with BPD have more affective instability and impulsivity.

Table 58–2. Health-related problem behaviors associated with personality disorders.

Criterion	Personality Disorder				
	Paranoid	**Schizotypal**	**Schizoid**	**Antisocial**	**Borderline**
Patient's perspective	People are malevolent; situation is dangerous.	Understanding of care may be odd or near delusional.	Illness will bring too much attention and invade privacy.	Threatened if unable to feel "on top"; illness presents opportunity for crime.	Fears abandonment. Overreacts to symptoms and situation.
Problem behaviors	Fearful; misconstrues events and explanations; irrational. Argumentative.	Odd health beliefs and behaviors. Poor hygiene. Avoids care.	Unresponsive to kindness; difficult to motivate. Avoids care.	Acts out to gain control; malingering; uses staff and physicians. Superficially charming. Drug seeking.	Idealizes, then devalues care; self-destructive acts. Splits staff.
Helpful physician responses and management strategies	Be empathic toward patient's fears, even when they seem irrational; carefully explain care plan. Provide advance information about risks. Protect patient's independence.	Communicate directly. Avoid misinterpreting patient as intentionally noncompliant; do not reject patient for oddness; honor patient's beliefs.	Manage personal frustration at feeling unappreciated; maintain a low-key approach. Appreciate patient's need for privacy.	Do not succumb to patient's anger and manipulation. Avoid punitive reactions to patients. Motivate by addressing patient's self-interest. Set clear limits that interventions must be medically indicated.	Manage feelings of hopelessness about patient. Avoid getting too close emotionally. Schedule frequent periodic checkups. Tolerate periodic angry outbursts, but set limits. Monitor for self-destructive behavior. Discuss feelings with coworkers.

Criterion	**Histrionic**	**Narcissistic**	**Avoidant**	**Dependent**	**Obsessive-Compulsive**
Patient's perspective	Illness results in feeling unattractive or presents an opportunity to receive attention.	Illness results in feeling inadequate or is an opportunity to receive admiration.	Illness is personal; fears exposure.	Fears abandonment. Intensifies feelings of helplessness.	Fears losing control of body and emotions. Feels shame.
Problem behaviors	Overly dramatic, attention-seeking; excessively familiar relationship. Not objective—overemphasis on feeling states.	Demanding and entitled attitude; will overly praise or devalue care providers to maintain sense of superiority.	Missed appointments. Delays seeking care. Extremely nonassertive.	Dramatic and urgent demands for medical attention; may contribute to or prolong illness to get attention.	Unable to relinquish control to healthcare team. Great difficulty and anger at any change. Excessive attention to detail.
Helpful physician responses and management strategies	Avoid frustration with patient vagueness. Show respectful and professional concern for feelings, with emphasis on objective issues. Avoid excessive familiarity.	Avoid rejecting the patient for being too demanding. Avoid seeking patient's approval. Generously validate patient's concerns, with attentive but factual response to questions. Protect self-esteem of patients by giving them a role in their care.	Provide empathic response to inadequacy. Be patient with timidity. Work toward clear treatment plans—must obtain patient's view. Treat anxiety disorder.	When exhausted by patient needs, avoid hostile rejection of patient. Give reassurance and consistency. Set limits to availability—schedule regular visits. Help patient obtain outside support.	Avoid impatience. Thorough history taking and careful diagnostic workups are reassuring. Give clear and thorough explanations. Avoid control battles; treat patient as a partner; encourage self-monitoring.

- Schizotypal PD patients have the micropsychotic symptoms of BPD, but are odder and lack the affective instability of BPD.
- Paranoid PD patients have volatile anger, but lack the self-destructive and abandonment issues of the BPD patient.
- Narcissistic PD patients have rages and reactive mood, but have a stable, idealized self-image in contrast to the patient with BPD, who has an unstable identity.
- Antisocial PD patients are often less impulsive than intentionally aggressive for materialistic gains. Patients with BPD act out when needy to gain support.

B. Other Mental Disorders

A PD diagnosis is not indicated if symptoms are explained by an axis I condition or substance use. Although PDs may share impulsivity, raging, and grandiosity with bipolar disorder, they seldom have the same intensity and rate of speech or irrationality of thought that a manic episode brings. Substance use disorders differ from antisocial PD when illegal behaviors are restricted to substance use and procurement. Dissociative identity disorder, formerly known as *multiple-personality disorder*, may have a more traumatic etiology similar to BPD. Patients with obsessive-compulsive disorder recognize that their behavior and thoughts are irrational, whereas patients with obsessive-compulsive PD are comfortable with their behavior. A diagnosis of PD does not apply when changes in behavior result from changes in brain function. For example, although personality changes are expected in dementia, a diagnosis of PD is not indicated. An axis I diagnosis "personality change due to a … [general medical condition]" is available when a change in personality characteristics is the direct physiologic consequence of a general medical condition. Because transient changes in personality are common in children and adolescents, diagnosis of a PD is not appropriate for a patient age <18 years unless the behavioral pattern has been present for at least 1 year.

C. Cultural Considerations

Culturally related characteristics may erroneously suggest PDs. Promiscuity, suspiciousness, and recklessness have different norms in different cultures. The degree of physical or emotional closeness sought and the intensity of emotional expression also differ. Manner of dress and health beliefs may seem strange to the conventional Western physician. Evaluate the patient's degree of acculturation. Passivity, especially with one's elders, is not a sign of dependence in most recent immigrants. Constricted affect is a normal response when entering a new environment. Asking someone from the culture if the behavior is extreme can help, as can checking for significant interpersonal difficulties.

▶ **Treatment**

Miller (1992) has described how experienced family physicians differentially and efficiently respond to visits that can be categorized as routine, ceremony, or drama. In some cases, good application of family medicine's care principles may be beneficial psychotherapeutically. (Compare the psychotherapy of PDs described in Section D with the patient-centered method of family practice.) Suggestions for helping patients with PDs in a nonpsychiatric medical setting appear in Table 58–2. Table 58–3 offers suggestions for helping patients who present with BPD.

Previously it was commonly believed that personality cannot be changed. However, increasingly specific psychopharmacologic and psychotherapeutic interventions have brought improved outcomes and some cures. The most effective treatments are multidisciplinary, combining medications, individual and group psychotherapies, and high coordination among providers. Comorbid substance dependence, violent acting out toward others, or severely

Table 58–3. Working with patients with borderline personality disorder in medical settings.

1. Recognize the characteristics. The patient fears abandonment and increases demands on the physician. May be noncompliant, manipulative, somatasize, or "split" the healthcare team.
2. Behavior is need-driven. Demands may be overt or covert. Identify needs and motivations. Patient has little insight into problems. Externalization is symptomatic.
3. Tolerate patient's behaviors. Speaking "harshly or strictly" will activate abandonment fears and worsen the situation. Use a nonconfrontational but an educational approach.
4. A long-term plan provides stability for the patient. Follow continuity of care principles. This may be curative for the patient.
5. Titrate closeness and visit frequency. Avoid extremes of constant availability.
6. Set limits. Make clear agreements about call and office visits. Point out to patients that you are almost always involved in solving some type of problem and are unable to give full attention to their problems without an appointment. Suggest that patients schedule fairly frequent visits so that a regular time is available to discuss the problems they are experiencing.
7. Foresee problems related to abandonment fears such as when the social situation is disturbed, when the patient is referred, or when there are changes in physician or staff.
8. Use a multidisciplinary approach. Involve a highly skilled clinical psychologist or clinical social worker in the care. Encourage communication and cooperation among the care team.
9. Monitor your and the staff's reactions. Frustration and anger may be expected. Discuss the situation. Help the staff to recognize that the etiology of the frustration might originate in the patient's personality, not in the crisis of the moment. Coordinate responses to patients.
10. Set personal limits for the number of these challenging patients that you accept into your practice.

self-harming behaviors must be addressed first, via inpatient care.

Angstman K, Rasmussen NH. Personality disorders: review and clinical application in daily practice. *Am Fam Physician.* 2011;84(11):1253–1260. [PMID: 22150659]

Miller WL. Routine, ceremony, or drama: an exploratory field study of the primary care clinical encounter. *J Fam Practice.* 1992;34:289–296. [PMID: 1541955]

A. Risk Management

Physicians should acknowledge the threats and challenges associated with PDs. General risk management considerations include the following:

- Having good collaboration and communication with a qualified mental health professional.
- Attention to documentation of communications and risk assessments.
- Attention to transference and countertransference issues, described earlier.
- Consultation with a colleague regarding high-risk situations.
- Careful management of termination of care, even when it is the patient's decision.
- Informed consent from the patient and, if appropriate, family members, regarding the risks inherent in the disorder and uncertainties in the treatment outcome.

B. Consultation or Referral

Consultation or referral should be considered when the following exist:

- The patient has several psychiatric diagnoses.
- The patient is experiencing depressive or anhedonic symptoms even if subthreshold (risk for suicide).
- The patient has significant problems with self-regulation.
- The patient has moderate to severe substance use disorder(s).
- The diagnosis is uncertain or the presentation is puzzling.
- Initial treatment by the family physician is ineffective.
- The physician or staff are unable to compensate for and are overwhelmed by the patient's personality problems.

Acceptance of treatment can be difficult. Symptomatically, patients with PD may externalize blame for their problems. PD behavioral patterns tend to be *egosyntonic*; that is, patients may consider their behavior reasonable, given their perception of the circumstances. Treatment may be perceived as an attempt to control the patient; referral may be experienced as devaluing or as abandonment. Thus, treatment and referral suggestions should be offered with an understanding of how patients with various PDs may perceive them. Table 58–2 describes common PD patient perspectives on care.

C. Pharmacotherapy

In many cases, medications are effective only as a means to manage stress-exacerbated symptoms. For example, under stress, paranoid, schizoid, or schizotypal patients may experience delusions, distress, and hallucinations, which can be managed with antipsychotic medications. When not stressed, the odd behavior and beliefs of these patients remain unresponsive to treatment.

Some PDs may be successfully treated with medications. Avoidant PD appears to be an alternative conceptualization of social phobia. It can be treated with selective serotonin reuptake inhibitors (SSRIs) and serotonin-norepinephrine reuptake inhibitors (SNRIs). Patients with obsessive-compulsive PD may become less irritable and compulsive with SSRIs. Rejection sensitivity seen in patients with dependent PD may be helped by SSRIs. Medications are not helpful for patients with narcissistic, antisocial, or histrionic PDs. Consider high rates of suicide attempts and completions when selecting medications to avoid those that are especially dangerous in overdose.

Not on the basis of diagnosis per se, Soloff (2000) has proposed three symptom-specific pharmacotherapy algorithms for PDs. They are based on differential medication effects on cognitive disturbances, behavioral dyscontrol, and affective dysregulation. Soloff's first algorithm is for treatment of PDs in which cognitive perceptual symptoms are most significant (ie, patients with suspiciousness, paranoid ideation, and micropsychotic symptoms). The second algorithm is for treatment of affective dysregulation (ie, patients with a depressed, angry, anxious, labile mood). The third algorithm is for treatment of impulsive behavioral symptoms (ie, patients with impulsive aggression, binging, or self-injuring behaviors). Practice guidelines largely in accord with Soloff's symptom-based approach were published for treatment of BPD by the American Psychiatric Association (APA) in October 2001 and again recommended in 2005. Recent systemic reviews continue to support a symptom-based approach and incorporate new studies of mood-stabilizing medications. It should be noted that current recommendations are based on a small database that lacks sufficient randomized controlled trials. Therefore, each treatment should be approached as an empirical trial, with the patient as a coinvestigator. Side effects, risk/benefit ratios, conjoint medications, and patient preferences should be considered carefully. Pharmacotherapy is an adjuvant to psychotherapy; medications do not cure character and will never be a substitute for the work of a therapist. Furthermore, some medications may worsen symptoms.

Both SSRIs and SNRIs are effective with affective dysregulation seen in cluster BPDs. Tricyclic antidepressants are no more effective than SSRIs and should not be used, given their cardiotoxic effects with overdose and a possibility of paradoxical worsening of symptoms. Monoamine oxidase inhibitors (MAOIs) proved useful in treating BPD prior to the advent of SSRIs and offer a second treatment option for affective dysregulation, including rejection sensitivity. Mood stabilizers offer an additional level of treatment, especially for anger. Valproate and carbamazepine may be offered alone, whereas lithium should be used in conjunction with an antidepressant, although lithium is the second choice, given its serious side effects. Although patients with BPD often complain of anxiety, benzodiazepines are contraindicated, as they have been shown to cause increased impulsivity. Clonazepam, a benzodiazepine with anticonvulsant and antimanic properties, is associated with increased serotonin levels and may be useful adjunctively for anxiety, anger, and dysphoric mood.

Antipsychotics are the most researched medications for the treatment of PDs and should be the first-line treatment when cognitive perceptual symptoms are significant. Low doses should be tried first. There is no evidence that antipsychotics are helpful for PD cognitive perceptual symptoms in the long term. Antipsychotics may also be used adjuvantly with antidepressants for affective dysregulation, particularly with anger. Antipsychotics such as risperidone may exacerbate or induce manic symptoms, although they produce symptom improvement in bipolar disorder when used in conjunction with mood-stabilizing medications. When the most recent guidelines were written, there was insufficient evidence that third-generation antipsychotics (eg, aripiprazole, risperidone, or olanzapine) would be effective with cognitive perceptual symptoms in BPD, but given the side effect profiles of conventional versus third-generation antipsychotics, the newer drugs are being used increasingly empirically. The atypical antipsychotic clozapine is effective in personality disturbances that are cognitive perceptual and impulsive but, given its risk for agranulocytosis, should be reserved until several trials of other medications have failed.

Risperidone appears to be superior to conventional antipsychotics in treatment of impulsivity and aggression, especially in BPD. However, SSRIs at low to moderately high doses should be tried first. If needed, low-dose antipsychotics may then be added to SSRIs or used more aggressively as a last line of treatment. Mood-stabilizing medications are indicated as midlevel treatment for impulsivity. Lithium is effective, perhaps because of its impact on serotonin levels. The anticonvulsant divalproex sodium has been used to treat irritability and impulsivity in patients with BPD who have not responded to SSRI therapy, apparently independent of the presence of abnormal electroencephalographic findings. Carbamazepine is also effective as a mood stabilizer. Use of mood stabilizers requires various laboratory tests to monitor metabolic functioning. Various antipsychotic medications

carry risks for extrapyramidal symptoms, tardive dyskinesia, weight gain, diabetes mellitus, extended QT intervals, and other problems.

Canadian Agency for Drugs and Technologies in Health. Aripiprazole for Borderline Personality Disorder: A Review of the Clinical Effectiveness. Rapid Response Report: Summary with Critical Appraisal. Ottawa, Ontario, Canada: Canadian Agency for Drugs and Technologies in Health; 2017.

Feurino L, Silk KR. State of the art in the pharmacologic treatment of borderline personality disorder. *Curr Psychiatr Rep.* 2011;13(1):69–75. [PMID: 21140245]

Oldham JM. Guideline Watch: Practice guideline for the treatment of patients with borderline personality disorder. Washington, DC: American Psychiatric Association; 2010. https://psychiatryonline.org/pb/assets/raw/sitewide/practice_guidelines/guidelines/bpd.pdf. Accessed October 31. 2018.

Soloff PH. Psychopharmacology of borderline personality disorder. *Psychiatr Clin North Am.* 2000;23:169–192. [PMID: 10729938]

Stoffers JM, Lieb K. Pharmacotherapy for borderline personality disorder—current evidence and recent trends. *Curr Psychiatry Rep.* 2015;17(1):534. [PMID: 25413640]

D. Psychotherapeutic Interventions

Some PDs are amenable to some forms of psychotherapy, but there is currently limited empirical support for the treatment of most PDs. One exception is BPD, where evidence suggests that psychotherapy alters neural activation and connectivity of regions subserving executive control and emotion regulation. Additionally, hypoactivation in prefrontal and cingulate regions has been shown to predict treatment response. Specific treatments described later may result in significant improvements over time, when compared to waitlist control or treatment as usual. Largest changes are observed in measures of self-reported distress or symptoms (eg, target complaints, level of depression). Measures assessing interpersonal problems and social functioning also show improvement, although to a smaller degree.

Treatments of <1 year in duration probably represent crisis interventions or treatments of concurrent axis I disorders rather than attempts to address core PD psychopathology. Psychotherapy for borderline and narcissistic personalities tends to take significantly longer. Even with extended duration, treatment goals tend to be for functional improvement such as decreased symptom severity and decreased acting out, rather than complete remission of symptoms. Anxiety-related PDs, such as avoidant and dependent PDs, are most amenable to psychotherapy, followed by BPD and then schizotypal PD. Cognitive behavioral psychotherapy, which challenges irrational beliefs, may be effective with avoidant, dependent, obsessive-compulsive, narcissistic, and paranoid PDs. Because individuals with antisocial PD are manipulative and seldom take responsibility for their behavior, psychotherapy is difficult and relatively rare, unless court-ordered interventions are counted as psychotherapy, which is questionable. Furthermore, persons showing characteristic psychopathy traits (eg, lack of remorse, aggressiveness) are the least amenable to treatment.

Successful treatment of borderline and narcissistic PDs requires high levels of therapist experience. Skills in managing the therapeutic alliance and creating a stable, trusting relationship are crucial. Psychotherapy for narcissistic PDs is highly specialized wherein the patient's hypersensitivity to slights is confronted after much trust building.

Group therapy and partial hospitalization are effective for patients with schizotypal and borderline PDs. Dialectical behavior therapy (DBT) is a unique form of psychotherapy that is efficacious for BPD. In DBT, patient beliefs, contradictions, and acting out are empathically accepted. Specifically, the patient's personhood is responded to positively, and dysfunctional behaviors are responded to matter-of-factly, neither sympathizing with, nor punishing, the patient. Sessions focus on learning to solve problems, control emotions, manage anxiety, and improve interpersonal relationships. After many months of this consistent and intensive treatment, limits are set on the patient's behavior.

Besides establishing a strong therapeutic alliance, several recommendations may be useful in the treatment of all PDs: (1) maintain a consistent and validating treatment process, (2) build motivation and reinforce commitment to change, (3) increase self-knowledge and foster new learning experiences, (4) target cognitive structures of personality/pathology, and (5) adopt a structured approach to treatment (eg, setting appropriate interpersonal boundaries, use of therapy contract).

Bartak A, Spreeuwenberg MD, Andrea H, et al. Effectiveness of different modalities of psychotherapeutic treatment for patients with cluster C personality disorders: results of a large prospective multicentre study. *Psychother Psychosom.* 2010;79(1): 20–30. [PMID: 19887888]

Beck AT, Butler AC, Brown GK, et al. Dysfunctional beliefs discriminate personality disorders. *Behav Res Ther.* 2001;39: 1213–1225. [PMID: 11579990]

Marceau EM, Meuldijk D, Townsend ML, et al. Biomarker correlates of psychotherapy outcomes in borderline personality disorder: a systematic review. *Neurosci Biobehav Rev.* 2018;94:166–178. [PMID: 30208302]

▶ Prognosis

Perhaps half of all patients with PDs never receive treatment. Several of the PDs, although pervasive in their negative effects, are perhaps not sufficiently impairing or distressing to warrant treatment. Treatment outcomes are improving for the PDs that are extremely debilitating, such as BPD. PDs with anxiety components have good potential for improvement. Debate remains as to whether any treatment other than incarceration can be effective for individuals with antisocial PD, and with this, whether effect seen comes with age (ie, the person becomes less disruptive as age 40 is approached). Patients with BPD appear to improve by age 40, as well. Patients with BPD who are in treatment improve at a rate of 7 times their natural course.

Sanislow CA, Marcus KL, Reagan EM. Long-term outcomes in borderline psychopathology: old assumptions, current findings, and new directions. *Curr Psychiatr Rep.* 2012;14(1):54–61. [PMID: 22139609]

59

Somatic Symptom Disorder (Previously Somatoform Disorder), Factitious Disorder, & Malingering

William G. Elder, PhD

▶ General Considerations

Somatic symptom disorder (SSD) involves unexplained physical symptoms that bring significant functional impairment. It presents one of the more common and most difficult problems in primary care. SSD is seldom "cured" and should be approached as a chronic disease. Recognition, a patient-centered approach, and specific treatments may help alleviate symptoms and distress. Factitious disorder and malingering, although not true SSD, are addressed separately in this chapter because of their similarity in the form of medically unexplained symptoms.

SSD is a new diagnostic term appearing in the fifth edition of the *Diagnostic and Statistical Manual of Mental Disorders* (*DSM-5*), the latest version of the diagnostic manual published by the American Psychiatric Association. SSD replaces *somatoform disorder* as used in the previous edition of *DSM*, and the diagnostic labels previously subsumed by somatoform disorders will also be subsumed by SSD in *DSM-5*. These disorders have specific courses, symptoms, complaints, and treatments, as listed in Table 59–1.

Features that characterize SSD include the following:

- Physical symptoms or irrational anxiety about illness or appearance, for which biomedical findings are not consistent with a general medical condition.

- Symptoms develop with or are worsened by psychological stress and are not intentional.

- Extensive utilization of medical care. Paradoxically, treatment and attempts to reassure patients can be counterproductive.

- Feelings of frustration on the part of the provider. Patients are often seen as "difficult patients."

Somatic expression of psychological distress can be normal, and degree of dysfunction determines whether the symptoms constitute a disorder. Furthermore, symptoms may be sufficient to suggest that the patient's condition is better described by a primary mental disorder (eg, somatic delusions) that may respond to specific therapies.

Designation of a symptom as somatic means that it appears to be a physical problem or complaint yet is medically unexplained. Presentations of illness without complete physical explanation have a significant impact on practice. For instance, 10% of all medical services are provided to patients with no organic disease, 26% of primary care patients meet criteria for somatic "preoccupation"; 19% of patients have medically unexplainable symptoms; and 25–50% of visits involve symptoms that have no serious cause. When true SSD is present, symptoms persist much longer and the cost of ambulatory care is 9–14 times greater than in controls. Patients with SSD undergo numerous medical examinations, diagnostic procedures, surgeries, and hospitalizations. They risk increased morbidity from these procedures, and up to 82% stop working at some point because of their difficulties. With appropriate recognition and treatment, costs of care may be reduced by 50%.

American Psychiatric Association. *Diagnostic and Statistical Manual of Mental Disorders*. 5th ed. Washington, DC: American Psychiatric Association; 2013. http://www.dsm5.org/Pages/Default.aspx. Accessed June 12, 2018.

Gerstenblith TA, Kontos N. Somatic symptom disorders. In: Stern TA, Rosenbaum JF, Fava M, et al, eds. *Massachusetts General Hospital Comprehensive Clinical Psychiatry*. 2nd ed. Philadelphia, PA: Elsevier; 2016:Chapter 24.

Kroenke K. Patients presenting with somatic complaints: epidemiology, psychiatric comorbidity and management. *Int J Methods Psychiatr Res*. 2003;12:34–43. [PMID: 12830308]

Voigt K, Nagel A, Meyer B, Langs G, Braukhaus C, Löwe B. Towards positive diagnostic criteria: a systematic review of somatoform disorder diagnoses and suggestions for future classification. *J Psychosom Res*. 2010;68(5):403–414. [PMID: 20403499]

▶ Pathogenesis

To some degree, somatic symptoms related to psychological and emotional states are common and should be considered normal.

Table 59–1. Somatic symptom disorders, factitious disorder, and malingering.[a]

Disorder	Symptoms Volitional	Symptom Presentation	Type of Symptoms	Symptom Duration	Treatment Modalities
Somatic symptom disorder (SSD)	No	Excessive concern about one or more physical complaints	Disproportionate and persistent thoughts about seriousness of symptoms High anxiety about health or symptoms Excessive time and energy devoted to symptoms	Chronic, recurring, and/or stable	Frequent visits, therapeutic relationship with provider, active listening, avoidance of excessive or invasive treatments, focus on management versus cure; consider CAM modalities
Conversion disorder	No	Onset after acute stress	Pseudoneurologic symptom or symptom complex such as strokelike weakness, sensory loss, or pseudoseizure	Sudden onset; short duration	Reassurance that symptom will resolve over days Avoid labeling as mental illness Cognitive behavioral therapy Trauma-focused therapy
Pain disorder	No	Preoccupation with pain; examination out of proportion with disease or injury	Pain insufficiently explained by any organic cause; frequently associated with disability, relationship disruptions, depression, anxiety	Sudden onset; worsens with time	Focus on functionality, symptom management, and nonopioid therapy Cognitive behavioral therapy
Illness anxiety disorder, also known as hypochondriasis	No	Intense fear of disease; preoccupied with symptoms; not reassured	Multiple symptoms over time; misinterpretation of normal sensations; may have unusual health and prevention behaviors	Long history, worsens after actual illness	SSRI may be beneficial, otherwise similar SSD
Body dysmorphic disorder	No	Excessive concern about imagined defect in appearance	Specific complaints of defect (other than obesity); behaviors to hide or avoid public exposure of "defect"	Usually several years	SSRI may be beneficial, otherwise similar to SSD
Factitious disorder with physical symptoms	Yes—motivation primary gain: sick role, attention	Unexplained fever, bleeding, injuries	Nonhealing and unremitting; tend to receive multiple procedures/operations over time; falsify records	Chronic; multiple admissions; remits with confrontation	Accurate diagnosis May remit with confrontation
Malingering	Yes—motivation secondary gain: money, disability, drugs, etc	Similar to above Protest; demand for medical help	Vague pain and/or paralysis common; belligerent with providers if need not met	Multiple episodes of same problem	Education regarding negative medical findings Confrontation

[a]All of these disorders are more common in the young, some beginning in the teens but most commonly in the 20s–30s. Similar symptoms presenting for the first time in the elderly should prompt more extensive investigations for organic cause. True factitious disorder is rare, whereas the prevalence of malingering is unknown. Supportive counseling may be considered in cases of factitious disorder and malingering if the patient does not have a personality disorder that would impede care.
CAM, complementary and alternative medicine; SSRI, selective serotonin reuptake inhibitor.

Examples include anger experienced through jaw tightening, tension through shoulder stiffening, loss or grief through chest discomfort, disappointment or fear through a "sinking feeling in the gut," and shame through a reddening of the face, and so on. Children often feel ill when they learn that a friend is sick or when family stress is high. An example of nonpathologic fear of having a disease is "student's syndrome," which is the common perception of medical students in pathology class that every symptom they experience could represent a serious diagnosis.

Genetic factors, demonstrated in adoption studies, appear to play a role in the development of somatic sensitivities and obsessive tendencies. Traumatic experiences in the form of sexual, physical, and emotional abuse and witnessing violence are predictive of SSD. Operant reinforcements and classically conditioned associations will also play a role, both in changes in perception of physical sensations and in pain-related behaviors. In particular, some individuals are susceptible to overexperiencing sensations. This phenomenon may occur through a difference in neuron gating, in which the threshold of firing is reduced by anxiety or psychological stress. Patients with hypochondriasis can experience a cycle of symptom amplification whereby obsession about the body focuses attention on sensations, which causes anxiety, increasing sensations, and further worsening obsessiveness. Other disorders, such as body dysmorphic disorder, may be related to obsessive-compulsive disorders or even a mild thought disorder.

Because families differ in how they respond to symptoms and illnesses, individual differences in health beliefs and illness-related behaviors are to be expected. Families also shape the tendency to experience, display, and magnify somatic symptoms; thus, SSD or malingering in children may be modeled or reinforced by adults. Social risk factors include single parenthood, living alone, unemployment, and marital and job difficulties.

Gender ratios and prevalence of SSD differ across cultures. In North America, somatization, conversion, and pain disorders are more frequent in women, whereas hypochondriasis and body dysmorphic disorder involve men and women equally. Somatic symptoms are more prevalent among Chinese American, Asian, and South American patients. These differences are most likely due to Western/empirical explanatory models contrasted with culturally based understandings in which ancient people's associations of phenomena and symptoms still affect the beliefs and expectations of modern populations.

Disorders with somatoform characteristics specific to certain cultures include the *dhat* syndrome in India, which is a concern about semen loss, and *koro* in Southeast Asia, a preoccupation that the penis will disappear into the abdomen. A sense of having worms in the head or burning hands is sometimes reported by people in Africa and Southeast Asia. Cultures influence how emotions should be expressed and sanction religious and healing rituals that may look like conversion disorders. Thus, somatoform-type symptoms should be evaluated for appropriateness to the patient's social context. Behaviors sanctioned by the culture are typically not considered pathologic.

Dimsdale JE, Dantzer R. A biological substrate for somatoform disorders: importance of pathophysiology. *Psychosom Med.* 2007;69:850–854. [PMID: 18040093]

Winfried R, Arthur JB. Psychobiological perspectives on somatoform disorders. *Psychoneuroendocrinology.* 2005; 30(10): 996–1002. [PMID: 15958280]

▶ Clinical Findings

A. Symptoms and Signs

Diagnosis of SSD involves both exclusion of general medical conditions and inclusion of somatoform features. The following features should increase suspicion of SSD:

- Unexplained symptoms that are chronic or constantly change.
- Multiple symptoms. Fainting, menstrual problems, headache, chest pain, dizziness, and palpitations are the symptoms most likely to be somatoform.
- Vague or highly personalized, idiosyncratic complaints.
- Inability of more than three physicians to make a diagnosis.
- Presence of another mental disorder, especially depressive, anxiety, or substance use disorders.
- Distrust toward the physician.
- Physician experience of frustration.
- Paradoxical worsening of symptoms with treatment.
- High utilization, including repeated visits, frequent telephone calls, multiple medications, and repeated subspecialty referrals.
- Disproportionate disability and role impairment.

B. Diagnostic Criteria

SSD is a mental disorder that involves physical symptoms or irrational anxiety about illness or appearance, and for which biomedical findings are not consistent with a general medical condition. Specific diagnosis requires that the symptoms have brought unneeded medical treatment or significant impairment in social, occupational, or other important areas of functioning. SSD cannot be caused by a general medical condition or by direct effects of substances. If the disorder occurs in the presence of a general medical condition, complaints or impairment must be in excess of what would be expected from the physical findings and history. Although SSD may occur concurrently with other mental disorders, other diagnoses such as depression or anxiety may be sufficient to supersede the SSD diagnosis.

1. SSD—Prior to *DSM-5*, formal diagnosis of somatization required identification (counts) of multiple symptoms from different body sites or functions. Current diagnosis focuses on the distress or disruption experienced by patients over somatic symptoms. Patients often do have multiple symptoms. Symptoms maybe specific or general (eg, fatigue) and may sometimes represent normal bodily sensations that do not signify significant disease. Patients with this disorder have the thoughts, feelings, or behaviors associated with the symptoms that are excessive, persistent, and dysfunctional.

2. Conversion disorder—This diagnosis consists solely of pseudoneurologic symptoms (ie, deficits affecting the central nervous system, voluntary motor or sensory functions). Psychological factors in the form of stressors or emotional conflicts are expected and precede the symptoms. Depending on the medical naiveté of the patient, symptoms are often quite implausible, not conforming to anatomic pathways or physiologic mechanisms. The symptoms, however, are not considered volitional. Symptoms may symbolically represent emotional conflicts, such as arm immobility as an expression of anger and impotence. Other clues indicating that the symptoms are pseudoneurologic include worsening in the presence of others; noninjuries despite dramatic falls; normal reflexes, muscle tone, and pupillary reactions; and striking inconsistencies on repeated examinations. Groups of symptoms also tend to not fit together physiologically. Symptoms may be experienced with a relative lack of concern (so-called *la belle indifference*), but dramatic presentations are more common. Course is an important consideration. Conversion disorder is rare before age 10 or after age 35 years. Symptoms are transient, rarely lasting beyond 2 weeks, and respond to reassurance, suggestion, and psychological support. Although primary and secondary gains may result from conversion disorder, these gains are not the motivating factor as they would be with factitious disorder or malingering.

3. Pain disorder associated with psychological factors—This disorder is the psychiatric equivalent of chronic nonmalignant pain syndrome, except that no minimum duration of symptoms is required. Psychological factors play a significant role in the pain picture, including its onset, severity, exacerbation, and maintenance. Physical pathologies are possible and frequent, but organic findings are insufficient to explain the severity of the pain. Functional deficits are common, including disability, increased use of the healthcare system, abuse of medications, and relational and vocational disruptions. Depression or anxiety may be secondary or may also be primary or comorbid, predisposing the patient to an increased experience of pain as well as a deficient ability to cope.

4. Hypochondriasis—The individual is preoccupied with fears of having a serious disease. The preoccupation may originate in an overfocus on and misinterpretation of normal physiologic sensations (eg, orthostatic dizziness), erroneous attributions about the body (eg, "aching veins"), or obsession about minor physical abnormalities. Patients are easily alarmed by contact with ill persons or media coverage of disease. Fears persist despite medical reassurance. More global symptoms may suggest a primary diagnosis of panic disorder, whereas more specific body-related concerns may be better explained by a diagnosis of body dysmorphic disorder. The key to this diagnosis is primary fear of disease rather than generalized worry or fear of a specific defect or disorder.

5. Body dysmorphic disorder—This disorder involves excessive preoccupation with a minor or imagined defect of one or more body parts, excluding the diagnosis of a primary eating disorder. Although many people are concerned about their appearance, the concerns and behaviors associated with this disorder are extreme, distressing, time-consuming, and debilitating. Self-consciousness is significant, and avoidance of public exposure, hiding of defects, and nondisclosure to the physician are common. Medical, dental, and surgical treatments are sought but may only worsen preoccupations. Concern cannot focus exclusively on a false belief that one is obese, which would indicate an eating disorder. Similarly, a belief that sexual characteristics are incorrect may be better represented in a diagnosis of gender identity disorder. Transient or more generalized concerns about appearance may indicate major depressive episodes. Patients who insist that an imagined defect is real and hideous will meet the criteria for delusional disorder, somatic type.

6. Malingering, factitious disorder, and factitious disorder by proxy—These are not SSDs; symptoms are voluntary and deceptive. Deception is obtained by feigning or self-inducing symptoms or by falsifying histories or laboratory findings. Common symptoms include fever, self-mutilation, hemorrhage, and seizures. Persons connected to health professions are common perpetrators. Malingering and factitious disorder differ by whether symptom gain is primary or secondary. In malingering, symptoms are produced to gain rewards or avoid punishments (secondary gains). Factitious disorder involves production of symptoms in order to assume the sick role (primary gain). Unlike malingering, factitious disorder is considered a mental disorder principally because the need to be in the sick role is abnormal. Factitious disorder by proxy occurs when illness is caused by a caregiver, typically to meet a need for drama and to be a rescuer of the patient. Signs of factitious disorder include direct evidence, such as inconsistent laboratory or physical findings or observations (eg, injection of bacteria), as well as vague clues, such as patients who are migratory or have no visitors; are comfortable with more aggressive treatments, including extended hospitalization; or whose presentation is exaggerated and quite dramatic (Munchausen syndrome).

C. Screening and Diagnostic Measures

Keeping SSD in the differential is the key to making the correct diagnosis over time. Valid diagnostic and screening questionnaires exist but often lack clinical utility because of the length and training required for interpretation. A directed interview with specific questions based on patient complaints is most effective for primary care providers. When doubts remain, referral to a specialist skilled in use of diagnostic questionnaires is indicated. Patients should be screened for depression.

▶ Differential Diagnosis

Diagnosis should be considered provisional until there is considerable external support. General medical conditions characterized by multiple and confusing somatic symptoms (eg, hyperparathyroidism, porphyria, multiple sclerosis, and systemic lupus erythematosus) should be considered. Conversion disorder, in particular, is often misdiagnosed. Daum and colleagues (2013) have described the high specificity of weakness, sensory, and gait symptoms in determining whether conversion presentations are pseudoneurologic. Onset of multiple physical symptoms in early adulthood suggests somatization disorder but, in the elderly, suggests a general medical condition. Primary or secondary depression should be considered in any patient suspected of having SSD. Personality disorders are also frequently associated with SSD. It is important to determine the primary disorder in order to choose effective treatment. Clinical factors, such as context, duration of symptoms, and age of the patient, may be able to distinguish SSD from other disorders.

Daum C, Hubschmid M, Aybek S. The value of "positive" clinical signs for weakness, sensory and gait disorders in conversion disorder: a systematic and narrative review. *J Neurol Neurosurg Psychiatr.* 2014;85(2):180–190. [PMID: 23467417]

▶ Complications

Failure to recognize and properly treat SSD can lead to excessive diagnostic procedures and treatments, which perpetuate patient preoccupations and place the patient at risk for iatrogenic harm. Use of unidentified, unconventional, or alternative treatments by SSD patients may interact negatively with prescribed medications. Dependences on sedative, analgesic, or narcotic agents are common iatrogenic complications.

▶ Treatment

Primary care patients who present with undifferentiated symptoms are best addressed with a comprehensive approach that includes continuity of care and attention to the physician-patient relationship. "Pathologizing" makes patients feel illegitimate, in itself a major source of distress, and produces stereotypes of patients as "crocks, whiners, or difficult." Patient characteristics considered as difficult

include extensive or exaggerated complaints, nonadherence with treatment recommendations, and behaviors that raise suspicion of seeking drugs. When patients are so labeled, the relevance of the patient's experience and the potential of partnership between patient and physician are both obviated. A patient-centered method, so important to family practice, becomes impossible. Even without attributions of a mental disorder, SSD presents one of the most difficult challenges in primary care. Uncertainties associated with the diagnosis, the sense that the focus is not medical and therefore the interaction is inappropriate, patient symptom amplification, and the sense that services are being overused inappropriately contribute to the perception that the patient is difficult.

A. General Recommendations

Symptoms of SSD exist on a continuum. Comprehensive, continuous, patient-centered care appropriately addresses most primary care patient presentations. The general recommendations as follows have been referred to as structured care. A Cochrane review suggests that they can be as effective as psychological interventions in adults.

1. First visits—A therapeutic alliance should be built by a thorough history and physical examination and a review of the patient's records. The physician should show curiosity and interest in the patient's complaints and validate the patient's suffering. Psychogenic attributions should be avoided. To appear puzzled initially is a good strategy. Delivery of a diagnosis is a key treatment step with SSD. Different disorders require different types of information.

2. Management—The disorder should be treated as a chronic illness, with the focus on functioning rather than cure. Gradual change should be expected, with periods of improvement and relapse. Physicians should try to avoid excessive and/or invasive diagnostics and treatment in order to minimize iatrogenic harm. When procedures or treatments are undertaken, they should be selected only on the basis of objective evidence, not subjective complaints. When new symptoms arise, at least a limited physical examination should be performed to avoid misdiagnosis and assure the patient that his or her concerns are taken seriously. The need for unnecessary tests and procedures can be avoided by having the patient feel "known" by the physician.

3. Management when controlled drugs are involved—Berland and colleagues (2012) have described a comprehensive approach for managing somatoform pain disorder where patient preferences for opioids complicate treatment. They recommend a structured approach that includes a comprehensive biopsychosocial evaluation and a treatment plan that encourages patients to set and reach functional goals.

4. Patient-centered care—Feelings of illegitimacy by patients and common physician attitudes toward patients contribute to power differentials and struggles. Physicians should speak with patients as equals, listen well, ask and answer many questions, explain things understandably, and allow patients to make decisions about their care. A collaborative relationship should be developed in which the physician works together with the patient to understand and manage patient problems. The "common ground" shared by the physician and the patient should be monitored and differences discussed.

5. Office visits—Regular, brief appointments should be scheduled, thus avoiding "as-needed" medications and office visits that render medical attention contingent on symptoms. Practical time-related strategies include negotiating and setting the agenda early in the visit, paying attention to the emotional agenda, practicing active listening through appropriate reactions and follow-up questions, soliciting the patient's attributions for the problems, and communicating empathetically.

6. Psychosocial issues—Reassurance should be provided to the patient, but not before a thorough exploration of symptoms. Psychosocial questions should be interspersed with biomedical ones to explore all issues: physiologic, anatomic, social, family, and psychological. The physician should inquire about trauma and abuse. As trust builds, the patient should be encouraged to explore psychological issues that may be related to symptoms. In this way, symptoms can be linked to the patient's life and feelings. Physicians should avoid using the term *stress* too liberally, as it may be misconstrued as the cause of the patient's symptoms or an excuse for an incomplete evaluation. Eventually and subtly, patients are likely to reveal their personal issues and concerns.

7. Family involvement—With the patient's permission, family members should be invited to participate in patient visits. An occasional family conference can be valuable. Each person's opinion about the illness and treatment can be solicited, and family members can be asked how family life would differ if the patient were without symptoms. Physicians should solicit and constantly return to the patient's and family's strengths and areas of competence.

Berland E, Rodgers P. Rational use of opioids for management of chronic nonterminal pain. *Am Fam Physician.* 2012;86(3): 252–258. [PMID: 22962988]

Heijmans M, Olde Hartman TC, van Weel-Baumgarten E, et al. Experts' opinions on the management of medically unexplained symptoms in primary care. A qualitative analysis of narrative reviews and scientific editorials. *Fam Pract.* 2011;28(4): 444–455. [PMID: 21368064]

Van Dessel N, den Boeft M, van der Wouden JC, et al. Non-pharmacological interventions for somatoform disorders and medically unexplained physical symptoms (MUPS) in adults. *Cochrane Database Syst Rev.* 2014;11:CD011142. [PMID: 25362239]

B. Pharmacotherapy

Because these patients may be extremely sensitive to side effects, psychopharmacologic agents generally should not be used unless the patient has demonstrated pharmacologically responsive mental disorder such as major depression, generalized anxiety disorder, panic disorder, or obsessive-compulsive disorder. (For further discussion of these disorders, see Chapters 56–58.) Selective serotonin reuptake inhibitors (SSRIs), other nontricyclic antidepressants, and benzodiazepines are the medications most frequently used for coexisting psychiatric conditions. Treatment should be initiated at subtherapeutic doses and increased very gradually, as described in Chapters 56–58. Exceptions to this general rule are hypochondriasis and body dysmorphic disorders. They are more similar to obsessive-compulsive disorder, and patients with these disorders may benefit from slow increases to higher doses of SSRIs if side effects are tolerated. Those with extreme but transitory dysmorphic concerns may benefit from temporary treatment with an atypical antipsychotic medication.

Gasparini S, Beghi E, Ferlazzo E, et al. Management of psychogenic nonepileptic seizures (PNES): a multidisciplinary approach. *Eur J Neurol.* 2019;26(2):e205–e215. [PMID: 30300463]

Somashekar B, Jainer A, Wuntakal B. Psychopharmacotherapy of somatic symptoms disorders. *Int Rev Psychiatr.* 2013;25(1): 107–115. [PMID: 23383672]

C. Consultation or Referral

Involvement of a mental health clinician may be helpful in diagnosing comorbid mental conditions, offering suggestions for psychotropic medications, and engaging some patients in psychotherapy. Patients, however, are unlikely to see the value of consultation or may experience referral as an accusation that their symptoms are not authentic. Pressuring the patient to accept a consultation is unlikely to be effective and may render the consultant encounter unproductive. Trust must first be established, and psychological issues must be made a legitimate subject for discussion. The idea of referral can be introduced later. When possible, it can be more effective to see the patient along with the mental health clinician so that a comprehensive approach continues to be emphasized, the patient does not feel abandoned, and worry that the patient's concerns are not taken seriously are alleviated. Extreme distress or preoccupations worsening to delusional levels may require inpatient hospitalization.

Jackson JL, Passamonti M, Kroenke K. Outcome and impact of mental disorders in primary care at 5 years. *Psychosom Med.* 2007;69(3):270–276. [PMID: 17401055]

Schweickhardt A, Larisch A, Fritzsche K. Differentiation of somatizing patients in primary care: why the effects of treatment are always moderate. *J Nerv Ment Dis.* 2005;193:813–819. [PMID: 16319704]

D. Psychotherapeutic Interventions

Standardized group or individual cognitive behavioral therapies can be an effective treatment for chronic somatoform disorders, reducing somatic symptoms, distress, impairment, and medical care utilization and costs. Cognitive interventions train the patient to identify and restructure dysfunctional beliefs and assumptions about health. Behaviorally, the patient is encouraged to experiment with activities that are counter to usual habits such as avoidance, "doctor shopping," or excess seeking of reassurance. In addition, patients can learn relaxation and meditation techniques to manage symptoms of anxiety. Patients with high emotional distress respond more rapidly to psychotherapy, and patients able to at least partially attribute symptoms to psychological factors show better therapeutic outcomes than patients who firmly believe that their physical symptoms have a physical cause.

For children, psychological interventions reduce symptom numbers and severity, disability, and school absence.

Bonvanie I, Kallesøe K, Janssens K, Schröder A, Rosmalen J, Rask C. Psychological interventions for children with functional somatic symptoms: a systematic review and meta-analysis. *J Pediatr.* 2017;187:272–281. [PMID: 28416243]

Gropalis M, Bleichhardt G, Hiller W, Witthöft M. Specificity and modifiability of cognitive biases in hypochondriasis. *J Consult Clin Psychol.* 2013;81(3):558–565. [PMID: 22563641]

Rosebush PI, Mazurek MF. Treatment of conversion disorder in the 21st century: have we moved beyond the couch? *Curr Treat Options Neurol.* 2011;13(3):255–266. [PMID: 21468672]

Sharma MP, Manjula M. Behavioural and psychological management of somatic symptom disorders: an overview. *Int Rev Psychiatr.* 2013;25(1):116–124. [PMID: 23383673]

E. Complementary and Alternative Therapies

It is to be expected that patients with somatoform symptoms often try alternative treatments such as herbal remedies, mind-body interventions, and other non-Western medical approaches. In these patients, conventional treatments appear to have failed, distrust of physicians may be high, and distress is great. Federal regulations require that label claims and instructions on herbal products and supplements address symptoms only; therefore, there are no specific herbal agents for SSD, per se. Given the plethora of symptoms that can exist in patients with SSD, it is not surprising that there are numerous alternative medications that patients may try.

Patients with pain disorder or primary or comorbid anxiety may benefit from body and mind-body interventions such as massage, movement therapies, manipulations, relaxation, guided imagery, and hypnosis. The placebo effect of various remedies may be helpful, particularly if the agents are largely inert, as bothersome side effects seen in conventional medicines may be avoided. Alternative therapies often include "nonspecific therapeutic effects" that go beyond the placebo effect and can be beneficial. Nonspecific effects include warmth and listening skills of the practitioner, empowerment that comes from legitimization of the patient's problem, and an egalitarian approach to care. Physicians may wish to recommend alternative treatments and collaborate with alternative practitioners but should also be prepared to protect the patient by cautioning against treatments that are potentially harmful, excessively expensive, or that circumvent conventional treatments that are needed for demonstrated medical conditions.

Elder WG, King M, Dassow P, Macy B. Managing lower back pain: you may be doing too much. *J Fam Practice.* 2009;58:180–186. [PMID: 19358795]

F. Patient Education

The American Academy of Family Physicians has developed a patient education page for somatoform disorders. The web address for the page is http://familydoctor.org/familydoctor/en/diseases-conditions/somatoform-disorders.html.

Substance Use Disorders

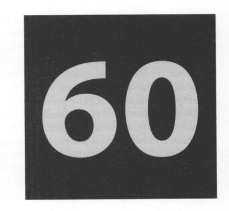

Kimberly Mallin, MD
Robert Mallin, MD

▶ General Considerations

The prevalence of alcohol and drug disorders in primary care outpatients is between 23% and 37%. Almost one-third of US adults meet the criteria for a form of alcohol use disorder during some point in their lives. The cost to society of these disorders is staggering. Each year in the United States, substance use disorders (SUDs) are associated with over 600,000 deaths and costs of approximately $250 billion. Of these deaths, 480,000 may be attributed to tobacco and 100,000 to alcohol. In 2016, drug overdoses alone accounted for 63,000 deaths, with >42,000 deaths due to opioids. The high prevalence of these disorders in primary care outpatients suggests that family physicians are confronted with these problems daily. These disorders rarely present overtly but are often found in conjunction with commonly seen illnesses such as hypertension, insomnia, depression, anxiety, and liver problems. The pediatric population is another area where diagnostic clues may be subtly present, with >10% of US children living with a least one parent with alcohol or drug problems. Patients in denial about the connection between their substance use and the consequences caused by it frequently minimize the amount of their use, and they rarely seek assistance for their substance use problem. One study exploring the care provided for patients with alcohol dependence found that only 11% of patients received recommended care in the primary care setting. The National Institute on Alcohol Abuse and Alcoholism (NIAAA) published a physician's guide, *Helping Patients Who Drink Too Much* (http://www.niaaa.nih.gov/guide) to help improve this discrepancy of care. Various tools are available to help integrate management of patients with SUDs into primary care offices, including SBIRT (Screening, Brief Intervention, Referral to Treatment) training (http://www.sbirteducation.com).

The epidemiology of alcohol and drug disorders has been well studied and is most often reported from data of the National Institute of Mental Health Epidemiologic Catchment Area Program (ECA). Lifetime prevalence rates for alcohol disorders from the ECA survey data were 13.5%. For men, the lifetime prevalence was found to be 23.8% and for women, 4.7%. The National Comorbidity Survey revealed lifetime prevalence of alcohol abuse without dependence to be 12.5% for men and 6.4% for women. For alcohol dependence, the lifetime prevalence was 20.1% in men and 8.2% in women. The ECA data yield an overall prevalence of drug use disorders of 6.2%. As with alcohol use disorders, drug use disorders occur more frequently in men (lifetime prevalence 7.7%) than in women (4.8%). Characteristics known to influence the epidemiology of SUDs include gender, age, race, family history, marital status, employment status, and educational status.

Boschloo L, Vogelzangs N, van den Brink W, et al. Alcohol use disorders and the course of depressive and anxiety disorders. *Br J Psychiatr.* 2012;200(6):476–484. [PMID: 22322459]

National Institute on Alcohol Abuse and Alcoholism/National Institutes of Health. Alcohol facts and statistics. https://www.niaaa.nih.gov/publications/brochures-and-fact-sheets/alcohol-facts-and-statistics. Accessed March 19, 2020.

Willenbring M, Massey S, Gardner M. Helping patients who drink too much: an evidence-based guide for primary care physicians. *Am Fam Physician.* 2009;80(1):44–50. [PMID: 19621845]

▶ Pathogenesis

The difference between mild, moderate, and severe SUD is an important one. With mild-moderate SUD, patients retain control of their use. This control may be affected by poor judgment and social and environmental factors and mitigated by the consequences of the patient's use. Patients who have severe SUDs no longer have full control of their drug use. Their brain has been "hijacked" by a substance that affects the mechanism of control over the use of that substance. This is far more than physical dependence. The need to use the drug becomes as powerful as the drives of thirst and hunger. There is significant evidence that the brains of addicted individuals are different from those of nonaddicted persons. Many of these abnormalities predate the use of the substance and are assumed to be inherited. In genetically predisposed individuals, substances of abuse cause changes in the dopaminergic mesolimbic system that result in a loss of control over substance use. These changes are mediated by several neurotransmitters: dopamine, γ-aminobutyric acid (GABA), glutamate, serotonin, and endorphins. The different classes of substances of abuse act through one or more of these neurotransmitters, ultimately affecting the level of dopamine in the mesolimbic system (otherwise known as the "reward pathway"). These changes in the brain are permanent and are the primary reason for relapse in the addicted patient trying to maintain abstinence, or control of use.

▶ Prevention

Although neurobiology plays a large role in addiction, the precursors of substance abuse are also environmental and include family, school, community, and peer factors (Table 60–1). These multiple factors make the design of effective prevention difficult. Primary prevention is designed to prevent the use of substances, thereby rendering abuse

Table 60–1. Environmental risk factors for substance abuse.

Family factors
Sexual or physical abuse
Parental or sibling substance abuse
Parental approval or tacit approval of child's substance use
Disruptive family conflict
Poor communication
Poor discipline
Poor supervision
Parental rejection
School factors
Lack of involvement in school activities
Poor school climate
Norms that condone substance use
Unfair rules
School failure
Community factors
Poor community bonding
Disorganized neighborhoods
Crime
Drug use
Poverty
Low employment or unemployment
Community norms that condone substance use
Peer factors
Bonding to peer group that engages in substance use or other antisocial behaviors

impossible. These programs are designed primarily for the young. Secondary prevention consists of screening programs to identify abuse early and to redirect the patient's behavior before addiction becomes overt. In tertiary prevention, the focus is on the treatment of addictive behavior in an effort to prevent the consequences of compulsive use. Prevention programs can be divided into those that address the four environmental areas of risk: family, school, peers, and community. Family physicians can support these efforts by including the following behaviors in their practice:

- Supporting efforts to strengthen parenting skills, family support, and communication.
- Providing patient and community education about drug and alcohol use, abuse, and treatment.
- Screening and assessing patients of all ages for SUDs in the office and hospital.
- Supporting community efforts in substance abuse prevention.
- Endorsing and promoting public policy that supports prevention, early detection, and treatment of SUDs.

Broning S, Kumpfer K, Kruse K, et al. Selective prevention programs for children from substance-affected families: a comprehensive systematic review. *Subst Abuse Treat Prev Policy.* 2012;7:23. [PMID: 22691221]
Newton NC, O'Leary-Barrett M, Conrold PJ. Adolescent substance misuse: neurobiology and evidence-based interventions. *Curr Top Behav Neurosci.* 2013;13:685–708. [PMID: 22057622]

▶ Clinical Findings

A. Symptoms and Signs

The signs and symptoms of substance abuse are varied and often subtle. This is complicated by the fact that most patients fail to recognize their substance use as the cause of their problems and are often quite resistant to that interpretation. Consequently, the family physician must have a high index of suspicion, recognizing that the prevalence of SUDs in outpatient primary care is high. A perspective that recognizes the prevalence of these disorders will enable physicians to interpret potential clues to substance use (Table 60–2).

The diagnosis of an SUD is based primarily on a careful history. However, substance-disordered patients may be deliberately less than truthful in their history, and often the patient's denial prevents the physician from seeing the connection between substance use and its consequences. Signs of sedative-hypnotic or alcohol withdrawal may be misinterpreted as an anxiety disorder. Chronic use of stimulants may present as a psychotic disorder. In fact, in the face of active substance abuse, other psychiatric diagnoses often must wait for detoxification before they can be accurately assessed.

Table 60–2. Clinical clues of alcohol and drug problems.

Social history
Arrest for driving under the influence of alcohol once (75% association
  with alcoholism) or twice (95% association)
Loss of job or sent home from work for alcohol or drug reasons
Domestic violence
Child abuse/neglect
Family instability (divorce, separation)
Frequent, unplanned absences
Personal isolation
Problems at work or school
Mood swings and psychological problems

Medical history
History of addiction to any drug
Withdrawal syndrome
Depression
Anxiety disorder
Recurrent pancreatitis
Recurrent hepatitis
Hepatomegaly
Peripheral neuropathy
Myocardial infarction at age <30 years (cocaine)
Blood alcohol level >300 or >100 without impairment
Alcohol on breath or intoxicated at office visit
Tremor
Mild hypertension
Estrogen-mediated signs (telangiectasias, spider angiomas,
  palmar erythema, muscle atrophy)
Gastrointestinal complaints
Sleep disturbances
Eating disorders
Sexual dysfunction

B. Screening Measures

The diagnosis of SUDs is most typically begun with a screening test that identifies a user at risk. The CAGE (**c**ut down,
annoyed, **g**uilty, and **e**ye opener) questionnaire (Table 60–3)

Table 60–3. CAGE questions adapted to include drugs.[a]

1. Have you felt you ought to **c**ut down on your drinking or drug use?
2. Have people **a**nnoyed you by criticizing your drinking or drug use?
3. Have you felt **g**uilty about your drinking or drug use?
4. Have you ever had a drink or used drugs first thing in the morning to
   steady your nerves or to get rid of a hangover or to get the day started?
   (**e**ye-opener)

[a]Two or more yes answers indicate a need for a more in-depth
assessment. Even one positive response should raise a red flag about
problem drinking or drug use.
Data from Graham AW, Shultz TK, eds. *Principles of Addiction Medicine*,
2nd ed. Chevy Chase, MD: American Society of Addiction Medicine;
1998.

is perhaps the most widely used screening tool for the identification of patients at risk for SUDs. When a patient answers
yes to two or more questions of the CAGE, the sensitivity is
60–90% and the specificity 40–60% for SUDs. Screening can
be as simple as this brief validated single-question screen:
How many times in the past year have you used an illegal
drug or used a prescription drug for nonmedical reasons?
(Nonmedical meaning use for the experience or feeling it
causes.) Because a screening test is more predictive when
applied to a population more likely to have a disease, clinical
clues to SUDs may be useful indicators to determine whom
to screen (see Table 60–2). Men age <65 years may be classified as at risk or heavy drinkers if they consume >4 drinks per
day or >14 drinks during a week. Women of any age and men
age >65 years are also considered at risk or heavy drinkers
if they consume >3 drinks daily or 7 drinks weekly. A *drink*
can be defined as a 12-oz can or bottle of beer, a 5-oz glass of
wine, or 1.5 oz of distilled spirits.

Miller MM, Goplerud E, Martin J, Ziedonis DM. New systems of
care for substance use disorders: treatment, finance, and technology under health care reform. *Psychiatr Clin North Am.*
2012;35(2):327–356. [PMID: 22640759]

C. Methods to Aid in Diagnosis of Substance Use Disorders

1. Diagnostic criteria—The *Diagnostic and Statistical
Manual of Mental Disorders,* fifth edition (*DSM-5*) came out
in 2013 and has made substantial changes. It no longer uses
the terms *substance abuse* and *substance dependence,* but
refers to *substance use disorders* (SUD), which are defined as
mild, moderate, or severe based on the number of diagnostic criteria endorsed by an individual. Two to three criteria
indicate a mild disorder; four to five criteria, a moderate
disorder; and six or more criteria, a severe disorder. SUDs
occur when the recurrent use of drugs and/or alcohol causes
clinically and functionally significant impairment, such
as health problems, disability, and failure to meet major
responsibilities at work, school, or home. According to the
DSM-5, a diagnosis of SUD is based on evidence of impaired
control, social impairment, risky use, and pharmacologic
criteria. Additional changes from the fourth edition of the
DSM are the inclusion of cannabis use disorders/withdrawal,
the addition of gambling as an SUD, and criteria changes
such as exclusion of legal problems and inclusion of craving.

2. Withdrawal syndromes—Although not always seen with
substance abuse, physiologic dependence suggests abuse
unless the patient is on long-term prescribed addictive
medicines. Table 60–4 contrasts signs and symptoms of
withdrawal from alcohol and other sedative-hypnotic drugs,
opiates, and cocaine and other stimulant drugs. Alcohol
withdrawal may be life threatening if not properly treated.
Opiate withdrawal is not life threatening (except for neonates);

Table 60–4. Symptoms and signs of withdrawal from alcohol, opioids, and cocaine.

Substance of Abuse	Manifestations of Withdrawal
Alcohol	Autonomic hyperactivity: diaphoresis, tachycardia, elevated blood pressure Tremor Insomnia Nausea or vomiting Transient visual, tactile, or auditory hallucinations or illusions Psychomotor agitation Anxiety Generalized Seizure activity
Opioids	Mild elevation of pulse rate, respiratory rate, blood pressure, and temperature Piloerection (gooseflesh) Dysphoric mood, drug craving Lacrimation or rhinorrhea Mydriasis, yawning, diaphoresis Anorexia, abdominal cramps, vomiting, diarrhea Insomnia Weakness
Cocaine	Dysphoric mood Fatigue, malaise Vivid, unpleasant dreams Sleep disturbance Increased appetite Psychomotor retardation or agitation

neither is withdrawal from marijuana, cocaine, or other stimulants, although they may be associated with morbidity and relapse to substance abuse.

In dealing with sedative-hypnotic, alcohol, or opiate withdrawal, assessment of the degree of withdrawal is important to determine appropriate use and dose of medication to reduce symptoms and, in the case of sedative-hypnotic drugs or alcohol, prevent seizures and mortality. The Clinical Institute Withdrawal Assessment of Alcohol Scale, Revised (CIWA-AR) allows quantification of the signs and symptoms of withdrawal in a predictable fashion that enables clinicians to discuss the severity of withdrawal for a given patient and thus choose intervention strategies that are effective and safe. This tool is available online and can be downloaded from the American Society of Addiction Medicine (ASAM) website (http://asam.org).

D. Laboratory Findings

Biochemical markers may help support the diagnostic criteria gathered in the history, or can be used as a screening mechanism to consider patients for further evaluation (Table 60–5).

American Psychiatric Association. *Diagnostic and Statistical Manual of Mental Disorders.* 4th ed (text revision). Washington, DC: American Psychiatric Association; 2000.

Hannuksela ML, Liisanantti MK, Nissinen AE, et al. Biochemical markers of alcoholism. *Clin Chem Lab Med.* 2007;45(8):953–961. [PMID: 17579567]

Hasin DS, O'Brien CP, Auriacombe M, et al. DSM5 criteria for substance use disorders: recommendations and rationale. *Am J Psychiatry.* 2013;170:834–851. [PMID: 23903334]

▶ Differential Diagnosis

Because substance abuse is a behavioral disorder, when considering a differential diagnosis, psychiatric disorders often come to mind. Indeed, there is a high comorbidity between SUDs and psychiatric disorders. Approximately 50% of psychiatric patients have a SUD. For patients with addictions, however, the rates of psychiatric disorders are similar to those of the general population. Problems such as substance-induced mood disorders (frequently noted in alcohol, opiate, and stimulant abuse) and substance-induced psychotic disorders (most frequently associated with stimulant abuse) complicate differentiation of primary psychiatric disorders from those that are primarily SUDs. Most clinicians agree that psychiatric disorders cannot be reliably assessed in patients who are currently or recently intoxicated. Thus detoxification and a period of abstinence are necessary before other psychiatric disorders may be effectively evaluated.

It may be necessary to examine a patient's behavior over an extended period of time, looking for evidence of past loss of control of use that may not currently be present. In addiction, a pattern of progressively increasing loss of control usually becomes evident as the consequences of chronic substance abuse unfold.

Table 60–5. Biochemical markers of substance use disorders.

Marker	Substance	Sensitivity (%)	Specificity (%)	Predictive Value (%)
Mean corpuscular volume (MCV)	Alcohol	24	96	63
γ-Glutamyltransferase (GGT)	Alcohol	42	76	61
Carbohydrate-deficient transferrin (CDT)	Alcohol	67	97	84

Complications

The medical complications of substance abuse are many and profoundly affect the health of our population (Table 60–6). The number of deaths attributed to the abuse of substances exceeds 600,000 yearly, with tobacco use accounting for 450,000 of these deaths. (For discussion of tobacco use, see Chapter 61.) Cardiovascular disease and cancer lead this list.

Table 60–6. Medical complications of substance abuse.

Drug	Medical Complication
Alcohol	Trauma
	Hypertension
	Cardiomyopathy
	Dysrhythmias
	Ischemic heart disease
	Hemorrhagic stroke
	Esophageal reflux
	Barret esophagus
	Mallory-Weiss tears
	Esophageal cancer
	Acute gastritis
	Pancreatitis
	Chronic diarrhea, malabsorption
	Alcoholic hepatitis
	Cirrhosis
	Hepatic failure
	Hepatic carcinoma
	Nasopharyngeal cancer
	Headache
	Sleep disorders
	Memory impairment
	Dementia
	Peripheral neuropathy
	Fetal alcohol syndrome
	Sexual dysfunction
	Substance-induced mood disorders
	Substance-induced psychotic disorders
	Immune dysfunction
Cocaine (other stimulants)	Chest pain
	Congestive heart failure
	Cardiac dysrhythmias
	Cardiovascular collapse
	Seizures
	Cerebrovascular accidents
	Headache
	Spontaneous pneumothorax
	Noncardiogenic pulmonary edema
	Nasal septal perforations
Injection drug use	Hepatitis C, B
	HIV infection
	Subacute endocarditis
	Soft tissue abscesses

Table 60–7. Neuropsychiatric complications of substance abuse.

Substance-induced mood disorder, depressed/elevated
Substance-induced anxiety disorder
Substance-induced psychotic disorder
Substance-induced personality change
Substance intoxication
Substance withdrawal
Delirium
Wernicke disease
Korsakoff syndrome (alcohol-induced persisting amnestic disorder)
Transient amnestic states (blackouts)
Substance-induced persisting dementia

Alcohol causes approximately 100,000 deaths yearly and is associated with motor vehicle and other accidents, homicides, cirrhosis of the liver, and suicide. Injection drug use is responsible for the fastest growing population of human immunodeficiency virus (HIV) infection. In addition to medical complications, substance abuse causes considerable neuropsychiatric morbidity, both as a primary cause (Table 60–7) and by exacerbating existing psychiatric disorders.

Acute substance-induced psychosis is often indistinguishable from a primary psychotic disorder such as schizophrenia in the setting of substance abuse. Neurocognitive states such as dementia may be substance induced and result in permanent brain damage. Depression, commonly diagnosed and treated in the primary care setting, may often be complicated by a substance-induced mood disorder. Often what appears to be treatment-resistant depression is actually the result of persistent substance abuse. Withdrawal syndromes often present as episodes of anxiety, sleep disorders, mood disorders, or seizure disorders.

Seltz R. Medical and surgical complications of addiction. In: Ries RK, Fiellin D, Miller S, et al, eds. *Principles of Addiction Medicine.* 4th ed. Philadelphia, PA: Lippincott Williams & Wilkins; 2009:945–969.

Treatment

Many SUDs resolve spontaneously or with brief interventions on the part of physicians or other authority figures in the workplace, legal system, family, or society. This occurs because patients with mild to moderate SUD continue to maintain control over their use, and when the consequences of that use outweigh the benefits of the drug, they choose to quit. Patients with moderate to severe disorders (addiction), on the other hand, have impaired control by definition. They rarely improve without assistance.

SUDs can be treated successfully. Brief interventions and outpatient, inpatient, and residential treatment programs reduce morbidity and mortality associated with addiction. Determining the type and intensity of treatment that is best for a given patient may be difficult. ASAM has developed guidelines for clinicians to help determine the level and intensity of treatment for patients (Table 60–8). Once patients have been adequately assessed, treatment can begin. Detoxification, patient education, identification of defenses, overcoming denial, relapse prevention, orientation to 12-step recovery programs, medical management of related health problems, and family services are the goals of substance abuse treatment.

A. Intervention

Once screening and diagnosis are complete, it is time for the physician to share the assessment with the patient. Because of the nature of substance abuse, patients rarely choose to seek help for their alcohol or drug problem until the consequences far outweigh the positive aspects of treatment. Intervention may be seen as a means of bringing these consequences to the attention of the patient. A wide range of approaches, some quite informal and others perhaps requiring careful orchestration and execution, can accomplish this task. Physicians or family members can often intervene simply by giving patients feedback about their behavior, describing the feelings that behavior generates, avoiding enabling behavior, and offering help.

The traditional intervention for alcohol or drug addiction is a formal process, best accomplished by an addictions

Table 60–8. American Society of Addiction Medicine placement criteria.

Levels of Service	
Level 0.5:	Early intervention
Level 1:	Outpatient services
Level 2:	Intensive outpatient/partial hospitalization services
Level 3:	Resident/inpatient services
Level 4:	Medically managed intensive inpatient services

Assessment Dimensions

1. Acute intoxication and/or withdrawal potential
2. Biomedical conditions and complications
3. Emotional, behavioral, or cognitive conditions and complications (eg, psychiatric conditions, psychological or emotional/behavioral complications of known or unknown origin, poor impulse control, changes in mental status, transient neuropsychiatric complications)
4. Readiness to change
5. Relapse, continued use, or continued problem potential
6. Recovery/living environment

Data from Mee-Lee D, Shulman GD, Fishman MJ, et al: *The ASAM: Treatment Criteria for Addictive, Substance-Related, and Co-Occurring Conditions*, 3rd ed. Carson City, NV: The Change Companies; 2013.

specialist trained in this process. This approach is often effective, resulting in positive results in approximately 80% of cases. Although effective, the traditional, formal model of intervention is often less than ideal for the family physician. Specialist involvement and orchestration of significant relationships of the patient are sometimes difficult to achieve. In addition, if the intervention fails, it may be difficult if not impossible for the physician to continue a relationship with the patient. Another approach to consider is that of the brief intervention. This highly effective approach to intervention is based on motivational interviewing and the stages of change model (also known as the *transtheoretical model*).

1. Stages of change—Underlying the strategy of the brief intervention is the *stages of change model*, developed by Prochascka and DiClementi. In this model, behavioral change is viewed as a process that evolves over time through a series of stages: precontemplation, contemplation, preparation, action, maintenance, and termination. The individual must progress through each of these stages to reach the next one and cannot leap past one to get to another.

Individuals in the *precontemplation* stage are not planning to take any action in the foreseeable future. This is the stage most often described as denial. Patients in this stage do not perceive their behavior as problematic. In the *contemplation stage*, people perceive that they have a problem and believe that they should do something about it. Many addicted patients who do not appear to be ready for traditional treatment programs are in this stage. They recognize that they have a substance problem, believe that they should stop using the addictive substance, but seem unable to do so. In the *preparation stage,* patients have decided to change and plan to do so soon, usually within the next month. These patients are ready to enter action-oriented treatment programs. *Action* in the present context refers to the stage of change during which patients make specific changes in their behavior. In the case of addiction, abstinence is the generally agreed-on behavior that signifies action. *Maintenance* is the period after action during which the changed behavior persists and patients work toward preventing relapse. Maintenance often requires a sustained effort longer than patients anticipate, and failure to continue with maintenance behavior is a common cause of relapse. *Termination* describes the stage in which there is no temptation, and there is no risk of returning to old habits. In the case of addiction, most patients must work toward a lifetime of maintenance rather than termination. The risk of relapse is such that few truly reach this final stage for the disease of addiction.

2. Brief interventions—Presenting the diagnosis of a SUD by itself may be viewed as a brief intervention. Most physicians who have worked with these patients will not be surprised to hear that as many as 70% of patients are in the precontemplation or contemplation stage when presented with the diagnosis. The resistance associated with these stages tends to force clinicians into one of two modalities—either avoiding the diagnosis or confronting and arguing with the patient. Both of these approaches are futile. One approach in presenting the diagnosis is to use the DEATH glossary, a list of pitfalls to avoid when presenting the diagnosis of addiction. On a more positive note, the SOAPE glossary (Table 60–9) describes suggestions to use when talking to patients about their addiction.

Even for patients in the precontemplative stage at presentation of the diagnosis, continued use of the brief intervention strategy will ultimately reduce the amount of drug use if not result in abstinence.

Brief interventions should include some of the elements of motivational interviewing. These elements include offering empathetic, objective feedback of data; meeting patient expectations; working with ambivalence; assessing barriers and strengths; reinterpreting past experience in light of current medical consequences; negotiating a follow-up plan; and providing hope.

B. Detoxification

Detoxification and treatment of withdrawal and any medical complications must have first priority. Alcohol and other sedative-hypnotic drugs share the same neurobiological withdrawal process. Chronic use of this class of drugs results in downregulation of the GABA receptors throughout the central nervous system (CNS). GABA is an inhibitory neurotransmitter and is uniformly depressed during sedative-hypnotic use. Abrupt cessation of sedative-hypnotic drug use results in upregulation of GABA receptors and a relative paucity of GABA for inhibition. The result is stimulation of the autonomic nervous system (ANS) and the appearance of the signs and symptoms listed in Table 60–4. Withdrawal seizures are a common manifestation of sedative-hypnotic withdrawal, occurring in 11–33% of patients withdrawing from alcohol.

Alcohol withdrawal seizures are best treated with benzodiazepines and by addressing the withdrawal process itself. Long-term treatment of alcohol withdrawal seizures is not recommended, and phenytoin should not be used to treat seizures associated with alcohol withdrawal. The cornerstones of treatment for alcohol withdrawal syndrome are the benzodiazepines. All drugs that provide cross-tolerance with alcohol are effective in reducing the symptoms and sequelae of alcohol withdrawal, but none has the safety profile and evidence of efficacy of the benzodiazepines. Table 60–10 summarizes recommendations in the treatment of alcohol withdrawal. Opiate withdrawal may not be life threatening, but the symptoms are significant enough that, without supportive treatment, most patients will not remain in treatment. Table 60–11 outlines recommendations for the treatment of opiate withdrawal. The symptoms of cocaine, methamphetamine, and other stimulant withdrawal are somewhat less predictable and much harder to improve. Despite multiple studies with many different drug classes,

Table 60–9. SOAPE glossary for presenting the diagnosis.

Support: Use phrases such as "We need to work together on this," "I am concerned about you and will follow up closely with you," and "As with all medical illnesses, the more people you work with, the better you will feel." These words reinforce the physician-patient relationship, strengthen the collaborative model of chronic illness management, and help convince the patient that the physician will not just present the diagnosis and leave.

Optimism: Most patients have controlled their alcohol or drug use at times and may have quit for periods of time. They may expect failure. By giving a strong optimistic message such as "You can get well," "Treatment works," or "You can expect to see improvements in many areas of your life," the physician can motivate the patient.

Absolution: By describing addiction as a disease and telling patients that they are not responsible for having an illness, but that now only they can take responsibility for their recovery, the physician can lessen the burden of guilt and shame that is often a barrier to recovery.

Plan: Having a plan is important to the acceptance of the illness. Using readiness to change categories can help in designing a plan that utilizes the patient's willingness to move ahead. Indicating that abstinence is desirable, but recognizing that all patients will not be able to commit to that goal immediately can help prevent a sense of failure early in the process. Ask "What do you think you will be able to do at this point?"

Explanatory model: Understanding the patient's beliefs about addiction may be important. Many patients believe that this is a moral weakness and that they lack willpower. An explanation that willpower cannot resolve illnesses such as diabetes or alcoholism may go a long way to reassure the patient that recovery is possible.

Data from Clark WD. Alcoholism: blocks to diagnosis and treatment. *Am J Med.* 1981 Aug;71(2):275–286.

Table 60–10. Treatment regimens for alcohol withdrawal.

Use the Clinical Institute Withdrawal Assessment of Alcohol Scale, Revised (CIWA-AR) for monitoring:
  Assess the patient using the CIWA-AR scale every 4 hours until the score is <8 for 24 hours
  For CIWA-AR >10:
    Give either chlordiazepoxide 50–100 mg, diazepam 10–20 mg, oxazepam 30–60 mg, or lorazepam 2–4 mg
  Repeat the CIWA-AR 1 hour after the dose to assess the need for further medication
Non–symptom-driven regimens:
  For patients likely to experience withdrawal, use chlordiazepoxide 50 mg, every 6 hours for four doses followed by 50 mg every 8 hours for three doses, followed by 50 mg every 12 hours for two doses, and finally by 50 mg at bedtime for one dose
Other benzodiazepines may be substituted at equivalent doses
Patients on a predetermined dosing schedule should be monitored frequently both for breakthrough withdrawal symptoms and for excessive sedation

Table 60–11. Treatment for opioid withdrawal.

Methadone: A pure opioid agonist restricted by federal legislation to inpatient treatment or specialized outpatient drug treatment programs. Initial dosage is 15–20 mg for 2–3 days, then tapered with a 10–15% reduction in dose daily guided by patient's symptoms and clinical findings.

Clonidine: An α-adrenergic blocker, 0.2 mg every 4 hours to relieve symptoms of withdrawal, may be effective. Hypotension is a risk and sometimes limits the dose. It can be continued for 10–14 days and tapered by the third day by 0.2 mg daily.

Buprenorphine: This partial μ-receptor agonist can be administered sublingually in doses of 2, 4, or 8 mg every 4 hours for the management of opioid withdrawal symptoms.

Naltrexone/clonidine: A rapid form of opioid detoxification involves pretreatment with 0.2–0.3 mg of clonidine followed by 12.5 mg of naltrexone (a pure opioid antagonist). Naltrexone is increased to 25 mg on the second day, 50 mg on day 3, and 100 mg on day 4, with clonidine given at 0.1–0.3 mg 3 times daily.

no medications have been shown to reliably reduce the symptoms and craving associated with cocaine withdrawal. Symptoms of cannabis withdrawal occur due to downregulation of brain cannabinoid CB1 receptors from heavy use and include multiple symptoms including irritability, anger, depression, anxiety, and most commonly, sleep difficulties. Synthetic cannabinoid withdrawal can cause clinically significant physiologic withdrawal symptoms, and a growing number of case reports suggest that serious life-threatening phenomena (eg, seizures, renal failure, cardiac arrhythmias) are not rare. Treatment of cannabis withdrawal includes cognitive behavioral therapy (CBT) and medications such as gabapentin or zolpidem.

Gorelick DA. Cannabis withdrawal: epidemiology, pathogenesis, clinical manifestations, course, assessment and diagnosis. In: Hermann R, ed, UpToDate. 2017. https://www.uptodate.com/contents/cannabis-withdrawal-epidemiology-pathogenesis-clinical-manifestations-course-assessment-and-diagnosis. Accessed December 3, 2019.

Manasco A, Chang S, Larriviere J, Hamm LL, Glass M. Alcohol withdrawal. *South Med J.* 2012;105(11):607–612. [PMID: 23128805]

Praveen KT, Law F, O'Shea J, Melichar J. Opioid dependence. *Am Fam Physician.* 2012;86(6):565–566. [PMID: 23062049]

C. Patient Education

Patients' knowledge and understanding of the nature of SUDs are the key to their recovery. For patients still in control of their use, education about appropriate substance use will help them to choose responsibly if they continue to use. For patients who meet the criteria for moderate or severe SUD (addiction), abstinence is the only safe recommendation. Once having made the transition to addiction, patients can never use addictive substances reliably again. The neurobiological changes in the brain are permanent, and loss of control may occur at any time when the brain is presented with an addictive substance. Loss of control can occur unpredictably; consequently, addicted patients may find that they can use the substance for a variable period of time with control, which gives them the false impression that they were never addicted in the first place or perhaps that they have been cured. Invariably, if they continue to use addictive substances, they will lose control of their use and begin to experience consequences at or above the level they did before. Understanding that the problem of addiction is a chronic disorder for which there is remission but not cure becomes essential. The question then becomes not whether, but *how* to remain abstinent.

D. Identification of Defenses and Overcoming Denial

During this phase of treatment, patients typically work in a group therapy setting and are encouraged to look at the defenses that have prevented them from seeking help sooner. Denial can best be defined as the inability to see the causal relationship between drug use and its consequences. For example, a patient who believes that he drank because he lost his job may be encouraged to consider the reverse scenario: that he lost his job because he drank.

E. Relapse Prevention

Once patients are educated to the nature of their disease and have identified destructive defense mechanisms, relapse prevention becomes the primary goal. In order to help patients maintain abstinence, it is important to help them identify triggers for alcohol and drug use, develop plans to prevent opportunities to relapse, and determine new ways to deal with problems. In most treatment programs, a relapse prevention plan is developed and individualized for each patient.

F. Twelve-Step Recovery Programs

It would be difficult to overstate the contribution that 12-step programs make to recovery. Despite millions of dollars in research and the efforts of a large segment of the scientific community, no treatment, medication, or psychotherapy has taken the place of the 12 steps.

Twelve-step recovery has its roots in Alcoholics Anonymous (AA), founded in 1935. Today >200 recovery organizations use the 12 steps with some modifications for patients with SUDs. These programs include Al-Anon, for friends and family of alcoholics; Narcotics Anonymous (NA), for those with drug problems other than alcohol; and Cocaine Anonymous, for those with cocaine addiction. At the heart of each of these fellowships is the program of recovery outlined in the 12 steps (Table 60–12). AA and related 12-step programs are spiritual, not religious, in nature. No one is

Table 60–12. The 12 Steps of Alcoholics Anonymous.

We:
1. Admitted that we were powerless over alcohol—that our lives had become unmanageable;
2. Came to believe that a power greater than ourselves could restore us to sanity;
3. Made a decision to turn our will and our lives over to the care of God as *we understood Him*;
4. Made a searching and fearless moral inventory of ourselves;
5. Admitted to ourselves, and to another human being, the exact nature of our wrongs;
6. Were entirely ready to have God remove all these defects of character;
7. Humbly asked Him to remove our shortcomings;
8. Made a list of all persons whom we had harmed, and became willing to make amends to them all;
9. Made direct amends to such people wherever possible, except when to do so would injure them or others;
10. Continued to take personal inventory and when we were wrong promptly admitted it;
11. Sought through prayer and meditation to improve our conscious contact with God as *we understand Him*, praying only for knowledge of His will for us and the power to carry that out;
12. Having had a spiritual awakening as the result of these steps, we tried to carry this message to alcoholics, and to practice these principles in all our affairs.

Note: The Twelve Steps are reprinted with permission of Alcoholics Anonymous World Services, Inc. ("AAWS"). Permission to reprint the Twelve Steps does not mean that AAWS has reviewed or approved the contents of this publication, or that AAWS necessarily agrees with the views expressed herein. A.A is a program of recovery from alcoholism *only*—use of the Twelve Steps in connection with programs and activities that are patterned after A.A, but that address other problems, or in any other non-A.A context, does not imply otherwise.

Table 60–13. Limitations of 12-step groups.

Alcoholics Anonymous (AA) does not solicit members; it will only reach out to people who ask for help.
AA does not keep records of membership (although some AA groups will provide phone lists for group members).
AA does not engage in research.
There is no formal control or follow-up on members by AA.
AA does not perform medical or psychiatric diagnoses. Each member needs to decide whether he or she is an addict.
AA as a whole does not provide housing, food, clothing, jobs, or money to newcomers (although individual members may do this).
AA is self-supporting through its own members' contributions; it does not accept money from outside sources.

Data from Alcoholics Anonymous. *A Brief Guide to Alcoholics Anonymous.* Akron, OH: Alcoholics Anonymous World Service Inc.; 1972.

required to believe in anything, including God. Agnostics and atheists are welcome in AA and are not asked to convert to any religious belief. Newcomers in AA are encouraged to attend meetings regularly (daily is wise initially), get a sponsor, and begin work on the 12 steps. A sponsor is usually someone of the same sex, who is in stable recovery and has successfully negotiated the steps. The sponsor helps guide the newcomer through the steps and provides a source of information and encouragement. At meetings, members share their experiences, relaying information about strategies for recovery. AA meetings vary in their composition and structure; consequently, if a patient feels uncomfortable at one meeting, another may be more acceptable. There are meetings for women or men only, those for young people, physicians, lawyers, and for virtually any special interest group in most large cities. There is often a great deal of confusion about what AA does and does not do. AA is not treatment. Despite the close connection that many treatment programs have with 12-step recovery fellowships, these fellowships are not affiliated with treatment centers by design. Table 60–13

lists some of the self-described limitations of AA and other 12-step groups.

From multiple sources, it appears clear that AA and other 12-step recovery programs are among the most effective tools to combat substance disorders. Approximately 6–10% of the population has been to an AA meeting during their lives, and this number doubles for those with alcohol problems. Although 50% of those who come to AA leave, of those who stay for a year, 67% remain sober; of those who stay for 2 years, 85% remain sober; and of those who stay sober for 5 years, 90% remain sober indefinitely. Outcome studies of 8087 patients treated in 57 different inpatient and outpatient treatment programs showed that those attending AA at 1-year follow-up were 50% more likely to be abstinent than those not attending. Adolescents studied were found to be 4 times more likely to be abstinent if they attended AA/NA when compared with those who did not. Finally, in an effort to identify which groups in AA did better than others, studies of involvement in AA (defined as service work, having a sponsor, leading meetings, etc) found that those who were involved maintained abstinence better than those who just attended meetings.

Having a list of AA members willing to escort potential new members to meetings is a powerful tool for physicians to help patients transition into recovery. Generally in every AA district, there is a person identified as the chair of the Cooperation with Professional Community Committee who can help physicians identify people willing to perform this service. Al-Anon and NA have similar contacts. These contacts can often supply physicians with relevant literature to help dispel some of the myths patients may hold regarding 12-step recovery. Patients often use these myths as excuses for why AA will not work for them, and understanding this as resistance and ambivalence about entering a life of recovery is important for the physician. Family physicians are in a unique position to encourage patients to invest in 12-step recovery. Recovering persons are keenly aware of this fact, and physicians are encouraged and welcomed at open AA and other 12-step meetings to become more familiar with the way they work.

G. Pharmacotherapeutic Treatment of Addiction

Agents useful in the treatment of withdrawal were discussed earlier (see section on detoxification). The agents discussed here are used to help prevent relapse into alcohol or other drug use. These drugs attempt to influence drug use by one of several mechanisms:

1. Sensitizing the body's response to result in a negative reaction to ingesting the drug, causing an aversion reaction such as with disulfiram and alcohol.

2. Reducing the reinforcing effects of a drug, such as the use of naltrexone in alcoholism.

3. Blocking the effects of a drug by binding to the receptor site, such as naltrexone for opiates.

4. Saturating the receptor sites by agonists, such as the use of methadone in opioid maintenance therapy.

5. Unique approaches, such as the creation of an immunization to cocaine.

Drug therapy for addiction holds promise. As our understanding of the neurobiology of addiction improves, so does the chance that we can intervene at a molecular level to prevent relapse. At the current level, however, pharmacotherapy to prevent relapse must be relegated to an adjunctive position. No drug alone has provided sufficient power to prevent relapse to addictive behavior. Still, in some patients, the use of appropriate medication may give them the edge necessary to move closer to recovery.

1. Pharmacotherapy for alcoholism—Disulfiram, naltrexone, possibly other opioid antagonists, selective serotonin reuptake inhibitors (SSRIs), and acamprosate are currently used in the prevention of relapse in alcoholism. Acamprosate appears to be the most promising of these medications. Although the goal of abstinence for patients addicted to alcohol cannot be met by medication alone at this time, in selected patients, it may improve their chances for stable recovery.

A. Disulfiram—Disulfiram inhibits aldehyde dehydrogenase, the enzyme that catalyzes the oxidation of acetaldehyde to acetic acid. Thus, if a patient taking disulfiram ingests alcohol, the acetaldehyde levels rise. The result is referred to as the *disulfiram-ethanol reaction*. This manifests as flushing of the skin, palpitations, decreased blood pressure, nausea, vomiting, shortness of breath, blurred vision, and confusion. The reactions are usually related to the dose of both disulfiram and alcohol. This reaction can be severe, and fatalities have been reported with doses of disulfiram of >500 mg and

2 oz of alcohol. Common side effects of disulfiram include drowsiness, lethargy, peripheral neuropathy, hepatotoxicity, and hypertension.

In the United States, doses of 250–500 mg are most commonly used. Because of individual variability in the disulfiram-ethanol reaction, often these doses do not produce a sufficient reaction to deter the patient from drinking. In the United Kingdom, it is common to perform an ethanol challenge test to determine the appropriate dose to produce an aversion effect. Whether disulfiram is actually effective in preventing relapse is the subject of some debate. Most studies have failed to show a statistically significant result. On closer examination, it appears that compliance with the medication is the most important factor. In a large Veterans Administration multicenter study, a direct relationship was found between compliance with drug therapy and abstinence. In addition, the involvement of a patient's spouse in observing the patient's consumption of disulfiram results in considerable improvement in outcome. It appears that disulfiram can be a useful adjunct for patients who have a history of sudden relapse and who have a social situation in which compliance may be adequately monitored. Because of its lack of effectiveness, potential adverse effects, and compliance issues, disulfiram is not recommended for use in the primary care setting.

B. Naltrexone—Naltrexone, an opioid antagonist, has been shown to reduce drinking in animal studies and in human alcoholics. It blocks euphoric and physiologic effects of opioid agonists without causing physical dependence or tolerance. Initial optimism over the potential of this discovery was tempered by several studies indicating that the effects of reducing drinking and preventing relapse diminished over time and overall failed to reduce relapse to heavy drinking. Still, the effect of naltrexone on alcohol craving is promising in that it suggests that the opioid system is involved in the craving for alcohol in alcoholism; this may open the door to the development of other opioid-active drugs that will have an impact on drinking. Studies are also showing promise with long-acting naltrexone in the form of injections or implantations as opposed to the oral route. The long-acting form has been found to be as safe and tolerable as the oral form with better patient compliance likely due to consistent blood levels of the drug.

C. Serotonergic drugs—Animal studies have consistently shown that SSRIs reduce alcohol intake in animal models. The data with respect to humans are less clear or consistent. It appears that the SSRIs reduce drinking in heavily drinking, nondepressed alcoholics, but probably only approximately 15–20% from pretreatment levels. When abstinence is the outcome studied, the results are not promising. However, the SSRIs may eventually find a place in concert with other anticraving medication. SSRIs appear to reduce drinking in a more robust fashion in alcoholics with comorbid depression.

D. Acamprosate (calcium acetylhomotaurinate)— Acamprosate has been shown to reduce craving for alcohol in alcoholics. While the overall mechanism of action is uncertain, it appears to affect both GABA and glutamine neurotransmission, both important in alcohol's effect in the brain. Unlike the effects of naltrexone, the effects of acamprosate on relapse appear to be greater and longer lasting. Twice as many alcoholics remained abstinent in a 12-month period while taking acamprosate compared with those who took placebo. The addition of disulfiram to the regimen appears to increase the effectiveness of acamprosate. Trials have also considered combining acamprosate with naltrexone, but the combination led to a higher rate of withdrawal from the trials because of adverse effects. Acamprosate alone has a very benign side effect profile and appears to be free of any effects on mood, concentration, attention, or psychomotor performance. Diarrhea is the only side effect that reached statistical significance in a review of 24 trials. Acamprosate has been used in Europe for >20 years and was approved by the US Food and Drug Administration (FDA) for use in the United States in 2004.

Overall evidence best supports the use of acamprosate and naltrexone along with counseling for the prevention of alcohol relapse. SSRIs are an option when a comorbid mood disorder is present.

Anton RF, O'Malley SS, Ciraulo DA, et al. Combined pharmacotherapies and behavioral interventions for alcohol dependence: the COMBINE study: a randomized controlled trial. *JAMA*. 2006;295:2003–2017. [PMID: 16670409]

Blondell RD. Ambulatory detoxification of patients with alcohol dependence. *Am Fam Physician*. 2005;71(3):495–502. [PMID: 15712624]

Cayley WE. Effectiveness of acamprosate in the treatment of alcohol dependence. *Am Fam Physician*. 2001;83(5):522–524. [PMID: 21391519]

Donaher P, Welsh C. Managing opioid addiction with buprenorphine. *Am Fam Physician*. 2006;73(9):1573–1578. [PMID: 16719249]

Kjome KA. Long-acting injectable naltrexone for the management of patients with opioid dependence. *Subst Abuse Res Treat*. 2011;5:1–9. [PMID: 22879745]

Willenbring M, Massey S, Gardner M. Helping patients who drink too much: an evidence-based guide for primary care physicians. *Am Fam Physician*. 2009;80(1):44–50. [PMID: 19621845]

Williams SH. Medications for treating alcohol dependence. *Am Fam Physician*. 2005;72(9):1775–1780. [PMID: 16300039]

2. Pharmacotherapy for cocaine addiction—The state of the art in the pharmacologic treatment of cocaine addiction makes it difficult to recommend any medication-based treatment with any confidence. Currently, only psychosocial interventions such as intensive outpatient therapy (IOT) and CBT have proven consistently efficacious in reducing stimulant use in patients with stimulant use disorder. Despite great interest and much activity devoted to finding an effective pharmacologic intervention for cocaine and other stimulant addiction, none has withstood the test of rigorous study. Heterocyclic antidepressants such as desipramine, SSRIs, monoamine oxidase inhibitors, dopamine agonists such as bromocriptine, neuroleptics, anticonvulsants, and calcium channel blockers have all been tried in cocaine addiction. Variable results, often positive in animal studies, have led to attempts to treat cocaine addicts with these drugs. As each potentially effective drug is studied more rigorously, however, little in the way of positive results is found. These drugs are used to try to ameliorate the craving for cocaine or to mediate the withdrawal symptoms of anhedonia and fatigue. An attempt to use stimulants such as methylphenidate or amphetamine for cocaine dependence in a way analogous to that of methadone maintenance for opiate addiction has produced disappointing results. One of the more interesting approaches to a pharmacologic answer to cocaine addiction has been the development of a "vaccine" for cocaine. In this approach, a cocaine-like hapten linked to a foreign protein produces antibodies that attach to cocaine molecules, preventing them from crossing the blood-brain barrier. Animal trials of the TA-CD vaccine have shown that it produces cocaine-specific antibodies and decreases self-administration of cocaine in rodents but has yet to be tested on humans.

3. Pharmacotherapy for opiate addiction—Agonist maintenance treatment with methadone has been the primary pharmacologic treatment for opioid treatment. The rationale for the use of methadone and its longer-acting relative, levo-α-acetylmethadol (LAAM), is to saturate the opiate receptors, thus blocking euphoria and preventing the abstinence syndrome. Methadone and LAAM treatment programs are highly regulated by the federal government; therefore, the average family physician would not be prescribing this drug but certainly might see patients who are on a maintenance program. Methadone programs and other similar programs with buprenorphine/naloxone are frequently referred to as "harm reduction programs" because the primary beneficiary of these programs is society. Reductions in crime and in the costs of active intravenous heroin abuse are clearly demonstrated as a result of these programs. The addict also benefits with a dramatic decrease in the risk of death due to addiction or contraction of HIV disease. There is social stabilization in the addict's life as well, especially when the maintenance program provides appropriate social services.

Antagonist maintenance with naltrexone was initially considered ideal, given its essentially complete blockade of opioid-reinforcing properties. Unfortunately, only 10–20% of patients remained in treatment when this approach was used. The most important use of naltrexone at this time appears to be in the management of healthcare professionals with opioid dependence. Compliance with a naltrexone regimen ensures abstinence and allows healthcare professionals to work in an environment where opioids may be accessible. Doses of 350 mg weekly divided into 3 days will provide complete protection from the effects of opioids.

Buprenorphine, a partial opioid agonist with K antagonist effects, is now being used as an alternative to methadone maintenance treatment. Dosing of this medication is problematic, with 65% of patients remaining abstinent at 16 mg/d compared with 28% abstinence at 4 mg/d. Suboxone, a combination of buprenorphine and naloxone, is another alternative that is effective for patients who do not require higher doses of methadone. Since naloxone has poor oral absorption but antagonizes opioid receptors when injected, its inclusion in suboxone make users less likely to crush and inject the drug (Donaher and Welsh 2006). Buprenorphine may decrease the use of cocaine in opioid-dependent patients. It also has less potential for diversion, making it an attractive alternative to methadone. The Drug Addiction Treatment Act of 2000 allows office-based maintenance treatment of opioid dependence by primary care physicians who have met the necessary requirements. This criterion includes licensure under state law, registration by the Drug Enforcement Administration, reasonable access and ability to refer patients to ancillary services if needed, and at least 8 hours of training in the management and treatment of opioid addiction from an approved association. The FDA approved the use of suboxone for treatment of opioid addiction in 2002. Treatment with suboxone has three phases, termed *induction*, *stabilization*, and *maintenance*. Therapy should start 12–24 hours after cessation of short-acting opioids or 24–48 hours after discontinuing use of long-acting opioids. Induction typically lasts 3–7 days. Day 1 consists of starting with a 4/1 mg (4 mg buprenorphine/1 mg naloxone) dose of suboxone, followed by a second dose 2 hours later if withdrawal symptoms persist. Over the next 6 days, this dose is titrated up to a maximum of 32/8 mg/d. Stabilization then begins and usually lasts 1–2 months. The goal of this stage of therapy is to find the minimal effective dose to decrease cravings, eliminate withdrawal, and minimize side effects of suboxone. Most patients require a daily dose between 12/3 mg and 24/6 mg to achieve these goals. Maintenance therapy is indefinite and focuses on monitoring for illicit drug use, minimizing cravings, and avoiding triggers to use.

As overdoses from opioids have increased, naloxone has become more readily available as an antidote for opioid overdose. It is currently carried by most first responders, and instruction in its use is included in Basic Life Support classes. As of March 2018, there were >115 deaths daily in the United States due to overdosing on opioids, including prescription pain medications, heroin, and synthetic opioids like fentanyl. About 25% of patients who are prescribed opioids for chronic pain misuse them, and about 10% of those patients develop an opioid use disorder, with about 5% of those transitioning to heroin. Naloxone is available in three formulations: injectable, autoinjectable, and nasal spray. It is available in many states without a prescription.

Blondell RD. Ambulatory detoxification of patients with alcohol dependence. *Am Fam Physician.* 2005;71(3):495–502. [PMID: 15712624]

Cayley WE. Effectiveness of acamprosate in the treatment of alcohol dependence. *Am Fam Physician.* 2001;83(5):522–524. [PMID: 21391519]

Donaher P, Welsh C. Managing opioid addiction with buprenorphine. *Am Fam Physician.* 2006;73(9):1573–1578. [PMID: 16719249]

Kampman K. Approach to treatment of stimulant use disorder in adults. In Hermann R, ed, UpToDate. March 2018. https://www.uptodate.com/contents/approach-to-treatment-of-stimulant-use-disorder-in-adults. Accessed December 4, 2019.

Litten RZ, Egli M, Heilig M, et al. Medications development to treat alcohol dependence: a vision for the next decade. *Addict Biol.* 2012;17(3):513–527. [PMID: 22458728]

Lobmaier PP, Kunoe N, Gossop M, Waal H. Naltrexone depot formulations for opioid and alcohol dependence: a systematic review. *CNS Neurosci Ther.* 2011;17(6):629–636. [PMID: 21554565]

Miotto K, Hillhouse M, Donovick R, et al. Comparison of buprenorphine treatment for opioid dependence in 3 settings. *J Addict Med.* 2012;6(1):68–76. [PMID: 22105061]

National Institute on Drug Abuse/National Institutes of Health. Opioid overdose reversal with naloxone. March 2018. https://www.drugabuse.gov/related-topics/opioid-overdose-reversal-naloxone-narcan-evzio. Accessed December 4, 2019.

Praveen KT, Law F, O'Shea J, Melichar J. Opioid dependence. *Am Fam Physician.* 2012;86(6):565–566. [PMID: 23062049]

Willenbring M, Massey S, Gardner M. Helping patients who drink too much: an evidence-based guide for primary care physicians. *Am Fam Physician.* 2009;80(1):44–50. [PMID: 19621845]

Williams SH. Medications for treating alcohol dependence. *Am Fam Physician.* 2005;72(9):1775–1780. [PMID: 16300039]

Websites

Alcoholics Anonymous (AA). www.aa.org

American Society of Addiction Medicine (ASAM). www.asam.org

Narcotics Anonymous (NA). www.na.org

National Institute on Alcohol Abuse and Alcoholism (NIAAA). niaaa.nih.gov

National Institute on Drug Abuse (NIDA). nida.nih.gov

Tobacco Cessation

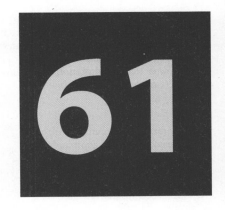

Martin C. Mahoney, MD, PhD, FAAFP

K. Michael Cummings, PhD, MPH

▶ Smoking Behavior & Disease Risk

Cigarette smoking, which is responsible for >480,000 deaths annually, represents the single most avoidable cause of premature death in the United States today. While the prevalence of smoking in the United States has declined since the early 1960s, as of 2016, >37 million adults are current smokers (15.5% prevalence among adults), ensuring that this behavior will continue to influence rates of premature morbidity and mortality for decades to come. Most people begin smoking during their teenage years and struggle to quit as adults. Clinicians need to view nicotine dependence as a chronic health condition with exacerbations and remissions.

There are benefits to quitting even among those who have already experienced health problems caused by smoking. Some of the benefits of smoking cessation occur shortly after quitting, while other smoking-related risks are not moderated for months or years. An individual's disease risk depends on previous duration and intensity of smoking, the presence of preexisting illnesses, and individual susceptibility. On a population-wide basis, it is now clear that progress achieved in extending life expectancy has been due in part to successful tobacco control, especially efforts to persuade and assist smokers to quit.

Cummings KM, Mahoney MC. Strategies for smoking cessation: what is new and what works? *Expert Rev Respir Med.* 2008; 2:201–213. [PMID: 20477249]

International Agency for Research on Cancer. *Tobacco Control: Reversal of Risk After Quitting Smoking.* Volume 11. Lyon, France: International Agency for Research on Cancer (IARC) Handbooks of Cancer Prevention; 2007.

Jamal A, Phillips E, Gentzke AS, et al. Current cigarette smoking among adults—United States, 2016. *MMWR Morb Mortal Wkly Rep.* 2018;67:53–59. [PMID: 29346338]

US Department of Health and Human Services. *The Health Consequences of Smoking: A Report of the Surgeon General.* Bethesda, MD: US Department of Health and Human Services, Centers for Disease Control and Prevention, National Center for Chronic Disease Prevention and Health Promotion, Office on Smoking and Health; 2004.

▶ Tobacco Dependence & Implications for Treatment

Most smokers report that they want to quit, and approximately 40–50% attempt to stop smoking annually. However, most quit attempts are unplanned, usually last only a few days or weeks, and are unsupported by the provision of pharmacotherapy and counseling support. Difficulty quitting is best predicted by how much one smokes on a daily basis and smoking within 30 minutes of waking up each day, both of which are measures of nicotine dependence.

Also, many smokers turn to methods with no proven efficacy to support sustained abstinence such as switching to so-called low-yield cigarettes, hypnotherapy, acupuncture, and various pharmacologic therapies (eg, selective serotonin reuptake inhibitors [SSRIs], tricyclic antidepressants [TCAs], anxiolytics, benzodiazepines, β-blockers, silver acetate, mecamylamine, appetite suppressants, caffeine, ephedrine, dextrose tablets, lobeline, moclobemide), further lowering quit success and contributing to a cycle of failed quit efforts, making the prospect of stopping smoking appear hopeless to many smokers.

The vast majority of current smokers (ie, 80–90%) are addicted to nicotine, which makes it difficult or impossible for some smokers to stop smoking cigarettes. Nicotine addiction is the fundamental reason why individuals persist in using tobacco products despite knowledge of the harms caused by tobacco use. Increasing evidence suggests that nicotine addiction is a hereditary characteristic. Those at higher genetic risk of smoking addiction were more likely to convert to daily smoking as teenagers, progress to heavy smoking as adults, and report failed quit attempts later in life. The reality is that smoking should be regarded as a chronic relapsing problem with exacerbations and remissions.

Baker TB, Piper ME, McCarthy DE, et al. Time to first cigarette in the morning as an index of ability to quit smoking: implications for nicotine dependence. *Nicot Tobac Res.* 2007;9(Suppl 4): 555–570. [PMID: 2933747]

Belsky DW, Moffitt TE, Baker TB, et al. Polygenic risk and the developmental progression to heavy, persistent smoking and nicotine dependence. *JAMA Psychiatr.* 2013;13:37–39. [PMID: 23536134]

National Cancer Institute. *Phenotypes and Endophenotypes: Foundations for Genetic Studies of Nicotine Use and Dependence.* Tobacco Control Monograph 20. Bethesda, MD: US Department of Health and Human Services, National Institutes of Health, National Cancer Institute. NIH Publication 09-6366; August 2009.

US Department of Health and Human Services. *How Tobacco Smoke Causes Disease: The Biology and Behavioral Basis for Smoking-Attributable Disease: A Report of the Surgeon General.* Atlanta, GA: US Department of Health and Human Services, Centers for Disease Control and Prevention, National Center for Chronic Disease Prevention and Health Promotion, Office on Smoking and Health; 2010. [PMID: 21452462]

▶ Use of Brief Interventions to Promote Smoking Cessation

Smoking cessation treatment often begins with a brief intervention, in which a physician or any other healthcare provider advises smokers to quit and may recommend methods for quitting. For many smokers, the only contact with the healthcare system may be through their family physician, and office visits often provide the impetus for smokers to attempt to stop smoking.

Meta-analyses report that brief counseling interventions have significant potential to reduce smoking rates, with even minimal brief interventions conferring an estimated 30% increased likelihood of cessation.

A Cochrane review evaluating the effectiveness of brief smoking cessation advice from a physician found that advice from a physician compared with no advice (or usual care) significantly increased the odds of being smoke free after 6 months and yielded an absolute improvement of 1–3% in the rate of smoking cessation.

The Public Health Service (PHS) guidelines for treating tobacco use and dependence, last updated in 2008, continue to recommend that healthcare workers screen all patients for tobacco use and provide advice and follow-up behavioral treatments to all tobacco users. Current users are advised to quit; those who are willing to make a quit attempt are given appropriate assistance, along with arrangements for a follow-up visit. In addition, those who are identified as former smokers are given advice to prevent relapse, and persons who have never used tobacco are encouraged to remain tobacco free.

Controlled studies have found that physician involvement, especially more extensive interventions, increases quit rates. This approach has also been found to be cost-effective since tobacco cessation interventions cost approximately $2500 per year of life saved, whereas mammography screening costs approximately $50,000 per year of life saved.

According to a comprehensive review of the efficacy of different smoking cessation treatments, the PHS has recommended that all smokers receive counseling and support to quit, preferably in combination with approved pharmacotherapy. Despite this treatment guideline, population-based surveys reveal that most tobacco users today are still not routinely receiving treatment assistance from their healthcare provider during visits. For example, a survey reported that tobacco counseling occurred in <25% of office visits by tobacco users, and cessation medications were prescribed on <3% of occasions. Studies have documented that utilization of evidence-based stop smoking treatments is lowest among those who are uninsured and have the greatest need for assistance in quitting tobacco (ie, those with mental health and other substance abuse problems). Encouraging smoking cessation is now recognized as a required part of good clinical practice.

The guideline continues to emphasize use of the "**5 As**" in clinical settings: **ask** about tobacco use, **advise** to quit, **assess** willingness to make a quit attempt, **assist** in quit attempt, and **arrange** for follow-up. The American Academy of Family Physicians has attempted to simplify this to "**2 As**": **ask** about tobacco use and **act** to advise smoker to quit, as well as assessing interest in quitting, assisting in organizing pharmacotherapy, and arranging for follow-up. These systematic approaches to tobacco dependence require <3 minutes to deliver with the potential to result in behavior change. Other key points from the 2008 PHS clinical guideline include the following:

- The need for all healthcare delivery systems to systematically identify and document tobacco use status and to offer treatment to every tobacco user.

- The importance of providing pharmacotherapy to all patients making a quit attempt.

- Counseling support is effective in a variety of settings (eg, individual, group, or via telephone), and effectiveness increases with treatment intensity. Counseling should address both practical issues (problem solving/skills training) and social support.

- While counseling and pharmacotherapy are each effective when used by themselves, the combination is more effective than either alone for treating tobacco dependence.

- Use of telephone quit lines should be promoted since counseling is effective with diverse populations and offers broad geographic reach.

Physician advice to stop smoking increases the likelihood that patients will try to quit and enhances the odds that those who do quit will remain off cigarettes. Long-term cessation rates approach 20% with counseling and increase to 30% when counseling is combined with pharmacotherapy.

Fiore MC, Jaén CR, Baker TB, et al. *Treating Tobacco Use and Dependence: 2008 Update.* Clinical Practice Guideline, US Department of Health and Human Services, Public Health Service; May 2008. https://www.ahrq.gov/professionals/clinicians-providers/guidelines-recommendations/tobacco/index.html. Accessed September 10, 2018.

Piper ME, McCarthy DE, Baker TB. Assessing tobacco dependence: a guide to measure evaluation and selection. *Nicot Tobac Res.* 2006;8:339–351. [PMID: 16801292]

Stead LF, Buitrago D, Preciado N, et al. Physician advice for smoking cessation. *Cochrane Database Syst Rev.* 2013;5:CD000165. [PMID: 23728631]

▶ Pharmacotherapy

Tobacco users have a physical dependence on nicotine, in addition to various reinforced psychological and social behaviors. The two-item Heaviness of Smoking Index (HSI) represents a reliable and valid way to assess the strength of someone's nicotine dependence. Those who use tobacco more frequently every day and find a need to use tobacco first thing when they wake up in the morning are scored as more dependent. Table 61–1 shows a strategy for identifying smokers and determining readiness to quit as well as actions to be completed at that visit.

The use of pharmacotherapy doubles the effect of any tobacco cessation intervention. A recent Cochrane review has validated the importance of providing counseling support, in addition to pharmacotherapy, among smokers attempting to quit. Studies with four or more sessions showed the greatest impact; counseling can be delivered either in person or by telephone.

The US PHS guideline on management of tobacco dependence recommends varenicline, sustained-release bupropion, and all forms of nicotine replacement (eg, resin or gum,

Table 61–1. Simplified model for addressing tobacco use and dependence: ask and act.

Ask:
Do you smoke?
How much do you want to quit? (1–10 scale)
How confident are you in your ability to quit? (1–10 scale)
Act:
Have you set a quit date?
Provide quit advice or referral
Provide pharmacotherapy prescription
Arrange for follow-up

Data from American Academy of Family Physicians. Ask and act. https://www.aafp.org/patient-care/public-health/tobacco-nicotine/ask-act.html.

inhaler, nasal spray, lozenges, and patch) as first-line agents. Patients should be queried about experiences with prior use of cessation medications and asked if they are interested in a particular agent. Clinicians are encouraged to apply appropriate clinical judgment when assessing contraindications to the use of a particular agent. The use of pharmacotherapy to support smoking cessation is summarized in Table 61–2.

A. Nicotine Replacement Therapy

Nicotine patches, lozenges, and resin (gum) are available over the counter (OTC), whereas nicotine nasal sprays and the nicotine inhaler systems both require prescriptions. Reduced-dose regimens of nicotine replacement therapy (NRT) might be considered for patients consuming <10 cigarettes daily or those weighing <100 lb (~45 kg). Using two forms of nicotine replacement (eg, patch plus resin or lozenges) results in higher quit rates and should be recommended if other forms of nicotine replacement have not been effective alone. Quit rates with use of NRT range between 20% and 24%; use of NRT is recommended for a minimum of 6–8 weeks; however, some patients elect to continue nicotine-containing therapy for the long term.

Nicotine medications appear to be safe for most people. Side effects of NRT mainly include local irritation (ie, mouth sores, skin rash, nasal and throat irritation) associated with the route of administration of the medication. Side effects are typically mild and transient. Studies show that only approximately 1 in 12 person reports discontinuing use of NRT because of side effects.

Nicotine-containing products are not associated with the occurrence of acute cardiac events. This finding is consistent with the observation that NRT is rarely able to achieve blood levels of nicotine associated with smoking. Nonetheless, NRT should be approached cautiously among patients who are within 2 weeks of an acute myocardial infarction, are known to have significant arrhythmias, and have significant or worsening symptoms of angina.

B. Bupropion (Zyban)

Sustained-release bupropion is started at a dose of 150 mg daily for 3 days before increasing to 150 mg twice daily on day 4. Treatment with bupropion begins 1–2 weeks before the anticipated quit date; its use is contraindicated among patients with a history of seizure disorders, current substance abuse, or other conditions that may lower the seizure threshold. The standard treatment course of bupropion (Zyban) in 8 weeks yields quit rates of approximately 30%.

C. Varenicline (Chantix)

This agent binds to $\alpha_4\beta_2$-nicotinic receptors in the central nervous system (CNS) to moderate symptoms of nicotine withdrawal, leading to reduced craving, decreased smoking

Table 61–2. Use of first-line adjunctive pharmacotherapy in smoking cessation.

Stop Smoking Medication	Contraindications	Side Effects	Rx Given (Dose/Frequency/Number)	Other Instructions Given
Nicotine patch (7, 14, or 21 mg/24 h for 4 weeks, then taper 2 weeks and 2 weeks)	Concurrent smoking	Local skin reaction Insomnia	7-, 14-, or 21-mg patch every 24 hours for 4 weeks, then taper every 2 weeks	Dosing, side effects reviewed Behavioral coaching/counseling and/or quitline referral Set quit date: _____ F/U appt: _____
Nicotine gum (1–24 cigs/day—2 mg gum or 25+ cigs/day—4 mg gum; max 24 pieces/day for up to 12 weeks)	Concurrent smoking	Mouth soreness Dyspepsia	2 mg or 4 mg gum Max 24 pieces/day for up to 12 weeks	Dosing, side effects reviewed Behavioral coaching/counseling and/or quitline referral Set quit date: _____ F/U appt: _____
Nicotine nasal spray (8–40 doses/day for 3–6 months)	Concurrent smoking	Nasal irritation	_____ doses/day for 3–6 months	Dosing, side effects reviewed Behavioral coaching/counseling and/or quitline referral Set quit date: _____ F/U appt: _____
Nicotine inhaler (6–16 cartridges/day for up to 6 months)	Concurrent smoking	Local irritation of mouth and throat	_____ cartridges/day for _____ months	Dosing, side effects reviewed Behavioral coaching/counseling and/or quitline referral Set quit date: _____ F/U appt: _____
Nicotine lozenges (if first cig smoked within 30 minutes of arising—4-mg lozenge; if first cig after 30 minutes of aris-ing—2-mg lozenge; max 5 loz/6 h or 20 loz/day for up to 12 weeks)	Concurrent smoking Contains phenylalanine	Mouth soreness Dyspepsia	2-mg or 4-mg lozenge Maximum 20 loz/day for up to 12 weeks	Dosing, side effects reviewed Behavioral coaching/counseling and/or quitline referral Set quit date: _____ F/U appt: _____
Zyban/bupropion SR	History of seizures History of eating disorder Currently treated for depression Used MAO inhibitor within past 14 days	Local skin reaction Insomnia	150 mg orally every day for 3 days, then 150 mg twice a day	Dosing, side effects reviewed Quit on day #8 Behavioral coaching/counseling and/or quitline referral Set quit date: _____ F/U appt: _____
Chantix/varenidine	Prior serious reaction	Nausea Insomnia, abnormal dreams GI symptoms	0.5 mg orally for 3 days, then 0.5 mg twice daily for 4 days, then 1.0 mg twice daily for 12 weeks or 24 weeks	Dosing, side effects reviewed Counsel on quit approach: "fixed," "flexible," or "gradual" and quit date Behavioral coaching/counseling Set quit date: _____ F/U appt: _____

appt, appointment; cig, cigarette; F/U, follow-up; GI, gastrointestinal; MAO, monoamine oxidase; Rx, prescription.

satisfaction, and diminished psychological reward. Varenicline (Chantix) is started 1 week prior to the identified quit date, titrating up from a dose of 0.5 mg daily for 3 days, to 0.5 mg twice daily for days 4–7, then to 1 mg twice daily beginning on day 8. Rates of continuous abstinence are 44%. A full treatment course of 12 weeks is recommended, and those who are abstinent at 12 weeks may continue with another 12 weeks of treatment. The most commonly encountered side effects are nausea, insomnia, and abnormal dreams; these are generally rated as mild and often resolve within several days or may be managed with a dose reduction as needed. Varenicline is minimally metabolized and is essentially excreted in the urine. There are no known drug interactions. Dose modification is necessary only with severe renal disease.

There are three approaches to using varenicline to help smokers to quit: with the "fixed" approach, smokers quit on day 8 of treatment; with the "flexible" quit approach, smokers select a quit date between day 8 and 35 of treatment; and with the "gradual" quit approach, a smoker reduces the amount smoked by 50% over each 4-week interval with the goal of achieving cessation by week 12 of treatment. The fixed and flexible quit approaches have a minimum 12-week course of treatment with an option to extend therapy for up to 24 weeks, whereas the gradual quit approach recommends a 24-week course of therapy.

A large placebo-controlled clinical trial of varenicline, bupropion, and NRT enrolled 8000 smokers, of whom about one-half had a history of a stable mental health condition, and was designed to examine both safety and efficacy end points. Rates of neuropsychiatric symptoms did not vary by therapy but were numerically increased among smokers with a history of a stable mental health condition. The highest rates of smoking cessation were observed among those treated with varenicline in both groups (with and without a history of a mental health condition) and were higher among those without a history of a mental health condition. Side effects were comparable to those noted in earlier studies. Clinicians should remember to support patient quit attempts by placing a follow-up call within 1–2 weeks of the quit date. Instruct patients to contact your office if they experience unusual thoughts or behaviors. Remind patients that irritability, mood swings, and drowsiness can result from nicotine withdrawal. These symptoms are most common immediately after a person stops smoking and typically lessen with time. In addition, patients should be counseled to use caution when driving, operating machinery, or using alcohol until they know how quitting smoking with varenicline may affect them.

Clinical experience with use of the pharmacotherapies for smoking cessation among pregnant women and adolescents is generally limited. Clinical judgment is advised regarding a comprehensive assessment of the risks and benefits associated with use of adjunctive pharmacotherapy in each of these settings.

On the basis of the observation that the number of past quit attempts is predictive of future quit attempts, clinicians should encourage smokers to continue to try to quit smoking. However, studies show that while motivation to quit is important in predicting whether someone makes a quit attempt, it does not necessarily predict ability to remain smoke free, which is more likely to be related to the strength of someone's nicotine dependence. Clinicians play a pivotal role in not only motivating patients to make a quit attempt, but also in offering evidence-based treatments to help them cope with craving and withdrawal symptoms that are the result of their nicotine addiction. Motivational interviewing can be used to enhance both level of motivation and the patient's self-efficacy to cope with the uneasy feelings that typically accompany smoking abstinence.

Electronic nicotine delivery systems (ENDS) are battery-powered devices that deliver nicotine in an aerosol to the user. Electronic cigarettes initially emerged in China in 2003 and since have become widely available in devices used to consume combusted tobacco. ENDS heat and vaporize a solution, often flavored, containing nicotine, and many are designed to outwardly resemble traditional tobacco cigarettes and have been touted by some as a smoking cessation aid for addicted smokers. At this time, the evidence supporting the efficacy of e-cigarettes as a cessation treatment for nicotine addiction is limited, although clearly smoking e-cigarettes appears to be less risky than smoking conventional cigarettes.

Anthenelli RM, Benowitz NL, West R, et al. Neuropsychiatric safety and efficacy of varenicline, bupropion, and nicotine patch in smokers with and without psychiatric disorders (EAGLES): a double-blind, randomised, placebo-controlled clinical trial. *Lancet.* 2016;387:2507–2520. [PMID: 27116918]

Borland R, Yong HH, O'Connor RJ, Hyland A, Thompson ME. The reliability and predictive validity of the Heaviness of Smoking Index and its two components: findings from the International Tobacco Control Four Country study. *Nicot Tobac Res.* 2010;12(Suppl):S45–S50. [PMID: 3307335]

Cobb NK, Abrams DB. E-cigarette or drug-delivery device? Regulating novel nicotine products. *N Engl J Med.* 2011;365(3): 193–195. [PMID: 21774706]

Ebbert JO, Hughes JR, West RJ, Rennard SI, et al. Effect of varenicline on smoking cessation through smoking reduction: a randomized clinical trial. *JAMA.* 2015;313(7):687–694. [PMID: 25688780]

Goniewicz ML, Knysak J, Gawron M, et al. Levels of selected carcinogens and toxicants in vapour from electronic cigarettes. *Tob Control.* 2014;23(2):133–139. [PMID: 23467656]

Gonzales D, Rennard SI, Nides M, et al. Varenicline, an alpha4beta2 nicotinic acetylcholine receptor partial agonist, vs sustained-release bupropion and placebo for smoking cessation: a randomized controlled trial. *JAMA.* 2006;296:47–55. [PMID: 16820546]

Heatherton TF, Kozlowski LT, Frecker RC, Rickert W, Robinson J. Measuring the heaviness of smoking: using self-reported time to the first cigarette of the day and number of cigarettes smoked per day. *Addiction.* 1989;84:791–800. [PMID: 2758152]

Henningfield JE, Fant RV, Buchhalter AR, Stitzer ML. Pharmacotherapy for nicotine dependence. *CA Cancer J Clin.* 2005; 55:281–299. [PMID: 16166074]

Jorenby DE, Leischow SJ, Nides MA, et al. A controlled trial of sustained-release bupropion, a nicotine patch, or both for smoking cessation. *N Engl J Med.* 1999;340:685–691. [PMID: 10053177]

Mallin R. Smoking cessation: integration of behavioral and drug therapies. *Am Fam Physician.* 2002;65:1107–1114. [PMID: 11925087]

Polosa R, Caponnetto P, Morjaria JB, Papale G, Campagna D, Russo C. Effect of an electronic nicotine delivery device (e-cigarette) on smoking reduction and cessation: a prospective 6-month pilot study. *BMC Public Health.* 2011;11:786. [PMC: 3203079]

Rennard S, Hughes J, Cinciripini PM, et al. A randomized placebo-controlled trial of varenicline for smoking cessation allowing flexible quit dates. *Nicotine Tob Res.* 2012;14(3):343–350. [PMID: 22080588]

Siegel MB, Tanwar KL, Wood KS. Electronic cigarettes as a smoking cessation tool: results from an online survey. *Am J Prev Med.* 2011;40(4):472–475. [PMID: 21406283]

Stead L, Lancaster T. Behavioural interventions as adjuncts to pharmacotherapy for smoking cessation. *Cochrane Database Syst Rev.* 2012;12:CD009670. [PMID: 23235680]

Tonstad S, Tønnesen P, Hajek P, et al. Effect of maintenance therapy with varenicline on smoking cessation: a randomized controlled trial. *JAMA.* 2006;296:64–71. [PMID: 16820548]

Payments for Cessation Services

Since 2005, the Centers for Medicare and Medicaid Services has provided reimbursement for smoking cessation counseling by clinicians as a preventive service provided that the patient is a Medicare beneficiary and has a disease or adverse health effect that is either caused or affected by tobacco use. Payment as a preventive service is based on two Healthcare Common Procedural Coding System (HCPCS) codes:

- G0375: Smoking and tobacco use cessation counseling visit; intermediate, >3 minutes and ≤10 minutes.

- G0376: Smoking and tobacco use cessation counseling visit; intensive, >10 minutes.

Reimbursement for tobacco cessation counseling is also available as a standard Part B Medicare benefit as Common Procedural Terminology (CPT) codes 99406 (intermediate, 3–10 minutes) and 99407 (intensive, >10 minutes), although the patient is responsible for both copayments and unmet deductible; payment varies by region. Additional payment may be received according to the evaluation and management service (99201–99215, including modifier –25) provided on that same day and separately identifiable from the smoking cessation counseling. Counseling that lasts <3 minutes is included in the standard physician visit and is not reported separately. Medicare beneficiaries are eligible for up to four counseling sessions for each quit attempt, and up to two quit attempts are covered over a 12-month interval. Resources to promote smoking cessation services within a medical office setting are available at https://www.aafp.org/patient-care/public-health/tobacco-nicotine/ask-act.html (accessed September 8, 2018).

Private health insurance plans are variable in their policies regarding reimbursement for smoking cessation counseling services. Alternative HCPCS codes include S9075 for smoking cessation treatment and S9453 for smoking cessation classes. The patient's health record should document all services provided. Medicare Part D has covered cessation US Food and Drug Administration (FDA)–approved drug therapies for eligible beneficiaries since 2006 as part of the prescription drug benefit, although OTC formulations of NRTs are sometimes excluded.

Pohlig C. Smoking cessation counseling: a practice management perspective. *Chest.* 2006;130:1231–1233. [PMID: 17035460]

Theobald M, Jaén CR. An update on tobacco cessation reimbursement. *Fam Practice Manage.* 2006;13:75–78. [PMID: 16736908]

Patients at the Precontemplation Stage of Quitting

For patients who are currently unwilling to make a quit attempt, clinicians should present a brief motivation intervention structured around the "5 Rs":

1. *Relevance*—make tobacco cessation personally relevant (personal medical history, family composition).

2. *Risk*—review the negative effects of quitting (include both immediate- and long-term risks).

3. *Rewards*—identify the benefits of quitting (improved sense of taste and smell, personal sense of accomplishment, money saved, and health benefits).

4. *Roadblocks*—identify perceived barriers to quitting and ways of overcoming these impediments (symptoms of withdrawal, weight gain, lack of social supports).

5. *Repetition*—repeat this intervention at all office visits.

Relapse

Although risk of relapse is greatest immediately following the quit attempt, it can occur months or even years following cessation. Because tobacco use status will be systematically determined for all patients at each visit, physicians should encourage all former tobacco users to remain abstinent and to express specific concerns or difficulties. Approaches can include reassurance, motivational counseling, extended pharmacotherapy, recommendations for exercise, or referral to supportive or behavioral therapy.

Future Approaches to Cessation

As a potent CNS modulator, nicotine stimulates various physiologic and behavioral effects through the release of various neurotransmitters. To date, therapeutic approaches to smoking cessation have tended to focus on nicotinic acetyl-choline receptors, which modulate the release of dopamine and other signaling substances, via use of nicotine replacement therapy or varenicline. In contrast, the mechanism of action for bupropion is poorly understood.

At the present time, no new FDA-approved therapies are anticipated to become available for the next several years. Initial studies examining the use of a nicotine vaccine did not yield anticipated results, although research continues using next-generation products. Cannabinoid receptor agonist agents as a potential cessation therapy have been abandoned because of unacceptable side effects. Additional potential candidate products for cessation therapy are focusing on central nervous neurotransmitter systems involving the actions of glutamate and γ-aminobutyric acid (GABA), as well as antagonists for selective glycine receptors, and N-methyl-D-aspartate (NMDA) receptors.

Additional research is examining treatment matching based on smoker genotype and phenotype information, combination therapy, and modified administration schedules in an effort to enhance the efficacy of currently available pharmacotherapies.

Henningfield JE, Fant RV, Buchhalter AR, Stitzer ML. Pharmacotherapy for nicotine dependence. *CA Cancer J Clin.* 2005; 55:281–299. [PMID: 16166074]

Pentel PR, LeSage MG. New directions in nicotine vaccine design and use. *Adv Pharmacol.* 2014;69:553–580. [PMID: 24484987]

Pidoplichko VI, DeBiasi M, Williams JT, Dani JA. Nicotine activates and desensitizes midbrain dopamine neurons. *Nature.* 1997;390:401–404. [PMID: 9389479]

▶ Summary

Nicotine dependence should be considered a chronic health condition with exacerbations and remissions. Identification of smokers and provision of pharmacotherapy to support a quit attempt can increase quit rates by 1.5- to 3-fold compared to placebo. NRT is favored based on cost and accessibility, whereas varenicline is favored based on efficacy; smokers benefit from linkage to counseling/coaching in addition to pharmacotherapy.

Each clinical encounter should include *asking* about tobacco use and *acting* to provide office-based or off-site counseling, as well as arranging linkages to quit lines, print and Internet-based educational materials, community-based cessation classes, and access to pharmacotherapy.

Smoking cessation treatments delivered by clinicians, whether physicians or nonphysicians (eg, psychologist, nurse, dentist, or counselor), can increase abstinence. Therefore, all members of the healthcare system should be empowered to provide smoking cessation interventions. Finally, it is important to emphasize that the combination of pharmacotherapy and behavioral counseling/coaching for each smoker will help to maximize the likelihood of achieving long-term abstinence.

Interpersonal Violence

Amy Crawford-Faucher, MD, FAAFP

▶ General Considerations

Family physicians must maintain a high index of suspicion for interpersonal violence in their patients. Despite growing public awareness, community advocacy, and education about this endemic public health problem, victims of interpersonal violence may be difficult to detect in the healthcare setting. Shame, fear, self-blame, and other cultural and social factors may limit the manner and nature of presentation and disclosure to the physician. Despite these challenges, the family physician is in a unique position to make a meaningful impact and potentially intervene before violence escalates.

Interpersonal violence includes the following:

- Emotional/psychological abuse
- Financial abuse
- Neglect (of dependent person)
- Physical violence
- Sexual violence
- Stalking, bullying, or cyberbullying/electronic aggression
- Homicide

Those at greatest risk for violence are children, the elderly, pregnant women, persons who are physically or mentally challenged, immigrants, and members of racial, cultural, or sexual minorities.

▶ Definitions

Emotional/psychological abuse includes humiliation, controlling behavior, repeated verbal assaults (name-calling), isolation (rejection, withholding attention and affection), threats, and public harassment, all of which can produce psychological trauma that reduces a person's self-worth perception, value, and sense of efficacy. Emotional/psychological violence often coexists with chronic physical or sexual violence but can also stand alone.

Financial abuse is when a person withholds resources such as money or transportation or limits freedom of movement or association (eg, domination, isolation) of another person—a tactic often found in abusive relationships. Financial abuse most often involves the inappropriate transfer or use of an elder's funds for the caregiver's purposes.

Neglect is the chronic failure of a person who is responsible for the physical and emotional needs of another person to provide for those needs. This form of abuse most often occurs in family relationships and is directed at children, elders, or disabled family members. However, caregivers in other social/community settings, including child and adult daycare, schools, group homes, nursing facilities, and hospitals, may be involved in neglect of a dependent person.

Physical violence, as defined by the Centers for Disease Control and Prevention (CDC), is the "intentional use of physical force with the potential for causing death, disability, injury, or harm." This includes, but is not limited to, scratching, pushing, shoving, throwing, grabbing, biting, choking, shaking, slapping, punching, or burning; or use of a weapon or use of restraints or one's body, size, or strength against another person. In the most extreme cases, physical violence may involve *homicide*.

Sexual violence, according to the CDC, is defined as "any sexual act that is perpetrated against someone's will." Sexual violence may include a completed nonconsensual sex act (ie, rape), an attempted nonconsensual sex act, abusive sexual contact (ie, unwanted touching), and noncontact sexual abuse (eg, threatened sexual violence, exhibitionism, verbal sexual harassment). It includes the following four types:

- "A *completed sex act* is defined as contact between the penis and the vulva or the penis and the anus involving penetration, however slight; contact between the mouth and penis, vulva, or anus; or penetration of the anal or genital opening of another person by a hand, finger, or other object."
- "*An attempted (but not completed) sex act.*"

- "*Abusive sexual contact* is defined as intentional touching, either directly or through the clothing, of the genitalia, anus, groin, breast, inner thigh, or buttocks of any person without his or her consent, or of a person who is unable to consent or refuse."

- "*Noncontact sexual abuse* does not include physical contact of a sexual nature between the perpetrator and the victim. It includes acts such as voyeurism; intentional exposure of an individual to exhibitionism; unwanted exposure to pornography; verbal or behavioral sexual harassment; threats of sexual violence to accomplish some other end; or taking nude photographs of a sexual nature of another person without his or her consent or knowledge, or of a person who is unable to consent or refuse."

Stalking, bullying, or *cyberbullying/electronic aggression* may involve harassment, threats, or physical violence and can lead to emotional or physical injury or death. The CDC defines *stalking* as repeatedly following a person; appearing at a person's home or place of business; making harassing phone calls or leaving objects or written, text, or internet messages; or vandalizing a person's property. *Bullying* can include spreading rumors, teasing, imposed social isolation, and influencing others to "gang up" on someone. These acts can occur in person or through increasingly frequent forms such as cyberbullying or electronic aggression—using cell phones, computers, and other electronic devices or the Internet. Cyberbullying can occur through email, texts, chat rooms, instant messaging, websites, videos, or photos.

Centers for Disease Control and Prevention. Preventing intimate partner violence. http://www.cdc.gov/ViolencePrevention/intimatepartnerviolence/definitions.html. Accessed December 3, 2019.

▶ Epidemiology

The prevalence of abuse and neglect vary with different populations. In general, young children and pregnant women are at highest risk of death from abuse. Child maltreatment is also more prevalent among racial/ethnic minority children whose families experience the highest levels of poverty.

A. Children

In the United States in 2017, there were >674,000 reported child victims of abuse and neglect. This likely significantly underestimates the true prevalence of child maltreatment. Of these reported cases:

- 74.9% of victims suffered neglect
- 18.3% suffered physical abuse
- 8.6% suffered sexual abuse
- 5.7% suffered psychological maltreatment

Childhood victimization is often a precursor to adult victimization—43% of female rapes and 51% of male rapes occur at or before age 18. In 2017, approximately 1720 children died as a result of abuse or neglect; 72% of the deaths occurred in children age <3 years. The victimization and mortality rates are highest for children age <1 year. Girls are maltreated at a slightly higher rate than are boys (9.5 vs 8.6 per 1000), but maltreatment-related deaths are higher for boys than girls (2.7 vs 2.0 per 100,000). Native American and Alaska Native children experience the highest rates of maltreatment and related death, followed by African Americans. Sadly, the vast majority of perpetrators of child abuse are parents (80.1%).

Bullying is a major public health problem among school-age children. Of a nationally representative sample, 13% of children reported being a bully, 11% reported being a victim of bullying, and 6% reported being both a bully and a victim. Boys are more likely to participate in physical aggression, whereas girls are more likely to engage in verbal aggression. In 2017, 14.9% of high school students reported being electronically bullied in the previous 12 months. Adolescents who bully are more likely to have other defiant or delinquent behaviors, whereas victims are more likely to have depression, anxiety, and isolation. Bullying is now a major risk factor for suicide among adolescents, with higher rates of bullying-related suicides among girls and youths who are both bully and victim of bullying. The emotional and behavioral problems associated with bullies and victims can continue into adulthood with long-term negative consequences.

B. Adults

Intimate partner violence is pervasive in the United States, where approximately 24 people per minute are victimized. This amounts to about 12 million women and men. Women are at increased risk of violent victimization by an intimate partner (or stranger). A 2015 CDC survey found the following:

- 1.5 million women were raped in the previous year.
- The lifetime risk for rape is about 1 in 5 women and 1 in 71 men.
- Severe physical assault by an intimate partner occurs in 1 in 4 women and 1 in 7 men.
- 1 in 6 women and 1 in 17 men are victims of stalking.

Stemming from these experiences are a host of co-occurring physical and mental health problems such as headaches, chronic pain, sleep difficulties, fear, and other symptoms related to posttraumatic stress disorder (eg, anxiety, flashbacks and nightmares, exaggerated startle response).

C. The Elderly

Elder abuse, like other forms of interpersonal violence, most often occurs in the context of the family. The primary perpetrators are spouses or companions or adult children or other family members who inflict physical, emotional/psychological, sexual, or financial abuse and neglect. Although the most recent estimate of elder abuse found that 14.1% of older adults in the general population experienced these forms of interpersonal violence, the US Government Accountability Office suggests that existing research underestimates the true prevalence of elder abuse. The National Center on Elder Abuse reports that older women are more likely than younger women to experience a longer period of violent victimization, to currently be in violent relationships, and to experience related health and mental health problems.

D. Persons with Disabilities

People with disabilities, including those with cognitive, hearing, vision, ambulatory, self-care, and independent-living deficits, are at higher risk for all types of abuse than are those without disabilities. At 48 per 1000, the rate of violence against those with disabilities is more than twice the rate for those who do not have disabilities (19 per 1000). Additionally, the rate of victimization increases for those with multiple disabilities. For 2015, the average age-adjusted (for 12 years to adult) rate of violent crime against those with a single disability type was 32 per 1000. Cognitively disabled individuals are at the highest risk for victimization compared to all other disabilities.

E. Lesbian, Gay, Bisexual, and Transgender Community

Historically, the national prevalence of intimate partner violence against lesbian, gay, and bisexual men and women has not been well studied; the National Intimate Partner and Sexual Violence Survey (NISVS) started reporting data from 2010 and is ongoing. NISVS found the following:

- Bisexual women have a significantly higher lifetime prevalence of rape and nonrape sexual violence by any perpetrator than do lesbian or heterosexual women.
  - Rape: 13.1% of lesbian women, 46.1% of bisexual women, 17.4% of heterosexual women
  - Other sexual violence: 46.4% of lesbian women, 74.9% of bisexual women, 43.3% of heterosexual women
- Bisexual women have a significantly higher lifetime prevalence of rape, physical violence, or stalking by an intimate partner compared to lesbian or heterosexual women.
- Although the prevalence of rape in men could not be estimated from the survey, the prevalence of nonrape sexual violence was higher for gay men (40.2%) and bisexual men (47.4%) compared to that for heterosexual men (20.8%).

Black MC, Basile KC, Breiding MJ, et al. *The National Intimate Partner and Sexual Violence Survey (NISVS): 2010 Summary Report.* Atlanta, GA: National Center for Injury Prevention and Control, Centers for Disease Control and Prevention; 2011.

Cooper GD, Clements PT, Holt KE. Examining childhood bullying and adolescent suicide: implications for school nurses. *J School Nurs.* 2012;28(4):275–283. [PMID: 22333524]

Hamburger ME, Basile KC, Vivolo AM. *Measuring Bullying Victimization, Perpetration, and Bystander Experiences: A Compendium of assessment Tools.* Atlanta, GA: Centers for Disease Control and Prevention, National Center for Injury Prevention and Control; 2011.

Harrell E. *Crime Against Persons with Disabilities, 2009-2015– Statistical Tables; July 2017, NCJ 250632.* Washington, DC: US Department of Justice Office of Justice Programs Bureau of Justice Statistics; 2017.

Kann L, McManus T, Harris WA, et al. Youth risk behavior surveillance—United States, 2017. *MMWR Surveill Summ.* 2018;67(No. SS-8):1–114. [PMID: 29902162]

US Department of Health and Human Services, Administration for Children and Families, Administration on Children, Youth and Families, Children's Bureau. Child Maltreatment 2017. https://www.acf.hhs.gov/cb/research-data-technology/statistics-research/child-maltreatment. Accessed December 3, 2019.

US Government Accountability Office. *Elder Justice: Stronger Federal Leadership Could Enhance National Response to Elder Abuse.* Washington, DC: USGAO; 2011. http://www.gao.gov/products/GAO-11-208. Accessed December 3, 2019.

Walters ML, Chen J, Breiding MJ. *The National Intimate Partner and Sexual Violence Survey (NISVS): 2010 Findings on Victimization by Sexual Orientation.* Atlanta, GA: National Center for Injury Prevention and Control, Centers for Disease Control and Prevention; 2013.

NATURAL HISTORY OF INTERPERSONAL VIOLENCE IN ADULTS

Interpersonal violence among known partners occurs in cycles, and similar cycles happen with elder abuse, child abuse, and sexual predatory behavior. Violence generally escalates; with each cycle, the victim is exposed to additional risk.

▶ Detection & Intervention

Refer to Chapter 43 for more detailed information about abuse in the elderly.

A. Adults

1. Identification and screening—Victims of abuse often feel ashamed, have low self-esteem, or are unable or afraid to share their circumstances readily. Creating an atmosphere that promotes a welcoming, frank, and professional discussion will allow patients the opportunity to bring their concerns forward to the physician. Actively listening, making eye contact, and giving full attention to the patient may facilitate more openness and trust between providers and at-risk patients.

The US Preventive Services Task Force (USPSTF) recently published updated guidelines on screening for intimate partner violence, giving a B recommendation (high

Table 62–1. Screening tests for interpersonal violence with the highest levels of sensitivity and specificity per the US Preventive Services Task Force.

1. Hurt, Insult, Threaten, Scream (HITS)—available in English and Spanish
2. Ongoing Abuse Screen/Ongoing Violence Assessment Tool (OAS/OVAT)
3. Slapped, Threatened, and Throw (STaT)
4. Humiliation, Afraid, Rape, Kick (HARK)
5. Modified Childhood Trauma Questionnaire–Short Form (CTQ-SF)
6. Woman Abuse Screen Tool (WAST)

certainty that the net benefit is moderate or moderate certainty that the net benefit is moderate to substantial) for screening asymptomatic women of childbearing age. The USPSTF recognized several validated screening tools that could identify past and current abuse or risk of future abuse (Table 62–1). It also found adequate evidence that effective interventions reduce violence, abuse, and physical or mental harm in this population. The USPSTF continues its I recommendation for screening and intervention in other groups, including the elderly and vulnerable adults, because of lack of adequate studies determining risks and benefits. (The I recommendation indicates that current evidence is insufficient to assess the balance of benefits and harms of the service; that evidence is lacking, of poor quality, or conflicting; and that the balance of benefits and harms cannot be determined.) The American Medical Association and American College of Obstetricians and Gynecologists recommend specific direct questioning of patients, when appropriate, in a nonthreatening manner. The policy of the American Academy of Family Physicians regarding family violence can be found at the association's website (https://www.aafp.org/about/policies/all/intimatepartner-violence.html) and advocates that family physicians be alert for risk factors as well as signs of family violence with each patient encounter. Much like screening for alcohol abuse or depression, low-threat questions can be incorporated to ascertain the possibility of abuse in the home situation (Table 62–2). The optimal frequency of screening has not been established.

Table 62–2. Screening questions for interpersonal violence in adults.

1. Do you feel safe in your current relationship?
2. Do you perceive any threats to your safety on a regular basis?
3. Have you been hit or hurt by someone in the past?
4. Would you care to share any concerns you might have regarding interpersonal violence in your home or among your friends?
5. Have you ever been or are you currently concerned about harming your partner or someone close to you?
6. Would you like information about interpersonal violence or substance abuse programs in our community?

2. Interventions—The abusive spouse, partner, or family member often accompanies the patient to the office visit to monitor the information being shared and the manner in which experiences are being portrayed by the victim. Although it is not abnormal for a spouse or significant other to attend a physician visit, the physician should be alert to cues, including nonverbal behaviors that might signal an abusive situation. In particular, physicians should carefully evaluate situations in which someone else does all the talking for a competent and able patient. If possible, the physician should attempt to interview the patient alone. However, as an abusive individual might revert to controlling behavior in the office or become aggressive, physicians must consider the safety of their staff when confronting such individuals.

Intensive therapy is often required for both the abuser and the victim, and referrals to appropriate resources should be readily available in medical practices. Referral to an appropriate safe house in the community and information on how to obtain a personal protective order from a judge can be important for the safety of the victim, and the patient should be encouraged to take these steps, if appropriate. Domestic violence programs can help victims follow through with these initial steps. During this period, therapy for the victim is aimed at improving objective decision making, reestablishing self-esteem, reversing the cycle of self-blaming, and addressing the reality of the situation. The abuser also requires therapy. Depending on the circumstance, this may occur in the penal system or be mandated by the courts to take place in a child welfare agency. Therapy is aimed at reordering the emotional responses of the abuser and improving self-esteem. Developing a new worldview and set of behaviors is very difficult and takes a great deal of effort on the part of the therapist and the abuser.

It is critical that the family physician be supportive of the therapist and encourage the patient to continue in therapy. "Relapse" rates (ie, returning to the abusive relationship) are high; physicians should not become judgmental about such reconciliations but rather should remain supportive of victims.

B. Children

1. Identification and screening—Emergency physicians and pediatricians advocate for specific and direct questioning about childhood injuries to determine their cause. Direct questioning of parents/caregivers should be done in private to maximize value, maintain confidence, and reassure family members of the physician's intent to help, not hurt, the child or the family. This may require or be best facilitated by a multidisciplinary team trained to assess and report child abuse, neglect, or other forms of child victimization.

There are specific cues that should heighten the physician's index of suspicion regarding domestic violence and child abuse. "Red flags" should be raised when

- One partner insists on accompanying the other parent and child and speaks for them.
- A parent is reluctant to talk with the other partner present.
- The child's history does not fit the injury or illness.
- A parent makes frequent appointments for vague, poorly defined complaints.
- A child has recurrent, medically unexplainable somatic problems (eg, failure to thrive, abdominal or genital pain or injuries, headaches, enuresis [wetting], encopresis [fecal soiling], problems eating or sleeping).
- Medical attention for injuries is sought later than would be expected.
- The family uses emergency department services more often than is usual.
- A parent attempts to hide the child's injuries with clothing.
- A parent or child has several injuries at various stages of healing.

Additional red flags are outlined at http://childabuse.stanford.edu/screening/children.html (accessed May 5, 2019). Family physicians should be alert to the symptoms and signs of potential child abuse or neglect listed in Table 62–3.

It is also important to recognize that children may have interpersonal violence experiences other than child abuse or neglect by family members that can manifest in similar ways in terms of physical or mental health and functional impairments. These include sexual exploitation; witnessing violence in their communities (eg, shootings, stabbings); bullying at or after school by peers, older children, or adults; and cyberbullying or electronic aggression.

2. Interventions—There is a need to strengthen the evidence base for primary care interventions addressing child maltreatment. Models of care that provide the best opportunities for prevention of child abuse and neglect in healthcare settings are those that involve a multidisciplinary team with a social worker, nurse, developmental specialist, or other staff member who can help families access resources to meet basic needs; involve caregiver screening for child maltreatment risk factors (eg, depression, interpersonal violence); and are brief and inexpensive. Although few interventions of this type exist and have been tested, these factors should be considered as many practices shift to a medical home or collaborative care approach. In practices that do not yet have provisions for integrated care, ensuring that all healthcare providers understand the necessity of addressing child abuse and neglect, and the mandate to report, is the bare minimum (see section on reporting later in this chapter). Family medicine practices that provide families with information on resources and opportunities to learn about healthy child development, healthy coping and stress reduction, and mental health prevention for children and caregivers may be aiding in the prevention of child abuse and neglect.

Dubowitz H, Feigelman S, Lane W, et al. Pediatric primary care to help prevent child maltreatment: The Safe Environment for Every Kid (SEEK) model. *Pediatrics*. 2009;123:858–864. [PMID: 19255014]

Table 62–3. Symptoms and signs of potential abuse and neglect in children.

Physical Abuse	Neglect	Emotional Abuse	Sexual Abuse
Burns	Malnutrition	Self-injury	Self-injury
School problems	Lack of supervision	Anger	Inappropriate sexuality for age/seductiveness
Self-destructive or suicidal behavior	Poor dental hygiene	Depression	Genital swelling, bruises, bleeding, sexually transmitted infections, yeast or urinary tract infections, pregnancy
Unexplained cuts, bruises, or welts	Inappropriate clothing	Apathy	Poor hygiene
Inappropriate fear of adults	Poor hygiene	Eating disorders	Eating disorders
Early-onset depression, alcohol or drug use	Extreme hunger	Anxiety	Sleep disorders
Bruises in the shape of objects		Anger	Excessive aggression
Injuries in uncommon locations			Fear of a particular person
Bite marks			Withdrawal Suicidal behavior

Zuckerman B, Parker S, Kaplan-Sanoff M, et al. Healthy steps: a case study of innovation in pediatric practice. *Pediatrics.* 2004;114(3):820–826. [PMID: 15342859]

C. Special Populations

Recent immigrants; ethnic and racial minorities; homeless people; people with disabilities; and lesbian, gay, bisexual, and transgendered (LGBT) persons may have additional challenges in gaining access to and communicating with their physicians. The USPSTF recognized that abuse in these populations is understudied. A wide range of social factors may contribute to underreporting of abuse in same-sex relationships. LGBT patients should be questioned, as all patients are, in a safe environment and in a nonthreatening manner. For additional discussion of LGBT issues, see Chapter 66.

Followers of some religious and cultural traditions may tolerate levels of behavior that are not accepted by the mainstream culture in the United States. The norms of acceptable or expected behaviors, including the sharing of intimate family details, child-rearing practices, discussion of mental health issues, and sexuality concerns, create additional challenges for the physician to discover abusive relationships. Understanding cultural influences is key to identifying abuse in these situations. Access to an advocate who has proper training and connection with the culture can be extremely helpful. This person may also play an important role in supporting the patient's decision making when seeking appropriate interventions.

Open-ended questions about a patient's cultural norms may provide an appropriate avenue and manner for inquiry into the presence or absence of interpersonal violence in the patient's life. Lack of trust in law enforcement may be a specific challenge in poor minority communities and among the homeless. The stigma associated with interpersonal violence may inhibit reporting or seeking of assistance. Additional information can be obtained from specific resources such as the University of Michigan Program for Multicultural Health, available at http://www.med.umich.edu/multicultural/index.html. A resource for the African American community is available at https://dawnrising.org/create-peace/dv-institute/, and a resource for the American Indian or Alaska Native community is available at https://store.samhsa.gov/system/files/sma08-4354.pdf.

▶ Prevention

Primary prevention of interpersonal violence is critically important in addressing this problem. The effectiveness of prevention programs remains an ongoing topic of study.

Family physicians should consider a routine discussion of interpersonal violence as part of the normal health maintenance routine. This can be part of the usual discussion of safety issues, including seat belt use, gun safety, and smoke detectors. In a matter-of-fact manner, the physician can introduce the discussion of interpersonal violence in a wide variety of contexts, including well-woman care, well-child visits, routine "physicals," and other health maintenance visits.

A routine discussion of parenting techniques, referral to appropriate parenting classes, and provision of printed information have all been shown to have a positive effect on families at risk for child abuse or neglect. A plan for abuse identification, prevention, and training can be part of the individual education plan and the transition plan for children with developmental and physical disabilities.

Living situations of elderly patients should be well documented and understood, especially if the caregivers are not well known or are not part of the physician's personal practice. Information obtained and communication established during calm, uneventful times may be useful later should an incident occur.

▶ Safety Instructions for Patients

Family physicians should be aware of local resources and update contacts with them annually to ensure a readily available system of referral for safe houses, therapeutic care or social services, and legal intervention. Although these options vary from community to community, local resources can usually provide assistance to physicians when dealing with complicated cases. The National Domestic Violence Hotline (www.thehotline.org) provides resources and 24/7 phone access.

▶ Reporting

Healthcare providers should familiarize themselves with the laws of their state regarding the required reporting of violent crimes. In general, acts of violence that involve lethal force or firearms and rape must be reported to the local police agency. Complete documentation of all encounter details—including quotations, details, and time requirements—is an important medicolegal requirement. Family physicians working in emergency departments should follow the policies and procedures of their institution in the management and reporting of such violent crimes.

The reporting of an individual's confidentially expressed intent to harm another person places the physician in a far more difficult ethical and legal position that may require legal advice. In emergencies, particularly when a patient is believed to be in danger, the patient should be told to call 911.

The reporting of child abuse to Child Protective Services is a requirement in all 50 states. Some states require reporting to the local police agency as well. It is important for physicians to know the laws in their state, as reporting requirements and processes vary (see Child Welfare Information Gateway website, listed at end of this chapter). To aid a physician's understanding and ease any anxiety associated with reporting, physicians should learn the process for reporting in their county or state and what happens after child victimization is reported to Child Protective Services.

Elder abuse is also covered by state laws, and physicians should report in accordance with the local law at the time of the suspected abuse. In general, Adult Protective Services should be notified of suspected neglect or abuse. Other agencies that may require notification, depending on the state, include the Area Agency on Aging and the County Department of Social Services.

Ahmad M, Lachs MS. Elder abuse and neglect: what physicians can and should do. *Cleve Clin J Med*. 2002;69:801–808. [PMID: 12371803]

Websites

American Bar Association Commission on Domestic Violence. https://www.americanbar.org/groups/domestic_violence/

Child Welfare Information Gateway. https://www.childwelfare.gov/organizations/?CWIGFunctionsaction=rols:main.dspList&rolType=Custom&RS_ID=5 (for state hotline numbers), https://www.childwelfare.gov/topics/systemwide/laws-policies/ (for state-specific policies), and http://www.childwelfare.gov/

Combat-Related Posttraumatic Stress Disorder & Traumatic Brain Injury

Evelyn L. Lewis, MD, MA, FAAFP, DABDA
Layne D. Bennion, PhD
Ronald J. Koshes, MD, DFAPA
Jeanette M. Witter, PhD

POSTTRAUMATIC STRESS DISORDER

ESSENTIALS OF DIAGNOSIS

The diagnosis of posttraumatic stress disorder (PTSD) requires that patients screen positive for experiences/symptoms in each of eight categories (Criteria A–H). The patient must meet at least one (or more) of the specified criteria in each category (*Diagnostic and Statistical Manual of Mental Disorders*, 5th edition [*DSM-5*], 2013). For example:

Criterion A (one is required): The patient must have or have had "exposure to actual or threatened death, serious injury, or sexual violence in one (or more) of the following ways:

▶ Directly experiencing the traumatic event.

▶ Witnessing, in person, the event(s) as it occurred to others.

▶ Learning that the traumatic event(s) occurred to a close family member or close friend (where the actual or threatened death was violent or accidental).

▶ Experiencing repeated or extreme exposure to aversive details of the traumatic event(s) (e.g., first responder collecting human remains, police officers repeatedly exposed to details of child abuse)."

▶ General Considerations

In the most recent edition of the *DSM-5* (2013), posttraumatic stress disorder (PTSD) is classified as a trauma- and stressor-related disorder, not as a disorder consisting primarily of anxiety alone. The criterion for the diagnosis conceptualizes trauma as the precipitating event where the person experiences, witnesses, or is confronted with an event or events that threaten death or serious injury or posed a threat to the physical integrity of self or others. The events are beyond the realm of usual and normal human experience and include traumatic events such as war or the Holocaust; natural disasters such as earthquakes, tsunamis, hurricanes, and volcanic eruptions; and anthropogenic disasters, including factory explosions, automobile crashes, and airplane crashes. Critical to understanding the diagnosis is the idea that the cause of the illness was a traumatic event that occurred outside of the individual and was not due to an inherent character or personality weakness of that person. An important revision in *DSM-5* is the removal of the requirement that the individual's reaction must include extreme fear or horror. This criterion was not empirically supported and was not found to increase diagnostic accuracy.

While this condition has likely existed since human beings have endured trauma, PTSD entered the medical diagnostic realm with the publication of the *DSM-3* in 1980. It was first brought to public attention in relation to war veterans and, depending on the time frame of the war, has been known by a number of different terms, including combat fatigue, gross stress reaction, post-Vietnam syndrome, shell shock, and battle fatigue. Currently, PTSD is described as a disorder of persistent reactivity in many areas of self-regulation, not just troubling memories and chronic anxiety. Distressing memories of past traumatic events and intense stress reactions to reminders of those events that occur in the person's current life are the cornerstone of chronic PTSD.

Combat-related PTSD is the result of traumatic experiences occurring in the context of active war zones whether directly experienced (eg, improvised explosive device [IED] attacks) or indirectly experienced (eg, body recovery after battle). Although all military personnel who are deployed in combat zones are exposed to traumatic events, not all develop PTSD.

Disclaimer: The opinions and assertions expressed herein are those of the author(s) and do not necessarily reflect the official policy or position of the Uniformed Services University or the Department of Defense. There are no conflict of interests to declare by either author.

The 2011 study by Ruzek and colleagues found that approximately 15% of military personnel exposed to combat eventually develop PTSD as a result of their experiences.

The brain is essentially a control system that regulates the body functions. Trauma forces the brain to make profound biological adaptations in how it operates. When the body is safe and working well, the brain puts its energy into the "higher" functions that enable one to function in today's society. However, when the brain detects serious threats to body survival or traumatic stressors such as severe accidents, disasters, violence, abuse, or betrayals, the neural alarm system is activated and overrides of the rest of the brain's operations, putting all systems in emergency mode until the threat is overcome or dissipates. In most cases, with nontraumatic threats as well as traumatic survival threats, the alarm reaction in the brain quickly subsides and resets automatically to its default mode. However, when the brain's alarm system does not automatically or rapidly reset itself and the alarm systems continue to signal danger, even though safety has been restored (ie, the person is no longer engaged in combat), the brain remains in a chronic stress response mode.

PTSD and traumatic brain injury (TBI) represent the largest portion of mental health–related diagnoses from the wars in Iraq and Afghanistan. Understanding the diagnosis and treatment of these conditions is important for healthcare providers, many of whom may not have clinical experience with war casualties whether they work in civilian or military clinic settings. There are many obstacles to the timely and proper diagnosis and treatment in the population of veterans, including overlapping symptoms as well as cultural factors affecting diagnosis and treatment. Family physicians, both military and civilian, are likely to encounter PTSD and TBI patients in their practices, and a knowledge of military culture, traditions, and war-related injuries and illnesses is important to master.

TRAUMATIC BRAIN INJURY

TBI as a diagnosis describes the acute and chronic aftermath of violent physical forces impinging on the brain. The resulting damage ranges from the cellular level to changes in hemostatic mechanisms to gross or localized pathology. If providers are not careful in their thinking, it is easy to oversimplify medical decision making about TBI to a yes or no decision. The reality can be much more complex, particularly for military members who sustain multiple concussions during active combat.

Unfortunately, there is not complete agreement on definitions of TBI (eg, *DSM-5* and the 10 revision of the International Classification of Diseases do not have exact concordance). The Departments of Defense and of Veterans Affairs have used Table 63–1 to specify differences between mild TBI (mTBI) and more severe forms (moderate and severe TBI). Moderate and severe TBI are generally more

Table 63–1. Traumatic brain injury (TBI).

	Mild	Moderate	Severe
Consciousness: alteration of consciousness (AOC), loss of consciousness (LOC)	AOC or LOC <30 min	LOC <6 hours	LOC <6 hours
Neuroimaging	Within normal limits CT/MRI	Abnormal CT or MRI	Abnormal CT or MRI
GCS score	GCS 13–15	GCS 9–12	GCS <9
Posttraumatic	PTA <24 hours	PTA <7 days	PTA >7 days

GCS, Glasgow Coma Scale; PTA, posttraumatic amnesia.

evident to service members and their families. These service members are typically taken out of routine duty roles and enrolled in intensive rehabilitation programs in an attempt to return the member to baseline (or near baseline) functioning. If rehabilitation is not successful, they are eventually medically discharged from the military. Moderate and severe TBIs can have a myriad of complicating and esoteric facets including, for example, *anosognosia* (impaired perception of limitations of their abilities), which is thought to be an outcome of disconnection syndromes. Many deficits resulting from moderate and severe TBI may be quite apparent to others in the social and occupational circle of the injured patient. Thus, interviews with significant others can be more helpful and accurate regarding the patient's day-to-day functioning than the patient's self-report may be.

mTBIs are not a single entity, do not have one outcome, and may or may not have been recognized by individual service members or even diagnosed by the military medical system (particularly prior to and during the early years of the Iraq and Afghanistan wars). An additional complicating factor is military cultural factors. That is, for many service members and veterans, a military cultural norm is to deny problems with functioning. Part of military training and culture is to always press forward despite personal difficulties, in part because each team needs each of its players to survive and be fully functional.

An important consideration in diagnosing mTBI, particularly for service members, is consideration of the cumulative nature of multiple-injury events. When interviewing service members who served (particularly in the recent wars in Iraq and Afghanistan), it is important to *not* assume there is a particular signature event as the sole or primary causative agent of reported symptoms. Recent research suggests the total number of concussive and subconcussive events as well as the time spacing between these events may be critical factors in longer term outcomes. Specifically, the greater the number of total concussions and the closer together these events are (or some of the events are), the greater is the potential for negative consequences and long-term symptoms.

Blast injuries such as IEDs are well publicized as a cause of mTBI (and moderate/severe TBI). Upon interview, many service members can easily describe "the big one." Unfortunately, medical professionals may stop there and neglect to also ask about other blast exposures as well as other common causes associated with concussions. For military members in primary combat roles, other potential causes of concussions or cumulative subconcussions include parachute or "jump" training (faster falls and harder landings than civilian parachutists), motor vehicle accidents in the combat zone (fast and aggressive driving), breacher training and breacher operations (close-quarters use of shaped charges to blow locked doors or create man-sized holes in walls), falls (including being blown off or jumping off of rooftops, walls, or large vehicles), repeated close-quarters exposure to blast waves from heavy artillery or shoulder-fired missiles, and close-quarters combatives training, among others. Careful interviewing with service members, particularly those who were directly involved in combat operation, often finds indications of many dozens of concussive or subconcussive events.

Making the assessment task even more challenging is that many service members equate concussions with complete loss of consciousness. Thus, unless specifically asked, they may not report episodes of altered consciousness such as memory gaps, nausea, vomiting, being dazed (often described as "bell rung"), slowed cognitive processing ("foggy thinking"), postevent persistent headaches, persistent light or sound sensitivity, sleep changes, and emotional changes following blast exposures.

The physiologic mechanisms of damage from mTBI are multifactorial and may include one or more of the following mechanisms: focal injury to brain tissue or vasculature, diffuse axonal injury, superimposed hypoxia or ischemia, changes in intracranial pressure, microvascular and cellular injury resulting in a biochemical cascade of changes including loss of autoregulation, and inflammatory responses (Table 63–2).

Based primarily on sports concussion research, the majority of individuals suffering an mTBI are expected to improve over days to several weeks, particularly if care is taken to include restful sleep, stress reduction, and a stepped approach to return to play or to academic or work environments. Some helpful websites are provided in the following references.

American Psychiatric Association. *Diagnostic and Statistical Manual of Mental Disorders* (DSM–5). www.dsm5.org. Accessed December 9, 2019.

Center for Deployment Psychology. http://deploymentpsych.org/. Accessed December 9, 2019.

Defense and Veterans Brain Injury Center. http://www.DVBIC.org. Accessed December 9, 2019.

Table 63–2. Anatomic and physiologic changes following traumatic brain injury.

Focal injury
Orbitofrontal and anterior temporal lobes (where brain lies next to bony edges)
Swelling contusion, or hematomas
Sequelae: attentional, memory, and behavioral abnormalities

Diffuse axonal injury
Axonal shearing may, in fact, be axonal retraction
Alterations in calcium metabolism may be delayed 12–24 hours, making early intervention critical

Hypoxia ischemia
Hippocampus and vascular border zones of brain are particularly susceptible

Microvascular changes
Cerebrovascular autoregulation disruption related to carbon dioxide, hypertension (catecholamines)
Endothelium-derived relaxing factor (EDRF), or nitrous oxide increasing brain blood flow
Superoxide radical formation causing microvascular constriction

Secondary tissue changes: cascade of biochemical and physiologic events
Arachidonic acid metabolites such as prostaglandins, leukotrienes
Formation of oxygen free radicals
Neuropeptide changes
Calcium and magnesium alterations
Neurotransmitter changes: acetylcholine and glutamate
Lactic acid formation
Kinin formation
Leukocyte response with release of lymphokines such as interleukin-1

Oxygen free radicals
Formed normally through mitochondrial respiration
Enhanced by leukocyte activation and arachidonic acid after trauma or ischemia
Combined with its own metabolite, hydrogen peroxide, it forms the hydroxyl radical and causes lipid peroxidation

Department of Defense. Directive Type Memorandum (DTM) 09-033. Policy Guidance for management of Concussion/Mild Traumatic Brain Injury in the Deployed Setting. Signed June 21, 2010. https://www.esd.whs.mil/Portals/54/Documents/FOID/Reading%20Room/Other/11-F-0369_DTM_09-033_Policy_Guidance_for_Management_of_Concussion_Mild_Traumatic_Brain_Injury_In_The_Deployed_Setting.pdf. Accessed December 9, 2019.

Psychology Today. PTSD becomes (more) complex in the DSM-5: part 1. http://www.psychologytoday.com/blog/hijacked-your-brain/201306/ptsd-becomes-more-complex-in-the-dsm-5-part-1. Accessed December 9, 2019.

US Department of Veterans Affairs. PTSD: National Center for PTSD. http://www.ptsd.va.gov/professional/pages/diagnostic_criteria_dsm-5.asp. Accessed December 9, 2019.

https://www.healthquality.va.gov/guidelines/Rehab/mtbi/mTBICPGFullCPG50821816.pdf under Policy and Guidance (Clinical Practice Guidelines and Decision-Tree for Management of Concussion in Deployed Environments). Accessed March 19, 2020.

PREVALENCE OF PTSD

The rates of PTSD after trauma or disaster show considerable variation. The lifetime prevalence of PTSD is 7–30%, and PTSD affects approximately 5–7.7 million American adults in any one year. Higher rates are found after traumas resulting in more severe damage, events that may have more personal meaning or loss, when people believe that the event hinged on acts of commission or omission and blame themselves for the trauma, or when they believe others have "let them down" (eg, friendly fire incidents).

High rates of PTSD in veterans can be found regardless of which war or conflict is examined. Rates of PTSD in Vietnam veterans, Persian Gulf War veterans, and Iraq War veterans are provided in the following sections.

▶ Vietnam Veterans

Following a congressional mandate in 1983, the US government conducted the National Vietnam Veterans Readjustment Study (NVVRS) to better understand the psychological effects of participating in the Vietnam War. Approximately 15% of male and 9% of female Vietnam vets were found to have PTSD at the time of the study, and approximately 30% of men and 27% of women developed PTSD at some point in their lives following their deployment(s) to Vietnam. As one might suspect, these rates were much higher than those found among non-Vietnam veterans and civilians. The rates are alarming since they indicate that, at the time of the study, there were approximately 479,000 cases of PTSD and 1 million lifetime PTSD cases associated with the Vietnam War.

▶ Persian Gulf War

Studies examining the mental health of Persian Gulf War veterans found that rates of PTSD ranged anywhere from almost 9% to approximately 24%. Although the Persian Gulf War was brief, the rates of PTSD were higher than what was found among veterans not deployed to the Persian Gulf. A complicating factor was that significant portions of veterans reported unusual physical health problems.

▶ Iraq War & Afghanistan

Although the current war in Iraq has somewhat subsided, the conflict in Afghanistan is ongoing. Thus, the full impact of these wars on the mental and behavioral health of US soldiers is not yet known. However, the results of one study examining members of four US combat infantry units (three army and one marine) that served in Iraq and Afghanistan showed that the majority of soldiers were exposed to various types of traumatic, combat-related situations, such as being attacked or ambushed (92%), seeing dead bodies (94.5%), being shot at (95%), and/or personally knowing someone who was seriously injured or killed (86.5%). Roughly 6–11% of veterans of the Afghanistan war and 12–20% of veterans of the Iraq War have been found to have PTSD.

▶ PTSD Risk

PTSD can occur in people of all ages. However, numerous vulnerabilities render a person more prone to develop PTSD after a traumatic event:

- History of experiencing other types of trauma, particularly early in life, such as childhood or adolescent abuse or neglect
- Being female
- Experiencing intense or long-lasting trauma
- Having other mental health problems, such as anxiety or depression
- Lacking a robust or healthy support system of family and friends
- First-degree relatives with mental health problems, including PTSD or depression

Risk factors for military personnel developing PTSD include combat experience, being wounded, witnessing death, serving in mortuary affairs roles or graves registration duties or handling human remains, being captured or tortured, being exposed to unpredictable and uncontrollable stress, and experiencing sexual harassment or assault. Higher rates of PTSD and depression are associated with longer deployments, multiple deployments, and greater time away from the protection and supports at base camp. Vehicular bombs, suicide bombers, IEDs, and the constant threat of missile and rocket-propelled grenade attacks whether during combat missions or at base camp asleep on a cot are all elements of the recent Iraq and Afghanistan conflicts and can exacerbate the intense stress of combat.

Women are at approximately twofold increased risk of PTSD because they are more likely to have experienced the historical traumas and stressors that can trigger the condition. Some research finds women at greater risk of PTSD particularly when considering rates of being victims of sexual assaultive violence. The probability of PTSD in women versus men exposed to assaultive violence was 36% versus 6%. Research has found that military women who are diagnosed with PTSD and have a history of military sexual trauma have poorer outcomes than women with PTSD who do not have a similar sexual trauma history.

Ethnic minorities (African Americans, Hispanics, and Native Americans) are more likely to develop PTSD than are whites or men (in general), and there is some evidence that there are genetic vulnerabilities for minorities. Some of above difference in risk is attributed to a tendency for ethnic minorities to harbor self-blame, to have less social support, and to have an increased perception of racial prejudice; in addition, ethnic minorities may express distress in a different manner and/or have higher rates of dissociation related to trauma events.

PREVALENCE OF COMBAT-RELATED MTBI

Prevalence of combat-related mTBI is a very difficult metric to assess in part because of the many types and causes of mTBI, the diverse range of on-the-ground missions military units have, and the differing tracking systems for active duty versus reservist or guardsman who deploy. Two recent studies found a 10–12% prevalence of mTBI in postdeployment service members using self-reported symptoms (eg, alteration of consciousness, loss of consciousness) and a 23% prevalence of mTBI in an army combat brigade using a mixture of self-report and clinician-confirmed mTBI. Certain military occupational specialties (eg, Combat Arms soldiers) have been found to have much higher prevalence rates; nearly half of these soldiers (48%) have a history of at least one mTBI during their most recent deployment.

PREVALENCE OF COMBAT-RELATED MTBI AND COMORBID PTSD

As noted earlier, estimations of prevalence are difficult for the reasons previously discussed. There is still much work to be done regarding whether a history of mTBI puts one at greater risk of developing PTSD or whether experiencing trauma sufficient to cause PTSD symptoms puts one at greater risk for a poor recovery if an mTBI occurs or both. A recent systematic review concluded that comorbid PTSD/TBI was found in 33–39% of service members. Obviously there is a massive confound when attempting to sort out the etiology of these disorders when both the trauma events and the concussive incidents are combat related. For example, a blast exposure that occurs in the context of active combat, by its nature, includes life-threatening danger with the potential of triggering PTSD-related symptoms as well as damaging the brain via blast wave exposure. Additionally, some long-term consequences to soldier may increase the risk of both disorders (eg, persistent sleep problems or chronic pain).

American Academy of Child and Adolescent Psychiatry. *Child and Adolescent Mental Health Statistics Resources for Families.* Washington, DC: American Academy of Child and Adolescent Psychiatry; 2007.

Hall-Clark BN, Kaczkurkin AN, Asnaani A, et al. Ethnoracial differences in PTSD symptoms and trauma-related cognitions in treatment-seeking active duty military personnel for PTSD. *Psychol Trauma.* 2017;9(6):741–745. [PMID: 28068141]

Loo CM. *PTSD among Ethnic Minority Veterans.* White River Junction, VT: National Center for PTSD; 2007.

MedicineNet. Posttraumatic stress disorder. http://www.medicinenet.com/posttraumatic_stress_disorder. Accessed December 9, 2019.

Sexton MB, Raggio GA, McSweeney LB, et al. Contrasting gender and combat versus military sexual traumas: psychiatric symptom severity and morbidities in treatment-seeking veterans. *J Womens Health (Larchmt).* 2017;26(9):933–940. [PMID: 28488917]

Steele M, Germain A, Campbell JS. Mediation and moderation of the relationship between combat exposure and PTSD symptoms in active duty military. *Mil Med.* 2017;182(5):e1632–e1639. [PMID: 29087905]

▶ Early Treatment That May Help Lessen Longer Term Symptoms of PTSD

Treatment that begins very soon (hours to days) after a life-threatening event may have a dampening effect on intensity of acute stress disorder symptoms as well as minimize later PTSD symptoms. It is important to note that recent careful research has called into question the efficacy of psychological debriefing strategies, such as critical incident stress management or debriefing (CISM or CISD), in the prevention of later PTSD after a traumatic event. Research findings indicated that, for some individuals, such interventions can actually make their symptomology and recovery worse.

In contrast to CISM or CISD, a successful military-initiated brief education-based intervention (BattleMind) has shown promise and focuses on normalizing trauma reactions and psychoeducation regarding the common aftermath of trauma. Cognitive behavioral therapy (CBT) and motivational interview–based treatment strategies have all shown significant positive effects in reducing later PTSD symptoms. Individualized behavioral activation strategies after a trauma, if spread over the course of changes in stepped care treatment, have been found to be beneficial in reducing later symptoms. Less beneficial is exposure to self-help booklets and general psychoeducation (eg, stress management).

Some pharmaceuticals administered within hours of the traumatic event have been shown to have some efficacy in reducing longer term symptoms. Hydrocortisone and glucocorticoid administration soon after an event has been associated with a reduction in PTSD-like symptoms in randomized controlled studies. Preliminary work with morphine and ketamine has raised the possibility of a beneficial effect related to later development of PTSD symptoms; however, randomized controlled studies have not yet been completed. Previous work suggested medications such as propranolol given acutely (eg, within 6 hours after the trauma) may help reduce physiologic reactivity. However, more recent carefully controlled studies with propranolol have failed to replicate this earlier finding. Similarly, use of escitalopram, temazepam, and gabapentin has not been found to be beneficial in the prevention of later PTSD symptoms.

Agency for Healthcare Research and Quality. Interventions for the prevention of posttraumatic stress disorder (PTSD) in adults after exposure to psychological trauma. http://effectivehealthcare.ahrq.gov/search-for-guides-reviews-and-reports/?pageaction=displayproduct&productID=1444#7302. Accessed December 10, 2019.

Fletcher S, Creamer M, Forbes D. Preventing post traumatic stress disorder: are drugs the answer? *Aust N Z J Psychiatr.* 2010;44(12):1064–1071. [PMID: 21080102]

Sijbrandij M, Kleiboer A, Bisson JI, Barbui C, Cuijpers P. Pharmacological prevention of post-traumatic stress disorder and acute stress disorder: a systematic review and meta-analysis. *Lancet Psychiatry.* 2015;2(5):413–421. [PMID: 26360285]

Sijbrandij M, Kleiboer A, Bisson JI, Barbui C, Cuijpers P. Corrections. Pharmacological prevention of post-traumatic stress disorder and acute stress disorder: a systematic review and meta-analysis. *Lancet Psychiatry.* 2015;2(7):584. [PMID: 26303542]

▶ Clinical Findings Associated with PTSD

A. Signs and Symptoms

PTSD symptoms typically start within 3 months of a traumatic event. However, in a small number of cases, symptoms may not appear until years after the event. The symptoms of PTSD are also known to appear and disappear sporadically. They may be plentiful or severe when a patient's life is more stressful or when reminders of the event are encountered. For example, hearing a car backfire may result in reliving combat experiences, or a news report about a rape may bring back memories of an assault. In addition to the *DSM-5* criteria noted at the beginning of this chapter, there are four categories or types of PTSD symptoms:

- **Reexperiencing the events:** Memories of the traumatic event that can return at any time (spontaneous memories of the traumatic event, recurrent trauma-related dreams, flashbacks, or other intense or prolonged psychological distress).

- **Heightened arousal:** Feeling anxious, jittery, and constantly on the lookout for danger. Sudden anger or irritability is not uncommon (aggressive, reckless, or self-destructive behavior; sleep disturbances; hypervigilance or related problems).

- **Avoidance:** Avoidance of situations, things, or people that bring back memories of the trauma (distressing memories, thoughts, feelings, or external reminders of the event).

- **Negative alterations in thoughts and mood or feelings:** Feelings may vary from a persistent and distorted sense of blame of self or others, to estrangement or disassociation from others or markedly diminished interest in activities, to an inability to remember key aspects of the event.

In addition to these symptoms, a patient must also meet the following criteria for at least a month:

- At least one recurring symptom
- At least three avoidance symptoms
- At least two hyperarousal symptoms
- And finally, the experienced symptoms must complicate daily life and make going to school or work, social contacts, and performing important tasks very difficult

Even with the assistance of the descriptive symptoms listed earlier, the assessment of PTSD can often be difficult for practitioners since most patients present with complaints other than anxiety associated with a traumatic experience. Those symptoms may include expression of disturbed body functions (somatization), depression, sleep problems, or substance misuse. Most studies of Iraq War veterans show they tend to display more physical symptoms than verbally describe the PTSD-associated emotional problems. In addition, the diagnosis of PTSD often occurs comorbidly with bipolar disorder (manic depression), eating disorders, and other anxiety disorders such as obsessive-compulsive disorder, panic disorders, social anxiety disorder, and generalized anxiety disorder.

American Psychiatric Association. *Diagnostic and Statistical Manual of Mental Disorders (DSM–5).* www.dsm5.org. Accessed December 10, 2019.

Mayo Clinic. www.mayoclinic.com. Accessed December 10, 2019.

National Institute of Mental Health. Post-traumatic stress disorder (PTSD). https://www.nimh.nih.gov/health/trials/post-traumatic-stress-disorder-ptsd.shtml. Accessed December 10, 2019.

US Department of Veteran Affairs. National Center for PTSD. www.ptsd.va.gov. Accessed December 10, 2019.

B. Neuroanatomic Features

Although mTBI, almost by definition, has a negative impact on neuronal functioning, recently there has been very interesting work focused on changes in cortical functioning associated with PTSD. Through the use of structural and functional brain imaging, characteristic changes in the brain structure and function of PTSD patients have been identified. Regions typically altered in patients with chronic or more severe PTSD include the hippocampus (volume reductions), prefrontal gray matter (volume reduction), amygdala (greater reactivity), and cortical regions involved in emotional management or inhibitory control (eg, hypoactivation of prefrontal cortex, hyperreactivity of dorsal cingulate and insula, changes in connectivity between cortical areas such as amygdala and hippocampus). The neural interconnectivity of these regions forms networks that mediate adaptation to stress and fear conditioning. It is the change in this circuitry that has been proposed to have a direct link to the development of PTSD.

Different experiential, psychophysiologic, and neurobiologic responses to traumatic symptom provocation in PTSD have been reported in the literature. Two subtypes of trauma response have been hypothesized, one characterized predominantly by hyperarousal of brain networks and the other primarily by dissociative or disconnection outcomes.

Butler O, Adolf J, Gleich T, et al. Military deployment correlates with smaller prefrontal gray matter volume and psychological symptoms in a subclinical population. *Transl Psychiatry.* 2017;7(2):e1031. [PMID: 28195568]

Hughes KC, Shin LM. Functional neuroimaging studies of post-traumatic stress disorder. *Expert Rev Neurother*. 2011;11(2):275–285. [PMID: 21306214]

Sripada RK, King AP, Garfinkel SN, et al. Altered resting-state amygdala functional connectivity in men with posttraumatic stress disorder. *J Psychiatry Neurosci*. 2012;37(4):241–249. [PMID: 22313617]

Stark EA, Parsons CE, Van Hartevelt TJ, et al. Post-traumatic stress influences the brain even in the absence of symptoms: a systematic, quantitative meta-analysis of neuroimaging studies. *Neurosci Biobehav Rev*. 2015;56:207–221. [PMID: 26192104]

C. PTSD Screening Tests

Screening measures of PTSD-related symptoms vary. One of the most important differences is the format of the measure (Table 63–3).

The PTSD screening instruments noted in Table 63–3 range from 4 to 17 self-report items. Selection of specific instruments depends on what is needed within a given provider's work setting. Elements to consider when selecting a measure include time required to complete the measure, reading level of the patient population, whether a patient's history is more likely to have a single traumatic event or multiple traumatic events, whether the assessed symptoms need to correspond to *DSM* criteria, the psychometric strengths

Table 63–4. Primary Care PTSD Screen (PC-PTSD).

In your lifetime, have you ever had any experience that was so frightening, horrible, or upsetting that, in the past month, you:	
Have had nightmares about it or thought about it when you did not want to?	YES/NO
Tried hard not to think about it or went out of your way to avoid situations that reminded you of it?	YES/NO
Were constantly on guard, watchful, or easily startled?	YES/NO
Felt numb or detached from others, activities, or your surroundings?	YES/NO

Data from Prins A, Ouimette P, Kimmerling R, et al. *The Primary Care PTSD Screen (PC-PTSD)*. White River Junction, VT: National Center for PTSD; 2003.

and weaknesses of the screen, and the per-use cost of the measure.

The Primary Care PTSD Screen (PC-PTSD) is a four-item screen administered by a medical provider or trained assistant and was designed for use in primary care and other medical settings. Administration begins with an introductory sentence, which cues patients to focus on traumatic events. For many outpatient clinic settings, the results of the PC-PTSD should be considered "positive" if a patient answers yes to any of the other three items. Those patients screening positive on the PC-PTSD should then be assessed more comprehensively with a structured interview for PTSD and/or by a specialist. This screen tool does not gather detailed information about potentially traumatic events (Table 63–4). The PC-PTSD is also available in Spanish.

The PC-PTSD has been adapted to *DSM-5* criteria (PC-PTSD-5), and research has found the revision to be useful, to be accepted by patients, and to have reasonable psychometrics.

Aside from screeners, there are of course, well-researched and more comprehensive measures of PTSD. Clinician-administered structured interviews are common in this category. The Clinician-Administered PTSD Scale (CAPS) is a 30-item structured interview that includes combined ratings of symptom frequency and intensity, has solid psychometrics, can include multiple trauma events, and is designed to assess both lifetime diagnosis of PTSD as well as recent/current PTSD symptoms. The process is rather lengthy given the schedules of many medical care providers (45–60 minutes), but appropriately trained paraprofessionals can use the tool.

Table 63–3. PTSD self-report screening instruments

Screens for PTSD	Number of Items	Time to Administer (minutes)	Allows Multiple Trauma	Corresponds to *DSM-4* Criteria
BAI-PC	7	3	Yes	N/A
Primary Care PTSD Screen (PC-PTSD)	4	2	Yes	N/A
Short form of the PTSD Checklist	6	2	Yes	N/A
Short Screening Scale for PTSD	7	3	Yes	N/A
SPAN	4	2	Yes	N/A
SPRINT	8	3	Yes	N/A
Trauma Screening Questionnaire (TSQ)	10	4	Yes	N/A
PTSD Checklist (PCL)	17	5–10	Yes	Yes

BAI-PC, Beck Anxiety Inventory–Primary Care; *DSM-4, Diagnostic and Statistical Manual of Mental Disorders*, 4th edition; N/A, not applicable; PSTD, posttraumatic stress disorder; SPAN, startle, physically upset by reminders, anger, and numbness; SPRINT, Short Posttraumatic Stress Disorder Rating Interview.

Prins A, Bovin MJ, Smolenski DJ, et al. The primary care PTSD screen for DSM-5 (PC-PTSD-5): development and evaluation within a veteran primary care sample. *J Gen Intern Med*. 2016;31(10):1206–1211. [PMID: 27170304]

Prins A, Ouimette P, Kimerling R, et al. The primary care PTSD screen (PC-PTSD): development and operating characteristics. *Primary Care Psychiatr.* 2003;9:9–14. [No PMID]

▶ Differential Diagnosis of PTSD & mTBI

Clinicians may have difficulty making the diagnosis of PTSD because the patient may have additional disorders. In particular, major depression and substance abuse are common comorbidities of PTSD. With military members, particularly those with a history of direct combat, mTBI is also very common, either as a comorbidity or as a complication.

Specific to military members, other common complications or comorbidities are sleep problems (including obstructive sleep apnea), chronic pain problems, chronic headaches, and subtle visual or hearing difficulties. Any of these can complicate and interfere with treatments for PTSD and mTBI.

▶ Complications

Patients with PTSD often initially present to their primary care physician with physical symptoms rather than psychological concerns. This is not unexpected as studies have shown that people with PTSD are at increased risk for a number of medical conditions, such as hypertension, diabetes, cardiovascular disease, and asthma. In addition, although specific mechanisms are not well understood yet, research indicates that mTBI and blast exposures can also negatively impact physiologic systems such as hormonal and endocrine systems and result in increased inflammatory responses.

Another complication in working with military members or veterans is pharmaceutical treatment. Specifically, service members and veterans with a wide range of complaints who are seen by different providers can be prescribed a surprising number of medications over time. Conversely, some patients are adverse to trying new medications or cannot tolerate side effects and may not take medications as prescribed.

When there is prolonged exposures or multiple traumas, some patients develop atypical patterns of behavior. These include difficulty in trusting others, irregular moods, impulsive behavior, increased shame, decreased self-esteem, and unstable relationships. Significant interpersonal difficulties are common in persons with PTSD, and the risk of interpersonal violence increases. Symptoms of estrangement, irritability, and anger, or associated depression, can severely stress relationships. Military members and veterans with PTSD may find it difficult to discuss their symptoms with those who have not experienced combat. Guilt about surviving while battle buddies were killed or guilt regarding actions taken in the fog of war can also cause increased isolation and tension in interpersonal relationships.

▶ Treatment

Empirically based treatments for PTSD typically include psychological and medical interventions, which are often used in combination. Each patient has a unique background and set of contributors; therefore, any treatment intervention should be well formulated and culturally appropriate to optimize clinical and functional outcomes. A starting point can be providing information about PTSD and what to expect in treatment, which helps to dispel inaccuracies and minimize any shame. This is particularly important in populations such as military personnel, who are frequently disadvantaged by the perceived and real stigma associated with seeing a mental health professional.

Empirically based treatments for mTBI are less well developed and understood, particularly when there is comorbid PTSD. Unfortunately, these conditions are often treated separately (eg, a particular treatment or program is focused on PTSD and a separate treatment or work focuses on adaptation after mTBI). Interdisciplinary and integrated treatment team programs treating both comorbidities as well as other complicating problems (eg, sleep problems and chronic pain) show promise.

A. Psychotherapy

PTSD has been shown to be effectively treated with CBT-based psychotherapy, particularly cognitive processing therapy and exposure therapy. Psychotherapies should share the following common elements:

- Therapy should always be individualized to meet the specific concerns and needs of each unique trauma survivor.
- A shared plan of therapy should be developed by the patient and therapist within an atmosphere of trust and open discussion.
- One goal is to enable the survivor to gain a realistic sense of self-esteem and self-confidence in managing bad memories.

More generally, CBT is widely accepted as useful for PTSD and is a relatively structured psychotherapy that involves teaching specific techniques (ie, exposure and cognitive restructuring, relaxation, self-talk, and assertiveness training) and generally involves fewer sessions. Cognitive restructuring involves identifying irrational patterns of thought, feeling, and behavior and gradually teaches the subject how to substitute new thoughts for the old and develop new emotional and behavioral patterns.

Exposure therapy targets the feared situations or triggers and, in a carefully designed, step-by-step approach, helps the patient face the fear and gain control of the accompanying distress. Some care is needed to avoid retraumatizing the patient.

Although the treatment has detractors and is controversial, eye movement desensitization and reprocessing can provide an avenue for patients to modify their memories of the trauma (including all of the negative thoughts, feelings, and sensations experienced at the time of the event) and guide patients through the work of minimizing reactions to triggering events.

Group psychotherapies, based in cognitive-processing therapy strategies and mindfulness-type therapies, have also shown effectiveness for military personnel with PTSD.

B. Complementary and Alternative Medicine

Complementary and alternative medicine (CAM) approaches to PTSD and mTBI employ a range of therapies that are not or may not be considered standard to the practice of medicine. Although the research base to support the effectiveness of CAM approaches is lacking, there is little evidence that use of these strategies is harmful. Patients who are reluctant to accept standard mental health labels or interventions may be more accepting of these innovative treatment approaches. Many CAM interventions are practiced in a manner that increases social support and reduces stress for the patient and family members. Thus, an active ingredient in some CAM interventions may be the promotion of greater resilience through an increased sense of control and social connectedness.

The CAM modality categories as delineated by the National Center for Complementary and Alternative Medicine include the following:

- **Natural products:** Including biologically based practices that include herbs, dietary supplements, vitamins, foods, and homeopathic remedies.
- **Mind-body medicine:** The goal is harmonization of mind-body function to promote health and wellness. Some approaches focus primarily on mental activity such as guided imagery, affirmations, and prayer. Some focus on activities designed to integrate the mind and body, such as yoga, meditation, tai chi, expressive art therapies, and breath-oriented therapies.
- **Manipulation and body-based practices (exercise and movement):** These modalities are based on practitioner manipulation of the patient's body parts or body systems. This includes disciplines such as chiropractic spinal and joint manipulation, osteopathic manipulation, massage therapy, reflexology, and acupuncture.
- **Energy medicine:** Practices that focus on theories of body energies look to balance energy fields that surround and penetrate the human body (qi gong, reiki, and therapeutic touch).

It has been estimated that 41% of service members and veterans have used one or more CAM treatments, a rate that is very similar to civilian populations. Furthermore, CAM is more often used by those who have a greater number of health symptoms (comorbid conditions). In one study, more than two-thirds of service members and veterans with a history of PTSD reported using one or more CAM treatments. Because many of the CAM modalities relate to particular cultural backgrounds, physicians and allied health professionals should pay particular attention to the values and desires of the patient and the family.

C. Medications

Several classes of medications are employed to help improve or eliminate symptoms of PTSD. They are nearly always used in conjunction with psychotherapy for PTSD, because although medications may minimize some of the symptoms commonly associated with the disorder, they will not relieve a person of the flashbacks, nor will the medication change the perceptions, cognitions, or feelings associated with the original trauma.

The selective serotonin reuptake inhibitor (SSRI) antidepressants are the most commonly prescribed class of medications for PTSD and the first class of drugs approved for PTSD by the US Food and Drug Administration (FDA). They include medications such as fluoxetine, sertraline, and paroxetine. Research shows that this group of medicines tends to decrease anxiety, depression, and panic associated with PTSD. These types of antidepressants may also help reduce aggression, impulsivity, and suicidal thoughts that can occur in people with PTSD. For combat-related PTSD, there is increasing evidence that prazosin can be particularly helpful. Depending on the severity of symptoms and degree of decline in functioning, antidepressants should be prescribed for at least a year. Many patients may need to try several types of antidepressants before finding one that meets their needs and helps relieve their symptoms.

The atypical antipsychotics are the next most common class of medications prescribed. They include medications such as risperidone, olanzapine, and quetiapine. These medicines seem to be most useful in the treatment of PTSD for those who suffer additional symptoms of agitation, dissociation, hypervigilance, intense suspiciousness, paranoia, or brief psychotic reactions. Although less effective for PTSD, the mood stabilizers such as lamotrigine, tiagabine, and divalproex sodium can be helpful for some individuals. Medicines that help decrease the physical symptoms associated with PTSD include drugs such as clonidine, guanfacine, and propranolol. Benzodiazepines are sometimes prescribed for certain symptoms because they provide rapid relief of anxiety, especially when reactions are trigged by specific, but infrequent, environments or situations. However, their long-term usefulness is limited because of their associated dependence. There is even a small sample of data indicating that, over time, they can exacerbate PTSD. Although other medications such as duloxetine, bupropion, and venlafaxine are sometimes used to treat PTSD, there is little research that has studied their effectiveness in treating this illness.

The current state of evidence suggests that if pharmaceuticals are used, the SSRIs remain the treatment of first choice for most patients. Currently there is minimal evidence to support the use of any specific SSRI over other SSRIs. Therefore, the differences in pharmacokinetic profile, individual tolerability, and drug interaction potential should be used to guide the selection. In the event that SSRI therapy has not provided adequate benefit, or where adverse effects or drug interactions mean that SSRI treatment is unsuitable, mirtazapine or venlafaxine can be regarded as reasonable alternatives.

Benedek D, Friedman MJ, Zatzick D, et al. Guideline watch: practice guideline for the treatment of patients with acute stress disorder and posttraumatic stress disorder. https://focus.psychiatryonline.org/doi/abs/10.1176/foc.7.2.foc204. Accessed December 10, 2019.

Cohen H. Treatment of PTSD. *Psych Central.* http://psychcentral.com/lib/an-overview-of-treatment-of-ptsd/0001612006. Accessed August 6, 2013.

National Center for Posttraumatic Stress Disorder. Treatment of PTSD. http://www.ptsd.va.gov/professional/pages/overview-treatment-research.asp. Accessed March 25, 2011.

Substance Abuse and Mental Health Services Administration. Pharmacologic guidelines for treating individuals with posttraumatic stress disorder and co-occurring opioid use disorder; May 2012. https://store.samhsa.gov/system/files/sma12-4688.pdf. Accessed December 10, 2019.

Ursano RJ, Bell C, Eth S, Friedman MJ, Norwood AE, Pfefferbaum B. Practice guideline for the treatment of patients with acute stress disorder and posttraumatic stress disorder [special issue]. *Am J Psychiatr.* 2004;161(Suppl):3–31. [PMID: 15617511]

VA/DoD Clinical Practice Guideline Working Group. *Management of Post-traumatic Stress.* Washington, DC: Veterans Health Administration, Department of Veterans Affairs and Health Affairs; Department of Defense; Office of Quality and Performance, publication 10Q-CPG/PTSD-03; Dec 2003. http://www.healthquality.va.gov/PTSD-FULL-2010c.pdf. Accessed December 10, 2019.

▶ **Prognosis of PTSD & mTBI**

The prognosis for PTSD depends primarily on the severity of symptoms and length of time that a person has suffered from the disorder. Symptom duration is variable and is affected by the proximity, duration, and intensity of the trauma, as well as comorbidity with other psychiatric disorders. The patient's subjective interpretation of the trauma also influences symptoms. In patients who are receiving treatment, the average duration of symptoms is approximately 36 months. In patients who are not receiving treatment, the average duration of symptoms increases to 64 months.

Overall, approximately 30% of people with PTSD eventually recover completely with proper treatment, and another 40% are functional, even though less intense chronic symptoms may remain. The majority of patients with PTSD respond to psychotherapy. More than one-third of PTSD patients never fully recover. These latter individuals are at risk for difficulty maintaining jobs and difficulty developing or retaining relationships and have a significant risk of suicide.

Both PTSD and mTBI are ongoing challenges for healthcare providers at every level of health care. Family physicians and other primary care clinicians will surely continue to be involved in the diagnosis and management of these patients. Although PTSD and mTBI may not be adequately diagnosed in the population of service members and veterans, any patient with combat experience should be considered at risk for both of these conditions. Screening for a history of blast injuries, concussions, and traumatic exposure should be part of the clinical workup of any former service member with a history of deployment into active combat areas. Family physicians are especially likely to encounter these patients at various stages of their illness progression, and a knowledge of how combat and deployment affect illness and health is essential.

Cultural & Linguistic Competence

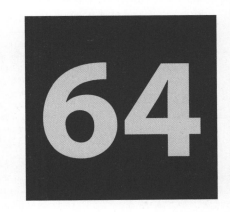

Kim A. Bullock, MD, FAAFP

Darci L. Graves, MPP, MA, MA

Family physicians are devoted to a holistic delivery of comprehensive health care across the lifespan from infancy to the end of life, all within increasingly diverse communities. The breadth of knowledge is focused on the individual within the context of the family and the greater community. The World Organization of Family Doctors specifies that the specialty provide personal, expansive and continuing care with consideration for the individual within the local as well as globally linked community. Many of these communities face existing and persistent health and healthcare disparities. Growing diversity and persistent disparities are among several arguments for the provision of care and services, which are patient centered as well as culturally and linguistically appropriate. This may include decisions and actions that are congruent with the patient's value systems and orientation to health and illness.

Every patient interaction is a unique cultural experience; each encounter is an opportunity to overcome the potential impediments in the exchange of information between physicians, patients, and their families. The American Academy of Family Physicians (AAFP) recognized the importance of culturally proficient and linguistically competent care in a 2014 position paper titled "Cultural Proficiency: The Importance of Cultural Proficiency in Providing Effective Care for Diverse Populations." The AAFP is not alone in its recognition of the crucial role of cross-cultural health in the effective delivery of health care. The list includes other influential groups such as the American Association of Medical Colleges, Liaison Committee on Medical Education, and the Centers for Medicare and Medicaid Services, and other national and international bodies, such as The Joint Commission, The Commonwealth Fund, and the World Health Organization (WHO).

The Institute of Medicine (IOM) produced a landmark report entitled *Crossing the Quality Chasm*, which crystallized the failures of the American medical system and asserted that the system must be changed to one that is equitable, patient-centered, safe, and effective. The following year, the IOM released *Unequal Treatment: Confronting Racial and Ethnic Disparities in Health Care*, which identified cross-cultural education as a possible intervention in the reduction of healthcare disparities. The documentary *Unnatural Causes* continued this narrative by examining how social determinants of health, including racism and class distinctions, created health inequalities within communities of color across the nation.

Agency for Healthcare Research and Quality. *2016 National Healthcare Quality and Disparities Report (NHDR)*. Rockville, MD: Agency for Healthcare Research and Quality; 2012. https://www.ahrq.gov/research/findings/nhqrdr/nhqdr16/index.html. Accessed December 10, 2019.

American Academy of Family Physicians. Cultural proficiency: the importance of cultural proficiency in providing effective care for diverse populations. https://www.aafp.org/about/policies/all/cultural-diverse-populations.html. Accessed December 10, 2019.

Institute of Medicine. *Crossing the Quality Chasm: A New Health System for the 21st Century*. Washington, DC: Committee on Quality of Health Care in America, National Academies Press; 2001.

Liaison Committee on Medical Education. *Functions and Structure of a Medical School: Standards for Accreditation of Medical Education Programs Leading to the M.D. Degree*. Washington, DC: Liaison Committee on Medical Education; 2018. http://lcme.org/publications/. Accessed December 10, 2019.

The Joint Commission. *Advancing Effective Communication, Cultural Competency, and Patient-and Family-Centered Care: A Roadmap for Hospitals*. Oakbrook Terrace, IL: The Joint Commission; 2010.

WHY CULTURALLY AND LINGUISTICALLY APPROPRIATE SERVICES ARE NECESSARY

▶ Emergent Diversity in American Communities

The changing demographics of the United States provide one of many compelling reasons for healthcare providers to

Box 64–1: Important terms to know.

Culturally and Linguistically Appropriate Services

Services that are respectful of and responsive to individual cultural health beliefs and practices, preferred languages, health literacy levels, and communication needs and employed by all members of an organization (regardless of size) at every point of contact. Over the past century, diversity within the United States has significantly increased, with 36% of the population, according to the 2010 census, represented by a mixed racial or ethnic nonmajority group. This figure will increase to 40% in 2030 (www.census.gov).

Health Disparities

A particular type of health difference that is closely linked with social, economic, and/or environmental disadvantage. Health disparities adversely affect groups of people who have systematically experienced greater obstacles to health based on their racial or ethnic group, religion, socioeconomic status, gender, age, sexual orientation, or other characteristics historically linked to discrimination or exclusion.

Health Equity

Attainment of the highest level of health for all people. Achieving health equity requires valuing everyone equally, with focused and ongoing societal efforts to address avoidable inequalities, historical and contemporary injustices, and the elimination of health and healthcare disparities.

consider the impact of cultural factors on health, disease, and health care. The population is increasingly diverse: aging, coming out, immigrating, and acculturating (Box 64–1). Currently, minorities represent one-third of the US population. Projections indicate that the United States will be a "majority-minority" nation by 2042, with the nation projected to be 54% minority in 2050 (Box 64–2).

Health & Healthcare Disparities

Health disparities refer to differences in health status between groups or populations, and although commonly interpreted to mean ethnic or racial distinctions, there are many dimensions of disparity that occur within this context. The performance of the US healthcare system reveals

Box 64–2: A cautionary word about the term *minority*.

The term *minority* is often used with little consideration for its connotations. People feel uncomfortable with this reference because of its implied status of inferiority. A clear example expressed by an Hispanic patient toward her caregivers is the following. She states, "I felt weak, small and irrelevant when they used the term to talk about me among themselves. It sounded like they were being derogatory, which made me feel more powerless than I already was." Alternative terms have emerged in both the medical and lay literature, such as people or communities of color, more defined country of origin delineations, or allowing patients to offer their own identification.

Data from Paniagua FA. *Assessing and Treating Culturally Diverse Clients.* 4th ed. Thousand Oaks, CA: Sage; 2014.

significant inequities across populations with missed opportunities in terms of preventing disease, disability, and morbidity and mortality indices. Disparities in health and health care are due to a complex interaction between many factors, from those that increase exposure to disease to those that decrease access to health care. The trends reveal that individuals from communities of color are in poorer health, face greater challenges in accessing care, experience significant navigation problems within the system, and receive a quality of care that is inferior to that of their nonminority peers. Individuals with limited English proficiency and low health literacy skills have also experienced lower quality health care.

Examples of disparities include the following:

- African Americans are 3 times more likely to die from asthma than non-Hispanic whites. Asian American adults are less likely than white adults to have heart disease; they are also less likely to die from heart disease.

- Lesbians are less likely to obtain preventive services for cancer.

Social Determinants of Health

Closely linked to health disparities are social determinants, which are the circumstances that influence where individuals work, play, pray, work, and conduct their lives. The varied economic and social factors play different roles in health, well-being, and overall risk of premature death. It has been documented that one's risk of premature death is broken down into 40% associated with individual behavior, 30% with genetics, 20% with social and environmental factors, and 10% with health care. It is with this understanding that medical organizations have publicly committed to addressing the social determinants of health in an effort to promote health equity. The WHO has expanded the definition to include inequity of financial resources on the global level, with leveraging of resources as a crucial action between majority and emerging countries in order to decrease the health gap. Other organizations, such as the National Academy of Medicine and the Robert Wood Johnson Foundation, have looked at life expectancy in relationship to census tracks or neighborhood-level data. This information can be used to identify disparities between city blocks, as well as between cities and states. Physicians can use these data to construct population health statistics, identify the socioeconomic status of their practice communities, and quantify structural barriers, such as number and location of public health centers, pharmacies, and hospitals that may not be easily accessible. Other factors to consider include access to fresh foods, transportation, adequate housing, and recreation, which also contribute to overall health and well-being. Box 64–3 illustrates six social determinants of health areas. These ecologic determinants influence health and disease prevalence but are rarely included in patient histories. Expanding the

Box 64–3: Social determinants of health.

Economic Stability	Neighborhood and Physical Environment	Education	Food	Community and Social Context	Healthcare System
Employment Income Expenses Debt Medical bills Support	Housing Transportation Safety Parks Playgrounds Walkability	Literacy (including health literacy) Language Early childhood education Vocational training Higher education	Hunger Access to healthy options	Social integration Support systems Community engagement Discrimination	Health coverage Provider availability Provider linguistic and cultural competency Quality of care
Health Outcomes: mortality, morbidity, life expectancy, healthcare expenditures, health status, functional limitations					

Reproduced with permission from Artiga S, Hinton E: *Beyond Health Care: The Role of Social Determinants in Promoting Health and Health Equity.* Kaiser Family Foundation. May 10, 2018. https://www.kff.org/disparities-policy/issue-brief/beyond-health-care-the-role-of-social-determinants-in-promoting-health-and-health-equity/.

biopsychosocial model to include ecologic factors provides a larger contextual model to evaluate a patient's health risks, susceptibilities, and health outcomes. Asking salient questions that reflect the patient's broader living situation is a more effective approach in guiding healthcare decisions and health interventions.

American Academy of Family Physicians. The Everyone Project: advancing health equity in every community. 2017. https://www.aafp.org/patient-care/social-determinants-of-health/everyone-project.html. Accessed January 26, 2019.

American Academy of Family Physicians. Research page into social determinants of health. https://www.aafp.org/media-center/kits/social-determinants-of-health/research-page-into-social-social-determinants-of-health.html. Accessed December 10, 2019.

Dilley JA, Simmons KW, Boysun MJ, et al. Demonstrating the importance and feasibility of including sexual orientation in public health surveys: health disparities in the Pacific Northwest. *Am J Public Health.* 2010;100(3):460–467. [PMID: 19696397]

Health Landscape. www.healthlandscape.org. Accessed December 10, 2019. (Health landscape tools for geomapping of communities that allows for community needs assessment, policy analysis to improve health care access in underserved areas.)

Hughes LS, Phillips RL, DeVoe JE, Bazemore A. Community vital signs: taking the pulse of the community while caring for patients. *J Am Board Fam Med.* 2016;29(3):419–422. [PMID: 27170802]

Like RC. Educating clinicians about cultural competence and disparities in health and health care. *J Contin Educ Health Prof.* 2011;31(3):197–207. [PMID: 21953661]

McCarthy D, How S, Ashley-Kay F, et al. *The Commonwealth Fund: Why Not the Best? Results from the National Scorecard on US Health System Performance. The Commonwealth Fund on a High Performance Health Care System.* October 2011. https://www.commonwealthfund.org/publications/fund-reports/2011/oct/why-not-best-results-national-scorecard-us-health-system. Accessed December 10, 2019.

Robert Wood Johnson Foundation. Could where you live influence how long you live? www.RWJF.org/en/library/interactives/whereyouliveaffectshowlongyoulive.html. Accessed December 10, 2019.

Schroeder S. We can do better: improving the health of the American people. *N Engl J Med.* 2007;357:1221–1228. [PMID: 17881753]

Sohn H. Racial and ethnic disparities in health insurance coverage: dynamics of gaining and losing coverage over the life-course. *Popul Res Policy Rev.* 2017;36(2):181–201. [PMID: 28366968]

► Theorizing Health & Illness Causation & Establishing the Therapeutic Relationship

Health and disease are interrelated dynamic processes. Definitions of both include biomedical, social, ecological, spiritual, and psychological constructs. Illness is a socially influenced condition and must be viewed within the socially recognized reality defined by the patient. Illness causation and etiologies influence the physician-patient interaction, and a culture-centered approach to care encourages physicians to offer solace and relief from the patient's viewpoint and experiences. There is a power differential with every clinical encounter, which impacts the physician-patient alliance. Medical and psychological problems are managed within this context and require the physician to mediate this imbalance through various techniques. These include affirmations and strengths that the patient may exhibit through healthy behaviors, lifestyle choices, beneficial existential cultural beliefs, and practices that advance health.

Family medicine offers helpful strategies through supportive and intentional counseling, such as motivational interviewing, which encourages affirmations and self-reflections that are patient directed. Other skills that empower patients include expressing empathy during the encounter and exhibiting a practice style that encompasses and appreciates diversity. Physician attributes such as eliciting the patient's goals and projecting a willingness to negotiate care options and patient preferences have been shown to increase visit satisfaction and adherence to treatment. Although time constraints create limitations on patient interactions, these activities do not add significantly to the length of the visit and do improve overall quality of care.

Implicit Bias

Implicit bias, also defined as social cognition, is the unconscious assignment of specific attributes ascribed to members of an identified socially racialized group. These perceptions are developed by learned associations assigned to certain groups and can produce in-group versus out-group associations. The in group has commonalities that shape one's worldview and beliefs, creating categorizations and potential "isms." These perceptions are usually influenced by stereotypes, which can be explicit (or conscious) or implicit (or unconscious). The latter are unrecognized during the clinical encounter but can influence the doctor-patient relationship, therapeutic decisions, and clinical outcomes. Implicit bias is malleable, and various methodologies and training techniques can be employed to minimize the impact and expression of bias thoughts and action.

Self-awareness and strong communication skills are key to establishing a strong therapeutic relationship and equality. Physicians must be aware of any implicit biases they may hold. As a society, we are conditioned to associate certain things with various demographic characteristics including gender, sex, age, race, and ethnicity. Historically, a bias has been documented regarding gender roles and science, with men being favored as the more equipped practitioners. Numerous studies have shown that physicians demonstrate similar levels of racial and ethnic bias as the general public. Resources such as Harvard's Project Implicit (https://implicit.harvard.edu/implicit/education.html) can assist individuals to identify biases they may not know they possess. Through increased self-reflection, cultural humility, and lifelong learning as it relates to diverse populations, change, and the relational dynamics between patients and physicians, a mutually effective partnership between patient, family, and provider can be put into practice.

Explanatory Models of Health, Illness, & Care

Patient-centered care focuses on engaging patients and their families in the care management plan and healthcare decision making. Health advocacy is linked to this model of care and encourages patients to be actively involved in the design and planning of their own healthcare delivery, in addition to the larger medical system. Attributes associated with patient-centered care mirror some of the tenets of culturally competent care. They include care that is "whole-person" focused; encourages patient empowerment and engagement; and emphasizes communication and coordination that is sensitive to the patient's linguistic level, personal preferences, cultural strengths, and values. The foundation for these principles is derived from Engel and Roman's biopsychosocial model, which maintains the patient's human dimension as the central focus to the medical encounter. Physicians are required to go beyond the traditional reductionist biomedical approach and incorporate cultural variables regarding family and community, health beliefs, and expectations in the therapeutic process.

Engel's biopsychosocial approach recognizes the complex interactions between healthcare delivery and the patient's beliefs and behaviors concerning wellness, illness, and disease. It is supported and enhanced by the clinical lessons offered by Kleinman's explanatory model, a tool for physicians to aid in providing culturally competent care. The model is elicited through open-ended questions, originally eight questions, focused on how patients perceive their illness state, their beliefs regarding causality, and perceived forms of treatment. This information provides contextual data, which strengthens the therapeutic alliance and informs the physician regarding diagnosis and management. The advantages in using this approach have been validated through qualitative and quantitative research that enriches medical practice as well as population health. Practical applications give physicians a living illness experience associated with their patients. It also provides information about sick roles and behaviors that are linked to care in various scenarios covering social health issues, including HIV/AIDS, domestic violence, and other community ills.

Mental & Behavioral Health

Mental health can be seen as the result of the complex interactions between biological, psychological, social, and cultural factors. The influence of any of these factors can be stronger or weaker depending on the illness or disorder. Cultural and social factors can affect patients' beliefs as to symptom causation and inform their reaction and reception to a diagnosis of mental illness.

Despite its prevalence in all cultures, mental health can carry with it a significant amount of shame and stigma around a diagnosis. In other cultures, acknowledging the illness can have consequences on the perception of the entire family. Cultural and religious communities have the power to demystify mental illness, while assisting and supporting individuals and their families.

Because of the complexities that exist around mental illness, numerous disparities exist and persist in culturally diverse communities. The US Surgeon General's report on mental health found the following:

- Minorities have less access to, have less availability of, and receive fewer mental health services.
- Minorities in treatment often receive a poorer quality of mental health care.
- Minorities are underrepresented in mental health research.
- Racial and ethnic minorities collectively experience a greater disability burden from mental illness than do

Box 64–4: LEARN model.

Listen to patients' perspectives.
Explain medical views.
Acknowledge similarities and differences.
Recommend a course of action.
Negotiate plans.

whites; this higher level of burden stems from minorities receiving less care and poorer quality of care, rather than from the fact that their illnesses are inherently more severe or prevalent in the community.

Application of Cultural Information & Skills in Clinical Interactions

Several tools that are available to family physicians can provide guidance in interacting with patients and incorporating cultural elements as part of the clinical assessment. Beginning with the Berlin and Fowkes' LEARN model (Box 64–4), others have been developed, including the BATHE, ESFT, ETHNIC, and CRASH frameworks. They provide the patient an opportunity to engage in and elaborate on signs and symptoms from their cultural perspective.

Betancourt JR, Carrillo JE, Green AR. Hypertension in multicultural and minority populations: linking communication to compliance. *Curr Hypertens Rep.* 1999;1(6):482–488. [PMID: 10981110]
Flores G, Abreu M, Pizzo-Barone C, Bachur R, Lin H. Errors of medical interpretation and their potential clinical consequences: a comparison of professional versus ad hoc versus no interpreters. *Ann Emerg Med.* 2012;60(5):545–553. [PMID: 22424655]
Hall W, Chaptman M, Lee K, et al. Implicit racial/ethnic bias among health care professionals and its influence on health care outcomes: a systematic review. *Am J Public Health.* 2015;105(12):e60–e76. [PMID: 26469668]
Institute of Medicine. *Speaking of Health: Assessing Health Communication Strategies for Diverse Populations. IOM, Committee on Communication for Behavior Change in the 21st Century: Improving the Health of Diverse Populations.* Washington, DC: Institute of Medicine; 2002.
Levin SJ, Like RC, Gottlieb JE. ETHNIC: a framework for culturally competent clinical practice. *Patient Care.* 2000;9(special issue):188. [No PMID]
Weiner SJ, Schwartz A, Sharma G, et al. Patient-centered decision making and health care outcomes. An observational study. *Ann Intern Med.* 2013;158(8):573–579. [PMID: 23588745]

ENGAGING IN CULTURALLY & LINGUISTICALLY APPROPRIATE CARE

Going Beyond the Clinical Interview

Fundamental to every clinical encounter is establishing a therapeutic relationship with a patient that is affirming, inclusive, and collaborative. This chapter provides information

for family physicians to assist in establishing that relationship. The information presented should be viewed as a starting point along the continuum of cultural and linguistic competency. This lifelong process begins with recognizing the inherent strengths and value of human diversity. The continuum also includes the confrontation of personal and societal bias, fosters the growth of cultural awareness and sensitivity, and develops the cross-cultural knowledge and skills that will improve clinical practice.

National Standards for Culturally & Linguistically Appropriate Services in Health & Health Care

The national culturally and linguistically appropriate services (CLAS) standards provide a blueprint with which to operationalize and institutionalize the concepts of cultural and linguistic competency and are intended to advance health equity, improve quality, and help eliminate healthcare disparities. The standards can assist physicians, small practices, and large hospitals plan and implement culturally and linguistically appropriate services geared toward improving care and services. Physicians need to be active members in clinics, hospitals, and medical societies in order to create culturally and linguistically competent institutions. Physicians can be powerful advocates for hiring bilingual-bicultural workers, employing trained interpreters, creating health education approaches for patients with limited English proficiency, ensuring quality translation, and engaging institutions in caring for diverse patients (Box 64–5). The national CLAS standards are referenced throughout the following case study to illustrate their application; however, to achieve the intended outcomes, the standards should be implemented in their entirety. The national CLAS standards and their accompanying guidance document, *A Blueprint for Advancing and Sustaining CLAS Policy and Practice,* are available through the Department of Health and Human Services, Office of Minority Health, Think Cultural Health website.

Box 64–5: Important terms to know.

Interpretation
The process of understanding and analyzing a spoken or signed message and reexpressing that message faithfully, accurately, and objectively in another language, taking the cultural and social context into account.

Translation
The conversion of a written text into a corresponding written text in a different language.

Data from Department of Health and Human Services, Office of Minority Health. National standards for culturally and linguistically appropriate services in health and health care: A blueprint for advancing and sustaining CLAS policy and practice. 2013. https://thinkculturalhealth.hhs.gov/assets/pdfs/EnhancedCLASStandardsBlueprint.pdf.

CASE 1

GT was a 42-year-old Spanish-speaking Latin American woman who presented at the family medicine center with headaches, malaise, nausea, one episode of vomiting, and weakness of 1 day's duration. The patient presented with several teenage children who appeared challenging to manage in the clinic. The constant interruptions made it difficult for the provider to obtain the history and conduct a physical exam. On initial presentation, the patient noted that the headaches were increasingly severe and unusual because of the intensity. Previous headaches had been relieved with over-the-counter medications. After a series of pointed questions through the use of a nurse interpreter who spoke Spanish, the patient was informed that the diagnosis was most likely the "flu," or exacerbation of stress-related tension headaches. The vital signs and examination were nonfocal, except for bradycardia of 55 bpm and a temperature of 99.8°F. The patient did not return to the clinic but presented later to the local emergency department because of worsening symptoms and was urgently evaluated and stabilized for toxic exposure to dried oleander leaves prepared for medicinal purposes. The leaves were obtained from a curandero local to the area where the patient lived.

In the current case, there are several points to consider.

▶ The Importance of Effective Communication

National CLAS standards 4, 5, 6, 7, 8, and 13 are just a few of the standards that can assist in providing effective communication for patients regardless of their English proficiency or communication needs (eg, deaf or hard of hearing).

The use of a lay or ad hoc interpreter is problematic and should not be acceptable in most settings (Box 64–6). A certified interpreter should be the standard for healthcare communications, and if unavailable, other modalities, such as phone banks and/or virtual interpreter programs should be

Box 64–6: From the literature.

> A cross-sectional error analysis was conducted to compare interpreter errors and their potential consequences in encounters with professional versus ad hoc versus no interpreters.
>
> Over a period of 30 months, emergency department visits in the two largest pediatric emergency departments in Massachusetts were audiotaped and analyzed.
>
> The resultant error rates for the three groups were as follows:
> - Professional interpreter: 12%
> - Ad hoc interpreter: 22%
> - No interpreter: 20%

Data from Flores G, Abreu M, Barone CP, et al: Errors of medical interpretation and their potential clinical consequences: a comparison of professional versus ad hoc versus no interpreters. *Ann Emerg Med.* 2012 Nov;60(5):545–553.

used. Physicians should be familiar with the different roles and types of interpreters. This includes video remote interpreting and telephonic or in-person interpreting. It is also important for physicians to appreciate the importance of using certified interpreters who have been assessed for their language proficiency and knowledge of medical terminology. The use of interpreters includes recognizing the importance of verbal and nonverbal cues, posture, and positioning with interpreters. In addition, the value of touch as therapeutic can be helpful in solidifying the physician-patient relationship, while the interpreter remains in the background.

Effective communication is fundamental to providing health care to diverse patients. Care that acknowledges and supports the patient's cultural beliefs and practices (eg, folk medicine, alternative treatments) allows patients to participate in negotiating a management plan. It may also reveal questionable or even harmful responses to the illness condition and provide a teachable moment for change. Care that includes cultural accommodations, when appropriate, builds trust in the professional's and patient's faith in the clinical process. Care that includes cultural negotiations and accommodations encourages patients and their families to participate in the clinical process and builds trust in the professional relationship.

Conversational styles vary across cultures and are challenging. For optimal communication, physicians must adapt their standard interviewing techniques to match patients' communication styles. Do not assume that one methodology will be effective for interviewing and relaying clinical information. In addition, appreciation for verbal-nonverbal cues is important. Although physicians may feel comfortable with a straightforward approach with direct eye contact, patients from various backgrounds and cultures may feel intimidated and threatened by this position. They may not answer questions, choose to change the subject, or simply remain silent. Misinterpretation of delivery of information can result in problems with adherence, follow-up, and outcomes.

Physicians can learn general approaches from community experts, such as bilingual-bicultural colleagues, and make adaptations as they are attuned to people's verbal and nonverbal cues.

▶ Recognizing the Important Roles of Traditional Medicine & Traditionalist Practitioners

National CLAS standards 4, 9, 11, 12, and 13 are a few of the standards that can assist in recognizing the important roles that traditional medicine and traditional practitioners serve as forms of community support.

Recognizing folk illness beliefs and interpretation of signs and symptoms is also linked with how patients respond to illness and disease. Culture influences help-seeking behaviors, which will be expressed in multiple ways, such as when and who is consulted first, treatment preferences, and expectations for healing. Indigenous practices and practitioners, such as herbalists, shamanists, and curanderos, may not be discussed during the family practice visit unless rapport is established and cultural sensitivity is demonstrated. Medicinal therapies may be taken alongside prescription medications and may be substituted because of side effects, the appearance of the pills, or confusion about the regimen. Family physicians should be familiar with some commonly used botanicals and herbs, since drug toxicities can present as chief complaints. Examples include ginseng and licorice, causing hypertension; chamomile tea, leading to anaphylaxis; ephedra (ma huang), causing a wide range of cardiovascular effects; and liver enzyme induction with eucalyptus oil, sassafras, and comfrey. In the present patient case, early signs of oleander toxicity could have been identified during the history-gathering process, instead of the premature diagnosis of "flu," viremia, or tension headache. Family physicians should sensitively ask their patients what they are taking and encourage them to bring their remedies into the office to discuss together.

A visit to the family medicine clinic or hospital may be the last resort when patients become ill. Patients may experience shame and humiliation by other family or community members if they seek care outside of normative practices or standards. Family physicians must therefore exhibit an open and nonjudgmental attitude, avoiding bias in evaluation and treatment. Family physicians should consider mobilizing additional resources and recognized community health experts in working with culturally diverse patients, especially where there may be knowledge gaps or other challenges.

▶ Use an Inclusive & Participatory Care Model

National CLAS standards 1, 10, 11, and 13 are a few of the standards that can assist in identifying, using, and maintaining an inclusive and participatory care model.

Encourage a participatory care model. Patient's and physician's information is interpreted through a cultural lens and influences the direction of the clinical questions leading to the diagnosis. Physicians who use a participatory framework allow patients to actively participate in the physician-patient exchange. Patients can offer explanatory models about their beliefs, perceptions of illness, and disease states, as well as offer information about their treatments. Patients allowed to engage and interject their health concepts and ideas will share more crucial information during the visit. The result will be a more accurate diagnosis, more appropriate management plan, and better adherence to treatment. Patient satisfaction leads to better patient follow-up, even if the diagnosis is inconclusive or, in this case, inaccurate. In this particular case, the patient most likely felt dissatisfied with the diagnostic explanation offered and sought care in the emergency department as a last resort. This was also

a missed learning opportunity for the physician, since the patient did not return for follow-up care.

Aboumater H, Cooper L. Contextualizing patient-centered care to fulfill its promise of better health outcomes; beyond who, what and why. *Ann Intern Med.* 2013;158(8):628–629. [PMID: 23588750]

Lorié Á, Reinero DA, Phillips M, Zhang L, Riess H. Culture and nonverbal expressions of empathy in clinical settings: A systematic review. *Patient Educ Couns.* 2017;100(3):411–424.

Flores G, Abreu M, Pizzo-Barone C, Bachur R, Lin H. Errors of medical interpretation and their potential clinical consequences: a comparison of professional versus ad hoc versus no interpreters. *Ann Emerg Med.* 2012;60(5):545–553. [PMID: 22424655]

Havranek EP, Hanratty R, Tate C, et al. The effect of values affirmation on race-discordant patient-provider communication. *Arch Intern Med.* 2012;172(21):1662–1667. [PMID: 23128568]

Riekert KA, Borreilli B, Bilderback A, et al. The development of a motivational interviewing intervention to promote medication adherence among inner-city African-American adolescents with asthma. *Patient Educ Couns.* 2011;82:117–122. [PMID: 20371158]

US Department of Health and Human Services, Office of Minority Health. *National Standards on Culturally and Linguistically Appropriate Services in Health and Health Care.* https://www.thinkculturalhealth.hhs.gov/clas/standards. Accessed June 9, 2018.

The quality of interpersonal care and interpersonal communications impacts all aspects of the health encounter. Research confirms that when physicians are more inclusive in their interactions and when patients are more involved as partners, consensus around treatment is more successful with increased satisfaction with care. A participatory model of caregiving that includes a biopsychosocioecological framework has a greater impact on positive behavior change and sustaining the physician-patient relationship. This has a direct effect on outcome rating scores and liability protection independent of diagnostic accuracy.

Providing cross-cultural care requires physicians to participate in lifelong learning both intellectually and experientially. Providing culturally competent care is a process requiring a deliberate study framework across a theoretical continuum of self-assessment and discovery. Continuous self-reflection, evaluation, and reevaluation are required if family physicians are to remain current in their understanding of changing demographics and emerging dominant populations regionally and nationally. Self-study, participation in discussion networks, and virtual community exchanges may be efficient strategies to engage in the learning process. Recently, the inclusion of evidence-based medicine has been added as a methodology to reduce health disparities as well as bias in clinical decision making. Integrating validated research and clinical guidelines and including patient values help to minimize unconscious or conscious bias in decision making and treatment strategies. Family physicians provide care in diverse clinical settings and therefore must continually nourish appreciation and sensitivity for their patient's cultural needs. This is a required educational journey if one is to partake in the universal goal to offer care that is personally meaningful and continues the ongoing search to address human sickness and healing in society.

The following sources are recommended for further information:

- American Board of Family Medicine: Cultural Competency Methods in Medicine Module. Five modules that qualify for Part IV recertification credit were released in fall 2010.
- American Muslim Health Professionals. http://amhp.us/
- Asian and Pacific Islander American Health Forum. http://www.apiahf.org
- Cross Cultural Health Care Program. www.xculture.org
- Ethnomed. www.ethnomed.org
- Gay and Lesbian Medical Association (GLMA). www.glma.org
- Department of Health and Human Services (HHS) Centers for Medicare and Medicaid Services, Office of Minority Health. go.cms.gov/omh
- HHS Health Resources and Services Agency (HRSA)
  - Toolkits, videos. http://www.hrsa.gov/culturalcompetence/index.html
- HHS Office of Minority Health, Think Cultural Health. https://www.thinkculturalhealth.hhs.gov
  - National Standards for Culturally and Linguistically Appropriate Services in Health and Health Care
  - A Physician's Practical Guide to Culturally Competent Care (9 CME)
- National Center for Cultural Competence (NCCC). http://nccc.georgetown.edu/
- National Coalition for LGBT Health. https://healthlgbt.org/
- National Council on Interpreting in Health Care. http://www.ncihc.org/
- National Health Law Program. http://www.healthlaw.org
- National Hispanic Medical Association. http://www.nhmamd.org/
- National Institutes for Health. Cultural respect. http://www.nih.gov/clearcommunication/culturalcompetency.htm
- National Medical Association. http://www.nmanet.org/
- Provider's Guide to Quality and Culture. https://innovations.ahrq.gov/qualitytools/providers-guide-quality-culture-0
- Resources for Cross-Cultural Health. www.diversityrx.org
- Society of Healthcare Professionals with Disabilities. http://www.disabilitysociety.org/
- W. K. Kellogg Foundation. http://www.wkkf.org

Health & Healthcare Disparities

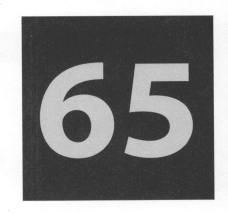

Jeannette E. South-Paul, MD, DHL (Hon), FAAFP

Evelyn L. Lewis, MD, MA, FAAFP, DABDA

BACKGROUND & DEFINITIONS

Health disparities are defined by the National Institutes of Health as "differences in the incidence, prevalence, mortality, and burden of diseases and other adverse health conditions that exist among specific population groups in the United States." Cardiovascular disease, cancer, and diabetes mellitus are the most commonly reported health disparities, followed by cerebrovascular diseases, unintentional injuries, and human immunodeficiency virus (HIV)/acquired immunodeficiency syndrome (AIDS). Assessing these differences requires that a wide variety of factors, including age, gender, nationality, family of origin, religiosity, education, income, geographic location, race or ethnicity, sexual orientation, and disability, be considered.

Healthcare disparities are defined by the Institute of Medicine (now called the National Academy of Medicine) as "differences in the quality of healthcare that are not due to access-related factors or clinical needs, preferences, and appropriateness of intervention." Causes of healthcare disparities most often relate to quality and include provider-patient relationships, provider bias and discrimination, and patient variables such as mistrust of the healthcare system and refusal of treatment. Although disparities in health and health care can be inextricably tied to one another, distinguishing between them increases our understanding of the complexity of the problem.

When considering health disparities from a population health perspective, the focus turns to an underrecognized determinant of health disparities described as the "Fundamental Causes" theory. This theory stipulates that when new health knowledge arises, those groups with higher socioeconomic status (SES) benefit more than groups with lower SES because of their greater material and nonmaterial resources. However, it is well known that various factors influence health. A helpful framework for understanding these factors is evident in the model described in the County Health Rankings where the percent contributions of a variety of factors can explain why there are disparities in health outcomes (Figure 65–1).

The Healthy People goals were initiated each decade beginning in the late 1990s as a way of setting goals to progressively address disparities. The changes in the demographics of the US population are reflected in changes in Healthy People goals. Healthy People 2000 goals were to reduce health disparities; Healthy People 2010 goals were to eliminate those disparities. Healthy People 2020 expands these goals further to focus on achieving health equity, eliminating disparities, and improving the health of all groups. The disparities evident in the health and/or health care of the US population reflect inconsistencies in implementing these principles.

Approximately one-third of Americans (slightly more than 100 million) self-identify as belonging to a racial or ethnic minority group, 51% of Americans (154 million) are women, 12% of Americans (36 million) not living in nursing homes or other residential care facilities have a disability, 70.5 million Americans (23%) live in rural areas and 233.5 million (77%) live in urban areas, and 4% of Americans identified themselves as lesbian, gay, bisexual, or transgender. Each of these groups experiences certain disparities in health or health care. (See Chapter 66 for a comprehensive discussion on the health disparities experienced by the LGBT community.) An estimated one in four Americans (almost 70 million persons) is classified as a member of one of the four major racial or ethnic minority groups: African American, Latino/Hispanic, Native American, and Asian/Pacific Islander. The US Census Bureau estimates that by the year 2050, people of color will represent one in three Americans. These populations bear a disproportionate burden of illness and disease relative to their percentage distribution in the population. Understanding the factors that contribute to inequities in health among these populations and the strategies that have resulted in improved health can inform and promote the delivery of quality health care.

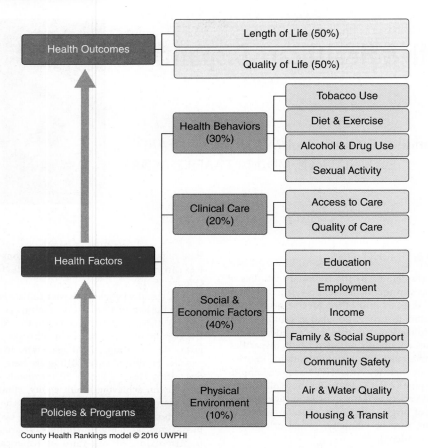

County Health Rankings model © 2016 UWPHI

▲ **Figure 65–1. County Health Rankings and Roadmaps.** (Reproduced with permission from County Health Rankings & Roadmaps. https://www.countyhealthrankings.org/explore-health-rankings/measures-data-sources/county-health-rankings-model.)

Burgoine T, Mackenbach JD, Lakerveld J, et al. Interplay of socioeconomic status and supermarket distance is associated with excess obesity risk: a UK cross-sectional study. *Int J Environ Res Public Health.* 2017;14:1290. [PMID: 29068365]

Smedley BD, Stith AY, Nelson AR, et al. *Unequal Treatment: Confronting Racial and Ethnic Disparities in Health Care.* Washington, DC: Institute of Medicine, Committee on Understanding and Eliminating Racial and Ethnic Disparities in Health Care; 2002.

US Department of Health and Human Services. *Healthy People 2010: National Health Promotion and Disease Prevention Objectives;* conference ed. in 2 vols. Washington, DC: Department of Health and Human Services; 2000.

US Department of Health and Human Services. Health People 2020. http://healthypeople.gov/2020/about/default.aspx. Accessed June 11, 2013.

Williams DR. Race, socioeconomic status, and health. The added effects of racism and discrimination. *Ann NY Acad Sci.* 1999;896:173–188. [PMID: 10681897]

APPROACHES TO DISPARITIES IN HEALTH OUTCOMES

In recent years, terms that had been used largely in academic settings such as *health equity* and *social determinants of health* have become more meaningful in establishing a framework to address modifiable factors for improving health. The Robert Wood Johnson Foundation released a series of issue briefs that began by establishing definitions: "Health equity means that everyone has a fair and just opportunity to be as healthy as possible. This requires removing obstacles to health such as poverty, discrimination, and their consequences, including powerlessness and lack of access to good jobs with fair pay, quality education and housing, safe environments, and health care. For the purposes of measurement, health equity means reducing and ultimately eliminating disparities in health and its determinants that adversely affect excluded or marginalized groups." The necessary actions that could remedy what this definition describes are founded on an understanding of the fundamental social determinants of health—nonmedical factors such as employment, income, housing, transportation, child care, education, discrimination, and the quality of the places where people live, work, learn, and play, which influence health. There must logically be measurement of progress toward health equity in order to assure positive change and accountability.

Braveman PA. Swimming against the tide: challenges in pursuing health equity today. *Acad Med.* 2019;94(2):170–171. [PMID: 30431455]

Braveman P, Arkin E, Orleans T, et al. *What Is Health Equity? And What Difference Does a Definition Make?* Princeton, NJ: Robert Wood Johnson Foundation; 2017.

HEALTHCARE DISPARITIES & THE LITERATURE

▶ Institute of Medicine Reports

In 1999, a report from the Institute of Medicine (IOM) entitled "Unequal Treatment: Confronting Racial and Ethnic Disparities in Health Care" was written in response to a request from Congress to address the extent of racial and ethnic disparities in health care. Following the review of >100 publications, the IOM study committee concluded that research findings consistently indicated that minorities were less likely than whites to receive needed services, including lifesaving procedures. The most commonly reported healthcare disparities were seen in cardiovascular disease, cancer, and diabetes. Other illnesses included cerebrovascular diseases, mental illness, and HIV/AIDS.

The IOM committee noted factors contributing to these complex healthcare disparities related to (1) minority patients' attitudes toward health care and preferences for and differing responses to treatment; (2) the operation of healthcare systems and regulatory environment in which they function (eg, lack of interpretation services for those with limited English proficiency, lack of resources for those with limited health literacy); and (3) factors derived from the clinical encounter. The committee suggested that provider bias, clinical uncertainty, and stereotyping or beliefs about the behavior of minorities may have a negative impact on the health outcomes of minorities. On the other side of the clinical encounter is the patient, whose reaction to the provider's biased or stereotyped behaviors may also contribute to disparities. In fact, a 2003 landmark report from the IOM highlighted the health casualties for minorities resulting from the intersection of implicit bias and the healthcare provided to them. The report documented that African Americans and other ethnic minority groups received fewer procedures and poorer quality of care than their white counterparts. These findings were consistent across the spectrum of simple to complex diagnostic and therapeutic interventions and persisted even after statistical adjustment for confounders that included elements of the social determinants of health, health insurance, stage and severity of disease, and comorbid conditions.

▶ National Healthcare Disparities Report

With a directive from the Healthcare Research and Quality Act of 1999 (Public Law 106-129) and guidance from the IOM (now National Academy of Medicine), the Agency for Healthcare Research and Quality (AHRQ) developed and produced two reports: the National Healthcare Disparities Report (NHDR) and the National Healthcare Quality Report (NHQR). The two reports were released simultaneously in 2003 to review the performance of the healthcare system as a step towards gaining future improvement. Since the original reports were released, reporting in one document has been available electronically every few years. The most recent National Healthcare Quality and Disparities Report published in 2017 revealed improvements in a number of areas while lags persisted in others.

Approximately 43% of access measures showed improvement (2000-2016), 43% did not show improvement, and 14% showed worsening. For example, from 2000 to 2017, there were significant gains in the percentage of people who reported having health insurance. In 2017, among adults ages 18-64, 69.3% had private health insurance, 19.3% had public coverage, and 12.8% were uninsured. After generally increasing, the percentage of adults ages 18-64 who were uninsured at the time of assessment generally decreased. In 2017, 24.4% of adults ages 18-64 who were poor, 23.8% who were near poor, and 8.2% who were not poor lacked health insurance coverage at the time of assessment.

Quality of healthcare improved overall from 2000 through 2015 but the pace of improvement varied by priority area. Metrics for quality care reflect trends towards person-centered care, patient safety, healthy living, effective treatment, care coordination, and affordable care. From 32% to 56% of disparities in healthcare quality have not improved in the past 10 years for African Americans, Latinos, Native Americans and Asian Americans. For example in 2016, the rate of new HIV cases per 100,000 population age 13 and over was worse for Blacks compared with Whites (52.9 vs 6.0). In 2015, the rate of adults with potentially avoidable hospital admissions for hypertension per 100,000 population was worse for Blacks than for Whites (170.3 admissions/100,00 compared with 33.9 admissions/100,000.

There were significant disparities for poor and uninsured populations in all priority areas. While some disparities were getting smaller from 2000 through 2015, disparities persist, especially among people in poor and low-income households and uninsured people. The National Healthcare Quality and Disparities Report (QDR) continues to track the nation's performance on healthcare access, quality, and disparities. The QDR data demonstrate progress in some areas while other areas merit more attention where wide variations persist.

U.S. Department of Health and Human Services (HHS) agencies are focusing on many of the priority areas, most notably opioid misuse, patient safety, effective treatment, and health disparities to include developing a strategy to address the ongoing opioid abuse crisis. The National Institute on Minority Health and Health Disparities now has an online data resource, *HDPulse*, for public health professionals and researchers that allows users to explore issues related to health disparities and access data, published reports, and public use files.

Website

2017 National Healthcare Quality and Disparities Report. Rockville, MD: Agency for Healthcare Research and Quality; September 2018. AHRQ Pub. No. 18-0033-EF. Accessed February 20, 2020.

HISTORICAL FACTORS

Original American citizens of color bear a historical legacy that affects all aspects of their integration into society today. American Indians make up a fraction of today's citizens (0.7% in the 2000 census) but have significant health and healthcare disparities. The prevalence of diabetes mellitus, obesity, alcoholism, and suicide is substantially greater in this population than in other US population groups. They are the one population with a health system that was established to help meet their medical needs. The availability of these services, however, is limited by distance for the many American Indians living in rural areas, and they may be completely inaccessible to those living in urban areas.

African Americans encompass several groups who came to the United States at different times. The impact of slavery on the original Africans cannot be minimized. Residual effects of this historical tragedy have been associated with discriminatory residential practices, educational disadvantages, and treatment practices in separate but unequal healthcare facilities. Later immigrants of African origin came to the United States from the West Indies, where slavery was abolished well before the Emancipation Proclamation in the United States. These differing experiences have influenced the views of Caribbean Americans and result in differences between them and African Americans who descended directly from slaves on the North American continent. The final group of immigrants from African countries chose to come to the United States in recent years for educational, economic, and political reasons. Cultural differences often exist among these three groups and include differences in customs, family roles, religious preferences, and their definition and experience of illness and disease.

Although the foundation of the United States was a union of indigenous groups and immigrants, the preceding groups along with new immigrants bear much of the burden of disease in the nation today. The number of immigrants entering the United States since the late 1990s has increased dramatically compared with the numbers seen in the previous four decades. Political crises, natural disasters, poverty, and hunger have forced population groups of significant size to leave their homes. These migrations have resulted in loss of homes and support systems, overcrowding and overexposure, decreased access to food and medical services, and contact with new infectious agents and other toxins.

IMMIGRANTS & REFUGEES

Globally, the largest ever recorded number of international migrants is underway at an estimated 244 million, although the percentage of the world's population who are migrants has remained relatively constant at approximately 3%. Migration occurs within countries as well as encompasses populations trapped within a country they planned only to transit while seeking a different destination. Scholars dispute the distinction between voluntary and involuntary migration, but approximately 66 million people worldwide are thought to have been forced from their homes. These distinctions are important because they can affect the health status of these populations and ultimately their access to care. Most articles published from 2000 forward and described in a 2015 annual review focused on behavioral and cultural factors, whereas the structural factors that typically restrict access to health care were limited.

The term *immigrant* has been applied to legal and illegal (undocumented) refugees and children adopted from other countries. As of 2011, nearly 40 million immigrants were residing in the United States, accounting for 13% of the total population. Most immigrants reside in linguistically isolated households (those in which no one >14 years old speaks English), which were identified for the first time in the 1990 census. Four percent of US households are in this category. This figure includes 30% of Asian households, 23% of Hispanic households, and 28% of all immigrant households with school-age children.

Immigrants enter the United States from many countries, but those coming from Mexico represent the largest group. California is home to approximately 4% of the 240 million people worldwide who are living outside of their countries of origin. Many Mexican immigrants arrive in the United States healthier than their white counterparts. However, their health deteriorates the longer they live here, possibly as a result of lifestyle changes (years of difficult labor, poverty, smoking, poor diet, and lack of attention to prevention) and a lack of health insurance. One study found that 2.6% of recent Mexican immigrants had diabetes mellitus, compared with 7.7% of Mexican immigrants who had lived in the United States for

15 years. More than two-thirds of recent Mexican immigrants and 44.8% of "long-term immigrants" have no health insurance, compared with 22.5% of Mexican-born Americans and 12.3% of US-born whites. Fewer than 10% of recent Mexican immigrants reported using emergency departments in 2000. Furthermore, >33% of Mexican women age 18–64 years who were recent immigrants had not had a Pap smear in 3 years. Approximately 37% of recent Mexican immigrants visited a health clinic instead of a physician for health care, compared with 15% of US-born whites.

Noncitizens are 3 times more likely than citizens to be uninsured and have more limited access to care than US-born citizens and are less likely to obtain recommended preventive services. Noncitizens are also subject to Medicaid and Children's Health Insurance Program (CHIP) eligibility restrictions—specifically, being subject to a 5-year waiting period for Medicaid or CHIP coverage even when lawfully present in the United States. This group will continue to face eligibility restrictions (eg, waiting periods) for health coverage options under the Affordable Care Act. Safety net providers will remain a major source of care for immigrants.

Pregnant women are of major concern because of risk for poor pregnancy outcomes. Despite these concerns, evidence suggests that infants of Mexican immigrants have favorable birth outcomes despite their high socioeconomic risks. These favorable outcomes have been associated with a protective sociocultural orientation among this immigrant group, including a strong family unit. However, one-fourth of infants of immigrants in predominantly Spanish-speaking households are at high risk for serious infectious disease despite using preventive care. As these children mature beyond the neonatal period, factors predisposing to illness are large households, poor access to care, and maternal characteristics, including smoking, pregnancy complications, and employment.

Lack of understanding by healthcare providers of cultural norms and traditional remedies for common ailments can result in negative interactions between patients and clinicians, misdiagnosis, and poor health outcomes. In one study, healthcare providers and the population of Vietnamese immigrants for whom they cared both identified misinterpretation of patient symptoms and healthcare provider recommendations as major issues. The special problems of unemployment, depression, surviving torture, and obtaining assistance are all made more difficult for refugees living in small communities that lack sufficiently large ethnic populations to facilitate culturally sensitive provision of health care.

With the exception of Southeast Asian refugees, there are few clinical studies on the health problems of refugees after arrival in the United States. Tuberculosis, nutritional deficiencies, intestinal parasites, chronic hepatitis B infection, lack of immunization, and depression are major problems in many groups. The great variation in health and psychosocial issues, as well as cultural beliefs, among refugees requires careful attention during the medical encounter. In addition to a complete history and physical examination, tests for tuberculosis, hepatitis B surface antigen, and ova and parasites, and hemoglobin measurement are advised for most groups.

American Academy of Pediatrics, Committee on Community Health Services. Health care for children of immigrant families. *Pediatrics.* 1997;100:153. [PMID: 9229707]

Castañeda H, Holes SM, Madrigal DS, et al. Immigration as a social determinant of health. *Annu Rev Public Health.* 2015;36(1): 375–392. [PMID: 25494053]

Chen J, Wilkins R, Ng E. Health expectancy by immigrant status, 1986 and 1991. *Health Rep.* 1996;8:29–38. [PMID: 9085119]

Gómez S, Castañeda H. Recognize our humanity: Immigrant youth voices on health care in Arizona's restrictive political environment. *Qual Health Res.* 2018;1:1049732318755580. [PMID: 29448885]

Mahoney FJ, Lawrence M, Scott C, Le Q, Lambert S, Farley TA. Continuing risk for hepatitis B virus transmission among Southeast Asian infants in Louisiana. *Pediatrics.* 1995;96: 1113–1116. [PMID: 7491231]

National Academies of Sciences, Engineering, and Medicine. *Immigration as a Social Determinant of Health: Proceedings of a Workshop.* Washington, DC: The National Academies Press; 2018.

National Academies of Sciences, Engineering, and Medicine. *The Integration of Immigrants into American Society.* Washington, DC: The National Academies Press; 2015.

Pew Research Center. *Modern Immigration Wave Brings 59 Million to U.S., Driving Population Growth and Change Through 2065: Views of Immigration's Impact on U.S. Society Mixed.* Washington, DC: Pew Research Center; 2015.

Power DV, Shandy D. Sudanese refugees in a Minnesota family practice clinic. *Fam Med.* 1998;30:185–189. [PMID: 9532440]

Stephens J, Artiga S. *Key Facts on Health Coverage for Low-Income Immigrants Today and under the Affordable Care Act.* Kaiser Commission on Medicaid and the Uninsured: Key Facts; March 2013. http://kff.org/disparities-policy/fact-sheet/key-facts-on-health-coverage-for-low. Accessed June 11, 2013.

Wallace S, Zuniga E. *Mexican Immigrants' Health Status Worsens after Living in US.* http://www.kaisernetwork.org/daily_reports/re-index. Accessed October 14, 2005.

POVERTY

A greater percentage of African Americans (53%) and Hispanics (59%) have incomes that are below 200% of the federal poverty line than non-Hispanic white Americans (25%) across their lifespans. Financial disadvantage has an impact on health and health care in that mortality rates around the world decline with increasing social class, a concept most easily associated with access to financial resources.

Poor, minority, and uninsured children are twice as likely as other children to lack usual sources of care, nearly twice as likely to wait ≥60 minutes at their sites of care, and use only about half as many physician services after adjusting for health status. Poverty, minority status, and absence of insurance exert independent effects on access to and use of primary care. Homelessness results in poor health status and high service use among children. Homeless children were reported to experience a higher number of acute illness symptoms, including fever, ear infection, diarrhea, and asthma. Emergency department and outpatient medical visits are also higher among the homeless group.

Urban Institute and Kaiser Commission on Medicaid and the Uninsured. Key facts: race, ethnicity and medical care. In: *Analysis of March 2002 Current Population Survey*. San Francisco, CA: Kaiser Family Foundation; 2003.

Weinreb L, Goldberg R, Bassuk E, Perloff J. Determinants of health and service use patterns in homeless and low-income housed children. *Pediatrics*. 1998;102:554–562. [PMID: 9738176]

UNINSURANCE & UNDERINSURANCE

A substantial portion of the US population is medically uninsured or underinsured, and a greater percentage of racial and ethnic minorities and immigrants are in this category. These numbers increase if individuals who have been without health insurance for ≥3 months in a given year are included. Underinsurance is the inability to pay out-of-pocket expenses despite having insurance and usually implies inability to use preventive services as well. The underinsured category includes unemployed persons age 55–64 years and those not provided health insurance coverage through their employment. These individuals are not eligible for Medicare and must pay high individual health premiums when they can obtain some form of group coverage. Lack of health insurance is associated with delayed health care and increased mortality. Underinsurance also may result in adverse health consequences. An estimated 8 million children from diverse groups in the United States are uninsured. Substantial differences in both sources of care and utilization of medical services exist between insured and uninsured children.

In 2005, 34% of all nonelderly adult Hispanics living in the United States lacked health insurance coverage (either private or public), compared with 21% of African American, 19% of Asian/Pacific Islander, 32% of American Indian, and 13% of non-Hispanic white nonelderly citizens. Because Hispanics are more likely to be uninsured than any other ethnic group and because they are the fastest growing minority group in the United States, it is likely that the number of uninsured in the US population will steadily increase.

There are marked discrepancies in access to and utilization of medical services, including preventive services, between uninsured and insured children, although both groups have similar rates of chronic health conditions and limitations of activity (evidence of the general health of the children being seen). The 2002 IOM report, "Unequal Treatment," documented the widespread evidence of racial and ethnic disparities in health care. However, only 5 of the 103 published studies cited in this report addressed health disparities in children. Yet there appear to be disparities of equivalent magnitude and persistence in children as are seen in adults. Substantial gaps in insurance coverage exist among children such that 37% of Hispanic, 23% of African American, and 20% of non-Hispanic white children have no health insurance. Children of color are more likely to be insured through public programs such as Medicaid and the State Children's Health Insurance Program (SCHIP).

Children eligible for Medicaid but who remain unenrolled are often younger than 6 years of age, live in female-headed single-parent families, or are African American or Hispanic. Not only do uninsured children lack routine medical care, but they also lack appropriate well-child care compared with insured children. Children who have a chronic disease, such as asthma, face difficulties of access to care and use substantially fewer outpatient and inpatient services.

Parents' utilization of healthcare services has a large impact on the services used by their children. Even if all children were universally insured, parental healthcare access and utilization would remain a key determinant in children's use of services. Neglecting financial access to care for adults who serve as caregivers for children may have the unintended effect of diminishing the impact of targeted health insurance programs for children.

The uninsured can manifest similar psychopathology as is seen in refugees. Rates of current psychiatric disorders (including major depression, anxiety disorders, and history of sexual trauma) are extremely high in ethnically diverse women who are receiving public medical assistance or are uninsured. These women also report behaviors that pose serious health risks, including smoking (23%) and illicit drug use (2%). Fewer than half have access to comprehensive primary medical care. Young, poor women who seek care in public-sector clinics would benefit from comprehensive medical care addressing their psychosocial needs.

In the United States, the cost of healthcare services is a major barrier to healthcare access. In addition, three-fourths of persons in the United States who have difficulty paying their medical bills have some type of health insurance. Although the affordability of health care among persons without health insurance has been described, few details regarding affordability among persons who are underinsured exist.

Investigators who looked at state programs offering subsidized coverage in commercial managed care organizations to low-income and previously uninsured people found no evidence of pent-up demand or an unusual level of chronic illness between people enrolled through large employer-benefit plans and previously uninsured patients. Similarly, there was little evidence of underutilization, although dissatisfaction and reported barriers to service were more frequent among nonwhite enrollees. In another study, undocumented immigrants had more complicated and serious diagnoses on admission but a lower adjusted average length of stay than native-born populations and those with permanent residency status (insured by Medicaid or of uninsured status) admitted to the same hospital.

Although generalist physicians appear to be more likely than specialists to provide care for poor adult patients, they may still perceive financial and nonfinancial barriers to caring for these patients. Nonwhite physicians were more likely to care for uninsured and Medicaid patients than were white physicians. In addition to reimbursement, nonfinancial factors played an important role in physicians' decisions not to care for Medicaid or uninsured patients. For example, perceived risks of litigation and poor reimbursement were cited by 60–90% of physicians as important in the decision not to care for Medicaid and uninsured patients.

Launch of the Affordable Care Act (ACA) following passage in 2010 was a significant step toward reducing disparities and a pathway to improve health and healthcare disparities for low- and moderate-income populations. People of color and low-income individuals have more barriers to care and receive poorer quality of care. The ACA established a new continuum of coverage options to include individual states' ability to expand Medicaid to a national eligibility floor of 138% of the federal poverty level (FPL) ($26,344 for a family of three in 2012) and the creation of new Health Benefit Exchanges with tax credits for individuals up to 400% of the FPL ($76,300 for a family of three in 2012). These expansions were designed to help reduce the wide variations in access to health coverage across states and increase availability of coverage for low- and middle-income populations, significantly impacting people of color who are disproportionately uninsured or low income.

Since 2016, there have been a number of actions instituted that directly impact the ACA law. These actions, which included scaling back the ACA outreach and education programs, decreased funding for navigators who helped consumers find the right coverage, and termination of reimbursement payments to insurers for reducing cost-sharing for low-income enrollees, all of which threaten the ACA markets, to access lower cost coverage. If the healthiest people shift to the alternative markets, the cost of ACA-compliant coverage will increase – also compromising overall cost of this system to patients who do participate. The creation of alternative individual health coverage markets independent of those that are a part of the ACA has also generated considerable concerns because they may not provide adequate protection for some who choose them. Efforts to eliminate the ban on preexisting condition exclusions, a benefit that is critical for the majority of Americans, would be devastating to the availability of coverage for low- and middle-income populations, especially people of color who are disproportionately uninsured, underinsured, or low income. Although the numbers of the uninsured have remained stable through 2018, unsubsidized enrollment has dramatically decreased.

The most recent Congressional Budget Office analysis showed that repealing these provisions of the ACA would increase the number of uninsured individuals by an estimated 18 million in the first year of enacting the repeal. By 2026, the number of uninsured individuals is projected to increase by an estimated 32 million people.

Avruch S, Machlin S, Bonin P, Ullman F. The demographic characteristics of Medicaid-eligible uninsured children. *Am J Public Health*. 1998;88:445–447. [PMID: 9518979]

Beal AC. Policies to reduce racial and ethnic disparities in child health and health care. *Health Affairs*. 2004;23(5):171–179. [PMID: 15371383]

Braveman P, Cubbin C, Egerter S, Williams DR, Pamuk E. Socioeconomic disparities in the United States: what the patterns tell us. *Am J Public Health*. 2010;100(1):S186–S196. [PMID: 20147693]

Eltorai AEM, Eltoral M. The risk of expanding the uninsured population by repealing the affordable care act. http://jamanetwork.com/pdfaccess.ashx?url=/data/journals/jama/0/ by University of Pittsburgh. Accessed February 27, 2017.

Hanson KL. Is insurance for children enough? The link between parents' and children's health care use revisited. *Inquiry*. 1998;35:294–302. [PMID: 9809057]

Holt JL, Szilagyi PG, Rodewald LE, et al. Profile of uninsured children in the United States. *Arch Pediatr Adolesc Med*. 1995;149:398–406. [PMID: 7704168]

Jost TS. The Affordable Care Act Under the Trump Administration. *To the Point* (blog), Commonwealth Fund, August 30, 2018. https://www.commonwealthfund.org/blog/2018/affordable-care-act-under-trump-administration. Accessed December 9, 2019.

Kaiser Family Foundation. *Focus on Health Care Disparities: Key Facts*. December 2012. http://kff.org/disparities-policy/issue-brief/health-coverage-by-race-and-ethnicity-the-potential-impact-of-the-affordable-care-act/. Accessed December 9, 2019.

Kaiser Family Foundation. Urban Institute and Kaiser Commission on Medicaid and the Uninsured: Key facts: race, ethnicity and medical care. In: *Health Insurance Coverage in America: March 2005 Current Population Survey*. Kaiser Family Foundation; 2005. www.kaiseredu.org/tutorials/REHealthcare/player.html. Accessed October 25, 2009.

Kilbreth EH, Coburn AF, McGuire C, et al. State-sponsored programs for the uninsured: is there adverse selection? *Inquiry*. 1998;35:250–265. [PMID: 9809054]

Komaromy M, Lurie N, Bindman AB. California physicians' willingness to care for the poor. *West J Med*. 1995;162:127–132. [PMID: 7725684]

Miranda J, Azocar F, Komaromy M, Golding JM. Unmet mental health needs of women in public-sector gynecologic clinics. *Am J Obstet Gynecol*. 1998;178:212–217. [PMID: 9500476]

Smedley BD, Stith AY, Nelson AR, et al. *Unequal Treatment: Confronting Racial and Ethnic Disparities in Health Care*. Washington, DC: National Academies Press; 2002.

Thamer M, Richard C, Casebeer AW, Ray NF. Health insurance coverage among foreign-born US residents: the impact of race, ethnicity, and length of residence. *Am J Publ Health*. 1997;87:96–102. [PMID: 9065235]

HOUSING & GEOGRAPHIC FACTORS

Racial residential segregation has been suggested as a fundamental cause of racial disparities in health. Although legislation exists to eliminate discrimination in housing, the degree of residential segregation remains extremely high for most African Americans in the United States. Williams and Collins (2001) argue that segregation is a primary cause of racial differences in SES by determining access to education and employment opportunities. Furthermore, segregation creates conditions that hamper a healthy social and physical environment. Levels of racial residential segregation grew dramatically from 1860 to 1940 and have been maintained since then.

Recent research has linked racial segregation to higher cancer risk, a risk that increases as the degree of segregation increases. Minorities living in highly segregated metropolitan areas are >2.5 times more likely to develop cancer from air pollutants when compared with whites. Hispanics who live in highly segregated areas are affected the most, with a risk 6.4 times that of whites. When neighborhood poverty indicators and population density are controlled, the disparities in cancer risk persist, although at lower levels.

Skinner and colleagues (2005) noted the contribution of community of residence to health disparities. The investigators suggested that African American patients are concentrated in a small number of poorly performing hospitals. In this study, nearly 70% of African American patients with myocardial infarctions were treated at only approximately 20% of regional medical centers. The majority of those with life-threatening cardiac conditions received care at smaller healthcare institutions that had less experience in treating these conditions. When >1 million Medicare recipients from 1997 to 2001 were examined, death rates for patients presenting with acute myocardial infarction were 19% higher at these hospitals than at facilities that saw only white patients. Because the factors contributing to health disparities are so complex, there is no one solution. However, these findings suggest that spending must be increased and quality improved at medical centers that primarily treat minorities and the poor.

Young to middle-aged residents of impoverished urban areas manifest excess mortality from several causes, both acute and chronic. African American youth in some urban areas face lower probabilities of surviving to 45 years of age than white youths nationwide surviving to 65 years of age. Minorities constitute 80% of residents of high-poverty, urban areas in the United States and >90% in the largest metropolitan areas. The lower the socioeconomic position held, the less ability the person has to gain access to information, services, or technologies that could provide protection from or modify risks.

For most Americans, housing equity is a major source of wealth. Residential segregation in such a fashion, therefore, directly influences SES. Income predicts variation in health for both white and African Americans, but African Americans report poorer health than whites at all levels of income. People residing in disadvantaged neighborhoods have a higher incidence of heart disease than people who live in more advantaged neighborhoods. The quality of housing is also likely to be worse in highly segregated areas, and poor housing conditions adversely affect health. For example, research reveals that a lack of residential facilities and concerns about personal safety can discourage leisure-time physical exercise.

Geronimus A. To mitigate, resist, or undo: addressing structural influences on the health of urban populations. *Am J Public Health*. 2000;90:867. [PMID: 10846503]

Morello-Frosch R, Jesdale BM. Separate and unequal: residential segregation and estimated cancer risks associated with ambient air toxics in U.S. metropolitan areas. *Environ Health Perspect*. 2006;114:386–393. [PMID: 16507462]

Skinner J, Chandra A, Staiger D, et al. Mortality after acute myocardial infarction in hospitals that disproportionately treat Black patients. *Circulation*. 2005;112:2634–2641. [PMID: 16246963]

Williams DR, Collins C. Racial residential segregation: a fundamental cause of racial disparities in health. *Public Health Rep*. 2001;116(5):404–416. [PMID: 12042604]

MENTAL HEALTH ISSUES

Disparities in mental health services have been known to exist among diverse communities for decades. Among these disparities is a high rate of misdiagnosis, lack of linguistically competent therapists, culturally insensitive diagnostic measures, and increased exposure to abuse.

The practice of psychiatry is heavily influenced by culture. The cultural identity of patients as well as providers, their perceptions of mental illness and appropriate treatment, their background, and their current environment potentially all have an impact on the psychiatric diagnosis, the therapy selected, and the therapeutic outcome. Mental illness has been diagnosed more frequently in African Americans and Hispanics than in non-Hispanic white Americans for >100 years. However, many of the studies reporting these data have been criticized for faulty methodology, cultural bias, and suspect racial theories.

There is some evidence that appropriate research and mental healthcare delivery for these populations are influenced by factors such as poor cultural validation of the *Diagnostic and Statistical Manual of Mental Disorders*, misdiagnosis of minority patients, and the unwillingness of many psychiatrists to acknowledge culturally defined syndromes and folk-healing systems.

General mental health screening is difficult in part because assessment of psychological health in non–English-speaking populations is impeded by lack of instruments that are language and population specific. Patients whose first language is not English usually undergo psychiatric evaluation and treatment in English. Cultural nuances are encoded in language in ways that are often not readily conveyed in translation, even when equivalent words in the second language are used. An appropriately trained interpreter will routinely identify these nuances for the monolingual clinician. When such an interpreter is not available, these nuances can be clarified through consultation with a clinician who shares the patient's first language and culture to maximize delivery of quality health care.

Alarcón RD. Cultural psychiatry. *Adv Psychosom Med.* 2013;33:15–30. [PMID: 23816859]

Collins JL, et al. Ethnic and cultural factors in psychiatric diagnosis and treatment. In: *Handbook of Mental Health and Mental Disorders among Black Americans.* Westport, CT: Greenwood Press; 1990.

Dassori AM, Miller AL, Saldana D. Schizophrenia among Hispanics: epidemiology, phenomenology, course, and outcome. *Schizophr Bull.* 1995;21:303–312. [PMID: 7631176]

Kirmayer LJ, Groleau D. Affective disorders in cultural context. *Psychiatr Clin North Am.* 2001;24:465–478. [PMID: 11593857]

Lewis-Fernandez R, Kleinman A. Cultural psychiatry. Theoretical, clinical, and research issues. *Psychiatr Clin North Am.* 1995;18:433–448. [PMID: 8545260]

DISCRIMINATION

In addition to cost, there are significant differences in how physicians make therapeutic decisions with respect to the minority status of the patient. Women, ethnic minorities, and uninsured persons receive fewer procedures than do affluent white male patients. Furthermore, the race and sex of a patient independently influence how physicians manage acute conditions such as chest pain. For example, women and minorities are less likely to be diagnosed with angina when presenting with comparable risk factors and the same symptoms as white men.

Illegal immigrants underuse health services, especially preventive services such as prenatal care, dental care, and immunizations, due to cost, language, cultural barriers, and fear of apprehension by immigration authorities. Further complicating efforts to provide access to health care for this group is fear for the well-being of family members who may be undocumented, even when the patient is here legally. The increasing number of immigrants entering the United States in recent years has resulted in more legislation seeking to restrict access of various refugee and immigrant groups to public services. Legislation such as Proposition 187, passed in California in 1994, prohibits people lacking legal residency status from obtaining all but emergency medical care at any healthcare facility receiving public funds.

This legislation has encouraged further obstacles to healthcare access for countless other people residing in the United States. For example, minorities who were born in the United States find that they are pressured to produce immigration documentation to receive care. Family physicians seeking to care for immigrants and refugees must recognize and effectively deal with problems in communication, establish trust regarding immigration concerns, understand cultural mores influencing the encounter, find the resources to provide necessary services, make an accurate diagnosis, and negotiate a treatment. Unfortunately, fear of these restrictive immigration laws and socioeconomic hardships combine to delay both seeking and obtaining curative care for these populations.

Title VI of the federal Civil Rights Act states that "no person in the United States shall, on the ground of race, color, or national origin, be excluded from participation in, be denied the benefits of, or be subjected to discrimination under any program or activity receiving Federal financial assistance." Current federal mandates ensuring access to emergency medical services and new restrictions on financing of health care for immigrants under federal programs such as Medicaid and Medicare appear to be in direct conflict. The Personal Responsibility and Work Opportunity Reconciliation Act and the Illegal Immigration Reform and Immigrant Responsibility Act specifically reaffirm federal law on delivery of emergency services without addressing the financing of that care. Unfunded mandates in an era of diminished ability to shift costs onto insured patients create a major dilemma for the institutions that provide uncompensated care. Medicaid is considered one form of insurance, although the level of reimbursement of providers has been so low that many providers will not treat patients with that coverage.

Leape LL, Hilborne LH, Bell R, Kamberg C, Brook RH. Underuse of cardiac procedures: do women, ethnic minorities, and the uninsured fail to receive needed revascularization. *Ann Intern Med.* 1999;130:183–192. [PMID: 10049196]

Schulman KA, Berlin JA, Harless W, et al. The effect of race and sex on physicians' recommendations for cardiac catheterization. *N Engl J Med.* 1999;340:618–626. [PMID: 10029647]

LANGUAGE & LANGUAGE LITERACY

The physician-patient relationship is grounded in communication and the effective use of language. One of the first principles taught in medical school is the importance of the patient's history. Along with clinical reasoning, observations, and nonverbal cues, skillful use of language establishes the clinical interview as the clinician's most powerful tool.

The 2000 census found that >46 million Americans speak a language different than that of their clinician. In the United States, the primary "other language" is Spanish. Approximately 25% of Hispanics were born outside of the United States and Puerto Rico, but >77% of them note speaking Spanish as their primary language at home. Contributing to the discrepancy, the demographic profiles of the nation's healthcare providers does not mirror population trends. In California, although 32% of the population is Hispanic, only 4% of nurses, 4% of physicians, and 6% of dentists are Hispanic.

Cultural competence is not necessarily associated with language fluency. The effectiveness of communication between a clinician and a patient is influenced by the cultural exposure that fosters command of the meaning of the words and phrases. A patient and clinician who do not share a common language face more challenges to quality care than those who share this foundation of communication.

Such language differences can have a negative impact on the clinical encounter. Parents, providers, hospital staff, and quality improvement professionals agree that language and cultural differences lead to communication issues that can have a pervasive, negative impact on the quality and safety of care that children receive. There is still disagreement regarding what needs to change to improve healthcare delivery in a language-discordant environment.

Thus, linguistic competence for an organization is critical to communicate effectively and convey information in a manner that is easily understood by diverse groups, including persons of limited English proficiency, those who have low literacy skills or are not literate, and individuals with disabilities. Linguistic competency requires organizational and provider capacity to respond effectively to the health literacy needs of populations served. The organization must have policy, structures, practices, procedures, and dedicated resources to support this capacity. Federal standards have been established for clinical practice when language discordance is present. To maintain quality of care and adhere to the federal guidelines defined in the National Standards for Culturally and Linguistically Competent Health and Health Care (CLAS), revised and published in 2013, clinicians must provide accommodation for patients in their chosen language.

▶ Cultural and Linguistic Competency Guidelines

It is important for health care organizations to engage in and improve on the federal CLAS (culturally and linguistically appropriate services) guidelines. AHRQ has developed a guide to assist health care organizations to improve their operations in this area. Part I is the CLAS assessment and details of the four aspects of this process:

- Preparing the CLAS Assessment and Planning Team.
- Assessing the Diversity of Members and the Community.
- Assessing the Managed Care Plan.
- Identifying Gaps, Determining Priorities, and Briefing Senior Leaders.

Part II is an overview of the areas of concentration for improving CLAS in their own organizations:

- Providing Linguistic Services (oral and written).
- Improving Cultural Competence.
- Developing a Diverse Workforce

Bethell C. Quality and safety of hospital care for children from Spanish-speaking families with limited English proficiency. *J Healthcare Qual.* 2006;28(3):W3-2–W3-16. [No PMID]

Dower C, McRee T, Grumbach K, et al. *The Practice of Medicine in California: A Profile of the Physician Workforce.* San Francisco, CA: UCSF Center for the Health Professions; 2001.

Duran DG, Pacheco G, eds. *Quality Health Services for Hispanics: The Cultural Competency Component.* DHHS Publication 99–21. Washington, DC: National Alliance for Hispanic Health; 2000. https://www.ahrq.gov/ncepcr/tools/cultural-competence/planclas.html

Morales LS, Elliott M, Weech-Maldonado R, Hays RD. The impact of interpreters on parents' experiences with ambulatory care for their children. *Med Care Res Rev.* 2006;63(1):110–128. [PMID: 16686075]

Woloshin S, Bickell NA, Schwartz LM, et al. Language barriers in medicine in the United States. *JAMA.* 1995;273:724–728. [PMID: 7853631]

Websites

National Center for Cultural Competence. Foundations of Cultural and Linguistic Competence, Definition of Linguistic Competence. https://nccc.georgetown.edu/foundations/framework.php

National Standards for Culturally and Linguistically Appropriate Services (CLAS) in Health and Health Care, Office of Minority Health Resource Center. https://minorityhealth.hhs.gov/omh/browse.aspx?lvl=2&lvlid=53

HEALTH CARE FOR THE DISABLED

Americans with disabilities are more than twice as likely to postpone needed health care because they cannot afford it. In addition, the National Organization on Disability has determined that people with disabilities are 4 times more likely to have special needs that are not covered by health insurance. Many nonelderly adults (46%) with disabilities note that they go without equipment and other items because of cost. More than a third (37%) postpone care because of cost, skip doses, or split pills (36%) because of medication costs and spend less on basics such as food, heat, and other services in order to pay for healthcare (36%). Those with Medicare alone (no supplemental coverage) report the highest rates of serious cost-related problems due to gaps in Medicare's benefit package. Those receiving Medicaid fare better because of the broad scope of benefits and relatively low cost-sharing requirements of Medicaid. However, >20% of adults with disabilities on Medicaid reported that physicians would not accept their insurance—more than twice the percentage of patients having private insurance or Medicare.

Current data suggest that health disparities among people with and without disabilities are as pervasive as those recognized among ethnic minority groups. People with disabilities were included in the Healthy People plan to provide a broad look at the health of this population. Of the 467 objectives listed in Healthy People 2010, 207 subobjectives address people with disabilities. Some of the subobjectives focus on areas outside of the usual scope of health care or healthcare services, such as education, employment, transportation, and housing—all of which have a direct impact on wellness and quality of life.

In addition to examining the health of all citizens with disabilities, particular focus is directed to evaluating the health status of women with disabilities. Regardless of age, women with functional limitations were consistently less likely to have received a Pap test during the past 3 years than women without functional limitations.

Although the Americans with Disabilities Act was enacted in 1990 in an effort to improve access to a broad range of services, women with physical disabilities continue to receive less preventive health screening than women with none. Furthermore, women with more severe disabilities undergo less screening than those with mild or moderate severity of disability.

Adults with developmental disabilities were more likely to lead sedentary lifestyles and 7 times as likely to report inadequate emotional support, compared to adults without developmental disabilities. Adults with physical and developmental disabilities were significantly more likely to report being in fair or poor health. Similar rates of tobacco use and overweight/obesity were reported. Adults with developmental disabilities had a similar or greater risk of having four of five chronic health conditions compared with nondisabled adults. Significant medical care utilization disparities were found for breast and cervical cancer screening as well as for oral health care. These women also had 40% greater odds of violence in the 5 years preceding the interview, and these women appeared to be at particular risk for severe violence.

The National Survey of SSI (supplemental security income) Children and Families (July 2001–June 2002) examined children with *disabilities* who were receiving SSI and their families. Children receiving SSI are more likely to live in a family headed by a single mother, and approximately 50% live in a household with at least one other individual reported to have had a disability. SSI support was the most important source of family income, accounting for nearly half of the income for the children's families, and earnings accounting for almost 40%.

Former US Surgeon General Richard H. Carmona, MD, MPH, released *The Surgeon General's Call to Action to Improve the Health and Wellness of Persons with Disabilities* on the 15th anniversary of the American with Disabilities Act in July 2005. The four goals of the *Call to Action* are to

1. Increase understanding nationwide that people with disabilities can lead long, healthy, and productive lives.

2. Increase knowledge among healthcare professionals and provide them with tools to screen, diagnose, and treat the whole person with a disability with dignity.

3. Increase awareness among people with disabilities regarding the steps they can take to develop and maintain a healthy lifestyle.

4. Increase accessible healthcare and support services to promote independence for people with disabilities.

FUTURE DIRECTIONS & CURRENT CHALLENGES

Multiple factors contribute to the persistence of health and healthcare disparities in the United States today. These factors originate from the patients, clinicians providing care, and the systems in which they must interact. Equitable, quality health care for all is achievable in an environment that values cultural competence. Cultural competence is necessary in multiple domains: values and attitudes; communication styles; community and consumer participation; physical environment, materials, and resources; policies and procedures; population-based clinical practice; and training and professional development. Only by assuming responsibility and accountability for this global problem at all levels of the healthcare system will there be any hope of narrowing the gap and ensuring health for all.

Brownridge DA. Partner violence against women with disabilities: prevalence, risk, and explanations. *Violence Against Women.* 2006;12(9):805–822. [PMID: 16905674]

Havercamp SM. Health disparities among adults with developmental disabilities, adults with other disabilities, and adults not reporting disability in North Carolina. *Public Health Rep.* 2004;119(4):418–426. [PMID: 15219799]

Hjern A, Angel B, Jeppson O. Political violence, family stress and mental health of refugee children in exile. *Scand J Soc Med.* 1998;26(1):18–25. [PMID: 9526760]

Hovey JD, King CA. Acculturative stress, depression and suicidal ideation among immigrant and second generation Latino adolescents. *J Am Acad Child Adolesc Psychiatr.* 1996;35: 1183–1192. [PMID: 8824062]

Johnson BL, Coulberson SL. Environmental epidemiologic issues and minority health. *Ann Epidemiol.* 1993;3(3):175–180. [PMID: 8269072]

Karter AJ, Ferrara A, Liu JY, et al. Ethnic disparities in diabetic complications in an insured population. *JAMA.* 2002;287: 2519–2527. [PMID: 12020332]

Lillie-Blanton M, Laveist T. Race/ethnicity, the social environment, and health. *Soc Sci Med.* 1996;43(1):83–89. [PMID: 8816013]

Marmot M. Inequalities in health. *N Engl J Med.* 2001;345: 134–136. [PMID: 11450663]

Mollica RE. Effects of war trauma on Cambodian refugee adolescents' functional health and mental health status. *J Am Acad Child Adolesc Psychiatr.* 1997;36(8):1098–1106. [PMID: 9256589]

Nickens HW. The role of race/ethnicity and social class in minority health status. *Health Serv Res.* 1995;30(1, Pt 2):151–162. [PMID: 7721589]

Pernice R, Brooks J. Refugees' and immigrants' mental health: association of demographic and post-immigration factors. *J Soc Psychol.* 1996;136(4):511–519. [PMID: 8855381]

Smeltzer SC. Preventive health screening for breast and cervical cancer and osteoporosis in women with physical disabilities. *Fam Commun Health.* 2006;29(1 Suppl):35S–43S. [PMID: 16344635]

Stephens DL. A longitudinal study of employment and skill acquisition among individuals with developmental disabilities. *Res Dev Disabil.* 2005;26(5):469–486. [PMID: 16168884]

66

Caring for LGBTQIA Patients

Steven R. Wolfe, DO, MPH, FAAFP, AAHIVS

OVERVIEW

▶ Who Is LGBTQIA?

The letters **LGBTQIA refer to lesbian, gay, bisexual, transgender, queer or questioning, intersex, and asexual or allied**. Initially starting as LGBT, the abbreviation has evolved over the years secondary to people feeling unheard under the LGBT nomenclature, which has now become more inclusive of sexuality, identity, and freedom of expression. *Transgender* (and gender nonconforming) individuals are those whose gender identity is not aligned with their sex assigned at birth. *Queer* is a controversial word given its past derogatory use. It is another term used to describe someone whose gender identity is outside the strict male/female binary. These are people whose gender identity and/or expression falls outside of the dominant societal norm for their assigned sex, who are beyond genders, or who are some combination of them. *Questioning* is used to describe people who are in the process of exploring their sexual orientation or gender identity. *Intersex* is a range of traits and conditions in an individual who is born with chromosomes, gonads, and/or genitalia that vary from what is considered typical for female or male bodies. *Asexual* people are those who lack sexual attraction to anyone. Finally, an *ally* is a person who shows support for LGBTQIA people and promotes their health and wellness in a variety of ways.

Most recent data report that 5–13% of men are gay, 3–7% of women are lesbian, and 2–5% of people are bisexual with high prevalence in women. In the 1940s, Alfred Kinsey, American sexologist and founder of the Institute for Sex Research at Indiana University, first reported these numbers at 10% for men and 2–6% for women. The US National Gay Task Force, led by Bruce Voeller, repeated an analysis in 1977 and found similar results. Approximately 1–3% of the population is transgender or gender nonconforming. Experts believe the actual prevalence to be upward of 5% of the population, although realistic estimates are challenging given most research only includes those easily identified as transgender. These numbers suggest physicians will care for LGBTQIA patients regardless of geographic location or the ethnic, religious, socioeconomic, or gender demographics of their practice, and perhaps without even knowing.

ESSENTIALS OF DIAGNOSIS

▶ The first step in providing high-quality health care to LGBTQIA patients is a thorough and sensitive sexual history.

▶ History forms can facilitate this, if including options relevant to LGBTQIA patients. For example, "marital status" should be revised to "relationship status," or for gender, forms can have an option for other or transgender.

▶ Comprehensive information about behavior is necessary as a foundation for optimal education and health screening.

Understanding patients' gender identity and sexual orientation is the most important part of providing quality care—even if patients do not self-identify as gay or bisexual but engage in same-sex sexual encounters. Accomplish this by taking a thorough and sensitive sexual history with all new patients and any time sexual behavior may be relevant to diagnosis and management.

▶ Sexual History

The process of taking a sexual history begins with creating a safe environment. As sexual and gender-variant minorities, many LGBTQIA people face discrimination and may fear sharing the details of their sexual lives with a healthcare provider. To further complicate matters, many healthcare providers may avoid discussing sexuality and sexual orientation details with patients, especially with adolescents, because they do not feel prepared to address issues of sexual orientation. By displaying sex-positive, LGBTQIA-relevant literature and positive, reassuring symbols (eg, a rainbow flag or the Human Rights Campaign equal sign) in the office, physicians can help their patients feel more at ease. History forms should include the full range of patient responses and not contain wording that ignores LGBTQIA patients' lives; such forms could facilitate conversation about sensitive topics. Physicians can overcome their own discomfort by routinely collecting sexual histories.

The goal of collecting a sexual history is to identify behaviors that can affect a patient's health. Whether a man who has sex with men (MSM) self-identifies as gay or bisexual is important for understanding his social and psychological situation, but less relevant in terms of screening for and treating organic disease processes. Before collecting a sexual history, clearly communicate the information will remain entirely confidential and help the patient understand that although questions may seem too personal or invasive, their complete and candid response helps physicians provide the best, most personalized care possible.

Physicians can help patients be forthcoming about behaviors by guaranteeing privacy, excusing family members and partners from the room (after first receiving the patient's consent to do so), and being mindful of the assumptions they make about patients. For example:

- Married heterosexual women may have sexual encounters with women.
- Self-identified lesbians have often had sexual encounters with men.
- Not all male-to-female transgender people are sexually active with men, or at all.
- Many elderly patients remain sexually active well into their senior years.

Compassionate, thorough discussion of a patient's behavior can help clarify and demystify assumptions healthcare providers make on the basis of superficial traits or stereotypes of LGBTQIA patients.

Many clinicians begin the sexual history by asking, "Are you sexually active?" This question is a good starting point but fails to address past behavior. In addition, patients may have variable definitions of what constitutes "being sexually active." These ambiguities should be addressed by carefully listening to patients' responses and following up with more specific questions.

The second question often used by providers is, "Are you sexually active with men, women, or both?" Asking this emphasizes behaviors over labels, making no assumption about sexual orientation. Providing a list of options instead of asking patients to fill in the blanks makes it easier to give voice to important medical information and communicates the physician's receptivity to hear any answer.

Regarding current and former partners, the patient's distinct sexual behaviors should be elucidated. It is these behaviors (eg, penile-vaginal intercourse, receptive or insertive anal intercourse, oral-vaginal intercourse, oral-anal intercourse), and the use of barrier protection during intercourse, that help determine screening and other management decisions. Without asking about specific behaviors, regardless of knowing their partners' gender(s), therapeutic decisions could be based on incorrect assumptions.

In addition, identifying the number of current and past partners may be useful for approximating risk of disease exposure and identifying ongoing risky behaviors that need attention, regardless of monogamy. In addition, asking about the use of barrier protection (keeping in mind condoms are often used improperly) and history of sexually transmitted infections is also important.

A physician must understand how a patient's sexual or gender identity affects their life at home, at work, and in the community. In addition, providers should ask all patients who are heterosexually active about their interest in birth control, regardless of their sexual identity. All LGBTQIA patients should be screened for experiences with violence of all forms—domestic violence, intimate partner violence, assault, rape, and molestation. Given increased rates of substance abuse in some LGBTQIA populations, the entirety of the social history should be completed, addressing the use of tobacco, alcohol, cocaine, methylenedioxymethamphetamine (MDMA; "Ecstasy" or "Molly"), methamphetamines ("crystal meth"), prescriptions (including opiates, benzodiazepines, and stimulants), hormones, hallucinogens, marijuana, and intravenous drugs.

Only by identifying behaviors can physicians appropriately screen, risk-stratify, effectively educate, and provide quality care for their patients. Individuals who are members of a sexual- or gender-variant minority group are often less obvious in their identity than those of other types of minority groups given behavior is less visible than, for example, someone's ancestry or skin color. Human behavior or gender expression does not always clearly align with societal gender norms of men and women.

The LGBTQIA population is heterogeneous, composed of individuals, couples, and families of all genders, ages, and socioeconomic, ethnic, religious, political, and geographic backgrounds. To represent this diversity, the rainbow flag was created as an LGBTQIA symbol. This diversity also serves as the complex social context of patients' lives that, in turn, shapes their experience of health and disease.

Centers for Disease Control and Prevention. Lesbian, gay, bisexual and transgender health. https://www.cdc.gov/lgbthealth/. Accessed April 29, 2019.

▶ Who is Gay? What is Bisexual?

The complexity of human sexual behavior defies simple categorization. Sexual orientation manifests as fantasies, desires, actual behavior, and self- or other-identified labels. For example, a man could think of himself and describe himself as heterosexual, engage in sex with men and women in equal numbers, and in his sexual fantasies focus almost exclusively on male images; a simple label fails to capture the reality of his sexuality. Even when considering only sexual behaviors, differences may exist between actual versus desired, past versus present, admitted versus practiced, and consensual versus forced.

In the medical setting, asking how a patient identifies (eg, "Are you gay or bisexual?") importantly assesses their self-perception but may fail to identify medically significant information. Many individuals who engage in same-gender, high-risk sexual behaviors do not identify as gay or bisexual. MSM may be at increased risk for sexually transmitted infections (STIs) compared with men who have sex with women only. Women who have sex with men and women (WSMW) may have an increased risk for STIs and substance abuse compared with either women who have sex with women (WSW) or women who have sex with men only. Differentiation would not be possible by asking a woman only if she identifies herself as lesbian, as both WSMW and WSW may identify themselves as lesbian.

Little specific literature exists describing the characteristics of bisexual men and women separate from either strictly heterosexual or homosexual persons. Research studies including bisexual-identified individuals typically group them with homosexual patients during statistical analysis, limiting information about bisexuality as distinct from heterosexuality or homosexuality. Historically, research focusing on LGBTQIA patients frequently suffers from definitional differences that limit cross-study comparisons, small sample size, population sampling bias, and other shortcomings. Changing societal attitudes, improved research methodology, and increased resources will improve our knowledge gaps.

▶ Homophobia, Heterosexism, & Sexual Prejudice

Homophobia is defined as an irrational fear of, aversion to, or discrimination against homosexuality or homosexuals. *Heterosexism* is the belief that heterosexuality is the natural, normal, acceptable, or superior form of sexuality. Sexual prejudice encompasses negative attitudes toward an individual because of their sexual orientation. In their most extreme manifestation, homophobia and sexual prejudice result in physical violence and homicide. Evolving societal attitudes may diminish such threats, but homophobia and its behavioral manifestations remain a significant threat to health.

Homophobia is dangerous. One survey of physicians found that 52% observed colleagues providing substandard care to patients due to sexual orientation. In another study, 37% of young gay men reported antigay harassment in the previous 6 months, resulting in increased suicidal ideation and diminished self-esteem. In human immunodeficiency virus (HIV)–seropositive gay men who were otherwise healthy, HIV infection advanced more rapidly, exhibiting a dose-response relationship, in participants who concealed their homosexual identity. A study of 1067 lesbians and gay men found that feelings of victimization resulting from perceived social stigma significantly contributed to depression. A study of 912 Hispanic men found that experiences of social discrimination strongly predicted suicidal ideation, anxiety, and depressed mood.

Overcoming prejudices and eliminating discriminatory practices are fundamental to health care for all patients. Bias against LGBTQIA individuals seems to respond more effectively to experiential interventions (eg, interaction with LGBTQIA individuals) than to rational interventions (eg, information dissemination). In a clinical setting, physicians can communicate acceptance and support with posters showing same-sex couples, stickers depicting a rainbow flag or equal sign, and a visible nondiscrimination statement stating that equal care is provided to all patients, regardless of age, race, ethnicity, physical ability or attributes, religion, sexual identity, and gender identity.

The perceived tolerance (or intolerance) strongly influences LGBTQIA patients' willingness to disclose sexual orientation and details of their personal lives. A patient's sexual practices affect risk for various diseases and can influence disease screening and diagnostic evaluation, so honest discussion of the patient's sexual and social life is vital to promote optimal health. A physician who fails to identify an LGBTQIA patient's sexual orientation may not adequately counsel or diagnose a patient and may compromise delivery of quality medical care. Incorrect assumptions about patients can have similar adverse outcomes (Table 66–1).

Websites

Gay and Lesbian Medical Association (GLMA). http://www.glma.org
Parents, Families, and Friends of Lesbians and Gays (PFLAG). http://www.pflag.org

HIV/AIDS

 ESSENTIALS OF DIAGNOSIS

▶ Not all LGBTQIA patients are at risk for HIV, but screening for HIV infection in adolescents and adults age 15–65 years is recommended. Younger adolescents and older adults who are at increased risk should also be screened (Grade A recommendation).

▶ Periodic screening using a fourth-generation serum HIV antigen/antibody test is recommended for all persons who are sexually active outside a mutually monogamous relationship and has a sensitivity and specificity of >99% (Grade A recommendation).

▶ Preexposure prophylaxis (PrEP) in HIV-negative person using Truvada (emtricitabine/tenofovir disoproxil) and maintaining an undetectable viral load in a HIV-positive person can substantially reduce the transmission of HIV (Grade A recommendation).

General Considerations

Any publication on LGBTQIA health that omitted mention of HIV would be incomplete, but thorough coverage of the topic is covered in a separate chapter.

Table 66–1. Pitfalls in caring for gay and lesbian patients.

Assumption	Solution
Assumption about sexual orientation: Many patients are neither exclusively heterosexual nor exclusively homosexual.	Learn to inquire about sexual orientation in a nonjudgmental manner that recognizes the range of human diversity and apply this learning to all patients.
Assumptions about sexual activity: Lesbian and gay male patients may have numerous different sexual partners, be in a monogamous relationship, be celibate, or vary in patterns of activity over time.	Take a specific, sensitive sexual history from all patients.
Assumptions about contraception: The need for contraception arises from a wish to prevent pregnancy from heterosexual intercourse, regardless of the patient's gender identity, sexual orientation, or label.	Inquire about need (rather than assuming need) or lack of need for all patients. Tailor recommendations to patient's needs.
Assumptions about marriage: Lesbians and gay men may have been, and may still be, married to persons of the opposite sex. In some states and countries, they may be married to same-gender partners and may use the terms *partner* or *husband/wife* to refer to their spouse.	Inquire about significant relationships for all patients. Use the same terminology that your patients choose.
Assumptions about parenting: Lesbian and gay male couples are often interested in becoming parents and choose to bear and raise children.	Inquire about parenting wishes and choices, and be prepared to discuss options.

Gay men constitute the largest number of acquired immunodeficiency syndrome (AIDS) cases in the United States. Recent literature suggests increased rates of unprotected anal intercourse ("barebacking") among certain gay populations. This trend may be due in part to decreased fear of HIV in the era of highly active antiretroviral therapy (HAART). Young gay men, those who use the internet or apps to meet sexual partners, or those with substance abuse problems, particularly those who use crystal meth, Ecstasy, and Viagra, are at greater risk. Increasingly, African American and Hispanic men are disproportionately affected. Another quickly growing HIV-positive population is African American women who have unprotected sex with African American men who identify as heterosexual but secretly have unprotected sex with men, often referred to as "on the down low." Increased stigma associated with homosexuality in ethnic minority communities may drive individuals at risk to hide behavior, complicating efforts at diagnosis and treatment.

Prevention

Behavioral interventions stop the spread of HIV most effectively. Physicians should screen all patients for risk behaviors (eg, unprotected intercourse, multiple partners, concurrent sex and substance use, injection drug use) and should intervene to reduce risk and test for HIV in patients with a positive risk history, repeating testing periodically if risk behaviors continue. Pursue a "harm-reduction" strategy if it is impossible to eliminate all risk (eg, stopping needle sharing until drug abuse can be stopped, keeping condoms available when sex with a new partner is possible). Because patients engaging in risky behaviors rarely volunteer information about their risk, physicians must proactively assess each patient's risk and intervene when needed.

In combination with behavioral intervention, two medication-related interventions prevent transmission of HIV. PrEP with Truvada (emtricitabine/tenofovir disoproxil) or soon to be approved Descovy (emtricitabine/tenofovir alafenamide) in appropriate selected HIV-negative individuals at higher risk of contracting HIV is an effective way of preventing HIV transmission. In addition, treatment-as-prevention by maintaining an undetectable viral load makes HIV nontransmittable.

Clinical Findings

Physicians should test for HIV in at-risk individuals who present with routine viral infection symptoms. Patients with acute HIV infection present with symptoms that are generally indistinguishable from common viral infections, including fever (96%), adenopathy (74%), pharyngitis (70%), rash (70%), and other nonspecific symptoms (see Table 14–2). HIV viral load tests (eg, polymerase chain reaction) become positive 1–2 weeks before routine (antibody-based) HIV tests and may be useful in diagnosis (as distinct from screening).

Latent HIV infection may remain essentially asymptomatic for years. Generalized lymphadenopathy may persist for years. Its disappearance may indicate clinically significant immune system decline, marked by nonspecific symptoms such as fevers, weight loss, and diarrhea. Early immune dysfunction results in diseases such as herpes zoster or persistent vaginal candidiasis. Without effective antiretroviral treatment, almost all patients will progress to one or more AIDS-defining illnesses.

▶ Treatment

Patients infected with HIV require a comprehensive care plan that involves skilled physicians, ancillary health services, pharmacologic therapy, and access to social and other support services. Excellent resources exist to guide physicians in the detailed management and care of patients with HIV/AIDS (see next section). The family physician's role in HIV care will be determined by the knowledge, skill, comfort level, and personal preferences of the physician, as well as the accessibility of referral physicians. Family physicians may serve primarily in case finding, by testing and referring patients found to be HIV positive, or may assume full responsibility for comprehensive management of HIV and its complications. Current research supports that all HIV-positive patients should immediately start HAART treatment regardless of CD4 count or viral load.

SEXUALLY TRANSMITTED INFECTIONS

ESSENTIALS OF DIAGNOSIS

▶ Many sexually active gay men are at increased risk for most STIs, which can often be asymptomatic, requiring routine periodic screening.

▶ Suspicion or diagnosis of one STI should routinely lead to testing for concomitant HIV and syphilis.

▶ Although generally at lower risk for STIs, lesbians have a higher incidence of bacterial vaginosis than heterosexual women.

▶ General Considerations

Human papillomavirus (HPV), leading to condyloma, genital warts, or epithelial dysplasia, is the most commonly transmitted STI.

Gonorrhea, chlamydia, and nonchlamydial nongonococcal urethritis (NGU) are common problems in sexually active gay men. As each of these may cause asymptomatic infection, periodic screening may be useful to detect clinically silent disease. Antibiotic resistance to *Neisseria gonorrhoeae* has become so ubiquitous that the only remaining first-line treatment is ceftriaxone, and fluoroquinolones are no longer recommended for treatment in MSM. Herpes simplex virus and syphilis most commonly cause genital ulcer disease in heterosexual and homosexual men.

Enteritis and proctocolitis may be caused by an STI via oral-anal contact. Enterobacteriaceae and *Giardia lamblia* are a common cause and should be included in the differential diagnosis of enteritis and proctocolitis in MSM, as well as cytomegalovirus in the HIV-positive patient. Unprotected receptive anal intercourse can lead to the tenesmus, rectal pain, and bleeding of proctitis, in which the most common pathogens are *N gonorrhoeae, Chlamydia trachomatis, Treponema pallidum,* and herpes simplex virus.

Oral stimulation of a man's penis, mistakenly thought to be a "safe" sexual practice, may be an independent risk factor for urethral and pharyngeal gonorrhea and nonchlamydial NGU; it has been implicated in HIV transmission and has been associated with localized syphilis epidemics in gay men. Syphilis epidemics have also been associated with high-risk sexual activity among HIV-positive men.

Some studies show comparable rates of STIs between lesbians and heterosexual women. Infections, including bacterial vaginosis (BV), candidiasis, herpes, gonorrhea, and HPV infections, can be contracted by lesbians. One series found a 2.5-fold increase in BV among lesbians compared to heterosexual women, often showing similar vaginal flora between female partners.

Human herpesvirus type 8 (HHV8) has been shown to predispose people to Kaposi sarcoma. Ten studies assessed the prevalence and correlates of HHV8, with most concluding that MSM have disproportionally higher HHV8 infection rates than do comparison groups.

Hepatitis C virus is a risk factor for non-Hodgkin lymphoma and hepatocellular carcinoma. Surveillance data suggest hepatitis B and C viral infections increased over time in MSM, while decreasing in the general population. In addition, hepatitis C is an emerging coinfection in HIV-infected MSM regardless of intravenous drug use.

▶ Prevention

Counseling reduces risk behaviors, and patients reporting high-risk behaviors or those diagnosed with an STI should receive counseling or be referred for individual or group counseling. In addition, MSM patients engaging in sex outside a mutually monogamous relationship should receive periodic STI screening, as should WSMW (see Chapter 14 for screening recommendations and other information about STIs). If not immune, gay men should be vaccinated against hepatitis A and hepatitis B.

▶ Patient Education

Patients diagnosed with or suspected to have an STI should be informed of transmission methods and how to reduce infection risk. Such patients should also be informed of specific treatment, if any, as well as potential coinfection with other sexually transmissible agents. Patients should be counseled to contact sex partners; in lieu of this, the health department may notify partners through anonymous partner notification systems.

Workowski K, Bolan G, Centers for Disease Control and Prevention. 2015 sexually transmitted diseases treatment guidelines. *MMWR Recomm Rep.* 2015;64(RR3):1–137. [PMID: 26042815]

HUMAN PAPILLOMAVIRUS INFECTION

 ESSENTIALS OF DIAGNOSIS

- ▶ HPV causes cervical cancer in all women; lesbians should be offered Papanicolaou (Pap) smear screening according to the same guidelines used for heterosexual women.
- ▶ HPV causes anal dysplasia and anal cancer. HIV-positive MSM should receive yearly anal Pap smears (Grade B recommendation). Research is unclear as to whether HIV-negative MSM who engage in anal-receptive intercourse would benefit as well.

General Considerations

HPV is a pervasive infection, manifesting in >100 viral types that infect various parts of the human body. Head and neck cancers can be caused by HPV, although current research shows that the risk of oral HPV infection did not differ by sexual orientation. HPV types infecting the genitalia carry varying risk for dysplasia and neoplasia. The types causing the most visually apparent warts are usually the types with least risk for dysplasia. Conversely, the types causing clinically unapparent disease carry high dysplastic risk.

Sexual orientation and receptive anal intercourse appear to be independent correlates of condyloma and anal intraepithelial neoplasia. Interestingly, one study even showed that anal HPV was more transient in men who have sex with women but more persistent in MSM. Most available evidence demonstrates that MSM have a higher prevalence of anal HPV infection than do comparison groups regardless of HIV status. In addition, both HIV infection and receptive anal intercourse are significant correlates of anal squamous intraepithelial lesions, and there is a higher prevalence of anal cancer in MSM with HIV than in women and heterosexual men.

Prevention

Secondary prevention via Pap smear remains the cornerstone of screening. One study of lesbians revealed that 25%

of respondents had not undergone a Pap test within the past 3 years and 7.6% never had. Lesbian patients may mistakenly believe themselves to be less susceptible to cervical cancer than heterosexuals or bisexuals, even though one study showed that 79% reported previous sexual intercourse with a man. Even in women reporting no prior sex with men, HPV DNA and squamous intraepithelial lesions may be found in ≤20% of patients. Thus, cervical Pap smears supplemented with HPV DNA testing should be performed routinely using the American Society of Colposcopy and Cervical Pathology guidelines. Individuals with abnormal screening tests should receive colposcopy or anoscopy and subsequent follow-up as indicated by findings.

A gay man's risk of anal dysplasia and squamous cell carcinoma is equivalent to the historical risk of cervical cancer women faced prior to the advent of Pap screening. Anal HPV DNA is very prevalent in gay men—one study detected it in 91.6% of HIV-positive and 65.9% of HIV-negative men. HIV exacerbates HPV effects and is associated with more prevalent HPV infection and higher grade squamous intraepithelial lesions. Screening HIV-positive homosexual and bisexual men for anal intraepithelial neoplasia and anal squamous cell carcinomas with anal Pap tests offers quality-adjusted life expectancy benefits at a cost comparable with other accepted clinical preventive interventions. Because the observed increased incidence of anal cancer does not appear to be due solely to HIV infection, high-resolution anoscopy and cytology screening of all MSM with anal condyloma and other benign noncondylomatous anal disorders is supported by current knowledge.

No consensus guidelines exist on screening for anal dysplasia and anal cancer in MSM, regardless of HIV status. Because of the ubiquity of HPV in the HIV-positive population, baseline cytology and yearly anal cancer screening using Pap smears for all HIV-positive MSM is recommended. Current research is conflicted on the cost-effectiveness of screening all MSM using anal Pap smear, although current expert recommendations suggest screening HIV-negative MSM every 3 years, similar to cervical cancer screening recommendations.

Taking an anal-rectal sample for cytology (ARC) is a simple procedure. It does not require the use of an anoscope. No special preparation is needed for the patient, although the patient may be advised to refrain from receptive anal intercourse or the use of intra-anal preparations before examination.

An ARC sample can be collected with the patient in the lateral recumbent position lying on one side, with the knees drawn up toward the chest. To collect an ARC sample, a tap water–moistened Dacron swab is used. The Dacron swab is inserted approximately 5–6 cm (or approximate length of your fifth finger) into the anal canal past the anal verge, into the rectal vault. This is done without direct visualization of the anal canal. Firm lateral pressure is applied to the swab handle as it is rotated and slowly withdrawn from the anal canal, inscribing a cone-shaped arc. Care should be taken to ensure the transition zone is sampled. A swab or smear of the perianal skin is an unsatisfactory sample for ARC. Avoid using cotton swabs on a wooden stick because the handle may break and splinter during collection.

For liquid-based cytology, the swab is then placed in the preservative vial and agitated vigorously several times to release the cellular harvest. If liquid-based cytology is not available, the swab can be smeared onto a glass slide and then spray-fixed as per the procedure for conventional cervical Pap smears. The lab requisition should be labeled as a rectal Pap smear.

The Centers for Disease Control and Prevention recommends routine vaccination for all male and female children at 11–12 years old. Gardasil 9 is licensed in the United States to prevent HPV, certain HPV-related cancers, and genital warts. Additional discussion of HPV appears in Chapter 14.

Petrosky E, Bocchini JA Jr, Hariri S, et al. Use of 9-valent human papillomavirus (HPV) vaccine: updated HPV vaccination recommendations of the Advisory Committee on Immunization Practices. *MMWR Morb Mortal Wkly Rep*. 2015;64(11): 300–304. [PMID: 25811679]

SUBSTANCE ABUSE

 ESSENTIALS OF DIAGNOSIS

▶ Substance use is more common in LGBTQIA patients than in the general heterosexual population.

▶ Gay, lesbian, and bisexual adolescents, especially females, are at heightened risk of engaging in polysubstance use.

▶ Methamphetamine use and addiction are particularly problematic in some gay male groups.

▶ General Considerations

Alcohol, psychoactive drug, and tobacco use appears to be more widespread in gay men and women than in the general heterosexual population. Several studies suggest lesbians and bisexual women consume more alcohol and use other psychoactive substances more often than heterosexual women. A meta-analysis found risk ratios of 4.0 and 3.5 for alcohol and substance dependence, respectively, among WSW and WSMW as compared to WSM. Another review of tobacco use found smoking rates among adolescent and adult lesbians, gays, and bisexuals to be higher than in the general population. A recent study published in April 2019 looked at 120,000 adolescents from 19 states in the 2015 Youth Risk Behavior Survey, which showed increased risk of multiple

types of polysubstance use. Methamphetamine use reached epidemic proportions in some gay male populations, and routine history taking should include a question regarding current and past use of this drug.

Alcohol use has been associated with high-risk sexual behavior (eg, unprotected anal and oral intercourse). Gay men who have unprotected anal intercourse are more likely to have a drinking problem than gay men who do not have unprotected intercourse, and unprotected intercourse after drinking is more common with casual sexual partners.

Drug use is also associated with increased high-risk sexual behaviors. Such drugs include hallucinogens, nitrate inhalants, cocaine, and other stimulants. Drug use during high-risk sex is common. However, associations between drug use and high-risk sexual behavior exist only for current use, not past drug or alcohol use. Providing adequate treatment to patients with substance abuse problems can diminish their subsequent risk of acquiring HIV and other STIs.

In some venues, the prevalence of illicit drug use and associated high-risk sexual activity is dramatic, with use of substances such as MDMA approaching 80% of the population. Men who attend "circuit parties"—a series of dances or parties held over a weekend attended by hundreds to thousands of gay and bisexual men—should be considered at high risk for concurrent illicit substance use and should be counseled accordingly.

Anabolic steroid use is a problem among a subset of gay men. One British study of >1000 gay men recruited from five gymnasiums found that 13.5% of the study population used anabolic steroids, and users were more likely than never users (21% vs 13%) to report engaging in unprotected anal intercourse, increasing their risk for HIV infection.

▶ Pathogenesis

Several theories propose explanations for the increased substance use in LGBTQIA patients:

• Maladaptive coping strategy to deal with societal bias against homosexuality

• Consequence of bars serving as a primary social gathering place for lesbians and gay men

• Genetic predisposition to substance abuse linked to genes coding for same-sex attraction

• Coping method for dealing with stresses such as coming to terms with self-identity, fear of HIV infection, lack of social support, fear of discrimination in housing or employment, and rejection by family or friends on the basis of sexual orientation

Research to date has not explained causation.

Reasons for steroid use are more straightforward: to modify the patient's musculature to conform more closely to an idealized male form according to some gay subcultures.

Significant social pressures may drive patients to resort to steroids to achieve an idealized masculine physique, and for these patients, substantial support and counseling may be required to overcome steroid abuse.

Prevention & Treatment

Prevention, clinical findings, complications, and treatment of substance abuse in LGBTQIA populations are similar to these management considerations in heterosexual populations (see Chapter 60 for further discussion). However, modification of standard treatment approaches to reflect LGBTQIA culture may enhance treatment effectiveness. Differences to consider with this population include the prevalence of methamphetamine use and its association with high-risk sexual behavior among some groups of gay men; concomitant use of sildenafil (Viagra) or other treatments for erectile dysfunction; and "club drugs" (eg, MDMA, amphetamines, γ-hydroxybutyrate [GHB], or ketamine). Erectile dysfunction treatments, either with or without other substance use, are associated with high-risk sexual behavior.

Coulter RWS, Ware D, Fish JN, et al. Latent classes of polysubstance use among adolescents in the United States: intersections of sexual identity with sex, age and race/ethnicity. *LGBT Health.* 2019;6(3):116–125. [PMID: 30822259]

Floyd SR, Pierce DM, Geraci SA. Preventative and primary care for lesbian, gay and bisexual patients. *Am J Med Sci.* 2016;352(6):637–643. [PMID: 27916220]

Goldbach JT, Tanner-Smith EE, Bagwell M, Dunlap S. Minority stress and substance use in sexual minority adolescents: a meta-analysis. *Prev Sci.* 2014;15(3):350–363. [PMID: 23605479]

DEPRESSION

 ESSENTIALS OF DIAGNOSIS

▶ Depression and anxiety are more prevalent in lesbians and gay men than in the general population.

▶ Suicidal ideation, attempts at suicide, and completed acts of suicide are more common in the LGBTQIA population than in their heterosexual counterparts.

▶ Suicide risk seems to be increased around the time that an individual "comes out" (reveals their gay or lesbian identity to others).

▶ Lack of social supports, lack of family support, and poor relationship quality are significant predictors of depression.

General Considerations

Feelings of stigmatization, internalized homophobia (the direction of society's negative attitudes and shame toward one's self), and actual experiences of discrimination or violence contribute to LGBTQIA distress. A study of HIV-infected men, which may be relevant to all gay men, found that men who did not demonstrate traditional gender identity were more likely to have current symptoms of anxiety and depression and a lifetime history of depression. Depression has also been linked to HIV diagnoses and the AIDS epidemic.

Well-designed studies with valid sampling techniques demonstrate suicidal ideation, attempts at suicide, and completed acts of suicide are more common in LGBT youth than their heterosexual counterparts. Population-based research demonstrates significantly higher rates of suicidal symptoms and suicide attempts among men who reported having same-sex partners than those who reported having exclusively opposite-sex partners. A recent meta-analysis indicates a fourfold increase in lifetime suicide-attempt prevalence among gay and bisexual men as compared to heterosexual men. Other investigators demonstrate similar findings (eg, in a study of twins in which one brother reported same-sex partners after age 18 and the other did not). Suicidality has been linked to the process of "coming out," or revealing one's homosexual orientation to others. Thus, physicians caring for gay adolescents or adults disclosing their sexual orientation to others should be especially sensitive to symptoms or signs suggesting any increase in suicide risk.

One study of lesbians considered predictors of depression and looked at relationship status, relationship satisfaction, social support from friends, social support from family, "outness" (degree to which the woman publicly shared her sexual orientation), and relationship satisfaction. Lack of social support from friends, poor relationship satisfaction, and lack of perceived social support from family were significant predictors of depression.

Prevention

Well-being is enhanced during later stages of gay identity development, which suggests that facilitation of an individual's synthesis of their gay identity may alleviate depressive symptoms. Conversely, in HIV-positive men, concealment of homosexuality is associated with lower CD4 counts and depressive symptoms, lending further support to the idea that facilitating gay identity development may alleviate or prevent depression in some patients and, in so doing, better equip them to maintain their health.

Clinical Findings

Symptoms and signs of depression in lesbian female and gay male patients are very similar to those in heterosexual populations (see Chapter 56). Although depression is often associated with decreased sexual activity, one study of gay men revealed that 16% had heightened sexual interest while depressed. Predictors of depression in lesbians (eg, lack of social support from friends, relationship status dissatisfaction, and lack of perceived social support from family) are similar to predictors for heterosexual women.

Floyd SR, Pierce DM, Geraci SA. Preventive and primary care for lesbian, gay and bisexual patients. *Am J Med Sci.* 2016;352(6):637–643. [PMID: 27916220]

OTHER HEALTH CONCERNS

▶ Cancer Screening

All LGBTQIA patients require the same age- and gender-appropriate cancer screening as heterosexual and non–gender-variant patients. As discussed earlier, cervical cancer screening should be offered to lesbian women, and anal cancer screening to men with a history of receptive anal intercourse, particularly if they are co-infected with HIV, although insufficient evidence exists to universally recommend the anal Pap at this time.

Because breast and ovarian cancers may be more common in nulliparous or uniparous women, it may be more common in lesbians, but well-designed, prospective studies are lacking. One study compiling survey data from almost 12,000 women found lesbians had greater prevalence rates of obesity and alcohol and tobacco use and lower rates of parity and birth control pill use. Another study confirmed higher prevalence of nulliparity and also found higher prevalence of other health risk factors, including high daily alcohol intake, higher body mass index, and higher prevalence of current smoking.

In transgender patients, it is important to screen according to current anatomy as well as use of hormonal therapy. For example, many male-to-female transgender patients are at risk for both prostate and breast cancers, and female-to-male transgender patients often require screening for breast, uterine, cervical, endometrial, and ovarian cancers. As in any patient population, tobacco and alcohol use among LGBTQIA patients increases risk for malignancy.

▶ Erectile Dysfunction

Studies have demonstrated that erectile dysfunction is more common in homosexual than in heterosexual men, although overall prevalence was still <4%. Related, gay men also report higher levels of performance anxiety (eg, more likely to agree with the statement "If I feel I'm expected to respond sexually, I have difficulty getting aroused") than do heterosexual men. This was true even when men reporting erectile dysfunction were excluded from analysis. Erectile dysfunction is more common in HIV-positive homosexual men than in HIV-negative homosexual men. Declines in serum testosterone have been associated with HIV infection, suggesting one possible etiology for this difference.

▶ Contraception & Reproductive Health

Assuming all women of reproductive age need contraception risks alienating lesbian patients, who may consequently decline to disclose their sexual orientation. However, lesbians who are sexually active with men may be interested in using contraceptives.

Lesbian patients may also be, or wish to become, mothers and may welcome a discussion of reproductive options. Parenthood options available to lesbians and gay men include adoption, artificial insemination, surrogacy, or heterosexual intercourse. Existing evidence suggests gay men and lesbians have parenting skills comparable to heterosexual parents. Special considerations that may arise for lesbian and gay parents include the children's awareness of lesbian and gay relationships, heterosexism, and homophobia. When compared with children of heterosexual parents, children of gay men and lesbians seem to be no different in significant variables measured, including their sexual or gender identity, personality traits, and intelligence. Despite this, gay men and lesbians may face unjustified barriers in their attempts to become foster and adoptive parents. Issues that warrant physician awareness include parental legal rights and durable power of attorney; gestation and pregnancy; choice of surrogate, sperm, or egg donor; possible HIV risk; and routine preconception and prenatal care. Physicians caring for lesbians and gay men wishing to become parents should maintain information about appropriate referrals to facilitate this process.

TRANSGENDER & GENDER NONCONFORMING PATIENTS

ESSENTIAL FEATURES

▶ Rather than assume, physicians should determine how patients wish to be addressed (name and pronouns) and understand how they conceptualize their gender.

▶ Transgender and gender nonconforming people are at high risk for marginalization and disparities, including violence and abuse directed at them; are more likely to be uninsured and have unmet health care needs; suffer prejudice in accessing services like housing, employment, and health care; and have disproportionate rates of HIV infection, mental health disorders, suicide attempts, cigarette smoking, and alcohol consumption.

▶ Medical management including hormone replacement therapy (HRT) can be managed by a trans-competent primary care physician. Gender-affirming surgery should be managed by multispecialty teams with experience caring for this population.

Terminology

Transgender and gender nonconforming individuals are those whose gender identity is not aligned with their sex assigned at birth or societal expectations for binary gender identities or expression.

Cisgender is a term for persons whose experience and expressed gender are congruent with their gender assigned at birth. *Gender-affirming surgeries* (GAS) are surgical procedures intended to alter a person's body to affirm their experienced gender identity (eg, sex reassignment surgery or gender reassignment surgery). *Genderqueer* is an individual whose experienced or expressed gender does not conform to the male/female binary or who rejects the gender binary. *Intersex individuals* are born with both male and female sexual characteristics and organs, such that unambiguous assignment of male or female sex at birth is not possible.

The term *male-to-female*, or the transgender community's preferred term *transwoman*, describes individuals born with male genitalia who presents as a female regardless of hormone or surgical intervention; the reverse is true for female-to-male individuals, or *transman*. Additional ways to characterize the biological, social, psychological, and legal identity of transgender individuals have been described. The best approach to caring for individual patients is to determine how they wish to be addressed and understand how they conceptualize their gender.

The *Diagnostic and Statistical Manual of Mental Disorders*, fifth edition (*DSM-5*) diagnosis of *gender dysphoria* communicates the emotional distress that can result from "a marked incongruence between one's experienced/expressed gender and assigned gender." Individuals who experience the strongest feelings of dissonance between their gender identity and their physical appearance believe the quest for full hormonal and surgical sex reassignment is vital because they actually feel "trapped" in an anatomically incorrect body. Gender dysphoria does not apply automatically to people who identify as transgender but is applied only to those who exhibit clinically significant impairment. Limited research into the etiology of gender dysphoria suggests that it may be multifactorial, including genetics, anatomic brain differences between transgender and nontransgender individuals, and differences in parental rearing. Regardless of etiology or classification, transgender patient needs are increasingly recognized as valid and deserving of attention from healthcare educators, researchers, policymakers, and clinicians of all types.

Treatment

A multidisciplinary team experienced with transgender care may be the most critical element in providing superior care and therapy. Some patients choose partial medical or surgical treatment, finding living with physical components of both genders best addresses the dissonance caused by their birth physiognomy. Others use extensive medical and surgical treatment to physically manifest their "internal" gender as fully as possible. Current literature on the health needs of transgender patients focuses on psychological and psychiatric evaluation and treatment, GAS, and hormonal therapy. Although common practice is to delay initiating GAS until the patient is at least 18 or 21 years of age, treatment in adolescence is well tolerated for carefully selected individuals, does not lead to postoperative regret, and may prevent psychopathology seen in individuals forced to delay therapy. Patients considering GAS should undergo psychological evaluation by a gender-affirming therapist experienced in working with this population.

Intensive gender-affirming counseling, hormonal treatment if desired and not contraindicated, and living in the role of the desired gender for a period of ≥1 year should precede surgical treatment. Surgical treatment can involve the face, breasts, genitalia, and larynx. The right to such treatment, even in health systems receiving government funding, has been sanctioned by courts. Because each patient is unique, surgical approaches must be tailored to individual patients, and patients seeking GAS should be referred to teams experienced with these procedures.

Primary care is an ideal setting for transgender health care, given primary care physicians are knowledgeable of and often experienced with the administration of estrogens (for menopausal care and contraception), testosterone (for androgen-deficient states, eg, as with HIV), and testosterone-blocking medications (for hirsutism and prostatic disease) and are aware of important mental and social health issues.

HRT is often used in both genders. Cross-sex HRT may have potential side effects, so the smallest doses needed to achieve the desired result should be used. For transgender females using estrogen therapy, outcome studies suggest that known complications of estrogen such as high-risk adverse events such as venous thromboembolism and moderate-risk events such as hyperprolactinemia, breast cancer, coronary artery disease, cerebrovascular disease, cholelithiasis, and hypertriglyceridemia do occur, but the incidence of complications can be held to acceptable levels with careful attention to regimens used. In transgender males, use of testosterone can result in high-risk adverse events such as erythrocytosis and moderate risk of severe liver dysfunction. Extensive experience with HRT in transgender persons indicates that hormonal therapy, particularly if transdermal formulations are used, does not cause increased morbidity or mortality; however, the most common formulations used are intramuscular (IM) or subcutaneous testosterone injections and IM or oral estrogen therapy.

Lapinski J, Covas T, Perkins JM, et al. Best practices in transgender health: a clinician's guide. *Prim Care Clin Office Pract.* 2018;45:687–703. [PMID: 30401350]

Websites

American Psychiatric Association. *Diagnostic and Statistical Manual of Mental Disorders*, fifth edition (*DSM–5*). http://www.dsm5.org/Documents/Gender%20Dysphoria%20Fact%20Sheet.pdf

Gay and Lesbian Medical Association (GLMA). http://www.glma.org

Parents, Families, and Friends of Lesbians and Gays (PFLAG). http://www.pflag.org

The World Professional Association for Transgender Health (WPATH). http://www.wpath.org

Transgender Law and Policy Institute. http://www.transgenderlaw.org

ADOLESCENTS

Lesbian and gay adolescents growing up in a loving, supportive environment develop and mature in a manner similar to their heterosexual counterparts. However, lesbian and gay adolescents may be vulnerable to parental wrath and withdrawal of support on disclosure or suspicion of their homosexual orientation. In certain instances, this can initiate a chain of events that leave the youth homeless and vulnerable. Lacking employable skills, some homeless gay youths may resort to prostitution or "survival sex" to support themselves.

Gay youths have an increased risk for suicide compared with their heterosexual peers. In addition, population-based surveys of adolescents indicate lesbian and gay adolescents report being physically abused ≤2 times as often as their heterosexual peers and sexually abused ≤10 times as often as heterosexual adolescents. Despite this, homosexual adolescents are generally more similar to than different from their heterosexual peers, face many of the same challenges, and have great potential to mature into healthy and happy adults.

Physicians caring for families need to be aware of the possibility that the typical adolescent struggle to establish identity may be compounded when a teen recognizes their sexual orientation, particularly when this occurs in a potentially hostile environment. Physicians can play a vital role in helping adolescents—and their families—find acceptance. Parental support can dramatically reduce the adverse effects of "coming out" and the potential risk for suicide and can increase the likelihood of healthy psychological development and maturation.

OLDER LGBTQIA PATIENTS

Older LGBTQIA people developed and matured in a different social milieu, when society was less tolerant of homosexuality or gender expression and the consequences of being LGBTQIA included even greater threats to the individual's social and family relationships, housing, and livelihood than exist today. Older patients are more likely to have experienced mistreatment and discrimination due to living a majority of their lives prior to recent advancements in acceptance and equal treatment. Thus, older patients may be even less willing to disclose their sexual orientation or gender expression to physicians and may have special healthcare needs that would go unrecognized if the physician did not take a thorough sexual history. Incorrect assumptions about geriatric patient sexuality may lead physicians to inaccurately identify risk behaviors and implement appropriate education or screening tests.

Yarns BC, Abrams JM, Meeks TW, et al. The mental health of older LGBT adults. *Curr Psychiatry Rep.* 2016;18(60):1–11. [PMID: 27142205]

FAMILY, COMMUNITY, AND MARRIAGE

One aspect of being gay or lesbian that may be overlooked in caring for a patient's medical needs is the role of family and social networks in providing support and sustenance to the LGBTQIA patient. In this context, family often includes individuals unrelated by biological ties. A useful concept is "family of origin," which consists of parents, siblings, and others with whom one shares a blood relation, contrasted with "family of choice," which includes those close friendship relationships enduring over time and incorporating the same types of support and emotions often associated with idealized views of the traditional family. The family of a lesbian or gay patient, including their partner, is a vital part of the individual's health and can serve as a source of both stress and support, just as with heterosexual patients. Physicians caring for gay men and lesbians need to assess the resources and stressors that exist within the family, as defined by the patient.

The American Academy of Pediatrics (AAP) has come out in support of gay marriage, saying that research indicates "there is no causal relationship between parents' sexual orientation and children's emotional, psychosocial and behavioral development." The AAP also endorses adoption and foster parenting by gays and lesbians.

Hospice & Palliative Medicine

Eva B. Reitschuler-Cross, MD

Robert M. Arnold, MD

INTRODUCING PALLIATIVE CARE & HOSPICE TO PATIENTS & FAMILIES

Patients with life-limiting, advanced illnesses need excellent symptom management, psychosocial and spiritual support, and guidance with decision making. Palliative care is a rapidly growing field that is meeting these needs in inpatient and outpatient settings. In addition, many providers of both general and specialty care embrace the philosophy of palliative care and incorporate its core principles into their practice. Whereas palliative care might be appropriate for patients of all stages of a life-limiting illness, hospice care is appropriate for patients in the terminal stage of their illnesses. Interdisciplinary team work is a core principle of palliative care and hospice, building on the expertise of clinicians, nurses, mental health providers, chaplains, social workers, and other care providers.

Patients with a serious illness are vulnerable and may have negative perceptions about palliative care and hospice care. Appropriate times to introduce palliative care are (1) at the time of diagnosis of a life-limiting illness; (2) at the time of an adverse change in clinical status (eg, disease progression, loss of function, or increased symptom burden); (3) at the time of a crisis (eg, hospitalization, intensive care unit admission, or consideration of advanced therapies such as left ventricular assist device, organ transplantation, renal replacement therapy, or artificial nutrition); or (4) when asked by patients or family members. Patients might confuse palliative care with end-of-life care. When they respond with anxiety or hesitancy to the idea of receiving palliative care, it is essential to ask what patients know and what they want to know and to explore their emotions. Clinicians can further ameliorate patients' concerns by explaining that palliative care is not intended to replace their current treatment plan but rather to augment it by being provided alongside disease-directed, life-prolonging therapies. Optimal symptom control can help patients to continue demanding therapies and achieve other goals patients might have.

A later transition in care that might elicit intense emotional responses is the transition to hospice care. Common concerns such as "giving up," feeling abandoned, or feeling "not ready to die" need to be carefully explored. The understanding that the adverse effects of further disease-directed therapies might outweigh their potential benefits often requires a cognitive and emotional process for which patients are not given enough time. A kind and patient approach can help these conversations to progress successfully.

Hospice provides medications necessary to address symptoms, care equipment, nursing, chaplaincy, and social work visits, as well as some home health aide visits. After a patient's death, bereavement services are provided. Most patients receive hospice care at home, and family members need to understand that they will be providing the bulk of day-to-day care. If severe symptoms cannot be controlled in the home setting, patients can be admitted to an inpatient hospice facility. Hospice care can also be provided in a nursing facility; however, most patients, depending on their insurance, would be financially responsible for room and board fees.

PAIN & SYMPTOM MANAGEMENT

Optimal symptom control is an important cornerstone of palliative medicine, because uncontrolled symptoms increase patients' and caregivers' distress. Poorly controlled symptoms often detract from patients' quality of life, impair their interactions with loved ones, and limit their ability to attend to important issues at the end of life. Many studies have documented the high frequency of symptoms in patients with serious illnesses and the tendency for symptoms to increase in intensity as a disease progresses. The following discussion reviews management of some common symptoms. As with most medical problems, successful management of symptoms starts with a careful history and physical examination, with therapy directed at identifiable underlying causes.

Table 67–1. Classification of pain.

	Nociceptive		Neuropathic
	Somatic	**Visceral**	
Etiology	Due to tissue damage—activation of nociceptors in cutaneous and deep tissues	Due to tissue damage—activation of nociceptors resulting from stretching, distension, or inflammation of visceral organs	Due to nervous system dysfunction ± tissue damage
Description of pain	Well localized, aching, throbbing, gnawing	Poorly localized, dull, crampy, squeezy, pressure	Burning, shooting, stabbing, tingling, electriclike, numb
Examples	Bone, soft tissues, muscle pain	Small bowel or ureteral obstruction, peritoneal carcinomatosis, hepatic distension	Peripheral neuropathy, plexopathy

▶ Pain

Pain can be classified physiologically as nociceptive (somatic or visceral) or neuropathic. (Table 67–1). Pain can occur directly from the underlying illnesses (eg, tumor involvement, cytokine release, or vasculopathy), as a consequence of therapy (particularly chemotherapy, radiation therapy, and invasive procedures), or from pathologies that are not directly related to the primary disease processes. It is important to remember that pain is a subjective experience, and it is essential to respect and accept the complaint of pain as characterized by the patient. Pain is influenced by psychosocial and spiritual issues, and effective pain management requires a multidisciplinary approach.

Unlike opioids, nonsteroidal anti-inflammatory drugs (NSAIDs) and acetaminophen have an analgesic ceiling effect. Therefore, the use of opioid-nonopioid combinations is limited by the dose of the NSAID or acetaminophen. Despite this fact, NSAIDs are effective pain medication, especially for inflammatory conditions. Their use can decrease the amount of opioids required and hence decrease the incidence of opioid side effects. Unless contraindicated, all pain protocols should include a NSAID or acetaminophen.

The general principles of pain management with opioids are as follows:

1. Assess pain using a standardized pain scale. Most commonly used is a 0–10 scale, where 0 indicates no pain and 10 represents the worst pain imaginable. Numerous validated scales can be used for patients who cannot communicate because they are intubated, are preverbal children, or are cognitively impaired adults.

2. In opioid-naive patients, start with a short-acting opioid (eg, morphine, oxycodone, or hydromorphone) to control acute, moderate to severe pain. Unless there are contraindications, morphine is the agent of choice given its low costs and variable routes of administration (oral, intravenous [IV], subcutaneous, intramuscular, or rectal). Short-acting opioids can be given as frequently as the time to peak onset of action: every 60–90 minutes

for oral immediate-release formulations and every 10–15 minutes for IV formulations. For severe pain, IV administration is recommended given the faster onset of action and greater ease of titration. Conversion to oral opioids can occur once the pain is controlled.

3. Determine whether the dose is adequate and adjust accordingly. The dose should be titrated at least every 24 hours if the pain is moderate and as often as every 4 hours if the pain is severe, particularly while using IV opioids. Dose increases should be made by 25–50% for moderate pain and by 50–100% for severe pain. There is no specific limit to opioid doses. These agents should be titrated until pain is controlled or side effects develop.

4. Further titration or rotation of opioids is achieved by first calculating the *oral morphine equivalent* (OME) of the previous 24 hours' worth of opioid use. Equianalgesic tables for opioids are readily available (Table 67–2); however, these tables often differ slightly. It is important to

Table 67–2. Opioid analgesic equivalences.

Opioid Agonist	Parenteral (mg)	Oral (mg)
Morphine[a]	10	30
Oxycodone		20–30
Hydromorphone	1.5	7.5
Fentanyl	0.1[b]	
Codeine	130	200
Hydrocodone		25–30
Oxymorphone	1	10

[a]The 24-hour oral morphine equivalent (OME) divided by 2 is equal to the fentanyl patch dose in micrograms per hour (eg, 24-hour OME is 100 mg, equivalent fentanyl patch dose is 50 µg/h).
[b]Equivalency of a one-time dose of intravenous fentanyl only.

remember that oral and parenteral doses are not equal because of oral medicines' first-pass hepatic metabolism; for example, 1 mg of IV morphine sulfate equals 3 mg of oral morphine sulfate, and 1 mg of parenteral hydromorphone equals 4 mg of oral hydromorphone.

5. Determine the dosing schedule. Chronic pain deserves scheduled pain medication, not just as-needed dosing: 66–75% of the patient's stable 24-hour OME needs should be given as a long-acting formulation.

6. Determine the breakthrough dose. *Breakthrough pain* is defined as a transitory exacerbation of pain that occurs on top of an otherwise stable persistent pain. An adequate breakthrough dose is calculated as 10–15% of the total daily long-acting opioid, and it should be given every 3 hours as needed. Whenever possible, the same opioid agent should be used for both short- and long-acting administration (eg, sustained-release morphine 150 mg orally every 12 hours and immediate-release morphine 30–45 mg orally every 3 hours, as needed).

7. During administration of opioid therapy, the patient's renal function should be closely monitored because toxic metabolites can accumulate with decreased kidney function, leading to alterations in mental status, myoclonic jerks, and seizures. Opioids that are safe to use in renal failure include hydromorphone, fentanyl, and methadone.

8. Reasons for rotating to a different opioid include renal failure, side effects, and a need to change the route of administration (eg, changing from oral morphine to transdermal fentanyl). When rotating to a different opioid, the dose should be reduced by 25–50% to account for incomplete cross-tolerance.

Fentanyl patches should not be used alone for acute severe pain. Because of the delayed onset of effect (12 hours) and long half-life of this formulation, which allows for titrations only every 48–72 hours, it cannot be titrated quickly for rapid pain control. If the pain is severe or unpredictable or if opioid requirements are unknown or increasing rapidly, patient-controlled analgesia (PCA) may be indicated. With PCA infusion pumps, opioids can be infused IV or subcutaneously at a continuous basal rate programmed by the care provider, while the administrations of bolus doses are controlled by the patient. There is theoretically no risk of overdose since the patient will fall asleep before serious signs of overdose occur, and for this reason, the patient's family or visitors should be carefully educated to avoid pushing the PCA button on the patient's behalf.

Guidelines on management of opioid-induced side effects are as follows:

1. **Nausea/vomiting:** Opioids can cause nausea and vomiting by decreasing gastrointestinal motility. Patients usually develop a tolerance to these side effects. It may be helpful to schedule an antiemetic for a few days and then change to as-needed administration. Dopamine receptor antagonists are most effective (haloperidol 0.5–2 mg every 6–12 hours or metoclopramide 10–40 mg every 6 hours).

2. **Sedation:** This is a commonly encountered side effect, although tolerance typically develops over time to this as well. Down-titration of opioids, rotation of opiates, and use of adjuvant, nonopioid pain therapies should be considered. Other sedating agents should be eliminated whenever possible. If sedation persists despite these interventions, the addition of a central nervous system stimulant can be helpful (methylphenidate 2.5–5 mg in the morning and at noon or modafinil 100–200 mg daily).

3. **Constipation:** This is one of the most common side effects. Since patients rarely develop tolerance, if at all, a bowel regimen must be started for most patients with initiation of opioid therapy. A bowel stimulant (senna) is the most commonly used agent. Methylnaltrexone is a peripherally acting opioid receptor antagonist that has been approved for refractory constipation in patients receiving opioid therapy. It does not reverse central analgesia.

4. **Delirium/confusion/hallucinations:** In this setting, opioid dose reduction, rotation to a different opioid, and initiation of neuroleptic therapy (haloperidol 0.5–1 mg 2–4 times a day or olanzapine 2.5–5 mg daily or twice a day) should be considered.

5. **Allergic reaction:** True allergic reactions are rare. Allergy-like symptoms are usually secondary to mast cell activation and subsequent histamine release.

6. **Respiratory depression:** Tolerance to the respiratory depressant effects occurs rapidly; thus, opioids can be used safely when titrated to pain control, even in patients with underlying emphysema. Naloxone administration is indicated if (1) the patient is somnolent and difficult to arouse or (2) respiratory rate is <8/min or oxygen saturation is <92% and the respiratory rate is <12/min. A dilution of 0.4 mg naloxone (one ampoule, 1 mL) in 9 mL of normal saline to yield 0.04 mg of naloxone per milliliter should be prepared, with administration of this diluted naloxone in 1- to 2-mL increments (0.04–0.08 mg) over 1- to 2-minute intervals until a change in alertness is observed. Giving naloxone in this way should not cause pain to return or opioid withdrawal. Remember that the half-life of naloxone is shorter than the half-life of most opioids, so respiratory depression may recur and a naloxone drip may be needed.

A challenge in prescribing opioid pain medications is to correctly differentiate a patient in pain from a patient with a substance abuse disorder. The key lies in understanding the specific characteristics of tolerance, physical and psychological dependence, and pseudoaddiction. *Tolerance* is a state of adaption in which exposure to a drug induces changes that result in a decreased effect of the drug dose over time. *Physical dependence* is a state of adaption that is manifested by a specific withdrawal syndrome when the drug is discontinued suddenly. Most patients on chronic opioids will develop physical dependence. If the need arises for a rapid decrease in opioid dose, administering 25–50% of the stable dose can prevent withdrawal symptoms. Both tolerance and physical dependence cannot be used to differentiate between a patient in pain and a patient with a substance abuse disorder. Psychological dependence or addiction is a primary, chronic, neurobiological disease with genetic and psychosocial factors influencing its development. It is characterized by certain behaviors, including loss of control, compulsive drug use, craving, and continued use of the drug despite harm. Research suggests that opioids used to treat pain rarely lead to psychological dependence. *Pseudoaddiction* describes a patient's behavior when the pain is undertreated. Some of these behaviors, such as "clock watching" or having "excessive pain," may mimic addiction. However, a distinguishing feature of pseudoaddiction not seen in true addiction is the resolution of these behaviors when pain is effectively treated.

It is especially important to be able to distinguish between a patient's true pain needs and opioid misuse in the contemporary clinical environment, in which palliative care is being used earlier in patients' disease processes, while there is concurrently increasing documentation of opioid misuse. To identify patients at risk, clinicians need to perform careful histories of all drug use, including past and present use of tobacco, alcohol, and recreational drugs, as well as misuse of prescription drugs. To further stratify risk of opioid misuse, a validated screening tool should be used. At initiation of therapy, an opioid agreement should be used to delineate safe practices and to identify when opioid therapy will be discontinued. All patients should routinely (including at initiation of therapy and at least annually) have urine drug testing. At the initiation of opioid therapy, the consequences related to the presence of illicit drugs on a urine drug screen, requests for early refills, or attempts to obtain controlled substances from other clinicians need to be explained. Furthermore, clinicians should review their patients' histories of use of controlled substances using state prescription drug monitoring program data to determine whether the patient is receiving opioid prescriptions from multiple providers or whether he or she is prescribed opioid dosages or combinations (eg, opioids and benzodiazepines) that increase the risk for overdose. Naloxone should be prescribed to patients who are at increased risk of opioid overdose, including patients with histories of previous drug overdose, substance abuse disorder, or concurrent use of benzodiazepines or other sedating drugs.

Patients with an active substance abuse disorder and chronic pain should be referred to an addiction medicine specialist.

A. Adjuvant Pain Therapies

Patients with neuropathic pain occasionally respond to opioids alone; however, many require the addition of adjuvant pain medications. Commonly used adjuvants for neuropathic pain include tricyclic antidepressants (TCAs), serotonin-norepinephrine reuptake inhibitors (SNRIs), anticonvulsants, and antiarrhythmics. The choice of an adjuvant is usually dictated by the individual drug side effect profile, the potential for drug interactions, and the previous drug therapy. The secondary amines, nortriptyline and desipramine, are generally better tolerated than amitriptyline. The analgesic effects of TCAs occur at lower doses and usually within several days, as compared with the antidepressant effects. Data on use of selective serotonin reuptake inhibitors (SSRIs) for neuropathic pain are not convincing; however, recent studies suggest that SNRIs may be as beneficial at tricyclic agents for pain control. Of the anticonvulsants, gabapentin, pregabalin, carbamazepine, and valproic acid are commonly used for neuropathic pain. Carbamazepine and valproic acid are cost-effective but have a higher risk of drug interactions and toxicity compared with gabapentin and pregabalin. Gabapentin requires more frequent dosing, slower titration secondary to sedation, and dose adjustments for renal insufficiency. Antiarrhythmics, topical lidocaine, and oral mexiletine have also been used successfully for neuropathic pain. For adjuvant pain medications, standard initial dosing and titration guidelines should be followed, although lower-than-usual doses have been effective for pain control. In elderly patients, it is generally safer to start at low doses and titrate at a slower rate.

Corticosteroids, benzodiazepines, and anticholinergics are also used as adjuvant pain medication. Corticosteroids, by decreasing tumor-associated edema and by their anti-inflammatory effects, are useful for pain because of multiple pathologies, including bone metastasis, liver capsule distention from metastasis, and conditions in which the tumor is compressing sensitive structures. Benzodiazepines and baclofen are indicated for pain from spasticity. Anticholinergics can relieve colic due to intestinal obstruction.

In addition to drug therapy for pain control, interventions such as palliative radiation therapy for bone metastasis, nerve blockage (eg, celiac plexus block for pancreatic cancer), palliative surgical resection, or immobilization of fractures should be considered. Before undertaking such interventions, the patient's overall prognosis and the effectiveness of less invasive measures should be considered. Complementary therapies are often used in hospice and palliative care for treatment of pain and other symptoms. Some of these therapies are described in Table 67–3.

Table 67–3. Complementary modalities used in palliative medicine.

Therapy	Brief Description	Recommendations
Acupuncture	Stimulation of defined points on the skin using a needle, electrical current (electroacupuncture), or pressure (acupressure). These points correspond to meridians, or pathways of energy flow with the intent to correct energy imbalances and restore a normal, healthy flow of energy in the body.	1. Acupuncture may provide pain relief in terminally ill patients with cancer pain. 2. Acupuncture may provide relief from breathlessness. 3. Acupressure may reduce chemotherapy- and radiation-induced nausea and vomiting.
Aromatherapy	Therapeutic use of essential oils, which are applied to the skin or inhaled. The impact on the emotional and psychological state is mediated through the olfactory nerve and the limbic system in the brain.	1. Aromatherapy may be used in conjunction with other complementary therapies, such as massage. 2. Aromatherapy may provide reduction in anxiety.
Massage therapy	Manipulation of the muscles and soft tissues of the body for therapeutic purposes.	1. Massage might provide short-term reduction in cancer pain. 2. Massage has been shown to reduce stress and anxiety and enhance feelings of relaxation.
Hypnosis	A state of increased receptivity of suggestion and direction.	1. Hypnotherapy can enhance pain relief. 2. Hypnotherapy may reduce nausea and vomiting in patients receiving chemotherapy.
Relaxation	The use of muscular relaxation techniques to release tension. These techniques are often used in conjunction with meditation, biofeedback, and guided imagery techniques.	1. Relaxation can reduce stress and tension. 2. Relaxation techniques can improve pain control in advanced cancer patients.
Therapeutic touch	A technique performed by physical touch and/or the use of hand movements to balance any disturbances in a person's energy flow.	1. Therapeutic touch may increase hemoglobin levels. 2. Therapeutic touch may relieve anxiety and tension and reduce the effects of stress on the immune system.
Music therapy	The use of music as a therapy to influence mental, behavioral, or physiologic disorders.	1. Music therapy may assist in the reduction of pain perception. 2. Music therapy may reduce anxiety and help persons cope with grief and loss.
Support group	The use of groups and psychosocial interventions to help persons learn how to cope better with their disease.	1. Support groups can enhance the quality of life. 2. Support group therapy can improve pain management and coping skills. 3. Support group therapy can reduce anxiety and depression.

▶ Nausea & Vomiting

Nausea and vomiting entail complex physiologic processes and are triggered by activation of one of four main pathways. An understanding of these pathways may aid in choosing an effective antiemetic regimen.

1. The *chemoreceptor trigger zone* is located at the area postrema of the medulla. It lies outside the blood-brain barrier and is therefore able to sample emetogenic toxins, drugs, or metabolic abnormalities such as uremia or hypercalcemia. It further receives input from the gastrointestinal tract. The main receptors involved include dopamine type 2 receptors (D_2), 5-hydroxytryptamine type 3 receptor (5-HT_3), and neurokinin type 1 receptor (NK1).

2. Pathways from the vestibular apparatus respond to vertigo and visuospatial disorientation. The main receptors involved include muscarinic acetylcholine receptors (m-Ach) and histamine type 1 receptors (H_1).

3. Peripheral pathways (vagus nerve and splanchnic nerves) mediate nausea triggered by activation of visceral chemoreceptors (local toxins) and serosal mechanoreceptors (stretch of organs and capsules). The main receptors involved include H_1 and m-Ach receptors. Enterochromaffin cells release 5-HT_3 when damaged by interventions such as chemotherapy or radiation therapy.

4. Cortical pathways respond to increased intracranial pressure, sensory stimuli (smell, pain), and psychogenic stimuli (anxiety, memory, conditioning).

Each of these pathways sends signals to the *vomiting center* (VC), which triggers nausea and vomiting when thresholds

Table 67–4. Commonly used antiemetics.

Drug	Receptor Activity/Effect	Common Indication	Dosage/Route	Side Effects
Haloperidol	D_2	Opioid-induced N/V	0.5–4 mg PO or SC or IV every 6 hours (Q6h)	EPS, QTc prolongation
Metoclopramide	Peripheral D_2	Opioid-induced N/V, delayed gastric emptying	5–20 mg PO or SC or IV before meals and at bedtime	EPS, esophageal spasm, colic in complete bowel obstruction
Prochlorperazine	D_2	Opioid-induced N/V, N/V of unknown etiology	5–10 mg PO or IV Q6h or 25 mg PR Q6h	EPS and sedation
Scopolamine	Ach, H_1	Vestibular dysfunction	1.5 mg transdermal patch every 3 days	Dry mouth, blurred vision, ileus, urinary retention, and confusion; patch starts being effective after 24 hours
Ondansetron	$5\text{-}HT_3$	Chemotherapy- or radiation therapy–induced N/V	4–8 mg PO as pill or dissolvable tablet or IV every 4–8 hours	Headache, fatigue, constipation
Dexamethasone	Decreases intracranial pressure	Increased intracranial pressure, capsular stretch	4–8 mg every morning or BID, PO (pill or liquid) or IV	Agitation, insomnia, hyperglycemia
Lorazepam	GABA receptor	Anticipatory N/V	0.5–2 mg PO or IV every 4–6 hours	Sedation, confusion, delirium
Aprepitant	NK1	Severe chemotherapy-induced N/V	125 mg PO on day 1, 80 mg PO on days 2–3	Somnolence, fatigue, may reduce warfarin levels

BID, twice per day; EPS, extrapyramidal symptoms; GABA, γ-aminobutyric acid; IV, intravenous; N/V, nausea/vomiting; PO, per mouth; PR, per rectum; SC, subcutaneous.

are reached. The main receptors involved at the VC are H_1, m-Ach, and $5\text{-}HT_3$.

Treatment should focus on correcting underlying causes as well as choosing antiemetics to target-specific receptors and pathways involved. Commonly used antiemetics are described in Table 67–4. If nausea or vomiting is persistent, severe, or refractory, it is recommended to schedule regular administrations of an antiemetic agent. A second or third antiemetic targeting a different receptor may be added (scheduled dosing or dosed as needed).

Nausea and vomiting also may be presenting symptoms of a malignant gastrointestinal obstruction. The patent should be evaluated for invasive procedures such as venting gastrostomy, intraluminal stent, or surgical diversion. With partial obstruction, the use of metoclopramide and dexamethasone along with a low-fiber diet can provide significant symptom relief for several weeks or longer. When an obstruction becomes complete, therapy is directed at decreasing intestinal motility and decreasing secretions using anticholinergics and somatostatin analogs. Metoclopramide is contraindicated in complete bowel obstruction as it increases gastrointestinal motility and leads to exacerbation of painful abdominal cramping.

▶ Dyspnea

Dyspnea, like pain, is a subjective experience and can be present with or without hypoxia. With a broad differential existing for dyspnea, reversible causes should always be considered first. The optimal therapy is aimed at the presumed etiology. Palliative therapy can involve chemotherapy, radiotherapy, thoracentesis, pericardiocentesis, and bronchial stent placement. General measures such as providing a fan, keeping the room temperature cool, use of relaxation techniques, or using a careful trial of supplemental oxygen (for hypoxic patients) can help dyspneic patients. Available palliative drug therapies include steroids, opioids, bronchodilators, diuretics, anxiolytics, antibiotics, and anticoagulants. All these drugs can be used in combination, depending on the etiology of dyspnea.

Opioids can relieve breathlessness, although the mechanism is unclear. Opioid administration, dose, frequency, and titration are the same as for pain control. The use of nebulized morphine sulfate is not more effective than placebo. Opioids can increase exercise tolerance and reduce dyspnea in patients with chronic obstructive airways. Fear of addiction or fear of respiratory depression should not preclude a trial of opioids in this population. Starting at low doses, carefully titrating the dose to achieve symptom control, and close monitoring allow for safe and effective use.

Steroids are useful for dyspnea from bronchospasm and tumor-associated edema. Specific indications include malignant bronchial obstruction, carcinomatous lymphangitis, and superior vena cava syndrome. Dexamethasone can be started at 4 mg twice daily and subsequently reduced to the lowest effective dose. Dexamethasone is more potent and has lower mineralocorticoid activity than other steroids, resulting in less fluid retention.

Some patients with dyspnea express disturbing fears of suffocation and choking. Understandably, anxiety often coexists with chronic dyspnea. Anxiety can heighten breathlessness, making symptom control more difficult. The use of anxiolytics such as benzodiazepines and phenothiazines can help treat dyspnea associated with a high component of anxiety. Lorazepam, 0.5–1 mg, can be tried initially. If patients show benefit, long-acting diazepam or clonazepam can then be prescribed. Low-dose chlorpromazine has also shown benefit in relieving both dyspnea and anxiety.

▶ Anorexia & Cachexia

Anorexia (poor appetite) and cachexia (involuntary weight loss regardless of caloric intake or appetite) are prevalent distressing symptoms in patients with advanced illnesses. Mechanisms of the anorexia-cachexia syndrome include an aberrant inflammatory response, generated by disease-host reactions, as well as neurohormonal dysfunction. Exacerbating factors include delayed gastric emptying, constipation, nausea, depression, mucositis, thrush, and even ill-fitting dentures.

Little effective drug therapy is available. Megestrol acetate, a progestin, has been shown to increase appetite and result in weight gain; however, weight gain is due largely to accumulation of adipose tissue and not lean muscle mass. Doses start at 160 mg/d and can be titrated to 800 mg/d if required. Side effects include thromboembolic events and adrenal insufficiency on abrupt cessation. Corticosteroids, such as dexamethasone, can be prescribed as appetite stimulants for patients in whom side effects of long-term steroid use are of less concern. Beneficial effects tend to be limited to several weeks. Significant weight gain is not seen with corticosteroids in this population. Dexamethasone can be started at 2–4 mg daily, with titration to 16 mg daily if required. The lowest effective steroid dose should always be used. Androgens, dronabinol, and growth hormones have been effective for patients with acquired immunodeficiency syndrome (AIDS)–associated anorexia and cachexia.

Nutritional support, parenteral and enteral, has not been shown to prolong survival in patients with advanced cancer who are not candidates for disease-specific therapy. Exceptions include patients with head and neck cancer undergoing radiation therapy or patients with gastrointestinal dysfunction and otherwise good performance status.

PSYCHIATRIC DIMENSIONS IN PALLIATIVE CARE

▶ Depression

There is a common assumption that symptoms of depression are normal or expected in patients facing life-threatening illness. This thought promotes the underdiagnosis of depression and, in turn, its undertreatment. Depressive states exist on a continuum from normal sadness that accompanies life-limiting disease to major affective disorders. It is important that clinicians differentiate among these levels of distress.

Besides a personal or family history of psychiatric illness, risk factors for depression in palliative care patients include young age, poor social support, worsening illness, high symptom burden, poor functional status, and the use of certain medications such as corticosteroids, interferon, interleukin-2, and some chemotherapeutic agents.

Diagnosing depression in physically healthy patients depends heavily on the presence of neurovegetative symptoms such as decreased appetite, loss of energy, insomnia, loss of sexual drive, and psychomotor retardation. Given that these symptoms are frequently present in patients with advanced illness, they are less reliable for diagnosing depression in this patient population. Elements of the history that can be helpful in diagnosing depression include anhedonia, feelings of hopelessness, worthlessness, helplessness, excessive guilt, and suicidal ideation. A quick and effective way to screen for depression is to ask the following two questions: "Have you been feeling down, depressed, or hopeless most of the time over the past 2 weeks?" and "Have you found that little brings you pleasure or joy over the past 2 weeks?"

Treatment of depression in the palliative care population is similar to the general population. Since antidepressants take as much as 4–8 weeks to show effect, it is reasonable to start treatment with a psychostimulant in patients with a prognosis of <6 months. Effects are usually felt within 1–2 days and include improved mood, energy, appetite, and cognition. Other effective treatment options include psychotherapeutic interventions.

It is important to differentiate depression from preparatory or anticipatory grief, which is defined as the "grief that a terminally ill person has to undergo in order to prepare himself for his final separation from this world" (Elisabeth Kübler-Ross). Features include withdrawal from loved ones, rumination about the past, sadness, crying, and anxiety. In contrast to depression, mood changes are typically transient, and patients maintain the capacity for experiencing pleasure. Further, patients' self-image is typically not disturbed, and they are able to maintain hope, although the focus of their hope may shift.

▶ Anxiety

Anxiety is a common symptom in patients facing serious illness. It is characterized by worries or fears stemming from one's perception of a threat in either the present or the future. Anxiety may be present as part of a primary psychiatric disorder, including generalized anxiety disorder, panic disorder, adjustment disorder, phobias, and acute or posttraumatic stress disorders. Anxiety may also be a secondary component of other symptoms, including pain, shortness of breath, or nausea. Furthermore, it can be a sign of drug withdrawal, including alcohol, opioids, benzodiazepines, antidepressants, and nicotine; and in addition, it can be an adverse drug reaction from medications such as corticosteroids, psychostimulants, and some antidepressants. Anxiety may have metabolic causes such as hyperthyroidism or syndromes of adrenergic or serotonergic excess. Often anxiety is also a sign of existential or psychosocial concerns about disease progression, disability, loss, dying, legacy, family, finances, and religion or spirituality.

Several formal screening tools for anxiety exist. The Edmonton Assessment Scale and the Hospital Anxiety and Depression Scale are most frequently used. Besides a thorough history and physical exam, the evaluation of a patient with anxiety should include an assessment of prior episodes of anxiety, depression, posttraumatic stress disorder, and alcohol and drug use. It is helpful to ascertain if there are specific thoughts or situations triggering anxiety. Symptoms that can be misdiagnosed as anxiety include agitated delirium, cardiac arrhythmias, or akathisia, which is a symptom induced by dopamine receptor–blocking agents such as metoclopramide or antipsychotics and manifests as an unpleasant sensation of restlessness.

The first step of treatment is active listening, with efforts to normalize the patient's experience and provide support. Pharmacologic treatment options include medications such as SSRIs and benzodiazepines. Longer-acting benzodiazepines such as clonazepam are usually preferred, as they are less likely to cause rebound anxiety. The patient's subjective level of distress is the primary indication for the initiation of pharmacologic treatment. Nonpharmacologic treatment options include psychotherapeutic interventions such as cognitive behavioral therapy or supportive expressive therapy. The use of relaxation techniques or guided imagery is also helpful.

For more detail on issues of depression and anxiety, please refer to Chapters 56 and 57.

▶ Delirium

Delirium is a frequently overlooked diagnosis, and it is associated with increased morbidity and mortality. It is characterized by an alteration of consciousness with a reduced ability to focus, sustain, or shift attention. Additional features are changes in cognition (eg, memory deficits, language disturbances, and disorientation) and the development of perceptual disturbances. These changes are acute in onset and typically fluctuate throughout the day. Further symptoms include changes in the sleep/wake cycle, altered psychomotor activity, or delusions. A formal diagnosis of delirium also requires evidence by history, physical exam, or laboratory data that the changes in consciousness and cognition are caused by the direct physiologic consequences of a medical condition.

The main differential diagnosis of delirium is dementia, which, unlike delirium, is characterized by little or no clouding in consciousness, an insidious onset, and a chronic, progressive course. Furthermore, hypoactive delirium may be mistaken for depression; conversely, early stages of hyperactive delirium may be mistaken for anxiety or extrapyramidal symptoms.

Treatment is focused on reversing or treating underlying causes, such as dehydration, infection, hypoxia, electrolyte disturbances (particularly hypercalcemia), metabolic disturbances, urinary retention, constipation, and brain metastases. The medication list should be reviewed for offending medications and drug-drug interactions. Benzodiazepines, anticholinergics, and antihistamines are often implicated in precipitating delirium and should be discontinued or decreased as much as possible. If opioids are suspected as the culprit agent and the treatment doses cannot be reduced because of pain needs, then rotation to a different opioid at a dose reduced by 25–50% is recommended.

Simple environmental measures are often underused and include frequent orientation (including use of clocks, calendars, caregivers, and pictures of loved ones), ample day/night indicators (well-illuminated rooms during the day and reduced noise and light at nighttime), and treatment of hearing and vision problems.

Pharmacologic interventions include the use of antipsychotics (Table 67–5). Haloperidol is most commonly used.

Frieden TR, Houry D. Reducing the risks of relief–the CDC opioid-prescribing guideline. *N Engl J Med.* 2016;374(16):1501–1504. [PMID: 26977701]

Goldstein N, Morrison RS. *Evidence-Based Practice of Palliative Medicine: Expert Consult: Online and Print.* Philadelphia, PA: Saunders-Elsevier; 2013.

McPherson ML. *Demystifying Opioid Conversion Calculations.* Bethesda, MD: American Society of Health-System Pharmacists; 2010.

Morrison RD, Meier DE. Palliative care. *N Engl J Med.* 2004;350:2582–2590. [PMID: 15201415]

National Institute for Health and Care Excellence. *Opioids in Palliative Care: Safe and Effective Prescribing of Strong Opioids for Pain in Palliative Care of Adults.* NICE guidelines, May 2012. https://www.ncbi.nlm.nih.gov/books/NBK115251. Accessed January 2019.

Palliative Care Network of Wisconsin. Fast facts and concepts. https://www.mypcnow.org/fast-facts. Accessed December 9, 2019.

Table 67–5. Pharmacologic treatment options of delirium.

Drug	Starting Dose (mg)	Dosing Interval	Maximum 24-Hour Dose (mg)	Comments
Haloperidol	0.5–1 (2 in ICU)	Every ½–1 hour for urgent symptoms, otherwise every 6–8 hours	20	Most commonly used; IV has less EPS than PO, but PO has less QTc prolongation than IV
Olanzapine	2.5–5	Daily or BID	20	Sedating, helpful in restoring day/sleep cycle when given at nighttime, less EPS
Quetiapine	12.5–50	Twice a day	800	At lower doses more sedating (antihistaminic) properties; antipsychotic effects at higher doses, less EPS
Risperidone	0.25–1	Twice a day or every ≤6 hours	6	Least sedating, caution with renal failure

EPS, extrapyramidal symptoms; ICU, intensive care unit; IV, intravenous; PO, per mouth.

SPIRITUAL DIMENSIONS IN PALLIATIVE CARE

Serious illness unavoidably raises fundamental questions about the meanings of life and death, as well as deep emotions often involving existential or spiritual angst, guilt, regret, hopelessness, feeling of being a burden, and sadness about broken relationships with loved ones, among others. Spiritual and existential suffering are prevalent, although they are often unrecognized by clinicians. When unrecognized and untreated, they may lead to anxiety and depression, and they may complicate symptom management. Clinicians may feel reluctant to explore issues that they do not have the expertise to solve. The goal of assessing spiritual and existential concerns is to provide a safe space for patients to share their fears and concerns and to facilitate involvement of care providers with expertise in spiritual suffering, such as hospital chaplains or clergy from the patients' own religious communities. The FICA spiritual history tool was developed to help clinicians explore spiritual issues with patients (Table 67–6). It is not intended to be used as a checklist, but rather as a guide to open and facilitate a conversation about spiritual and existential concerns.

Berry M, Brink E, Harris, et al. Supporting relatives and carers at the end of a patient's life. *BMJ.* 2017;356:j367. [PMID: 28154119]

Martin J, George R. What is the point of spirituality? *Palliat Med.* 2016;30:325–326. [PMID: 26992803]

Pearce MJ, Coan AD, Herndon JE, et al. Unmet spiritual care needs impact emotional and spiritual well-being in advanced cancer patients. *Support Care Cancer.* 2012;20:2269–2276. [PMID: 22124529]

The FICA Spiritual History Tool. https://smhs.gwu.edu/gwish/clinical/fica/spiritual-history-tool. Accessed January 2019.

COMMUNICATION SKILLS IN PALLIATIVE CARE

Physicians treating patients with serious illness encounter several difficult conversations with the patients and their families. These conversations span the entire disease course, from the diagnosis through the disease progression and, finally, end-of-life care. Challenging aspects of these conversations include the breaking of serious news and discussions of prognosis, goals of care, and advance directives. These conversations often culminate in the emotionally challenging decision to transition from curative or life-prolonging therapies to hospice care. While easing difficult situations, effective communication also results in improved patient adjustment to illness, increased adherence to treatments, lessened pain and other physical symptoms, reduced anxiety, decreased conflict, and avoidance of ineffective, often invasive treatments.

Table 67–6. FICA spiritual history tool.

F: Faith, believe, meaning	"Do you consider yourself spiritual or religious?" "Do you have spiritual beliefs that help you cope with stress?" If the patient answers "No," a clinician may ask, "What gives your life meaning?"
I: Importance and Influence	"What importance does your faith or belief have in your life?" "Have your beliefs influenced you how you handle stress?" "Do you have specific beliefs that might influence your healthcare decisions? If so, are you willing to share those with your healthcare team?"
C: Community	"Are you part of a religious or spiritual community?" "Is this of support to you and how?" "Is there a group of people you really love and/or who are important to you?"
A: Address/action in care	"How should I address these issues in your health care?"

Responding to Emotions

Difficult conversations are very complex and elicit a wide range of emotions and reactions in patients and their families. These responses may include shock, withdrawal, sadness, crying, denial, fear, anger, and acceptance. During difficult conversations, clinicians tend to focus on objective, medical data; however, it is crucial to notice and respond to emotions. Understandably, difficult conversations represent a form of danger to patients. When facing danger, we usually respond with a fight-or-flight reaction, while more cognitive, analytical responses get shifted into the background. This is the reason why patients commonly report that they "did not hear anything" after their clinician conveyed serious news. The key at this point in the conversation is to slow down and respond to emotions so the "system can cool down" and patients are able to cognitively process important medical data.

Empathy is the process of recognizing and responding to emotions in others. It starts with noticing and identifying the patient's emotion; clinicians should importantly not try to fix or quiet a patient's emotion. The next step includes acknowledging the emotion. This can be done nonverbally (eg, through eye contact, changes in body position, or touch) or through explicit statements. The acronym NURSE summarizes ways to respond verbally to emotions (Table 67–7).

Another powerful way to respond to emotions is to normalize the experience. Examples include "Anyone receiving such news would feel anxious and sad," or, "It is completely expected to feel devastated when one's life changes so dramatically."

Breaking Serious News

Conversations in which serious news is delivered by the clinician to the patient and family occur not only at the time of diagnosis but also when the illness progresses to the point at which it no longer responds to therapies. The SPIKES (set up, perception, invitation, knowledge, emotion, summarize/strategy) protocol is a six-step protocol that can be used in these stressful situations:

1. Set up—prepare for the conversation. Prior to the conversation, all medical data and information about possible treatment options need to be reviewed. The conversations should take place in a quiet place where everybody who is attending can sit down. Pagers and cell phones need to be silenced, and tissues should be in the patient's reach.

2. Assess the patient's perception. This step can provide an important window into the patient's perspective, especially if a clinician is meeting the patient for the first time. It may guide how much more information the patient may need. A simple way to assess a patient's understanding is to ask, "What have other doctors told you so far about your illness?" This step may not be necessary if the clinician knows the patient very well.

3. Ask for an invitation to talk about the news. This is a very valuable step, as patients in these situations can often feel out of control. Simply asking the question, "Are you ready to talk about this?" gives patients a little bit of control and signals an intent to work cooperatively. It is also important to assess how much the patient wants to know, taking into account cultural, religious, social, or personal issues.

4. Knowledge—disclose the news. Information needs to be communicated in a way that helps the patient to process and understand. It is helpful to preface serious news with a warning statement, such as, "The test result came back, and there is some serious news that we need to talk about" or "I am sorry to tell you that . . . ." Clear language without medical jargon should be used. The information needs to be provided in small, understandable amounts; details can be filled in later.

5. Respond to the patient's emotions. A wave of emotions will follow hearing the news. Ways on how to respond have been described earlier.

6. Summarize the conversation and discuss the strategy (treatment plan).

7. It is important to ask for questions, summarize what has been discussed, and outline next steps. Providing information also in writing can reduce confusion and anxiety.

Discussing Goals of care

Addressing goals of care (GoC) is an essential skill when taking care of patients with serious illnesses. As these conversations can feel overwhelming, they are often deferred until late

Table 67–7. Responding to emotions: NURSE.

N	Name the emotion	"It sounds like this has been frustrating." "I can see you are feeling sad."
U	Understand the emotion	"It must be so hard to be in pain like this." "I understand that you are feeling lonely."
R	Respect (praise) the patient	"I am very impressed that you have been able to keep up with your treatments while experiencing all these side effects."
S	Support the patient	"My team and I will be here to support you." "No matter what happens next, I will be there for you."
E	Explore the emotion	"Tell me more why you are feeling frustrated." "Tell me more how this pain has been interfering with your life."

in the disease process, when the difficulty of the conservation may be even greater. The framework REMAP can help guide these conversations.

1. **Reframe:** Before a patient can participate in any meaningful GoC conversation, it is essential that the patient understands the current medical situation. During this step, a clinician tries to the assess a patient's understanding about his or her illness trajectory; shares new information when needed, such as news that previous treatments are no longer working; and possibly includes information about prognosis. Sometimes this step can resemble a "giving serious news" conversation, and based on the patient's ability to cope with the news, further steps of the GoC conversation may need to be postponed.

2. **Expect and address emotions:** Most patients will have an emotional reaction when being informed about changes in their illness trajectory. See Table 67–7 on how to address emotions.

3. **Map patient values:** Instead of focusing on specific treatment options, a clinician should at this point in the conversation take a step back and explore a patient's values, concerns, and hopes. This step is necessary to develop a patient-centered treatment plan. An easy way to start is to ask if the patient has a living will or if the patient has ever thought about what would be important when his or her underlying illness progresses. Further possible questions to ask are outlined in Table 67–8. At times, patients' values can be conflicting. In order to get a clear understanding about what is important to a patient, it helps to explore values with several different questions, to reflect them back to the patient, and to see if certain values can be prioritized.

4. **Align with values:** The clinician summarizes what he or she has learned about a patient's values, distills what a patient says into a specific statement of what is important, and allows for the patient to further clarify and elaborate, if needed, on the description of his or her values.

5. **Propose a plan:** It is the clinician's responsibility to propose a plan that is based on a patient's values, as well as on the feasibility of medical treatment options. The proposed plan should be clearly linked to previously explored values. A clinician might say, "Given that time is short and you would like to spend that time with your family and not in the hospital, I recommend hospice care." It is helpful to first discuss what will be done to achieve a patient's goals, and later to discuss which available treatment options would not help to achieve these goals and therefore should be either discontinued or withheld. This needs to be immediately followed by asking the patient about his or thoughts about the proposed plan. If a patient disagrees, values need to be further discussed so the plan can be adjusted.

Table 67–8. REMAP: addressing goals of care.

Reframe why the status quo is not working	"Given these new findings, I would like to talk about what to do next." "You have been through a lot. I wonder if it makes sense to reevaluate what we are doing. I am concerned that more treatments might do more harm than good." "You have been fighting very hard over the past few years. You tell me that you are getting increasingly tired, and you struggle to do the things you enjoy. We are in a different place now."
Expect and respond to emotions	"What are you most concerned about?" "I can see this is a shock. This is not what you expected." "This is difficult stuff to talk about."
Map patient values	"Given that time is short, what is important to you?" (After an answer is given: "And what else is important to you?") "What do you enjoy doing? What gives your life meaning?" "What would you like to avoid?" (After an answer is given: "And what else would you like to avoid?") "When you think about your future, are there things you hope to do?" "When you think about the future, what concerns you?"
Align with patient values	"As I listen to you, it sounds like it is important to you to . . . ."
Propose a treatment plan	"Since you are hoping to make it to your granddaughter's wedding in 2 months, I propose we enroll you in a clinical trial. Should you experience significant side effects from the treatment and should your weakness significantly worsen, I recommend that we stop the trial and rather focus on controlling your symptoms very aggressively." "You want to focus on being comfortable. If your heart stops, we will not use machines to try to keep you going and rather let you pass peacefully." "What do you think about all of this?"

▶ Discussing Prognosis

Discussing prognosis is difficult; telling patients that they will die from their illness may feel, at its worst, like handing down a death sentence. It may often seem easier to defer these conversations and instead focus on symptoms and other care-related issues. For this reason, clinicians may have conflicting feelings about these conversations because they understand that, although difficult and challenging, conversations that provide information about prognosis will allow the patient and family to prepare appropriately. Patients may also have contradictory wishes for their care. Most patients report that they want to be included in decision making and receive as much information as possible. However, they also want their care providers to support their wishes.

Having conversations about prognosis has been shown to impact advance care planning, particularly with regard to do-not-resuscitate orders and timely referrals to hospice. However, physicians are poor prognosticators and tend to be overly optimistic. The accuracy of prognostication improves with experience, but it worsens as the duration of the patient-physician relationship increases.

Prognostication is not commonly taught in medical school or during postgraduate training. In addition to observational data culled from patients with specific diseases, several models and scales are available to aid in forming prognoses. Some of these models are disease specific, such as the Seattle Heart Failure Model, a 6-month mortality calculator for patients on maintenance hemodialysis, and the Mortality Risk Index for patients with dementia. An example of a non–disease-specific tool to assess prognosis is the Palliative Performance Scale (PPS; Table 67–9). Several studies showed correlations of PPS scores with survival in palliative care patients (including patients with different diagnoses and in different care settings).

A conversation about prognosis entails four steps: (1) negotiating the content, (2) providing information, (3) acknowledging the patient's and family's reaction to the news, and (4) checking for understanding.

1. **Negotiating the content:** Even though most patients are interested in hearing about prognosis, not all want the same level of detail. Therefore, it is helpful to start the conversation by asking, "How much do you want to know about your prognosis?" A clinician can further explain the range of possible information provided by saying, "Some people want to hear every detail, some want to focus on the big picture, and others may rather not discuss prognosis at all. What would be best for you?" If a patient is interested in talking about prognosis, it is recommended to ask if the patient would like to hear specific statistics or rather be informed about the best, worst, and most likely case scenarios.

2. **Providing information:** The information needs to be given straightforwardly and slowly, in digestible pieces and with sufficient pauses to allow the patient to absorb it and then react and ask relevant questions. Information about time should be given in ranges, such as hours to days, days to weeks, weeks to months, or months to years.

3. **Acknowledging the patient's and family's reaction to the news:** The patient and family will most likely have an emotional reaction of some considerable intensity. Ways to respond verbally to emotions have been outlined in Table 67–6. Acknowledging the emotion can lead to a deepening of the conversation.

4. **Checking for comprehension:** Given the complexity of these conversations, patients and families may hear only the good or bad aspects. Ways to check in and ascertain what information was understood include, "Tell me what you are taking away from this conversation," or, "Tell me what you will tell your spouse/friend about this conversation."

Back A, Arnold R, Tulsky J. *Mastering Communication with Seriously Ill Patients—Balancing Honesty with Empathy and Hope.* Cambridge. United Kingdom: Cambridge University Press; 2009.

Baile WF, Buckman R, Lenzi R, Glober G, Beale EA, Kudelka AP. SPIKES: a six-step protocol for delivering bad news: application to the patient with cancer. *Oncologist.* 2000;5(4):302–311. [PMID: 10964998]

Campbell TC, Carey EC, Jackson VA, et al. Discussing prognosis: balancing hope and realism. *Cancer J.* 2010;16(5):461–466. [PMID: 20890141]

Childers JW, Back AL, Tulsky JA, Arnold RM. REMAP: a framework for goals of care conversations. *J Oncol Pract.* 2017; 13(10):e844–e850. [PMID: 28445100]

Smith AK, Williams BA, Lo B. Discussing overall prognosis with the very elderly. *N Engl J Med.* 2011;365(23):2149–2151. [PMID: 22150033]

Vitaltalk. https://www.vitaltalk.org. Accessed January 2019.

CARE OF THE DYING PATIENT

Family members may turn to care providers to help them understand what to expect when their loved one is dying. Patients who are very close to the end of life display a series of signs that predict the closeness of their deaths. One of the first signs is a decrease in engagement with one's surroundings and in communication. As the body is preparing to die, the patient decreases his or her oral intake. This is often the most difficult change for family members, as they may become concerned that their loved one is suffering and starving. Often it is enough to explain to them that this is part of the normal dying process. Most of the time, patients do not report being hungry or thirsty, although they may complain of a dry mouth. In this case, effective mouth care with moistened sponges and a lip balm is sufficient.

As the dying process continues, the patient will become progressively somnolent, with fewer and shorter awake

Table 67–9. Palliative Performance Scale.

%	Ambulation	Activity Level/Evidence of Disease	Self-Care	Intake	Level of Consciousness	Estimated Median Survival in Days[a]		
						A	B	C
100	Full	Normal No disease	Full	Normal	Full	N/A	N/A	108
90	Full	Normal Some disease	Full	Normal	Full			
80	Full	Normal with effort Some disease	Full	Normal or reduced	Full			
70	Reduced	Can't do normal job or work Some disease	Full	Normal or reduced	Full	145		
60	Reduced	Can't do hobbies or housework Significant disease	Occasional assistance needed	Normal or reduced	Full or confusion	29	4	
50	Mainly sit or lie	Can't do any work Extensive disease	Considerable assistance needed	Normal or reduced	Full or confusion	30	11	41
40	Mainly in bed	Can't do any work Extensive disease	Mainly assistance	Normal or reduced	Full or drowsy or confusion	18	8	
30	Bedridden	Can't do any work Extensive disease	Total care	Reduced	Full or drowsy or confusion	8	5	
20	Bedridden	Can't do any work Extensive disease	Total care	Minimal	Full or drowsy or confusion	4	2	6
10	Bedridden	Can't do any work Extensive disease	Total care	Mouth care only	Drowsy or coma	1	1	
0	Death							

[a]Key:
(A) Survival postadmission to an inpatient palliative unit, all diagnoses.
(B) Days until inpatient death following admission to an acute hospice unit, diagnoses not specified.
(C) Survival postadmission to an inpatient palliative unit, cancer patients only.
N/A, not applicable.

periods. Sometimes the patient may become confused or restless. The clarity of hearing and vision is also often seen to decrease. Family members sometimes ask if their loved one is still able to hear them. Hearing is the last one of the five senses to be lost, and family members should be invited to continue talking to their loved one.

As oral intake decreases and metabolic changes continue, urine output will decrease and the urine will be more concentrated. When very close to death, patients may develop urinary and bowel incontinence. Other physical changes include alterations in body temperature and blood pressure, increased perspiration, and skin changes, such as mottling or a pale, yellowish pallor. Breathing changes also occur, including increased, decreased, or irregular respirations, as well as periods of apnea. As the patient is becoming weaker and more

somnolent, he or she is no longer able to clear the throat or cough. Secretions begin to pool in the throat directly above the vocal cords. As air is passing by these secretions, the sound produced may be loud and rattling, often referred to as "death rattle." Family members who never have witnessed somebody dying may become concerned and wonder if the patient is "drowning." Very often, comparing the death rattle to snoring can comfort them; like snoring, this sound may be disturbing to the person hearing it, but is not uncomfortable to the person producing it. Measures to decrease the death rattle include simply repositioning the head or the use of anticholinergic medications (Table 67–10). Deep suction is not recommended, as it is uncomfortable and can lead to bleeding.

Medical care should be simplified as much as possible. Laboratory tests, radiologic procedures, and other

Table 67–10. Drugs used to control symptoms in the dying patient.

Symptom	Drug Class	Drug	Route	Dose
Pain	NSAID	Ketorolac	IV/SC	15–30 mg every 6 hours
	Opioid	Morphine	IV/SC	4 mg every 4 hours
			PO/PR	15 mg every 4 hours
"Death rattle"	Anticholinergic	Scopolamine	TD	1 patch every 3 days
		Atropine	IV/SC	0.2–0.4 mg every 2 hours
		Glycopyrrolate	IV/SC	0.2 mg every 4 hours
		Hyoscyamine	SL	0.125–0.25 mg every 4 hours
Dyspnea	Opioid	Morphine	IV/SC	4 mg every 4 hours
			PO/PR	15 mg every 4 hours
Restlessness/anxiety	Benzodiazepine	Midazolam	SC	2–5 mg every 2 hours
		Lorazepam	IV/SC/SL	0.5–1.0 mg every 4 hours
Agitation/hallucinations	Antipsychotic	Haloperidol	IV/SC	1–2 mg every ½ hour to effect
		Thorazine	IV	12.5–25 mg every 6 hours
			PR	25–50 mg every 6 hours

IV, intravenous; NSAID, nonsteroidal anti-inflammatory drug; PO, oral; PR, per rectum; SC, subcutaneous; SL, sublingual; TD, transdermal.

interventions should be done only if they will result in improvement of the patient's comfort. Nonessential medications should be discontinued. Artificially provided hydration and nutrition are seldom necessary or helpful for the dying patient. Administration of parenteral fluids may result in progressive edema, lung congestion, increased oral secretions, and frequent urination with attendant discomfort and distress. Experienced hospice professionals note no increase in discomfort or suffering with the naturally occurring dehydration that accompanies the dying process. Frequently used medications to address symptoms of the dying patient are listed in Table 67–10.

Additionally, of great importance are nursing interventions, such as daily bathing, good mouth care, and application of artificial tears and lubricating ointment to the eyes, as well as comfortable positioning in the bed with pillows placed under the calves or other areas of support. Family members may be instructed in these nursing interventions and participate in the care of their loved one. This often is very meaningful and comforting to both the patient and family members.

Sleeman KE, Collis E. Caring for a dying patient in hospital. *BMJ.* 2013;346:f2174. [PMID: 23596214]

BEREAVEMENT

Grief, which is a normal reaction to loss, is the process of adjusting to a difficult reality. Both patients and families experience grief prior to and in anticipation of death; families and friends, of course, grieve after the death of a loved one. Attention to grief and bereavement is an often neglected

part of excellent end-of-life care. Clinicians can play an important role in facilitating healthy grief and assessing for complicated grief.

Grieving individuals experience a variety of difficult emotional reactions, which usually occur in waves. Grief is triggered or exacerbated predictably by new losses, such as decline in functional status, as well as significant life events, including anniversaries and holidays. But grief can also worsen unpredictably by seemingly trivial events. Elisabeth Kübler-Ross first described five stages of grief—denial, anger, bargaining, depression, and acceptance—which may occur in any order and usually peak within 6 months following a loss. Somatic symptoms of grief include insomnia, dizziness, anorexia, nausea, restlessness, generalized weakness, and shortness of breath.

The death of a loved one is likely one of the most stressful human experiences, yet most people cope without needing professional interventions. A few individuals have more pronounced symptoms and may experience a persistent, debilitating phenomenon referred to as *complicated grief* (CG). The symptoms of CG include longing for the loved one; trouble accepting the death; feeling uneasy about moving on with one's life; inability to trust others after the death; excessive bitterness or anger about the death; persistent feeling of being shocked, stunned, or numb; intense feeling of loneliness; feeling that life is empty or meaningless without the deceased; and frequent preoccupying thoughts about the deceased. These symptoms persist after 6 months, and they cause impairments in daily function. Predisposition to CG seems related to insecure attachment styles, an unstable sense of self, weak parental bonding in childhood, female gender, low perceived social support, death in an intensive care unit, and insufficient preparation for the loss (eg, after an unexpected, traumatic death). Bereavement after the death of a child should always be considered CG. No interventions have been shown to prevent CG, but there is evidence from a recent meta-analysis that it is responsive to cognitive behavioral or group therapy.

Clinicians can play an important role in facilitating a healthy grieving process. They can assess patient and family risk factors for difficulties in grieving, and they can provide psychosocial resources as needed. Factors that have been associated with better bereavement outcomes include effective symptom management and open and honest communication about the course of the illness, prognosis, and advance care planning. Timely hospice enrollment has also been shown to positively affect bereavement outcomes.

Even after a patient's death, clinicians can facilitate healthy grieving. Throughout the course of a serious illness, clinicians become an integral part in patients' and families' lives. Therefore, it is a very appreciated and meaningful act of kindness to not end this relationship suddenly when a patient dies, and rather to make a condolence call, write a condolence letter, or even attend the funeral or memorial service. Screening for insomnia, hypertension, and substance abuse, as well as complicated grief and other psychiatric illnesses, is indicated.

Palliative Care Network of Wisconsin. Fast facts. https://www.mypcnow.org. Accessed January 2019.

Shear MK, Ghesquiere A, Glickman K. Bereavement and complicated grief. *Curr Psychiatry Rep.* 2013;15(11):406. [PMID: 24068457]

RESOURCES

Books

American Medical Association. *Participant's Handbook and Trainer's Guide for Education for Physicians on End-of-Life Care (EPEC).* http://www.epec.net/item-products.php?type=3. Accessed December 9, 2019.

Cherny N, Fallon M, Kaasa S, et al. *Oxford Textbook of Palliative Medicine.* 5th ed. Oxford, United Kingdom: Oxford University Press; 2017.

Goldman A, Hain R, Liben S. *Oxford Textbook of Palliative Care for Children.* 2nd ed. Oxford, United Kingdom: Oxford University Press; 2012.

Goldstein N, Morrison RS. *Evidence-Based Practice of Palliative Medicine: Expert Consult: Online and Print.* Philadelphia, PA: Saunders-Elsevier; 2013.

Lynn J, Harrold J. *Handbook for Mortals: Guidance for People Facing Serious Illness.* 2nd ed. Oxford, United Kingdom: Oxford University Press; 2011.

Quill TE, Bower KA, Holloway RG, et al. *Primer of Palliative Care.* 6th ed. Chicago, IL: American Academy of Hospice and Palliative Medicine; 2014

Journals

Journal of Pain and Symptom Management. Portenoy RK, ed. Elsevier Science Publishers, New York.

Journal of Palliative Medicine. Weissman DE, ed. Mary Ann Liebert, Inc, Larchmont, NY.

Palliative Medicine, The Research Journal of the EAPC. Geoffrey Hanks, ed. Sage Publications, London, United Kingdom.

Supportive Care in Cancer. Senn HJ, ed. Springer-Verlag, Heidelburg, Germany.

Websites

American Academy of Hospice and Palliative Medicine. http://www.aahpm.org

American Board of Hospice and Palliative Medicine. http://www.abhpm.org

Canter to Advance Palliative Care. http://www.capc.org

End-of-Life Nursing Education Consortium. https://www.aacnnursing.org/ELNEC

National Comprehensive Cancer Network guidelines for supportive care. https://www.nccn.org/professionals/physician_gls/default.aspx#supportive

National Consensus Project for Quality Palliative Care. https://www.nationalcoalitionhpc.org

National Hospice and Palliative Care Organization. http://www.nhpco.org

Palliative Care Network of Wisconsin. Fast Facts. https://www.mypcnow.org/fast-facts

Vitaltalk. https://www.vitaltalk.org/

Apps

Vitaltalk Tips. Free app for communication skills

Palliative Care Fast Facts. Free app for broad range of palliative care topics

68

Telemedicine

Charles R. Doarn, MBA, FATA, FAsMA

INTRODUCTION

Imagine managing your patients with virtual technology—technology that permits patients access to health care from their home or wherever they may be; technology that provides you, the clinician, with better ways to manage your patient's chronic disease. Telemedicine and telehealth are tools that have enabled a new approach and perhaps a fundamental change in addressing your needs as a clinician and, more importantly, the needs of your patients. These tools are focused on enabling more efficient and better health care.

Over the past 100 years or so, medical care has evolved as a direct result of innovation. This innovation will continue to push the boundaries of what is possible. Sensors, robotics, artificial intelligence, high-speed communications, massive storage systems, computing power, informatics, and smart medical systems are but a few of the tools you will use in clinical practice in the coming years.

This chapter provides a summary of what telemedicine and telehealth are and how they are being integrated into clinical practice and medical education. It lays out an historical timeline, defines terms, highlights empirical evidence, discusses challenges and barriers and clinical applications, and presents an update on the patient-centered healthcare system.

BACKGROUND

In the 19th century, innovation in electricity and telephony changed the way we all lived and worked. The introduction of these two technologies led to better medical care. Lighting in the operating theater (Figure 68–1) and patient examination room, tools for individuals to communicate with one another across some distance, and many other applications of these new technologies led to modernization of health care. Röntgen's discovery of x-rays in 1895 changed how we diagnose and treat our patients. Laparoscopic surgery,

developed at the beginning of the 20th century and perfected in the 1980s, helped lead the way to robotic surgery. William Osler's work in the early 20th century led medicine into a new paradigm in education, training, and clinical practice.

These and a myriad of technologies laid the foundation for our healthcare systems today. Some of these changes did not come about overnight, and some challenged the very foundation of medicine at the time. For example, it took several decades for Laennec's stethoscope to become a standard tool. Most of his colleagues thought he was not following the standard of care. The same can be said for hand washing. In 1847, Ignaz Semmelweis was severely ridiculed by his contemporaries for his efforts to institute handwashing between the cadaver lab and the delivery room and between patients, thus reducing puerperal fever (*Streptococcus pyogenes*) and lessoning the burden of mortality in delivering mothers and their infants. The thinking at the time was "Gentlemen don't have dirty hands." An interesting point here is that midwives of this period did not see mortality of birthing mothers at as high a rate as physicians. These two examples amplify the lack of understanding and the fear of change, which are still part of the belief system of many in the medical community in the 21st century.

Other significant issues globally include access to health care, increasing demands on limited resources, an aging population, and a growing shortage of physicians and nurses. These issues must drive change, and innovation in delivery models is one approach that has been shown and continues to show great promise in alleviating some of these challenges.

FOUNDATIONS FOR TELEMEDICINE & TELEHEALTH

Innovation often comes about because of an unmet need or as a result of simply applying a new gadget to an old problem. In the 1920s, physicians in Australia were linked to researchers on the ice in the Antarctic, where there was literally no

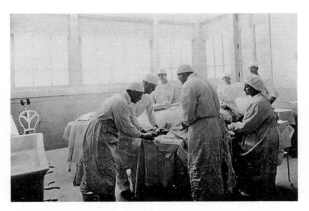

▲ **Figure 68–1.** Operating theater in the late 19th century.

way to definitive care. In 1924, the publication *Radio News* ran a thought-provoking and futuristic story, "The Radio Doctor – Maybe!" (Figure 68–2). The image depicts a young patient being seen by his physician via television. This was

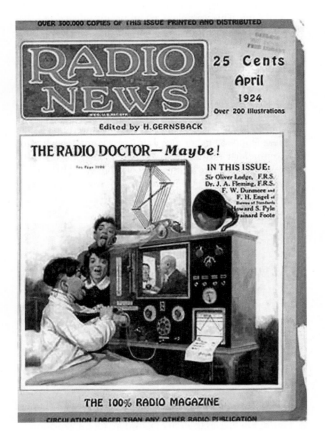

▲ **Figure 68–2.** Cover of the 1924 issue of *Radio News*.

quite futuristic and laid the foundation of what might be possible in the coming decades. It took several decades for this concept to become a reality.

In the mid-1950s, psychiatrists in Nebraska linked physicians, patients, and students together via telemedicine for consultative services, educational initiatives, and training and research efforts. Using closed circuit television, telepsychiatry was simplified and implemented. Similarly, the Massachusetts General Hospital integrated a telemedicine solution for assessing patients at Boston's Logan Airport in the early 1960s. These two early applications demonstrated the need to increase access using television and communication networks. They also demonstrated the utility of addressing a patient's needs when the patient and physician were separated.

In the late 1950s and with the birth of the space age in 1958, wireless communication, sensors, and remote monitoring systems were developed to monitor cosmonauts and astronauts in space flight. The systems developed to support these programs have led to a wide variety of technologies that we use today, including advanced diagnostic tools, communication tools, and computing power. This is an example of how technologic development occurred as a direct result of an unmet need and significant investment by governments. The healthcare industry continues to benefit from this investment today.

In the early 21st century, investment in healthcare technologies, computing power, and telecommunications has been enabled more by individuals and companies than by large government programs. Evidence of this can be seen in companies such as Apple, Tesla, Google, SpaceX, Amazon, and Epic.

In all the aforementioned examples, telecommunications technologies and information technologies were adopted, adapted, and integrated into patient care. Those early events did not have the inexpensive and ubiquitous tools we have available to us today. Today, the penetration of mobile telephony and the wide distribution of smart phones concomitant with an ever-growing collection of health-related apps are changing the way we manage our lives and those of our patients.

A NEW PARADIGM

The fundamentals of telemedicine and telehealth are neither onerous nor challenging to integrate into practice. Simply put, the integration of telecommunications, computer systems, and devices is the foundation for telemedicine and telehealth. These terms are often used interchangeably but are actually different (see later section titled "Definition of Terms").

When thinking about addressing a patient's needs, one must also think about them comprehensively. As a family physician, you manage patients' conditions, but they also have other challenges in their lives, including family and work. We often have patients travel to our offices rather than bringing health care to them. This is a key tenant of telemedicine and telehealth. Why not manage patients in their familiar surroundings by taking health care to them if possible? A patient who lives some distance from the physician incurs travel costs, parking costs, lost wages, and so on, all of which can be avoided. Therefore, a fundamental question is: What is best for our patients? If we neglect these issues when we have the proven capability to ameliorate them, are we negligent in our care? This is a fundamental challenge we face today as clinicians. Clearly, innovation has been shown to be a disruptor. But is our answer to make patients wait for us to see them in clinic, or can we begin to enable tools that will benefit the patient, physician, and the healthcare system? The 19th century doctor will return to his or her patient with 21st-century technology (Figure 68–3). This approach does not imply a reduction in face-to-face interaction nor does it imply everything can be done via telemedicine or telehealth. This paradigm is but a tool that can be employed when it makes sense for both patient and physician.

For example, telemedicine and telehealth through e-visits can be an efficient way to manage a chronic disease, wound healing, and dermatologic issues, among others. Even surgery has been done remotely, albeit in a research setting.

However, there will always be a need for face-to-face contact where you are in the same room as your patient. The real challenge in the coming decades will be when the robot or avatar is the one interacting with the patient. This situation is not that far in the future, and it will change the foundation of medical education and clinical practice.

DEFINITION OF TERMS

There are a wide variety of terms and tools used in telemedicine and telehealth. The following list provides short definitions or descriptions of each. Some figures are used to further illustrate these terms.

Asynchronous—This term implies that an interaction is not in real time. Information can be stored and forwarded for review at a later time. This type of telemedicine is used when bandwidth is an issue (availability and/or expense). If the bandwidth is limited, real-time interaction is not desirable or possible. Examples include web-based tools, file transfers, e-mail, and transfer of digitized files (Figure 68–4). It is ideal for moving large data files, videos, and images that are not needed in real time. This approach has some advantages and disadvantages. Advantages include less technical support, lower communications costs, and better data security. Disadvantages include limited capabilities with regard to the specialist, no real-time feedback, and limited reimbursement.

Bandwidth—This term is used to describe the speed and quantity of data that can be moved or transmitted across a cable or wireless system and is measured in kilobits per second (Kbps) or megabits per second (Mbps). Most commercial entities have *broadband*, which is a significantly larger bandwidth and is often referred to as high-speed Internet. The challenge for most home owners is

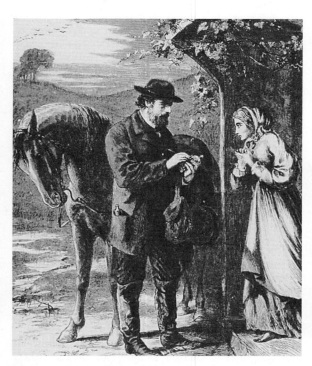

▲ **Figure 68–3.** Nineteenth-century physician.

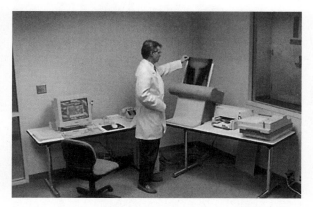

▲ **Figure 68–4.** Digitization of x-ray film for transmission asynchronously.

(1) the internet service provider (ISP) and (2) the last mile—the distance from the ISP line to the customer's location. ISPs vary across regions within a country, and upload and download speeds can vary. The higher the bandwidth, the faster large files can be transmitted or downloaded and the more activities that it can support. Remember how slow dial-up was using a modem?

DSL—Digital subscriber line uses the phone line at a higher frequency to transmit voice and data. Bandwidth range is 128 Kbps to 8 Mbps.

e-Health (electronic health)—This term encompasses many of the concepts of telemedicine, telehealth, mobile health, and so on, where certain types of information technology systems and telecommunications tool are employed to support health care.

e-Visits (electronic visits)—This is a capability where a patient can interact with his or her physician or allied health provider via a web-based portal.

Home health care—The ability to monitor the health and well-being of patients wherever they may be. Usually, this implies the patients are in their residence (or home).

Hub and spoke—Like a wagon wheel, where the center (hub) is linked to many outlying facilities.

Internet protocol (IP)—This is a communication protocol for transmission of data across the Internet.

ISDN—Integrated services digital network is a circuit-switched network for digital telephony and transmission of data and voice over the telephone system's copper wire. It is limited in bandwidth at 1.544 Mbps.

LAN—Local area network is a network that connects computers within a discrete location (eg, office building, clinic, academic setting).

m-Health (mobile health)—This implies that a patient can gain access to health information and interact with a physician or allied health provider using a mobile device, such as a smartphone or computing device (eg, laptop, tablet computer).

Patient-centered medical home (PCMH)—Also called the medical home, this refers to a team-based approach to the delivery of health care through care coordination. See also the American Academy of Family Physicians website (www.aafp.org/fpm/topicModules/viewTopicModule.htm?topicModuleId=94).

Plain Old Telephone Systems (POTS)—This is a term you might hear from time to time. It simply implies the use of the telephone to interact with someone. It is considered a legacy system.

Remote monitoring—The ability to monitor patients wherever they are using different tools and a telecommunications link.

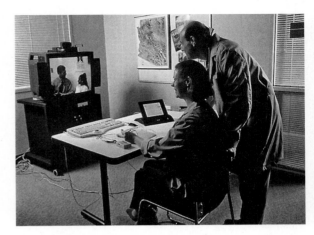

▲ **Figure 68–5.** Synchronous telemedicine via video teleconferencing.

Synchronous—This term means that interaction is in real-time. It can support video teleconferencing (VTC), where individuals are using tools on their computers or mobile phones (Figure 68–5). Examples of this include not only VTC but also all technologies that permit real-time interaction. The limiting factor is bandwidth. Examples include programs like Skype, WebEX, and Zoom.

Telehealth—This term, often intertwined with telemedicine, is actually a broader term that includes the concepts of telemedicine, remote monitoring, mobile health, and electronic health.

Telemedicine—There are many definitions for this term. It simply means the delivery of healthcare services where patient and physician are separated by some distance using a computer system or a mobile device connected via a telecommunication link.

VoIP—Voice over Internet Protocol uses the Internet as a delivery mechanism for voice.

VPN—A virtual private network is a private network that enables transfer of voice, data, and other information across a public network that ensures privacy via a point-to-point connection.

WAN—Wide area network is a network that connects computers across a much larger area (eg, communities).

CHALLENGES AND BARRIERS

There are a number of challenges and barriers to deployment and integration of telemedicine and telehealth (Table 68–1). While some have been addressed by legislative action, technology, and training, significant obstacles remain. These include leadership, or lack thereof, robust infrastructure, reimbursement, cross-state licensing, access to technology,

Table 68–1. Barriers to adoption and integration of telemedicine (not inclusive).

Access
Attitude
Culture
Digital divide
Distance and geography
Education and training: competencies and skills
Financial
Legislation
Licensing
Policies
Political
Privacy and security
Reimbursement

socioeconomic impact/influences, and concerns over security. Although this list is not comprehensive, it is illustrative of the issues we face in American medicine.

Access—Access to healthcare services is vitally important for health and well-being. Often access is limited by several factors, including geography, transportation, distance, limited telecommunications, access to the Internet, and socioeconomic status. All of these characteristics can be barriers in rural and urban settings.

Attitude—Sometimes an individual's understanding of how telemedicine and telehealth can be integrated is solely based on the attitude of management, the provider, and/or the patient. Often, administrators and physicians have said they do not believe in this change. Younger physicians tend to be more willing to integrate innovative approaches as their education and residency have more likely included some form of telemedicine or telehealth. A wide variety of senior physicians, who were trained decades ago, may not embrace the integration because they have concerns regarding interference with care or the physician-patient interaction.

Culture—Although culture can mean many different things to many different people, the use here is related to the culture of the organization in which the clinician functions. Some organizational culture is all about embracing change and pushing the limits of what is possible. Others are recalcitrant to change and are uncomfortable with or fear innovation. Governments at all levels can reflect the same attitudes.

Digital divide—As technology penetrates a market, there are often gaps in capabilities and resources. Figure 68–6 illustrates a composite photograph of the Earth with all the population centers lit up at night. What is telling about this image is not who has electricity and, therefore, the potential for Internet access, but who does not have access. This digital divide can also be observed between high-, middle-, and low-income countries and

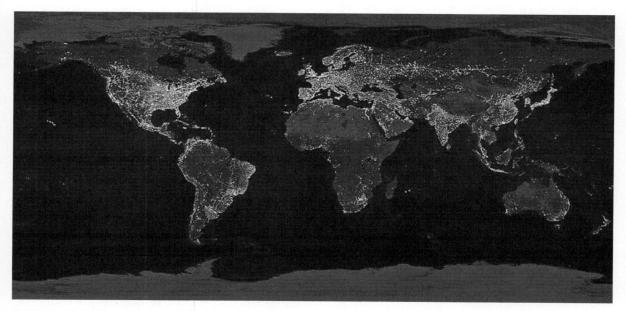

▲ **Figure 68–6.** The entire world illuminated at night. (Reproduced with permission from Earth at Night: Our Planet in Brilliant Darkness. National Aeronautics and Space Administration.)

can be simplified to zip codes anywhere in the world. Consider a map of a leading wireless provider; there is a lot of coverage in a metropolitan area, but in the middle of nowhere, there may be limited or no access. Thus, this digital divide actually mirrors unequal access to medical care globally.

Distance and geography—Referring back to Figure 68–6, the Earth is a large place, and often we may find our patients in unique places—on airplanes, on oil rigs, on ships at sea, or in buildings within walking distance from our clinical site.

Education and training: competencies and skills—Medical education has undergone changes over the past century or so. To meet the growing shortage of physicians, there is a need to train physicians faster. Concomitant with medical education needs, innovations in simulation and computer-based training have evolved. Each physician, based on the time since completion of his or her education, may have experienced different approaches. Figure 68–7 illustrates a painting from the University of Pittsburgh (*The Agnew Clinic 1889*) that depicts Dr. Hayes Agnew performing a partial mastectomy.

This image portrays a knowledgeable professor instructing his students on how to perform this procedure. Each student can be seen observing, but alas, they are actually not visualizing the surgical field in the same way. Today, technology can bring each student into the operating theater to see what everyone else sees, thereby increasing pedagogical interchange for all. Furthermore, Osler's work at McGill University in Montreal and his sentinel work at Johns Hopkins provided the foundation of medical education that we use today.

Technologies in digital textbooks, digital pathology specimens, digital imaging, virtual anatomy, informatics, and so on have led medical education in a new direction. Telemedicine and telehealth use technology to train individuals regardless for their location. The tenets of medical education can be achieved virtually, although we may miss that occasional large lecture hall.

Financial—This barrier has several components. The first is the capital expense of investing in technology and personnel. This barrier can be imposed at many different levels and is dependent on available resources and leadership. A second is identifying the incentives a health system may have to integrate telemedicine and telehealth. Often the business manager may be looking for an immediate return on investment, which may not accurately reflect the true financial impact. Opportunity costs—those costs that are thought of as missed if an action is or is not taken—are often not considered when a breakeven analysis is conducted. Fixed and variable costs are used, but those aforementioned costs to the patient are not inclusive in this analysis.

Legislation—At various levels of government, laws are developed to address a public need, provide safety, security, or taxation, and so on. Often legislative action impacts the delivery of health care. Consider that physicians must be licensed in the state where they practice medicine. States regulate all healthcare personnel within the boundaries of that state. The only facilities that are outside of this legality are federal facilities. This is a significant barrier today as 21st-century technologies provide patients and physicians the opportunity to interact with one another regardless of location. Beginning in the early part of the 21st century, the laws in countries, territories, and state have evolved. In the United Sates, there are compacts, where state law recognizes licensed physicians from other states (Interstate Medical Licensure Compact; https://imlcc.org/).

Policies—The laws established within a nation, territory, or state provide the foundation from which regulations and policies are formulated. Policies in health care are influenced by evidence-based medicine and the environment in which health care is to be provided, but can be influenced by other factors such as population needs, human resource capability, access, equity, governance models, technology, innovation, and knowledge. Technical capability has advanced significantly in public health and health care to a point where our legacy systems have not kept pace. This means we have the ability and capability to enable better health care by changing the law and the subsequent development of policies and regulations. Policies are assessed for effectiveness and are modified accordingly.

Political—Politics play a role in everything we do. This could be in the workplace and health systems and on local, state, national, and international levels. Often, nascent technologies and new paradigms in care disrupt the status quo. Recall the earlier examples of Laennec and

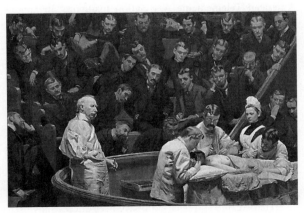

▲ **Figure 68–7.** Thomas Eakins: *The Agnew Clinic 1889*.

Semmelweis. They were trying to change the very foundation of what physicians of that period had learned in their medical training. Politicians are no different. There are some who literally do not believe in change by integrating technology. Dr. Michael DeBakey once quipped that when he was trained in medical school to listen to a patient's heart and lung sounds, he was 25 years old. Over his nearly 100 years of life, his hearing and eyesight were not the same. While he could still auscultate a patient's chest sounds, he was keenly aware that technical innovation provided a much better alternative. Yet, there are some who remain obstinate to change.

Privacy and security—Privacy and security are two distinct challenges where information is available. From the simplest form to complex, data must remain private and it must remain secure. Over the past several decades, our ability to collect, store, retrieve, manipulate, and use data to treat and manage our patients has been absolutely amazing. Electronic health records are now embedded in all we do. We have devices on our body and in our hands that can do all manner of things. Each step of the way, we must remain vigilant regarding both privacy and security. Often people at all levels of the healthcare continuum concern themselves with this. Some actually have posited that computer systems are not as secure as the patient's paper file in the clinical setting. As technology in storage and retrieval systems continues to be developed, the security systems, with dual authentication, including passwords and biometrics, continue to be developed in concert. Of course, we must remain cognizant of cybersecurity breaches from nefarious characters attempting to steal patient records and probably, more importantly, identification numbers.

Reimbursement—The reimbursement of telemedicine and telehealth continues to evolve and is often dependent on where you are practicing. Federal law drives state law, and some states can reimburse for certain types of services, whereas others cannot. There are Current Procedural Terminology (CPT) codes from Medicare. These codes are updated each year and can be found at the Centers for Medicaid and Medicare Services website (see https://www.cms.gov/Medicare/Medicare-General-Information/Telehealth/Telehealth-Codes.html). Medicare reimbursement for telehealth will be based on the service and where it is conducted. There are fee structures for the originating site (where the patient is) and the distant site (where provider is). Table 68–2 illustrates a few examples of Healthcare Common Procedural Coding System and CPT codes as of 2018. The same is true of International Classification of Diseases, 10 revision, codes. Keep in mind this list is updated annually.

Billing for telemedicine and telehealth services is driven by state laws and regulations, which only frustrates the

Table 68–2. Sample CPT codes that Medicare reimburses in 2018.

Service	HCPCS/CPT Code
Telehealth consultations, emergency department of initial inpatient	HCPS G0425-G0427
Office or other outpatient visits	CPT 99201-99215
Individual and group health and behavior assessment and intervention	CPT 96150-96154
Individual psychotherapy	CPT 90832-90384 and 90836-90383

Note: This is only a very small sample for illustration purposes. Visit the Centers for Medicaid and Medicare Services website for more detailed information.
CPT, Current Procedural Terminology; HCPCS, Healthcare Common Procedural Coding System.

further integration across the entire healthcare enterprise. Over the past several years, chronic care management uses CPT 99487 and CPT 99489 to help shift the burden from inpatient to outpatient care. The services can be billed by physicians, certified nurse midwives, clinical nurse specialists, nurse practitioners, and physician assistants. Chronic conditions include such conditions as Alzheimer disease and related dementia, arthritis, asthma, atrial fibrillation, autism spectrum disorder, cancer, chronic obstructive pulmonary disease, depression, diabetes, heart failure, hypertension, ischemic heart disease, and osteoporosis.

Each of the challenges and barriers discussed earlier continues to slowly be ameliorated. This has been driven by technology, consumer demand, evidence-based medicine, changing attitudes, and market share. For a state-by-state review of how telemedicine and telehealth are used, the American Telemedicine Association maintains an annual analysis (https://www.americantelemed.org/policy-page/state-telemedicine-gaps-reports). This analysis, performed annually, discusses what is done in each state and provides a grading of performance in comparison to other states.

CLINICAL APPLICATIONS

The concepts of telemedicine and telehealth can literally be applied to every clinical discipline. The ability to transmit pathology slides and radiology films across secure networks has given rise to new industries of teleradiology and telepathology. Often digital films are sent abroad to American-trained and American board-certified clinicians for review and decision making, usually at a significantly lower cost.

Telemedicine and telehealth have been successfully used in a patient's home to monitor all manner of chronic disease.

In addition to radiology and pathology, telemedicine and telehealth have been used in global health, disaster response, dermatology, rural health, stroke, rehabilitation, pediatrics, remote monitoring, ophthalmology, trauma, psychiatry, obstetrics/gynecology, pharmacy, nursing, and education, among others. Integrating computers, sensors, and telecommunication tools no longer has boundaries in care.

Over the past several decades, research in surgery at a distance has established new tools and new approaches. Figure 68–8 displays an early 20th-century physician interacting with a patient who is at a distant site. The tools we have today in our "traditional black bag" provide us an opportunity to see our patients virtually. We can monitor them and manage them with synchronous and asynchronous interaction. We have smart medical systems such that each patient has a digital footprint. From the moment of birth, we have 1s and 0s attached to us. These numerical objects are the basis of how a computer works—1 is on and 0 is off, which is the same as a circuit (open or closed). Everything we do now in our lives is linked to computers and their ability to interact with one another.

TELEMEDICINE IN PRIMARY CARE

Over the past several years, several research efforts have resulted in significant empirical evidence. Much of this has been driven by leaders in the field and the professional societies that continue to guide our discipline. Over the past

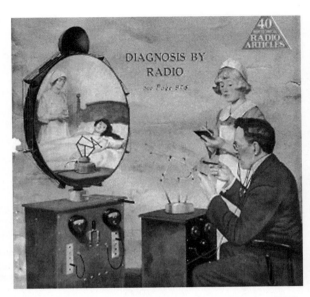

▲ **Figure 68–8.** Cover of *Science and Invention* circa 1925.

several years, a National Library of Medicine scholar has developed a series of empirical evidence manuscripts that lay out the evidence of telemedicine and telehealth as a significant tool in health care. Table 68–3 lists these manuscripts.

Table 68–3. Empirical evidence in various disciplines.

Title	Authors	Discipline	Year; Volume (Issue); Page Numbers[a]
The Empirical Foundations of Telemedicine Interventions for Chronic Disease Management	Shannon GW, Smith BR, Alverson DC, Antoniotti N, Barsan WG, Bashshur N, Brown EM, Coye MJ, Doarn CR, Ferguson S, Grigsby J, Krupinski EA, Kvedar JC, Linkous J, Merrell RC, Nesbitt T, Poropatich R, Rheuban KS, Sanders JH, Watson AR, Weinstein RS, and Yellowlees P	Chronic disease management	2014;20(9):769–800
The Empirical Evidence for the Telemedicine Intervention in Diabetes Management	Bashshur RL, Shannon GW, Smith BR, and Woodward MA	Diabetes	2015;21(5):321–354
The Empirical Foundations of Teledermatology: A Review of the Research Evidence	Bashshur RL, Shannon GW, Tejasvi T, Kvedar JC, and Gates M	Dermatology	2015;21(12):953–979
The Empirical Evidence for Telemedicine Interventions in Mental Disorders	Bashshur RL, Shannon GW, Bashshur N, and Yellowlees PM	Mental health	2016;22(2):87–113
The Empirical Foundations of Telemedicine Intervention in Primary Care	Bashshur RL, Howell JD, Krupinski EA, Harms KM, Bashshur N, and Doarn CR	Primary care	2016;22(5):342–375
The Empirical Foundations of Teleradiology and Related Applications: A Review of the Evidence	Bashshur RL, Krupinski EA, Thrall JH, and Bashshur N	Radiology	2016;22(11):868–898
The Empirical Foundations of Telepathology: Evidence of Feasibility and Intermediate Effects	Bashshur RL, Krupinski EA, Weinstein RS, Dunn MR, and Bashshur N	Pathology	2017;23(3):155–191

[a]All manuscripts came from *Telemedicine and e-Health Journal*, published by Mary Ann Liebert, Inc Publishers.

Furthermore, the American Academy of Family Physicians has also studied telemedicine and telehealth to determine their utility and applicability. There is a plethora of evidence in the literature about telemedicine and telehealth. Although all of these references cannot be listed in the "References" section, a fairly comprehensive summary list is provided. Searching PubMed using the term *telemedicine in family medicine* yielded 1053 results from 1992 to 2019; the term *telehealth in family medicine* yielded 1119 results from 1992 to 2019; the term *telemedicine in primary care* yielded 3478 results from 1977 to 2019; and finally, the term *telehealth in primary care* yielded 3940 results from 1977 to 2019.

Several studies are notable to cite here from research undertaken by the American Academy of Family Physicians. Moore and colleagues reported in 2018 that >50% of family medicine residencies incorporate the use of telehealth services. Moore and colleagues reported in 2017 that family medicine physicians have considerable interest in telehealth but also reported limited use. There is a plethora a reference material in the form of published books, government-managed websites, federal reports, and peer-reviewed manuscripts that elucidate the evidence. Some resources are delineated here, and the reference materials are alphabetically listed in the "References" section.

RESOURCES

Beginning in 1993, the research community established a professional society, the American Telemedicine Association (ATA; http://www.americantelemed.org/home), and in

Table 68–4. Practice guidelines for telemedicine and telehealth established by the American Telemedicine Association.

Discipline	Title
Mental health	Best Practices in Videoconferencing-Based Telemental Health
Telemedicine lighting	Let There Be Light: A Quick Guide to Telemedicine Lighting
Dermatology	Quick Guide to Store-Forward and Live-Interactive Teledermatology for Referring Providers
Pediatrics	Operating Procedures for Pediatric Telehealth
Rehabilitation	Principles for Delivering Telerehabilitation Services
Telestroke	Practice Guidelines for Telestroke
Mental health for children and adolescents	Practice Guidelines for Telemental Health with Children and Adolescents
Burns	Practice Guidelines for Teleburn Care
Dermatology	Practice Guidelines for Dermatology
Human factors	A Concise Guide for Telemedicine Practitioners Human Factors: Quick Guide Eye Contact
Urgent care	Practice Guidelines for Live, On Demand, Primary and Urgent Care
Pathology	Clinical Guidelines for Pathology
Intensive care unit (ICU) operations	Guidelines for TeleICU Operations
Operations	Core Operational Guidelines for Telehealth Services Involving Provider-Patient Interactions
Mental health	A Lexicon of Assessment and Outcome Measures for Telemental Health
Mental health	Practice Guidelines for Video-Based Online Mental Health Services
Operations	Videoconferencing-Based Telepresenting Expert Consensus Recommendations
Diabetic retinopathy	Telehealth Practice Recommendations for Diabetic Retinopathy
Mental health	Practice Guidelines for Videoconferencing-Based Telemental Health
Mental health	Evidence-Based Practice for Telemental Health

Data from American Telemedicine Association. ATA practice guidelines.

1994, two peer-reviewed scientific journals were established, the *Telemedicine and e-Health Journal* (https://www.liebertpub.com/loi/tmj) and the *Journal of Telemedicine and Telecare* (https://journals.sagepub.com/home/jtt). Over the past three decades, tens of thousands of research articles have been published in these journals as well as in a wide variety of clinical discipline journals. The specialty associations have recently weighed in on definitions and guidelines. The notable organizations include the following: (1) American College of Physicians, (2) American Academy of Pediatricians, (3) American Medical Association, (4) American Psychological Association, (5) American Psychiatric Association, (6) American Academy of Family Physicians, (7) American Academy of Dermatology, and (8) American Medical Informatics Association. Each of these organizations and many others define and support telemedicine and telehealth as a method to improve patient-physician interaction and improve health outcomes.

In addition to the robust and influential peer-reviewed literature, the ATA works closely in the development of federal policy and, through a wide network of subject matter experts, has laid out a series of informative guidelines. These are listed in Table 68–4 and have been published in the *Telemedicine and e-Health Journal*. These documents serve as wonderful tools for establishing a telemedicine and telehealth operation.

The US Department of Health and Human Services established the Office for the Advancement of Telehealth (OAT; https://www.hrsa.gov/rural-health/telehealth/index.html). OAT has funded a variety of research efforts since the early 1990s. The have also created the telehealth resource centers (TRCs; https://www.telehealthresourcecenter.org/) (Figure 68–9). As the figure depicts, the country is divided into regions, and each region has its own TRC to provide support for telemedicine and telehealth in the region.

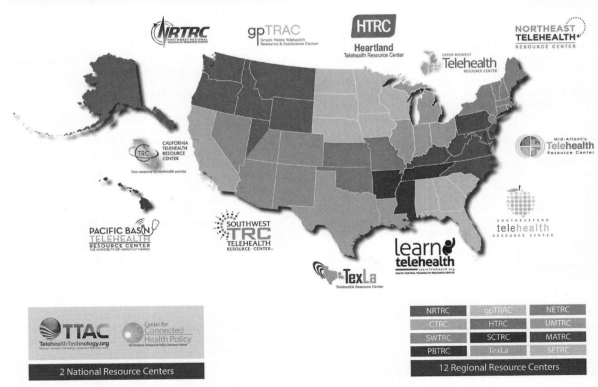

▲ **Figure 68–9.** Telehealth resource centers, 2019.

CONCLUSION

This chapter could have been hundreds of pages long. There are entire textbooks on this subject and the various disciplines associated with it. The objective was to lay out what telemedicine and telehealth are and what challenges and barriers exist and to provide significant resources that will be of great value to you and your work moving forward.

Prior to the beginning of the 21st century, science fiction seemed to be everywhere—books, film, television, and magazines. The very foundation on which we stand today is based on individuals pushing the envelope. As mentioned earlier, those pioneers pushed medicine and, more importantly, society forward. It is no longer science fiction. Much of what we can dream up, we can actually do today. Healthcare knowledge and delivery can be accessed from our mobile phones. Computer systems are intelligent enough to help us make decisions. We are no longer isolated as individuals or as medical teams. Robotics and artificial intelligence will be significant adjuncts to our work, and we must remain vigilant that they are tools that serve us. As we continue to march forward, we will try our best to assimilate to nascent technologies but also reinforce our commitment to our patients and to that ancient oath!

REFERENCES

Abdolahi A, Scoglio N, Killoran A, Dorsey ER, Biglan LM. Potential reliability and validity of a modified version of the Unified Parkinson's Disease Rating Scale that could be administered remotely. *Parkinsonism Relat Disord*. 2013;19:218–221. [PMID: 23102808]

American Academy of Child and Adolescent Psychiatry (AACAP) Committee on Telepsychiatry and AACAP Committee on Quality Issues. Clinical update: telepsychiatry with children and adolescents. *J Am Acad Child Adolesc Psychiatry*. 2017; 56(10):875–893. [PMID: 28942810]

American Telemedicine Association Guidelines. https://www.americantelemed.org/search?executeSearch=true&SearchTerm=guidelines&l=1. Accessed January 22, 2019.

Ashwood JS, Mehrotra A, Cowling D, et al. Direct-to-consumer telehealth may increase access to care but does not decrease spending. *Health Aff*. 2017;36(3):485–491. [PMID: 28264950]

Aucar JA, Doarn CR, Sargsyan AE, Samuelson BA, Odonnell MJ, DeBakey ME. Case report: use of the internet for international post-operative follow-up. *Telemed J*. 1999;4(4):371–374. [PMID: 10220478]

Bashi N, Karunanithi M, Fatehi F, et al. Remote monitoring of patients with heart failure: an overview of systematic reviews. *J Med Internet Res*. 2017;19(1):e18. [PMID: 28108430]

Bashshur RL. On the definition and evaluation of telemedicine. *Telemed J*. 1995;1(1):19–23. [PMID: 10165319]

Bashshur RL, Howell JD, Krupinski EA, Harms KM, Bashshur N, Doarn CR. The empirical foundations of telemedicine interventions in primary care. *Telemed J E Health*. 2016;22(5):342–375. [PMID: 27128779]

Bashshur RL, Krupinski EA, Thrall JH, Bashshur N. The empirical foundations of teleradiology and related applications: a review of the evidence. *Telemed J E Health*. 2016;22(11):868–898. [PMID: 27585301]

Bashshur RL, Krupinski EA, Weinstein RS, Dunn MR, Bashshur N. The empirical foundations of telepathology: evidence of feasibility and intermediate effects. *Telemed J E Health*. 2017; 23(3):155–191. [PMID: 28170313]

Bashshur RL, Shannon GW, eds. *History of Telemedicine: Evolution, Context, and Transformation*. New Rochelle, NY: Mary Ann Liebert, Inc. Publishers; 2009.

Bashshur RL, Shannon GW, Bashshur N, Yellowlees PM. The empirical evidence for telemedicine interventions in mental disorders. *Telemed J E Health*. 2016;22(2):87–113. [PMID: 26624248]

Bashshur RL, Shannon GW, Krupinski EA, et al. National telemedicine initiatives: essential to healthcare reform. *Telemed J E Health*. 2009;15(6):600–610. [PMID: 19534591]

Bashshur RL, Shannon G, Krupinski EA, Grigsby J. Sustaining and realizing the promise of telemedicine. *Telemed J E Health*. 2013;19(5):339–345. [PMID: 23289907]

Bashshur R, Shannon GW, Krupinski E, Grigsby J. The taxonomy of telemedicine. *Telemed J E Health*. 2011;17(6):484–494. [PMID: 21718114]

Bashshur RL, Shannon GW, Smith BR, et al. The empirical foundations of telemedicine interventions for chronic disease management. *Telemed J E Health*. 2014;20(9):769–800. [PMID: 24968105]

Bashshur RL, Shannon GW, Smith BR, Woodward MA. The empirical evidence for the telemedicine intervention in diabetes management. *Telemed J E Health*. 2015;21(5):321–354. [PMID: 25806910]

Bashshur RL, Shannon GW, Tejasvi T, Kvedar JC, Gates M. The empirical foundations of teledermatology: a review of the research evidence. *Telemed J E Health*. 2015;21(12):953–979. [PMID: 26394022]

Biagio L, Swanepoel DW, Adeyemo A, et al. Asynchronous video-otoscopy with a telehealth facilitator. *Telemed J E Health*. 2013;19(4):252–258. [PMID: 23384332]

Brown FW. Rural telepsychiatry. *Psychiatr Serv*. 1998;49(7): 963–964. [PMID: 9661235]

Chen A, Hollander J, Doarn CR. Telemedicine point/counterpoint: the future of healthcare or the end of personal medicine. *Health Trans*. 2016;1(1):33–43. [No PMID]

Coffman M, Moore M, Jetty A, Klink K, Bazemore A. Who is using telehealth in primary care? Safety net clinics and health maintenance organizations (HMOs). *J Am Board Fam Med*. 2016;29(4):432–433. [PMID: 27390373]

da Costa CA, Pasluosta CF, Eskofier B, da Silva DB, da Rosa Righi R. Internet of health things: toward intelligent vital signs monitoring in hospital wards. *Artif Intell Med*. 2018;89:61–69. [PMID: 29871778]

Daniel H, Snyder Sulmasy L. Policy recommendations to guide the use of telemedicine in primary cares: an American College of Physicians position paper. *Ann Intern Med*. 2015;163(10): 787–789. [PMID: 26344925]

Doarn CR. Editor's note: innovative biomedical equipment for diagnosis and treatment. *J Bioeng Biomed Sci*. 2017;6(5):e215. [No PMID]

Doarn CR. Invited commentary: telehealth: a very useful tool that enables and improves patient access. *J Am Board Fam Med*. 2016;29(4):430–431. [PMID: 27390372]

Doarn CR. Invited editorial: telemedicine and psychiatry—a natural match. *mHealth*. 2018;4:60. [PMID: 30701178]

Doarn CR. Telemedicine in tomorrow's operating room: a natural fit. *Semin Laparosc Surg*. 2003;10(3):121–126. [PMID: 14551654]

Doarn CR, Dorogi A, Tikhtman R, Pallerla H, Vonder Meullen MB. Opinions of the role of telehealth in a large Midwest academic health center: a case study. *Telemed J E Health.* 2019;doi: 10.1089/tmj.2018.0259. [PMID: 30625029]

Doarn CR, Latifi R. Telementoring and teleproctoring in trauma and emergency care. *Curr Trauma Rep.* 2016;2(3):138–143. [No PMID]

Doarn CR, Nicogossian AE, Merrell RC. Application of telemedicine in the United States Space Program. *Telemed J.* 1998; 4(1):19–30. [PMID: 9599070]

Doarn CR, Pruitt S, Bott DM, et al. Federal efforts to define and advance telehealth-a work in progress. *Telemed J E Health.* 2014;20(5):409–418. [PMID: 24502793]

Doarn CR, Yellowlees P, Jeffries D, et al. Societal drivers in the application of telehealth. *Telemed J E Health.* 2008;14(9): 998–1002. [PMID: 19035816]

Dorsey ER, Topol EJ. State of telehealth. *N Engl J Med.* 2016; 375(2):154–161. [PMID: 27410924]

Durner G, Durner J, Dunsche H, et al. 24/7 live stream telemedicine home treatment service for Parkinson's disease patients. *Mov Disord Clin Pract.* 2017;4(3):368–373. [PMID: 30363378]

Ferguson EW, Doarn CR, Scott JC. Survey of global telemedicine. *J Med Systems.* 1995;19(1):35–40. [PMID: 7790806]

Ferrandiz L, Ojeda-Vila T, Corrales A, et al. Internet-based skin cancer screening using clinical images alone or in conjunction with dermoscopic images: a randomized teledermoscopy trial. *J Am Acad Dermatol.* 2017;76(4):676–682. [PMID: 28089728]

Fierson WM, Capone A Jr. Telemedicine for evaluation of retinopathy of prematurity. *Pediatrics.* 2015;135(1):e238–e254. [PMID: 25548330]

Gough F, Budhrani S, Cohn E, et al. ATA practice guidelines for live, on-demand primary and urgent care. *Telemed J E Health.* 2015;21(3):233–241. [PMID: 25658882]

Haselkorn A, Coyle M, Doarn CR. The future of remote health services: summary of an expert panel discussion. *Telemed J E Health.* 2007;13(3):341–347. [PMID: 17603837]

Jetty A, Moore MA, Coffman M, Petterson S, Bazemore A. Rural family physicians are twice as likely to use telehealth as urban family physicians. *Telemed J E Health.* 2018;24(4):268–276. [PMID: 28805545]

Krupinski E, Burdick A, Pak H, et al. American Telemedicine Association's practice guidelines for teledermatology. *Telemed J E Health.* 2008;14(3):289–302. [PMID: 18570555]

Latifi R, ed. *Telemedicine for Trauma, Emergencies and Disaster Management.* Boston, MA: Artech House Publishers; 2010.

Latifi R, Merrell RC, Doarn CR, et al. "Initiate-Build-Operate-Transfer": a strategy for establishing sustainable telemedicine programs in developing countries: initial lessons from the Balkans. *Telemed J E Health.* 2009;15(10):956–969. [PMID: 19832055]

Le Fanu J. Rise and fall of modern medicine. *Lancet.* 1999; 354(9177):518. [PMID: 10465212]

Lin CC, Dievler A, Robbins C, Sripipatana A, Quinn M, Nair S. Telehealth in health centers: key adoption factors, barriers, and opportunities. *Health Aff.* 2018;37(12):1967–1974. [PMID: 30633683]

Lundberg T, de Jager LB, Laurent C. Diagnostic accuracy of a general practitioner with video-otoscopy collected by a health care facilitator compared to traditional otoscopy. *Int J Pediatr Otorhinolaryngol.* 2017;99:49–53. [PMID: 28688565]

Majumder S, Mondal T, Deen MJ. Wearable sensors for remote health monitoring. *Sensors.* 2017;17(1):130. [PMID: 28085085]

Mashima PA, Doarn CR. Overview of telehealth activities in speech-language pathology. *Telemed J E Health.* 2008; 14(10):1101–1117. [PMID: 19119834]

McKoy K, Antoniotti NM, Armstrong A, et al. Practice guidelines for teledermatology. *Telemed J E Health.* 2016;22(12):981–990. [PMID: 27690203]

McLaren P, Ball CJ, Summerfield AB, Watson JP, Lipsedge M. An evaluation of the use of interactive television in an acute psychiatric service. *J Telemed Telecare.* 1995;1(2):79–85. [PMID: 9375124]

Moore MA, Coffman M, Jetty A, Klink K, Petterson S, Bazemore A. Family physicians report considerable interest in, but limited use of, telehealth services. *J Am Board Fam Med.* 2017;30(3):320–330. [PMID: 28484064]

Moore MA, Coffman M, Jetty A, Petterson S, Bazemore A. Only 15% of FPs report using telehealth; training and lack of reimbursement are top barriers. *Am Fam Physician.* 2016;93(2):101. [PMID: 26926405]

Myers K, Nelson EL, Rabinowitz T, et al. American Telemedicine Association practice guidelines for telemental health with children and adolescents. *Telemed J E Health.* 2017;23(10):779–804. [PMID: 28930496]

Myers K, Turvey CL. *Telemental Health: Clinical, Technical and Administrative Foundations for Evidence-Based Practice.* Waltham, MA: Elsevier Insight; 2013.

Nair U, Armfield NR, Chatfield MD, Edirippulige S. The effectiveness of telemedicine interventions to address maternal depression: a systematic review and meta-analysis. *J Telemed Telecare.* 2018;24(10):639–50. [PMID: 30343660]

Neufeld JD, Doarn CR. Telemedicine spending by Medicare a snapshot from 2012. *Telemed J E Health.* 2015;21(8):686–693. [PMID: 25839672]

Neufeld JD, Doarn CR, Aly R. State policies influence Medicare telemedicine utilization. *Telemed J E Health.* 2016;22(1):70–74. [PMID: 26218148]

Ohta H, Kawashima M. Technical feasibility of patient-friendly screening and treatment of digestive disease by remote control robotic capsule endoscopes via the Internet. *Conf Proc IEEE Eng Med Biol Soc.* 2014;2014:7001–7004. [PMID: 25571607]

Osler W. *Evolution of Modern Medicine.* DevCom; 1921.

Powell RE, Henstenburg JM, Cooper G, et al. Patient perceptions of telehealth primary care video visits. *Ann Fam Med.* 2017;15(3):225–229. [PMID: 28483887]

Rathbone AL, Prescott J. The use of mobile apps and SMS messaging as physical and mental health interventions: systematic review. *J Med Internet Res.* 2017;19(8):e295. [PMID: 28838887]

Rathi S, Tsui E, Mehta N, Zahid S, Schuman JS. The current state of teleophthalmology in the United States. *Ophthalmology.* 2017;124(12):1729–1734. [PMID: 28647202]

Rheuban KS, Krupinski EA. *Understanding Telehealth.* New York, NY: McGraw-Hill; 2018.

Roguin A. Rene Theophile Hyacinthe Laënnec (1781–1826): the man behind the stethoscope. *Clin Med Res.* 2006;4(3):230–235. [PMID: 17048358]

Russell LB. Opportunity costs in modern medicine. *Health Aff.* 1992;11(2):162–169. [PMID: 1500048]

Ryan MC, Ostmo S, Jonas K, et al. Development and evaluation of reference standards for image-based telemedicine diagnosis and clinical research studies in ophthalmology. *AMIA Annu Symp Proc.* 2014;2014:1902–1910. [PMID: 25954463]

Sanchez Gonzales ML, McCord CE, Dopp AR, et al. Telemental health training and delivery in primary care: a case report of interdisciplinary treatment. *J Clin Psychol.* 2019;75(2):260–270. [PMID: 30589440]

Satou GM, Rheuban K, Alverson D, et al. Telemedicine in pediatric cardiology: a scientific statement from the American Heart Association. *Circulation.* 2017;135(11):e648–e678. [PMID: 28193604]

Schulze N, Reuter SC, Kuchler I, et al. Differences in attitudes toward online interventions in psychiatry and psychotherapy between health care professionals and nonprofessionals: a survey. *Telemed J E Health.* 2019;25(10):926–932. [PMID: 30412450]

Shore JH, Yellowlees P, Caudill R, et al. best practices in video-conferencing-based telemental health April 2018.*Telemed J E Health.* 2018;24(11):827–832. [PMID: 30358514]

Shortliffe EH, Millet LI, eds. *Strategies and Priorities for Information Technology at the Centers for Medicare and Medicaid Services.* Washington, DC: The National Academies Press; 2012.

Simmons S, Alverson D, Poropatich R, D'Iorio J, Devany M, Doarn CR. Applying telehealth in natural and anthropogenic disasters. *Telemed J E Health.* 2008;14(9):968–971. [PMID: 19035809]

Speedie S, Ferguson S, Sanders J, England W, Doarn CR. Telehealth: the promise of new care delivery models. *Telemed J E Health.* 2008;14(9):964–967. [PMID: 19035808]

Sood S, Mbarika V, Jugoo S, et al. What is telemedicine? A collection of 104 peer-reviewed perspectives and theoretical underpinnings. *Telemed J E Health* 2007;13(5):573–590. [PMID: 28704442]

Spatz M. *The Medical Library Association Guide to Providing Consumer and Patient Health Information.* Lanham, MD: Rowman and Littlefield; 2014.

Sprenger M, Mettler T, Osma J. Health professionals' perspective on the promotion of e-mental health apps in the context of maternal depression. *PLoS One.* 2017;12(7):e0180867. [PMID: 28704442]

Tatsioni A, Zarin DA, Aronson N, et al. Challenges in systematic reviews of diagnostic technologies. *Ann Intern Med* 2005; 142(12 Pt2):1048–1055. [PMID: 15968029]

Theurer L, Bashshur R, Bernard J, et al. American Telemedicine Association guidelines for teleburn. *Telemed J E Health.* 2017;23(5):365–375. [PMID: 28287905]

Thiele JS, Shore JH, Doarn CR. Locum tenens and telepsychiatry: filling critical holes in psychiatric care. *Telemed J E Health.* 2015;21(6):510–513. [PMID: 25764147]

Torous J, Wisniewski H, Liu G, Keshavan M. Mental health mobile phone app usage, concerns, and benefits among psychiatric outpatients: comparative survey study. *JMIR Ment Health.* 2018;5(4):e11715. [PMID: 30446484]

Vegesna A, Tran M, Angelaccio M, et al. Remote patient monitoring via non-invasive digital technologies: a systematic review. *Telemed J E Health.* 2017;23(1):3–17. [PMID: 27116181]

Wadsworth HE, Dhima K, Womack KB, et al. Validity of teleneuropsychological assessment in older patients with cognitive disorders. *Arch Clin Neuropsychol.* 2018;33(8):1040–1104. [PMID: 29329363]

Weinstein RS, Krupinski EA, Doarn CR. Clinical examination component of telemedicine, telehealth, m-health, and connected health practices. *Med Clin North Am.* 2018;102(3): 533–544. [PMID: 29650074]

Weinstein RS, Lopez AM, Joseph BA, et al. Telemedicine, telehealth, and mobile health applications that work: opportunities and barriers. *Am J Med.* 2014;127(3):183–187. [PMID: 24384059]

Wittson CL, Benschoter R. Two-way television: helping the Medical Center reach out. *Am J Psychiatry.* 1972;129(5):626–627. [PMID: 4673018]

Wolf JA, Moreau JF, Akilov O, et al. Diagnostic inaccuracy of smartphone applications for melanoma detection. *JAMA Dermatol.* 2013;149(4):422–426. [PMID: 23325302]

Wootton R. Twenty years of telemedicine in chronic disease management: an evidence synthesis. *J Telemed Telecare.* 2012; 18:211–220. [PMID: 22674020]

Zangbar B, Pandit V, Rhee P, et al. Smartphone surgery: how technology can transform practice. *Telemed J E Health.* 2014; 20(6):590–592. [PMID: 24693938]

Index

Note: Page numbers followed by *f* and *t* indicate figures and tables.